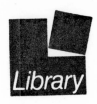
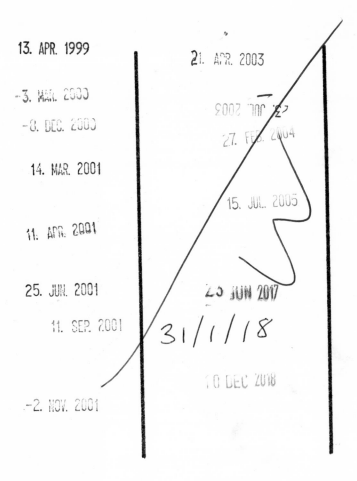

SURGERY OF THE
COLON &
RECTUM

Edited by

R. JOHN NICHOLLS, B.A., M.CHIR., F.R.C.S. (ENG.), F.R.C.S. (GLASG.)
Honorary Senior Lecturer
Imperial College of Science, Technology, and Medicine
University of London
Dean
St. Mark's Academic Institute
Consultant Surgeon
Department of Surgery
St. Mark's Hospital
London, England

ROGER R. DOZOIS, M.D., M.S., F.A.C.S., F.R.C.S. (GLASG.) (HON.)
Professor of Surgery
Mayo Medical School
Emeritus Chair and Consultant
Division of Colon and Rectal Surgery
Mayo Clinic and Mayo Foundation
Rochester, Minnesota

With illustrations by Gillian Lee, F.M.A.A., Hon. F.I.M.A., A.M.I., R.M.I.P.

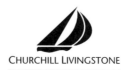

CHURCHILL LIVINGSTONE

New York, Edinburgh, London, Madrid, Melbourne, San Francisco, Tokyo

CHURCHILL LIVINGSTONE

Medical Division of Pearson Professional Limited

Distributed in the United States of America by Churchill Livingstone Inc., 650 Avenue of the Americas, New York, N.Y. 10011, and by associated companies, branches, and representatives throughout the world

First published 1997

ISBN 0-443-05565-3

British Library Cataloguing in Publication Data
A catalogue record for this book is available from the British Library

Library of Congress Cataloging in Publication Data
A catalog record for this book is available from the Library of Congress

Medical knowledge is constantly changing. As new information becomes available, changes in treatment, procedures, equipment and the use of drugs become necessary. The editors/authors/contributors and the publishers have, as far as it is possible, taken care to ensure that the information given in this text is accurate and up to date. However, readers are strongly advised to confirm that the information, especially with regard to drug usage, complies with the latest legislation and standards of practice.

The Publishers have made every effort to trace the copyright holders for borrowed material. If they have inadvertently overlooked any, they will be pleased to make the necessary arrangements at the first opportunity.

Acquisitions Editor: *Deborah Russell*
Project Editor: *John Hindmarch*
Production Editor: *Paul Bernstein*
Production Supervisor: *Sharon Tuder*
Cover design: *Andrew Jones* and *Robert Britton*

Printed in the United States of America

To Stella and Celia and our children

CONTRIBUTORS

ANJAN BANERJEE, M.Sc., D.M., M.S.
Senior Clinical Lecturer, Department of Surgery, Leeds University, Leeds, England; Consultant Surgeon, Department of Surgery, Halifax Royal Infirmary, Halifax, England

MICHAEL P. BANNON, M.D.
Assistant Professor of Surgery, Mayo Medical School; Consultant, Department of Surgery, Mayo Clinic and Mayo Foundation, Rochester, Minnesota

CLIVE I. BARTRAM, F.R.C.P., F.R.C.R.
Honorary Senior Lecturer, Imperial College of Science, Technology, and Medicine, University of London; Consultant Radiologist, Intestinal Imaging Centre, St. Mark's Hospital; Honorary Consultant Radiologist, Department of Radiology, Hammersmith Hospital, London, England

THERESA BERK, M.S.S.A.
Clinical Co-ordinator, Steve Atenas Stavro Familial Gastrointestinal Cancer Registry, Mount Sinai Hospital, Toronto, Ontario, Canada

LISA BOARDMAN, M.D.
Fellow, Division of Gastroenterology, Department of Internal Medicine, Mayo Medical School; Gastroenterology Fellow, Division of Gastroenterology, Department of Internal Medicine, Mayo Clinic and Mayo Foundation, Rochester, Minnesota

WILLIAM S. BRENNOM, M.D.
Clinical Assistant Professor, Department of Surgery, University of Minnesota Medical School, Minneapolis, Minnesota; Surgeon, Department of Surgery, Children's Hospital-St. Paul, St. Paul, Minnesota

KEITH E. BRITTON, M.D., M.Sc., F.R.C.R., F.R.C.P.
Professor, Department of Nuclear Medicine, St. Bartholomew's and the Royal London Hospitals School of Medicine and Dentistry, University of London; Physician, Department of Nuclear Medicine, Nuclear Medicine Group, Imperial Cancer Research Fund, St. Mark's Hospital, London, England

DOUGLAS W. BURDON, M.B., B.S., F.R.C.PATH.
Senior Clinical Lecturer, Department of Infection, University of Birmingham; Consultant Microbiologist, Department of Microbiology, The Queen Elizabeth Hospital, Birmingham, England

MICHAEL CAMILLERI, M.D., M.PHIL. (LOND.), F.R.C.P. (LOND.), F.R.C.P. (EDIN.), F.A.C.P., F.A.C.G.
Professor of Medicine, Mayo Medical School; Consultant in Gastroenterology and Physiology and Biophysics, Mayo Clinic and Mayo Foundation, Rochester, Minnesota

LEO KAI-MING CHIU, M.B.B.S., F.R.C.S. (EDIN.), F.C.S.H.K., F.H.K.A.M.
Chief Medical Officer, Department of Surgery, Kwong Wah Hospital, Hong Kong

YANEK S. Y. CHIU, M.D.
Associate Clinical Professor, Department of Surgery, University of California, San Francisco, School of Medicine; Private Practice, Colon and Rectal Surgery, California Pacific Medical Center, San Francisco, California

JUDY CHO, M.D.
Instructor, Department of Medicine, University of Chicago Division of the Biological Sciences Pritzker School of Medicine, Chicago, Illinois

ZANE COHEN, M.D., F.R.C.S. (C.)
Professor, Department of Surgery, University of Toronto Faculty of Medicine; Surgeon in Chief, Department of Surgery, Mount Sinai Hospital, Toronto, Ontario, Canada

PHILLIP A. DEAN, M.D.
Assistant Professor, Department of Surgery, University of Alabama School of Medicine, University of Alabama at Birmingham, Birmingham, Alabama

KEMAL I. DEEN, M.D.
Research Fellow, Division of Colon and Rectal Surgery, Department of Surgery, University of Minnesota Medical School, Minneapolis, Minnesota

N. M. DE SOUZA, M.D., F.R.C.R.
Senior Lecturer, Department of Radiology, Royal Postgraduate Medical School; Consultant Radiologist, Robert Steiner MRI Unit, Hammersmith Hospital, London, England

RICHARD M. DEVINE, M.D., F.A.C.S.
Assistant Professor of Surgery; Mayo Medical School; Consultant, Division of Colon and Rectal Surgery, Mayo Clinic and Mayo Foundation, Rochester, Minnesota

ROGER R. DOZOIS, M.D., M.S., F.A.C.S., F.R.C.S. (GLASG.) (HON.)
Professor of Surgery, Mayo Medical School; Emeritus Chair and Consultant, Division of Colon and Rectal Surgery, Mayo Clinic and Mayo Foundation, Rochester, Minnesota

CHARLES O. ELSON, M.D.
Professor and Chairman, Division of Gastroenterology, Department of Medicine, University of Alabama School of Medicine, University of Alabama at Birmingham, Birmingham, Alabama

MICHAEL J. G. FARTHING, M.D., F.R.C.P.
Professor, Digestive Diseases Research Centre; Clinical Dean, St. Bartholomew's and the Royal London Hospitals School of Medicine and Dentistry, London, England

PAUL J. FINAN, M.D., F.R.C.S.
Honorary Senior Clinical Lecturer, University of Leeds; Consultant General and Colorectal Surgeon, Department of Surgery, General Infirmary at Leeds, Leeds, England

ALASTAIR FORBES, B.Sc., M.D., F.R.C.P.
Honorary Clinical Senior Lecturer, Imperial College of Science, Technology, and Medicine, University of London; Subdean, St. Mark's Academic Institute; Consultant Gastroenterologist, Department of Gastroenterology, St. Mark's Hospital, London, England

ROBERT GILLILAND, M.S.
Research Fellow, Department of Colorectal Surgery, Cleveland Clinic Florida, Fort Lauderdale, Florida

BENGT GLIMELIUS, M.D., PH.D.
Associate Professor, Departments of Oncology and Radiotherapy, Uppsala University, University Hospital. Uppsala, Sweden

HAK-SU GOH, B.Sc. (HON.), M.B., B.S., F.R.C.S.
Consultant Surgeon, Goh Hak-Su Colon and Rectal Centre, Gleneagles Medical Centre, Singapore, Republic of Singapore

STANLEY M. GOLDBERG, M.D., F.A.C.S., (HON.) F.R.A.C.S., (HON.) F.R.C.S. (ENG.)
Clinical Professor, Division of Colon and Rectal Surgery, Department of Surgery, University of Minnesota Medical School, Minneapolis, Minnesota

PHILIP H. GORDON, M.D., F.R.C.S.(C.), F.A.C.S.
Professor, Departments of Surgery and Oncology, McGill University Faculty of Medicine; Director, Colon and Rectal Surgery, McGill University and Sir Mortimer B. Davis Jewish General Hospital, Montreal, Quebec, Canada

MARIE GRANOWSKA, M.D., M.Sc.
Reader in Nuclear Medicine, St. Bartholomew's and the Royal London Hospitals School of Medicine and Dentistry; Honorary Consultant, Department of Nuclear Medicine, Nuclear Medicine Group. Imperial Cancer Research Fund, St. Mark's Hospital, London, England

TH. GROSS, M.D.
Chief Resident, Department of Surgery, Triemli Hospital, Zurich, Switzerland

STEPHEN HALLIGAN, M.B., B.S., M.D., M.R.C.P., F.R.C.R.
Honorary Senior Lecturer, Imperial College of Science, Technology, and Medicine, University of London; Consultant Radiologist, Intestinal Imaging Centre, St. Mark's Hospital, London, England

STEPHEN B. HANAUER, M.D.
Professor, Departments of Medicine and Clinical Pharmacology, University of Chicago Division of the Biological Sciences Pritzker School of Medicine, Chicago, Illinois

JACQUES HEPPELL, M.D., F. R. C. S. (C.)
Associate Professor of Surgery, Mayo Medical School, Rochester, Minnesota; Head and Consultant, Division of Colon and Rectal Surgery, Mayo Clinic and Mayo Foundation, Scottsdale, Arizona

H. P. HONEGGER, M.D.
Associate Professor of Oncology, University of Zurich; Head, Division of Oncology, Triemli Hospital, Zurich, Switzerland

LEIF HULTÉN, M.D., PH.D.
Professor, Institute of Surgical Sciences, Göteborg University; Professor, Colorectal Unit, Department of Surgery, Sahlgrens University Hospital, Göteborg, Sweden

C. DANIEL JOHNSON, M.D.
Professor of Radiology, Mayo Medical School; Consultant, Diagnostic Radiology, Mayo Clinic and Mayo Foundation, Rochester, Minnesota

MICHAEL A. KAMM, M.D., F.R.C.P., F.R.A.C.P
Honorary Senior Lecturer, Imperial College of Science, Technology, and Medicine, University of London; Consultant Gastroenterologist and Director, Physiology Unit, St. Mark's Hospital, London, England

WILLIAM E. KARNES, JR., M.D.
Assistant Professor of Medicine, Mayo Medical School, Mayo Medical School; Consultant, Division of Gastroenterology and Internal Medicine, Mayo Clinic and Mayo Foundation, Rochester, Minnesota

DARLENE G. KELLY, M.D., PH.D.
Adjunct Assistant Professor of Nutrition, University of Minnesota Medical School; Assistant Professor of Medicine, Mayo Medical School; Consultant, Division of Gastroenterology and Internal Medicine, Mayo Clinic and Mayo Foundation, Rochester, Minnesota

KEITH A. KELLY, M.D., M.S., F.A.C.S. (EDIN.) (HON.)
Professor of Surgery, Mayo Medical School; Chair and Consultant, Department of Surgery, Mayo Clinic and Mayo Foundation, Scottsdale, Arizona

MICHAEL L. KENNEDY, B.SC. (HON.)
Research Fellow, Department of Colorectal Surgery, St. George Hospital, Sydney, Australia

DONALD G. KIM, M.D.
Clinical Fellow, Division of Colon and Rectal Surgery, Department of Surgery, University of Minnesota Medical School, Minneapolis, Minnesota

W. A. KMIOT, M.S., F.R.C.S.
Senior Lecturer, Department of Colorectal Surgery, Royal Postgraduate Medical School; Consultant Colorectal Surgeon, Hammersmith Hospital, London, England

OLE KRONBORG, M.D.
Professor, Department of Surgery, Odense University Hospital; Consultant and Chief, Colorectal Services, Department of Surgery, Odense University Hospital, Odense, Denmark

ADRIAN FRANCIS PENG-KHEONG LEONG, M.D.
Consultant Surgeon, Department of Colorectal Surgery, Singapore General Hospital, Singapore, Republic of Singapore

DAVID Z. LUBOWSKI, F.R.A.C.S.
Consultant Colorectal Surgeon and Director, Anorectal Physiology Laboratory, Department of Colorectal Surgery, St. George Hospital, Sydney, Australia

PETER J. LUNNISS, B.SC., M.S., F.R.C.S.
Senior Lecturer, St. Bartholemew's and the Royal London Hospitals School of Medicine, University of London; Consultant Surgeon, Homerton Hospital, London, England

JOHN M. MACKEIGAN M.D., F.R.C.S. (C.), F.A.C.S.
Associate Clinical Professor, Department of Surgery, Michigan State University College of Human Medicine, East Lansing, Michigan; Staff Surgeon, Department of Colon and Rectal Surgery, Ferguson Clinic, Grand Rapids, Michigan

ROBERT D. MADOFF, M.D.
Clinical Associate Professor and Director of Research, Division of Colon and Rectal Surgery, Department of Surgery, University of Minnesota Medical School, Minneapolis, Minnesota

PETER W. MARCELLO, M.D.
Clinical Fellow, Department of Colon and Rectal Surgery, Lahey Hitchcock Medical Center, Burlington, Massachusetts

RAOUL MAYER, M.D., PH.D.
Fellow, Division of Colon and Rectal Surgery, Department of Surgery, University of Minnesota Medical School, Minneapolis, Minnesota

U. METZGER, M.D.
Associate Professor of Surgery, University of Zurich; Head, Department of Surgery, Triemli Hospital, Zurich, Switzerland

NEIL MORTENSEN, M.A., M.BCH.B., F.R.C.S. (ENG.)
Consultant Surgeon and Reader in Colorectal Surgery, University of Oxford Clinical Medical Centre; Department of Colorectal Surgery, John Radcliffe Hospital, Oxford, England

VANDANA NEHRA, M.D.
Instructor, Department of Medicine, Mayo Medical School; Senior Associate Consultant, Division of Gastroenterology, Department of Internal Medicine, Mayo Clinic and Mayo Foundation, Rochester, Minnesota

HEIDI NELSON, M.D., F.A.C.S.
Associate Professor, Department of Surgery, Mayo Medical School; Consultant and Chair, Division of Colon and Rectal Surgery, Mayo Clinic and Mayo Foundation, Rochester, Minnesota

R. JOHN NICHOLLS, B.A., M.CHIR., F.R.C.S. (ENG.), F.R.C.S. (GLASG.)
Honorary Senior Lecturer, Imperial College of Science, Technology, and Medicine, University of London; Dean, St. Mark's Academic Institute; Consultant Surgeon, Department of Surgery, St. Mark's Hospital, London, England

SANTHAT NIVATVONGS, M.D., F.A.C.S.
Professor of Surgery, Mayo Medical School; Consultant, Division of Colon and Rectal Surgery, Mayo Clinic and Mayo Foundation, Rochester, Minnesota

SVANTE NORDGREN, M.D., PH.D.
Associate Professor, Department of Surgery, Institute of Surgical Sciences, Göteborg University; Consultant Surgeon, Colorectal Unit, Department of Surgery, Sahlgrens University Hospital, Göteborg, Sweden

JOHN NORTHOVER, M.S., F.R.C.S. (ENG.)
Senior Lecturer, Imperial College of Science, Technology, and Medicine, University of London, Honorary Director, Colorectal Cancer Unit, Imperial Cancer Research Fund; Consultant Surgeon and Chairman Emeritus, Department of Surgery, St. Mark's Hospital, London, England

DENIS C. N. K. NYAM, F.R.C.S. (ED.)
Academic Fellow, Division of Colon and Rectal Surgery, Department of Surgery, Mayo Medical School, Rochester, Minnesota; Consultant Surgeon, Department of Colorectal Surgery, Singapore General Hospital, Singapore, Republic of Singapore

TOM ÖRESLAND, M.D., PH.D
Associate Professor, Department of Surgery, Institute of Social Sciences, Göteborg University; Consultant Surgeon, Colorectal Unit, Department of Surgery, Sahlgrens University Hospital, Göteborg, Sweden

LARS PÅHLMAN, M.D., PH.D.
Associate Professor, Colorectal Unit, Department of Surgery, Uppsala University, University Hospital, Uppsala, Sweden

JOHN H. PEMBERTON, M.D., F.A.C.S.
Professor, Department of Surgery, Mayo Medical School; Consultant, Division of Colon and Rectal Surgery, Department of Surgery, Mayo Clinic and Mayo Foundation, Rochester, Minnesota

ROBIN K. S. PHILLIPS, M.S., F.R.C.S. (ENG.)
Honorary Senior Lecturer, Imperial College of Science, Technology, and Medicine, University of London; Dean-Elect, St. Mark's Academic Institute; Consultant Surgeon and Chairman, Department of Surgery, St. Mark's Hospital, London, England

SIDNEY F. PHILLIPS, M.D.
Professor of Medicine, Mayo Medical School; Karl F. and Marjory Hasselmann Professor of Research, Consultant, Division of Gastroenterology, Mayo Clinic and Mayo Foundation, Rochester, Minnesota

JOHN ROMANOS, M.D.
Research Fellow, Department of Colorectal Surgery, John Radcliffe Hospital, Oxford, England

DAVID A. ROTHENBERGER, M.D.
Clinical Professor and Chief, Division of Colon and Rectal Surgery, Department of Surgery, University of Minnesota Medical School, Minneapolis, Minnesota

PETER M. SAGAR, B.Sc., M.D., F.R.C.S. (ENG.)
Consultant Surgeon, Department of Surgery, Leeds General Infirmary, Leeds, England

BRIAN P. SAUNDERS, M.B.B.S., M.R.C.P. (LOND.)
Senior Lecturer in Endoscopy, Imperial College of Science, Technology, and Medicine, University of London; Consultant Endoscopist, Endoscopy Unit, St. Mark's Hospital, London, England

DAVID J. SCHOETZ, JR., M.D., F.A.C.S.
Chairman, Department of Colon Rectal Surgery, Lahey Hitchcock Medical Center, Burlington, Massachusetts

PHILIP F. SCHOFIELD, M.D., F.R.C.S. (ENG.)
Visiting Professor, Department of Surgery, University of Manchester; Honorary Consultant, Department of Surgery, Christie Hospital, Manchester, England

FRANCIS SEOW-CHOEN, M.B.B.S., F.R.C.S. (ED.), F.A.M.S.
Head and Senior Consultant Surgeon, Department of Colorectal Surgery and Director, Endoscopy Unit, Singapore General Hospital, Singapore, Republic of Singapore

NEIL A. SHEPHERD, M.B., B.S., F.R.C. PATH.
Consultant Histopathologist, Department of Histopathology, Gloucestershire Royal Hospital, Gloucestershire, England

W. ROSS STEVENS, M.D.
Clinical Assistant Professor, Department of Radiology, Southern Illinois University School of Medicine; Radiologist, Department of Radiology, St. John's Hospital, Springfield, Illinois

SCOTT A. STRONG, M.D.
Staff Surgeon, Department of Colorectal Surgery, Cleveland Clinic Foundation, Cleveland, Ohio

IAN C. TALBOT, M.D., F.R.C.PATH.
Professor of Histopathology, Imperial College of Science, Technology, and Medicine, University of London; Consultant Histopathologist, Department of Histopathology, St. Mark's Hospital, London, England

ROBERT L. TELANDER, M.D.
Clinical Professor, Department of Surgery, University of Minnesota Medical School, Minneapolis, Minnesota; Director, Department of Surgery, St. Paul's Hospital; Partner, Pediatric Surgical Associates, Ltd., St. Paul, Minnesota

JOE J. TJANDRA, M.D., F.R.A.C.S., F.R.C.S., F.R.P.C.S.
Senior Lecturer, Department of Colorectal Surgery, University of Melbourne; Consultant Colorectal Surgeon, Colorectal Unit, Royal Melbourne Hospital, Parkville, Victoria, Australia

STEVEN D. WEXNER, M.D.
Chairman and Residency Program Director, Department of Colorectal Surgery, Chairman, Division of Research and Education, Cleveland Clinic Florida, Fort Lauderdale, Florida

CHRISTOPHER B. WILLIAMS, B.M., B.CH. F.R.C.P.
Honorary Senior Lecturer, Imperial College of Science, Technology, and Medicine, University of London; Consultant Physician, Endoscopy Unit, St. Mark's Hospital, London, England

W. DOUGLAS WONG, M.D., F.A.C.S.
Clinical Associate Professor and Director, Residency Program, Division of Colon and Rectal Surgery, Department of Surgery, University of Minnesota Medical School, Minneapolis, Minnesota

A. P. ZBAR, M.D., F.R.C.S.
Clinical Research Fellow, Department of Colorectal Surgery, Royal Postgraduate Medical School; Clinical Associate, Surgical Directorate, Hammersmith Hospital, London, England

FOREWORD

For many years, John Goligher's *Surgery of the Anus, Rectum and Colon* was the surgical "bible" for anyone interested in colorectal surgery. The fifth and last edition of this wonderful text was published in 1984. Since then there have been a number of new texts dealing with this topic. Such a multitude of texts has probably been necessary to keep up with all the changes in this rapidly evolving discipline. Those of us with an interest in the field have appreciated the efforts of these authors to keep us up to date. But the field has changed a great deal; physiologic studies have evolved, sexually-transmitted diseases have become a significant part of colorectal surgery, and continence-preserving operations have become the icon of our specialty. Our understanding of the physiologic principles of the surgical management of colorectal disease has mandated a revolution in the training and practice of colorectal surgeons. I, perhaps more than most, was not inclined to relish the appearance of yet another textbook in this field. But for a number of reasons I welcome the publication of *Surgery of the Colon and Rectum* and am pleased to introduce this text.

First and foremost, the editors of this book, R. John Nicholls and Roger R. Dozois, are treasured friends. They are recognized both as leaders in their countries and as consummate clinicians. They have kindly guided my own understanding and shared their insight as I evolved my own practice of colorectal surgery. Both of these men have dedicated themselves to further the understanding of the care of the patient with colorectal disease and tried to develop means to provide better care. Their text is a tribute to their efforts and to their desire to share with us their understanding of colorectal surgery.

Intrinsic to their understanding is the recognition that colorectal surgery has evolved further than any single physician can comprehend. Physicians throughout the world are bound together, not by their common understanding of how to treat diseases, but by their common experiences in confronting threats from disease and anatomic problems. We need to know how physicians have interpreted these common experiences and devised various methods of treatment. As the first international multi-author text in its field, *Surgery of the Colon and Rectum* brings together the breadth of experience in the various aspects of colorectal surgery that has accumulated in recent years. The international list of contributors, which includes physicians from North America, Europe, Asia, and Australia, is no accident; the editors clearly recognize the worldwide nature of the advances that have been made in the last decade. By creating such a comprehensive overview the editors have produced the standard work in this field.

Second, the editors have distinguished themselves throughout their careers; I welcome a text that shares their insight. Imitation might well be the most sincere form of flattery, but it is also the most secure route to success by the imitator. We would all do well to imitate those dedicated clinicians who contributed to this book as revealed in their various chapters.

I am particularly pleased to see the extent of fundamental science that is included in this volume. The clinician today needs this background to understand current management of colorectal disease. I do not mean this foreword to be a book review, but this text will provide the student, as well as the teacher, with the fundamental understanding that is mandatory to function fully in this field.

We can anticipate that colorectal surgery will continue to evolve rapidly, just as it has over the past decade. It is truly an exciting time to be part of this specialty. This book cannot help but stimulate excitement over what we are now able to do and what we will be able to do in the near future.

I am grateful for the efforts that the editors expended to create this book, which I personally know were extraordinary. It raises the standards by which we will judge future texts to a new level. By emphasizing a practical clinical approach, comprehensive referencing, clear diagrams and technical descriptions, a comprehensive physiologic review, and a unique readability with a user-friendly format, *Surgery of the Colon and Rectum* is the benchmark work in its field.

Robert W. Beart, Jr, M.D.
Professor
Center for Colorectal Disease
Department of Surgery
University of Southern California School of Medicine
Los Angeles, California

PREFACE

Surgical practice changes gradually, but in the last few years rapid developments in technology and basic science understanding have accelerated this process. In addition to the technical consequences of laparoscopic and other forms of minimally invasive surgery, advances such as those in the understanding of tumor spread or in molecular genetics have led surgeons to reconsider strategies for treatment and for postoperative surveillance. Integrated care involving internists, diagnosticians, nurse specialists, and psychologists has become a framework for management of the patient with cancer and inflammatory bowel disease as well as functional bowel disorders. The surgeon is no longer in a position to treat complex diseases isolated from this input. The team structure requires the surgeon to have knowledge of other specialties and to have a working understanding of what is known of the pathophysiology of the disease and where basic science stands regarding etiology. It is a hard task to become familiar with all these disciplines and yet the surgeon must do so if he or she is to offer the best treatment to patients.

Surgery of the Colon and Rectum is intended to supply this information. Only a multi-author work can do justice to covering the wide range of knowledge and experience now necessary for surgical practice. Its contributors have been carefully chosen for their expertise in their respective fields. Their clinical experience and personal involvement in research have allowed them to deliver authoritative accounts of the present state of clinical practice, surgical technique, and the extent of knowledge of causation and current research strategy. The book includes detailed reviews of normal anatomy and physiology, including digestion, absorption, motility, and immunology. It deals systematically with diseases of the anus, rectum, and colon, with a full account of pathology, etiology, and medical management, as well as detailed descriptions of surgical treatment. It includes a chapter on iatrogenic aspects of large bowel surgery in recognition of this increasingly important consideration. An attempt has been made to provide comprehensive references that include many of the classic publications as well as up-to-date sources.

We hope that this comprehensive text will be valuable to practitioners of colorectal surgery, including trainees. It will also be useful for general surgeons who are involved with the treatment of large bowel disease, for internists and diagnosticians, and, perhaps, for basic scientists as a useful general summary of the field.

We gratefully acknowledge the tremendous help given by our secretaries, Ms. Jill Grimsey and Ms. Jennifer Anderson.

R. John Nicholls, B.A., M.Chir., F.R.C.S. (Eng.),
F.R.C.S. (Glasg.)

Roger R. Dozois, M.D., M.S., F.A.C.S., F.R.C.S.
(Glasg.) (Hon.)

CONTENTS

1

TOPOGRAPHIC ANATOMY

Peter M. Sagar
John H. Pemberton

THE COLON

The colon measures 120 to 200 cm in length. Its diameter gradually decreases from 7.5 cm at the cecum to 2.5 cm at the distal sigmoid colon. Three features distinguish the colon from the small intestine: three long muscular bands (the taenia coli), haustral sacculations, and small fatty appendages (appendices epiploicae).

Cecum

The cecum forms a blind-ending recess of the large intestine that hangs down from the ascending colon inferior to the ileocecal junction. The ileocecal junction is marked by the ileocecal valve, the lips of which lie transversely several centimeters above the most dependent part of the cecum. The pouting upper lip overhangs the lower lip. At colonoscopy, the ileocecal valve is usually viewed from the side and appears as a straight fold. It is a lobular, soft anatomic structure the mucosa of which has a more velvety appearance than the surrounding colonic mucosa. It moves rhythmically, and bile-stained effluent may be seen to flux intermittently through the orifice. Reflux through the ileocecal junction is prevented in part by the superior and inferior ileocecal ligaments. They are made of fibrous tissue and maintain the angulation between the ileum and cecum.

The cecum itself can be identified at colonoscopy by the convergence of the taenia coli; its cul-de-sac appearance, which allows retroflexion of the scope; and the presence of the appendiceal orifice, which has a slight fold that partly closes the orifice. The taenia coli lie anterior, posteromedial, and posterolateral and converge onto the base of the appendix. Although the cecum is conical in infancy with the appendix extending down from the apex, the medial wall grows slower than the lateral wall, which comes to hang down from below the base in the adult. The base of the appendix therefore comes to lie on the posteromedial wall of the cecum. The terminal 2 to 4 cm of ileum are often adherent along with its fatty pad to the medial aspect of the cecum.

The front and sides of the cecum are covered with peritoneum. This coat continues up partly behind the cecum before being reflected downwards to cover the floor of the right iliac fossa. The depth of this retrocecal space varies according to the distance of the peritoneal fold from the bottom of the cecum. Two cecal folds are usually present, and they form a retrocecal recess within which the appendix may be found. Further recesses are formed by peritoneal folds in the region of the cecum. An anterior fold lies in front of the terminal ileum between the base of the mesentery and the anterior wall of the cecum. This fold contains the anterior cecal artery (the vascular fold of the cecum). A second fold runs from the terminal ileum to the base of the appendix and frequently contains small blood vessels (the ileocecal fold). The openings of the paracecal recesses all face away from each other, unlike the openings of the paraduodenal recesses, where a hernia in one may spread to involve the others.

Usually the cecum does not possess a significant mesentery and mobility is limited. The cecum can on occasion possess a very long mesentery, in which case it may twist upon its axis and form a volvulus.

Ascending Colon

The ascending colon extends from the ileocecal valve to the hepatic flexure, a distance of about 15 cm. It overlies, and is fixed to, the iliac fascia and lumbar fascia, while the hepatic flexure lies on the inferior pole of the right kidney. It is separated from the kidney by the perirenal fascia of Gerota. Mobilization of the right colon in the course of a right hemicolectomy returns the ascending colon on its hinge-like mesentery to the midline and exposes the ureter, gonadal vessels, and duodenum on the posterior abdominal wall. The front and sides of the ascending colon are covered with peritoneum, which continues

1

laterally to form the right paracolic gutter. This sulcus is well marked and forms a relatively bloodless plane for initial mobilization of the ascending colon.

As with the rest of the colon, the ascending colon possesses three taenia coli, haustra, and small pouches of peritoneum filled with fat, the appendices epiploicae. The taenia coli are anterior, posteromedial, and posterolateral, and are shorter in length than the bowel itself. This results in a saccular appearance. Division of the taenia coli allows the sacculations to be stretched apart and the bowel flattened.

Hepatic Flexure

The hepatic flexure marks the colic depression on the inferior surface of the right lobe of the liver. Anteriorly, it is often in contact with the gall bladder, to which it may be attached by adhesions. It is completely retroperitoneal. Posteriorly lies the perirenal fascia. The hepatocolic ligament is an inconstant finding but when present represents a continuation of the lesser omentum. The hepatic flexure has a vertical range of movement with respiration of 2.5 to 7.5 cm.

Transverse Colon

The transverse colon is draped between the hepatic and splenic flexures, from which it hangs on the transverse mesocolon to a variable degree. It is usually greater than 45 cm in length; a particularly long and redundant transverse colon can cause difficulties during colonoscopy, when ''looping'' of the instrument can be a nuisance. In some subjects, the degree of its pendulousness may allow it to extend inferiorly to below the umbilicus and even down into the pelvis. It is connected to the greater curvature of the stomach by the gastrocolic omentum. Because the transverse mesocolon, greater omentum, and transverse colon are fused, the greater omentum appears to hang down from the transverse colon and thereby covers loops of small intestine.

The line of attachment of the transverse mesocolon to the posterior abdominal wall runs from the inferior pole of the right kidney across the second part of the duodenum, to the head, body, and tail of the pancreas, to the hilum of the left kidney. The transverse mesocolon forms a partition between the lesser sac and structures of the supracolic compartment from those of the infracolic compartment, and acts as an effective barrier to the spread of infection between these two areas. The duodenal-jejunal junction lies immediately below the root of the transverse mesocolon. Some rotation of the colonic wall occurs at the flexures such that the anterior taenia of the ascending colon comes to lie posteriorly while the other two lie anteriorly.

Splenic Flexure

The transverse colon rises towards the inferior edge of the spleen. Here it is attached to the diaphragm by the phrenicocolic ligament. It runs directly posterior then turns downwards upon itself to form the descending colon. The splenic flexure lies

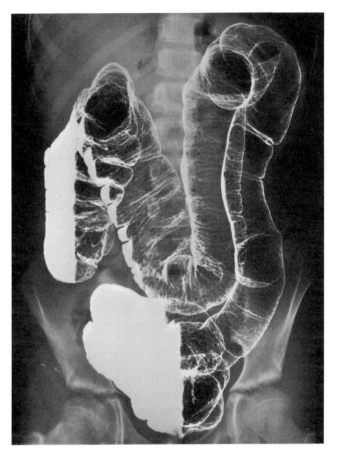

Figure 1-1. A double-contrast barium enema. The splenic flexure is higher than the hepatic flexure and the haustra are clearly evident.

higher than the hepatic flexure (Fig. 1-1) under cover of the costal margin, and apart from the rectum is the most fixed part of the large intestine. The splenic flexure may be directly attached to the spleen by a number of congenital adhesions. Minimal traction on this flexure during surgery may result in these adhesions tearing off the splenic capsule, and bothersome bleeding may ensue.

Descending Colon

The descending colon is about 30 cm in length and extends from the splenic flexure to the pelvic brim. It is entirely retroperitoneal by virtue of being plastered to the posterior abdominal wall by the peritoneum. It overlies the left kidney, separated by the perirenal fascia, and runs over the groove between psoas major and quadratus lumborum and then onto iliacus. The positions of its three taenia coli mirror those of the ascending colon. As the midline dorsal mesocolon of the embryo hinged to the left, it became fused with the parietal peritoneum of the posterior abdominal wall. The right leaf of this embryonic dorsal mesocolon thus forms the floor of the left infracolic compartment. The descending colon ends by curving inferomedially in the left iliac fossa to the pelvic brim.

Sigmoid Colon

The sigmoid colon begins at the pelvic brim, curves inferiorly along the pelvic side wall, loops superiorly and medially over the bifurcation of the left common iliac vessels, and finally runs inferiorly to the midline. The sigmoid mesocolon begins at the pelvic brim and becomes longer to the midpoint of the sigmoid colon, which then decreases in length to a point at the end of the sigmoid. This attachment thus forms an inverted V. The sigmoid colon is four times longer than its mesocolon. Congenital adhesions between the sigmoid colon and the pelvic side wall can be divided to expose the intersigmoid recess. This is a small funnel-shaped pouch into which a loop of bowel may insert itself, forming an internal hernia. Further incision of the peritoneum along the white line of Toldt and mobilization of the sigmoid colon will allow exposure of the ureter and gonadal vessels as they cross in front of the bifurcation of the common iliac artery.

Like the transverse colon, the sigmoid colon is completely invested in peritoneum, and again its length (usually about 45 cm) and mobility may vary enormously. The taenia coli are wider here than in the rest of the colon and they gradually meet to invest the sigmoid in a complete longitudinal coat. The sigmoid colon is usually found within the pelvis arranged in close proximity to the rectum, bladder, and uterus.

Colonic Blood Supply and Venous Drainage

Arterial Supply

The cecum, ascending colon, and proximal two thirds of the transverse colon represent part of the embryonic midgut and are therefore supplied by branches of the superior mesenteric artery. The superior mesenteric artery is a midline aortic branch at the level of L1. It emerges from the undersurface of the pancreas to cross the third part of the duodenum. It runs between the two layers of the small bowel mesentery with branches supplying the whole of the small intestine and midgut portion of the large intestine.

The anterior and posterior cecal vessels arise from the ileal branch of the ileocolic artery and are distributed over the respective sides of the cecum. The posterior cecal artery is the more significant artery supplying most of the cecum. It also gives off the appendicular artery. The ileal branch of the ileocolic artery anastomoses with the distal end of the main stem of the superior mesenteric artery, and in so doing completes a loop of all of the branches from the right side of this major vessel. The mesenteric arcades become modified in the last part of the terminal ilium to form a marginal vessel. This is of practical value when constructing a terminal ileostomy (Fig. 1-2).

The ascending colon is supplied by the ileocolic and right colic arteries. The transverse colon is supplied in its proximal two thirds by the middle colic artery, which has right and left branches and forms a significant series of arcades. The right colic artery arises from the superior mesenteric artery in about 40% of subjects, the middle colic in 30%, the ileocolic artery in 12%, and is absent in 18% of subjects.[1] The middle colic artery arises from the concave surface of the superior mesenteric artery just before it enters the mesentery of the small bowel.

The descending colon receives blood from the left colic artery, a branch of the inferior mesenteric artery, which supplies the derivatives of the embryonic hindgut. The left colic artery divides into an ascending and a descending branch. The ascending branch runs anterior to the left kidney before entering the transverse mesocolon to supply the distal third of the transverse colon and the splenic flexure. An anastomotic arch is formed with the left branch of the middle colic artery. The descending branch supplies the descending colon and anastomoses with the highest of the sigmoid arteries.

The sigmoid arteries are branches of the inferior mesenteric artery and run in the sigmoid mesocolon, where they anastomose with each other to form another series of arcades. However, the lowermost sigmoid artery does not usually anastomose with the superior rectal artery.

Marginal Artery

A marginal artery runs around the medial margin of the whole colon from the colic branch of the ileocolic artery to the arcades of the sigmoid arteries. It is effectively an amalgamation of anastomotic branches of both superior and inferior mesenteric arteries. A collateral blood supply is therefore available. The weakest point in this functional artery lies at the junction of the mid- and hind-gut vessels near the splenic flexure. Inadequacy of the marginal artery in this region may compromise the blood supply to the descending colon from the middle colic artery if the inferior mesenteric artery is ligated. The regional distribution of blood flow also explains the finding that two regions are anatomically vulnerable to ischemic disease: Griffith's point at the junction of the superior mesenteric and inferior mesenteric arteries and Sudeck's critical point at the midportion of the sigmoid at the junction of the inferior mesenteric artery and the hypogastric arteries. Adequate collateral circulation is probably maintained more often than would be suggested by some anatomic studies.[2-4] In these situations, placement of ligatures in relation to the bifurcation of the left colic artery may be important. Ligation of the left colic artery proximal to the bifurcation can permit adequate flow.

Venous Drainage

The venous drainage of the cecum and colon corresponds to the arteries and reaches the portal vein by superior or inferior mesenteric tributaries. Generally, venous blood from the right colon drains via the superior mesenteric vein to the portal vein and blood from the left half drains via the inferior mesenteric vein into either the splenic or superior mesenteric vein and then into the portal vein.

Lymph Drainage

Lymph from the appendix and cecum drains to ileocolic nodes via appendicular and cecal nodes. Lymph from the ascending, transverse, and descending colons drains to nodes along the right, middle, and left colic vessels respectively, while lymph from the sigmoid colon drains first to nodes along the sigmoid arcades. Lymphatics draining the transverse colon communicate

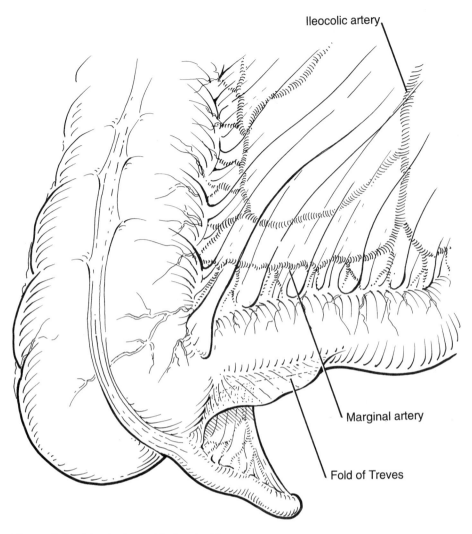

Figure 1-2.   Marginal vessel in terminal ileum.

with those of the greater omentum and can also drain into nodes at the hilum of the spleen. There appears to be no communication, however, between the lymph vessels of the transverse colon and those of the stomach.[5]

Lymph drains from the various regional nodes to the superior or inferior mesenteric nodes along the blood vessels. From these nodes, lymph is channeled upward to the coeliac nodes. The abdominal confluence of lymph trunks join the paired lumbar lymph trunks to form the thoracic duct.

Nerve Supply of the Colon

Parasympathetic Innervation

The colon receives preganglionic parasympathetic nerve fibers from the vagi and pelvic splanchnic nerves. The fibers run from the coeliac and superior mesenteric plexi along branches of the coeliac and superior mesenteric arteries. The vagal branches supply parasympathetic innervation to a point two thirds of the way along the transverse colon, after which pelvic splanchnics from S2–4 take over. These latter nerves run in the superior

hypogastric plexus and then along branches of the inferior mesenteric artery. Preganglionic parasympathetic nerves synapse with their postganglionic counterparts in the wall of the colon and innervate the smooth-muscle and glands. Stimulation increases peristalsis and glandular secretion while blood vessels are dilated.

Sympathetic Innervation

The sympathetic nerve supply is from postganglionic nerve fibers, which originate in spinal cord segments T10 to L2 and follow blood vessels to the colon. Stimulation results in vasoconstriction, inhibition of peristalsis, and constriction of smooth muscle sphincters. Pain fibers accompany these nerves, and as a rule result in pain being referred to the periumbilical area when the source lies in a derivative of the midgut and to the suprapubic region if it originates from a derivative of the hindgut. The exceptions to this rule are the cecum, where pain is referred to the right iliac fossa, and the hepatic flexure, where pain is referred to the right upper quadrant. Pain from fixed parts of the colon tends to be better localized than pain from the more mobile sections.

THE RECTUM, ANUS AND PELVIC FLOOR

Rectum

The sigmoid colon becomes the rectum in front of the third sacral segment at the level at which the sigmoid mesentery ends and the appendices epiploicae disappear. The taenia coli become more diffuse around the rectum and form a complete outer layer of longitudinal muscle. Strands of fibers from the anterior and posterior rectal walls pass to the perineal body and coccyx.[6] The longitudinal muscle merges with muscle bundles of pubococcygeus, and this conjoined muscle splits to pass both sides of the external anal sphincter.

The rectum is both longer and wider than the sacrum, which tapers and is related posteriorly to the fascia over the posterior pelvic wall. The rectum is 15 to 18 cm in length. Proximally, it is of a similar diameter to the sigmoid colon, but it widens to the infraperitoneal ampulla, which is capable of significant distension. The ampulla of the rectum lies upon the anococcygeal ligament and the levator ani muscles.

The transverse crescentic folds of the mucosa of the sigmoid become smooth at the top of the rectum. There are no haustra. The mucosa is folded longitudinally when the rectum is empty, but these folds disappear as the rectum distends and two or three transverse folds then appear (valves of Houston; Fig. 1-3). These rectal folds are produced by the circular muscle of the rectum and are not confined to the mucous membrane, un-like the circular folds of the upper small intestine. The middle fold is the most prominent, and it has been suggested that this fold acts to functionally separate the rectum into an upper part able to distend and store feces and a lower part that only contains feces during defecation. It may also provide a shelf-like support for feces while flatus is passed.

Although the Latin word *rectus* means straight, the rectum actually follows two curves in the sagittal plane (a forward curve in the concavity of the lower sacrum followed by a backward curve as the rectum passes through the pelvic floor) and three curves in the coronal plane (an upper curve convex to the left, a middle one convex to the right, and a lower one convex to the left). The upper third of the rectum is covered by peritoneum anteriorly and at the sides, the middle third is only covered anteriorly, and the lower third is devoid of a peritoneal covering. The peritoneum is reflected forwards to the upper bladder in the male or the upper vagina to form the rectovesical or rectouterine pouch of Douglas. This pouch forms the most dependent part of the peritoneal cavity that is well within reach during a digital rectal examination.

Rectal Dissection and Fascial Planes

Safe mobilization of the rectum can be achieved by ''anatomic'' dissection. The sigmoid loop is elevated firmly to put stretch on the superior rectal artery. Tissue adherent to this vessel is swept backwards, thereby clearing presacral and hypogastric nerves. A window in the sigmoid mesentery is opened and the retrorectal space entered. Sharp dissection develops this space first downward and then forward to the rectosacral fascia at the

Figure 1-3. The valves of Houston.

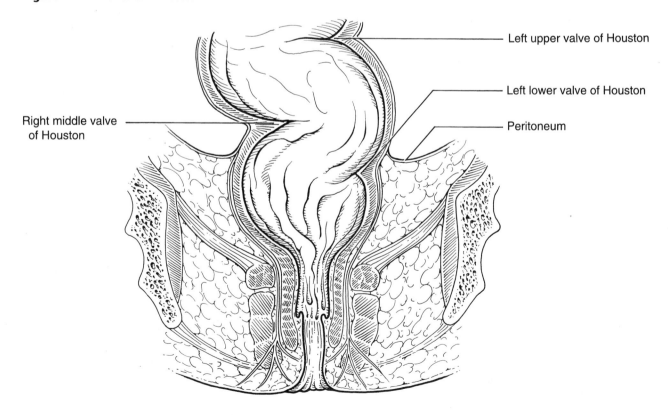

Right middle valve of Houston

Left upper valve of Houston

Left lower valve of Houston

Peritoneum

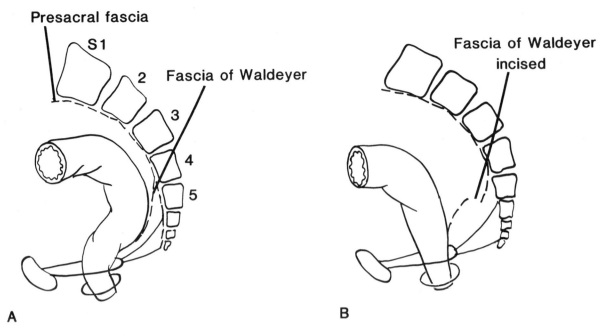

Figure 1-4. The position of the rectum before and after incision of Waldeyer's fascia.

level of S4. The rectum is inversed by the fascia propria. This delicate structure is continuous with the fascia of Denonvilliers anteriorly.

The lower part of the rectum is attached to the sacrum by Waldeyer's fascia (Fig. 1-4), which blends into the rectal longitudinal muscle at the level of the puborectalis. It has a gray-white color and covers the presacral vessels. To mobilize the rectum fully this fascia has to be incised. This should be done with sharp scissor dissection and not bluntly with fingers as this can tear vessels beneath the fascia and cause troublesome presacral venous bleeding. The existence of several venous connections to the vertebrobasilar system can make such bleeding very difficult to control. Moreover, blunt dissection of Waldeyer's fascia can breach the mesorectum.

The peritoneum over the sides of the rectum is incised and the incisions are continued round to meet in the midline. Gentle rotation of the rectum loosens the perirectal tissue and elevates the rectum out of the pelvis.

Anterior to the lower rectum lie the base of the bladder, seminal vesicles, prostate, ureters, and ductus deferens. The rectum is separated from these structures by the rectovesical fascia of Denonvilliers (Fig. 1-5) This structure is continuous laterally with the fascia propria of the rectum and inferiorly with the pelvic fascia covering the levator ani muscle. It extends downwards from the peritoneal reflection to the urogenital diaphragm, between the rectum and urogenital structures. Laterally, it is attached to the lateral ligaments of the rectum. Denonvilliers' fascia is of variable thickness but is often a tough fibrous membrane that provides a firm barrier to the early stages of cancerous spread. Sharp rectal dissection proceeds in the plane between fascia and rectum, and this offers protection to the prostatic plexus of veins, which lie anterior. The rectovaginal septum is the corresponding structure in the female. Both form a useful guide to the anterior mobilization of the rectum during proctectomy.

Finally, there are two lateral condensations of tissue containing the nerves and vessels to the rectum. These are the lateral rectal ligaments and can best be identified after completion of the anterior and posterior parts of the dissection. Traction on the rectum tents the ligaments, which may be defined by pinching beneath the ligaments with the thumb and index finger. The ligaments are divided close to the rectum in benign disease but more laterally in malignant disease. The pelvic nerve plexus lies well lateral and is unlikely to be damaged. Division of these ligaments increases the mobility and "length" of the rectum (by about 5 cm) and is essential in low anterior resection of the rectum.

Anal Canal

The surgical anal canal differs from the anatomic anal canal. The anatomist defines the anal canal as the area from anal valves to anal verge (about 2 cm), whereas the surgeon considers the anal canal to extend from anorectal ring (the level where the rectum passes through the pelvic floor) to anal verge.[7] The average length of the surgical canal is 4 cm (range, 3 to 5 cm) and tends to be shorter in women than in men.[8] The anal canal lengthens when the anal sphincter squeezes and shortens during straining. The anorectal ring at the commencement of the anal canal can be accurately palpated on digital rectal examination because of the prominent fibers of the puborectalis sling. There is no relationship between the length of the anatomic anal canal and that of the surgical anal canal.[8]

The junction of the rectum and anal canal lies at the pelvic floor, where puborectalis pulls the rectum forward (Fig. 1-6). From here, the anal canal runs downwards and backwards. The angulation between anal canal and rectum needs to be remembered when performing anoscopic and proctoscopic examinations.

The muscles of the anal sphincter form a tube within a funnel.

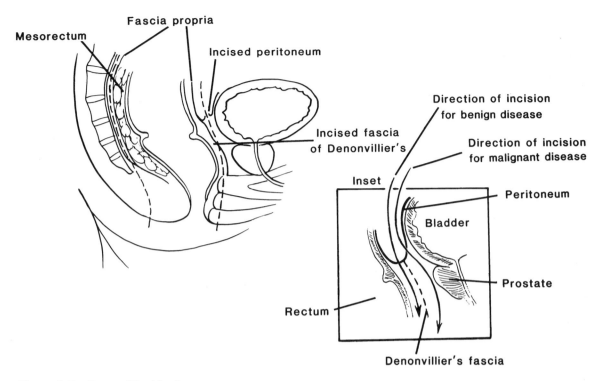

Figure 1-5. Denonvilliers' fascia.

The sides of the upper part of the funnel are levator ani with the external sphincter making the stem of the funnel. The tube within the funnel includes the lower rectal muscularis propria and the internal sphincter (Fig. 1-7).

The circular muscle of the rectum becomes thicker (1 to 5 mm) as it forms the internal anal sphincter. The lower border is quite distinct. The smooth muscle fibers form dense bundles in an oblique arrangement[9] that forms a concentric high-pressure zone. The conjoint longitudinal coat is a thin fibroelastic sheet that passes between the internal and external sphincters. It is formed by fusion of the outer longitudinal layer of rectal muscle with the fibrous components of puborectalis. The presence of this coat separates the two sphincters creating the intersphincteric space.

The external anal sphincter, made of striated muscle, is probably best considered as a continuous, circumferential mass[10] rather than being divided into superficial and deep components or the more conventional description of three components: subcutaneous, superficial, and deep.[11] It is 6 to 10 mm thick[12] and is surrounded by the superficial fascia of the ischiorectal fossae and perianal subcutaneous tissue. The external sphincter is attached to the coccyx posteriorly by the anococcygeal raphe and to the perineal body anteriorly.

Lining of the Anal Canal

The anal canal forms a slit in the sagittal plane with the walls closely opposed and with longitudinal mucosal folds (columns of Morgagni) extending proximally from the anal valves located at the dentate line. Anal glands that secrete mucus empty into small pockets above the valves called anal crypts (Fig. 1-8). The glands are mostly submucosal and some penetrate into the internal sphincter (Fig. 1-9). Infection within these glands may result in perianal or ischiorectal abscesses and fistulae in ano.

Below the dentate line (also known as the pectinate line) is the pecten, which is smooth. The pecten extends down to the intersphincteric groove, and below this lies the perianal skin.

The epithelial lining of the anal canal is in three parts. In the pecten—that is, from the anal margin to the dentate line—the anal canal is lined with a stratified squamous epithelium, which

Figure 1-6. Puborectalis—a sling-like muscle. The anorectal angle is indicated.

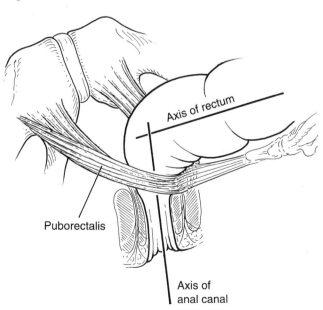

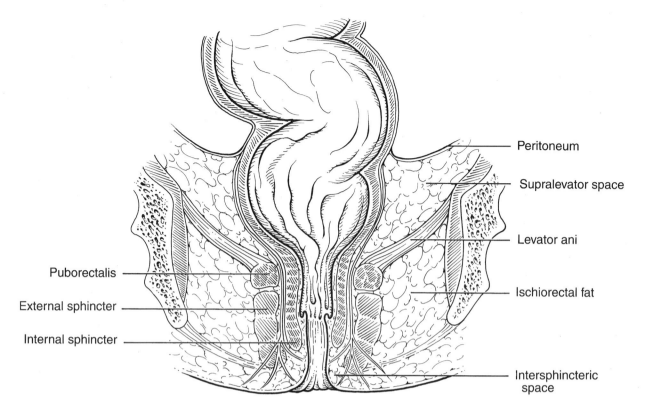

Figure 1-7. The relationship of the rectum to the pelvic floor and anal canal.

Figure 1-8. The anal canal.

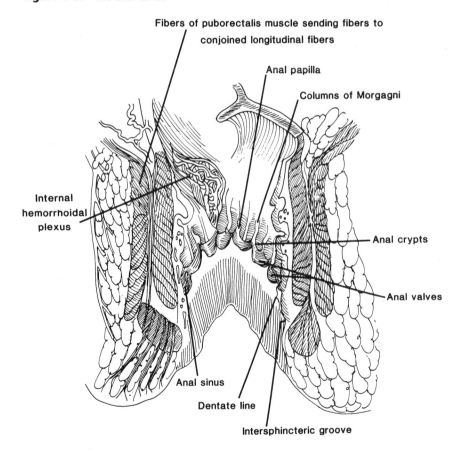

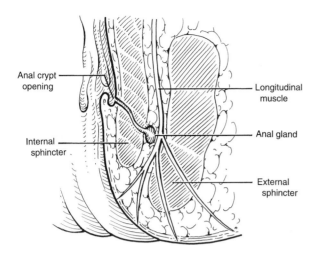

Figure 1-9. Anal glands and crypts.

is keratinized in its lowest portion and contrary to traditional belief contains hair follicles and sweat and apocrine glands. At the level of the anal valves, the epithelium becomes transitional in type with a modified form of columnar epithelium. This anal transitional zone (ATZ) extends for 1.5 to 2 cm.[13] It contains overlapping distributions of endocrine cells from above and melanin-containing cells from below.[14] Rectal columnar mucosa is present above the ATZ. The junction between the ATZ

and the columnar mucosa of the lower rectum is irregular, with tongues of columnar mucosa interdigitating with the ATZ. Frequently, these tongues extend all the way down to the level of the dentate line.[15] This zone, between uninterrupted rectal mucosa and uninterrupted squamous epithelium, plays a critical role in the sensory function of the anal canal.

The anal lining is important in continence, as it fills the lumen of the anal canal, which cannot be fully achieved by the sphincter musculature. The vascular cushions of the anal canal form a dynamic component to the anal lining, as abdominal straining shuts off venous flow from these spaces, which thus act as a gasket to hermetically close the anal canal. Indeed, the cushions may account for up to 15% of resting anal pressure.[16] When the mucocutaneous junction is in its correct position in the high-pressure zone of the anal canal, it acts as an effective barrier against mucus and fecal material. If this junction prolapses, as in patients with hemorrhoids, such that it comes to lie outside the high-pressure zone, then this barrier function fails and patients experience fecal spotting.[17]

Pelvic Floor

The pelvic floor consists of two symmetrical muscular sheets collectively referred to as the pelvic diaphragm or levator ani muscles (Fig. 1-10). Their function is to lend support to pelvic viscera and abdominal contents and to prevent excessive descent of the perineum. The postural reflex of the pelvic floor

Figure 1-10. The muscles of the pelvic floor.

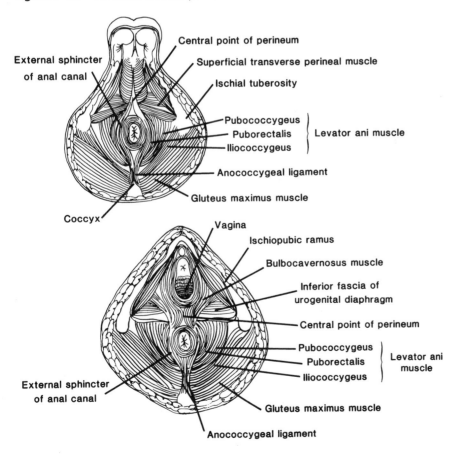

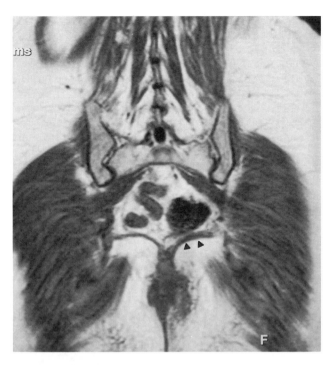

Figure 1-11.   MRI of pelvis demonstrating levator ani sheet (*arrows*).

maintains these muscles in a state of tonic contraction.[18] This muscular sheet is closely related to muscles of the anal canal, vagina, and urethra, as these structures pass through the pelvic floor in the midline. The pelvic floor anterior and posterior to the anorectum is reinforced by the perineal body and anococcygeal body, respectively. The perineal body forms a fibromuscular wedge while the anococcygeal body is a layered structure of muscle, fascia, and tendon.

The levator ani muscles can be divided into four parts: puborectalis, pubococcygeus, iliococcygeus, and ischiococcygeus (Fig. 1-11). The fibers run medially, downwards, and backwards to form a funnel. The puborectalis muscle, at the outlet of this funnel, forms a muscular sling around the anorectal junction and helps create the anorectal angle by pulling this junction towards the pubis. The anorectal angle is about 90 degrees at rest and 135 degrees when straining.[19] Puborectalis arises from the pubic bone and forms a sling around the gut tube creating the anorectal junction. Some fibers fuse with the anococcygeal body and insert into the anterior surface of the coccyx. It is intimately related to the deep part of the external anal sphincter. Some of its fibers enter the wall of the anal canal and strengthen the longitudinal muscle. Iliococcygeus arises from the arcus tendineus between the ileum and ischium, contiguous with, and partly overlapping, pubococcygeus, and inserts into the tip of the coccyx. Finally, ischiococcygeus originates from the ischial spine and inserts into the lateral aspect of the lower sacrum. It appears to be vestigial.

Blood Supply

Rectum

The inferior mesenteric artery becomes the superior rectal (hemorrhoidal) artery as it crosses the pelvic brim. This artery bifurcates, and each branch descends and passes laterally to its respective side of the rectum. It is the principal source of blood for the rectum, with some additional contributions from the middle and inferior rectal arteries and the median sacral artery. The middle rectal arteries arise from the internal iliac arteries and reach the rectum from the side usually on the pelvic floor or, less likely, along the lateral ligaments of the rectum. The symmetrical distribution of a middle rectal artery on each side is seen in only about 20 to 30% of individuals. The inferior rectal (hemorrhoidal) arteries run in the walls of the anal canal directly into the rectum (Fig. 1-12). The rectum will remain viable after division of the superior and middle rectal arteries at least to the level of the peritoneal reflection, surviving solely on the contribution from the inferior rectal arteries.

The rectal veins form an internal rectal plexus in the submucosa that drains to the external rectal plexus outside the rectal wall. Venous blood drains mainly by the superior and inferior rectal veins to the portal and systemic systems. The middle rectal vein is usually insignificant.

Anal Canal

The upper anal canal is supplied by the superior rectal artery, the middle by the middle rectal and middle sacral arteries, and the lower part by the inferior rectal arteries.

Venous drainage corresponds to the arteries. The veins are continuous with the rectal venous plexuses. The upper part of the anal canal drains via the superior rectal and inferior mesenteric veins to the portal system; the lower part drains via the inferior and middle rectal veins to the internal iliac veins and thus to the systemic circulation. An anastomosis between the portal and systemic circulation therefore exists in the region of the anal columns.

Lymphatic Drainage

Rectum

Lymphatic drainage runs along the superior rectal and then inferior mesenteric artery, in the curve of the sacrum with the median sacral artery, and on the side wall of the pelvis with the middle rectal artery (Fig. 1-13). Although the rectum does not have a true mesentery, these nodes are irregularly distributed throughout the loose pelvic fascia in the presacral space. All of this tissue needs to be removed with the rectum in the course of a radical resection for rectal cancer. Lymphatic drainage to iliac nodes on the lateral pelvic wall is an important potential route of spread in tumors of the middle and lower rectum.

Anal Canal

Above the dentate line, lymph drains to the internal iliac nodes. Below the dentate line, lymph drains to the superficial inguinal lymph nodes. Note then that the lymphatic drainage of the lower third of the anal canal is unusual in that it does not follow the vessels. From the superficial inguinal nodes, lymph flows to the external iliac nodes and on to the lumbar trunks.

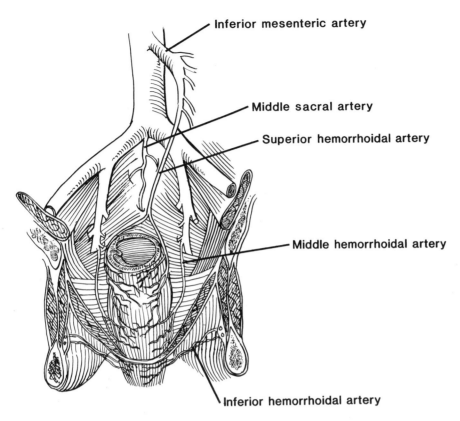

Figure 1-12. Arterial supply to the rectum.

Nerve Supply

Rectum

The parasympathetic nerve supply is motor to rectal muscle and arises from S2 and 3 (or 3 and 4) via the pelvic splanchnic nerves (nervi erigentes; Fig. 1-14). The sympathetic supply is by branches from the hypogastric plexuses, which form the presacral nerve on each side, and by fibers running along the inferior mesenteric and superior rectal arteries.

Sensory Innervation

Ganglion cells are distributed throughout the rectum in three plexuses: Auerbach's myenteric, deep submucous, and superficial plexuses.[20] Intraepithelial receptors, however, are sparse in the rectum.[21] Nerve fibers, myelinated and nonmyelinated, can be seen close to the rectal mucosa, but none are connected to the epithelium. This absence of receptors in the rectal mucosa explains the limited discrimination of rectal sensation. Although the rectum is insensitive to painful stimuli, it is sensitive to distension. It is unknown whether this is a response to stretching of the rectal wall, reflex contraction, or distortion of the rectal "mesentery" or nearby structures. The rectum has a lower threshold to distension than the colon.[22] Until relatively recently, it was assumed dogmatically that receptors capable of detecting distension were located within the rectal wall and that preservation of the rectum was essential if normal fecal continence was to be maintained. The development of restora-

tive proctocolectomy, in which the rectum is replaced by a neorectum fashioned from ileum, and the operation of coloanal anastomosis have shown that normal continence with "recto"-anal reflexes can be preserved in the absence of the rectum.[23-26] These patients experience normal sensations of fullness and need to evacuate. They also recover the ability to discriminate flatus from feces. Therefore, such receptors must lie outside the rectal wall, perhaps in the pelvic floor. This suggestion receives support from observations in children with congenital absence of the anal sphincter mechanism in whom a colonic pull-through operation is performed with colon drawn through the puborectalis sling and anastomosed to the perianal skin. Discrimination of rectal contents is achieved.[27]

Afferent signals from the rectum travel either in sympathetic fibers to ganglion cells at the level of L1 and L2[28] or in parasympathetic nerves to S2–4. Rectal-type sensation is completely abolished by parasympathetic blockade,[22] which appears to be the major pathway.

Innervation of the Pelvic Floor Muscles and Anal Sphincter

The striated muscles of the pelvic floor are innervated by motor neurons that lie in the ventral gray matter of the second and third sacral cord segments. The motor fibers travel in the pudendal nerves that run in Alcock's canal at the level of the sciatic notch. The external anal sphincter is innervated by inferior hemorrhoidal branches of the pudendal nerve, although one in three subjects also has an additional branch directly from the fourth

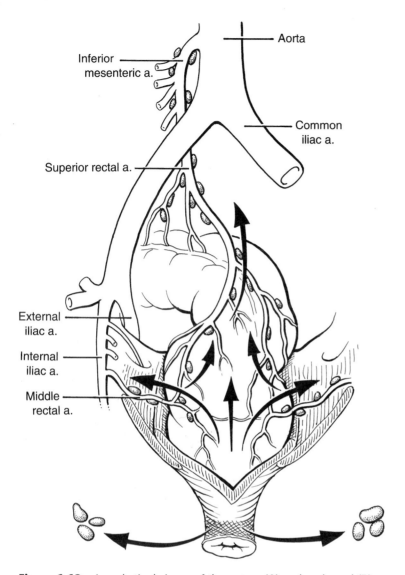

Figure 1-13. Lymphatic drainage of the rectum (**A**) and anal canal (**B**).

sacral nerve (Fig. 1-15). This finding is significant because it explains why a bilateral pudendal nerve block does not completely paralyze the external anal sphincter in all cases.[29] Puborectalis may be innervated by perineal branches of the pudendal nerve from below or by branches of the sacral plexus from above.

The integrity of the pudendal nerve and sacral plexus can be tested by eliciting the anocutaneous reflex by stroking the perianal skin, which normally causes transient contraction of the external anal sphincter. It may be absent in fecal incontinence.

The internal anal sphincter is under inhibitory as well as excitatory control,[30] with cholinergic, adrenergic, and peptidergic nerve fibers present between the smooth muscle cells.[31] Sympathetic fibers are excitatory while parasympathetic nerves are inhibitory. The internal anal sphincter is innervated by postganglionic sympathetic nerves traveling in the hypogastric nerves,[29] and receives preganglionic parasympathetic innervation via the sacral nerves.[32] In vitro studies of isolated internal anal sphincter muscle suggest excitatory α-adrenergic recep-

tors, while β-adrenergic, muscarinic cholinergic, and noncholinergic, nonadrenergic receptors are all inhibitory.

The cell bodies of the motor fibers to the striated sphincter muscles lie at S2 in the ventral horn of the spinal cord (Onuf's nucleus)[33] and are under voluntary control by way of the corticospinal pathways. An extrapyramidal component to control of anal sphincter function is implied by the frequent observation of disturbances in this control in patients with Parkinson's disease.[34] Motor neurons of Onuf's nucleus differ from alpha motor neurons because they are tonically active during sleep[35] and are affected in autonomic diseases such as Shy-Drager syndrome[36] but are resistant to motor neuron disease.[37]

Sensory Innervation of the Anal Canal

The mucosa of the upper anal canal, in contrast to the rectal mucosa, has a rich sensory nerve supply with both free and organized nerve endings such as Krause end-bulbs, Meissner's

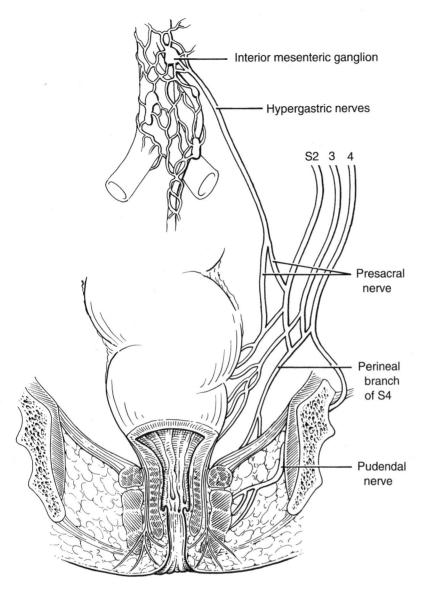

Interior mesenteric ganglion

Hypergastric nerves

S2 3 4

Presacral nerve

Perineal branch of S4

Pudendal nerve

Figure 1-14. Innervation of the rectum, anal canal, and pelvic floor.

corpuscles, and Golgi-Mazzoni bodies. The nerve endings are most concentrated near the anal valves.[38]

The perianal skin is innervated much like hairy skin found elsewhere on the body. Although there are no organized nerve endings, intraepithelial free nerve endings are plentiful. Krause end-bulbs, closely applied to hair follicles, are evident in the skin of the anal margin.

Touch, hot and cold, and pin-prick sensations are all perceived in the anal transitional zone (ATZ), where there are free nerve endings beneath the epithelium. The sensitivity of this region is similar to that of the tip of the index finger. Some nerves form sensory end-knobs. Krause end-bulbs are numerous and respond to temperature. Meissner's corpuscles, although relatively few in number, are sensitive to light touch. Golgi-Mazzoni bodies are plentiful and may respond to alterations in tension and pressure within the anal canal, as do Pacinian corpuscles located near the internal anal sphincter. Muscle spindles have also been identified in this region of the anal canal

as would be predicted by the integrated response of the anal sphincter to increased intra-abdominal pressure.[38]

Sensory impulses from the anal canal travel via the inferior hemorrhoidal branches of the pudendal nerve to S2–4. The main sensory input is below S2.[39]

Ischiorectal Fossa

The ischiorectal fossa is wedge shaped and filled with fat (Fig. 1-7). The base of this wedge is formed by the perianal skin, the medial wall by the anal canal and levator ani muscles, and the lateral wall by the ischial tuberosity and obturator internus. The medial and lateral walls meet at the apex of the fossa with levator ani being attached to the obturator fascia. Anterior to the base lies the perineal body and urogenital diaphragm and posteriorly is the sacrotuberous ligament and the lower border of gluteus maximus. The anococcygeal body separates the two fossae only toward the bases and higher up, behind the anal

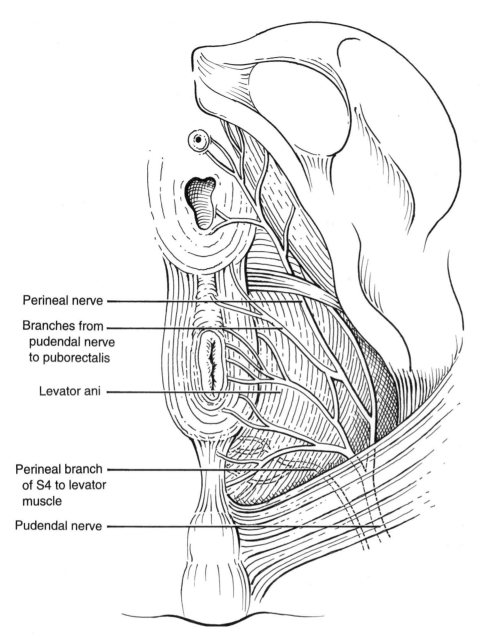

Perineal nerve

Branches from pudendal nerve to puborectalis

Levator ani

Perineal branch of S4 to levator muscle

Pudendal nerve

Figure 1-15. Innervation of puborectalis and external anal sphincter.

canal, there is free communication. This permits the tracking of infection and the potential development of complex horseshoe fistulae.

Alcock's canal runs along the lower lateral wall of the fossa and contains the pudendal nerve and internal pudendal vessels. The nerve can be easily accessed in this canal for physiologic tests.

Perineal Body

The perineal body is an elongated midline fibromuscular mass between the perineal membrane in front and anal canal behind. It acts to stabilize perineal and pelvic structures.

Functional Anatomy of the Anorectum With Reference to Normal Continence and Defecation

Rectoanal Inhibitory Reflex and Sampling

At rest, the anal sphincter is at maximum length and excludes rectal contents from the sensitive mucosa of the ATZ.[40] As the rectum distends, activity in the internal anal sphincter decreases, with a consequent drop in the sphincter pressure,[41] a reflex that is independent of cerebral influence.[42] This reflex is termed the *rectoanal sphincter inhibition response*. The anal canal becomes more funnel shaped and shortened. Intraluminal rectal pressure equals the pressure in the upper anal canal and rectal contents come into contact with the sensitive epithelium of the upper anal canal. The lower part of the anal canal is kept closed by the external sphincter so that continence is maintained. The external anal sphincter shows a burst of EMG activity as the rectum distends, which is abolished by blockade of the pudendal nerve.[29] This burst is followed by sustained contraction of the external anal sphincter. This contractile response (the inflation reflex) is achieved by the recruitment by the external sphincter of muscle activity in the distal anal canal[43] and is heavily influenced by conscious mechanisms.[44]. The internal sphincter recovers spontaneously.

The reflex may be elicited by as little as 5 ml of water or air and most subjects will show a positive response to 20 ml.[29] With 50 ml of air, the rectoanal inhibitory reflex usually lasts for about 20 seconds. Increased distension is associated with increased depth and duration of relaxation.[43] Electrical stimulation of the rectal wall will elicit a similar response,[45] as will instillation of cold water into the rectum.[32] The reflex can be abolished by covering the rectal wall with a local anesthetic gel.[32] This reflex, apparently mediated by enteric nerves, although the exact nerve pathways and transmitters have yet to be identified, was originally demonstrated in static patients lying in the left lateral position, but its presence has recently been confirmed in ambulatory patients and it correlates with episodes of passage of flatus. It occurs about 7 times per hour and lasts 10 to 30 seconds.[46] As rectal distension increases, internal anal sphincter relaxation also increases and eventually, when the external sphincter becomes fatigued, evacuation is inevitable. Chronic inhibition of the anal sphincter complex, as in patients with fecal impaction, leads to a patulous anus with stool in the anal canal and seepage and soilage.[30] Treatment of fecal impaction allows anal tone to return to normal and continence to be regained.

The rectoanal inhibitory reflex is lost after restorative proctocolectomy unless a long rectal muscular cuff is preserved. The reflex may return with time if the ATZ is preserved, but this is less likely if it is sacrificed. Intramural rectal ganglia are critical to the function of this reflex as it is absent in patients with Hirschsprung's disease.[47]

Although this sampling reflex plays a major role, the exact mechanism that allows discrimination between gas, liquid, and solid within the rectum remains to be determined. Temperature change may be important. Although the rectum is insensitive, the anal canal is very sensitive to small changes in temperature along its entire length.[48] Changes as small as 0.6°C are detectable. It is likely that complex integration of sensory input from several modalities is involved in this discriminatory process.

Mechanism of Defecation

Events leading to defecation start when the volume of content in the sigmoid becomes large enough to initiate contractions that empty the stool into the rectum. Conscious awareness of a full rectum is brought about by receptors in the rectal wall, pelvic floor, and upper anal canal by way of the rectoanal inhibitory reflex. Rectal filling is recognized at a volume of about 50 ml. If the rectum continues to fill, a temporary sensation of an urge to defecate is elicited, followed by a constant urge and eventually pelvic discomfort—the maximal tolerable volume. Puborectalis is stretched by rectal pressure waves, and the amplitude of these waves increases[49] as the rectum distends. The urge to defecate is probably mediated by stretch receptors in the pelvic floor because tugging a small balloon against puborectalis will produce this feeling.[50] The precise influences of the rate of rectal filling and the nature of its content on conscious awareness are unknown. Distension of the rectum leads to relaxation of the internal anal sphincter and sampling of the contents. The external sphincter contracts. If it is socially convenient, then the pressure within the rectum must be made to exceed

Figure 1-16. Normal structures that can be palpated on digital examination.

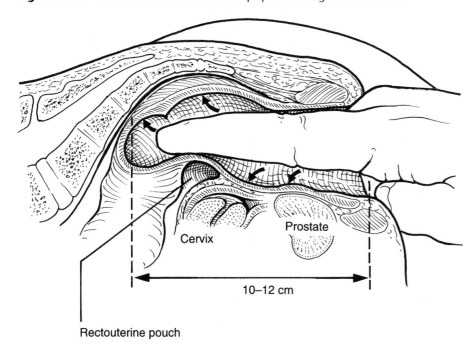

Cervix

Prostate

10–12 cm

Rectouterine pouch

that of the anal canal. This is largely achieved by increasing the intra-abdominal pressure by contraction of the diaphragm, abdominal muscles, and performance of the Valsalva maneuver. It is not known if contraction of the rectal wall occurs during defecation. Relaxation of puborectalis allows the anorectal angle to become less acute, increasing from a mean of 92 degrees to a mean of 111 to 137 degrees,[51] and this is helped if the subject adopts the squatting position, which increases the anorectal angle more than that achieved by flexion of the hips to 90 degrees alone. Inhibition of pelvic floor activity allows descent of the pelvic floor by about 2 cm, which further straightens out this angle.[52,53] As the rectum evacuates, there is prolonged inhibition of the internal and external anal sphincters and anal pressure falls. Conversely, if it is not socially convenient, then brief conscious contraction of the external sphincter allows the internal sphincter to recover and the rectal contents are propelled in an oral direction by forceful contraction of puborectalis and the rest of the pelvic floor musculature. Internal anal sphincter tone returns to normal.

Defecation is influenced by the size and consistency of the stool. The time required to expel a single solid sphere is inversely proportional to its diameter.[54] More effort is required to evacuate small, hard stools. The ideal stool diameter is about 2 cm.

Straining at defecation is associated with the co-contraction of laryngeal, respiratory, and abdominal muscles and the inhibition of anal sphincter muscles, and this patterned recruitment is closely linked to the extrapyramidal system. Paradoxical contraction of puborectalis and the external anal sphincter during defecation is seen in patients with Parkinson's disease.[55] Higher control is needed for appropriate defecatory responses, as illustrated by patients with damage to the frontal lobes.[56] Defecation will occur without any warning in these patients.

Digital Examination

The normal structures that can be palpated in digital examination per anus are shown in Figure 1-16. Essentially they include the lining of the rectum and anal canal, extrarectal pelvic structures, the pelvic floor, and the anal sphincter. Normally, palpable extrarectal structures include the bony confines of the pelvis, the uterus in the female, and the prostate in the male. Occasionally the sigmoid colon or the ovary may be palpable—the pouch of Douglas. It is possible to examine the rectum to a distance of about 12 cm from the anal verge in most patients. Stool may resemble a pathologic mass but can be diagnosed by its indentibility.

REFERENCES

1. Rankin FW, Steward AJ (1932) p. 30. In Rankin FW, Bargen JA, Buie LA (eds): The Colon, Rectum & Anus. WB Saunders Philadelphia
2. Ault GW, Castro AF, Smith RS (1952) Clinical study of ligation of the inferior mesenteric artery in left colon resections. Surg Gynecol Obstet 94:223–228
3. Goligher JC (1954) The adequacy of the marginal blood supply to the left colon after high ligation of the inferior mesenteric artery during excision of the rectum. Br J Surg 41:351–353
4. Griffiths JD (1956) Surgical anatomy of the blood supply of the distal colon. Ann R Coll Surg Engl 19:241–256
5. Jamieson JK, Dobson JF (1909) The lymphatics of the colon. Proc R Soc Med 2:149
6. Wesson MB (1951) Rationale of prostatectomy. Am J Surg 82:714–719
7. Milligan ETC, Morgan CN (1934) Surgical anatomy of the anal canal with special reference to anorectal fistulae. Lancet 2:1150–1156
8. Nivatvongs S, Stern HS, Fryd DS (1981) The length of the anal canal. Dis Colon Rectum 24:600–601
9. Goligher JC, Leacock AG, Brossy JJ (1955) The surgical anatomy of the anal canal. Br J Surg 43:51–61
10. Dalley AF II (1987) The riddle of the sphincters. Am Surg 53:298–306
11. Thompson P (1899) The Myology of the Pelvic Floor: A Contribution to Human and Comparative Anatomy. McCorquodale, London
12. Nielson MB, Hauge C, Rasmussen OO et al (1992) Anal sphincter size measured by endosonography in healthy volunteers. Acta Radiol 33:453–456
13. Fenger C (1979) The anal transitional zone. APMIS 87:379–386
14. Fenger C, Lyon H (1982) Endocrine cells and melanin containing cells in anal canal. Histochem J 14:631–639
15. Ambroze WL, Pemberton JH, Dozois RR et al (1993) The histologic pattern and pathologic involvement of the anal transition zone in patients with ulcerative colitis. Gastroenterology 104:514–518
16. Lestar B, Pennickx F, Kerremans R (1989) The composition of anal basal pressure. Int J Colorect Dis 4:118–122
17. Eyers AA, Thomson JP (1979) Pruritus ani: is anal sphincter dysfunction important in aetiology? Br Med J 2:1549–1551
18. Parks AG, Porter NH, Melzak J (1962) Experimental study of the reflex mechanism controlling the muscles of the pelvic floor. Dis Colon Rectum 5:407–414
19. Mahieu P, Pringot J, Bodart P (1984) Defecography: I. Description of a new procedure and results in normal patients. Gastrointest Radiol 9:247–251
20. Aldridge RT, Campbell PE (1968) Ganglion cell distribution in the normal rectum and anal canal. J Pedatr Surg 3:475–490
21. Duthie HL, Gairns FW (1960) Sensory nerve endings and sensation in the anal region of man. Br J Surg 47:585–595
22. Goligher JC, Hughes ESR (1951) Sensibility of the rectum and colon. Its role in the mechanism of anal continence. Lancet 1:543–547
23. Lane RHS, Parks AG (1977) Function of the anal sphincter following colo-anal anastomosis. Br J Surg 64:596–599
24. Beart RW, Dozois RR, Wolff BG et al (1985) Mechanisms of rectal continence: lessons from the ileoanal procedure. Am J Surg 149:31–34
25. Sagar PM, Holdsworth PJ, Johnston D (1991) Correlation between laboratory findings and clinical outcome after restorative proctocolectomy: serial studies in 20 patients after end-to-end pouch-anal anastomosis. Br J Surg 78:67–70

26. Ferrara A, Pemberton JH, Hanson RB (1992) Preservation of continence after ileoanal anastomosis by the coordination of ileal pouch and anal canal motor activity. Am J Surg 163: 83–89

27. Stephens FD, Durham-Smith E (1971) Ano-rectal Malformations in Children. Year Book Medical Publishers, Chicago

28. Gask GE, Ross JP (1937) The Surgery of the Sympathetic Nervous System, 2nd Ed. Bailliere Tindall, London

29. Freckner B, von Euler C (1975) Influence of pudendal block on function of the anal sphincters. Gut 16:482–489

30. Denny-Brown D, Robertson GE (1935) An investigation of the nervous control of defaecation. Brain 58:256–310

31. Penninckx F (1981) Morphological and Physiological Aspects of Anal Continence. Acco, Leuven, Belgium

32. Meunier P, Mollard P (1977) Control of the internal anal sphincter (manometric study with human subjects). Pflugers Arch 370:233–239

33. Onuf B (1901) On the arrangement and function of cell groups of the sacral region of the spinal cord in man. Arch Neurol Psychopath 3:387–412

34. Pallis CA (1971) Parkinsonism: natural history and clinical features. Br Med J 3:683–690

35. Floyd WF, Walls EW (1953) Electromyography of the sphincter ani externus in man. J Physiol 122:599–609

36. Sung JH, Mastri AR, Segal E (1979) Pathology of Shy-Drager syndrome. J Neuropathol Exp Neurol 38:353–367

37. Mannen T, Iwata M, Toyokura Y et al (1982) The Onuf's nucleus and external anal sphincter muscles in amyotrophic lateral sclerosis and Shy-Drager syndrome. Acta Neuropath 58:255–260

38. Gould RP (1960) Sensory innervation of the anal canal. Nature. 187:337–338

39. Gunterberg B, Kewenter J, Petersén I et al (1976) Anorectal function after major resections of the sacrum with bilateral or unilateral sacrifice of sacral nerves. Br J Surg 63:546–554

40. Duthie HL, Bennett RC (1963) The relation of sensation in the anal canal to the functional anal sphincter: a possible factor in anal continence. Gut 4:179–182

41. Gowers WR (1878) The automatic action of the sphincter ani. Proc R Soc Lond 26:77–84

42. Gaston EA (1948) The physiology of fecal continence. Surg Gynecol Obstet. 87:280–290

43. Bannister JJ, Read NW, Donely TC et al (1989) External and internal anal sphincter responses to rectal distension in normal subjects and in patients with faecal incontinence. Br J Surg 76:617–621

44. Whitehead WE, Orr WC, Engel BT et al (1982) External anal sphincter response to rectal distension: learned response or reflex. Psychophysiology 19:57–62

45. Kamm MA, Lennard-Jones JE, Nicholls RJ (1989) Evaluation of the intrinsic innervation of the internal sphincter using electrical stimulation. Gut 30:935–938

46. Miller R, Lewis GT, Bartolo DCC (1988) Sensory discrimination and dynamic activity in the anorectum: evidence using a new ambulatory technique. Br J Surg 75:1003–1007

47. Lawson J, Nixon HH (1967) Anal canal pressures in the diagnosis of Hirschsprung's disease. J Pediatr Surg 2:544–552

48. Miller R, Bartolo DCC, Cervero F et al (1987) Anorectal temperature sensation: a comparison of normal and incontinent patients. Br J Surg 74:511–515

49. Haynes WG, Read NW (1982) Anorectal activity in man during rectal infusion of saline: a dynamic assessment of the anal continence mechanism. J Physiol 330:45–56

50. Scarli AF, Kiesewetter WB (1970) Defecation and continence. Dis Colon Rectum 13:81–107

51. Womack NR, Williams NS, Holmfield JH et al (1985) New method for the dynamic assessment of anorectal function in constipation. Br J Surg 72:994–998

52. Barkel DC, Pemberton JH, Phillips SF et al (1986) Scintigraphic assessment of the anorectal angle in health and after operation. Surg Forum 37:183–186

53. Womack NR, Williams NS, Holmfield JHM (1987) Anorectal function in the solitary rectal ulcer syndrome. Dis Colon Rectum 30:319–323

54. Ambroze WL, Pemberton JH, Bell AM et al (1991) The effect of stool consistency on rectal and neorectal emptying. Dis Colon Rectum 34:1–7

55. Christmas TJ, Kempster PA, Chapple CR (1988) Role of subcutaneous apomorphine in Parkinsonian voiding dysfunction. Lancet 2:1451–1453

56. Andrew J, Nathan P (1964) Lesions of the anterior frontal lobes and disturbances of micturition and defaecation. Brain 87:233–262

2

INTESTINAL FUNCTIONS

Sidney F. Phillips

Patients can lead productive and healthy lives after total procto-colectomy; clearly, the human colon is not an essential organ. However, a healthy large intestine is essential for normal intestinal metabolism of water, electrolytes, and some nutrients; moreover, colorectal function needs to be normal if defecation is to be socially convenient. Thus, the large bowel, being the final conduit for chyme and digestive residues, offers the last chance for the gut to reduce fecal volumes and to package stools for programmable evacuation. In this regard, the colon salvages any chyme that escapes digestion and/or absorption in the small bowel, and reabsorbs endogenous secretions. Although the human large intestine is highly efficient in performing these functions, its proficiencies rely heavily on cooperative interactions with the small bowel. Flow through the ileocolonic junction determines what the colon receives, and the rate at which it is received. The colon's function is also much dependent upon the resident flora, which have important digestive functions. Without intraluminal digestion by bacterial enzymes, the colon would not be able to achieve its full potential. Fortunately, the healthy colon is adaptable and is able to handle widely variable loads, by increasing absorption considerably, before diarrhea occurs.[1–3]

This textbook is directed towards the large bowel, and is intended for a primary readership of colorectal surgeons. The role of this chapter is to provide a background for the combined digestive and absorptive functions of the small and large intestines; attention is therefore directed to similarities and differences among the jejunum, ileum, and colon. This is appropriate, for the functions demanded of the colon result largely from what is accomplished, and what is left undone, by the small bowel. Thus, review of digestion and absorption in the small bowel is pertinent background to an understanding of what the colon is called upon to achieve.

Some of the first experiments that quantified human colonic absorption in vivo measured rates of fluid and electrolyte absorption in healthy volunteers.[3] On a normal diet, between 1 and 2 L of fluid were absorbed each day, representing more than 90% of the water and salts transferred from the ileum into the colon. In a later experiment, the large intestine was systematically overloaded (by cecal infusions of fluid) up to and beyond its capacity[2]; these studies showed that the healthy colon could increase its basal rate of absorption several-fold, up to 5 to 6 L daily. Diarrhea due to incomplete reabsorption of fluid in the small bowel thus requires an overwhelming increase in the colon's inflow volume. Such a major load, as a result of small bowel failure, has been documented only in severe examples of small bowel diarrhea, such as with Asiatic cholera, major small bowel disease, or resection. In perhaps the clearest clinical example, cholera, the function of the colon is thought to be largely unchanged, yet debilitating diarrhea is usual; ileal volumes are in the range of 5 to 10 liters.[4]

Fortunately, severe small bowel diarrheas are unusual; but a number of circumstances are known to reduce the colon's normal capacity to compensate even for normal volumes of inflow. These include changes in the composition of chyme entering from the ileum. Thus, colonic epithelial transport is impaired by high luminal concentrations of bile salts or fatty acids,[5–9] and numerous clinically relevant examples are well documented.[1,9,10] Other possible reasons for inadequate compensation by the colon include motility patterns that do not provide conditions for optimal storage and reabsorption.[11] Indeed, attention has been drawn previously to the important role played by ''colonic salvage'' in normal bowel function and the pathogenesis of diarrhea.[1]

Do the reverse circumstances apply to the symptom of constipation? Can constipation result from ''hyperabsorption''? Decreased flow from the ileum into the colon in constipated persons is possible, but no data are available. Certainly, persons on restricted or elemental diets pass small stools, presumably in association with lesser inputs to the large bowel. Disordered motility of the proximal gut, and slow transit of chyme to the colon, has been said to accompany, and perhaps be implicated in, the pathophysiology of simple constipation.[12] However, the presence of motor disorders of the stomach and/or small bowel in patients with constipation more likely raises the possibility of a generalized disorder of motility, such as intestinal pseud-obstruction. Increased mucosal uptake of solutes and fluids (''hyperabsorption'') was not demonstrated in constipated persons, except as a phenomenon secondary to slow transit.[13] Thus, although altered absorption/secretion are possible pathophysiologies in constipated patients, disorders of colonic transit and/or rectal evacuation[14,15] are more likely the primary etiologies of constipation. This chapter reviews mucosal function, intraluminal metabolism, and transit in the healthy human small bowel and colon, and addresses abnormalities that might apply to patients with colonic disease.

PROPERTIES OF SMALL AND LARGE BOWELS AS ABSORBING ORGANS

Secretion, Digestion, and Absorption in the Small Bowel

The major functions of the small intestine are (1) secretion, whereby fluids of widely differing composition are added to foods; (2) digestion, the physiochemical reactions that break down dietary components to simpler compounds; and (3) absorption of the products of digestion, electrolytes, and water. Motility, which propels and mixes foodstuffs with secretions, facilitates all of these functions.

Most of these phenomena are relatively quiescent under basal circumstances. They are variably stimulated by sensory (cephalic) stimuli and evoked specifically by the ingestion of food. The concept that the different functions are normally integrated by hormonal, paracrine, and neural mechanisms into a precisely coordinated whole is central to an understanding of how disease and surgical operations might derange these functions.[16]

Secretion

In addition to specific glandular fluids, mucosal secretion and absorption can greatly influence body water and electrolyte content, because a normal intake of fluid added to the endogenous secretions of the upper gut amounts to 8 to 10 L daily (Table 2-1). The secreted fluid comes largely from the extracellular space. For example, in a 70-kg adult, a volume equal to about half of the extracellular fluid is secreted into the upper gastrointestinal tract daily, a far larger volume than is added normally from the diet.

Food entering the upper gastrointestinal tract promotes the simultaneous or sequential secretion of saliva, gastric juice, bile, and pancreatic juice. These fluids, although being isotonic, contain widely varying concentrations of sodium, potassium, chloride, bicarbonate, and hydrogen ions (Table 2-1). Mixing, propulsion, digestion, and progressive equilibration toward the physiologic extracellular pH and osmolality occur in the stomach and duodenum. In the small intestine, isotonic, neutral fluid (succus entericus) is added to chyme; this fluid is rich in chloride in the jejunum but, in the ileum, bicarbonate is the predominant anion.

Absorption of fluid begins in the duodenum and peaks in the proximal jejunum. Reabsorption in the proximal bowel conserves 6 to 8 L of water, more than 500 mEq of sodium and chloride, 200 mEq of bicarbonate, and 100 mEq of potassium. Absorption of water and electrolytes continues in the ileum and is completed in the colon, where each day 1 to 2 L of semiliquid material is progressively desiccated to feces. Absorption is so efficient that 200 mL or less is excreted as feces per day.[16]

Digestion

Gastric emptying is slowed postprandially, mainly by the stimulation of receptors in the duodenum that are sensitive to the initial emptying of fat, acid, and hyperosmolar foods. The meal is retained in the stomach until solids are triturated by the antrum to a mean size of approximately 1 mm, and peptic digestion of proteins has proceeded. Emptied chyme is then mixed with pancreatic, biliary, and intestinal juices. Starch is broken down, mainly to oligosaccharides, by pancreatic amylase. Lipids are hydrolyzed into fatty acids and monoglycerides by lipase; proteins are broken down into small peptides and amino acids by trypsin, chymotrypsin, and carboxypeptidases.

The processes of luminal digestion set the stage for the final hydrolytic steps, which occur at the brush border and microvilli of enterocytes. Oligosaccharides accumulate at the brush border, where they are hydrolyzed to monosaccharides by sucrase, lactase, and maltase. Oligopeptides are similarly broken down to amino acids by peptidases. High concentrations of the final digestive products at the brush border of epithelial cells facilitate passive and active absorption. Micelles, composed of bile salts, monoglycerides, fatty acids, and phospholipids, constitute an aqueous phase from which dietary fats are absorbed.

Absorption

Absorption moves nutrients, ions, and water from the lumen of the bowel into portal venous blood and the abdominal lymphatics, utilizing a variety of passive and active transport systems.

Table 2-1. Approximate Composition of Diet and Gastrointestinal Secretions Per 24 Hours

	Content (mEq)				Concentration (mEq/L)				
	Fluid (L)	Na⁺	K⁺	Cl⁻	HCO₃⁻	Na⁺	K⁺	[Cl⁻]	[HCO₃⁻]	pH
Diet	2–3	150	50	200	—	—	—	—	—	—
Saliva	1	50	20	40	50	20–80	10–20	20–40	20–60	7.0–8.0
Gastric juice	1–2	40–160	15	200	—	60–130	5–10	120–130	—	1.0–7.0
Bile	1	100	5	40	40	150–250	5–10	40–80	20–40	7.0–8.0
Pancreatic juice	1–2	150	5	40	120	160	5–10	20–100	30–100	7.0–8.0
Succus entericus	1–2	140–280	5–10	Variable	Variable	140	5	Variable	Variable	7.0–8.0

Most important nutrients are absorbed by active mechanisms, which require specific mucosal "carriers." Passive transport of ions is determined by relative chemical (concentration) and electrical (mucosal-serosal potential difference) forces across the mucosa. Active transport is defined as movement not explicable by, and sometimes against, electrochemical gradients. Absorption may be modified also by "solvent drag," that is, the incorporation of solute into the bulk flow of water. Solvent drag is determined by the particulate size of solutes in solution relative to water-filled "pores" through which the solvent (water) moves.

Absorption of sodium is considered central to the absorption of water, other electrolytes, and certain nutrients. Sodium transport is active throughout the small and large intestine. Inhibition of active sodium absorption leads to net accumulation of sodium in the lumen, which in turn creates an osmotic gradient along which water flows. An ATP-dependent "sodium pump," which normally transports sodium from lumen to blood across the basolateral surface of enterocytes, is sensitive to a variety of toxic, humoral, or mechanical insults.[6,7] Inhibition of active sodium transport unmasks a simultaneous mechanism for loss of sodium from extracellular fluid into the lumen. There is evidence that mucosal villi are the prime site of fluid absorption and that crypts are the source of the endogenous secretion.

Amino acids, simple sugars, glycerol, and short- and medium-chain fatty acids pass directly into the portal venous blood, while long-chain fatty acids are refashioned within enterocytes into triglycerides that are incorporated into chylomicrons that pass first into the intestinal lymphatics and only later into the systemic circulation via the thoracic duct.

In the jejunum, sodium is absorbed actively and also moves with bulk flow of water through relatively large mucosal pores. Glucose, other actively absorbed monosaccharides, amino acids, and bicarbonate ions all enhance sodium absorption. Sodium in turn augments glucose and amino acid transport, a process called facilitated active transport. Water transport is considered to be passive and dependent on osmotic forces. Potassium also moves across the mucosa, following its concentration gradient between the lumen and blood, modified by the small negative electric potential of jejunal mucosa. Chloride mostly follows sodium to preserve electrical neutrality in the lumen. Bicarbonate disappears rapidly from the lumen by mechanisms that involve active ionic absorption and neutralization of bicarbonate by hydrogen ions present in chyme.

Each day, 2 to 3 L of neutral, isotonic chyme passes into and through the ileum. The ileal mucosa is less permeable than the jejunum to simple diffusion of ions; however, sodium is absorbed actively against large electrochemical gradients, and water follows (Table 2-2). Movement of potassium across the mucosa of the ileum can be explained by electrochemical gradients, but the mechanisms of anion movement are more complex. Absorption of chloride and secretion of bicarbonate are coupled to a process that involves active transport of one or both ions. It follows that pH and bicarbonate concentrations increase in the distal small bowel, and losses from the distal small bowel are more likely to result in metabolic acidosis. The ileum actively absorbs bile salts and vitamin B_{12}, provided that the vitamin is complexed to gastric intrinsic factor. Some of these gradations of function from jejunum to ileum continue

Table 2-2. Comparative Absorption Characteristics of Small Bowel and Colon

	Jejunum	Ileum	Colon
Water absorption	Isotonic	Isotonic	Hypertonic
Mucosal permeability	+ + +	+ +	+
Active Na transport	±	+	+ +
Active Cl transport	±	+ +	+ + +
Mucosal PD	< 10 mV	< 10 mV	30–40 mV
Response to mineralocorticoids	±	+	+ +
Stimulation by glucose/amino acid	+ +	+	±

into the large intestine. One of the striking changes is in the mucosal permeability (Table 2-2).

Colonic Mucosa as a "Tight" Epithelium: Contrasts With the Small Bowel

The absorptive properties of colonic epithelium reflect in large part its structure as a bilayer phospholipid membrane, which readily allows diffusion of lipophilic solutes across it while restricting the movement of water and hydrophilic molecules. Small, water-soluble molecules therefore require specific carrier proteins for active transport, or water filled pores for passive movement, if they are to cross the membrane. The pores are probably located in the tight junction region between epithelial cells, and pores of this type have indeed been classified as tight or leaky.[17] The colon, unlike the small intestine, has a tight mucosa, one that restricts the passive fluxes of ions and thereby minimizes water and electrolyte loss in the stool. The basic knowledge of these features has focused on three concepts: pore size, mucosal permeability, and transepithelial potential difference (Table 2-2).

Effective pore size in the colon has been estimated as less than 23 nm, smaller than the urea molecule; comparable values for the jejunum and ileum are 80 and 40 nm, respectively. These differences are important determinants of in vivo function. Thus, permeability studies have demonstrated that the human colon can absorb water even in the face of large osmotic gradients, whereas transport in the small bowel is isotonic. In addition, the colon restricts the movement of molecules such as polyethylene glycol (PEG) to a much greater degree than do the ileum and jejunum, as evidenced by studies of urinary excretion of these substances after their colonic instillation.[18]

The functional consequence of these membrane properties, when combined with active sodium (Na) absorption, is a spontaneous, transepithelial potential difference (PD), with the mucosa being negative to the serosa.[6,7] The voltages generated as low in the small bowel, high in the colon (Table 2-2). The PD of the colonic mucosa is increased by exogenous mineralocorticoids and in hypercortisonism (endogenous). Though possible in theory, more efficient absorption of Na leading to a greater negative PD and contributing to hyperabsorption of fluids in constipation, has never been reported.

Intestinal permeability can be measured by noninvasive, simple, and relatively inexpensive methods[18,19] that have been applied to a wide range of clinical conditions including Crohn's disease, intestinal injury by nonsteroidal anti-inflammatory drugs and sprue. The commonest methods use test molecules given by mouth,[19] so that it is the permeability of the small intestine (predominantly jejunum) that is assessed. Convenient methods have not been developed for the measurement of colonic permeability in clinical practice. Test solutions would probably need to be instilled directly into the colon, as has been done experimentally.[18] Abnormalities of permeability have been implicated in the pathogenesis of Crohn's disease (see ref. 19 for a review).

Colonic Absorption of Inorganic Ions and Water

In most mammalian species, the colonic mucosa actively absorbs Na and chloride (Cl) whereas bicarbonate (HCO_3) accumulates on the mucosal side. Net movements of ions follow the same general principles in humans, but the major mechanisms for ionic transport vary in relative importance from the proximal to the distal colon. Sodium is absorbed actively, against electrical and concentration gradients, such that a linear relationship is maintained between the rate of Na absorption and luminal concentrations of Na, from 25 to 150 mmol/L.[20] Both active electrogenic (giving rise to PD) and electroneutral processes move Na out of the lumen, but mechanisms accounting for all of Na transport across the colonic mucosa have not yet been described.

Three absorptive membrane pumps are important.[6,7] The first is a ouabain-sensitive sodium-potassium (Na-K) ATPase located at the basal surface of colonic epithelial cells; this pump actively extrudes Na into the extracellular fluid, thereby lowering the intracellular Na concentration. The second operates at the apical surface of colonocytes, is electrogenic, and can be blocked by amiloride. This pump is more important in the distal colon. Electrogenic Na absorption thus exhibits a gradient from proximal to distal bowel and contributes most to Na absorption in distal segments. The third mechanism accomplishes electroneutral Na and Cl absorption by parallel Na-H and Cl-HCO_3 exchange and has been localized to the brush border of colonocytes. Exchangers of sodium and hydrogen ions are not unique to the colon but are found in almost all cells, are probably driven by sodium gradients established by Na-K ATP-ase, but are particularly prominent in the large bowel. In contrast to the small bowel, addition of glucose or amino acids to solutions in contact with colonic mucosa does not augment sodium uptake (Table 2-2).

Chloride, like Na, is actively absorbed against large concentration gradients. Indeed, chloride continues to be absorbed even when the flow of water is into the lumen. At equal concentrations of Na and Cl, Cl absorption exceeds that of Na, the difference being accounted for by HCO_3 secretion.[20] Cl-HCO_3 exchange has been estimated to provide for approximately 25% of total Cl absorption in the human colon. Thus, the colon acts to conserve chloride; it is conveniently exchanged for bicarbonate ions, which can be generated metabolically. Carbonic anhydrase is involved in the process, because Cl absorption and HCO_3 secretion are reduced by acetazolamide. Failure of Cl-HCO_3 exchange is important clinically; the dramatic loss of this mech-

anism has been demonstrated in the diarrheal syndrome of infants, congenital chloridorrhea.[21]

Several mechanisms regulate the movement of K in and out of the lumen. Luminal concentrations of K and the total levels of body K both appear to influence the balance between absorption and secretion. K accumulates in the lumen when luminal fluid contains less than 15 mmol/L, but K is absorbed when greater concentrations are present.[20] These findings are consistent with passive K movement along electrochemical gradients. However, other mechanisms also operate, including a secretion of K that is dependent on luminal Na.[6,7]

Calcium, magnesium, and zinc are largely absorbed in the small intestine and there is very little information on the role of the colon in their homeostasis. Hypermagnesaemia has been described after the administration of enemas that contain magnesium sulphate and, during colonic perfusion experiments, magnesium can be absorbed and calcium secreted. Radioactive magnesium and calcium were absorbed and readily detectable in the blood of healthy volunteers after rectal instillation. Zinc deficiency may occur with prolonged parenteral nutrition, but its metabolism by the human colon is unknown.[6,7]

Secretion of Ions and Water

A net accumulation of fluid in the intestine could result from inhibition of absorption, especially if a basal state of secretion was thereby "unmasked." Conversely, fluid would also accumulate in the lumen if ions and water were actively secreted. The relative contribution of either mechanism is not clear. Active secretion requires that ions move from the serosal to mucosal fluids against electrochemical gradients. The phenomenon fundamental to intestinal secretion is now thought to be an active secretion of chloride ions; thus, most basic studies focus now on the control of chloride channels. Chloride secretion can be stimulated in colonic mucosa by the phosphodiesterase inhibitor theophylline, thus implicating cyclic nucleotides. Secretion can be inhibited by both serosal ouabain and furosemide. Presumably by blocking Na-K ATP-ase, ouabain interferes with sodium-chloride exchange at the basolateral membrane, thus making chloride unavailable for apical secretion.[6,7]

A number of stimuli have been shown to elicit net secretion in the intact colon; several of these are of particular relevance. They include the laxatives castor oil or ricinoleic acid,[5] bisacodyl,[22,23] dioctyl sodium sulfosuccinate,[24] dihydroxy bile acids,[8] and prostaglandins.[25] Secretagogues provoke secretion by stimulating a flux of chloride into the lumen, although some also act as mucosal irritants, causing epithelial damage and increases in permeability (Fig. 2-1).

To explain the diarrhea of diffuse colitis, the mechanisms most likely responsible are abnormalities in fluid and electrolyte absorption and secretion, although disorders of motility should also be implicated. The absorptive/secretory processes found in colitis have been reviewed elsewhere.[9] In vivo perfusion studies of diseased colons have shown a net decrease in the absorption of sodium, chloride, and water, although it is not clear whether these findings represent a primary defect in sodium transport or an increase in mucosal permeability. Administration of glucocorticoids appears to increase sodium absorption in these patients. An in vitro study showed a net secretion of sodium and potassium in diseased colon. Other observers

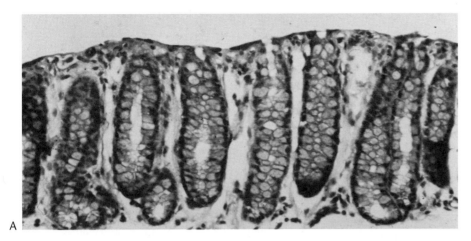

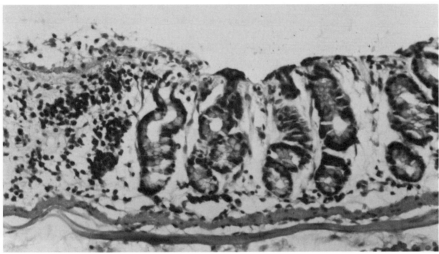

Figure 2-1. **(A)** Light microscopic appearance of rabbit colon after 4 hours of perfusion with 5 mmol/L ursodeoxycholic acid. The appearances are not different from those seen after perfusion with saline. **(B)** Rabbit colon after 4 hours of perfusion with 5 mmol chenodeoxycholic acid. The surface layer has been disrupted and there is an infiltration of the mucosa with inflammatory cells.

have reported decreased sodium absorption through a primary defect in sodium transport, increased mucosal permeability, or both. Thus, inflamed colonic mucosa shows evidence of reduced absorption of electrolytes and water.

On the other hand, it seems likely that fluid and electrolyte absorption in the small intestine and proximal colon is normal in patients with proctosigmoiditis.[9] Potassium to sodium ratios in stools from patients with proctosigmoiditis were normal or only slightly elevated, and fecal volumes are often not greatly increased. Indeed, a syndrome of "fecal stasis" in proctosigmoiditis has been described[26]; thus, patients may evacuate only mucus and blood from the rectum, and pass fecal matter only every few days.

Control of Absorption and Secretion

Humoral Control

Both mineralocorticoids and glucocorticoids regulate electrolyte transport in the colon; these activities are found in aldosterone and also in glucocorticoids considered to have little or no mineralocorticoid action. Crossover effects may result from specific ligand-receptor interactions or may be produced by partial binding of one ligand to the receptor of the other, if the interaction is less restricted.[6,7] Moreover, ligand-receptor binding may augment an existing membrane transport process or induce new mechanisms. For example, aldosterone, which has only modest effects in the small intestine, increases electrogenic Na transport in rabbit distal colon where amiloride-sensitive absorption occurs under basal conditions. In contrast, the rat distal colon does not exhibit any baseline electrogenic Na transport, but rather absorbs Na and Cl by an electroneutral Na-Cl absorption. Thus, in the rat, aldosterone apparently induces a new Na transport mechanism and inhibits the existing Na-Cl absorption pathway. Complexity is further added because the physiologic responses vary with the segment of the colon being studied.[6] Unlike its effects in the rat distal colon, aldosterone in the rat proximal colon increases electroneutral absorption of Na-Cl and does not induce a new amiloride-sensitive process of electrogenic Na transport.

Overall, therefore, aldosterone increases Na-Cl absorption in the colon; however, pure glucocorticoids also augment Na-Cl absorption, and they do so by both electrogenic and electroneutral mechanisms. The increase by glucocorticoids of electrogenic Na absorption is mediated by binding of the glucocorticoid to the aldosterone receptor, and is thus an example of overlap of gluco- into mineralocorticoid activity. On the other hand, the increase in electroneutral Na-Cl absorption is mediated by the glucocorticoid receptor.[6] Note needs to be drawn again to the comparative lack of response of the small intestine to corticoid stimulation. The jejunum and ileum respond very little to potent mineralocorticoids, explaining the relatively fixed losses of sodium from ileostomies.[27,28] On the other hand, the healthy colon can reduce fecal losses of sodium to a few milliequivalents per day.

The net effect of aldosterone on K transport is secretion, but this is achieved by a combination of increased absorption and secretion of K, the latter effect being the greater. These changes are mediated by binding to the aldosterone receptor. Similarly, glucocorticoids enhance net K secretion by partial binding to the aldosterone receptor.[6]

Neural Control

The gastrointestinal tract contains billions of neurones, referred to as the enteric nervous system (ENS). Indeed, it has been estimated that the ENS contains as many neurones as does the spinal cord, leading to the term, ''mini-brain in the gut.'' Overall, the ENS is composed of myenteric, submucosal, and mucosal components. In the simplest possible terms, most neurons of the myenteric plexus project to smooth muscle in the tunica muscularis, whereas most submucosal plexus neurons project to the mucosa, where they serve to modulate ion transport and other epithelial functions.[6,7,29] Neuropeptides are shared intermediates, participating in the humoral and neural regulation of mucosal and muscular function.

Submucosal neurons contain many neuropeptides and neuromodulators, including vasoactive intestinal polypeptide (VIP), galanin, neuropeptide Y (NPY), somatostatin, substance P, and nitric oxide. Although most experimental observations have been gathered from the guinea pig small bowel,[29] comparable principles must apply to the colon and to other species. Some investigators have studied colonic tissues specifically.[30] Thus, in the guinea pig colon, electrical stimulation of submucosal neurons evoked a serosal to mucosal flux of Cl. In comparable experiments with human tissue, cecal mucosa responded by Cl secretion and reduced Na absorption; the transverse colon did not respond, and the sigmoid colon showed reduced Cl absorption only.[30] It is clear that mucosal transport can be modulated, and may be ultimately controlled, by the ENS. This system of nervous mediation also orchestrates motility and blood flow.[29]

Relevant to the possible neurogenic pathogenesis of constipation are the putative toxic effects of laxatives on the ENS, a concept based on the work of Smith.[31] Thus, stimulatory laxatives have been proposed to perpetuate colonic inertia by interrupting the nervous control of smooth muscle function by the ENS. Although still widely accepted, the experimental data on which the concept was based originally must now be questioned.[32,33] Indeed, it is now generally accepted that neural degeneration, often seen in the ENS of colons removed for chronic

constipation, and first documented by Schuffler and Zonak,[34] is a primary pathology and is not due to the toxicity of laxatives.

Prostaglandins and leucotrienes are derived from long-chain unsaturated fatty acids present in the plasma membrane of all cells. Many are intestinal secretagogues.[25] In parallel with the growing understanding that the healthy gut exists in a dynamic state of balanced inflammation, it is clear that there is a baseline level of prostaglandin and leucotriene production throughout the intestine.[7] Thus, the concept is that even the healthy intestine may exhibit a low, basal level of inflammation leading to a background secretory state. Because there is much overlap in the functions of these inflammatory-secretory molecules, their study in vivo is difficult. It is clear, however, that leucotrienes such as LTB4 amplify the inflammatory response by stimulating and recruiting polymorphs, which in turn impair the barrier function of the colonic epithelium and facilitate net secretion. In addition, prostaglandins exert a mucosal protective effect, to varying degrees, in different regions. Yet another layer of complexity has been discerned with the expanding knowledge of the connections between prostaglandins and other systems that mediate inflammation, such as the mast cells and the cytokine network.[7]

Short-Chain Fatty Acids

Short-chain fatty acids (SCFAs) constitute the major fecal anions of all herbivores and most omnivores. The three principle SCFAs of stool water are acetic, propionic, and butyric acids. SCFAs are produced by the anaerobic fermentation by colonic bacteria of undigested carbohydrate and they are present in the colon almost completely in the form of nonprotonated anions; their average pKa is 4.8 and the pH of colonic fluid is 6.0 to 7.0 SCFAs are the preferred energy source for colonocytes[35] and have been shown to increase the bacterial mass in the lumen (that is, they are important substrates for the flora). They also affect the proliferation of colonic epithelial cells; it has also been suggested that deficiencies of intraluminal SCFAs contribute to the pathogenesis of colonic disease, specifically ulcerative colitis.[36] In support of the hypothesis that colitis is an ''energy-deficient'' state, local treatment with enemas of SCFAs has been shown to reduce the inflammation of ulcerative[37,38] and diversion[39] colitis.

Absorption rates of sodium and water are augmented by the absorption of SCFA. The mechanisms by which SCFA[40] are absorbed (and how they stimulate sodium absorption) have been controversial until recently. Previously, two theories were proposed; nonionic diffusion and anion exchange. It now seems clear that nonionic diffusion accounts for the major proportion of SCFA absorption and that this is dependent upon availability of hydrogen ions for the protonation of SCFAs to their nonionic forms. There is evidence that the electroneutral NaCl absorption that results from Na-H exchange allows butyrate to be protonated, followed by nonionic diffusion of the SCFA into the colonocyte.[6] H-butyrate then dissociates and butyrate anion is exchanged for luminal Cl. The question of whether SCFAs cross the basolateral membrane of the colonic epithelial cell or are used exclusively as a fuel source by the cell is not resolved.

Consequences of Colectomy

Fecal Outputs After Proctocolectomy

After colectomy and *any* form of ileostomy, the capacity of the colon to reabsorb electrolytes and water is lost. Usually, this creates no major clinical problems, but important principles should be remembered. A normal colon absorbs at least 1 L of water and 100 mEq of sodium choride daily.[3] These amounts can be augmented; when overloaded progressively, the healthy colon absorbs more than 5 L daily.[2] Also, the colon responds to salt depletion by conserving NaCl avidly, but the small intestine has a lesser capacity to so adapt. For example, under conditions of extremely low salt intake, fecal losses of sodium in normal stools can be reduced to 1 or 2 mEq/day, whereas patients with ileostomies have obligatory losses of sodium of 30 to 40 mEq/day.[27]

Well-functioning conventional ileostomies discharge 300 to 800 g of material daily; 90% of this is water. Continent ileostomies and ileal pouch-anal anastomoses have similar volumes of effluent. Foods containing much absorbable residue increase the total output by increasing the amount of solids discharged. However, overall the effects of foods on the volume and consistency of effluents are usually minimal.[41]

Functional Sequelae

When oral intakes of sodium, chloride, and fluid are adequate, patients with ileostomies do not become depleted; however, negative sodium balance may follow periods of diminished oral intake, vomiting, or excess loss in perspiration.[28] In addition, chronic oliguria should be anticipated because normal stools contain approximately 100 ml of water, whereas ileostomies lose 500 to 600 ml daily. These patients also have lower Na^+ K^+ ratios in urine owing to compensatory renal conservation of sodium and water. These changes in the composition of urine presumably contribute to the increased frequency of urolithiasis (probably about 5%) after colectomy.

When ileostomy is accompanied by resection of terminal ileum, abnormalities of bile acid reabsorption and malabsorption of vitamin B_{12} may result.[9] Steatorrhea and greater daily losses of fluid (1 L/day or more) also may be seen. However, these abnormalities do not occur in the usual circumstances when colectomy is performed for inflammatory disease of the colon or polyposis coli; the ileum, being free of disease, is usually preserved.

Lack of a colon also reduces the exposure of bile acids to the metabolic effects of the fecal flora. After ileostomy, secondary bile acids largely disappear from bile,[42] but no metabolic consequences of significance have been recognized. The flora of ileostomy effluents has quantitative (10^4 to 10^7 organisms/ml) and qualitative characteristics that are intermediate between those of feces and those of normal ileal contents.[43] The presence of a reservoir, Kock pouch or IPAA, predisposes to a more fecal-like flora.

Pathophysiologic sequelae are therefore mainly the potential consequences of a salt-losing state; patients should be advised to use salt liberally and to increase their fluid intake, especially at times of stress, in extremely hot weather, and with vigorous exercise. Unfortunately, the limited ability of the small intestine to absorb sodium and water means that stomal volumes also increase when the oral intake is increased.

FUNCTION OF THE ILEOCOLONIC JUNCTION

Ileocolonic Sphincter

The junction between the small and large bowels represents an ecologic and physiologic transition of considerable biologic importance.[44,45] The subject was widely written on by early anatomists and surgeons of the late 19th and early 20th centuries. Consensus about the major mechanism of the sphincter fluctuated between the relative contributions of a "mechanical valve" and a "functional sphincter," and now appears to encompass both concepts. Hurst[46] crystallized many of these ideas, by terming the junction (ICJ) an "intestinal stomach", he proposed that the ileum stored and mixed chyme until distension initiated a wave of contraction that emptied the contents into the colon. Almost a century later, indirect evidence still supports this view (Fig. 2-2).

Taking this further, and drawing an analogy with other junctional zones, such as the gastric cardia and pylorus, a general hypothesis can be proposed that the function of crucial intestinal "gates" is too important to be entrusted to only one mechanism of control.[45] Thus, these regions appear to depend not only on intrinsic sphincters but also on specialized motility in the adjacent bowel. The ICJ appears to fit this mode very well. That a sphincter exists at the ICJ is clear, but equally apparent is the variable magnitude of the high-pressure zone. In humans, the sphincter is poorly developed anatomically and functionally; the pressure barrier is low.[44] Even a low-pressure barrier, however, may be able to compartmentalize the ileum from the colon against weak retropulsive forces. On the other hand, the second part of the hypothesis is that the resistance to reflux also includes mechanical barriers; these may be necessary to resist greater heads of colonic pressure. In these terms, "flap-valve" at the ICJ would be useful; this possibility has been examined, and such a mechanism appears to be present.[44] A third protection against coloileal reflux would be a means whereby the breaching of competence is sensed and corrected. In this regard, the analogy can be drawn between SCFA in the ileum and HCl in the esophagus; both may act as chemical stimuli for "secondary peristalsis." Certainly, reflux of SCFA into the ileum evokes strong motor forces that empty the ileum.[44]

The propulsive forces that normally empty the ileum of food residues are less clear. Fasting (or postprandial) ileal motility, tone at the ICS, and colonic receptivity of the bolus are coordinated, but the mechanisms mediating this are still largely unexplored. The ileum exhibits frequent bursts of phasic pressure waves fasting and postprandially, and high-amplitude, peristaltic sequences are recorded from the ileum more often than from the jejunum. The peristaltic sequences are thought to empty the ileum; they are provoked by ileal influence of SCFA.

Entry of Residue Into the Colon

Observations using breath excretion of H_2 (Fig. 2-2) support the concept of Arthur Hurst[46] that the distal ileum can store and later propel dietary residues. Hydrogen excretion serves as a signal that fermentable dietary residues have reached the fecal

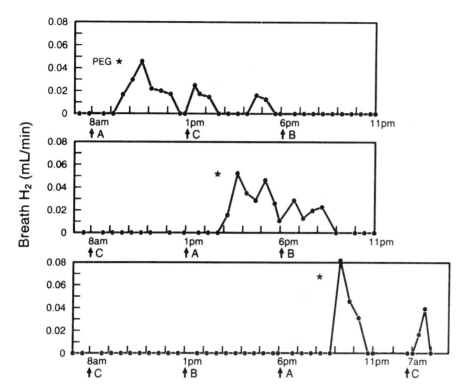

Figure 2-2. Breath hydrogen excretion measured at 30-minute intervals in 3 subjects. Times of ingestion of meals are indicated by arrows. Study meal A contained polyethylene glycol (PEG 4000) and baked beans as a source of hydrogen, but meals B and C generated no hydrogen. Peak concentration of liquid marker PEG 4000 is shown by asterisk. *Upper two panels:* meals B and C "flush" residue into colon and provoke a peak of hydrogen excretion. *Lower panel:* meal C was taken again for breakfast next morning. Despite negative breath H_2 excretion before breakfast, meal C was followed by an increase in breath H_2 excretion. (From Kerlin and Phillips,[92] with permission.)

flora. Using various meals it was shown that residue was stored in the ileum. Scintigraphy has also been used to explore these phenomena; thus, when radiolabeled residue was stored in the distal ileum (Fig. 2-3), transit to the cecum occurred largely in the form of bolus transfers.[47–49] A steady trickle of isotope counts was also noted, the proportion of bolus and steady transfer being on the order of 50–50.

Scintigraphy has also been applied to ileocolonic transfer, after the anatomy of the ICJ had been altered surgically. Transit of residue down to, and through, the colon was not greatly different in patients after right hemicolectomy (who had little disturbance of bowel habit), from that in healthy, age-matched controls[50] (Fig. 2-4). Thus, the new terminal ileum, the ileocolectomy, and the transverse colon were able to compensate for resection of the ileocolonic junction and the proximal colon.

Effects of Ileal Resection

The ileum has specialized absorptive functions, notably for vitamin B_{12} and bile acids. The active reabsorption of bile acids in the healthy ileum protects the colon against the consequences of exposure to excessive concentrations of irritant (secretory) bile acids.[8] On this basis it is not surprising that diarrhea is usual after ileal resection, when the bile acid pool gains greater access to the colon. In fact, two major mechanisms account for

the diarrhea that accompanies severe ileal disease or follows ileal resection. By one, diarrhea is induced primarily by malabsorbed bile acids and in the other by malabsorbed fat. When ileal function is only moderately impaired, wastage of bile acids is also small, and their increased hepatic synthesis is sufficient to compensate for the increased fecal losses. Luminal concentrations of bile acids in the small intestine are maintained within the micellar range; thus when steatorrhea is present, it is of mild degree. The excess of bile acids that enters the colon impairs electrolyte and water absorption.[8] The term bile acid diarrhea has been applied to this circumstance.

On the other hand, when the ileal resection is extensive, hepatic compensation for wastage of bile acids is incomplete and the concentration of bile acids in the lumen of the small bowel is too low for adequate micellar solubilization of fat. Steatorrhea is moderate to severe in extent. In this circumstance, malabsorbed fat is responsible primarily for the diarrhea, and excessive amounts of fatty acids in the colon are known to impair electrolyte and water absorption.[5] Consistent with these mechanisms are the therapeutic observations that a reduction in the dietary intake of long-chain fats reduces the severity of diarrhea in the second instance. Sequestrants of bile acids (cholestyramine or aluminum hydroxide) are effective in bile acid diarrhea.

These basic concepts require some modification. Cummings,[51] Arrambide,[10] and their associates emphasized the role

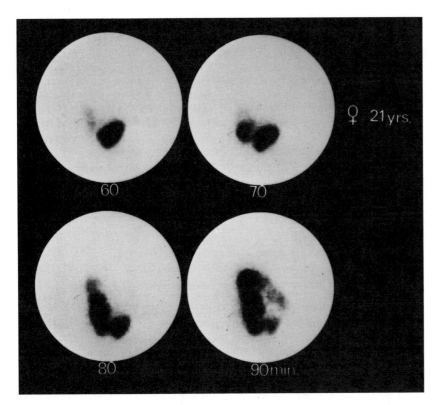

Figure 2-3. Scintiscans of ilecolonic junction in a healthy adult. The four scans cover a period of 30 minutes during which almost all of a test meal moved from the terminal ileum (60-minute scan) into the ascending and transverse colons (90-minute scan).

of the colon in the diarrhea that follows ileal resection. These investigators reasoned that variable portions of the large bowel are removed in association with resection of the ileum. They independently examined the role of missing segments of the small and large intestines. The amount of colon removed was an important determinant of the severity of diarrhea, whereas the length of ileal resection was not. On the other hand, fecal excretion of fat correlated well with the length of ileum removed but not with the proportion of the colon resected.

Intracolonic pH has been shown to influence greatly the solubility of secretory bile acids.[52] Because the potential of bile acids to impair sodium, chloride, and water absorption in the

Figure 2-4. Scintiscans of food residues passing through the bowel, taken at the same time point postprandially. (**A**) Healthy intact colon, filling to the midtransverse region. (**B**) A patient after right hemicolectomy, showing loops of ileum, the ileocolostomy and transverse and descending colons. (From Fich et al.,[50] with permission.)

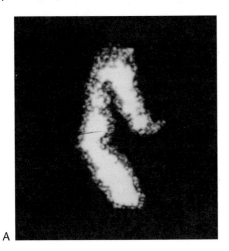
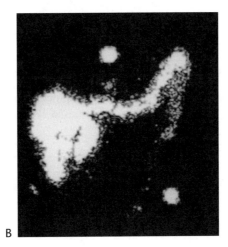

A

B

colon depends on their ability to enter the aqueous phase, factors that modify the solubility of bile acids influence the propensity of bile acids to provoke diarrhea. Thus, aqueous concentrations of the secretory bile acids, deoxycholic and chenodeoxycholic acids, are related to fecal pH; the higher the intraluminal pH, the more dihydroxy bile acids pass into solution and the more should be their secretory potential.

INTEGRATION OF TRANSIT, STORAGE, AND ABSORPTION BY THE COLON

Site of Colonic Storage

The rate at which materials move through the human colon varies widely, from hours to weeks. Thus, colonic storage covers a wide time frame, and it becomes important to know where solids and liquids can be stored, often for long periods. Mechanisms whereby the human colon accommodates fluids have been explored experimentally, by simulating diarrhea with experimental infusions of fluid into the cecum.[2,11] When subjected to slow, continuous fluid overload (1 to 2 ml min^{-1}), the human colon absorbed up to 5 L/day. However, briefer but faster infusions (500 ml) overloaded the colon's compensatory mechanisms and fecal weight increased.[2] When these studies were extended, 15 years later,[11] the further refinement of scintigraphy was used to assess regional flow and storage in response to simulated diarrhea.

Solids of small particle size were placed in the cecum of healthy persons, accompanied by infusions of saline, at various rates.[11] Fast rates of infusion accelerated the emptying of both liquids and solids from the ascending colon (Fig. 2-5); subsequently, liquids and solids were stored equally in the transverse colon, even after the fastest infusions of saline. Thus, it appeared that the transverse colon was a site for storage, even under conditions of simulated diarrhea. Later, in the same experiments, when contents had reached the distal colon, liquids and solids were stored together in the rectosigmoid, often for many hours. Indeed, prolonged rectal storage was able to allow solid stools to be formed in the rectum, even when rapid initial transit had moved liquid contents quickly to the rectum. These experiments were interpreted as highlighting the potential of the rectosigmoid to compensate for rapid transit through the more proximal regions of the colon.

Transit and absorption can be changed markedly by the nature of colonic contents. Long-chain fatty acids have been well substantiated as colonic secretagogues[5]; excess fat in the colon also influences transit. Oleic acid is a C-18 fatty acid that is abundant in the diet and also is found in steatorrheal stools. When this fat was infused into the ascending colon of healthy volunteers, steatorrhea was simulated, the volume of the proximal colon decreased, and distal transit was accelerated.[48,53] High-amplitude, propagated pressure waves (giant migrating contractions) were recorded manometrically; they were associated with rapid distal transit of contents and abdominal cramps (Fig. 2-6).

Despite information on the colonic transit of liquids, the segments in which solids are normally stored has been debated. In one series of scintigraphic studies,[47,54,55] segmental colonic transit was assessed with a noninvasive method, using a solid-phase marker released from a capsule into the distal ileum or proximal colon. The isotope labelled the fecal mass and 12 hours later, radioactivity was most obvious in the ascending colon. By 24 hours, counts were equally distributed between the ascending and transverse colons and the stools. It was concluded that the proximal colon was the usual site of storage and that the descending colon and rectosigmoid segments contributed little. When solids and *small* volumes of liquids were given together and their transits compared, they largely moved together.[55] However, when large volumes of fluids were injected into the cecum, fluids initially moved rapidly and preferentially into the transverse colon; solids then caught up with the liquids in the transverse colon.[11] Krevsky and associates[56] introduced liquid scintigraphic markers into the cecum with a thin nasocecal catheter; their studies concluded that the transverse colon was most likely the major site for storage. In summary, the ascending and, perhaps even more so, the transverse colon are important for the initial storage of both liquids and solids.

With emphasis emerging on the proximal colon as the major site for storage, it was intriguing that bowel habit usually changes so little after proximal colectomy, so long as ileal segment removed concomitantly is short. Thus, severe diarrhea is rare after right hemicolectomy; the genesis of any diarrhea that does occur has been thought to be related to a decrease in transit time. This, in turn, should be determined by the length of colon resected. We tested the potential of distal remnants of colon to compensate well for loss of storage function and absorbing surface. In patients with right hemicolectomy in whom bowel habits had changed little postoperatively,[50] radioisotopic markers given by mouth remained for long periods in the transverse colon, and the fractions of isotope that moved into the distal colon was increased only slightly above those recorded for the intact bowel. Thus, the transverse colon remaining after hemicolectomy functioned almost as well as did the intact proximal colon.

Colonic Responses to Eating

It is well recognized that manometric and myoelectric activities of the right, left, and rectosigmoid colons are enhanced *immediately* by eating.[57,58] Also, when the tone of the colon was recorded by a barostat, colonic tone increased soon after food in dogs and humans.[58a,59,60] Wiley et al.[61] investigated the stim-

Figure 2-5. Residence time of solids and liquids in the human colon. Solids were introduced into the cecum together with liquids infused at rates that varied from 1 to 14 ml/min^{-1}. The rate at which liquids were infused influenced their emptying, but not that of solids, from the ascending colon. Infusions did not influence storage time of liquids and solids in the transverse colon. (From Hammer and Phillips,[11] with permission.)

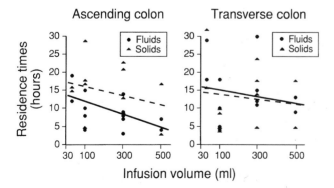

RELATIONSHIP BETWEEN MOTILITY TRACING AND TRANSIT

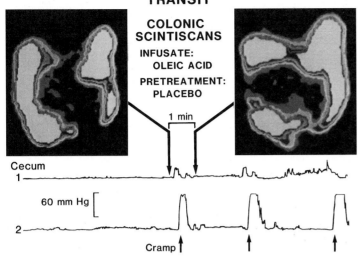

Figure 2-6. Scintiscans of human colon and simultaneous intraluminal manometry. Oleic acid evoked high pressure waves, abdominal cramps, and rapid movement of isotope from the cecum-ascending colon to the descending colon-rectum. (From Kamath et al.,[53] with permission.)

uli that generated this early motor response to food. Gastric distention with water or a balloon induced a dose-related increase in rectosigmoid motility. Motility also increased after duodenal perfusion of lipids, but not after saline, glucose, or amino acids. Thus, mechanical distension of the stomach was a trigger, although calories augmented the strength of the signal. Extrinsic nerves appear to be involved in the early response to food because none was observed in extrinsically denervated canine loops.[62] Humoral factors, especially cholecystokinin (CCK), have been postulated as mediators of the gastrocolonic response, but a CCK-A antagonist did not block the response, and these CCK receptors therefore do not appear to be involved.[63] Whatever the mechanism, well before chyme reaches the colon, colonic motility and tone increase, an effect possibly mediated by extrinsic nerves, though the mediation of the response has not been fully defined.

Does this early "gastrocolonic response" induce movement of contents already in the colon? This question has been addressed with gamma scintigraphy. Radionuclide markers have been instilled at the splenic flexure by a tube through the rectum[64] or into the proximal and distal colons through a nasocolonic tube.[65] After eating, radioactivity in the cecum-ascending colon regions and at the hepatic flexure moved aborally. Radioactivity instilled at the splenic flexure moved both orally and aborally; counts in the descending colon did not move appreciably. However, when markers were delivered to the cecum without use of a colonic tube,[66] their aboral transfer from the proximal colon after the meal was less impressive. Thus, the magnitude and clinical significance of the proximal colon's response to a meal is still uncertain. The "gastrocolic response" is potentially more important in the distal colon. Defecation is often prompted by food especially in patients with fecal urgency (proctitis, irritable bowel syndrome). These people are often greatly distressed postprandially, and control of this "reflex" by novel pharmacologies would be useful.

The colon's motility also responds to local stimulation associated with the arrival of chyme in the late postprandial period. In dogs, cyclical patterns of colonic motility were different early (0 to 2 hours) and late (2 to 8 hours) after a meal.[67] The arrival of chyme in the large bowel stimulated motility; perfusion of isolated canine loops of colon with chyme or saline reestablished the postprandial pattern seen in the intact bowel. Based on these studies in the dog, the large intestine responds to eating immediately ("gastrocolonic reflex," possibly mediated neurally), early (during small bowel transit of the meal), and late, when dietary residues reach the large bowel.

Carbohydrate Metabolism in the Colon

In the proximal colon, dietary residues (mainly carbohydrate) that escape digestion and absorption from the diet, together with endogenous secretions (such as glycoproteins), are metabolized by the fecal flora to SCFA. These organic ions (acetate, butyrate, propionate) are the major anions of fecal water. They are well absorbed by the colon and their absorption also facilitates the reabsorption of sodium, chloride and water. Some SCFAs escape salvage in the colon and are excreted in the stools.

Although dietary fiber has received most attention as the source of biodegradable carbohydrate in the colon, starch is also an important component (Fig. 2-7). Indeed, the dietary intake of starch (up to several hundred grams daily) is much greater than that of fiber and, even in health, substantial quantities of starch escape digestion and absorption in the small bowel.[68,69] Unabsorbed dietary residue, with starch probably playing the major role, is necessary if the fecal bacterial mass, which constitutes 50% of stool weight, is to be maintained.[70] These interactions among dietary residues, the fecal flora, and the absorptive epithelium are of prime importance to colonic function.

As examples of subtle bacterial-substrate interactions, the

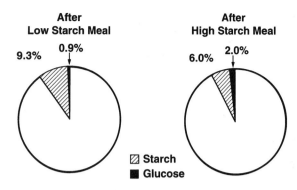

Figure 2-7. Amounts of glucose and starch recovered by aspiration of the human ileum after two test meals. Total carbohydrate reaching the colon, mainly as starch, after these meals was 8 to 10% of the amount eaten (see reference 69 for details).

quantities of lactulose (a nonabsorbable disaccharide) or wheat starch that were metabolized by the fecal flora were defined, as were the threshold loads of these substrates that needed to be surpassed before diarrhea occurred.[71,72] Further, bacterial enzymes were shown to be inducible. When lactulose was fed chronically to healthy persons, the efficiency with which the bacteria metabolized lactulose was increased. These balances between the diet, fecal metabolism, the composition of stools and bowel function are thus finely set. These issues, in turn, raise other possibilities, such as whether starch-deficient diets lead to lesser fecal bulk, possibly slower transit, and constipation.

SCFAs, and butyrate in particular, are thought to supply calories for use by colonic epithelium. The concept is attractive teliologically. Readily absorbable sugars do not reach the hindgut in quantities likely to be important metabolically. Adaptation of the energy pathways in colonocytes to use a fuel (SCFAs) that is produced locally has obvious advantages. The role of butyrates as a colonic nutrient has been the basis of the proposal that the etiology of colonic inflammation, as with chronic ulcerative colitis, involves a mucosa undergoing energy deprivation.[36] Beneficial effects of SCFA enemas were observed in ulcerative and diversion colitis.[37-39]

Few observations have been made as to how the motor and metabolic functions of the colon are integrated. When oroanal transit time, which mainly reflects colonic transit, was modified pharmacologically, the volumes of stools and their microbial activity changed concomitantly.[70] Speeding up of colonic transit reduced the digestibility of cellulose, and increased the stool weight and bacterial mass. Thus, any variation in the colonic residence time can be expected to affect the metabolic function and growth of the microbial mass. In a scintigraphic study, the ingestion of lactulose changed stool water and electrolyte composition and accelerated colonic transit,[73] thus providing additional insights into bacterial metabolism, colonic transit, and the laxative action of lactulose.

Nervous Integration of Colonic Motility and Transit

Classical neurophysiology proposed that the prevertebral ganglia were merely relay stations in the sympathetic pathways that supply inhibitory signals to the hindgut. The cell bodies of the system (for the colon) were localized to the dorsal roots of the corresponding spinal segments, and relay in the prevertebral ganglia was thought to be obligatory and unmodified by external stimuli. For a period, discussion centered on whether or not central pathways needed to be involved. With the advent of newer experimental preparations, especially ones in which the colon could be separated from the spinal cord, while still maintaining continuity with the prevertebral ganglia and connecting nerves, it became clear that the colon and the prevertebral ganglia are an autonomous system.[74] Thus, in these isolated preparations, the colon was able to "talk to itself" very effectively. Distension of one segment of the colon provoked a motor response at another level. Moreover, the signals were shown to pass through the intermesenteric nerves; their transsection abolished the "message."

Description of these pathways of control through the mesenteric nerves and prevertebral ganglia prompted more detailed analysis of the system. Subsequent experiments demonstrated that stimulation of mechanoreceptors in the wall of the colon aroused a feedback signal from the ganglia that caused other segments of the colon to relax. Control of this system has been since shown to involve not only the classical neurotransmitters but also nonadrenergic, noncholinergic agents.[74]

The influence of prevertebral innervation on the intact canine colon was reported by Brugere et al.[75] Cylical patterns of motility during fasting[57] were not dependent upon input from the inferior and superior mesenteric ganglia. Loss of sympathetic input from the inferior mesenteric ganglion resulted in an exaggerated, presumably uninhibited, motor response to a meal, with rapid transit and diarrheal stools.

The overall message is very clear; the prevertebral ganglia and the mesenteric nerves constitute an important mechanism whereby colonic function is controlled. Just as the enteric nervous system within the wall of the gut has only recently been fully appreciated as a vital, and discrete, element of control, so must the prevertebral ganglia be recognized as being not merely passive relay stations. An interesting clinical observation of how the colon may be self-regulatory, presumably mediated by these reflexes, was made by Klauser et al.[76] They showed that transit in the human proximal colon of healthy volunteers was slowed when they distended the rectum chronically, by the voluntary retention of stools.

Rectoanal Function

Accommodation of dietary and/or fecal residue in the rectosigmoid represents the last possible reserve for the storage of residue. Prolonged recordings of anorectal motility have shown that the human rectum exhibits periodic motor activity (rectal motor complex), particularly at night[77]; no physiologic function has yet been assigned to this phenomenon, although it usually coincides with activity in the anal sphincters and possibly contributes to sleep-time continence. Manometric activity of the rectosigmoid increases with the arrival of food residue (the "head" of the meal) in the proximal colon[58]; moreover, rectal tone, as measured by a barostat, increases consistently after meals. Failure of the rectosigmoid to react to the ingestion of food or to stimulation of the proximal colon by food residues may be relevant to disturbances of evacuation and constipation syndromes.

MEASUREMENTS OF COLONIC TRANSIT

Historical Perspectives

Cannon reported, almost a century ago, on the movement of bismuth subnitrate in the feline colon.[78] Since that time, it has been clear that contents do not leave the colon in the same order in which they enter. Thus, in healthy humans, glass beads of different colors given on successive days appeared in the stool around 24 to 72 hours from the time of ingestion, but they were mixed together. Differences in passage of these different particulate markers, as judged by their appearance in the stools, appeared to be proportional to their specific gravity; heavier material passed more slowly than did lighter contents.

Cinefluorography of barium-impregnated contents[79,80] demonstrated mixing, storage, and propulsion in the colon. Interhaustral shuttling, propulsion, retropulsion, and movements to and fro were found to thoroughly mix the colonic contents. Propulsion and retropulsion appeared to be achieved by similar mechanisms. Contents moved from one haustrum to the next, through multihaustral segments and by interhaustral propulsion. During multihaustral propulsion, three or more haustral segments became contiguous and the mass of contents moved to the next segment, while the original haustration was reformed. Interhaustral propulsion and peristalsis appeared to be similar, but peristaltic contractions usually started as interhaustral constrictions, travelled further along the colon, and were able to propel feces distally. Defecation emptied the distal colon, but colonic contents orad to those that were actually emptied appeared to be relatively undisturbed by the act of defecation.[79] The rectum was usually the only region that emptied completely, although at times material from the distal transverse colon could be eliminated.

Methodology for Colonic Transit

Although cinefluorography describes the movements of contents impregnated with barium, it does not quantify the colonic transit of dietary residues. Moreover, radiation exposure is high and the methodology is now no longer feasible. Nevertheless, the widespread use of barium in contrast radiographs of the gut led to the clinical use of barium as a marker of intestinal transit. When barium is ingested with food, the arrival of the head of the column and the disappearance of all barium from the colon has been used to quantify transit from the mouth to various colonic segments or to the anus. After 24 hours, barium reaches the rectum in 60% of normal subjects, 84% of patients with diverticulosis, and 90% of patients with irritable bowel syndrome. Approximately 4 days are necessary for 70 to 80% of the barium to leave the colon. However, only the progress of the head of the barium column and the disappearance of contrast can be observed; thus, transit times probably reflect the mixing of contents as much as they do the aborad propulsion of fecal matter.

Quantification of transit requires the measurable marker, the appearance of which in the feces, or its imaging in segments of the colon, can be analyzed mathematically. Marker substances can be taken orally, but they have also been introduced directly into the cecum; they can be given as a single bolus, repeated boluses, or continuously. The differences relate merely to how the data are analyzed mathematically. Observing the appearance and disappearance of markers in stools (mouth to anus transit) approximates total colonic transit, but does not assess changes in transit through colonic segments (segmental transit). Whole gut or segmental colonic transit can be expressed simply as the time taken for a proportion of the marker to pass by the location of interest (for example, emptying of a colonic segment). Another approach is to describe transit in terms of segmental or whole colonic half-emptying times ($T_{1/2}$). The latter method takes into account the exponential emptying of markers from one colonic segment to the next. The subject has been reviewed before in more detail.

Whole Gut Transit

Dyes (such as carmine red) and chemicals (chromium sesquioxide, copper thiocyanate) have been used experimentally but they have no advantages, and quantitation of their recovery in feces is sometimes difficult. Chromium-51, given as chromic oxide powder or sodium chromate solution, can be measured in the stool by scintillation counting; again, there are no important advantages, and segmental transit is not assessed.

Discrete, barium-impregnated polythene markers, having a specific gravity close to that of stools, move with the colonic contents. Hinton et al.[81] measured gastrointestinal transit times using solid, 2- to 5-mm polythene pellets impregnated with barium sulphate. These inert radiopaque markers were completely recoverable in the stool and had a specific gravity similar to gut contents. When followed by either abdominal radiographs or radiographs of stools, the movement of such markers can be taken to represent the transit of meal residues through the gut. No significant differences were found in their transit when they were given immediately before or with a meal. In 25 healthy men, all but one had passed 80% of the markers by the fifth day after ingestion, but none had passed 80% by the end of the first day. All subsequent work with radio-opaque markers has been directed at refining this range of normality, reducing x-ray exposure and minimizing inconvenience (such as stool collections).

Methods involving many radio-opaque markers (15/day) taken over a long period (6 weeks) were compared to the single-dose method. The technique of repeated ingestion depends on the appearance of markers in stool during "steady state," and data were transformed mathematically from the number of markers in stool to a time for colonic transit, in hours. Calculation of the colonic transit time utilized the turnover of markers accumulated in the colonic pool at equilibrium, that is, when daily elimination equaled the number ingested.

Segmental Transit

The rate of disappearance of radio-opaque markers from defined colonic segments was monitored with daily abdominal radiographs after a single dose of radio-opaque markers.[82] Right and left colonic, sigmoid, and rectal segments were defined by simply drawing lines between bony landmarks (vertebral column and pelvis), and by confirming the validity of the segments using gas shadows. Two days after administration, markers were found in all colonic segments; over the succeeding days markers moved from the right to the left colon with exponential emptying of markers from each segment. In a study of 114 healthy adults and children, none retained markers after 8 days.[82] It was then possible to develop a calculation of actual segmental transit times, rather than the rate of disappearance of markers from colonic segments. A mathematical expression, based on the time interval between serial abdominal radiographs, was established to describe the continuous change in the numbers of markers at any location in the colon. The original method involved repeated abdominal radiographs with considerable exposure to radiation and the inconvenience of repeated visits to the radiology department.

Metcalf et al.[83] simplified this method so that only one x-ray exposure, using a fast film, high-kilovoltage technique, was necessary; radiation exposure was therefore minimized. The protocol now requires radiopaque markers to be ingested in fixed numbers (24/day), at the same time (arbitrarily, 9:00 AM), for each of 3 days. Instead of daily radiographs, on the fourth day, again at the same time, an abdominal radiograph is taken. Assuming that the colon handles all markers in the same way, the number of markers present on a single radiograph taken on the fourth day is equivalent to the total number of markers present on the first three sequential radiographs after a single bolus of markers. The results obtained from this technique correlated very well with the daily radiograph approach. Both this method and the repeated radiographic method assume that a 24-hour sampling interval (either for daily radiographs or daily markers) *approximates* a continuous set of observations. For persons with slow-transit constipation, the assumption may well be justified. However, the more rapid colonic transit is, the less valid is the assumption. Thus, very rapid transit could cause all of the markers to be lost in the feces before the day 4 film. Conversely, if transit is very slow, all 72 markers may still be present at day 4. A later film, such as on day 7, can then give more information in the constipated patient. At present, the technique is a robust and simple way of measuring segmental and total colonic transit in clinical practice, with particular application to the constipated patient.[83]

Scintigraphic Assessment of Transit

In contrast to radiographic methods, scintigraphy offers the advantage of more frequent observations of transit of an isotope, for long periods, without increasing the exposure to radiation. If resources are available, very frequent scans can approach a continuous set of observations. The advantages over radiography are several; images can be quantified precisely using scintillation counts; the transit of solids and liquids can be measured simultaneously, if different isotopes are used to label liquid and solid contents; any intestinal region of interest is available for study, and dynamic (continuous) scanning is possible. Importantly, the volume of radioisotopes needed for satisfactory images is negligible. Isotopes can be given mixed together with food and, when bound to suitable carrier molecules (such as diethylene triamine pentacetic acid, or DTPA), are poorly absorbed and biologically inert. Gamma scintigraphy had earlier been applied successfully to the quantification of gastric emptying, and such methods are now in regular clinical use. Application of scintigraphy to the large intestine has been slower to develop, and although now generally accepted, is not used routinely by many centers.

When isotopes are given by mouth, one consequence of orocecal transit is that the markers could disperse broadly within the small bowel, leading to prolonged transfer of isotope from ileum to colon. Therefore, methods using direct instillation of isotope into the colon were the first approach.[48,49,56] Krevsky et al.[56] used a thin, orocecal tube to instill small volumes of isotopically labelled fluid into the cecum; later, Spiller et al.[48,49] used the same approach to study experimental steatorrhea, induced by infusing fatty acids and isotope directly into the cecum. Proano et al.[54,55] provided a novel approach; they developed a noninvasive method whereby labeled solids could be followed across the ileocolonic junction and into the colon. A solid-phase carrier (small, 1-mm, polystyrene beads) was labeled with an isotope (^{111}In or ^{99m}Tc); the label was recovered quantitatively in stool, and it was still in the solid phase.[54] Beads could also be confined within a medication capsule that was coated with a pH sensitive polymer. The properties of the polymer were such that it dissolved in the distal ileum and/or proximal colon. This offered a method of delivering isotope, as a bolus, directly to the distal small bowel and/or colon.

Meanwhile, Spiller et al.[48,49] and Camilleri et al.[47] studied the ways in which ileal contents, liquids and solids, moved into the colon. Direct injections of liquids into the ileum, or solids taken by mouth, filled the colon by a series of bolus movements of isotope, separated by "plateaus" during which little isotope moved from the small to the large bowel (Fig. 2-3). This finding raised the possibility that if a bolus of isotope could be delivered to the distal ileum, it would enter the colon over a relatively short time span. Thus, the filling of the proximal colon would represent an acceptable "zero-time," from which could be established emptying curves for regions of the colon. By this approach, it became possible to image the unprepared colon, and to develop mathematical expressions of segmental transit, without the use of intubation.

The best way to analyze colonic scintigraphy is still debated. Dividing the colon into anatomic regions of interest, and producing time-activity graphs for each region, is the most direct approach, but a simpler summary of segmental transit is also useful. Thus, the weighted averaging of counts from different colonic regions of interest is an attractive alternative[56]; this yields a "geometric center" (GC) of radioactivity, which can be followed along the colon in sequential images. The GC summarizes multiple observations very conveniently, and this is the method now used most commonly.[84]

Radioscintigraphy can be further extended, so that a single test that quantifies gastric emptying, small bowel transit, and segmental colonic transit has now been validated for clinical use.[84] Radiolabeled beads (^{99m}Tc) that are *not* encapsulated are mixed with a meal; these are used to assess gastric emptying and small bowel transit. The encapsulated beads, labeled with ^{111}In, are used to quantify colonic transit. By reducing the number of scans to a minimum number, the test has been made cost effective, for use in a clinical department of nuclear medicine.[84] The technique offers a 24-hour test suitable for patients with slow or rapid transit; it provides a convenient alternative to the radio-opaque approach.[85,86]

PHARMACOLOGY OF COLONIC FUNCTION

The list of commonly prescribed drugs that feature constipation as a side effect is long, The mechanisms by which constipation results from the action of many of these agents are not well

Table 2-3. Common Constipating Drugs

Class	Action
Anticholinergics: tricyclic antidepressants	Muscarinic blockade (nonspecific receptors)
Antiparkinsonian drugs/ antihistamines	Muscarinic blockade?
Sympathomimetics	Sympathetic inhibition
Opiates, antidiarrheals	Increased motility: tonic and segmental
Calcium channel blockers	Reduced contractility
Antacids containing calcium and aluminum	Binding to bile acids?
Nonsteroidal anti-inflammatory agents	Uncertain

known, although some information is available (Table 2-3). Thus, many drugs have antimuscarinic side effects; best recognized among agents prescribed frequently are the tricyclic antidepressants. Opiate analgesics act as antidiarrheals or have constipating effects because of their agonism for μ receptors in the colon. Most calcium channel blockers have at least some depressant effects on intestinal smooth muscle.

The constipating effects of opium have been used therapeutically for centuries; most narcotics that are used for analgesia also affect the colon, and the side effects of these agents on the gut ("narcotic bowel") are often reasons for referral to gastroenterologists. Indeed, narcotic bowel is one of the important clinical differential diagnoses of idiopathic constipation, intestinal pseudo-obstruction, and megacolon, and it is vital that medications be discontinued before these patients are evaluated. The clinical circumstances often involve a history of multiple abdominal operations, questions of recurrent partial bowel obstruction, and narcotics for pain, leading to dysmotility syndromes and constipation.

There are paradoxes as to the pharmacologic effects of opiates on the colon. Morphine increases wall tone and the numbers of contractile events in the colon; however, it is the repetitive, rhythmic, nonpropagating contractions that are particularly stimulated. These contractile events are thought to be nonpropulsive and they may even retard the movement of contents. Although morphine increased basal tone in the human[60] and canine[59] colon, it did not impair the colon's activity to relax ahead of peristaltic contractions. On the other hand, when painful and propulsive colonic contractions were stimulated in healthy volunteers by luminal fatty acids (Fig. 2-6), the proximal colon decreased its volume (presumably by an increase in tone) and contents moved quickly to the rectum. Under these circumstances, morphine blocked the high-pressure contractions and relaxed the bowel.[53]

At the other end of the spectrum, several of the agents commonly used to treat constipation have powerful effects on colonic function.[5,8,53,87] Thus, fatty acids such as ricinoleic acid (castor oil) and bile acids (a component of several folk purgatives) are of particular interest. Closely related molecules are common in the average diet (oleic and other long-chain fatty acids) or are normal components of endogenous secretions (bile acids). Both molecular species (fatty acids and bile acids) can

effect the colon profoundly, stimulating secretion and rapid transit. Structure-activity profiles vary widely among individual molecules. For example, the trihydroxy bile acid, cholic acid, is a less potent colonic secretagogue[8] than is its dihydroxy analogue (deoxycholic acid), and the C-18 dietary fatty acid, oleic acid, is less potent than is its monohydroxylated analogue, ricinoleic acid.[5] However, most molecules belonging to these classes have dose-related effects. Secretagogues reduce absorption of electrolytes and water; greater concentrations evoke a net secretion of fluid. Effects on colonic motility and transit have been less well documented and the results are sometimes inconsistent. However, the overall response of the colon to bile and fatty acids is an increase in motor activity and rapid transit.

Also in this group of secretagogues should be included the traditional "vegetable laxatives" (cascara, senna, phenolphthalein) and the commonly used drug, bisacodyl.[22–24,88] Literature on these individual agents cannot be reviewed here in detail, but certain general principles apply. In sufficient doses, all are secretogogues and they also produce superficial inflammatory changes (Fig. 2-1) that can be confused with acute colitis. Even "stool softeners," sometimes assumed to be relatively inert agents acting only by physiochemical interactions with feces, alter mucosal function and structure.[24] The motor response of the colon to stimulant laxatives has also been well defined. Hardcastle and Mann[88] demonstrated that bisacodyl or oxyphenisatin stimulated active peristaltic activity of the healthy human colon.

The controversy surrounding the question as to whether long-term exposure of the colon to stimulant laxatives damages the myenteric ganglia has been mentioned. It was proposed, based on the work of Smith[31] that chronic laxative use destroys myenteric neurons, leads to further disturbances of motility, and produces the "cathartic colon"; however, these concepts have been challenged.[32–34] The observations of Schuffler et al.[34] have now been well confirmed by others, that the myenteric neurones of colons removed from patients with chronic constipation regularly show pathologic changes. These are now considered to be primary lesions of an enteric neuropathy and are not thought to result from laxative abuse.

ASSESSMENT OF ABNORMAL COLONIC FUNCTION: CONSTIPATION AND DIARRHEA

Departure from the orderly and planned production and excretion of stools prompts many patients to seek medical care, but the frequency of defecation, stool consistency, fecal volume, and the wet and dry weights of stools are highly variable. Thus, altered bowel habits are of only limited specificity for any particular diagnosis, and any changes must be evaluated in context only for that individual. When faced with patients with altered bowel habits, the prevalence and great importance of mucosal disease (neoplasia, inflammation) obliges the clinician first to rule out structural diseases. If intestinal (structural) and systemic (biochemical) disorders can be eliminated, functional diagnoses, such as idiopathic constipation or the irritable bowel syndrome, need to be entertained. However, it now becomes even more important to keep in mind that patients define symptoms variably. Constipation may imply infrequent, hard, or small stools; on the other hand, frequency and consistency may be "normal" and the term used to describe unsatisfied defecation (common in functional disorders), excessive straining, or pain. Comparable uncertainties apply to ''diarrhea,'' and the importance of a careful, and specific, history cannot be overemphasized. For example, it is well recognized that many patients use the term diarrhea to mask the more embarrassing one of incontinence.

Disorders of transit can be evaluated most simply by noting the form and consistency of fecal matter. Heaton and colleagues[89] first related stool consistency, as judged on a 7-point scale, to total gut transit; they compared fecal form with the timed appearance of radiopaque markers in stools. Looser stools were associated with rapid mouth-to-anus transit, and vice versa. A further step was taken when stool consistency was recorded during studies in which colonic transit was altered experimentally[11]; a strong relationship was noted between co-lonic transit time and stool form. Further observations in our laboratory have featured healthy volunteers, eating normal diets and studied on two occasions. We confirmed that the range of colonic transit times in health is wide, within and between individuals. We also reaffirmed the close relationships among stool frequency, stool form, and colonic transit.[90]

Although loose stools contain high proportions of water,[11] the relationships among stool form, fecal solids, and percent water content are not simple. Solids are present even in loose stools, and their water-holding capacity contributes importantly to the rather complex physicochemical relationships that ultimately determine stool consistency.[91] Nevertheless, it is reasonable to generalize that looser stools reflect the incomplete degree to which water has been reabsorbed by the colon. Conversely, the small, hard stools of constipation reflect slower transit and greater degrees of water absorption.

References

1. Basilisco G, Phillips SF (1993) Colonic salvage in health and disease. Eur J Gastroenterol Hepatol 5:777–783
2. Debongnie JC, Phillips SF (1978) Capacity of the human colon to absorb fluid. Gastroenterology 74:698–703
3. Phillips SF, Giller J (1973) The contribution of the colon to electrolyte and water conservation in man. J Lab Clin Med 81:733–746
4. Phillips SF (1986) Asiatic cholera: nature's experiment? (editorial). Gastroenterology 91:1304–1307
5. Ammon HV, Phillips SF (1973) Inhibition of colonic water and electrolyte absorption by fatty acids in man. Gastroenterology 65:744–749
6. Binder HJ, Sandle GI, Rajendrum VM (1991) Colonic fluid and electrolyte transport in health and disease. pp. 141–168. In Phillips SF, Pemberton JH, Shorter RG (eds): The Large Intestine: Physiology, Pathophysiology and Disease. Raven Press, New York
7. Chang EB, Rao MC (1994) Intestinal water and electrolyte transport: Mechanisms of physiological and adaptive responses. pp. 2027–2082. In Johnson LR (ed): Physiology of the Gastrointestinal Tract. 3rd Ed. Raven Press, New York
8. Mekhjian HS, Phillips SF, Hofmann AF (1971) Colonic secretion of water and electrolytes induced by bile acids: perfusion studies in man. J Clin Invest 50:1569–1577
9. Sandborn WJ, Phillips SF (1995) Pathophysiology of symptoms and clinical features of inflammatory bowel disease. pp. 407–428. In Kirsner JB, Shorter RG (eds): Inflammatory Bowel Disease. 4th Ed. Williams & Wilkins, Baltimore
10. Arrambide KA, Santa Ana CA, Schiller LR et al (1989) Loss of absorptive capacity for sodium chloride as a cause of diarrhea following partial ileal and right colon resection. Dig Dis Sci 34:193–201
11. Hammer J, Phillips SF (1993) Fluid loading of the human colon: Effects of segmental transit and stool composition. Gastroenterology 105:988–998
12. Reynolds JC, Ouyang A, Lee CA et al (1987) Severe chronic constipation. Prospective motility studies in 25 consecutive patients. Gastroenterology 92:414–420
13. Devroede GJ, Soffie M (1973) Colonic absorption in idiopathic constipation. Gastroenterology 64:552–561
14. Devroede GJ (1993) Constipation in gastrointestinal disease. pp. 837–887. In Sleisenger MH, Fordtran JS (eds): Gastrointestinal Disease, 5th Ed. W. B. Saunders, Philadelphia
15. Pemberton JH, Rath DM, Ilstrup DM (1991) Evaluation and surgical treatment of severe chronic constipation. Ann Surg 214:403–411
16. Phillips SF (1987) Small and large intestinal disorders: associated fluid and electrolyte conplications. pp. 865–878. In Maxwell MH, Kleeman CR, Narins RC, eds. Clinical Disorders of Fluid and Electrolyte Metabolism. McGraw-Hill, New York
17. Diamond JM (1974) Tight and leaky junctions of epithelia: a perspective on kisses in the dark. Feder Proc 33:2220–2224
18. Chadwick VS, Phillips SF, Hofmann AF (1977) Measurements of intestinal permeability using low molecular weight polyethylene glycols (PEG 400). II. Application to normal and abnormal permeability states in man and animals. Gastroenterology 73:247–251
19. Bjarnason I, MacPherson A, Hollander D (1995) Intestinal permeability: An overview. Gastroenterology 108:1566–1581
20. Devroede GJ, Phillips SF (1969) Conservation of sodium, chloride and water by the human colon. Gastroenterology 56:101–109
21. Holmberg C, Perheentupa J, Launiala K (1975) Colonic electrolyte transport in health and in congenital chloride diarrhea. J Clin Invest 56:302–310
22. Ewe K, Hoker B (1974) Einfluss eines diphenolischer Laxars Bisacodyl auf den Wasser- und Elektrolyttransport im menschilichen Colon. Klinische Wochenschrift 52:827–833
23. Saunders DR, Sillery J, Rachmilewitz D (1977) Effect of bisacodyl on the structure and function of the rodent and human intestine. Gastroenterology 72:849–856
24. Saunders DR, Sillery J, Rachmilewitz D (1975) Effect of dioctylsodium sulfosuccinate on structure and function of rodent and human intestine. Gastroenterology 69:380–386
25. Racusen LC, Binder HJ (1980) Effect of prostaglandin on ion transport across isolated colonic mucosa. Dig Dis Sci 25:900–903
26. Lennard-Jones JE et al (1962) Observations on idiopathic proctitis. Gut 3:201
27. Kramer P (1966) The effect of varying sodium loads on the

ileal excreta of human ileostomized subjects. J Clin Invest 45: 1710

28. Pemberton JH, Phillips SF (1993) Ileostomy and its alternatives. pp. 1331–1339 In Sleisenger MH, Fordtran JS (eds): Gastrointestinal Disease. Pathophysiology/Diagnosis/Management, 5th Ed. W.B. Saunders, Philadelphia

29. Cooke HJ (1991) Regulation of colonic transport by autonomic nervous system. pp. 169–180. In Phillips SF, Pemberton JH, Shorter RG (eds): The Large Intestine: Physiology, Pathophysiology and Disease. Raven Press, New York

30. Hubel KA, Renquist KS, Shirazi S (1987) Ion transport in human cecum, transverse colon and sigmoid colon in vitro: baseline and response to electrical stimulation of intrinsic nerves. Gastroenterology 92:501–507

31. Smith B (1968) Effect of irritant purgatives on the myenteric plexus in man and the mouse. Gut 9:139–143

32. Dufour P, Gendre P (1984) Ultrastructure of mouse intestinal mucosa and changes observed after long term anthraquinone administration. Gut 25:1358–1363

33. Kiernan JA, Heinicke EA (1989) Sennosides do not kill myenteric-neurons in the colon of the rat or mouse. Neuroscience 30:837–842

34. Schuffler MD, Zonak A (1982) Chronic idiopathic intestinal pseudoobstruction caused by a degenerative disorder of the myenteric plexus: the use of Smith's method to define the neuropathology. Gastroenterology 82:476–486

35. Roediger WEW (1982) Utilization of nutrients by isolated epithelial cells of the rat colon. Gastroenterology 83:424–429

36. Roediger WEW (1980) The colonic epithelium in ulcerative colitis: an energy-deficiency disease? Lancet 2:712–715

37. Breuer RI, Buto SK, Christ ML et al (1991) Rectal irrigation with short-chain fatty acids for distal ulcerative colitis: preliminary report. Dig Dis Sci 36:185–187

38. Vernia P, Marcheggiano A, Caprili R et al (1995) Short-chain fatty acid topical treatment in distal ulcerative colitis. Aliment Pharmacol Ther 9:309–313

39. Harig JM, Soergel KH, Komorowski RA et al (1989) Treatment of diversion colitis with short-chain fatty acid irrigation. N Engl J Med 320:23–28

40. Ruppin H, Bar-Meir S, Soergel KH et al (1980) Absorption of short-chain fatty acids by the colon. Gastroenterology 78: 1500–1507

41. Kramer P, Kearney MS, Ingelfinger FJ (1962) The effect of specific foods and water loading on the ileal excreta of ileostomized human subjects. Gastroenterology 42:535

42. Gadacz TR, Kelly KA, Phillips SF (1977) The Kock ileal pouch: absorptive and motor characteristics. Gastroenterology 72:1287

43. Gorbach SL, Nahas L, Weinstein L (1967) Studies of intestinal microflora, IV. The microbiology of ileostomy effluent: A unique microbial ecology. Gastroenterology 53:874

44. Phillips SF, Quigley EMM, Kumar D et al (1988) Motility of the ileocolonic junction. Gut 29:390–406

45. Phillips SF (1992) Sphincters of the gastrointestinal tract: functional properties. pp. 7–27 In Daniel EE, Tomita T, Tsuchida S et al (eds). Sphincters: Normal Function—Changes in Diseases. CRC Press, Boca Raton

46. Hurst AF (1931–1932) Discussions on the functions of the sympathetic nervous system. Proc R Soc Med 25:1597–1599

47. Camilleri M, Colemont LJ, Phillips SF et al (1989) Human gastric emptying and colonic filling of solids characterized by a new method. Am J Physiol 257: G284–G290

48. Spiller RC, Brown ML, Phillips SF (1986) Decreased fluid tolerance, accelerated transit, and abnormal motility of the human colon induced by oleic acid. Gastroenterology 91: 100–107

49. Spiller RC, Brown ML, Phillips SF (1987) Emptying of the terminal ileum in intact man—influence of meal residue and ileal motility. Gastroenterology 92:724–729

50. Fich A, Steadman CJ, Phillips SF et al (1992) Ileocolonic transit does not change after right hemicolectomy. Gastroenterology 103:794–799

51. Cummings JH, James WPT, Wiggins HS (1973) Role of the colon in ileal resection diarrhea. Lancet 1:344

52. McJunkin B, Fromm H, Serva RP et al (1981) Factors in the mechanism of diarrhea in bile acid malabsorption: fecal pH—a key determinant. Gastroenterology 80:454

53. Kamath PS, Phillips SF, O'Connor MK et al (1990) Colonic capacitance and transit in man: modulation by luminal contents and drugs. Gut 31:443–449

54. Proano M, Camilleri M, Phillips SF et al (1990) Transit of solids through the human colon: regional quantification in the unprepared bowel. Am J Physiol 258:G856–G862

55. Proano M, Camilleri M, Phillips SF et al (1991) Unprepared human colon does not discriminate between solids and liquids. Am J Physiol 260:G13–G16

56. Krevsky B, Malmud LS, D'Ercole F et al (1986) Colonic transit scintigraphy. A physiologic approach to the quantitative measurement of colonic transit in humans. Gastroenterology 91: 1102–1112

57. Dapoigny M, Trolese JF, Bommelaer G et al (1988) Myoelectric spiking activity of right colon, left colon, and rectosigmoid of healthy humans. Dig Dis Sci 33:1007–1012

58. Kerlin P, Zinsmeister A, Phillips S (1983) Motor responses to food of the ileum, proximal colon, and distal colon of healthy humans. Gastroenterology 84:762–770

58a. Basilisco G, Phillips SF, Cullen JJ, Chiravuri M (1995) Tonic responses of the canine proximal colon: effects of eating nutrients and simulated diarrhea. Am J Physiol 268:G95–G101

59. Neri M, Phillips SF, Fich A (1991) Measurement of tone in canine colon. Am J Physiol 260:G505–G511

60. Steadman CJ, Phillips SF, Camilleri M et al (1992) Control of muscle tone in the human colon. Gut 33:541–546

61. Wiley J, Tatum D, Keinath R et al (1988) Participation of gastric mechanoreceptors and intestinal chemoreceptors in the gastrocolonic response. Gastroenterology 94:1144–1149

62. Shibata C, Sasaki I, Matsuno S et al (1991) Colonic motility in innervated and extrinsically denervated loops in dogs. Gastroenterology 101:1571–1578

63. Niederau C, Faber S, Karays M (1992) Cholecystokinin's role in regulation of colonic motility in health and in irritable bowel syndrome. Gastroenterology 102:1889–1898

64. Moreno-Osset E, Bazzocchi G, Lo S et al (1989) Association between postprandial changes in colonic intraluminal pressure and transit. Gastroenterology 96:1265–1273

65. Picon L, Lemann M, Flourié B et al (1992) Right and left colonic transit after eating assessed by a dual isotopic technique in healthy humans. Gastroenterology 103:80–85

66. Jian R, Najean Y, Bernier JJ (1984) Measurement of intestinal progression of a meal and its residues in normal subjects and

patients with functional diarrhoea by a dual isotope technique. Gut 25:728–731

67. Flourie B, Phillips S, Richter H III et al (1989) Cyclic motility in canine colon: responses to feeding and perfusion. Dig Dis Sci 34:1185–1192

68. Levitt MD (1983) Malabsorption of starch: a normal phenomenon. Gastroenterology 85:769

69. Stephen AM, Haddad AC, Phillips SF (1983) Passage of carbohydrate into the colon. Direct measurements in humans. Gastroenterology 85:589–595

70. Stephen AM, Wiggins HS, Cummings JH (1987) Effect of changing transit time on colonic microbial metabolism in man. Gut 28:601–609

71. Florent C, Flourie B, Leblond A et al (1985) Influence of chronic lactulose ingestion on the colonic metabolism of lactulose in man (an in vivo study). J Clin Invest 75:608–613

72. Flourie B, Florent C, Jouany JP et al (1986) Colonic metabolism of wheat starch in healthy humans. Effects on fecal outputs and clinical symptoms. Gastroenterology 90:111–119

73. Barrow L, Steed KP, Spiller RC et al (1992) Scintigraphic demonstration of lactulose-induced accelerated proximal colon transit. Gastroenterology 103:1167–1173

74. Szurzewski JH, King BF (1989) Physiology of prevertebral ganglia in mammals with special references to the inferior mesenteric ganglia. In Shultz SG, Wood JP (eds): Handbook of Physiology, The GI System, I. American Physiological Society, Bethesda

75. Brugere HB, Ferre JP, Ruckebusch Y (1991) Colonic motility and transit after inter mesenteric nerve transection and mesenteric ganglinectomy in dogs. J Gastrointest Motility 3:107–116

76. Klauser AG, Vonderholzer WA, Heinrich CA et al (1990) Behavioral modification of colonic function: Can constipation be learned? Dig Dis Sci 35:271–175

77. Orkin BA, Hanson RB, Kelly KA (1989) The rectal motor complex. J Gastrointest Motility 1:5–8

78. Cannon WB (1902) The movements of the intestines studied by means of the roentgen rays. Am J Physiol 6:251–277

79. Edwards DAW, Beck LR (1971) Movement of opacified feces during defecation. Dig Dis 16:709–711

80. Ritchie JA (1968) Colonic motor activity and bowel function, I. Normal movement of contents. Gut 9:442–456

81. Hinton JM, Lennard-Jones JE, Young AC (1969) A new method for studying gut transit times using radiopaque markers. Gut 10:842–847

82. Arhan P, Devroede G, Jehannin B et al (1981) Segmental colonic transit time. Dis Colon Rectum 24:625–629

83. Metcalf AM, Phillips SF, Zinsmeister AR et al (1987) Simplified assessment of segmental colonic transit. Gastroenterology 92:40–47

84. Charles F, Camilleri M, Phillips SF et al (1995) Scintigraphy of the whole gut: clinical evaluation of transit disorders. Mayo Clinic Proc 70:113–118

85. Stivland T, Camilleri M, Vassallo M et al (1991) Scintigraphic measurement of regional gut transit in severe idiopathic constipation. Gastroenterology 101:107–115

86. Vassallo M, Camilleri M, Phillips SF (1992) Transit through the proximal colon influences stool weight in irritable bowel syndrome. Gastroenterology 102:102–108

87. Karaus M, Sarna SK (1987) Giant migrating contractions during defecation in the dog colon. Gastroenterology 92:925–933

88. Hardcastle JD, Mann CV (1968) Study of large bowel peristalsis. Gut 9:512–520

89. Heaton KW, Ghosh S, Bradton FEM (1991) How bad are the symptoms and bowel dysfunction of patients with irritable bowel syndrome? A prospective, controlled study with emphasis on stool form. Gut 32:73–79

90. Degen, LP, Phillips SF (1996) How well does stool form reflect colonic transit? Gut 39:109–113

91. Wenzl HH, Fine KD, Schiller LR et al (1995) Determinants of decreased fecal consistency in patients with diarrhea. Gastroenterology 108:1729–38

92. Kerlin P, Phillips SF (1983) Differential transit of liquids and solid residue through the human ileum. Am J physiol 8: G38–43

3

LARGE BOWEL MOTILITY

Svante Nordgren
Tom Öresland
Leif Hultén

With the exception of the pelvic floor muscles and the external anal sphincter, motility of the large bowel is controlled by the autonomic nervous system. Several different nervous centers, such as autonomic parts of the central nervous system (CNS), extraintestinal autonomic ganglia, and the enteric nervous system (ENS), are involved (Fig. 3-1). Although controversial and less well clarified, mental activity, via supraspinal centers, also has an impact on the motility of the large bowel (Fig. 3-2). Sleep has convincingly been shown to depress motility, while hostility and anger may increase motor activity.

The ENS is often referred to as the "brain of the gut" and has the ability to control large bowel motility without any external input. The ENS may be compared to a computer that processes information from intestinal and extraintestinal sources, by means of "software" contained within the system itself. From the ENS nerve impulses are distributed to the effector cells, which constitute the smooth muscle coat of the large intestine, the vascular bed, and the cells of the mucosa.

Furthermore, humoral factors, systemic as well as local, also modify the smooth muscle motor response to nervous stimulation, although these mechanisms are still poorly known.[1]

The principal pattern of colonic motility is segmental contractions, the overall effect of which is to promote mixing of the bowel contents. Withdrawal of the resistance caused by segmental contractions is required for propulsion to occur. Little force is then needed to achieve transit.

HISTORICAL REMARKS

The present concept of the extrinsic nervous control of large bowel motility is largely derived from the comprehensive works of Langley and Andersen[2,3] and of Bayliss and Starling.[4] Cannon[5] demonstrated that the bowel, even when deprived of connections with the central nervous system, still could perform characteristic movements, but that severing of extrinsic nerves immediately resulted in an impairment of the normal function. In the middle of this century an exhaustive synthesis by Al-

varez[6] gave an overview of the extrinsic nervous control of the large bowel.

With the advent of "modern" physiology, from 1950, the nervous control of the gastrointestinal tract was investigated in more detail both with respect to motility and regional blood flow. The basic impact of the sympathetic and the parasympathetic nervous systems on the GI tract were clarified and an understanding of the ENS and receptor pharmacology evolved.[7–10]

The distal extreme of the gastrointestinal tract, the anus, has attracted great interest from physiologists. Anal sphincter pressure has been studied in detail,[11] while the motility of the rectum has not attracted much attention until quite recently. Improved laboratory techniques including radiology, ambulatory manometry, and electromyography, and the increasing use of restorative sphincter-preserving surgery for colorectal disease, have contributed to a great revival of interest in colorectoanal physiology and pathophysiology.

In recent decades methods for the detailed investigation of intestinal motility have been developed and applied in research. Knowledge of intestinal physiology increased further with methods allowing for intracellular analysis of biochemistry, administration of drugs in vitro and in vivo, as well as recording of electrical events. The identification of peptide hormones involved in control of intestinal motility has increased enormously. Presently small molecules, like NO or CO are investigated for possible involvement in nervous transmission. Motility research today involves not only mechanical and electrical techniques for recording of dynamic events but also modern techniques of neuroanatomy, including the use of fluorescent dyes, immunohistochemistry, and immunoradiography.

DEFINITION OF MOTILITY

The concept of bowel motility comprises different aspects of mechanical activity of the intestines. First, motility is understood as movements of the individual muscular elements. Sec-

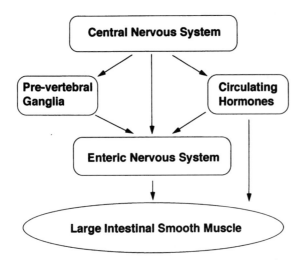

Figure 3-1. The effector organ for large intestinal motility, the smooth muscle coat of the bowel, is under nervous and hormonal influence.

ond, motility also implies the mechanical activity of the colonic wall as recorded from intra- or extraluminal sensors. Third, motility is understood as the work produced by the intestine, that is, the transport of its contents. These three aspects of colonic motility are basically different ways to describe the same mechanical, physiologic events. Electrical events, recorded from the intestinal smooth muscle cells, are sometimes used in the analysis of motility. Although electromyography does bear a relationship to mechanical activity of the bowel, electrical activity should not be referred to as equivalent to motility.

From a clinical and experimental point of view there are few if any instances where the three different aspects of motility meet and information from one can be used for conclusions about another. It is also important to stress that any information concerning intestinal motility must be appreciated knowing the precise technology that has been used to document the event. Similar techniques, even apparently identical techniques, may not justify direct comparison of observations. Minute differences in technical details (e.g., compliance of recording systems, infusion dynamics in perfused systems, or different computer programs in the ambulatory systems) make comparison unreliable and irrelevant.

EXTRINSIC INNERVATION OF THE LARGE BOWEL

It has been deduced from analogy with laboratory results that the extrinsic nervous supply to the colon in humans may be organized according to a principle similar to what is known in the cat.[8]

While the vagal nerves may well reach the colon, also in humans their influence on colon motility is still a matter of dispute. The sacral parasympathetic supply is anatomically better defined in humans. The innervation is derived from the second, third, and fourth sacral spinal segments and reaches the colon via the pelvic nerves. These nerves are located extrafascially on the pelvic side walls, in the lateral ligaments, and on the surface of the pelvic part of the large bowel (Fig. 3-3). Extensions from the pelvic nerves travel in an oral direction on the large bowel. While the pelvic nerves extend orally supplying almost the entire colon in the cat,[8] their extension in humans seems to be limited mainly to the left colon.[12]

The sympathetic division of the autonomic nervous system in humans is more complex. Efferent preganglionic axons leave the spinal cord via the ventral roots from ThX to LII, pass uninterrupted through the sympathetic ganglia, and synapse in the prevertebral (preaortic) ganglia. Postganglionic sympathetic fibers form a network around the superior and inferior mesenteric arteries and ramify all over the large bowel. From the root of the inferior mesenteric artery these fibers form a plexus, the hypogastric plexus, from which the bilateral hypogastric nerves originate (Fig. 3-3). The hypogastric nerves (or presacral nerves) traverse the pelvis and join with parasympathetic fibers to form the pelvic plexus,[13] located on the lateral and posterior aspects of the rectum. The hypogastric nerves supply the rectum and the internal anal sphincter as well as the genitourinary pelvic organs. The periarterial nerves along the inferior mesenteric artery (the lumbar colonic nerves) also project as distally as the internal anal sphincter.[14]

The sacral ventral roots also contain somatic efferent axons that innervate the striated muscles of the pelvic floor. These nerves (the pudendal nerves) can be demonstrated both on the rostral and the caudad side of the pelvic floor muscles.[15] An extensive review of the extrinsic nervous control of the large bowel was published by Gonella and co-workers.[16] The function of the striated muscles of the pelvic floor and the external anal sphincter will be discussed in a separate section.

Figure 3-2. Example of emotional influence on large bowel motility (volume recording). At the arrow the normal subject is told: "We will now give you an injection." Note the disappearance of spontaneous contractions.

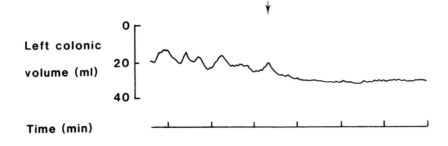

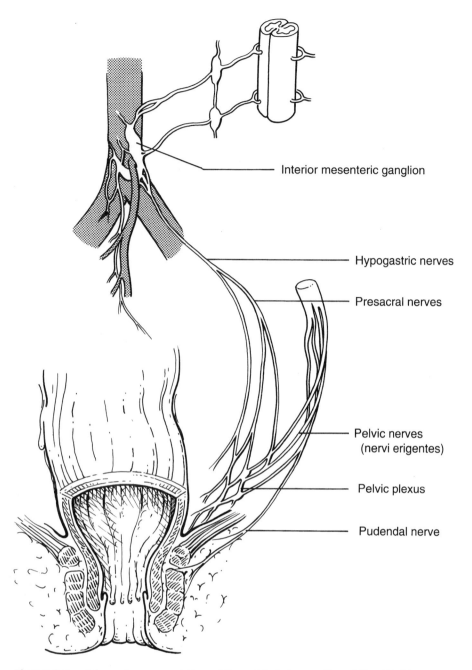

Figure 3-3. Schematic representation of the extrinsic innervation of the distal large bowel.

Interior mesenteric ganglion

Hypogastric nerves

Presacral nerves

Pelvic nerves
(nervi erigentes)

Pelvic plexus

Pudendal nerve

EVIDENCE FOR A FUNCTIONAL DIVISION OF THE COLON

The distributions and projections of the autonomic nerves to the large bowel are not known precisely. Much knowledge is gained from studies in animals. Considerable species differences exist, however.[8,17]

A detailed study of the extrinsic nervous control of colonic motility and blood flow in the cat[8] showed strong evidence that that both the parasympathetic excitatory and sympathetic inhibitory control of colonic motility are organized to form two different but partly overlapping antagonistic fiber systems. Thus, the vagal and splanchnic nerve supply affects only the proximal third while the pelvic and lumbar colonic nerves affect almost the entire colon—also that part to which the vagal and splanchnic sympathetic supply is restricted. The double control of the proximal colonic part appears to be functionally different in important respects. Vagal activation induces a response characterized by motility waves of increasing amplitude and frequency, superimposed on a slightly elevated tone. This is a motility pattern that favours mixing of contents. Pelvic nerve activation, on the other hand, excites the entire colon in a way that is different both with the respect to its effect on the proximal and distal colonic sections and especially in comparison with a vagal influence on the proximal section. Volume recordings show that the pelvic nerves produce a sustained luminal reduction in the entire colon favoring expulsion. The response in the proximal part starts as pronounced and frequent annular constrictions, but soon these fuse into a sustained overall contraction that greatly reduces the lumen.

The sympathetic supply appears to exert its inhibitory influence on colonic motility at the intramural ganglionic level. The splanchnic fiber supply appears to be distributed almost identically with the vagal supply, while the lumbar colonic nerves follow the same distribution as the pelvic nerves. Therefore the proximal colonic part appears to have a double supply of sympathetic fibers with respect to the motility control.

Simultaneous recording of the regional colonic blood flow lends further evidence for a differentiated proximal and distal colon function. Selective activation of the splanchnic vasoconstrictor fibers blanches the mucosa of the proximal third, and the remaining two thirds are similarly affected only when the lumbar colonic nerves are subsequently activated. Simultaneous stimulation of the two sets of sympathetic vasoconstrictor fibers led to an intense and uniform blanching of the entire colonic mucosa. With respect to the parasympathetic supply, even intense vagal stimulation over a wide range of frequencies had no effect on colonic blood flow, suggesting that these nerves do not convey any specific vasodilator fibers to the colon or do not in other indirect ways significantly affect blood vessel tone. In contrast, pelvic nerve stimulation produced an intense flush of the colonic mucosa but mainly in its distal two-thirds, that is, largely corresponding to the part supplied with vasoconstrictor fibers via the lumbar colonic nerves. Concomitantly with the mucosal vasodilatation there was also a pronounced secretion of mucus.

It may be argued that the observation that two sets of colonic vasoconstrictor fibers control different parts of vascular bed does not mean that these parts should be functionally differentiated. The nervous anatomy could as well be explained by the embryologic development of the colon, the proximal part being derived from the midgut and consequently supplied by fibers from the thoracic sympathetic outflow. The distal part is developed from the hindgut and controlled by the lumbar sympathetic outflow. However, the absence of the vagal vasodilator influences combined with the fact that the pelvic nerves produce mucosal vasodilator essentially confined to the distal colon suggests that the two parts may be functionally differentiated.

INNERVATION OF THE INTERNAL ANAL SPHINCTER

The sympathetic nervous system exerts a continuous excitatory effect on the internal anal sphincter. This is clinically significant, and sympathetic tone accounts for approximately 50% of internal anal sphincter tone.[18] The influence of the parasympathetic pelvic nerves on anal motility is complex and includes excitatory as well as inhibitory activity.[14,19] From a pharmacologic point of view the pelvic nerves seem to control at least three different internal anal sphincter motor activities:

A contraction of the internal anal sphincter, which is transmitted via a noradrenergic transmission step and probably involves modulation of release of an adrenergic transmittor.

An inhibition with nonadrenergic, noncholinergic characteristics, possibly involving activation of the nitric oxide pathway.[20]

An excitatory effect, which is partly sensitive to ganglionic blockade with hexamethonium, indicating a postganglionic character of the activated neurone or preganglionic with atypical transmission, but sensitive to atropine, indicating a muscarinic transmission step.[19]

The act of defecation involves several cholinergic steps, including a forceful contraction of the rectal wall and a concomittant contraction of anal longitudinal muscle, which shortens the anal canal and facilitates expulsion of feces. The muscarinergic excitatory mechanism in the internal anal sphincter, as mentioned, may be the result of a contraction of the longitudinal muscle.[21] Continence, on the other hand, is preserved by events mediated via the sympathetic nervous system.

METHODOLOGIC ASPECTS

From what has been said it is clear that a detailed knowledge of methodology is of great importance in understanding motility. Any study aiming at investigation of intestinal motility must first define a method that is accurate for the current conditions, to be able to record appropriate data.

A few standard concepts on recording techniques have evolved in the clinical motility laboratory: intraluminal pressure, intraluminal volume, and transit. Furthermore, deformation of the bowel wall may be recorded with the use of strain-gauge sensors, implanted during laparotomy onto the intestinal wall, a technique best suited in experimental studies. In vitro methods for the recording of motility or motility equivalents and measurement of deformation of surface belong to the research laboratory.

Pressure changes within the bowel are recorded with intraluminal balloons (as volume or pressure) (Fig. 3-4), perfused open-tip catheters (as resistance to flow) (Fig. 3-5), and by means of microtransducers (as pressure) (Fig. 3-6). Intestinal tone (volume to a given pressure) is recorded with a mechanical isobaric volume recording device (Fig. 3-7) or an electronically controlled barostat. Measurement of transit involves recording of propagation of feces, preferably with the use of isotopes or radiologic methods. It is a complex procedure with risk of numerous artifacts and errors.

Techniques for Recording Colonic Motility

The relative inaccessibility of the colon makes recording of mechanical and electrical activity difficult. Until recently, most information has been collected from the rectosigmoid area because of the ease with which this part of the bowel can be intubated. However, positioning of probes for manometry in the proximal colon via endoscopic intubation is presently being developed.[22] A systematic overview of methodology in motility recording was presented by Wingate[23] and others.[24,25]

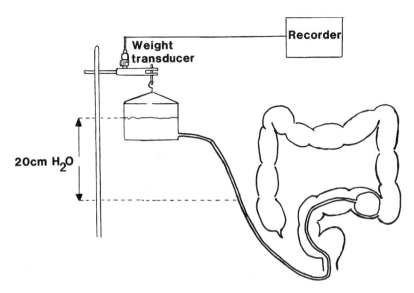

Figure 3-4. Experimental setup for intraluminal volume recording. The volume of the dynamic displacement water is recorded.

The perfused open-tip system has been the dominating method for pressure recording during several decades. In principle these systems consist of a pressure source for fluid perfusion, a fine-bore catheter with high intrinsic compliance, and a pressure transducer connected via a T-piece. Perfusion should be of constant speed and generated by a pressure significantly higher than maximal pressure to record. Recording medium has evolved from the smoked drum, over ink and paper, to the computer, with data processed via an analog/digital exchanger.

Figure 3-5. Multilumen catheter for pressure recordings at various distances from the tip of the assembly. Each catheter in the assembly is perfused with saline. Pressure is recorded as resistance to flow.

The parameter that is recorded is resistance to flow of the perfusion fluid. This makes the system sensitive to the local geometry at the point of opening of the catheter. Fragments in the lumen of the intestine may obstruct the flow and cause false high recordings. This may also be the result of pressure exerted on the bowel wall by the catheter from its inherent stiffness, particularly likely to occur in narrow bends of the organ. Uneven flow of the perfusion fluid is also reflected in the record, often identified as sudden changes of pressure (sawtooth appearance). The experienced investigator has the ability to discern many artifacts from the true record by ocular trial, something that is rarely possible in computerized systems.

Figure 3-6. Catheter with pressure-sensitive membrane close to the tip (microtip transducer) and solid-state memory box.

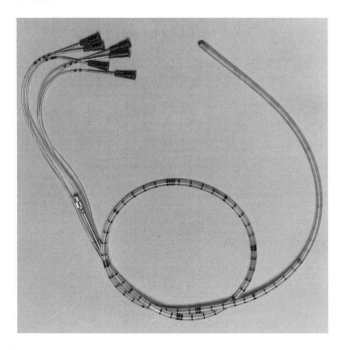

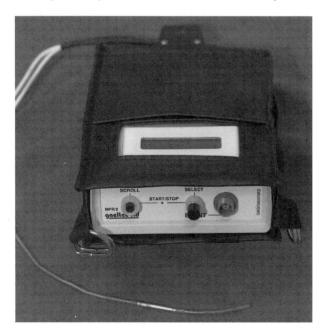

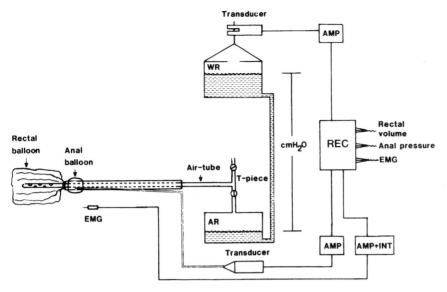

Figure 3-7. Schematic design of a system for anorectal manovolumetry. The rectum is distended with a preset pressure. By interposition of the lower reservoir, air is used as distension medium. This allows for a rapid distension. Also shown is the cylindrical cuff used for recording of anal pressure and needle electrode for recording of EMG.

The microtip transducers lodge the pressure-sensitive part (the transducer membrane) at the tip of or along the catheter (Fig. 3-6). No perfusion fluid is necessary. However, technical problems are common and records are often difficult to interpret. The systems are manufactured by several different companies and the various systems are not compatible. Most of the models comprise catheters of different shapes and with varying numbers of pressure-sensitive ports, a solid-state memory box, and a computer for processing and permanent storage of information (Fig. 3-8). The solid-state box has a memory capacity of more than 24 hours of recording and may be used in the ambulatory patient. In computer-based systems the pressure record is stored in a digital form. Of crucial importance, therefore, is the velocity of sampling of pressure data. This may be preset by the investigator or varied by the computer program according to the dynamics of pressure changes. High sampling frequency gives a more accurate recording but short recording time (memory consuming); a low frequency of sampling makes long-term records possible but with inferior precision.

It was appreciated in the 1960s that recording of pressure did not fully mirror all mechanical events in the gastrointestinal tract.[10] Particular, reduction of tone, relaxation/inhibition, was not possible to record with the current systems for pressure recording.[26] This led to the development of systems for volume recording. In principle these systems act as plethysmographs and record changes of volume to a constant, preset pressure. In its most simple design such a system consists of a fluid-filled balloon connected to a fluid reservoir. This reservoir is suspended on a weight recorder, and shifts of fluid to and from the balloon is recorded as changes of weight (Fig. 3-4). To allow for rapid shifts of large volumes, fluid as distension medium can be replaced by air, by the interposition of an air reservoir (Fig. 3-7). It may be argued that any shift of fluid will change the preset pressure, but by keeping the area of the reservoirs wide, changes will be insignificant. The error is systematic and can be

Figure 3-8. Setup for pressure recording with a digital system (Gaeltec). From top: Video screen for display, processing unit, memory box (compare to Fig. 3-6), keyboard, and printer.

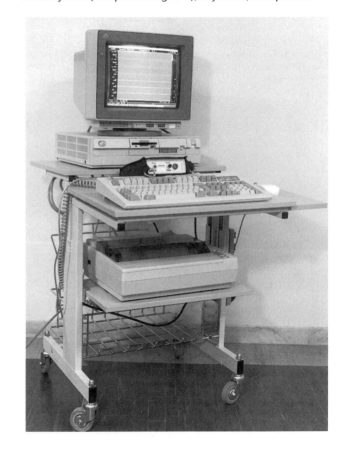

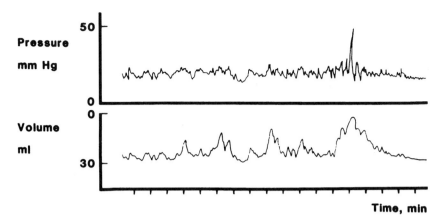

Figure 3-9. Example of pressure and volume recording from the sigmoid colon. Upper panel shows pressure, lower panel volume. Recording sites 5 cm apart.

corrected.[27] In the electronically controlled barostat this small change of pressure is compensated.

Differences between pressure- and volume-sensitive systems (Fig. 3-9) were pointed out and analyzed in a study by von der Ohe et al.[28] Differences between pressure curves from computerized microtip transducers and perfusion systems are less obvious but nonetheless equally important.

Intraluminal transport of contents is measured by the use of radio-opaque or isotope-labeled markers.[29,30] A strong wish to avoid handling of feces has made it necessary to rely on radiologic methods. In most protocols markers are ingested and disappearance is determined. To reduce the dose of radiation the number of exposures has to be kept low. Under these circumstances the saturation method described by Abrahamsson appears particularly attractive.[29]

It is claimed that selective study of motility in different regions of the colon is possible by use of radiographic and isotope methods. However, this opinion should be regarded with great caution, remembering that fecal stasis in one segment inevitably will affect transit in adjacent areas of the large bowel. Moreover, as stated, comparison of results from different recording systems should be pursued with great caution. Transit time will be further discussed in a separate section.

ELECTRICAL ACTIVITY

Contractions of the large bowel are controlled, as in other parts of the intestine, by electrical oscillations of the membrane potentials of the cells of the muscle layers. However, this myogenic electrical control mechanism of colonic motility is different from that of the upper intestine. In vitro studies have shown that the stomach and the small intestine exhibit a well-defined electrical control activity that is stable in amplitude and frequency, also called slow waves. In the colon, similar types of slow waves were found only intermittently. The human colon also exhibits oscillations that resemble slow waves, but these oscillations show further differences. In human colon circular muscle the frequency ranges from 4 to 60 cpm and in the longitudinal muscle from 20 to 40 cpm.[31] Thus, the frequency of the human colon slow waves is variable in time. Furthermore, colonic electrical activity needs stimulation in order to occur;

in the absence of an appropriate stimulus, like distension or nervous stimulation, the electrical oscillations decrease in amplitude and may disappear. Slow waves are supposed to be generated by the circular muscle layer in the colon of animal species.[32,33]

Myoelectrical activity recorded in vivo has been obtained from serosal electrodes implanted during surgery. Such studies in humans have shown that slow waves from the large bowel can be recognized only intermittently, ranging from 25% to about 50% of the time. There seems to be a frequency gradient along the large bowel, although the major drop in frequency occurs in the distal part of the bowel (Fig. 3-10).[34]

In addition to slow waves, spike activity can also be recorded from colonic smooth muscle. Two patterns of spike activity may be differentiated in the large intestine of humans: the long spike burst (LSB) and short spike burst (SSB) (Fig. 3-11).[35] SSBs are supposed to originate in the circular muscle layer; they are stationary, and phasic contractions of low amplitude have been recorded in association with this type of electrical activity.[36] LSBs last for 10 to 30 seconds, are associated with prolonged contractions, and may be propagated.[35] Propagation in the aborad direction is most commonly seen but occasionally they may also migrate towards the cecum. LSBs increase during hours following a meal and decrease during sleep.[37] Propagated LSBs may be the electrical equivalent of mass movements (discussed later), as seen radiologically. The myoelectrical equivalent to receptive relaxation is poorly described.

QUANTITATIVE ASPECTS OF COLONIC MOTILITY

Because of the great variability of colonic motility it is obvious that some means of objective standard for documentation of motility is needed. Several different methods for quantification of colonic motility have been used,[38] including measuring the frequency of contractions, the duration of contractions, the amplitude of contractions, the percentage of total recorded time during which contractions occur, and the area under the pressure curve. The most commonly used means for quantification is a combination of several parameters, known as a motility index. A motility index can be produced in different ways, but most often includes a product of pressure and time; for example, mean (amplitude $\times$ duration) $\times$ activity percentage.[39]

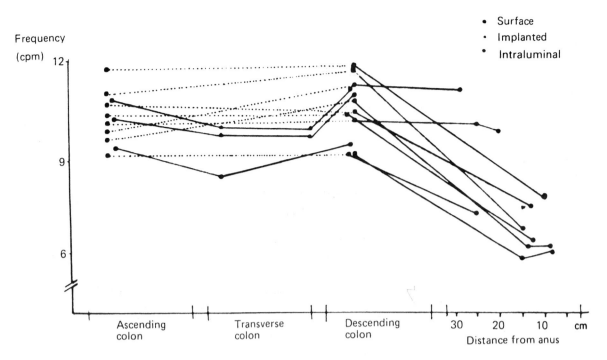

Figure 3-10.   Mean frequency of slow waves throughout the human colon and rectum. Recordings obtained with surface, luminal and implanted electrodes. (From Taylor et al.,[34] with permission.)

Figure 3-11.   Example of electromyogram from the large bowel. 1: right colon, 8: rectosigmoid junction. The diagram shows various types of electrical spike activity pattern, stationary short spike bursts (SSBs), large spike bursts (LSBs), and migrating long spike bursts (MLSBs). (From Frexinos et al.,[35] with permission.)

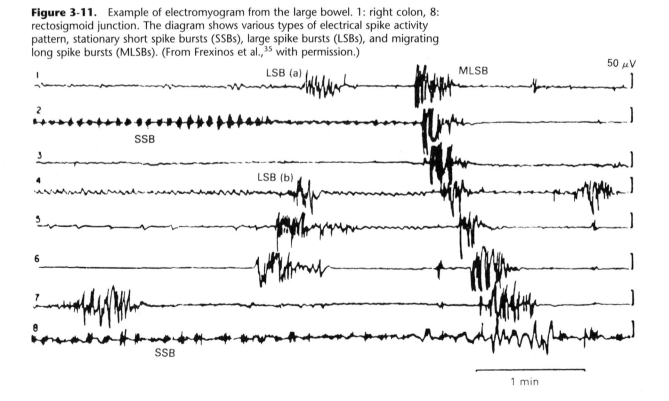

Modern computerized systems for long-term recording of motility have introduced computer software for an automated analysis of pressure records. This has made it possible to investigate events that occur only rarely and that are believed to be affected by the artificial milieu of the physiology laboratory. These computer programs perform a wave analysis according to basic criteria that may be determined in advance by the investigator. Specific modules are introduced to the program to identify and avoid inclusion of artifacts from breathing, coughing, and so forth. Criteria are defined to identify baseline pressure. For extended purposes, particularly to be used in clinical research, it is necessary to obtain a much deeper knowledge of the impact of wave criteria on the results. This is particularly true when comparison of various records is intended. An initiative to penetrate the impact of various computer software programs on the analysis of upper GI motility has been undertaken. Prior to purchasing a system the characteristics of the wave-analysis program should be defined.

NORMAL COLONIC MOTILITY

Components of Normal Motility

Approximately 90% of total intestinal transit time is accounted for by the large bowel. This enables the colon to fulfil one of its main tasks, to absorb fluid and electrolytes. This process necessitates a motor activity that delays transport along the colon. Cannon[40] reported observations on colonic motility from radiologic observations of radiopaque feces. A classification of colonic movements was suggested that in principle is still accepted. This included rhythmic segmentation, receptive relaxation, antegrade and retrograde peristalsis, and mass movements.

Rhythmic segmentation, causing mixing of the contents, has been documented throughout the colon but prevails in the oral part of the large bowel, as described. Antegrade peristalsis is said to be the dominating type of movement in the right colon, although studies on segmental transit time[41] have shown no significant difference in transit time between the right and the left colon. Receptive relaxation has been recorded from the cecum and the rectum. This is manifested by an increase in volume without concomitant pressure increase.[26] During a mass movement a contraction is propagated over a longer colonic segment, delivering feces distally, and is often associated with a desire to defecate. These contractions occur rarely.[42] An association with migrating motor complexes (MMCs) transmitted from the small bowel past the ileocecal junction has been suggested but not proven.

Studies on colonic motility using intraluminal manometry have shown significant increases of motor activity in the postprandial periods. At night the motor activity is reduced.[22] During activity a mixture of phasic short-lasting periods of contractions and quiescent periods are seen. With a period of about 4 to 5 hours during the day mass contractions are observed traveling in an aborad direction. Mean amplitude has been reported between 127 ± 0.7 and 158 ± 21 mmHg and mean propagation velocity between 0.9 ± 0.4 and 1.2 ± 0.7 cm/sec.[22,43] Colonic motility is extremely variable, and "normal" colon motility is not defined. Studies of colon motility therefore cannot as yet be used in the diagnosis of colonic motility disorders.

This is a disappointing fact in the management of colonic pathology.[44]

Few studies have investigated the relation between pressure changes and transport. Except for the peristaltic reflex,[4] which provides the physiologic ground for distal transport of solids, it has been assumed that propulsion follows pressure gradients. Support for this hypothesis was published by García-Olmo et al.[45]

The Colonic Response to Eating

Colonic motility is significantly increased in the postprandial periods. A cephalic phase was suggested and demonstrated by Welch and Plant.[46] A gastric phase was also considered likely, although gastric distension alone does not elicit a colonic response.[47] Evidence for a nervous basis for the colonic segmenting response to eating is equivocal. It is doubtful whether the vagal nerves have any direct influence on the colon and the motor response to eating persists after vagotomy. Because the postprandial motility increase is not clearly neural and the stimulus is not confined to the stomach, use of the term "gastrocolic reflex" should be abandoned. The failure to find a clear nervous pathway for the response has led to the search for a possible humoral mechanism. Hormones such as secretin, serotonin, gastrin, and CCK have been considered possible mediators but the mechanisms involved are still unknown.

An intestinal phase was postulated on the observation that the response does not require the presence of a stomach, acid, antral gastrin, or an intact vagal innervation.[48] The effect in humans has been shown to require an intact cholinergic innervation, and the effect is blocked by naloxone.[49] This implies that the response requires muscarinic and opiate receptors.

Apart from neurohumoral factors, the composition and quantity of food and eating habits also influence bowel transit to a considerable extent.[50,51] The possible influence of bile and pancreatic juice released in this context has attracted particular interest. The important role of bile acids as regulators of gastrointestinal transit has been demonstrated both in animals and humans. Thus bile acids, in a physiologic concentration (1 to 5 mmol/L), have been shown to reverse net fluid absorption to net secretion in the human ileum, influencing the consistency of postprandial ileal content. The excitatory effect of bile acid on colonic motility is well known and the ancient Egyptians used ox bile as a cathartic. The fat component of the food has been demonstrated to be a powerful stimulus for postprandial increase in colonic motility. Even a small amount of intraduodenal fat provokes a considerable increase of ileal output in ileostomy patients, temporally related to the motility response of feeding.[52] The concentration of bile acids in the ileal effluent was similar to postprandial levels collected from the lower ileum by intubation (2 to 10 mmol/L).

Duodenal fat administration in patients in whom terminal ileum has been excluded or resected causes an increase of ileal flow that appears earlier and reaches higher peak values.[52] In the clinical situation this is reflected in the postprandial watery diarrhea and defecation urge occurring in patients with a terminal ileopathy. Patients with Crohn's disease, patients who have had radiotherapy to the pelvis, and those who have had an ileal resection will develop this functional disturbance. Increased spillover of bile acids to the colon interfering with water absorption and colonic motility is probably the main cause of this disturbance.[53] The cholerheic diarrhea can be managed by a low-fat diet, and similar beneficial effects are described when using cholestyramin, a bile acid-binding resin.[54] In the experimental setting,[52] pretreatment with intraduodenal cholestyramin, before instillation of fat, completely abolished the ileostomy flow response.

Intraduodenal fat instillation induced a significant increase in sigmoid colonic motility, while this motor response failed to appear when the small bowel contents were prevented from reaching the colon by means of a diverting ileostomy.[55] The observation suggests that an intact small bowel continuity is a prerequisite for the colonic motility response to feeding, and that propulsive motility both in the small and large bowel is mainly and in a sequential fashion dependent on activation of short intramural reflexes elicited by intraluminal factors (Fig. 3-12).

COLON MOTILITY AND EPIDURAL ANESTHESIA

Epidural anesthesia is a significant positive contribution to surgery. Reduction of postoperative sympatho-adrenergic response and improved patient comfort is documented. However, concern has been raised as to the possibility of negative effects on a colonic anastomosis. Experimental studies have shown that blockade of the sympathetic outflow to the colon caused a significant increase of intracolonic pressure and a reduction of rectal volume (contraction). There is also a concommittant reduction in anal pressure (Fig. 3-13). This increase of colonic motility may, from a theoretical point of view, be harmful to a recently constructed colorectal anastomosis. Several studies have been directed to the question whether epidural anesthesia may induce a risk of leak to a colorectal anastomosis. Increased contractions of the circular muscle layer may create closed segments of the colon, allowing intraluminal pressure to rise to a

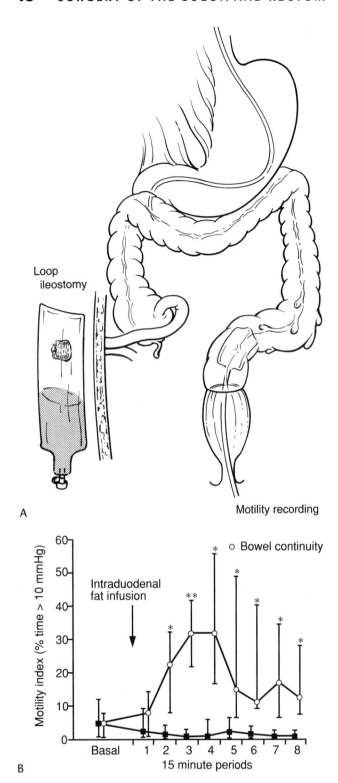

Figure 3-12. (**A**) The experimental setup. Experiments were done twice with and without the covering loop-ileostomy. (**B**) Relative phasic motility, median and interquartile range as compared with basal values $^*P < 0.05;^{**} P < 0.01$.)

Figure 3-13. The effects of epidural anesthesia on rectal volume and anal pressure in humans. (From Carlstedt et al.,[18] with permission.)

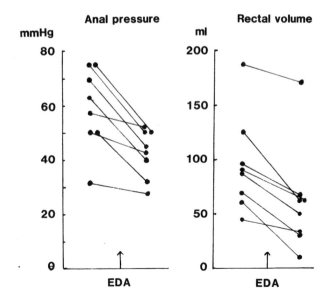

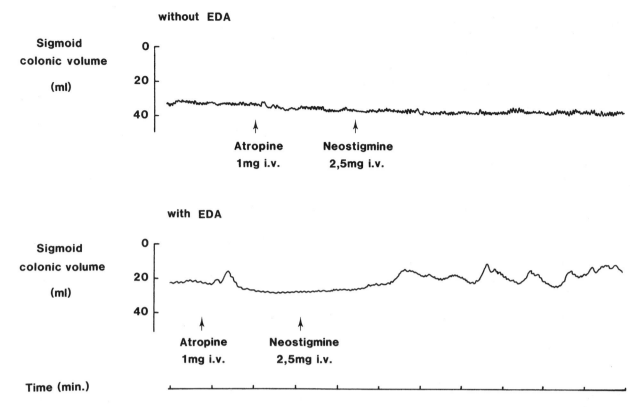

Figure 3-14.   Record showing the effect of neostigmine on left colonic volume in man before and after epidural anesthesia was given. Atropine was given according to anesthesiologic routines. Note the contractions during epidural anesthesia.

level that may cause disruption of an anastomosis with fecal leak through the suture line. Moreover, such pressure increase may also interfere with regional blood perfusion, and shortening of the longitudinal smooth muscle layer may increase the tension over the anastomosis. This sequence of events could be convincingly demonstrated in an experimental study in humans during epidural anesthesia. Increased intraluminal pressure and excessive shortening of the bowel was clearly documented and the response was particularly strong after administration of neostigmine, used by the anesthetist for reversal of the muscle relaxant. (Figs. 3-14, 3-15).[56] In a porcine model intestinal transit was significantly increased after epidural bupivacain and morphine, but anastomotic bursting strength on day 7 was not altered.[57] Clinical studies are difficult to interpret, but great caution is justified using neostigmine in combination with epidural analgesia in patients with a low colorectal anastomosis.[56,58]

DISORDERED COLONIC MOTILITY

Diverticular Disease

Diverticular disease of the colon is a clinical entity that appears to be caused partly or entirely by disordered motility. Although the etiology remains obscure it appears reasonable to accept that the characteristic pseudodiverticula are developed by herniation of colonic mucosa through openings in the muscular coat, caused by an increase of intraluminal pressure (Fig. 3-16). Patients with diverticular disease exhibit considerable in-

Figure 3-15.   The effect of neostigmine, in the presence of atropine, on left colonic volume in humans, as in Figure 3-14. Results from 8 patients.

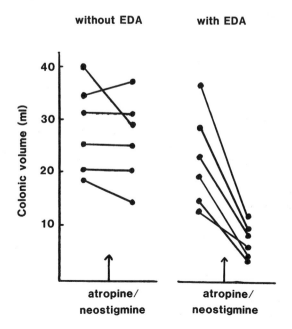

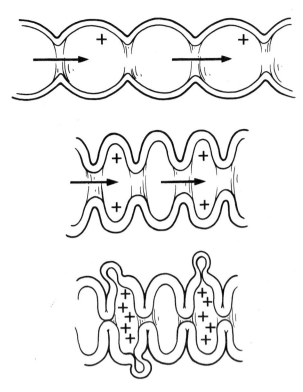

Figure 3-16. Present concept of the pathogenesis of colonic diverticular disease. Increased muscular work causes raised intraluminal pressure. When closed segments of the bowel are formed, the pressure may increase in excess of 100 mmHg.

crease in postprandial intraluminal pressure[59] and pathologically increased pressure has been demonstrated even in the resting state.[60] The underlying pathology is not known.

Irritable Bowel Syndrome

In the irritable bowel syndrome (IBS) an underlying motor disturbance has also been suggested. It appears that the colonic response to eating is significantly delayed in patients with IBS.[61] An early observation that disordered colonic motility in these patients could be diagnosed by means of frequency analysis[62] could not be confirmed in further studies.[36] However the impact of CNS on the colonic function is obvious. Strong emotions and psychologic conflicts are known to cause considerable gastrointestinal disturbances in general, and in fact the color of the colorectal mucosa may reflect emotions as expressively as the blanching and flushing of the face. The motility disorder in IBS may well reflect an exaggerated visceral reflex response in a situation of centrally elicited increases of autonomic discharge. An overview of intestinal motor function in IBS was recently published by Gorard and Farthing.[63] IBS will be further discussed in a separate section.

CONSTIPATION

Drugs, metabolic and endocrine disturbances, injuries to the spinal parasympathetics, multiple sclerosis, and various forms of aganglionosis are associated with constipation. Constipation

is also a common symptom of the irritable bowel syndrome. In the elderly, immobility, inadequate toilet facilities, poor diet, and mental and physical decline may often contribute to constipation. Although disordered motility may play a role in constipation in general, it is best defined in slow-transit constipation.

IDIOPATHIC SLOW-TRANSIT CONSTIPATION

Patients with idiopathic slow-transit constipation (ISTC) are invariably women of childbearing age. They may open the bowel once every 2 to 3 weeks. They suffer from abdominal distension, and often pain, and have no urge to defecate. Symptoms mostly date from adolescence and the condition has progressively deteriorated with the passage of time. They have to rely on increasing amount of laxatives to induce defecation. Apart from those who cannot relate their constipation to any recognizable event there are women who more clearly attribute the onset of the condition to childbirth or a pelvic operation such as hysterectomy. Others associate their problems with a drastic slimming cure. Many women often have a confusing mixture of ISTC and pelvic floor dyssynergia.

Since ISTC is almost exclusively seen in women of reproductive age, particular attention has been focused towards sex hormone levels. The exact role of hormones remains to be established. Reduced levels of vasoactive intestinal peptide (VIP) have been demonstrated,[64,65] and VIP-containing nerves proved to be absent from the circular smooth muscle.[66] Hypothetically these observations might imply a central role for VIP in the pathophysiology of ISTC. Histologic abnormalities demonstrated in ISTC are circular smooth muscle hypertrophy and reduction in the number of axons and neurons with Schwann cell hyperplasia. Later studies have failed to support some of these findings, however. Recently abnormalities in the extrinsic colonic nerve supply have been more clearly demonstrated by means of a special antibody staining technique.[67] Whether neuropathology in such studies represent primary or secondary pathology is not known.

Many of these women relate the constipation to a previous pelvic operation, and there is evidence that damage of the autonomic supply to the rectum and left colon may be responsible for the malfunction. Experimental work confirms that degeneration and subsequent regeneration may contribute to colorectal dysfunction. A comparative study between patients with slow transit constipation and patients after hysterectomy failed to prove the hypothesis, however.[68]

Similar to the IBD syndrome, the impact of central nervous stimuli on colon motility may at least to some extent explain the large bowel motility pattern in slow-transit constipation.[69] Constipation in these young women might have a psychologic background. These women are often emotionally labile, sometimes "hysterical and quite aggressive," demanding instant cure to their "life-long" problem. There may be a long complex history, sometimes with sexual assault or sexual child abuse, and a high incidence of anxiety and depression has been demonstrated on psychometric testing.

In constipation in general the number of contractions in the left colon appears to be increased whereas the opposite is found in patients with diarrhea.[70] In ISTC, however, motility appears to be very scarce[71] and not readily elicited by stimulant laxatives[72] and mass movements appear to occur significantly less often in patients compared to controls.[73] Prolonged ambulatory recording has been suggested as a discriminatory test for the diagnosis of slow-transit constipation, although further experience is needed.[74]

In chronic constipation, various features of obstructed defecation are often found. Subtotal colectomy and an ileorectal anastomosis is the suggested surgical treatment, but a less than optimal alternative when pelvic floor function is impaired. It appears to be of great importance to rule out any component of obstructed defecation before surgery is undertaken.[75] Medical means of treating slow-transit constipation may emerge from future prostaglandin research.[76] Diarrhea and constipation will be further discussed in Chapter 21.

RECTOANAL MOTILITY

General Features of Rectoanal Motility

Defecation and maintenance of continence are the main features of rectal motility. The rectum has a significant adaptive capacity to distension (Fig. 3-17). The rectal wall accommodates when distended by fecal residues and intraluminal pressure remains low. Similarities to the receptive relaxation of the stomach has been demonstrated in experimental animal studies,[10] and evidence for a central control has been put forward.[26]

Pressure recordings from the anal canal have been obtained for more than a century. It is particularly the rectoanal reflex, absent in Hirschsprung's disease, that has been the object of investigation.[11]

Methodology in Rectoanal Motility

Due to the specific properties of rectal motility, pressure-sensitive systems are not appropriate for the correct recording of rectal motor activity.[26] For detection of relaxatory mechanisms various systems for isobaric volume recording (techniques for assessment of volume to distension with a given pressure) have been developed.[27,77] To obtain correct data it is essential to use a rectal balloon with a low compliance. For this purpose the

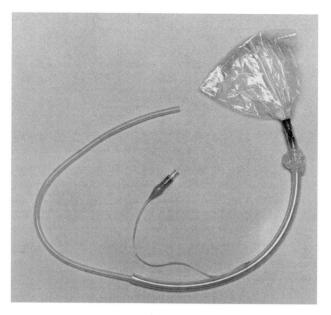

Figure 3-18. By the use of a plastic bag, the pressure at rectal distension is transmitted entirely to the rectal wall, provided the volume of the bag is not exceeded. Also note the endotracheal tube used as an anal probe for single use.

polyethylene plastic bag with a volume in excess of 600 ml is useful. The rectal distension pressure is entirely transmitted to the rectal wall as long as the inflated volume does not exceed the volume of the balloon (Fig. 3-18). In these systems rectal volume to a constant and predetermined pressure is recorded (isobaric volumetry, Fig. 3-19). This concept has given the term ''rectal tone'' a specific meaning. In this situation tone can be defined as compliance, or resistance to stretch, of the rectal muscular wall. Measurement of rectal compliance necessitates the definition of the pressure range within which resistance to stretch is tested. It is likely that the volume recorded during rectal distension from zero pressure to some extent reflects plain ''unfolding'' of the rectal wall, whereas distension within an interval not including zero more accurately identifies rectal wall properties. By means of simultaneous rectoanal manovolumetry (Fig. 3-20) the relationship between volume and pressure with respect to compliance, sensory functions, and rectoanal reflexes has been studied (Fig. 3-21). There is a close association between level of first sensation of filling and the threshold for eliciting the rectoanal inhibitory reflex.[78]

A great variety of techniques have been used for recording of anal sphincter activity. The types of probes that have been used can be subdivided according to the geometry of the probe and the magnitude of distension of the anal canal that is caused by the recording system. The geometry determines the area of the anal canal that is reflected in the pressure record. A small ''area of interest'' (≤ 1 mm^2) is obtained from open-tip catheters, an intermediate area (1 to 6 mm^2) from microtransducers, and a large area from microballoons and cylindrical anal probes. A large area of pressure sensitivity implies less accuracy to detect regional differences within the anal canal, a disadvantage offset by the advantage of less sensitivity for axial dislocation.[27] Among these probes various cylindrical cuff and membrane sensors can be found, including the Dent sleeve catheter.[79]

Figure 3-17. The effect of rapid distension (30 cm H$_2$O), of the colon and rectum, volume recording. Note the receptive relaxation in the rectum, spontaneous contractions are aborted.

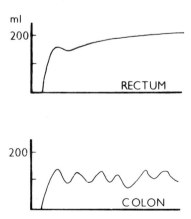

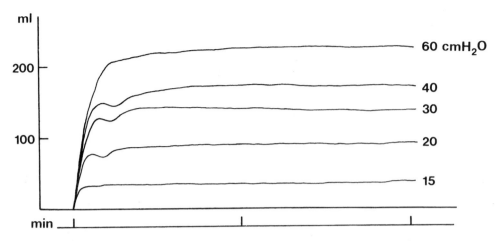

Figure 3-19. Rectal volumetrogram showing rectal compliance as a function of time and applied pressure. Note the rapid volume increase on distension, the aborted rectal contraction, and the steady state obtained after less than 1 minute.

Pull-through techniques with multiple side-hole catheters have made it possible to create a three-dimensional view of the anal pressure on the computer screen. It should be noted, however, that these systems are liable to express artifacts from lateral pressure exerted by the stiffness of the catheter on the side wall of the anal canal.

Normal Rectal Motility

A physiologic sphincterlike area seems to exist in the rectosigmoid junction and is supposed to be caused by the gradient in the inherent muscle activity between the distal colon and rectum.[44,80] Feces are propelled into the rectum as a conse-

Figure 3-20. Rectoanal manovolumetry and EMG in humans. The effects of rectal distension (40 cm H_2O) on the rectum, anal canal, and the striated sphincter are depicted. The increase of EMG activity reflects voluntary movements, elicited by sensations from the rectal area.

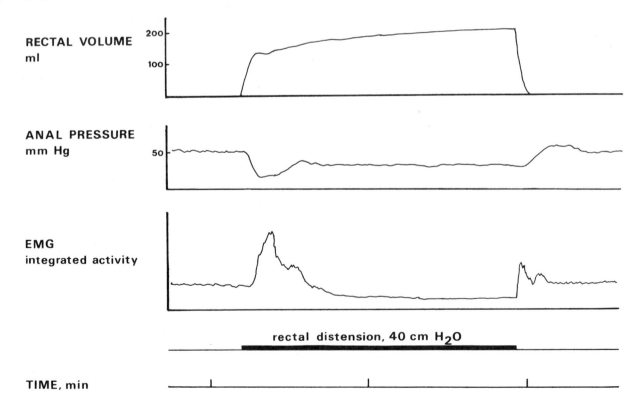

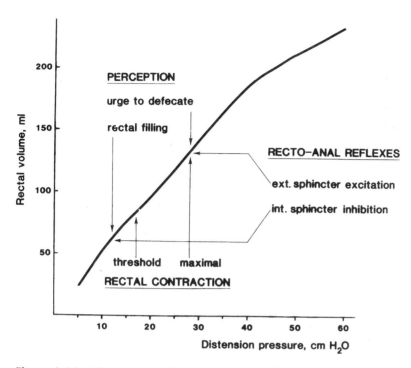

Figure 3-21. Thresholds to elicit sensations and reflexes by rectal distension in humans. Mean thresholds are denoted on the rectal compliance curve (pressure/volume at 4 seconds of distension). Note the association between rectal sensation and rectoanal inhibition and between perception of urge and external sphincter reflex contraction.

quence of the colonic mass contraction. This is normally followed by a desire to defecate. If not convenient, the desire may be voluntarily suppressed, a receptive relaxation occurs, and the rectal contraction subsides. It appears likely that lifelong neglect of the call to defecation leads to numbness of this reflex and probably to more or less continuous storage of feces in the rectum.

Twenty-four hours pressure recordings with modern solid-state technology from the rectum have shown that overall contractile activity is reduced during sleep. This is in concert with what is described for the colon.

Earlier balloon studies have shown that an increase in rectal tone occurs in response to a meal, rendering the rectum less compliant,[81] and feeding also increases rectal contractions.[82] Neostigmine also caused a prompt and steady increase in rectal tone.[81]

Resting Anal Pressure

Resting anal sphincter pressure is the sum of basal myogenic contraction and the superimposed tone induced by nervous activity. The myogenic component consists of the contraction of the smooth and striated muscles and tension in elastic tissue. It is obvious, therefore, that recorded anal pressure is dependent on the magnitude of distension that is caused by the recording probe itself.[83] The great variability of recording systems for anal pressure necessitates careful evaluation of each system before it is used, and also indicates the risks and difficulties in extrapolating and comparing data. Another possible source of error in the recording of anal pressure is the possible influence

of a simultaneously recording device in the rectum. This may initiate a rectoanal inhibitory reflex that may cause an underestimation of the true anal pressure.

Anal resting pressure in the left lateral position, as measured with a cylindrical probe (external diameter 10 mm) amounts to 59 (11) mmHg (mean, SD) in men and 56 (11) mmHg in women.[84] An inverse correlation has been found between age and resting anal pressure, with a drop measuring 0.4 mmHg $\times$ year^{-1}. This implies a 23% reduction from 30 to 70 years.[84]

About 15% of anal tone is contributed by the external striated sphincter in the resting state.[85] This means that resting anal pressure reflects the tone of the internal sphincter whereas the maximal squeezing pressure reflects the performance of the external anal sphincter.

The voluntarily controlled external sphincter may introduce another error to the recording of resting anal pressure. Any sensation from the anal and perianal area elicits a reflex contraction in the awake subject. Adjustment to the probe is necessary, which may take up to 8 to 10 minutes.[27] This is also a problem in pull-through recordings, and it should therefore be stated whether this is performed as a continuous or a station pull-through.

Normal Anal Motility

Long-term ambulatory recordings of anal pressure have revealed that there is a continuous activity during the day as well as at night.[86] Ultra-slow pressure changes (frequency, 0.5 to 1.5 per minute) have been observed. Although these pressure waves have been associated with pathologic conditions in the anal canal, such as anal fissures and hemorrhoids, similar pressure oscillations can also be demonstrated in normals.

During long-term recording of anal pressure sudden and precipitous drops in anal pressure are recorded intermittently. It appears as these are associated with passage of feces into the rectum, passage of flatus, or a rectal contraction. Most likely these anal pressure drops may be regarded as anal inhibitory responses to rectal contractions.[11] In the analysis of anal pressure records it should be remembered that anal pressure is a function of motor activity in the internal smooth muscle anal sphincter as well as in the external striated sphincter. This makes interpretation of recordings from the anal area particularly difficult to analyze in the ambulatory patient. During sleep, however, reduced activity from the external sphincter facilitates interpretation of the records.

The Rectoanal Inhibitory Reflex

The rectoanal inhibitory reflex is one of the earliest autonomic reflexes to be studied from a scientific point of view.[11] This reflex is regarded as the aboral extreme of the descending inhibitory component of the peristaltic reflex by Bayliss and Starling.[4] It is elicited by distension of the rectum and is expressed as a precipitous reduction in anal pressure.[27] This is followed, on continuous distension, by a "steady state" phase of less pronounced reduction of anal pressure (Fig. 3-22). The pressure reduction, particularly during the steady state phase, shows a relationship to the applied distension pressure. The rectal volume threshold (the minimal volume required to elicit the rectoanal inhibitory reflex) in humans varies greatly. The reflex is normally elicited by distension with a spherical balloon of less than 20 ml volume. In patients with a megarectum, however, the volume threshold may be increased tenfold.

The rectal pressure threshold, as measured in an isobaric system, is quite well defined at 12 ± 3 cm H_2O[79] and coincides with the threshold of rectal subjective perception.

The rectoanal inhibitory reflex persists after complete division of all extrinsic nerves to the anorectum. It is abolished by sectioning of the anorectal junction or by local destruction of the nervous elements in this area. The absence of the reflex is considered typical of Hirschsprung's disease, which is charac-

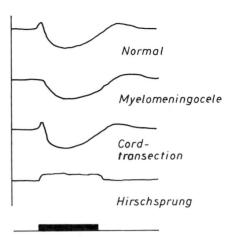

Figure 3-23. The appearance of the rectoanal inhibitory reflex in various neurologic conditions and in Hirschsprung's disease. Note that the inhibitory reflex is independent of connections with the CNS. Black bar denotes rectal distension.

terized by absence of the myenteric plexus in distal bowel wall (Fig. 3-23). The rectoanal inhibitory reflex is therefore considered an exclusively intramural reflex. However, in several experimental animal models evidence is presented indicating an external nervous influence over the reflex.

DEFECATION

On rectal filling the rectoanal inhibitory reflex induces a relaxation, that is, a widening of the upper end of the anal canal. This allows for a close contact between the rectal contents and the densely innervated mucosa of the anal canal, the sampling reflex.[87] A "sampling" of the contents of the distal rectal ampulla is performed, and the appropriateness of defecation is judged. When inappropriate, defecation urge is suppressed and receptive relaxation occurs. The external sphincter is contracted, which forces fecal contents back up in the rectum. If the opportunity is convenient and defecation can occur, the external sphincter relaxes and the rectum empties by reflex contraction (if present) or by straining.

Figure 3-22. Anal pressure during rectal distension with increasing pressure in humans. Note that the rectoanal inhibitory reflex is proportional to applied rectal pressure and that spontaneous anal motility is aborted on distension with 60 cm H_2O.

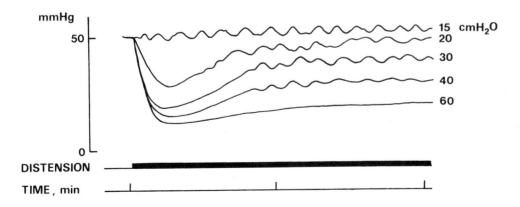

Reflex defecation caused by an expulsive rectal contraction probably occurs in less than 50% of the population. These subjects normally experience an urge to defecate after a meal, most often after breakfast. In the appropriate situation only a short episode of moderate straining is required. However, in most subjects this rectal contraction is too weak to allow for reflex evacuation, or it may be absent, and defecation requires straining of varying intensity and duration. This condition may be due to long-lasting neglect of the urge to defecate and may cause damage to the normal function of the pelvic floor structures. Disordered defecation is a great clinical problem and will be further elaborated in a separate section.

References

1. Sarna SK (1993) Colonic motor activity. Surg Clin North Am 73:1201–1223
2. Langley JN, Anderson HK (1895) On the innervation of the pelvic and adjoining viscera, I. The lower portion of the intestine. J Physiol (London) 18:67–105
3. Langley JN, Anderson HK (1896) The innervation of the pelvic and adjoining viscera. J Physiol (London) 20:372–406
4. Bayliss WM, Starling EH (1900) The movements and the innervation of the large intestine. J Physiol (London) 26:107–118
5. Cannon WB (1901/1902) The movements of the intestines studied by means of the Röntgen rays. Am J Physiol 6:251–277
6. Alvarez WC (1948) An Introduction to Gastroenterology. P. B. Hoeber, New York
7. Celander O (1959) Are there any centrally controlled sympathetic inhibitory fibres to the musculature of the intestine? Acta Physiol Scand 47:299–309
8. Hultén L (1969) Extrinsic nervous control of colonic motility and blood flow — an experimental study in the cat. Acta Physiologica Scand 335:1–116
9. Kewenter J (1965) The vagal control of the jejunal and ileal motility and blood flow. Acta Physiol Scand 65 (suppl 251): 1–68
10. Martinsson J (1965) Studies on the vagal control of the stomach. Acta Physiol Scand 65 (suppl 255):1–24
11. Gowers WR, Sandersons JSB (1877) The automatic action of the sphincter ani. Proc R Soc London 26
12. Telford ED, Stopford JSB (1934) Autonomic nerve supply of the distal colon; anatomical and clinical study. Br Med J 1: 572–580
13. Pearl R, Monsen H, Abcarian H (1986) Surgical anatomy of the pelvic autonomic nerves. Am Surg 52:236–237
14. Carlstedt A, Nordgren S, Fasth S et al (1989) The influence of the pelvic nerves on anorectal motility in the cat. Acta Physiol Scand 135:57–64
15. Percy JP, Parks AG (1981) The nerve supply of the pelvic floor. Schweizerische Rundschau für Medizin Praxis 70: 640–642
16. Gonella J, Bouvier M, Blanquet F (1987) Extrinsic nervous control of motility of the small and large intestines and related sphincters. Physiol Rev 67:902–961
17. Jule Y (1975) Modifications de l'activité electrique du côlon proximal de lapin, in vivo, par stimulation des nerfs vagues et splanchhniques. J Physiol (Paris) 70:5–26
18. Carlstedt A, Nordgren S, Appelgren L et al (1988) Sympathetic nervous influence on the internal anal sphincter and rectum in man. Int J Colorectal Dis 3:90–95
19. Buntzen S, Hultén L, Delbro D et al (1995) The effect of the pelvic nerve stimulation on recto-anal motality in the cat. J Autonom Nerv Syst
20. Buntzen S, Hultén L, Delbro D et al (1996) The role of nitric oxide for the acetylcholine-indiced relaxation of the feline internal anal sphincter, in vitro. Scand J Gastroenterol 31: 1189–1194
21. O'Kelly TJ, Brading AF, Mortensen NJ (1993) In vitro response of human anal canal longitudinal muscle layer to cholinergic and adrenergic stimulation: evidence of sphincter specialization. Br J Surg 80:1337–1341
22. Narducci F, Basotti G, Gaburri M et al (1987) Twenty-four-hour manometric recording of colonic motor activity in healthy man. Gut 28:17–25
23. Wingate DL (1983) Methodology of motility. pp. 2215–2219. In Christensen J, Wingate DL (eds): A Guide to Gastrointestinal Motility. Wright, London 1983
24. Cann P (1993) Sensors for direct measurement of gastrointestinal motility. Eur J Gastroenterol Hepatol 5:129–131
25. Nordgren SR, Abrahamsson H (1990) Methods for the investigation of colonic motility. Eur J Surg 564 (suppl):63–72
26. Fasth S, Hultén L, Nordgren S (1980) Evidence for a dual pelvic nerve influence on large bowel motility in the cat. J Physiol 298:159–169
27. Åkervall S, Fasth S, Nordgren S et al (1988) Manovolumetry: a new method for investigation of anorectal function. Gut 29: 614–623
28. Von der Ohe MR, Hanson RB, Camillieri M (1994) Comparison of simultaneous recordings of human colonic contractions by manometry and a barostat. Neurogastroenterol Motility 6: 213–222
29. Abrahamsson H, Antov S, Bosaeus I (1988) Gastrointestinal and colonic segmental transit time evaluated by a single abdominal X-ray in healthy subjects and constipated patients. Scand J Gastroenterol 23(suppl 152): 72–80
30. Kamm MA (1992) The small intestine and colon: scintigraphic quantitation of motility in health and disease. Eur J Nucl Med (Heidelburg) 19:902–912
31. Huizinga JD, Stern HS, Chow E et al (1986) Electrical basis of excitation and inhibition of human colonic smooth muscle. Gastroenterology 90:1197–1204
32. Christensen J, Caprilli R, Lund GF (1969) Electric slow waves in circular muscle of the cat colon. Am J Physiol 217:771–776
33. El-Sharkawy TY (1983) Electrical activities of the muscle layers of the canine colon. J Physiol 342:67–83
34. Taylor I, Duthie HL, Smallwood R et al (1975) Large bowel myoelectrical activity in man. Gut 16:808–814
35. Frexinos J, Bueno L, Fioramonti J (1985) Diurnal changes in myoelectric spiking activity of the human colon. Gastroenterology 88:1104–1110
36. Sarna S, Latimer P, Campbell D et al (1982) Effects of stress, meal and neostigmine on rectosigmoid electrical control activ-

ity in normals, and in irritable bowel syndrome patients. Dig Dis Sci 27:582–591

37. Furukawa Y, Cook IJ, Panagopolus V et al (1994) Relationship between sleep patterns and human colonic motility motor patterns. Gastroenterology 107:1372–1381

38. Loening-Bauke V, Anuras S (1983) Effects of a meal on the motility of the sigmoid colon nad rectum in healthy adults. Am J Gastroenterol 78:393–397

39. Weinreich J, Andersen D (1976) Intraluminal pressure in thee sigmoid colon, I. Method and results in normal subjects. Scand J Gastroenterol 11:577–580

40. Cannon WB (1912/1913) Peristaltic segmentation and the myenteric reflex. Am J Physiol 30:114–128

41. Metcalf AM, Phillips SF, Zinsmeister AR et al (1987) Simplified assessment of segmental colonic transit. Gastroenterology 92:40–47

42. Ritchie JA, Truelove SC, Ardran GM et al (1971) Propulsion and retropulsion of normal colonic contents. Dig Dis Sci 16:697–704

43. Garcia D, Hita G, Mompean B et al (1991) Colonic motility: electric and manometric description of mass movement. Dis Colon Rectum 34:577–584

44. Dinoso VP, Murthy SNS, Goldstein J et al (1983) Basal motor activity of the distal colon: A reappraisal. Gastroenterology 85:637–642

45. García-Olmo D, García-Picazo D, Lopez-Fando J (1994) Correlation between pressure changes and solid transport in the human left colon. Int J Colorectal Dis 9:87–91

46. Welch PB, Plant OH (1926) A graphic study of the muscular activity of the colon, with special reference to its response to feeding. Am J Med Sci 172:261–268

47. Tansy M, Kendall FM, Murphy JJ (1972) The reflex nature of the gastrocolic propulsive response in the dog. Surg Gynecol Obstet 135:404–410

48. Holdstock DJ, Misiewicz JJ (1970) Factors controling colonic motility: colonic pressures and transit after meals in patients with total gastrectomy, pernicious anemia and duodenal ulcer. Gut 11:100–110

49. Sun EA, Snape WJ, Cohen J et al (1982) The role of opiate receptors and cholinergic neurones in the gastrocolonic response. Gastroenterology 82:689–693

50. Gill RC, Kellow JE, Wingate DL (1987) The migrating motor complex (MMC) at home. Gastroenterology 92:1405

51. Higham SE, Read NW (1990) Effect of investigation of fat on ileostomy effluent. Gut 31:435–438

52. Hallgren T, Öresland T, Andersson H et al (1994) Ileostomy output and bile acid excretion after intraduodenal administration of oleic acid. Scand J Gastroenterol 29:1017–1023

53. Hoffman AF (1967) The syndrome of ileal disease and the broken enterohepatic circulation:cholerheic enteropathy. Gastroenterology 52:752–757

54. Andersson H (1976) Effects of fat-reduced diet in faecal excretion of radioactivity following administration of ^{14}C-cholic acid and on the duodenal concentration of bile salt in patients of ileal disease. Nutr Metab (Basel) 20:254–263

55. Hallgren T, Öresland T, Cantor P et al (1995) Intestinal intraluminal continuity is a prerequisite for the distal bowel motility response to feeding. Scand J Gastroenterol 30:554–561

56. Carlstedt A, Nordgren S, Fasth S et al (1989) Epidural anaesthesia and postoperative colorectal motility—a possible hazard to a colorectal anastomosis. Int J Colorectal Dis 4:144–149

57. Schnitzler M, Kilbride M, Senagore A (1992) Effect of epidural analgesia on colorectal anastomotic healing and colonic motility. Regional Anaesthesie (Berlin) 17:143–147

58. Bredtman RD, Herden HN, Teichmann W (1990) Epidural analgesia in colonic surgery: results of a randomized prospective study. Br Surg 77:638–642

59. Arfwidsson S (1964) Pathogenesis of multiple diverticula of the sigmoid colon in diverticular disease. Acta Chir Scand (Stockholm) 342:1–68

60. Trotman IF, Misiewiecz JJ (1988) Sigmoid motility in diverticular disease and the irritable bowel syndrome. Gut 29:218–222

61. Sullivan MA, Cohen S, Snape WJ (1978) Colonic myoelectrical activity in irritable bowel syndrome-effect of eating and anticholinergics. N Engl J Med 298:878–883

62. Snape WJ, Carlson GM, Cohen S (1976) Colonic myoelectric activity in the irritable bowel syndrome. Gastroenterology 70:326–330

63. Gorard DA, Farthing MJG (1994) Intestinal motor function in irritable bowel syndrome. Dig Dis 12:72–84

64. Koch T, Carney J, Go L et al (1988) Idiopathic chronic constipation is associated with decreased colonic vasoactive intestinal peptide. Gastroenterology 34:300–310

65. Milner P, Crowe R, Kamm M et al (1990) Vasoactive intestinal polupeptide levels in sigmoid colon in idiopathic constipation and diverticular disease. Gastroenterology 99:666–675

66. Krischnamurthy S, Schuffler M, Rohrman C et al (1985) Severe idiopathic constipation is associated with a distinctive abnormality of the colonic myenteric plexus. Gastroenterology 88:26–34

67. Sjölund K, Sanden G, Håkanson R et al (1983) Endocrine cells in human intestine: an immunocytochemical study. Gastroenterology 85:1120–1130

68. Roe AM, Bartolo DCC, Mortensen NJM (1988) Slow transit constipation. Comparison between patients with or without previous hysterectomy. Dig Dis Sci 33:1159–1163

69. Stanghellini V, Malageda J, ZXinsmeister A et al (1984) Effect of opiate and adrenergic blockers on the gut motor response to central acting stimuli. Gastroenterology 87:1104

70. Conell AM (1962) The motility of the pelvic colon, II. Paradoxical motility in diarrhea and constipation. Gut 3:342–348

71. MacDonald A, Baxter JN, Finlay IG (1993) Idiopathic slow transit constipation. Br J Surg 80:1107–1111

72. Preston DM, Lennard-Jones JE (1985) Pelvic motility and response to intraluminal bisacodyl in slow transit constipation. Dig Dis Sci 30:289–293

73. Basotti G, Gaburri M, Imbimbo BP et al (1988) Colonic mass movements in idiopathic chronic constipation. Gut 29:1173–1179

74. Ferrara A, Pemberton JH, Grotz RL et al (1994) Prolonged ambulatory recording of anorectal motility in patients with slow transit constipation. Am J Surg 167:73–79

75. Åkervall S, Fasth S, Nordgren S et al (1988) The functional results after colectomy and ileorectal anastomosis for severe constipation (Arbuthnot Lanes's disease) as related to rectal sensory function. Int J Colorect Dis 3:96–101

76. Soffer EE, Metcalfe A, Launspach J (1994) Misoprostol is

effective treatment for patients with severe chronic constipation. Dig Dis Sci 39:929–933

77. Azpiroz F, Malagelada JR (1985) Physiological variations in canine gastric tone measured by an electronic barostat. Am J Physiol 248:G229–237

78. Åkervall S, Fasth S, Nordgren S et al (1989) Rectal reservoir and sensory function studied by graded isobaric distension in normal man. Gut 30:496–502

79. Dent J (1976) A new technique for continous sphincter pressure measurement. Gastroenterology 71:263–267

80. Kerlin P, Zinsmeister A, Phillips S (1983) Motor responses to food of the ileum, proximal colon, and distal colon of healthy humans. Gastroenterology 84:762–770

81. Ritchie JA (1968) Colonic motor activity and bowel function, II. Distribution and incidence of motor activity at rest and after food and carbachol. Gut 9:502–511

82. Ferrara A, Pemberton JH, Hanson RB (1991) Motor response of the sigmoid colon, rectum, and anal canal in health and in patients with slow transit constipation. Gastroenterology 100: A441. Abstract

83. Gregersen H, Sørensen S, Rittig S et al (1991) Measurement of anal cross-sectional area and pressure during anal distension in healthy volunteers. Digestion 48:61–69

84. Åkervall S, Nordgren S, Fasth S et al (1990) The effects of age, gender and parity on recto-anal functions in adults. Scand J Gastroenterol 25:1247–1256

85. Frenckner B, Ihre T (1976) Influence of autonomic nerves on the internal anal sphincter in man. Gut 17:306–312

86. Ferrara A, Pemberton JH, Levin KE et al (1993) Relationship between anal canal tone and rectal motor activity. Dis Colon Rectum 36:337–342

87. Duthie HL, Bennett RC (1963) The relation of sensation in the anal canal to the functional anal sphincter: a possible factor in anal continence. Gut 4:179–182

4

IMMUNOLOGY

Phillip A. Dean
Charles O. Elson

The enormous surface area of the intestinal mucosa makes it the major interface between the host and the environment, and antigenic challenge to the host from this environmental source is massive. This challenge is most intense in the colon, where the number of resident microbial cells alone exceeds the total number of cells in the body.[1] Added to this are antigens from ingested food and nutrient particles, and challenge from invasive or pathogenic infectious agents. The mucosa is responsible for adapting to this challenge by appropriately responding to the need for host defense while maintaining the ability to absorb nutrients and maintain an appropriate enteric flora. To accomplish this a unique system of protective mechanisms has evolved.

Exactly how the mucosal surface of the colon deals with this enormous luminal challenge is unknown, but it clearly involves the combined effects of the epithelial barrier protection, the innate (nonspecific) immune system, and the specialized antigen-specific mucosal immune system found in the gut-associated lymphoid tissue (GALT). The epithelium of the colon provides the first line of defense, and acts as a strong and effective barrier against most organisms and other antigenic macromolecules.[2] When the epithelial barrier is broken down by invading organisms or disease, protection of the host is left to nonspecific and specific inflammatory responses under the coordination of the specific mucosal immune system.[3] This mucosal immune system has evolved under the pressure for a variable response that can be tolerant to the normal array of harmless products of ingestion and digestion and to the wide variety of resident intestinal flora, yet provide for a vigorous local immune and inflammatory response against locally invading pathogens, and contribute to an effective systemic immune response to pathogens that invade through the mucosa (Fig. 4-1). Thus, a critical function of the mucosal immune system is to balance protective, but potentially destructive immune responses toward pathogenic organisms with a tolerant response toward normal enteric flora and food antigens in order to maintain normal mucosal homeostasis.

This complex and highly regulated mucosal immune response will be the focus of this chapter. Individual components and compartments of the mucosal immune system will be considered separately, although in reality they represent a dynamic and integrated system of host defense with the flexibility for adaptation and regulation at many points. The purpose of this chapter is to provide a framework for understanding the mucosal immune system as a basis for continued advances into the understanding and treatment of diseases such as ulcerative colitis and Crohn's disease, which are intimately linked to the mucosal immune system.

MUCOSAL IMMUNE COMPONENTS

An effective immune response depends on the ability to discriminate between endogenous "self" proteins and foreign or "nonself" proteins, referred to as antigens. For initiation of the immune response, exogenous antigen is typically endocytosed as a large particle or whole infectious organism by professional antigen-presenting cells (APCs) such as monocytes, macrophages, and dendritic cells.[4,5] Antigen is then internally processed within endosomes into small peptide fragments that fit into the peptide-binding groove on a major histocompatability complex (MHC) class II molecule and transported to the cell surface. Antigens expressed as endogenous proteins are processed through a similar mechanism but bind to MHC class I molecules for delivery to the cell surface.[6] The intestine is populated with a variety of potential APCs, including "professional" APCs such as macrophages and dendritic cells as well as less traditional APCs such as epithelial and endothelial cells.[7] This variety of APCs enhance the ability of the mucosa to generate a number of specific immune responses against the variety of different antigens to which it is exposed.

Effector cells central to the mucosal immune response are

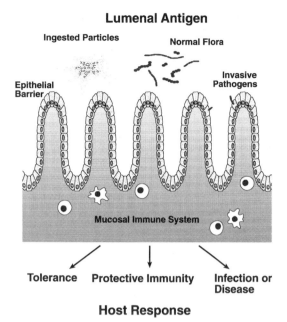

Host Response

Figure 4-1. Protective challenge of the mucosal immune barrier. The colonic mucosa is continuously exposed to a massive antigenic load and has developed unique protective mechanisms capable of preventing infection and injury from potential pathogenic organisms and toxins, yet permitting immunologic tolerance against the variety of food antigens and commensal bacteria of the normal colonic flora. This complicated mucosal immune system is dependent on an intact epithelial barrier and a highly regulated innate and acquired immune response. Disruption of this balance can result in acute or chronic inflammation and may be involved in the pathogenesis of inflammatory bowel disease.

the T and B lymphocytes. Both cells originate in the bone marrow, and while B cells can migrate directly to the mucosa, the majority of T cells undergo thymic education to eliminate self-reactive T cells and then migrate to the mucosa. T-cell receptors (TCRs) are incapable of recognizing antigen free in solution, but recognize the complex of peptide antigen associated with a MHC molecule.[8] The majority of T cells express either CD4 or CD8 surface markers in association with the TCR. CD4 + T cells recognize antigen presented by MHC class II, and therefore respond to exogenous foreign antigen. They produce a unique pattern of cytokines that regulates the immune response. CD8 + T cells, on the other hand, recognize antigen in the context of MHC class I and therefore respond to endogenously produced foreign antigen such as viral proteins.[9] These CD8 + T cells may in some situations serve a regulatory function, but their major role is cytolysis.

Cytokines produced by regulatory T cells and macrophages induce B cells to mature into antibody-producing plasma cells. In contrast to systemic lymphoid tissue, where immunoglobulin G (IgG) and IgM are predominant, the hallmark of mucosal immunity is unique mechanisms that allow mucosal B cells to differentiate into plasma cells producing primarily IgA.[10] IgA is the predominant immunoglobulin produced in the mucosa,[11] and has a variety of functions at mucosal surfaces, including the ability to limit absorption of protein antigens, inhibit the attachment of bacteria, and neutralize a broad spectrum of vi-

ruses.[12] This antibody provides the first antigen-specific line of defense in colonic mucosa, and provides a major mechanism for controlling potentially harmful environmental agents.

Over 25% of the cells in the intestine are lymphoid cells, and approximately 80% of the immunoglobulin-producing cells are in the gut, making it the major lymphoid organ.[11] The mucosal immune system is a highly organized yet flexible arrangement of several interconnecting compartments with specific functions (Fig. 4-2). Peyer's patches and isolated lymphoid follicles in the submucosa of the intestine serve as a primary site for induction of mucosal immune responses. Lymphocytes stimulated by antigen leave the Peyer's patches via draining lymphatics and travel through mesenteric lymph nodes, eventually entering the systemic circulation through the thoracic duct. Lymphocytes activated in the mucosa preferentially recirculate to mucosal sites, including the breast, lacrimal glands, salivary glands, bronchial and genitourinary mucosa as well as the intestinal mucosa, suggesting a common cross-protective mucosal immune system.[13] Thus, lamina propria and intraepithelial lymphocytes, and lamina propria plasma cells appear to be derived from lymphocytes exposed to antigen in lymphoid follicles or Peyer's patches.[14,15] The unique interactions that occur within each compartment of this system provide for regulation of the mucosal immune response, and will be discussed in detail.

INDUCTION SITES: LYMPHOID FOLLICLES AND PEYER'S PATCHES

Organized lymphoid aggregates specialized for the uptake and presentation of antigens occur throughout the human gastrointestinal tract.[16] These single lymphoid follicles or groups of lymphoid follicles, termed *Peyer's patches*, occur with increasing frequency in the terminal ileum and the colon.[17] Unlike peripheral lymph nodes, there are no afferent lymphatics in these mucosal follicles. Instead, antigen enters the follicle through a specialized epithelium, follicle-associated epithelium (FAE), which is characterized by a lack of goblet cells and the presence of the unique M, or membrane cell (see Fig. 4-2).[7]

M Cells

M cells of the FAE are specialized for transepithelial transport of particles from the gut lumen into the follicle. A unique feature of M cells is the lack of polymeric IgA receptors on the basolateral surface, suggesting that unlike other epithelial cells, the M cell does not secrete IgA into the lumen.[18] The luminal surface of the M cell is particularly suited for uptake and transport of particulates.[19] They lack a brush border as seen on typical gut epithelial cells, and express large endocytic domains for invagination. Macromolecules and particles adherent to the luminal surface are taken up and transported rapidly and efficiently into a pocket underlying the M cell.[7] A variety of pathogenic organisms exploit this route to rapidly cross the epithelial barrier and infect the mucosa or spread systemically.[20,21] Although MHC class II can be demonstrated on the M-cell membrane, whether the M cell actively presents antigen or simply functions as a portal of antigen entry into the follicle is unknown.[22]

Specific populations of both T and B lymphocytes are present within the M-cell pocket in humans.[23] T cells are primarily CD4 + (in contrast to normal intraepithelial lymphocyte popu-

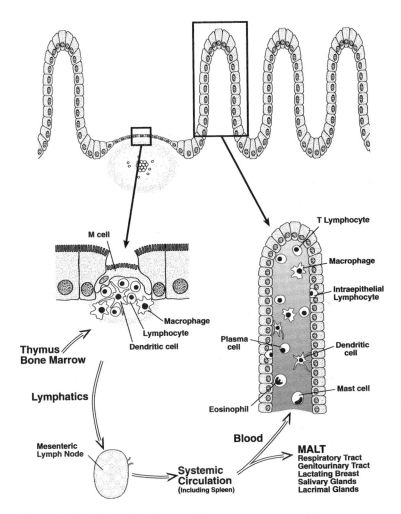

Figure 4-2. Schematic diagram of the common mucosal immune response elements in humans. Lymphoid cells arrive from the bone marrow (B cells) or thymus (T cells) via the systemic circulation and enter isolated lymphoid follicles or Peyer's patches. Lumenal antigen enters these organized lymphoid structures through specialized epithelium containing M cells, and is presented to lymphocytes by a variety of accessory cells. These activated lymphocytes leave the follicle via the mesenteric lymphatics and enter the systemic circulation, where they have a tendency to selectively migrate back to the lamina propria of the gastrointestinal tract and to other common mucosal associated lymphoid tissue (MALT) effector sites. These antigen-primed B (plasma cells) and T lymphocytes are primed for a widespread antigen-specific mucosal immune response at many mucosal surfaces.

lation, which is primarily CD8 +), and express surface markers characteristic of memory cells. B cells, on the other hand, are primarily naive precursor B cells similar to those in the underlying follicle. An extensive network of macrophages and dendritic cells is also intimately associated with the M-cell pocket, and can serve as professional APCs for the transcytosed antigen particles.[24] Particles taken up from the lumen can be identified within these macrophages, and it is likely that such antigens are processed and presented both within the mucosal follicles and within draining mesenteric lymph nodes. Dendritic cells also appear near this M-cell pocket, and are particularly effective at presenting oral antigens to naive Peyer's patch T cells.[25]

M cells are derived from the same crypt epithelial stem cell as other epithelial cell types. These M cells differentiate from other epithelial cells in the region of an underlying lymphoid follicle.[18,26] The stimulus for differentiation of M cells, however, is unclear. The fact that stem cells on the follicle side of a crypt develop into M cells, while those on the opposite side of the same crypt become standard columnar epithelial cells, suggests that factors associated with the underlying follicle lead to this differentiation.[26] The presence of T and B lymphocytes is clearly required for development of M cells over a follicle,[27] but normal lumenal bacterial flora also appears to play a role.[28] These findings suggest that gut epithelial cells can differentiate along different pathways due to signals from the underlying mucosal immune system.

Lymphoid Follicles

Lymphoid follicles and Peyer's patches contain all the cells required for immune induction: B cells, T cells, and APCs. These lymphocytes leave the systemic circulation through the postcapillary high-endothelial venules (HEVs) through a selective homing process,[29] and segregate into distinct B-cell and T-cell zones in the Peyer's patch.[30] In Peyer's patches, B cells predominate in the lymphoid follicles, whereas T cells are found primarily in the interfollicular regions and beneath the FAE.[30] Macrophages and dendritic cells are scattered both beneath the FAE and throughout the follicles.[7]

B cells make up the majority of lymphocytes in these follicles (60 to 70% of total cells), with approximately 20% of the cells being T cells.[31] IgA is the major immunoglobulin produced at mucosal sites, and Peyer's patch lymphocytes are enriched for IgA B-cell precursors relative to other lymphoid tissues.[32] Both CD4+ and CD8+ T cell subsets are found in the interfollicular regions.[30] Although T cells make up only a small percentage of the population they appear to be critical for Peyer's patch function[31] and M-cell differentiation.[27] A unique feature of the Peyer's patch and mucosal lymphoid follicles is that many of the B and T cells are precursor cells rather than functional effector cells. These precursor cells are presumed to leave the follicle after antigen exposure and migrate to effector sites in the gut or other mucosal sites where they differentiate into functional effector cells (Fig. 4-2).

MUCOSAL LYMPHOCYTE MIGRATION

As in other lymphoid tissue, mature lymphocytes in the mucosal immune system continuously recirculate through blood and tissue in a pattern that is not random, but highly regulated by a series of endothelial cell-lymphocyte interactions mediated by adhesion molecules.[33] The expression of adhesion molecules on the surface of both lymphocytes and endothelial cells in a reciprocal receptor-ligand relationship is tightly regulated to signal the circulating lymphocytes to adhere to the endothelial surface and leave the blood vessel at specific sites in a multistep process regulated by the local environment.[34] Most of these adhesion interactions occur on postcapillary high endothelial venules where constitutive or inducible expression of endothelial cell adhesion molecules is a dynamic process regulated by cytokines and other environmental factors.[35–37] Expression of adhesion molecules on lymphocytes is dependent on cell type, but can also depend on their activation state, which further facilitates selective targeting of lymphocyte subsets to tissue sites.[38] Lymphocyte adhesion molecules and their respective endothelial cell ligands important for recirculation to the gut include LFA-1/ICAM-1 and ICAM-2, L-selectin/MAdCAM-1, $\alpha_4\beta_7$ MAdCAM-1, and CD44/VAP-1.[33]

Lymphocytes leave the mucosal follicle via efferent lymphatic ducts to mesenteric lymph nodes, but the recirculation pattern from there is variable depending on the lymphocyte population. Naive lymphocytes (which have not recognized antigen) continue to recirculate through the thoracic duct and blood to secondary lymphoid tissues such as lymph nodes, Peyer's patches, spleen, and tonsils until they recognize antigen or die.[33] Antigen-primed lymphocytes are capable of recirculating through extralymphoid effector sites including not only the gut

lamina propria but other common mucosal immune system sites such as the breast, pulmonary interstitium, and reproductive tract (see Fig. 4-2).

Central to this theme of a common mucosal immune system is that lymphocytes can preferentially recirculate between different mucosal tissues.[13] Activated IgA precursors in the mesenteric lymph node can migrate to the lamina propria or to the lactating mammary gland as antibody-producing plasma cells.[39] The latter route is an important mechanism for providing specific IgA antibodies in mother's milk to protect the infant against microbial organisms with which the mother is colonized.[40] These tissue-selective recirculation mechanisms provide a means of focusing antigen-primed effector lymphocytes to the mucosal surface where exposure to a particular antigen is most likely. It also allows exposure at one mucosal site to extend immunity to other mucosal sites, which is important for regulation of host response to the environment and can be exploited for the development of effective mucosal vaccines.

MUCOSAL LYMPHOCYTES

The colon mucosa is a rich collection of B cells, plasma cells, T cells, and macrophages along with occasional eosinophils, mast cells, and dendritic cells within a complex vascular and lymphatic-rich stroma (Fig. 4-2). The majority of lymphocytes are located beneath the basement membrane of the epithelium, but a significant number are within the epithelium. The latter are referred to as intraepithelial lymphocytes (IELs).

B/Plasma Cells

The intestinal lamina propria is the only site in the body where large numbers of plasma cells are constitutively present. Up to 40% of cells isolated from the lamina propria are of B-cell lineage.[41] The majority of these antibody-producing cells secrete IgA (70 to 90%), though IgM and IgG are produced by 5 to 10% of plasma cells each.[11] IgE and IgD-producing plasma cells are rare or absent. Whereas the upper gastrointestinal tract and small bowel produce predominantly IgA1, IgA2 is the predominant isotype produced in the colon and rectum.[42] These plasma cells are terminally differentiated and non-replicating, with an estimated half-life of 5 days, suggesting that there is continuous repopulation of the lamina propria with B cells. Peyer's patch B cells are a prime source of IgA-producing plasma cells in the lamina propria[43] in a cycle that may require as little as 3 days to complete.[44]

Lamina Propria T Cells

The majority of lymphocytes in the lamina propria display the CD3/TCR complex characteristic of T cells.[45] These T cells differ in a number of functional and phenotypic characteristics from circulating blood T cells as summarized in Table 4-1. As in circulation, approximately two-thirds of lamina propria T cells are CD4+, with one-third CD8+. Unlike circulating lymphocytes, however, lamina propria T cells express a memory phenotype (high CD45RO) and markers of T-cell activation (IL-2Rα, MHC class II, HML-1) suggesting that these cells have been exposed to antigen and are functionally active.[46–48]

Functionally these lamina propria T cells are distinctively

Table 4-1. Phenotypic and Fucntional Differences Between Circulating and Mucosal T Lymphocytes

	Lamina Propria	Circulation
Surface Markers		
CD4+/CD8+	2/1	2/1
Memory	High	Low
Activation	High	Low
Function		
Proliferation—CD3/TCR	Low	High
Proliferation—CD2, CD28	High	Low
Cytokine production	High	Low

different than the circulating T-cell pool. T cells from the lamina propria have a diminished proliferative response to conventional stimulation through the CD3/TCR complex, but respond well to stimulation via CD2 or CD28.[49,50] This property appears to be mediated by factors in the local mucosal environment,[51] and may represent an important local regulatory mechanism for the activated T cells. Upon activation, lamina propria T cells also produce higher levels of cytokines such as IL-2, IL-4, IL-5, TNF-α and IFN-γ, particularly with stimulation via CD2 or CD28, which is consistent with the predominant helper role of these T cells in the local immune response.[51,52] Cytotoxic T-cell function is also present in the lamina propria.[53] The overwhelming evidence suggests that lamina propria T cells, through a variety of regulatory mechanisms, are responsible for primary control of the immune response to antigens from the colonic lumen.[54]

Intraepithelial Lymphocytes

Intraepithelial lymphocytes (IELs), a unique subset of mucosal lymphocytes, reside entirely above the basement membrane, between columnar epithelial cells of the villi. Most IELs express the CD3/TCR complex, and while most are CD8+, some are CD4+, CD8+/CD4+, or even CD8−/CD4−.[55] Though most IELs in humans are CD8+ and have an α/β-type TCR, 5 to 10% express the γ/δ TCR. Significant differences between small and large bowel IEL have been identified,[56] with a higher percentage of CD4+ IEL in human colon.[57] IEL demonstrate increased activation and memory markers similar to other mucosal lymphocytes.[58,59] They also respond poorly to activation through the CD3/TCR complex, but activate well with stimulation through CD2.[60]

The location of IELs make these lymphocytes the first cellular mucosal defense against luminal antigen, which has generated much interest in the function of this population, though their exact role in mucosal immunity remains obscure. Unlike most peripheral T cells, certain IEL subsets develop independent from the thymus,[61] and in some cases do not respond to antigens presented through traditional MHC molecules,[62] suggesting that they may respond to nontraditional antigens. Although γ/δ TCR IELs are found in germ-free mice, indicating that bacterial antigens and mitogens are not required for their development and maturation,[63] α/β TCR IELs are greatly reduced in germ-free mice and do not express activation markers, suggesting that this T-cell subset is activated in response to the

intestinal flora.[59] IELs have strong cytolytic activity in vitro, which may be important in host defense against some pathogens, or could be involved in removing senescent, injured, or infected epithelial cells.

REGULATION OF THE MUCOSAL IMMUNE RESPONSE

The mucosal immune system in the colon is constantly challenged with an enormous number of antigens from the lumen, and forced to differentiate between "helpful" food particles, innocuous commensal bacteria, or "harmful" invasive or pathogenic organisms (Fig. 4-1). Though the epithelial barrier, including mucus and the IgA coat prevent the majority of luminal antigens from exposure to the subepithelial mucosal immune system, penetration by even a small fraction of these antigens could provide constant stimulation for a potential immune response. To protect against the development of an inappropriately aggressive or damaging response to "helpful" antigens, yet respond with swift destruction to eliminate "harmful" invasive pathogens and toxins, a variety of complex regulatory mechanisms are present within the mucosal immune system to balance the response.

T lymphocytes orchestrate the acquired immune response to this wide variety of helpful or harmful agents.[3] The crucial role for T cells in mucosal immune regulation in the colon can be seen in a number of experimental models of colitis,[64] in which disruption of normal T-cell regulatory processes has resulted in an inappropriate and damaging chronic inflammation in the colon.[54] These various models have helped to elucidate a number of local mechanisms critical to normal mucosal immune regulation.

Initial activation of the acquired antigen-specific immune system occurs when peptide antigen complexed with an MHC molecule on the surface of an APC binds TCR on a T cell (Fig. 4-3). The type of APC can be a crucial determinant of the magnitude of an immune response.[5] Dendritic cells are the most potent APCs for T cells[65] and are present both in the Peyer's patches and lamina propria of the intestine,[7,66] though macrophages are also effective, and are active scavengers in the mucosa. A number of other factors, including amount of antigen and avidity for the TCR, the local environment, timing of antigen presentation, and the presence and character of a required "second signal" or costimulation of the T cell by APC are critical for determining the initial response of triggered T cells.[67] Local mucosal factors also influence the type of initial T-cell response, where continuous and dynamic antigen exposure alters some of the normal TCR-mediated activation pathways.[68,69]

Following initial activation (primary response), T cells mature into effector cells along a number of different pathways, leading to distinct immunologic outcomes (Fig. 4-3). This is particularly evident with CD4+ T cells, which differentiate into specialized patterns of response after prolonged stimulation.[70] As mentioned previously, the particular pattern of T-helper (T_h) response is determined at the time of primary T-cell activation and is dependent on the APC, the mucosal environment, and the nature of the antigen. For example, IL-12 production by macrophage APCs at the time of antigen presentation favors a $T_h 1$ response.[71] $T_h 1$ responses lead primarily

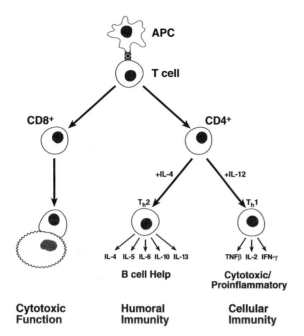

Figure 4-3. T-cell differentiation pathways in control of the mucosal immune response. Antigens are presented to T cells by MHC class I or II molecules on APCs. Recognition of antigen by the T-cell receptor leads to activation of the T cell. CD8 + T cells recognize antigen presented by MHC class I molecules, and are primarily involved in cytolysis of damaged or infected cells. CD4 + T cells recognize antigen presented by MHC class II and tend to differentiate into T_h1, T_h2, or a combination of T_h cells depending on the cytokine milieu of the local environment during antigen stimulation (particularly IL-4 and IL-12). These T_h subsets are distinguished by their production of characteristic cytokine patterns as shown. T_h2 cells primarily provide help for humoral (antibody) immunity, and are particularly important in allergic and antiparasitic immune responses. T_h1 cells mediate classic delayed-type hypersensitivity responses, and are particularly effective against intracellular pathogens.

to macrophage phagocytosis and cytotoxic responses, and are characterized by the production of IFN-γ and TNFα in addition to IL-2. They are often associated with an aggressive cellular response and tissue damage. T_h2 responses, on the other hand, are mediated primarily by IL-4, IL-5, IL-6, IL-10, and IL-13, which collectively mediate the growth and activation of mast cells and eosinophils, and promote B-cell maturation and immunoglobulin production. These two types of T_h response regulate one another, with IFN-γ acting to inhibit a T_h2 and promote T_h1 responses, and IL-4 promoting a T_h2 response coupled with IL-10 inhibition T_h1 responses. In humans, the exact role of each of these responses is unclear, and overlap between T_h1 and T_h2 cell types is common; but this framework provides a convenient mechanism for understanding the complex cross-regulation involved in local immune response. Establishing the proper balance between T_h1 and T_h2 responses is likely to be important for balancing the protective mucosal host defense against pathogens with a more permissive response to food antigens and endogenous flora.[54]

The enteric nervous system may contribute to the local mucosal environment, which plays such a critical role in defining the pattern and type of immune response generated. The lamina propria is richly innervated, with neural elements in close proximity to lymphocytes throughout the lamina propria.[72] Lymphoid cells have receptors for the major neuropeptides of the enteric nervous system, including VIP, substance P, and somatostatin,[73] and each are capable of affecting lymphocyte function in vitro. The regulatory role for these peptides in vivo has yet to be defined, but is likely to be important for coordination of local stimuli and immune response.

Exposure to antigens by oral feeding generally induces little or no detectable systemic or mucosal immune response and induces a state of systemic unresponsiveness to subsequent parenteral immunization known as oral tolerance.[74] Oral tolerance is likely to be crucial in preventing a massive immune and inflammatory response to the enormous dietary and endogenous flora antigen load in the colon. For example, oral tolerance is nearly complete for most dietary antigens, but the extent tolerance to complex bacterial and viral antigens may vary depending on the route of antigen presentation.[71] A number of different mechanisms for oral tolerance have been demonstrated, but the role for each in human mucosal immune responses remains unclear. Oral tolerance in humans can be demonstrated for T cells but not B cells after oral antigen feeding.[75] One mechanism for development of oral tolerance is clonal anergy, or lack of responsiveness to TCR stimulation with antigen.[76] Suppression of T- or B-cell responses may also be important, and CD8 + suppresser cells can be demonstrated in the mucosal immune system.[77] Suppression of T-cell responses, which appears to be most effective for T_h1 responses, is dependent on cytokines such as TGF-β and IL-4.[77–79] Other mechanisms such as deletion of antigen-specific T-cell clones may also be important, but have not been systematically evaluated. Similarly, factors that determine whether tolerance or effective immunity occurs after exposure to endogenous antigens of the bacterial flora remain to be identified, though such regulation may play a central role in mucosal immune diseases such as inflammatory bowel disease.[80] These mechanisms of mucosal immune regulation are critical for understanding intestinal disease as well as the design and implementation of mucosal vaccines, and represent an area of active basic and clinical research.

SECRETORY IgA-MUCOSAL IMMUNE DEFENSE

The primary product of the antigen-specific mucosal immune system is the continuous secretion of IgA onto the external surface. This secretory IgA is the end result of a number of complex molecular and cellular interactions that begin with recognition of foreign antigen in the Peyer's patch, continue with production of a specific, protective IgA by lamina propria plasma cells, and end with the transport of secretory IgA through epithelial cells into the intestinal lumen, where these antibodies bind and neutralize foreign antigen, including toxins and viral and bacterial antigens (see Fig. 4-2).[81] As previously mentioned, IgA is produced in two subclasses in humans IgA1 and IgA2. IgA2 production predominates in the colon and rectum, which is significant for host defense against enteric pathogens because IgA1 but not IgA2 is susceptible to degradation by bacterial IgA proteases, which may limit appropriate biologic function.[42]

Differentiation of B lymphocytes into plasma cells occurs

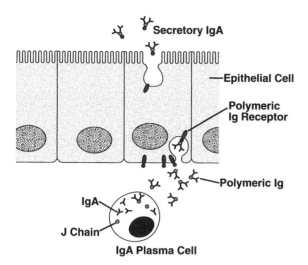

Figure 4-4. Secretory IgA is the combined product of plasma cells and mucosal epithelial cells. Lamina propria plasma cells produce primarily dimeric IgA, which is covalently bound to the J chain within the plasma cell. Dimeric or polymeric IgA secreted into the lamina propria is bound by polymeric Ig receptors on the basolateral membrane of epithelial cells, endocytosed, and transported to the apical membrane, where the polymeric Ig receptor is cleaved, releasing secretory IgA into the intestinal lumen.

under the influence of IL-5, IL-6, IL-10, and TGF-β derived from both T_h2 CD4+ T cells and epithelial cells.[82] Plasma cells in the lamina propria produce IgA in its polymeric form (Fig. 4-4), with individual IgA molecules linked by the glycoprotein J chain within the plasma cell prior to secretion into the stroma.[83] Dimeric or tetrameric IgA is capable of binding to the polymeric immunoglobulin receptor/secretory component on the basolateral surface of columnar epithelial cells, which transports the IgA into endocytic vesicles.[84] After transport to the apical (luminal) membrane, the polymeric receptor is cleaved, releasing IgA into the lumen with a portion of the polymeric immunoglobulin receptor attached. This molecule is known as secretory IgA.[85] Expression of both J-chain and polymeric immunoglobulin receptor/secretory component is regulated by local production of IL-2, IL-4, IL-5, and IL-6, as well as T_h1 cytokines IFN-γ and TNF-α.[83] While similar pathways for IgA secretion are found in other mucosal sites such as salivary glands, liver/biliary tract, and lactating breast, IgA synthesis in the gastrointestinal tract predominates, and is the major front-line immune response against lumenal antigen.[81]

MUCOSAL IMMUNE FUNCTION AND GASTROINTESTINAL DISEASE

As evidence of complexity in mucosal immune responses accumulates, the importance of appropriate regulation in maintaining mucosal homeostasis is becoming clear. Any alteration in the mucosal immune defense mechanisms tends to result in either decreased protective immunity or damaging immune hy-

perreactivity. Deficiencies in IgA or other immunoglobulins, accessory immune cells, or T cells impair the host response to pathogens and result in clinical disease characterized by increased bacterial, viral, or parasitic infections, demonstrating the crucial role of the mucosal immune response in protection from enteric pathogens.[86]

Regulation of appropriate balance in the mucosal T-cell response is particularly important in maintaining homeostasis. With application of molecular biology tools to selectively disrupt a number of immunoregulatory pathways, chronic colitis has developed in experimental animals when critical control mechanisms for the immune response are altered.[87] Alteration of T-cell regulation by disruption of normal T-cell populations, T-cell development, or T-cell regulatory cytokines leads to the development of colitis.[54] It appears that there are distinct populations of T cells in normal animals that are capable of either inducing or suppressing the development of chronic inflammation in the colon if normal regulatory mechanisms are disrupted.[88] Increasing evidence suggests that chronic colonic inflammation is due to a dysregulated response to normal enteric flora,[54,80,89] emphasizing the importance of mucosal immune regulation in response to resident colonic bacteria.

These pathologic conditions demonstrate the importance of the mucosal immune response in the host's interaction with gut luminal antigens. Appropriate mucosal protection involves an intimate interaction between the epithelial barrier, innate immune mechanisms, and a highly regulated antigen-specific immune response. When well orchestrated, this system provides constant protection from invading enteric pathogens, while avoiding a deleterious immune response to the massive antigenic challenge from ingested antigens and resident enteric flora. Disruption in regulatory mechanisms that control the host immune response to enteric antigens may be significant in the pathogenesis of inflammatory bowel disease and a number of enteric infections. Understanding differential response mechanisms of the mucosal immune system may allow for manipulation of intestinal and/or systemic immune responses by enteric antigen administration in the future. This ability to manipulate

---

Mucosal Immune Components Important in Gastrointestinal Disease

Infection

Secretory IgA deficiency
Eosinophil deficiency
Mast cell deficiency
Common variable immunodeficiency
CD4+ T-cell deficiency (AIDS)
Mucosal barrier breakdown

Chronic Inflammation

Mucosal barrier breakdown
IL-2
IL-10
TGF-β
T-cell selection/maturation disruption
CD4+ T-cell dysregulation

the immune response has important implications for vaccine development and disease prevention, and for therapy of allergic, autoimmune, neoplastic, and inflammatory diseases in the colon and elsewhere. A priority for the future is to define the molecular and cellular mechanisms underlying this complex mucosal immune regulation.

References

1. Savage DC (1977) Microbial ecology of the gastrointestinal tract. Annu Rev Microbiol 31:107–121
2. Sanderson IR, Walker WA (1994) Mucosal barrier. pp. 41–51. In Orga PL, Mestecky J, Lamm ME et al (eds): Handbook of Mucosal Immunology, Academic Press, San Diego
3. Fearon DT, Locksley RM (1996) The instructive role of innate immunity in the acquired immune response. Science 272:50–54
4. Unanue ER, Allen PM (1987) The basis for the immunoregulatory role of macrophages and other accessory cells. Science 236:551–557
5. Constant S, Sant'Angelo D, Pasqualini T et al (1995) Peptide and protein antigens require distinct antigen-presenting cell subsets for the priming of CD4+ T cells. J Immunol 154:4915–4923
6. Neefjes JJ, Momberg F (1993) Cell biology of antigen presentation. Curr Opin Immunol 5:27–34
7. Neutra MR, Pringault E, Kraehenbuhl J (1996) Antigen sampling across epithelial barriers and induction of mucosal immune responses. Annu Rev Immunol 14:275–300
8. Schwartz RH (1985) T lymphocyte recognition of antigen in association with gene products of the major histocompatibility complex. Ann Rev Immunol 3:237–261
9. Engleman EG, Benike CJ, Grumet FC, Evans RL (1981) Activation of human T lymphocyte subsets: helper and suppressor/cytotoxic T cells recognize and respond to distinct histocompatibility antigens. J Immunol 127:2124–2130
10. Strober W, Harriman GR (1991) The regulation of IgA B cell differentiation. Gastroenterology Clin North Am 20:473–94
11. Brandtzaeg P (1994) Distribution and characteristics of mucosal immunoglobulin-producing cells. pp. 251–26 In Orga PL, Mestecky J, Lamm ME et al (eds): Handbook of Mucosal Immunology, Academic Press, San Diego
12. Kilian M, Mestecky J, Russell MW (1988) Defense mechanisms involving Fc-dependent functions of immunoglobulin A proteases. Microbiol Rev 52:296–303
13. Phillips-Quaggliata JM, Lamm ME (1994) Lymphocyte homing to mucosal effector sites. pp. 225–234. In Orga PL, Mestecky J, Lamm ME et al (eds): Handbook of Mucosal Immunology, Academic Press, San Diego
14. Craig SW, Cebra JJ (1971) Peyer's patches: an enriched source of precursors for IgA-producing immunocytes in the rabbit. J Exp Med 134:188–200
15. Guy-Grand D, Griscelli C, Vassalli P (1978) The mouse gut T lymphocyte, a novel type of T cell. Nature, origin, and traffic in mice in normal and graft-versus-host conditions. J Exp Med 148:1661–1667
16. Owen RL, Ermak TH (1992) Structural specializations for antigen uptake and processing in the digestive tract. Springer Semin Immunopathol 12:139–152
17. Langman JM, Rowland R (1986) The number and distribution of lymphoid follicles in the human large intestine. J Anat 194:189–194
18. Pappo J, Owen RL (1988) Absence of secretory component expression by epithelial cells overlying rabbit gut-associated lymphoid tissue. Gastroenterology 95:1173–1177
19. Ermak TH, Dougherty EP, Bhagat HR et al (1995) Uptake and transport of copolymer biodegradable microspheres by rabbit Peyer's patch M cells. Cell Tissue Res 279:433–436
20. Owen RL (1983) And now pathophysiology of M cells: good news and bad news from Peyer's patches. Gastroenterology 85:468–470
21. Jones BL, Pascopella L, Falkow S (1995) Entry of microbes into the host: using M cells to break the mucosal barrier. Curr Opin Immunol 7:474–478
22. Allan CH, Mendrick DL, Trier JS (1993) Rat intestinal M cells contain acidic endosomal-lysosomal compartments and express class II major histocompatibility complex determinants. Gastroenterology 104:698–708
23. Farstad IN, Halstensen TS, Fausa O Brandtzaeg P (1994) Heterogeneity of M cell-associated B and T cells in human Peyer's patches. Immunology 83:457–464
24. Spaulding DM, Koopman WJ, Eldridge JH et al (1983) Accessory cells in murine Peyer's patch, I. Identification and enrichment of a functional dendritic cell. J Exp Med 157:1646–1659
25. Kelsall BL, Strober W (1996) Distinct populations of dendritic cells are present in the subepithelial dome and T cell regions of the murine Peyer's patch. J Exp Med 183:237–247
26. Bye WA, Allan CH, Trier JS (1984) Structure, distribution and origin of M cells in Peyer's patches of mouse ileum. Gastroenterology 86:789–801
27. Savidge TC, Smith MW (1995) Evidence that membranous (M) cell genesis is immunoregulated. pp. 239–241. In Mestecky J (ed); Advances in Mucosal Immunology, Plenum, New York
28. Smith MW, James PS, Tivey DR (1987) M cell numbers increase after transfer of SPF mice to a normal animal house environment. Am J Pathol 128:385–389
29. Bargatze RF, Jutila MA, Butcher EC (1995) Distinct roles of L-selectin and integrins alpha-4-beta-7 and LFA-1 in lymphocyte homing to Peyer's patch-HEV in situ: the multistep model confirmed and refined. Immunity 3:99–108
30. Miura SY, Tsuzuki Y, Fukumura D et al (1995) Intravital demonstration of sequential migration process of lymphocyte subpopulations in rat Peyer's patches. Gastroenterology 109:1113–1123
31. Guy-Grand D, Griscelli C, Vassalli P (1975) Peyer's patches, but IgA plasma cells and thymic function: study in nude mice bearing thymic grafts. J Immunol 115:361–364
32. Tseng J (1981) Transfer of lymphocytes of Peyer's patches between immunoglobulin allotype congenic mice: repopulation of the IgA plasma cells in the gut lamina propria. J Immunol 127:2039
33. Butcher EC, Picker LJ (1996) Lymphocyte homing and homeostasis. Science 272:60–66
34. Springer TA (1994) Traffic signals for lymphocyte recircula-

tion and leukocyte emigration: the multistep paradigm. Cell 79:301–314

35. Dean PA, Ramsey PS, Donohue JH, Nelson H (1994) Microvascular expression of MALA-2 correlates with in vivo lymphocytes trafficking and is preferentially enhanced in tumors by tumor necrosis factor-α and interleukin-1α. Int J Cancer 59:1–7

36. Girard JP, Springer TA (1995) High endothelial venules (HEV): specialized endothelium for lymphocyte imigration. Immunol Today 16:449–457

37. Haraldsen G, Kvale D, Lein B et al (1996) Cytokine-regulated expression of E-selectin, intercellular adhesion molecule-1, and vascular cell adhesion molecule-1 in human intestinal microvascular endothelial cells. J Immunol 156:2558–2565

38. Picker LJ (1994) Control of lymphocyte homing. Curr Opin Immunol 6:394–406

39. Croitoru K, Bienenstock J (1994) Characteristics and functions of mucosa-associated lymphoid tissue. pp. 141–149 In Orga PL, Mestecky J, Lamm ME, et al (eds): Handbook of Mucosal Immunology, Academic Press, San Diego

40. Goldblum RM, Ahlstedt S, Carlson B (1975) Antibody forming cells in human colostrum after oral immunization. Nature 257: 797–799

41. Bull DM, Bookman MA (1979) Isolation and functional characterization of human intestinal mucosal lymphoid cells. J Clin Invest 59:966–974

42. Kett K, Brandtzaeg P, Radl J, Haaijman JF (1986) Different subclass distribution of IgA-producing cells in human lymphoid organs and various secretory tissues. J Immunol 136: 3631–3635

43. Hilbert DM, Anderson AO, Holmes KL, Rudikoff S (1994) Long-term lymphoid reconstitution of SCID mice suggests self-renewing B and T cell populations in peripheral and mucosal tissues. Transplantation 58:466–475

44. Kramer DR, Cebra JJ (1995) Role of maternal antibody in the induction of virus specific and bystander IgA responses in Peyer's patches of suckling mice. Immunology 7:911–918

45. Goodacre R, Davidson R, Singal D, Bienenstock J (1979) Morphologic and functional characteristics of human intestinal lymphoid cells isolated by a mechanical technique. Gastroenterology 76:300–308

46. Schieferdecker HL, Ullrich R, Weiss Breckwoldt AN et al (1991) The HML-1 antigen of intestinal lymphocytes is an activation antigen. J Immunol 144:2541–3549

47. Zeitz M, Schieferdecker HL, Ullrich R et al (1991) Phenotype and function of lamina propria T lymphocytes. Immunol Res 10:199–206

48. De Maria R, Fais S, Silvestri M et al (1993) Continuous in vivo activation and transient hyporesponsiveness to TcR/CD3 triggering of human gut lamina propria lymphocytes. Eur J Immunol 23:3204–3208

49. Pirzer UC, Schurmann G, Post S et al (1990) Differential responsiveness to CD3-Ti vs. CD2-dependent activation of human intestinal T lymphocytes. Eur J Immunol 20: 2339–2342

50. Qiao L, Schurmann G, Betzler M, Meuer S C (1991) Activation and signaling status of human lamina propria T lymphocytes. Gastroenterology 101:1529–1536

51. Targan SR, Deem RL, Liu M et al (1995) Definition of a lamina propria T cell responsive state. J Immunol 154:664–675

52. Zeitz M, Quinn TC, Graeff AS, James SP (1988) Mucosal T cells provide helper function but do not proliferate when stimulated by specific antigen in lymphogranuloma venereum proctitis in nonhuman primates. Gastroenterology 94:353–366

53. Shanahan F, Brogen M, Targan S (1987) Human mucosal cytotoxic effector cells. Gastroenterology 92:1951–1957

54. Powrie F (1995) T cells in inflammatory bowel disease: protective and pathogenic roles. Immunity 3:171–174

55. Jarry A, Cerf-Bensussan N, Brousse N et al (1990) Subsets of CD3+ (T cell receptor α/β or γ/δ) and CD3- lymphocytes isolated from normal human gut epithelium display phenotypical features different from their counterparts in peripheral blood. Eur J Immunol 20:1097–1103

56. Beagley KW, Fujihashi K, Lagoo AS et al (1995) Differences in intraepithelial lymphocyte T cell subsets isolated from murine small versus large intestine. J Immunol 154:5611–5619

57. Trejdosiewicz LK, Smart CJ, Oakes DJ et al (1989) Expression of T cell receptors Tcrl (γ/δ) and Tcr2 (α/β) in human intestinal mucosa. Immunology 68:7–12

58. Ullrich R, Schieferdecker HL, Ziegler K et al (1990) Gamma delta T cells in the human intestine express surface markers of activation and are preferentially located in the epithelium. Cell Immunol 128:619–927

59. Huleatt JW, Lefrancois L (1995) Antigen-driven induction of CD11c on intestinal intraepithelial lymphocytes and CD8+ T cells in vivo. J Immunol 154:5684–5693

60. Ebert EC (1989) Proliferative responses of human intraepithelial lymphocytes to various T-cell stimuli. Gastroenterology 97:1372–1381

61. Mosley RL, Styre D, Klein JR (1990) Differentiation and functional maturation of bone marrow derived intestinal epithelial T cells expressing membrane T cell receptors in athymic radiation chimeras. J Immunol 145:1369–1375

62. Fujiura Y, Kawaguchi M, Kondo Y et al (1996) Development of CD8$\alpha\alpha$+ intestinal intraepithelial T cells in β_2-microglobulin- and/or TAP1-deficient mice. J Immunol 156:2710–2715

63. Bandeira A, Mota-Santos T, Itohara S et al (1990) Localization of gamma/delta T cells to the intestinal epithelium is independent of normal microbial colonization. J Exp Med 172: 239–244

64. Elson CO, Sartor RB, Tennyson GS, Riddell RH (1995) Experimental models of inflammatory bowel disease. Gastroenterology 109:1344–1367

65. Steinman RM, Swanson J (1995) The endocytic activity of dendritic cells. J Exp Med 182:283–288

66. Maric I, Holt PG, Perdue MH, Bienenstock J (1996) Class II MHC antigen-bearing dendritic cells in the epithelium of the rat intestine. J Immunol 156:1408–1414

67. Goodnow C (1996) Balancing immunity and tolerance: Deleting and tuning lymphocyte repertoires. Proc Nat Acad Sci USA 93:2264–2271

68. Qiao L, Schurmann G, Autschbach F et al (1993) Human intestinal mucosa alters T cell reactivities. Gastroenterology 105: 814–819

69. Jung HC, Eckman L, Suk-Kyun Y et al (1995) A distinct array of proinflammatory cytokines is expressed in human colon epithelial cells in response to bacterial invasion. J Clin Invest 95:55–65

70. Mosmann TR, Coffman RL (1989) T$_h$1 and T$_h$2 cells: different

patterns of lymphokine secretion lead to different functional properties. Annu Rev Immunol 7:145–174

71. Song F, Matsuzaki G, Mitsuyama M, Nomoto K (1996) Differential effects of viable and killed bacteria on IL-12 expression of macrophages. J Immunol 156:2979–2984

72. Stead RH (1992) Innervation of mucosal immune cells in the gastrointestinal tract. Regional Immunol 4:91–99

73. Pascual DW, Stanisz AM, Bost KI (1994) Functional aspects of the peptidergic circuit in mucosal immunity. pp. 203–216. In Orga PL, Mestecky J, Lamm ME et al (eds): Handbook of Mucosal Immunology, Academic Press, San Diego

74. Mowat AM (1994) Oral tolerance and regulation of immunity to dietary antigens. pp. 185–201. In: Orga PL, Mestecky J, Lamm ME et al (eds): Handbook of Mucosal Immunology. Academic Press, San Diego, 185–201

75. Husby S, Mestecky J, Moldoveanu Z et al (1994) Oral tolerance in humans. T cell but not B cell tolerance after antigen feeding. J Immunol 152:4663–4670

76. Takahashi I, Nakagawa I, Kiyono H et al (1995) Mucosal cells induce systemic anergy for oral tolerance. Biochem Biophys Res Commun 206:414–420

77. Miller A, Lider O, Roberts AB (1992) Suppressor T cells generated by oral tolerization to myelin basic protein suppress both in vitro and in vivo immune responses by the release of transforming growth factor beta after antigen-specific triggering. Proc Nat Acad Sci USA 89:421–425

78. Burstein HJ, Abbas AK (1993) In vivo role of interleukin 4 in T cell tolerance induced by aqueous protein antigen. J Exp Med 177:457–463

79. Galliaerde V, Desvignes C, Peyron E, Kaiserlian D (1995) Oral tolerance to haptens: intestinal epithelial cells from 2,4-dinitrochorobenzene-fed mice inhibit hapten-specific T cell activation in vitro. Eur J Immunol 25:1385–1390

80. Duchmann R, Kaiser I, Hermann E et al (1995) Tolerance exists towards resident intestinal flora but is broken in active inflammatory bowel disease. Clin Exp Immunol 102:448–455

81. Childers NK, Bruce MG, McGhee JR (1989) Molecular mechanisms of immunoglobulin A defense. Annu Rev Microbiol 43:503–546

82. Beagley KW, Elson CO (1992) Cells and cytokines in mucosal immunity and inflammation. Gastroenterol Clin North Am 21:347–366

83. Mestecky J, Lue C, Russel MW (1991) Selective transport of IgA. Cellular and molecular aspects. Gastroenterol Clin North Am 20:441–471

84. Mostov KE, Friedlander M, Blobel G (1984) The receptor of transepithelial transport of IgA and IgM contains multiple immunoglobulin-like domains. Nature 308:37–38

85. Ahnen DJ, Brown WR, Kloppel TM (1985) Secretory component: the polymeric immunoglobulin receptor. Gastroenterology 89:667–682

86. Levine MM, Nataro JP (1994) Intestinal infections. pp. 505–512. In Mestecky J, Lamm ME, Strober W et al (eds): Handbook of Mucosal Immunology, Academic Press, San Diego

87. Strober W, Ehrhardt RO (1993) Chronic intestinal inflammation: an unexpected outcome in cytokine or T cell receptor mutant mice. Cell 75:203–205

88. Powrie F, Leach MW, Mauze S et al (1993) Phenotypically distinct subsets of CD4+ T cells induce or protect from chronic intestinal inflammation in C. B-17 scid mice. Int Immunol 5:1461–1471

89. Videla S, Vilaseca J, Guarner F et al (1994) Role of intestinal microflora in chronic inflammation and ulceration of the rat colon. Gut 35:1090–1097

90. Kramer DR, Cebra JJ (1995) Role of maternal antibody in the induction of virus specific and bystander IgA responses in Peyer's patches of suckling mice. Int Immunol 7:911–918

5

CLINICAL ASSESSMENT

Raoul Mayer
Robert D. Madoff
Stanley M. Goldberg

The diagnosis of the great majority of patients seen in the colorectal clinic can be established on the spot following a careful clinical evaluation. This assessment should include a detailed history and a thorough but focused examination, including, as appropriate, such procedures as anoscopy, rigid sigmoidoscopy, and flexible sigmoidoscopy. Furthermore, the surgeon should be prepared to perform such diagnostic and therapeutic office procedures as anorectal biopsy, hemorrhoidal banding, infrared coagulation of hemorrhoids, perianal abscess drainage, and excision or ablation of small anal lesions. Thus, many patients presenting with colorectal complaints can undergo complete diagnostic evaluation and often curative therapy at the time of their initial office visit.

INSTRUCTIONS TO PATIENTS

Patients requiring evaluation for anorectal symptoms are usually and understandably anxious about their office visits. Anxiety can be alleviated by adequate explanation of anticipated studies, both at the time of scheduling the appointment and by the examining physician. It is important to ensure appropriate patient preparation prior to the office visit. Patients requiring sigmoidoscopy are instructed to administer two prepackaged phosphate enemas 1 hour prior to their appointments. Patients with painful anorectal conditions should not be instructed to prepare, as this is unnecessarily painful, and endoscopy is contraindicated in the evaluation of acute pain.

FACILITIES

A satisfactory clinical facility is the essential basis for adequate examination and efficient clinical function. Space must be adequate with ample provision for privacy. Clinic efficiency is greatly enhanced when more than one examination room is available. Satisfactory illumination of the anorectum is best achieved with a headlight (Fig. 5-1). The examining table should be capable of accommodating the left lateral (Sims), knee-chest, and prone jackknife positions, and works best with electric foot controls (Fig. 5-2). Each examination room should have its own full complement of equipment to maximize efficiency. Well-trained ancillary staff is mandatory to provide assistance to the surgeon and to avoid medicolegal liability.

HISTORY OF PRESENT ILLNESS

Because the diagnosis of many anorectal disorders is so characteristic, often the patient's diagnosis is highly suspected by the completion of the patient interview. Physical examination thus very frequently serves only to confirm the initial diagnostic impression. After completion of the history of the present illness, a concise history of other pertinent information should be obtained, including other medical conditions, medications, allergies, sexual and infectious exposures, significant family history, and bleeding tendencies. This information serves as a framework for subsequent evaluations.

SYMPTOMS

Bleeding

Bleeding is one of the most common symptoms encountered in the colorectal clinic. Clues to the source of bleeding come from its characteristics: bleeding emanating from the anal canal is typically bright red in color, often is seen only on the toilet paper, and may drip or spurt into the toilet bowl. Colonic bleeding is variable in color and is less prone to have the appearance of fresh red blood that is typical of anal bleeding. Blood mixed in the stool and passage of clots also suggest a colonic source.

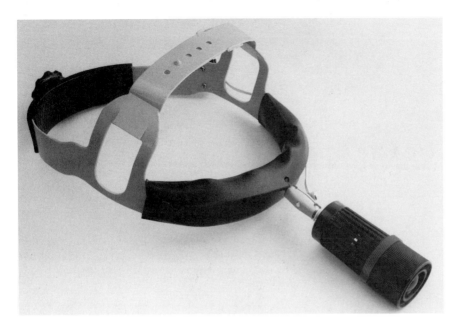

Figure 5-1. Welch & Allen headlight for office examination.

Black, tarry stools are highly suggestive of a proximal gastrointestinal bleeding source. Bloody stools combined with mucus, diarrhea, and nonspecific abdominal pain suggest inflammatory bowel disease, although distal rectal carcinomas or prolapsed internal hemorrhoids can also present with blood or mucus in the stool. The presence of occult bleeding in the stool requires complete colonic evaluation to rule out neoplasia.

The extent of evaluation for rectal bleeding should be dictated by the risk status of the individual patient. Young patients with no significant risk factors for colorectal neoplasia can be evaluated using anoscopy and sigmoidoscopy (preferably flexible); these patients rarely need a full colonoscopic evaluation. Internal hemorrhoids can be promptly treated by alteration of stool consistency, ligation, injection, or coagulation. Fissures, when

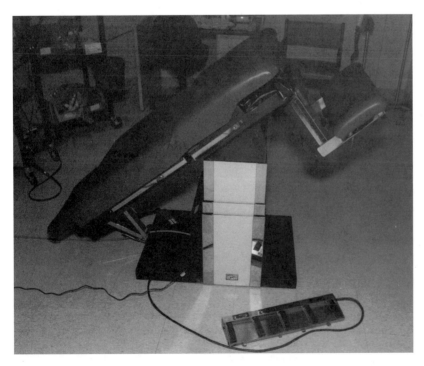

Figure 5-2. Electrically powered Ritter examination table.

demonstrated, should be initially treated conservatively, unless there is severe prolonged pain or internal sphincter muscle fibers are clearly visible, in which case surgical intervention is usually necessary. The algorithm for the evaluation of the patient with severe lower gastrointestinal hemorrhage is beyond the scope of this chapter, and may involve several diagnostic tests, including tagged red blood cell scans, angiography, and colonoscopy. Patients whose bleeding is unexplained by distal large bowel evaluation and patients at high risk for colorectal cancer should have complete colonoscopic evaluation.

Pain

Anorectal Pain

Anorectal pain is another very common symptom seen in the colorectal clinic. When pain is associated with passage of stool, a fissure is usually the cause. Severe throbbing pain associated with a palpable perianal lump is most often due to a thrombosed external hemorrhoid. Thrombosed external hemorrhoids may occur following strenuous exertion and may frequently complicate pregnancy. The diagnosis of perianal abscess is obvious when anal pain is accompanied by erythema, tenderness, fever, chills, and a fluctuant mass. Occult abscesses are suggested by a history of constant throbbing pain that is exacerbated by coughing or sneezing. Both tiny intersphincteric and large, deep postanal abscesses can be present without obvious external signs. Proctalgia fugax and related ''levator syndromes'' are characterized by fleeting pains that are typically localized by the patient to the rectum or pelvis. Proctalgia fugax pain is generally unrelated to the passage of stool and often awakens patients at night.

Occasionally, severe fecal impaction may present with rectal pain. Pain that is not associated with the passage of stool is commonly caused by pathology located outside the anatomic anorectum. Retrorectal tumors, iliac artery aneurysms, inflammation of the prostate gland, and pelvic and coccygeal abnormalities can all cause pain in the area of the rectum. Some patients with spinal stenosis may have pain referred to the anorectal region.

Acute anorectal pain should be assessed in the clinic by physical examination alone. Needless instrumentation, including anoscopy and sigmoidoscopy, are rarely diagnostic and only serve to aggravate the patient's discomfort. Occasionally, more sophisticated diagnostic measures are necessary. For example, complex fistulas and occult abscesses can be evaluated by use of endoanal ultrasonography and magnetic resonance imaging (MRI) scanning using a rectal coil. Endorectal ultrasonography can also be used for evaluation of low rectal tumors. It has proved to be more accurate than computed tomography (CT) scanning to stage these lesions.

Many painful conditions can be addressed in the clinic at the time of diagnosis. Thrombosed external hemorrhoids should be excised and perianal abscesses should be drained under local anesthesia. Severe rectal impaction should be treated by breaking up the fecal bolus with cotton-tipped applicators and repeated use of tap water (rather than irritant) enemas. Inter-

sphincteric and large perirectal abscesses generally require operating room drainage under general anesthesia.

Abdominal Pain

Abdominal pain tends to be poorly localized unless the parietal peritoneum is involved. Pain originating in the proximal colon is frequently referred to the hypogastrium, whereas rectal irritation is generally referred to the sacral region. Pain originating in the sigmoid colon may be referred to the flank or low back. When the pain is diffuse and is seen with distension, nausea, and vomiting, an obstructing process, such as neoplasm or stricture, should be suspected. Occasionally, patients with colonic obstructions complain of right lower quadrant pain due to cecal distension. Chronic intermittent episodes of partial small bowel obstruction can cause poorly localized pain. These episodes sometimes cause only mild nausea, no vomiting, and only minimal abdominal distension.

Abdominal pain is a surprisingly frequent symptom of colorectal neoplasm. This pain is typically described as nonspecific, dull, and poorly localized. Chronic diverticular disease can lead to abdominal pain due to a spasm of the hypertrophied colonic smooth muscle. During acute episodes of diverticulitis, the inflammatory process results in irritation of the parietal peritoneum with resultant well-localized left lower quadrant pain. On occasion, an inflamed loop of sigmoid lying to the right of the midline may mimic an attack of acute appendicitis. Rarely, supralevator abscesses may cause pelvic and lower abdominal pain, again due to local irritation of the pelvic peritoneum.

Abdominal pain suspected to be of colonic origin can be investigated in the clinic by use of flexible sigmoidoscopy. If acute diverticulitis is suspected, contrast radiography is the procedure of choice. A contrast enema using a water-soluble dye, such as Gastrografin, is generally the most expeditious available test and the least expensive. Barium should not be used in this setting as its presence in the peritoneum, should a perforation be present, leads to an intense chemical peritonitis. CT scanning with rectal contrast is a useful diagnostic test because it establishes the diagnosis, stages the severity of disease, and permits percutaneous drainage of any associated abscesses. It is important to stress that diverticulitis and left-sided carcinomas are sometimes difficult to distinguish by contrast study. Accordingly, endoscopic evaluation of the colon should be performed after the acute attack has been treated if colonic resection is not planned. A CT scan is generally the diagnostic test of choice when a supralevator abscess is suspected, and full colonoscopy should be used when a mucosal lesion is suspected proximal to the range of the flexible sigmoidoscope.

Change in Bowel Habits

There is a great deal of variation of the ''normal'' bowel pattern, but most authorities accept a range of one to four bowel movements per day to three bowel movements per week as being normal. Only changes from the usual bowel frequency must be investigated. Left-sided carcinomas may present with a gradual change in bowel habits. If tenesmus is present, inflammatory bowel disease or distal large bowel lesions should be suspected. Consistent decreases in stool caliber must be viewed with suspicion for distal colonic or rectal neoplasm. Medications (iron, antibiotics, antihypertensives), surgical procedures (including among others vagotomy, bowel resection, gastrectomy, jejunoileal bypass, cholecystectomy, gastrojejunostomy), and alterations in diet can all contribute to abnormal bowel frequency.

Constipation

Constipation is a common complaint but a vague term. In order to understand the problem, the surgeon must clarify exactly what the patient means: infrequent bowel movements? difficult bowel movements? incomplete bowel movements? painful bowel movements? During assessment, one should note stool frequency, consistency, changes in stool caliber, and new difficulties with evacuation. The chronicity of symptoms should be determined. Patients with severe chronic symptoms should be assessed further using colonic marker studies. Patients who expel more than 80% of their markers after 5 days are considered normal and generally require no further evaluation. Patients with abnormal transit times and patients with symptoms of difficult or incomplete evacuation can be referred to the anorectal physiology laboratory for further testing that includes electromyography (EMG) muscle recruitment, anal manometry, assessment of the rectoanal inhibitory reflex, and cinedefecography.

Diarrhea

Diarrhea is a common symptom of many gastrointestinal diseases. A careful history should be obtained regarding recent travel, food exposures, previous operations, and antibiotic use. The frequency, chronicity, and character of the diarrhea should be determined. Bloody diarrhea is common with colitis, whereas a clear, watery diarrhea may be due to a secretory rectal villous adenoma. Any recent antibiotic use associated with the onset of diarrhea must be viewed with suspicion for pseudomembranous colitis due to overgrowth of *Clostridium difficile*.

Incontinence

Incontinence is defined as the inability to control passage of stool or flatus. Common causes of incontinence include advanced age with debility, obstetric injuries, anorectal surgery (especially fistulotomy), neurologic disorders, trauma, and diabetes mellitus with neuropathy. The severity, chronicity, and onset of symptoms must be established. Severity of symptoms should also be evaluated. Loss of solid stool denotes the most severe incontinence, followed by loss of liquid stool. Loss of gas only denotes mild incontinence. Diurnal pattern of accidents is also important. Daytime loss of control is more serious than loss of control that occurs during sleep, when normal reflex mechanisms are not fully active. Patients with diarrheal states of any cause may develop incontinence, and patients with inflammatory bowel disease may become incontinent during disease flares. Long-standing rectal prolapse may eventually cause incontinence by stretching of the anal sphincter mechanism and pudendal nerves. Patients with large rectal villous adenomas may develop incontinence to liquid mucus. Passage of gas and/ or stool *per vaginam* suggests the presence of an enterovaginal, colovaginal, or rectovaginal fistula.

Anal incontinence is assessed by digital examination and documentation of resting and squeeze anal pressures. Further assessment for patients with significant incontinence includes formal anorectal physiology testing, including anal manometry, pudendal nerve latency studies, and cinedefecography. Endoanal ultrasonography provides an excellent anatomic depiction of both the internal and external anal sphincter mechanisms. The decision for surgical versus medical treatment is based on the patient's level of disability, overall medical condition, and diagnostic findings. If corrective surgery is contemplated, the patient's degree of incontinence should be documented preoperatively. Specific points, such as the nature and timing of incontinent episodes, the need to wear protective pads, and the impact on the patient's daily life, should be addressed.

Tenesmus

Patients may present with the sensation of a painful spasm of the sphincter, an urgent feeling to evacuate, and involuntary straining, which results in little, if any, evacuation. When present, tenesmus is usually associated with low rectal cancers, inflammatory bowel disease, or diarrheal states.

Discharge

Mucus is secreted by the mucosal goblet cells of the large bowel. Clear mucus may be encountered due to a rectovillous adenoma. Patients with ulcerative colitis or rectal neoplasms may leak bloody mucus. Patients with chronically prolapsed hemorrhoids and anal ectropion may also experience mucus discharge. The patient with severe pruritis ani with weeping perianal skin may give a history of discharge as a major complaint.

Purulent discharge is usually due to a draining abscess or fistula. A prior history of an abscess suggests the presence of a chronic fistula-in-ano. Purulent material in the stool is seen in patients with spontaneously draining abscesses or gonococcal proctitis. Patients presenting with discharge should be assessed with digital examination, anoscopy, and flexible sigmoidoscopy.

Perianal Swelling and Masses

A variety of masses can be seen in the perianal region. In general, unless they clearly represent prolapsing hypertrophied anal papilla or thrombosed external hemorrhoid, these masses should be removed and sent for pathologic analysis. When a painful swelling is associated with fever or chills, it usually represents an abscess. A painful swelling that has spontaneously drained represents either an abscess or an anal fistula; the latter is to be suspected if the drainage is persistent or recurrent. Anal cancer frequently presents as a painless anal mass. Perianal Crohn's disease is characterized by multiple abscesses, fistulas (often complex), and large perianal skin tags. A chronic nonhealing wound following excision of a skin tag or drainage of an abscess suggests the diagnosis of Crohn's disease.

The treatment of abscesses is by prompt drainage. Temporizing delay using antibiotics is inappropriate and only leads to extension of the infectious process. Inadequately treated abscesses can progress to severe necrotizing perineal infections, particularly in diabetic and immunocompromised patients. A thrombosed external hemorrhoid should be treated by excision of the hemorrhoidal tissue and not just by simple drainage to prevent early "recurrence," which is often just residual untreated thrombus. Prompt excision under local anesthesia is the treatment of choice for thrombosed external hemorrhoids that occur during pregnancy. When large prolapsing hemorrhoids are present, proctoplasty and hemorrhoidectomy should be considered in the immediate postpartum period.

Pruritis

Pruritis ani is a common condition that can be caused by a variety of conditions. Most often, it is caused by local irritation due to inadequate hygiene, excessive sweating, or skin breakdown by excessive scratching. Various dermatologic diseases, such as psoriasis, Paget's disease, Bowen's disease, and parasites (pinworms) can all induce pruritis. The treatment of this condition is focused on removal of the causative factors. Most "idiopathic" cases respond to simple measures of improved anal hygiene, topical treatment with 1% hydrocortisone cream, cessation of scratching, avoidance of potential allergens, and use of a skin barrier cream. Occasionally, the condition is aggravated by secondary fungal infection.

Anal Protrusion

External prolapse of tissue from the anus can represent either rectal mucosal prolapse, which is associated with internal hemorrhoids, or a full-thickness rectal prolapse. These conditions can be differentiated by a physical examination. Full-thickness rectal prolapse is associated with circular rectal folds versus the radial folds typical of rectal mucosal prolapse. Full-thickness prolapse is frequently larger than mucosal prolapse, which rarely exceeds 4 to 5 cm in size. Finally, a palpable sulcus between the protruding tissue and the anal verge is present in full thickness but not mucosal prolapse.

Occasionally, rectal polyps may be the cause of prolapsing tissue. In children, these are typically juvenile polyps; prolapsing polyps in adults tend to be large villous adenomas. Chronic mucosal prolapse frequently results in squamous metaplasia of the mucosal surface, which may give the tissue a neoplastic appearance. Biopsies should be obtained when there is any doubt as to the diagnosis.

Prolapsing hemorrhoids can usually be treated in the clinic by fixation techniques, such as Barron ligature or injection. Surgery is necessary when the hemorrhoids are very large, have a significant external component, or require manual reduction. Hypertrophied anal papillae can easily be removed if they produce significant symptoms. Full-thickness prolapse should be treated by surgical repair in the operating room.

Flatulence

Excessive passage of flatus is often due to diets that contain an excessive quantity of carbohydrates, especially nonabsorbable, nondigestible oligosaccharides typically found in certain vegetables. These substances, which are not broken down in the human small bowel, are digested by colonic bacteria by fermentation, which produces hydrogen and methane gas. A similar pathophysiology explains the excessive flatulence seen in pa-

tients with lactose deficiency, who are unable to break down lactose in the small bowel, and therefore provide this undigested sugar to the colonic bacteria. Flatulence can be exacerbated by ingestion of carbonated drinks and poor eating habits (rapid eating, eating while talking) that lead to aerophagia. Treatment of flatulence consists of dietary adjustments and patient education.

Miscellaneous Symptoms

Weight loss is a nonspecific symptom often associated with malignancy or inflammatory bowel disease. Passage of flatus or stool through the vagina or the urinary tract is almost always due to a fistula from the gastrointestinal tract. Common causes of these fistulas include complicated diverticular disease, carcinoma, trauma (operative and otherwise), and Crohn's disease. Extraintestinal manifestations of Crohn's disease can cause a wide variety of symptoms, including arthritis, iritis, ankylosing spondylitis, sacroiliitis, erythema nodosum, pyoderma gangrenosum, and ulcers of the mouth. Anorexia may be related to chronic illness, neoplasia, medication use, or psychological causes.

HISTORY

A wide variety of general conditions are pertinent to patients with anorectal disease. Patients with diabetes mellitus may develop incontinence due to autonomic neuropathy. Patients with severe atherosclerotic vascular disease may suffer from mesenteric ischemia, characterized by postprandial abdominal pain, diarrhea, or vomiting. Patients with advanced liver disease may develop rectal or peristomal varices. Patients with ileal inflammation or resection are prone to develop kidney stones. Patients with a family history of colon cancer or a personal history of extracolonic cancers (including endometrial, genitourinary, and others) are at increased risk for developing colorectal neoplasia.

Medications

A complete list of all medications must be obtained and should include over-the-counter drugs. Laxative, stool softener, and analgesic use should be specifically queried. A wide variety of other medications, such as antihypertensives, antidepressants, antipsychotics, iron preparations, antibiotics, antineoplastics, and thyroid drugs may also alter bowel function. Nonsteroidal antiinflammatory drugs and warfarin are frequent causes of bleeding.

Allergies

All drug allergies and intolerances should be recorded in the patient's record.

Travel and Sexual History

Recent travel history should be obtained, particularly travel to areas of endemic disease. A sexual history should be elicited when appropriate, particularly when there is evidence of sexually transmitted disease.

Family History

Patients with a family history of colon cancer in a first-degree relative are at increased risk for the development of neoplasia. This is particularly true when multiple relatives are involved or the involved relative developed cancer at an early age. A history of multiple relatives with colorectal cancer raises the question of a familial cancer syndrome, such as familial adenomatous polyposis (or one of its variants) or a Lynch syndrome. Numerous cancers, including endometrial and genitourinary, raise the possibility of Lynch syndrome type 2. Crohn's disease and ulcerative colitis can be seen to cluster in families about 10% of patients.

PHYSICAL EXAMINATION

At the completion of the interview and prior to the physical examination, it is often helpful to reassure the patient (when appropriate) that their symptoms are most likely due to a benign condition. This simple step decreases the anxiety bred from the widespread misconception that, for example, rectal bleeding is invariably a sign of cancer. The surgeon should spend a few moments explaining all the steps of the examination to reassure the patient and avoid unnecessary surprises. The liberal use of drawings, anatomic charts, and short, focused pamphlets is reassuring to patients and highly desirable.

The examination room must have adequate privacy and heating. A commode must be present in close proximity for patient comfort. The surgeon should wear a headlight and gloves for protection. Lubricant jelly is used for all examinations and anesthetic jelly may be helpful in patients with skin level discomfort. All instruments, such as biopsy forceps, anoscopes, sigmoidoscopes, fistula probes, hemorrhoid ligators, wire snares, and suction catheters must be kept within easy reach but out of the sight of patient entering the room. Excellent suction is mandatory.

Abdomen

The patient is placed in the supine position. The abdomen should be inspected from the xyphoid to the pubis. Masses, scars, pulsations, and distended veins will be apparent when present. Auscultation reveals the presence and quality of bowel sounds, as well as bruits that may be present due to visceral arterial disease. All four quadrants are gently and carefully palpated, including the liver and spleen. Any abnormal masses must be evaluated for size, mobility, and direct to transmitted pulsations. The groin should be palpated for hernias, enlarged lymph nodes, or other masses. Patients with chronic constipation often have palpable stool in their colon, which must be distinguished from other masses.

Position and Table

A variety of endoscopic examining tables are commercially available, but an adjustable table with electrical controls is optimal. The Ritter table is ideal because it allows examination of the patient in both the left lateral and prone jackknife positions. The Sims left lateral position is probably the most comfortable position for the patient, but the prone position provides easier access for the examiner and permits the best examination of the anorectum. The two positions are equivalent for visualizing the anus and the lower rectum. Elderly and obese patients in particular find the jackknife position difficult, and the left lateral position is often the only option for these patients.

Inspection

Many of the diseases of the anorectal region are diagnosed easily by careful inspection alone. The examiner can appreciate the function or dysfunction of the external anal sphincter and puborectalis muscles by observing voluntary contraction. A patulous anus is frequently associated with full-thickness rectal prolapse.

With simple gentle separation of the buttocks, masses, such as warts, prolapsing hemorrhoids, and anal papillae, can be readily visualized; any asymmetric swelling and redness due to an abscess can be appreciated. The external openings of anal fistulas can readily be seen as small buds of granulation tissue. Scars from previous anorectal surgery, obstetric injury, and trauma should be noted. Anal fissures, typically located in the posterior or anterior midline, are diagnosed by opposing lateral traction of the perianal skin. Their presence is often indicated by that of an associated "sentinal" skin tag. The position of the anus and the quality of the perineal body in women should be noted.

Perineal descent, procidentia, rectocele, cystocele, and rectal mucosal prolapse can be further evaluated by having the patient perform a Valsalva maneuver. When the patient offers a history of anal protrusion and a diagnosis is not obvious, the patient should be instructed to strain while seated on a commode. The prone jackknife position is particularly disadvantageous for demonstrating rectal prolapse due to the force of gravity.

Palpation

Palpation of the perianal areas must be done in a gentle fashion and should precede the digital examination. A painful fullness or mass is characteristic of an abscess. When the patient with an abscess is in significant discomfort, the remainder of the examination should be conducted under anesthesia or during a follow-up visit after the abscess has been drained. When evaluating a fistula, the characteristically indurated fistula tract can often be appreciated. Gentle external pressure may demonstrate the presence of purulent material, expressed from either the internal or external fistula opening. Circumferential palpation of the sphincter mechanism should be performed when an intrasphincteric abscess is suspected in an attempt to make the diagnosis and localize the abscess.

Digital Examination

Digital examination should commence only after the patient has been informed that it is about to begin. The gloved examining finger must be well lubricated with a water-soluble jelly. Application of slight pressure on the sphincter mechanism itself facilitates the gentle insertion of the index finger. Digital examination should not be performed when patient comfort does not permit it. Patients with mild anal stenosis can continue to be examined if the examination is not painful. Further examination of a tight sphincter is possible by use of a well-lubricated, cotton-tipped applicator. Very tight anal stenoses require assessment and treatment under anesthesia. Forceful anal dilatations are both painful and ineffective, and are mentioned only to be condemned.

Once the examining finger is in the anal canal, resting sphincter tone should be noted. Next, the examiner should ask the patient to strain, which should result in reflex relaxation of the internal sphincter and puborectalis muscles. This maneuver may also demonstrate the presence of an occult prolapse. The patient next is asked to squeeze the sphincter muscle, which establishes the function of the puborectalis and the external sphincter muscles. Puborectalis contraction is appreciated as a strong anterior pull of the posteriorly based muscle sling.

The examining finger should next palpate the anal canal circumferentially. In the anterior region, the prostate gland should be assessed in men and the cervix and uterus in women. An anterior sphincter defect in women can often be appreciated by bidigital examination of the perineal body with the index finger in the anal canal and the thumb in the posterior fourchette. Bidigital rectovaginal examination (index finger in rectum, middle finger in vagina) is also useful in patients with suspected enterocele, which is often palpable when the patient is instructed to strain.

If a neoplasm is detected, the surgeon should determine its level, with particular reference to the distance from its distal margin to the anal verge. The texture of the mass (hard, nodular, soft, or velvety), approximate size, mobility, and position within the anal canal (anterior versus posterior or lateral) should all be determined.

DIAGNOSTIC PROCEDURES

Anoscopy

Visual evaluation of the anal canal is best achieved by use of an anoscope. The instruments may be disposable, lighted, and bivalved, or they may have obturators. In our practice, we prefer to use the pediatric Ives anoscope, which is small and has a

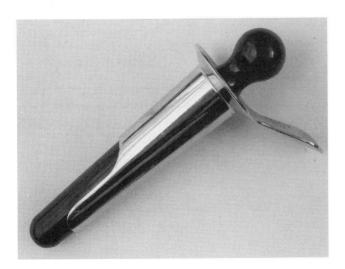

Figure 5-3.   Ives anoscope.

slot that permits a side view of the anal canal (Fig. 5-3). After the instrument is well lubricated, it is gently advanced into the anal canal and is rotated in order to visualize the entire anal circumference. Fissures are easily visualized on inspection alone; anoscopy in the presence of a fissure is unnecessary, painful, and contraindicated. The patient is instructed to strain to demonstrate internal hemorrhoids and rectal mucosal prolapse, which can easily be seen bulging into the anoscope slot. Carcinomas and polyps of the lower rectum can occasionally be evaluated and biopsied with the aid of an anoscope.

Rigid Sigmoidoscopy

Since its introduction, the flexible sigmoidoscope has largely replaced the rigid sigmoidoscope. The rigid sigmoidoscope, however, still presents adequate evaluation of the midrectum and allows the biopsy or snare removal of lesions located in this area. Furthermore, distance of a lesion from the anal verge is estimated more accurately using the rigid than flexible instrument. The average length of insertion is between 17 and 20 cm. The instruments are 25 cm in length and have diameters of 11, 15, or 19 mm. The smaller instruments are used in patients with strictures whereas the larger instruments are preferred when stool or blood in the rectum needs to be irrigated or a large polyp is present. For most examinations, the 15-mm instrument is recommended.

The sigmoidoscope should be advanced only under direct vision with clear delineation of the lumen. Because the rectosigmoid junction represents an acute angulation, particular care must be given when attempting to advance the scope in this area, and one should always remember that this is not possible in all patients. Moderate air insufflation facilitates the examination but excessive insufflation is painful and counterproductive. The mucosa should be carefully visualized. Irrigation, suction, and electrocoagulation may be used through the instrument. In order to avoid possible explosions when fulgurating or using cautery snare through the rigid sigmoidoscope, special care must be exercised to adequately remove bowel gas prior to applying electrical current. Rigid sigmoidoscopy is the examination of choice for patients with suspected sigmoid volvulus.

Flexible Sigmoidoscopy

The flexible sigmoidoscope is very similar to the initial 60-cm fiberoptic instruments developed as colonoscopes in the 1960s. Studies have demonstrated that the flexible sigmoidoscopic exam is better tolerated and more sensitive in detecting distal large bowel lesions than rigid sigmoidoscopy. This is due to the magnification, ability to angulate, and superior optics of the flexible sigmoidoscope. The instrument can be advanced to above 50 cm in the majority of cases. However, there is no shame in terminating an examination that is unduly painful and difficult; indeed, to do otherwise violates common sense, safety and decency. The examiner should remember that more complete evaluation remains possible at a later date using contrast radiography or colonoscopy under sedation. The procedure usually takes 3 to 5 minutes and no anesthesia is required. Small lesions or polyps may be biopsied or removed using biopsy forceps and snares. Flexible sigmoidoscopy is extremely useful for the evaluation of diverticulitis, colitis, ischemia, anastomoses, and all mucosal lesions. Occasionally, it may be useful for the reduction of sigmoid volvulus or removal of foreign bodies.

CONCLUSION

Colorectal disease is almost uniformly well suited to office diagnosis. Careful and systematic evaluation with adequate illumination and appropriate equipment will lead to early, accurate diagnosis in most patients, and to simple office treatment in many.

6

FLEXIBLE ENDOSCOPY

Christopher B. Williams
Brian P. Saunders

Flexible endoscopy and radiology by double-contrast barium enema (DCBE) have, in the past two decades, reversed their positions in first-line role for colonic investigation. Endoscopy has the obvious advantages over radiography of color view and the ability to irrigate away any residue or biopsy uncertain lesions, and also has therapeutic potential. It is generally regarded as considerably more accurate, especially for smaller polyps[1,2] or flat lesions such as mild inflammatory disease[3] or vascular anomalies and other causes of blood loss.[4] Even large polyps or malignancies can be missed by the radiologist or mistaken as fecal residue,[2,5] but will generally only escape the endoscopist if he or she fails to perform a complete examination.[3,6] On the other hand colonoscopy has, especially in inexpert hands, a higher complication rate than radiography (1:1,500 vs 1:25,000)[1,7,8]; localization of stenosing or obstructing lesions may be incorrect[9,10]; and extracolonic impressions or communications can be missed. Endoscopy is usually better regarded by patients who have been through both it and DCBE, mainly because of the sedation that endoscopists usually employ.[11]

Having a (double-contrast) barium enema available beforehand is not essential for the endoscopist, because the radiologic appearances are not predictive of the technical ease of colonoscopy, except that a redundant transverse colon on radiograph or severe diverticular disease in the sigmoid colon do make it more likely that endoscope insertion will be difficult.[12] On the other hand, it is well accepted that the sigmoid colon is, because of tortuosity, the most inaccurate area for radiologic interpretation, so that it has been recommended by some that DCBE should always be supplemented by flexible sigmoidoscopy.[13-15]

INDICATIONS AND CONTRAINDICATIONS

Colonoscopy is the "investigation of choice" for most intracolonic symptomatology and conditions, because fine focus vision, histology, or color appreciation are important; for confirmation or exclusion of blood loss or inflammatory disease these factors are especially relevant. Many other patients, although their presentation suggests symptomatology of "dysfunction" or "irritable bowel" (pain, altered habit, etc.) are in the 50 or older age range where endoscopy gives a valuable opportunity to screen for small polyps, and to destroy them if present. Effectively, presupposing an adequately skilled endoscopist, the clinical question is more of the rare contraindications to flexible endoscopy. The main contraindication to colonoscopy, or reason for discontinuing it once started, is the appreciation that there may be a potential for perforation. On this ground an acute episode of diverticulitis within the previous 2 weeks, abdominal tenderness in a patient with acute colitis, or endoscopically visible deep ulceration in a colitic or, rarely, gangrene in ischemic colitis, all contraindicate starting colonoscopy or suggest abandoning it at once. Otherwise any patient well enough to tolerate bowel preparation or at risk for surgery is appropriate for colonoscopy.

COMPLICATIONS

Literature reviews suggest the complication rate of diagnostic colonoscopy to be 1:1,500 examinations, with potential for bleeding or perforation in 1:100 colonoscopic polypectomies and a mortality rate around 1:10,000.[7,16-18] These figures are, however, highly questionable, being based on survey evidence, often dating back to the days when endoscopes were considerably less mobile and endoscopic technique more aggressive than currently. No complication has occurred during diagnostic colonoscopy in our hospital during the last 20,000 diagnostic colonoscopies, no mortality in 30,000 colonoscopies of all types, and complications have been limited to therapeutic procedure with delayed hemorrhages 1 to 10 days after polypectomy (see below) or perforations (threatened or actual) after dilatation of strictures.

Nonetheless colonoscopy is sometimes unavoidably physical, so that there is potential for hypotensive, vasovagal, or cardiac dysrhythmic episodes; transient bacteremia (dangerous in immunosuppressed subjects, and those with valve prostheses or ascites); or trauma to the bowel wall, mesenteries, or their visceral attachments. Avulsion or capsular tears to the spleen have been reported,[19–21] as have air-pressure perforations or even sometimes "pneumoperitoneum" from diverticulosis or sometimes localized to the proximal colon when colonoscope insertion has been limited to the sigmoid.[22,23]

The message to the endoscopist is to be cautious and kind, to avoid oversedation and overaggression. Any maneuver that a lightly sedated patient can tolerate is unlikely to be hazardous, but unexplained pain should always be taken seriously, the colon deflated, the instrument straightened back, and, if pain continues or if in doubt the procedure abandoned. The unexpected can happen, such as the instrument tip becoming looped and incarcerated in an unexpected hernia,[24,25] but there will also be accompanying protests from the patient to warn the endoscopist to take corrective action. Minor events, which cannot be classified as complications, do occur after colonoscopy. Many patients are transiently hypotensive or "vasovagal" immediately after colonoscopy, but recover after 10 to 15 minutes recumbent; others experience wind distension pains for some hours after the procedure (which is avoidable by using CO_2 insufflation).[26,27]

FLEXIBLE SIGMOIDOSCOPY

Flexible sigmoidoscopy is performed 20 to 30 minutes after an evacuant enema (hypertonic sodium phosphate or contact laxative), although good results and patient compliance have also been reported after oral preparation.[28] Conventionally no sedation is given for flexible sigmoidoscopy, although in a few nervous patients or others with a fixed or sensitive colon both extent and patient acceptance can be improved by a small-dose intravenous sedation or inhaled nitrous oxide/oxygen mixture.[29] The choice of instrument used for flexible sigmoidoscopy is of little importance, for limited examinations can be performed with a full-length colonoscope (or even a gastroscope). The most comfortable, and therefore easiest, examinations will be performed with a small (1-cm) diameter 70-cm long sigmoidoscope or 130-cm long pediatric colonoscope; these instruments allow maximum maneuverability, with minimum tendency to cause pain in stretching up the sigmoid loop. The only contraindication to flexible sigmoidoscopy (as for colonoscopy) is acute abdominal tenderness suggesting a potential for perforation.

Insertion technique is straightforward, given the need to withdraw every time the luminal view is lost, to insufflate a reasonable minimum of air, and to pull back from time to time to avoid any excessive forced looping of the sigmoid colon. Flexible sigmoidoscopy is unpredictable in extent. The main rule is that insertion should be terminated if it is unreasonably painful, for the whole object is that the flexible instrument should be more comfortable for the patient than the rigid proctosigmoidoscope. On the other hand the diagnostic yield of flexible sigmoidoscopy is greater with greater distance examined,[30] and skilled endoscopists may therefore try to insert to the descending colon or even the splenic flexure. In practice insertion is often limited by a combination of fecal residue (making further examination unrewarding) and increasing discomfort. The length of instrument used may be the limiting factor, but should be of little importance; a skilled examiner may coax the instrument up to the descending colon with 40 to 45 cm of shaft inserted, whereas the less skilled examiner can have inserted the whole 70 cm of the instrument without reaching the proximal part of the looped sigmoid colon.

Visual inspection, biopsies, and video prints can all be made during flexible sigmoidoscopy but electrosurgical polypectomy should not be undertaken unless due care is taken about the potential for explosive gas mixtures (hydrogen or methane) either by repeatedly deflating or re-insufflating, or by using CO_2 "Cold-snaring" smaller polyps without current[31] will avoid this potential hazard.

COLONIC ANATOMY AND ENDOSCOPIC LOCALIZATION

Between the fixed points of the rectum and the ileocecal valve bulge, both anatomy and endoscopic localization can be highly variable and uncertain.[32] The distal colon is generally thicker walled and circular in outline, whereas the thinner transverse colon is characteristically triangular in shape (due to the longitudinal muscle bands of the taenia coli), which can indent visibly in the proximal colon but also be seen more distally in particularly large colons. In close-up the arclike circular muscle indentations and fixed haustral infoldings give useful clues as to luminal direction, and when a taenia coli is visible on a bend it is also a useful pointer to the midline axis.

The retroperitoneal attachments (Fig. 6-1) of the descending and ascending colon expected at 3 months of intrauterine fetal development do not occur in approximately 10% of subjects.[32,33] Furthermore in about 20% of patients, especially women, the colon can be remarkably long with the transverse colon looping down to the symphysis pubis.[12] It is therefore perhaps not surprising that some colonoscopies are remarkably

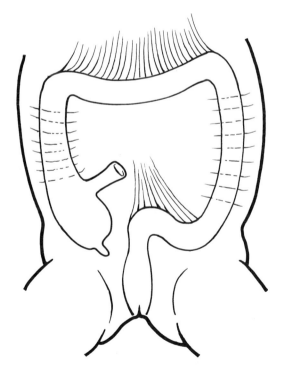

Figure 6-1. By the third month of fetal life the ascending and descending "mesocolons" become fixed retroperitoneally in 90% of subjects.

uncontrollable and difficult and that even experts can be grossly disoriented as to what loops are forming, or where the tip of the instrument is. Serious errors of localization are possible when a cancer or obstructing lesion is present and the endoscopist cannot reach the cecum, at which point it becomes possible to straighten out all loops, orient, and thereafter make distance-based judgments on withdrawal.

Clues as to anatomic localization include transillumination through the abdominal wall (with the room lights turned off if necessary), finger indentation, use of fluid levels (horizontal in the descending and ascending colon with the patient in lateral position), and distance on the shortened endoscope. Both distance and extracolonic blue viscera (usually liver, but spleen and other adjacent organs can sometimes be seen) are variable and subjective, except taken in context with other judgments. It is remarkable how often even an experienced endoscopist can be mistaken between the proximal sigmoid and splenic flexure, or between splenic and hepatic flexures, so everyone (especially the surgeon) needs to be aware of the possibility of errors in endoscopic localization.[9]

BOWEL PREPARATION

For many patients bowel preparation is the most unpleasant part of colonoscopy, and, if it fails, the result is just as unpleasant for the endoscopist and greatly reduces the accuracy of examination. Difficulty in bowel preparation is predictable in those with chronic constipation or obstructive features but, more surprisingly, the colon of some patients with active or healed extensive inflammatory disease can also be difficult to clear. Compliance with the suggested preparation is another limiting factor, so that the best preparation regimens are those that are palatable, easy to drink, and do not result in colic or nausea. The traditional combination of castor oil (which has a disgusting aftertaste) and nurse-administered enemas now has few supporters.[34] The 4-L volume and salty taste of polyethylene-glycol (PEG)-electrolyte mixture[35,36] causes at least 10% of patients to stop drinking too early, [37] with appalling clearance as a result—although successful PEG electrolyte preparation gives a perfectly clear colon. "Split administration" of PEG-electrolyte into two 2-L aliquots some hours apart (or on the evening before and morning of examination) helps acceptance considerably.[38] A magnesium citrate-purgative combination (Picolax) is inexpensive, effective, and has had a following in Europe,[39] although its bitter taste is disliked by some and it can cause severe colic in older subjects. A well-tolerated and reportedly effective alternative is the small-volume oral sodium phosphate solution (Phospho-soda),[40,41] although significant electrolyte shifts can occur with it, including hypokalemia.[42]

To help the endoscopist avoid difficulties in aspirating particulate matter any preparation regimen should be preceded by 24 hours of soft diet (no fruit, vegetables, whole-grain cereal, nuts, mushrooms, etc.). Constipating medication should be stopped but any normally taken purgatives continued; iron preparations cause foul black discoloration of colon contents (iron tannates) and should be discontinued 5 to 7 days before. Apart from these restrictions, the key to successful endoscopic bowel preparation is to cause profuse watery diarrhea in the hours before examination, while permitting the patient some sleep and the ability to travel for the procedure without incontinence. Depending on

whether colonoscopy is to be in the morning or the afternoon, this usually means taking all the preparation on the preceding evening (in two doses) or drinking the second dose early on the morning of the examination. Copious intake of clear fluids up to the last moment before examination (including tea, coffee, or alcoholic drinks) is good for clearance and makes aspiration of any residue easy; it also helps morale.

MEDICATION AND MORALE

Many first-time patients are scared, either about the possibility of cancer or the indignity and possible trauma of the event itself. They may have heard negative reports from acquaintances, or have understood that it is normal to receive an anesthetic for the experience. The answer is to individualize management to some extent, but to ensure that all staff are, from first contact, kind and understanding to each patient.[43] An opportunity to talk for some minutes to a staff member beforehand should be reassuring and also allows a checklist of important matters such as allergies, relevant medications (nonsteroidal anti-inflammatory drugs [NSAIDs], anticoagulants), or medical conditions (heart valve prostheses, previous surgery, etc.). Informed consent is important, but mainly in relationship to possible therapy (where the main potential risks lie) and permission for sedative medication to be used as necessary.

Medication requirements for colonoscopy vary widely, according to endoscopist or patient preference, hospital or national routines, and the relative ease or difficulty of a particular individual's anatomy. Patients having previous sigmoid colectomy frequently need no sedation at all; others with negative previous experience may insist on being "knocked out." We strongly favor an adaptable regimen combining, in most cases a low-dosage intravenous sedation/analgesia combination,[44] increased as necessary during the procedure but normally leaving the patient in verbal communication with the endoscopist and able to change position on command (conscious sedation). A typical initial dose, according to the body configuration, anxiety level, and preference of the patient, would combine benzodiazepine (diazepam 2.5 to 5 mg, alone or in fat emulsion, or midazolam 2 to 4 mg) with pethidine (meperidine) 25 to 50 mg, each given slowly through an indwelling cannula. The amnesic properties of midazolam are an advantage for some patients, especially if the procedure proves to be traumatic, although with the disadvantage that the patient has to be re-interviewed afterward to remember anything. General anesthesia (propofol) is semiroutinely given in some countries,[45] but we believe this approach encourages heavy-handed insertion technique and should only be used by an experienced endoscopist for special reasons and very rarely—perhaps in around 1:1,000 colonoscopies, whether in adults or children.

This flexible attitude toward medication, none for some examinations and rarely rendering the patient incoherent or asleep, partly reflects the fact that it is difficult for an observer to assess a patient's response to pain. A degree of pain is tolerable by almost anyone for 20 to 30 seconds, and, as colonoscopic pain is invariably due to looping or angulation, and almost instantly removable by straightening the shaft again, it is easy to "forgive and forget." Recurrent or prolonged visceral pain, with its unpleasant gnawing distension quality, is best suppressed by extra analgesia, and it is for this that opiates are especially effective.

Pethidine has the bonus of being "mood enhancing," with a pleasant euphoriant effect. If additional medication is required extra doses of pethidine are usually the best option, with midazolam available for amnestic purposes if the situation cannot be properly controlled. Antidote medication (naloxone intravenously or intramuscularly for opiates, flumazenil by slow intravenous injection for benzodiazepine overdose) are occasionally valuable, both for safety reasons and for the logistics of recovery management.

INSERTION TECHNIQUE

The principles for flexible colonoscope insertion (as for sigmoidoscopy) are to steer under direct vision, to avoid excessive air insufflation, and to keep the instrument as straight as possible.[46] In practice this is frequently less easy than it sounds. The tip may easily abut against the mucosal surface, losing the view; when this happens pulling back to disimpact and reorient is usually the quickest and best course. Overinsufflation is all too easy, especially during a difficult insertion or polypectomy; but, even though the view may be worse, the partially deflated colon is shorter, more malleable, and easy to manage compared to the distended one. Inexperienced or aggressive endoscopists easily forget that a good view *ahead* of the tip is irrelevant and misleading if the shaft behind is unproductively looped or angulated (Fig. 6-2); this is usually immediately apparent, either from the patient's complaints or from the fact that the shaft and/or angling controls are affected by increasing friction and become unresponsive and "snarled up." A straight or nearly

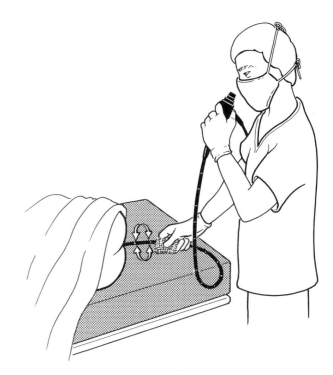

Figure 6-3. For "single-handed" colonoscopy the right hand is used mainly for shaft push-pull and twist, while the left hand alone manages the angulation wheels and buttons of the control body.

straight endoscope within a favorable configuration of colon will slide easily without significant pain, and respond easily and immediately to control knob angling or to gentle in-out or rotational movements of the shaft. It is important to learn this feeling of subtlety in the sigmoid colon, managing the scope in the fingers (not the clenched fist) and avoiding clumsy or erratic steering. Proximal to the sigmoid colon it is almost inevitable that there will be moments of shaft looping (usually in the sigmoid colon, but sometimes in the transverse) for which much larger-scale movements in or out, and much more forcible twisting forces must be applied to make progress, before subsequently straightening out, regaining control, and returning to "subtle mode" once again.

The most common mistake in colonoscopy is to push too hard and too long; this produces loops that the endoscopist never quite dares to pull back to reduce adequately for fear of "falling out" and, as a result, becomes too accustomed to needing forceful maneuvers (and heavy sedation) most of the time. Slow and careful steering, frequent and substantial instrument withdrawals, and a reluctance to use force are the keys to good technique. A corollary to this approach is the apparent paradox that an endoscopist who takes time inserting through the sigmoid colon will usually be quicker and more certain to the cecum thereafter, compared to the extrovert whose "crash and dash" approach from the outset simply results in unmanageable knots in the distal colon.

"Single-handed" colonoscopy is the procedure in which the endoscopist manages the angling controls and air, water, and suction buttons in the left hand, keeping the right hand mainly on the shaft in order to keep precise control of push-pull and twisting movements (Fig. 6-3). Although more difficult to cope

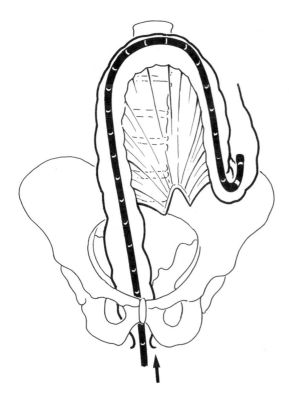

Figure 6-2. A looped colonoscope results in mesentery stretch and pain for the patient, as well as less responsive instrument control.

with initially, this is the key to coordinated colonoscope control, whereas ''two-man'' colonoscopy can too easily result in over-enthusiastic pushing by the assistant and unnecessary loops. The rotational elements of colonoscope control are important, both in the economic ''corkscrew'' steering movements that it allows around bends, especially in the sigmoid colon, and for the torsional control that is often possible so as to minimize loop formation. The three dimensional, often spiral, nature of clonic looping has been described above, and it is inherent in a spiral loop that torsion one way will tend to straighten it, whereas the other way will worsen the loop. Because the sigmoid colon classically spirals clockwise to reach out of the pelvic brim in the midline and across to the descending colon in the left side of the abdomen, a clockwise twist (called torque when sustained) is predictably the most often useful, both in propelling the instrument tip into the descending colon and in avoiding excessive sigmoid colon looping as the instrument pushes inward. Obviously once torque is applied to the shaft to help control a loop, corkscrewing movements of the tip for steering purposes (especially if in the opposite direction to the required torque) will be counterproductive and allow relooping.

A good measure of ''single-handed'' expertise is to be aware of the number of times that the lateral control knob is used—the less the better, for this means that the right hand is successfully managing rotational steering movements so that the three-dimensional potential of colonoscope control will become apparent, and the endoscopist will start to *feel* the shaft. The ability of the endoscopist to feel with the right hand the colonoscope shaft as it loops or straightens against colonic attachments and, simultaneously, with the left hand to appreciate the degree of control knob angulation brings a new level of feedback subtlety to the technique. Those that believe they cannot manage ''single-handed'' colonoscopy are usually holding the control body wrong, often failing to use the left middle finger as ''helper'' to the thumb in angulation (Fig. 6-4) or mistakenly using both

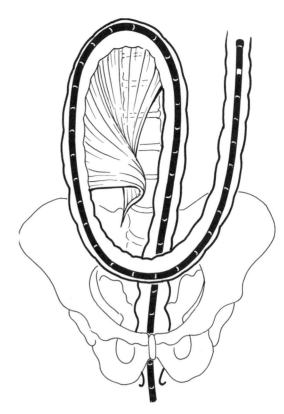

Figure 6-5. The ''alpha'' loop is a beneficial clockwise spiral configuration because it allows the instrument to reach the splenic flexure without acute bends.

the forefinger and the middle finger unnecessarily to activate the air, water, and suction buttons (rather than the forefinger alone).

Shaft-looping and straightening of the sigmoid colon, usually of a spiral nature, can always be straightened out and controlled when the proximal descending colon or splenic flexure are reached, and often before then. The most extreme spiral loop is the ''alpha'' configuration (Fig. 6-5), which can occur spontaneously if the sigmoid colon is long enough. Alpha loop formation can be guessed-at if the instrument is obviously looping, but there is no acute angulation, so no hold-up or excessive pain while the tip runs up into the fluid-filled descending colon to the splenic flexure, which is reached at 90 cm with the loop in position. If the sigmoid colon is less generous, or if the colonoscope tip happens not to deviate across toward the cecum, a modified spiral or ''N'' loop will result, the prime consequence being an acute iatrogenic ''hairpin'' bend at the sigmoid-descending colon junction (Fig. 6-6). Trying to force through this acute bend with the N loop in position, rather than having the patience and dexterity to straighten out the colonoscope by withdrawal or to maneuver it into a more favorable configuration, is the most frequent mistake in this most difficult area for the colonoscopist.

The splenic flexure, once reached, is the halfway stage of colonoscopy. This is the moment to regain control of the instrument by pulling back the shaft to 50 cm insertion—sometimes only to 40 cm if the splenic flexure is mobile on its attachments. This vigorous pullback movement, usually with a simultaneous

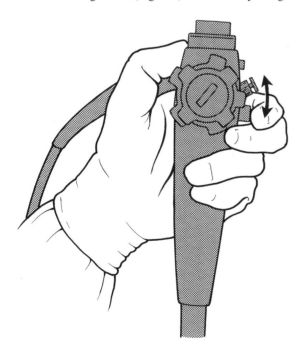

Figure 6-4. The middle finger has an important role as ''helper'' to the thumb on the angulation wheels.

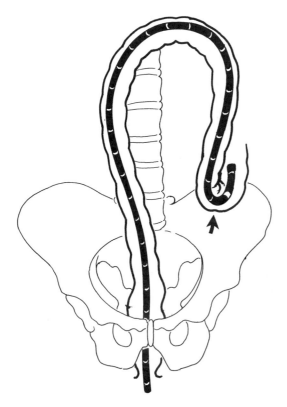

Figure 6-6. The "N" spiral loop causes an acute iatrogenic hairpin bend at the sigmoid-descending colon.

clockwise twist, straightens the shaft and can be felt to restore the subtlety of control, which is essential before passing to the proximal colon. If a sigmoid loop remains it will usually make things increasingly difficult and friction limited for the rest of the procedure.

Position change from left lateral to supine or right lateral position, smoothes out the splenic flexure usefully[46] if it proves too acutely angulated to pass easily. Conversely, change back to left lateral position will usually help somewhat in passing from the proximal transverse into the hepatic flexure, partly by causing the transverse and hepatic flexure to flop downward and also by allowing air aspiration to collapse and shorten the capacious proximal colon. Position changes are particularly, sometimes unpredictably, helpful in patients with "difficult" and long colons, where small gravitational changes in configuration can greatly improve the interaction between endoscope and colon, which is the basis of gentle colonoscopy.

Abdominal pressure is another very useful adjunct during colonoscopy.[46,47] Often it is simply used to reduce the antero-posterior diameter of the lower abdominal cavity, so reducing the space available in which the sigmoid colon can loop, or compress the loop somewhat ("nonspecific pressure"). At other times the assistant or the examiner can feel the shaft looping and oppose it, or empirically press against different sites in the abdomen until the tip is seen to advance, and then select the best site for continued "specific" pressure. Generally speaking hand pressure is only effective in colons with a markedly three-dimensional configuration in which the sigmoid and transverse loop anteriorly against the anterior abdominal wall. Such colons

are usually also among the most difficult to intubate and even modest help from assistant hand pressure can be very helpful.

The hepatic flexure is frequently a problem to those who have not straightened out the distal colon, who are forced to use aggression in order to try to pass through the grossly looped colon. If, by contrast, the sigmoid colon has been straightened there may still be a deep "down and up" loop through the transverse colon, requiring some force, but this will rapidly be straightened out on pulling back again. Several quite vigorous push and pull movements may be required to pass through a long transverse colon, almost akin to the movements used by a trombonist. Once the tip has nearly reached the hepatic flexure however, a combination of aspiration, assistant hand pressure (often in the left hypochondrium or epigastrium, an example of "specific" hand pressure),[47] and careful steering will usually reach to and pass the hepatic flexure more rapidly and easily than any amount of force. Useful adjunctive measures at this point include *counter*clockwise twist (to raise the splenic flexure anteriorly) and patient inspiration (to lower the diaphragm transiently).

The ileocecal region, not infrequently somewhat poorly prepared and requiring irrigation because it is a "cul de sac," is the endoscopists' goal in colonoscopy. The ileocecal valve is often best located from afar, as a slight bulge or flattening on the last fold, which is accentuated into a more obvious bulge or even bubbles as the colon is deflated. Angling carefully toward the valve bulge and aspirating further, preferably with the forceps already in position if histology is needed, will either allow the instrument tip to enter through the slit and into the ileum, or at least give a blind biopsy. The most common error at this stage is to thrash around too near the cecal pole, for the valve slit is several centimeters back from the pole and often best entered as the angulated tip is pulled backward; the villi of the ileal mucosa in close-up appear granular compared to the shiny colon surface. This appearance is the indication to insufflate a little and cautiously search out the luminal direction of the ileum.

EXAMINATION OF THE COLON

Even the 130° wide-angle lens of modern endoscopes cannot see all areas of the colon surface without active steering by the endoscopist, not least because of the haustral folds, acute angulations, and convolutions in the colon, but also due to the pools of fluid or bubbles that remain. Suitable use of irrigating fluid, silicone-particle "antifoam" suspension, and aspiration will help to clear the surface, but changes of posture are also useful. Turning the patient to supine or partially to the right side, gives much better views of the splenic flexure and descending colon (as is routine for the radiologist during barium enema). The principal requirement for accurate examination is commitment to quality and mental discipline on the part of the endoscopist; it requires integrity, dexterity, and effort to scour around with the instrument tip in order to see the numerous potential "blind spots" as well as possible, and even so probably 5% to 10% of the mucosal surface is not seen.[48]

Retroversion of the tip is often possible in a capacious ascending colon, as well as in the rectum, which can be important in patients with multiple polyps or unexplained blood loss. Naked eye examination alone is insufficient to exclude inflammatory disease in those with bowel frequency or diarrhea; both active "microscopic" colitis (ulcerative or Crohn's)[49] or the burnt-out equivalent "collagenous colitis"[50] are absolutely invisible to the endoscopist, but obvious to a skilled histopathologist on biopsy. Similarly it is possible to have any degree of cellular atypia (dysplasia) present even in normal-looking mucosa after long-standing ulcerative colitis; therefore, biopsies are essential.[51,52]

With these exceptions, however, most endoscopic interpretation is reasonably obvious, even though histopathologic confirmation and video print or video tape documentation are wise. Certain appearances are visually diagnostic, such as bright red telangiectases or angiodysplasia. The discrete "aphthoid ulcers" of Crohn's disease, on a background of normal submucosal vessel pattern, cannot be mistaken for the more general mucosal abnormality in ulcerative colitis—although when there is chronic extensive damage and some surface ulceration it may be impossible for the endoscopist to differentiate between the two. Sometimes physical characteristics are important; shiny soft mucosal tags or a wide-open atrophic ileocecal valve are evidence of previous inflammatory disease; firmness or fixity of a polyp (to prodding with the forceps or closed polypectomy snare) warn of possible infiltration or malignancy. Appearances can also be misleading; endoscope tip or stretch trauma, sometimes transmitted between loops, can mimic inflammatory change and mucosal redness may be due to hyperemic blood vessels of healed colitis rather than active inflammation.

POLYPS AND POLYPECTOMY

Most polyps require removal,[53,54] but there are exceptions. Post-inflammatory mucosal tags have been mentioned, and are harmless. Soft, shiny lipomas in the proximal colon show the typical "cushion sign" when prodded with forceps, and a yellow-white fatty interior if biopsied repeatedly at the same point or partially snared; full-snare polypectomy of lipomas is unnecessary and potentially hazardous.[55,56] The 1 to 3 mm typical "dew drop" or "disappearing" hyperplastic (metaplastic) polyps of the distal rectum are a normal finding[57] of no more consequence than freckles on the skin. Polypoid bumps in the terminal ileum are lymphoid aggregations of hypertrophic follicles, and are normal, especially in younger subjects.

Small polyps from the midrectum to the cecum usually need to be destroyed and removed.[58–60] Snaring is mechanically the most efficient way and the "minisnare" most convenient for polyps under 1 cm. Some endoscopists remove those under 5 mm by physical "cold snaring"[31] to avoid the small possibility of delayed hemorrhage. For polyps up to 5 mm in diameter (with the exception of patients taking aspirin or NSAIDs, whose greater bleeding tendency[61,62] indicates snaring) we prefer the convenience of simultaneous destruction and sampling using hot-biopsy forceps.[58,63] The principle of hot biopsy is to obtain a satisfactory biopsy because the forceps' low-resistance metallic jaws are unheated, whereas, because the polyp has been tented-up onto a "pseudo-pedicle", a 1 to 2-second low-power current selectively heats and destroys the feeding vessels to the remnant. Only brief heating and minor whitening (the "Mount Fuji" effect) is needed, because any heat subsequently causes a remarkably large necrotic ulcer and a danger of substantial

bleeding 1 to 10 days later if there happens to be an arteriole underneath.

If 10 or more small polyps are visible it is sensible to think of the possibility of familial adenomatous polyposis (FAP) and to look for (and biopsy) other even smaller polyps. These can be seen as bumps against the shiny "light reflex" of the transparent mucosal surface, or can be more obviously highlighted for biopsy or imaging purposes by surface dyeing[64] with a nonabsorbable color contrast agent such as indigo-carmine (0.1%) or diluted washable blue pen ink. With dye-spray any polyps will show up as small pink islands, but lymphoid follicles also stand out, so biopsy confirmation is important before diagnosing FAP.

Large-stalked polyps (2 cm or greater) require care to avoid bleeding, or full-thickness damage, either of which can be immediate or delayed.[65,66] Thick-stalked pedunculated polyps are less of a problem, unless the stalk is very short, in which case they are sometimes best treated as sessile and removed piecemeal for safety's sake. Longer stalks give the potential, before or after transection as judged appropriate, to reduce the chance of bleeding by adrenaline injection, placement of a nylon self-retaining loop (Endo loop, Olympus), or simply by resnaring lower down the stalk to recoagulate without transection in order to maximize local heat effect, swelling, and resultant vessel compression. If bleeding does occur from a stalk, the snare loop should rapidly be closed over the basal remnant and the snare handle physically taped shut for approximately 5 minutes, by which time coagulation is likely to have occurred. Local adrenaline injection can also be made, with a separate endoscope passed alongside the first one on the rare occasion that the snare loop cannot be released without bleeding.

Sessile polyps up to about 1 cm in diameter will usually bunch up in the snare as it closes, and can then be removed as if stalked. Between 1 and 1.5 cm there is still a potential to remove a sessile lesion in one portion, but the trick is to preinject into the submucosa below it with saline or saline-adrenaline mixture so as to elevate the polyp onto a "safety cushion."[67] When polyp diameter is more than 1.5 cm "injection polypectomy" may still be a good option to avoid full-thickness damage and the "post polypectomy syndrome" of threatened or actual perforation.[18,66] When trying to ring a larger sessile polyp with submucosal injections for this purpose, the trick is to start injection proximal to the polyp, so that the view is not lost when the polyp margin elevates; insert the needle into the margin of each successive bleb until 10 to 30 cc have been introduced underneath the polyp. Thereafter actual piecemeal removal should be cautious, because it is better to end up with 5 to 15 smaller bits than to risk complications. Equally it is better to stop snaring and complete polypectomy at a subsequent visit if there seems to be difficulty, excessive heat effects, or the patient experiences any warning peritoneal heat pain. On the rather rare occasions that threatened or actual perforation occurs an endoscopically aware surgeon should be involved; there is no need for "knee-jerk" surgery, conservative management often being adequate if the defect is likely to be small.[68]

The limit for endoscopic removal of large sessile polyps depends on a number of factors, including the expertise (and motivation) of the endoscopist, in relation always to the clinical state and interests of the patient. As a general rule it is unlikely that a lesion over about 5 cm diameter will be endoscopically removable, but it has also been said that involvement of more than one-third of the bowel circumference or extension over two haustral folds is a contraindication in practice.[54] The possible interrelationship with laparoscopic management could change criteria, however, because endoscopy has the obvious disadvantages of usually requiring multiple visits, as well as producing multiple fragmented specimens.

Recovery of specimens can be with a wire "polyp retrieval basket," or by catching a few of the larger fragments in the polypectomy snare, filling the colon proximal to the area with at least 500 ml of tap water (and extra air as judged safe) before withdrawing the instrument, administering a phosphate enema, and recovering fragments from the commode or bed pan.

Tattooing the area adjacent to a sessile or possibly malignant polyp with 1-ml aliquots of India ink[69] can be invaluable for quick and accurate subsequent location or localization. By pre-injecting to raise a saline bleb, and then switching syringes to 10% dilution of water-soluble black ink (carbon particles in aqueous suspension, preferably sterilized) messy leakage can be minimized. If surgery or laparoscopic management are likely several larger tattoos should be made to ensure an obvious view from the serosal aspect.[70]

Other therapeutic maneuvers are possible during colonoscopy. Tube placement can relieve ileus or pseudo-obstruction (transchannel, over a guide wire,[71] or pulled up alongside with a breakable and releasable thread beside the endoscope).[72] Angiodysplasias can be coagulated with argon beam, heater probe, laser, or careful use of hot forceps (no biopsy).[73-75] Balloon dilatation of strictures with water-filled balloons,[76] usually through-the-scope (TTS), which ideally requires a large-channel instrument, should use generous silicone fluid prelubrication and a carefully deflated and furled balloon to allow good "feel" as the balloon passes in. A 5-cm balloon is ideal and 1.8-cm diameter is generally safe and effective; smaller and shorter balloons may be needed for awkward strictures or small-channel instruments. For longer, uncertain, or awkwardly placed strictures combined management with a radiologist is wise, allowing soluble-contrast views and use of a guide wire if a necessary for added safety. Some weblike anastomotic narrowings can be cut with a "needle-knife"[77] or the point of the snare and some low strictures can be managed with dilating bougies inserted over a guide wire.[78,79]

FUTURE STRATEGIES

As flexible endoscopy is increasingly used for mass screening and "walk in-walk out" well-patient surveillance, there are implications for logistics and quality control. Logistically it is inevitable that more doctors must become adept and probably that nurse-endoscopists will have a role for flexible sigmoidoscopy at least. Teaching and certifying hand skills should be on a more objective basis than at present and we believe that micro computer simulation will be useful for this.[80,81]

Another probably useful adjunct should be the electromagnetic imager,[82,83] in which small electrical position-sensing coils within the endoscope give real-time images of tip position and shaft-looping on-screen. Preliminary experience[84] suggests that this technology will help experts in difficult cases and speed skills acquisition in the learning phase for less-experienced endoscopists. It will also eliminate errors of diagnostic localization.

Computer databases are widely used to administer surveillance and audit performance overall but image archiving should provide another means of quality control. Endoscopists aware that the videotaped record of the quality and extent of any examination may be randomly selected for review, and compared to the report issued, are likely to keep their standards high.

Combining the technologies for audit and assessment purposes it should be apparent which endoscopists oversedate, overloop, or underreport. Theoretically it should even be possible to retrain (and certify) those that need it in "virtual reality."

REFERENCES

1. Dodd G D (1991) Imaging techniques in the diagnosis of carcinoma of the colon. Cancer 67:1150–1154
2. Norfleet R G, Ryan M E, Wyman J B et al (1991) Barium enema versus colonoscopy for patients with polyps found during flexible sigmoidoscopy. Gastrointest Endosc 37:531–534
3. Lindsay D C, Freeman J G, Cobden I, Record C O (1988) Should colonoscopy be the first investigation for colonic disease? BMJ 16:167–169
4. Irvine E J, O'Connor J, Frost R A et al (1988) Prospective comparison of double contrast barium enema plus flexible sigmoidoscopy versus colonoscopy in rectal bleeding: barium enema versus colonoscopy in rectal bleeding. Gut 29:1188–1193
5. Anderson N, Cook B H, Coates R (1991) Colonoscopically detected colorectal cancer missed on barium enema. Gastrointest Radiol 16:123–127
6. Waye J D, Bashkoff E (1991) Total colonoscopy: is it always possible. Gastrointest Endosc 37:152–154
7. Habr-Gama A, Waye J D (1989) Complications and hazards of Gastrointestinal endoscopy. World J Surg 13:193–201
8. Hart R, Classen M (1990) Complications of diagnostic gastrointestinal endoscopy. Endoscopy 22:229–233
9. Hancock J H, Talbot R W (1995) Accuracy of colonoscopy in the localisation of colorectal cancer. Int J Colorect Dis 10:140–141
10. Frager D H, Frager J D, Wolf E L, Beneventano T C (1987) Problems in the colonoscopic localization of tumours: continued value of the barium enema. Gastrointest Radiol 12:343–346
11. VanNess M M, Chobanian S J, Winters C et al (1987) A study of patient acceptance of double-contrast barium enema and colonoscopy—which procedure is preferred by patients? Arch Intern Med 147:2175–2176
12. Saunders B P, Halligan S, Jobling C, et al (1995) Can barium enema indicate when colonoscopy will be difficult? Clin Radiol 50:318–321
13. Rex D K, Weddle R A, Lehman G A et al (1990) Flexible sigmoidoscopy plus air contrast barium enema versus colonoscopy for suspected lower gastrointestinal bleeding. Gastroenterology 98:855–861
14. Eckardt V F, Kanzler G, Willems D (1989) Same-day versus

separate-day sigmoidoscopy and double contrast barium enema: a randomised controlled study. Gastrointest Endosc 35: 512–515

15. Saito Y, Slezak P, Rubio C (1989) The diagnostic value of combining flexible sigmoidoscopy and double contrast barium enema as a one-stage procedure. Gastrointest Radiol 14: 357–359

16. Nivatvongs S (1988) Complications in colonoscopic polypectomy: lessons to learn from an experience with 1576 polyps. Am Surg 54:61–63

17. Keefe E B (1994) Determinants of safe endoscopy. Gastrointest Endosc 40:379–382

18. Macrae F A, Tan K G, Williams C B (1981) Towards safer colonoscopy: a report on the complications of 5000 diagnostic or therapeutic colonoscopies. Gut 24:376–383

19. Colarian J, Alousi M, Calzada R (1991) Splenic trauma during colonoscopy. Endoscopy 23:48–49

20. Merchant A A, Cheng E H (1990) Delayed splenic rupture after colonoscopy. Am J Gastroenterol 85:906–907

21. Rockey D C, Weber J R, Wright T L, Wall S D (1990) Splenic injury following colonoscopy. Gastrointest Endosc 36: 306–309

22. Ehrlich C P, Hall F M, Joffe N (1984) Postendoscopic perforation of normal colon in an area remote from instrumentation—with secondary tension pneumoperitoneum. Gastrointest Endosc 30:190–211

23. Rossini F P, Ferrari A, Spandre M, Coverlizza S (1982) Colonoscopic polypectomy in diagnosis and management of cancerous adenomas: an individual and multicentric experience. Endoscopy 14:124–217

24. Koltun W A, Coller J A (1991) Incarceration of colonoscope in an inguinal hernia ''pulley'' technique of removal. Dis Colon Rectum 34:191–193

25. Saunders M P (1995) Colonoscope incarceration within an inguinal hernia: a cautionary tale. Br J Clin Pathol 49:157–158

26. Phaosawasdi K, Cooley W, Wheeler J, Wheeler (1986) Carbon dioxide-insufflated colonoscopy: an ignored superior technique. Gastrointest Endosc 32:330–333

27. Hussein A M T, Bartram C I, Williams C B (1984) Carbon dioxide insufflation for more comfortable colonoscopy: Gastrointest Endosc 30:68–70

28. Hickson D E G, Cox J G C, Taylor R G, Bennett J R (1990) Enema or Picolax as preparation for flexible sigmoidoscopy? Postgrad Med J 66:210–211

29. Saunders B P, Elsby B, Boswell A M et al (1995) Intravenous antispasmodic and patient-controlled analgesia are of benefit for screening flexible sigmoidoscopy. Gastrointest Endosc 42: 123–127

30. Smith L E (1985) Flexible fiberoptic sigmoidoscopy: an office procedure. Can J Surg 28:233–236

31. Tappero G, Gaja E, Degiuli P et al (1992) Cold snare excision of small colorectal polyps. Gastrointest Endosc 38:310–313

32. Saunders B P, Phillips R K S, Williams C B (1995) Intraoperative measurement of colonic anatomy and attachments with relevance to colonoscopy. Br J Surg 82:1491–1493

33. Saunders B P, Masaki T, Sawada T et al (1995) A peroperative comparison of Western and Oriental colonic anatomy and mesenteric attachments. Int J Colorectal Dis 10:216–221

34. Kolts B E, Lyles W E, Achem S R et al (1993) A comparison of the effectiveness and patient tolerance of oral sodium phosphate, castor oil and standard electrolyte lavage for colonoscopy or sigmoidoscopy preparation. Am J Gastroenterol 88: 1218–1223

35. Davis G R, Santa-Ana C A (1979) Development of a lavage solution with minimal water and electrolyte absorption and secretion. Gastroenterology 78:991–995

36. Fordtran J S, Santa-Ana C A, Cleveland M B (1990) A low-sodium solution for gastrointestinal lavage. Gastroenterology 98:11–16

37. Mark J S, Spiro H (1990) Informed consent for colonoscopy: a prospective study. Arch Intern Med 150:777–780

38. Rosch T (1987) Fractional cleansing of the large bowel with 'Golytely' for colonoscopic preparation: a controlled trial. Endoscopy 19:198–200

39. Roe A M, Jamieson M H, Maclennan I (1984) Colonoscopy preparation with Picolax. J R Coll Surg Ed 29:103–114

40. Golub R W, Kerner B A, Wise JNR et al (1995) Colonoscopic bowel preparations—which one? Dis Colon Rectum 38: 594–599

41. Cohen S M, Wexner S D, Binderow S R et al (1994) Prospective, randomised, endoscopic-blinded trial comparing precolonoscopy bowel cleansing methods. Dis Colon Rectum 37: 689–696

42. Clarkston W K, Tsen T N, Dies D F et al (1996) Oral sodium phosphate versus sulfate-free polyethylene glycol electrolyte lavage solution in outpatient peparation for colonoscopy: a prospective comparison. Gastrointest Endosc 43:42–48

43. Salmon P, Shah R, Berg S, Williams C B (1994) Evaluating customer satisfaction with colonoscopy. Endoscopy 26: 342–346

44. Keeffe E B (1995) Sedation and analgesia for endoscopy. Gastroenterology 106:932–933

45. Carlsson U, Grattidge P: (1995) Sedation for upper gastrointestinal endoscopy: a comparative study of propofol and midazolam. Endoscopy 27:240–243

46. Cotton P B, Williams C B (1996) Practical Gastrointestinal Endoscopy. 4th Ed. Blackwell Scientific, Oxford

47. Waye J D, Yessayan S A, Lewis B S, Fabry T L (1991) The technique of abdominal pressure in total colonoscopy. Gastrointest Endosc 37:147–151

48. Waye J D, Braunfeld S (1982) Surveillance intervals after polypectomy. Endoscopy 14:79–81

49. Kingham J G C, Levison D A, Ball J A, Dawson A M (1982) Microscopic colitis—a cause of chronic watery diarrhoea. BMJ 285:1601–1604

50. Danzi J T, McDonald T J, King J (1988) Collagenous colitis. Am J Gastroenterol 83:83–85

51. Connell W R, Lennard Jones J E, Talbot I C et al (1994) Factors affecting the outcome of endoscopic surveillance for cancer in ulcerative colitis. Gastroenterology 107:934–944

52. Grandqvist S, Granberg-Ohman I, Sundeline P (1990) Colonoscopic biopsies and cytological examination in chronic ulcreative colitis. Mater Med Pol 283–328

53. Winawer S J, Zauber A G, May Nah Ho M S (1993) Prevention of colorectal cancer by colonoscopic polypectomy. N Engl J Med 329:1977–1981

54. Waye J D (1991) Endoscopic treatment of adenomas. World J Surg 15:14–19

55. Pfeil S A, Weaver M G, Abdul-Karim F W, Yang P (1990)

Colonic lipomas: outcome of endoscopic removal. Gastrointest Endosc 36:435–438

56. Renda A, Coppola L, Lepore R et al (1990) Lipoma of the sigmoid: late perforation following polypectomy. Colo-Proctology 6:374–376

57. Waye J D, Bilotta J J (1990) Rectal hyperplastic polyps: now you see them, now you don't—a differential point. Am J Gastroenterol 85:1557–1559

58. Williams C B (1991) Small polyps—the virtues and dangers of hot biopsy. Gastrointest Endosc 37:394–395

59. Church J M, Fazio V W, Jones I T (1988) Small colorectal polyps: are they worth treating? Dis Col Rectum 31:50–53

60. Waye J D, Lewis B S, Frankel A, Geller S A (1988) Small colon polyps. Am J Gastroenterol 83:120–122

61. Dyer W S, Quigley E M M, Noel S M et al (1991) Case report: major colonic haemorrhage following electrocoagulating (hot) biopsy of diminutive colonic polyps: relationship to colonic location and low-dose aspirin therapy. Gastrointest Endosc 37: 361–364

62. Wadas D D, Sanowski R A (1987) Complications of the hot biopsy forceps technique. Gastrointest Endosc 33:32–37

63. Williams C B (1973) Diathermy-biopsy: a technique for the endoscopic management of small polyps. Endoscopy 5: 215–228

64. Tada M, Katoh S, Kohli Y, Kawai K (1976) On the dye spraying method in colonofiberoscopy. Endoscopy 8:70–74

65. Nivatvongs S (1986) Complications in colonoscopic polypectomy. An experience with 1555 polypectomies. Dis Col Rectum 29:825–830

66. Waye J D, Lewis B S, Yessayan S (1992) Colonoscopy: a prospective report of complications. J Clin Gastroenterol 15: 1–4

67. Waye J D (1994) Saline injection colonoscopic polypectomy. Am J Gastroenterol 89:305–306

68. Christie J P, Marrazzo J (1991) "Mini-perforation" of the colon—not all postpolypectomy perforations require laparotomy. Dis Colon Rectum 34:132–135

69. Ponsky J L, King J F (1975) Endoscopic marking of colonic lesions. Gastrointest Endosc 22:42–43

70. Hyman N, Waye J D (1991) Endoscopic four quadrant tattoo for the identification of colonic lesions at surgery. Gastrointest Endosc 37:56–58

71. Messmer J M, Wolper J C, Loewe C J (1984) Endoscopic-assisted tube placement for acute colonic pseudo-obstruction. Endoscopy 16:135–216

72. Sariego J, Matsumoto T, Kerstein M D (1991) Colonoscopically guided tube decompression in Ogilvie's syndrome. Dis Colon Rectum 34:720–722

73. Kheterpal S (1991) Angiodysplasia: a review. J R Soc Med 84:615–618

74. Gupta N, Longo W E, Vernava III A M (1995) Angiodysplasia of the lower gastrointestinal tract: an entity readily diagnosed by colonoscopy and primarily managed nonoperatively. Dis Colon Rectum 38:979–982

75. Danesh B J Z, Spiliadis C, Williams C B, Zambartas C M (1987) Angiodysplasia—an uncommon cause of colonic bleeding; colonoscopic evaluation of 1,050 patients with rectal bleeding and anaemia. Int J Colorect Dis 2:218–222

76. Couckuty H, Gevers A M, Coremans G et al (1995) Efficacy and safety of hydrostatic balloon dilatation of ileocolonic Crohn's strictures: a prospective longterm analysis. Gut 36: 577–580

77. Oz M C, Forde K A (1990) Endoscopic alternatives in the management of colonic strictures. Surgery 108:513–519

78. Bedogni G, Ricci E, Pedrazzoli C (1987) Endoscopic dilation of anastomotic colonic stenosis by different techniques: an alternative to surgery? Gastrointest Endosc 33:21–24

79. Fregonese D, Di Falco G, Di Toma F (1990) Balloon dilatation of anastomotic intestinal stenoses: long-term results. Endoscopy 22:249–253

80. Baillie J, Jowell P, Evangelou H et al (1991) Use of computer graphics simulation for teaching of flexible sigmoidoscopy. Endoscopy 23:126–129

81. Rey J-F, Romanczk T (1995) The development of experimental models in the teaching of endoscopy: an overview. Endoscopy 27:101–105

82. Bladen J S, Anderson A P, Bell G D, Heatley D J: (1996) Non radiological technique for three-dimensional imaging of endoscopes. Lancet 341:719–722

83. Williams C B, Guy C, Gillies D F, Saunders B P (1993) Electronic three-dimensional imaging of intestinal endoscopy. Lancet 341:724–725

84. Saunders B P, Bell G D, Williams C B et al (1995) First clinical results with a real-time electronic imager as an aid to colonoscopy. Gut 36:913–917

7

IMAGING

CONTRAST STUDIES AND ULTRASOUND

Clive I. Bartram
Stephen Halligan

CONTRAST STUDIES

Soft tissue differentiation is limited on plain films, so that the colon is visualized only by gas remaining within the lumen, or trapped in fecal residue. Some radiopaque agent is needed to outline the mucosa surface to visualize colonic detail. Since about 1910, barium sulfate has been the contrast agent of choice for this purpose. There are two methods of examination: single or double contrast. In the single-contrast barium enema (SCBE) a low concentration suspension is used to fill the colon. Views in different projections demonstrate the configuration of the colon. Fine mucosal detail may be seen at the edge of the bowel, where the beam is tangential to the barium suspension. Lesions are visible en face only when large enough to reduce absorption of the beam sufficiently to register on the film. This limitation may be overcome to a certain extent by compressing the bowel where possible, and by taking an after-evacuation film of the emptied contracted colon. The double-contrast barium enema (DCBE), developed in the 1960s, uses gas, which is radiolucent, to distend the barium-filled bowel. This leaves a thin coating of barium suspension on the mucosal surface (Fig. 7-1), which gives fine mucosal detail both tangential and en face of both sides of the bowel wall.[1]

DOUBLE-CONTRAST BARIUM ENEMA

Double contrast is more accurate than single contrast for the diagnosis of small polyps and early colitis. Whatever technique is used, good bowel preparation is essential[2] because retained residue degrades the accuracy of the DCBE. The colon also needs to be relatively dry for double contrast, as retained fluid impairs coating. Purgation should therefore be undertaken some hours beforehand, with a short period of fluid restriction prior to examination.

The examination takes only 15 minutes. The patient is given an intravenous smooth muscle relaxant, such as 20 mg of hyoscine butylbromide, barium is run into the transverse colon, and the colon is distended by gas, preferably carbon dioxide. This is reabsorbed rapidly, preventing abdominal cramps and prolonged distension.[3] The patient is turned under fluoroscopic guidance to manipulate the barium column around the bowel under gravity, and gas insufflated for adequate colonic distension. Multiple digital spot films of bowel segments in double contrast without excess barium pooling enable a composite picture of the colon to be built up. This may be supplemented by overhead films, such as the lateral decubitus views where the x-ray tube is horizontal and the patient lies on his or her side. Barium pooling is unavoidable. With the patient supine/prone, the suspension may spread along long lengths of bowel, and the x-ray beam will always be directed down onto the barium surface. It is only in the erect and decubitus views that the beam cuts across the barium/gas level. This allows double-contrast views of parts of the bowel that may be impossible to obtain in other positions. Digital technology has allowed a dramatic reduction in radiation dosage[4] compared with conventional films, with the result that the DCBE is no longer a high-dose examination.

In the DCBE the barium layer coating the mucosa is only about 0.2 mm thick. The thin line, where the x-ray beam strikes the bowel wall tangentially, is called the *mucosal line*. En face the coating should be smooth and even. Normal variants sometimes seen are the innominate groove pattern or lymphoid follicles. Abnormal patterns reflect the presence of either depressed (ulcers) or elevated (polyps) mucosal lesions.

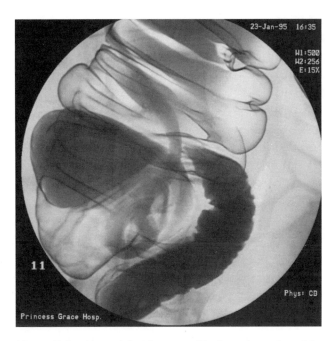

Figure 7-1. Normal double-contrast barium enema view of the cecum. Note the smooth even coating over the mucosa, with the mucosal line visible tangentially. There is a little pooling of barium in between dependent haustral folds. Reflux has occurred into a normal terminal ileum and appendix. This is a digital spot view, where barium has been set to be black instead of white as it is on normal radiographs.

Superficial erosions in early colitis create a granular surface (Fig. 7-2). Larger mucosal defects (i.e., ulcers), create defined depressed areas that fill with barium. Ulcers vary in configuration. Aphthoid ulcers (Fig. 7-3) have a thin black ring where the barium coats poorly over the erythematous surrounding, and a rather dense center where barium precipitates in slough at the ulcer base. The intervening mucosa is normal and the lesions so shallow that there is no projection from the mucosal line. As the ulcer enlarges, barium tends to just the rim of the crater, as it falls out of the center unless the ulcer is on the dependent

Figure 7-2. Granular mucosa in ulcerative colitis.

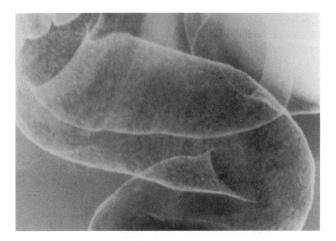

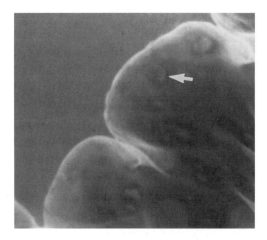

Figure 7-3. Aphthoid ulcers in Crohn's disease.

wall (Fig. 7-4). Ulcers may be longitudinal or transverse in orientation, and linear, serpiginous, or rounded in shape. Tangentially the ulcer is seen projecting into the bowel wall from the mucosal line, often undercutting the mucosa to produce a "T" shape (Fig. 7-5).

Elevated lesions, such as polyps, create a meniscus around the base of the lesion. The meniscus has a sharp inner border where it abuts the edge of the polyp, and a poorly defined outer border where it tapers out into the normal mucosal coating (Fig. 7-6). This is clearly seen when the polyp is viewed end on. When viewed obliquely, the meniscus with a thin layer coating the surface of the polyp produces the classic "bowler hat" sign. The stalk of a pedunculated polyp may be seen as two parallel lines (Fig. 7-7). Irregularity at the base of a sessile polyp suggests early malignancy (Fig. 7-8). An irregular menisceal line denotes the edge of an elevated lesion, such as a plaquelike carcinoma. Distinguishing abnormal lines from the normal ones

Figure 7-4. Larger ulcers in Crohn's disease. The barium has fallen out of the ulcer crater, which is outlined by the rim only (arrow).

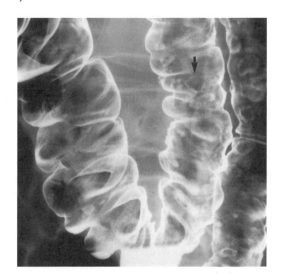

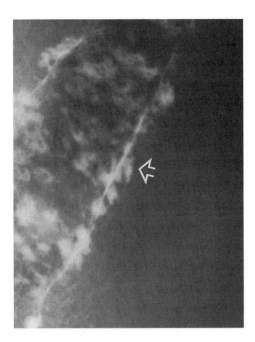

Figure 7-5. Ulcerative colitis in an acute attack with ulceration. Note the undercutting of the ulcers projecting from the mucosal line (arrowhead).

Figure 7-6. Small flat villous adenoma in the descending colon. Meniscus at the edge of the elevated lesion is clearly visible (arrowhead).

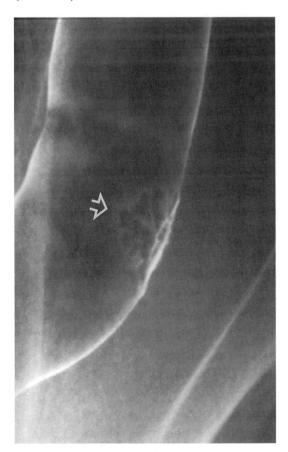

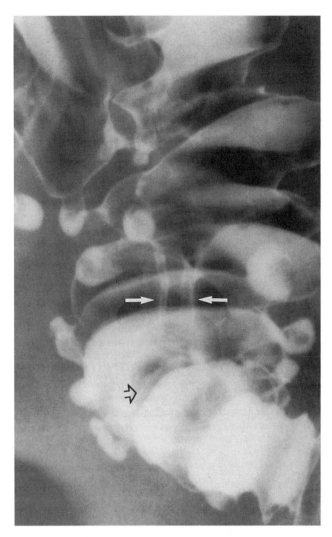

Figure 7-7. Pedunculated polyp in diverticular disease with parallel lines along the stalk (white arrows) and the head creating a filling defect in the barium pool (black arrow).

at flexures or haustral folds is the key to the diagnosis of neoplasia (Fig. 7-9).

Some excess barium is unavoidable, and will pool in the dependent segments of bowel. Small polyps on the dependent wall will be hidden within the pool; larger lesions on the nondependent wall may be outlined in double contrast, but obscured by the radiographically dense pool on the dependent side. Conversely, where compression is possible, as in the sigmoid and cecum, the barium pool may be used to confirm that a lesion is intraluminal (Fig. 7-10).

The two components of diverticular disease, thickened pleated folds in the sigmoid and diverticula, are demonstrated. Diverticula may fill completely or partially with barium, when fluid levels will be seen on erect or decubitus views. Smooth muscle tone affects opening of the necks of the diverticula. It is common for more diverticula to fill as the examination progresses.

Mural lesions, such as lipoma, leiomyoma, or pneumatosis coli (Fig. 7-11), have a smooth surface because the covering is

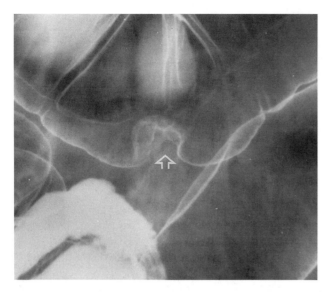

Figure 7-8. Malignant sessile polyp 1 cm in size with an irregular indrawn base (arrowhead).

normal mucosa. There is no meniscus as the lesion tapers into normal bowel.

Extrinsic disease, such as secondary carcinoma (Fig. 7-12) or endometriosis, produces a mass effect deforming the bowel wall. A desmoplastic response within the bowel wall to cellular infiltration produces localized contraction with pleating of mucosal folds.

The accuracy of the DCBE has been the subject of a number of studies. It is not as accurate as colonoscopy in detecting early colitis, as vascular changes may be present endoscopically

Figure 7-9. Irregular lines (arrows) around the edge of polypoid carcinoma in the transverse colon.

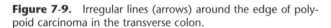

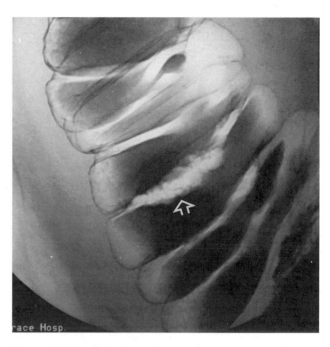

Figure 7-10. Flat villous adenoma running along a haustral fold (arrow) seen as a filling defect in the shallow barium pools within the haustral folds.

Figure 7-11. Pneumatosis coli. Smooth mural gas cysts present in the redundant sigmoid. Air within the cysts is seen tangentially (arrow), confirming pneumatosis.

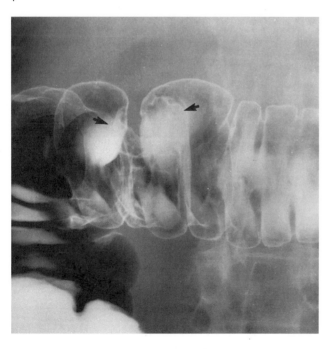

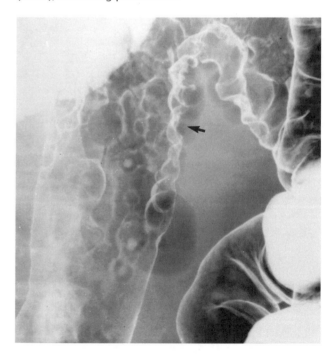

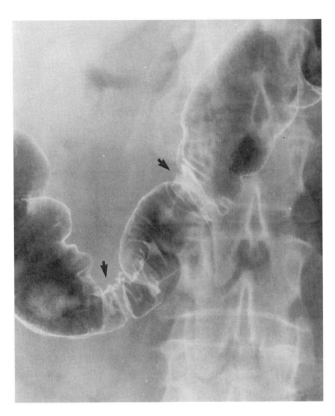

Figure 7-12. Extrinsic involvement of the transverse colon from a gastric carcinoma. Note the mass effect and mucosal deformity from the desmoplastic response (arrows).

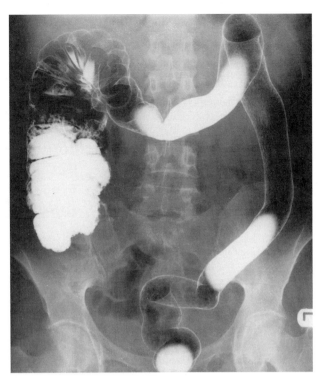

Figure 7-13. Instant enema in extensive ulcerative colitis. There is a granular mucosa extending into the proximal transverse colon. Some residue is present in the ascending colon, where the mucosal surface is normal and haustration present.

before the surface coating is sufficiently altered to be apparent radiologically.[5] In a review of the literature on colon cancer detection, Stevenson[6] concluded that the sensitivity of DCBE in cancer detection was 65% to 99%, compared with 70% to 95% in colonoscopy, and for detecting polyps smaller than 1 cm the best results radiologically were 85% to 90%, compared with 90% for colonoscopy. For diminutive polyps, DCBE was only 40% to 60% accurate, whereas colonoscopy was 60% to 75% accurate.

Instant Enema

Instant enema was designed to show the extent and severity of the colitis when the upper limit was not visible sigmoidoscopically.[7,8] The examination is a modified DCBE, without any bowel preparation. An intravenous smooth muscle relaxant is helpful to reduce spasm. Barium is run in until either the transverse colon or formed residue is reached. A little gas is then insufflated and a few spot digital films or a prone overhead film taken. The residue defines normal bowel, and the absence of residue where the bowel is inflamed allows good double-contrast visualization (Fig. 7-13). The technique works best in ulcerative colitis, where the colitis is in continuity, but is still useful in Crohn's colitis.[9]

The examination is very safe, and after a total experience of several thousand studies, only a few patients have shown any deterioration attributable to the instant enema. It is contraindicated in toxic megacolon or perforation.

Plain films often give adequate information in an acute attack, but if there is conflict between the clinical state and plain film appearances, an instant enema may be helpful to document the colitis accurately. If there is any localized tenderness, transabdominal ultrasound should be performed prior to a contrast study to exclude a localized sealed perforation. The "air enema" is an alternative to using barium,[10] where gas is gently insufflated to outline the entire colon. An irregular mucosal edge with loss of haustration indicates ulceration.

Relationship to Endoscopy

The DCBE is a very safe examination. At St. Mark's the perforation rate is less than 1 in 25,000. Balloon retention catheters are seldom used, and misuse of these is the most common cause of perforation.[11]

The DCBE provides a simple, safe, and economic method for detecting major colonic pathology. The images are complementary to endoscopy[12] with some advantages: the entire colon is examined in almost every case; anatomic representation and localization are exact; the depth of mucosal defects is demonstrated so that fistula, deep ulcers, and diverticula are shown clearly; and it is more sensitive for mural deformity, such as strictures or extrinsic masses. The disadvantages stem from the lack of direct visualization of the mucosa in color, so that vascular changes in early colitis, angiodysplasia, or telangiectasia are not seen, and fecal residue cannot be distinguished from a small polyp. The inability to biopsy the mucosa further limits the value of the DCBE in colitis. Interventional procedures, apart from the reduction of intussusceptions, are obviously the prerogative of endoscopy.

The indications for either DCBE or colonoscopy as the initial investigation have been debated. A radiologic viewpoint suggests the following:

1. Suspected irritable bowel disease to exclude major pathology or diverticular disease. Confirmation may be obtained when typical pain is simulated either during colonic distension or contraction.
2. Rectal bleeding when the likely cause has been identified, such as hemorrhoids, and the clinical concern is to exclude major pathology.
3. Change in bowel habit. Any neoplastic lesion responsible is likely to be large and easily visible. Diverticular disease may be present. Any extrinsic mass will be better demonstrated. Gross colonic redundancy may not be of direct therapeutic significance, but is useful to know about.
4. Suspected diverticular disease. This is more clearly depicted on DCBE. Stricture or pericolic abscess will be revealed, and diverticular disease is a risk factor in colonoscopy.
5. Acute colitis. The instant enema is very safe and informative in an acute attack.
6. Chronic colitis, where cancer is not suspected. The DCBE maps the colitis, with an overview of gross mucosal disease, depth of ulceration, possible fistula formation, or colonic deformity that is difficult to match endoscopically.

DCBE indicates those cases where total colonoscopy may be difficult. Increased rectosigmoid or total colonic length, transverse colon mobility and redundancy, and moderate to severe diverticular disease are significant factors[13] that allow appropriate planning of future endoscopy, either transferring the case to a more experienced endoscopist, or allowing more time for total examination.

There is another factor in the argument of DCBE versus total colonoscopy. Flexible sigmoidoscopy is increasingly replacing rigid sigmoidoscopy for initial clinical assessment. This may alter which is the more appropriate examination to follow sigmoidoscopy. If a polyp is found on flexible sigmoidoscopy, total colonoscopy with polypectomy is the obvious choice. However, if results from flexible sigmoidoscopy are normal, there are advantages in performing a DCBE. If the bowel has been prepared fully, it is possible to do this soon afterward, without detracting from the quality of the examination.[14] DCBE is cheaper and safer than colonoscopy, and invariably provides a complete examination of the colon. Colonoscopy is frequently incomplete, and the significance of this is shown by 39% of endoscopically missed cancers being in the proximal colon.[15] Complete double-contrast views of the sigmoid colon may be difficult. Flexible sigmoidoscopy examines the weakest link in the DCBE, so that the combination should enhance polyp detection. An accuracy of 72% for DCBE and 86% endoscopically was increased to 94% for both examinations,[16] demonstrating how sigmoidoscopy supports DCBE, and to a lesser extent vice versa, to improve polyp detection. DCBE is complementary to limited flexible endoscopy in the diagnosis of polyps, inflammatory bowel disease, and diverticular disease.[17]

Negative flexible sigmoidoscopy followed by DCBE may have a useful role in cancer detection. In the study of 66 patients[18] having flexible sigmoidoscopy, total colonoscopy, and DCBE, 4 cancers, 11 polyps larger than 5 mm, and 11 smaller than 5 mm were diagnosed. The DCBE was modified with limited views concentrating on the colon proximal to the sigmoid. The combined technique missed only 4 polyps, all smaller than 5 mm. Using this algorithm, 24 patients (36%) would have been spared total colonoscopy without loss of diagnostic efficacy.

WATER-SOLUBLE CONTRAST STUDIES

Peritoneal contamination with barium sulfate requires careful peritoneal lavage to avoid subsequent adhesion formation, and water-soluble contrast agents are much safer whenever there is a risk of perforation. These are absorbed from the peritoneal cavity and excreted systemically, so that no residue is left to cause a peritoneal reaction. or interfere with subsequent computed tomography (CT).

For colonic examination, Gastrografin (Schering AG, Berlin, Germany) diluted 3:1 with water, or Urografin 150 (Schering AG, Berlin, Germany) are suitable. These are hypertonic and draw in fluid, reducing the circulating blood volume. The recommended maximum volume of 500 ml causes minimal circulatory disturbance in the adult. Diarrhea is usual afterward, but if a large volume becomes trapped proximal to a stricture there is the risk of colonic overdistension with perforation.[19] The contrast is a mucosal irritant that may have some therapeutic value in pseudo-obstruction.[80] The lower viscosity of water-soluble agents is also an advantage in demonstrating fistulas, and outlining a very loaded colon to distinguish megarectum (Fig. 7-14) from Hirschsprung's disease.[21] No bowel preparation is required, and in most circumstances would be contraindicated. Contrast is run in under screening control with spot and overhead films as required. There may be minimal holdup at a stricture, so it is important to image all the filled bowel particularly when investigating suspected pseudo-obstruction.[22]

A water-soluble contrast enema will demonstrate a higher incidence of anastomotic dehiscence than expected clinically,[23] although the clinical significance of a small track may be questioned.[24] Anastomotic breakdown may be delayed, so that in a series of 233 examinations performed 7 days postoperatively, there was a false-negative rate of 4.7%.[24] Patients with pyrexia and suspected anastomotic breakdown should have ultrasound or CT to exclude an extramural collection, and a water-soluble contrast enema to demonstrate any anastomotic breakdown, and if present the extent of extraluminal tracking, size of cavity, and drainage into bowel.

POUCHOGRAPHY

In the development of pouch surgery, radiology showed that long distal segments prevented spontaneous evacuation (Fig. 7-15), and were associated with a greater need for catheterization, with its attendant risks of ulceration and stenosis.[25] With current pouch designs, most referrals for pouchography are to check anastomotic integrity prior to closing a covering ileostomy. Evacuation pouchography is sometimes requested to investigate patients with difficult pouch function, although anal stricture has been shown to be the only consistent factor associated with poor emptying.[26]

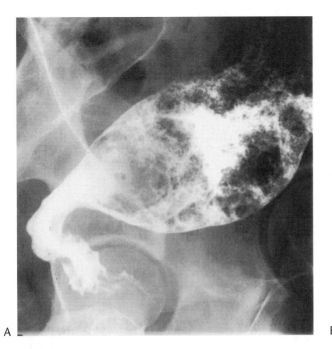 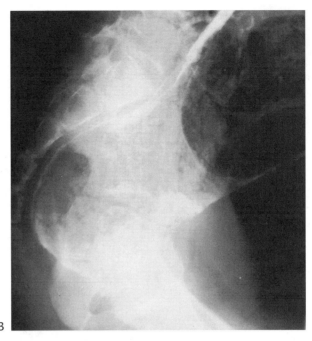

Figure 7-14. (**A**) Unprepared Gastrografin enema showing a short segment Hirschsprung's. (**B**) Megarectum. Note that the distended rectosigmoid extends down the pelvic floor.

Figure 7-15. Pouchogram with a long distal segment (between arrows).

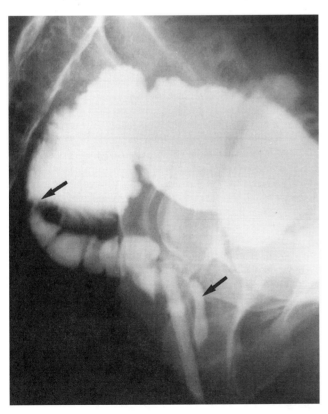

A simple technique for pouchography is to insert a 16 French Foley catheter gently into the pouch without inflating the balloon, and fill the pouch with a water-soluble contrast agent such as Gastrografin diluted 3:1 with water. Initially the patient should be screened posteroanterior (PA) with the head elevated, until the pouch is distended and contrast refluxes into the distal small bowel. This ensures adequate filling of the ileoanal anastomotic region; otherwise small tracks may not fill, or an underfilled part of pouch may be mistaken for a large presacral cavity.[27] The patient is then turned onto the left lateral, with lateral (Fig. 7-16), PA, and oblique spot films taken. If the pouch has been stapled, the position of the clips should be noted, because abnormal displacement suggests anastomotic breakdown.[28]

The most common problem, seen in 11% to 14% of cases,[27,29] is extravasation from the ileoanal anastomosis (Fig. 7-17). The clinical significance of short tracks may be questioned, but the incidence of anastomotic stricturing requiring dilatation is much greater following radiographic evidence of any anastomotic dehiscence.[30] The lateral view of the pouch shows the presacral space. Widening of this may be related to surgical technique, although in 71% of cases where it was greater than 4 cm a significant abnormality, such as a large hematoma or abscess, was present.[27] This is an indirect sign of a pelvic collection. CT is the preferred examination[31] to image a noncommunicating abscess. In females transvaginal ultrasound is an alternative method to interrogate the pouch and posterior pelvic compartment in detail. Transabdominal scanning is less accurate. It may be helpful to delineate the pouch with a water infusion while scanning. Pouchitis is an endoscopic diagnosis, but may be detected by scintigraphy in 80% of cases.[31]

Examination of the Kock continent pouch requires a different

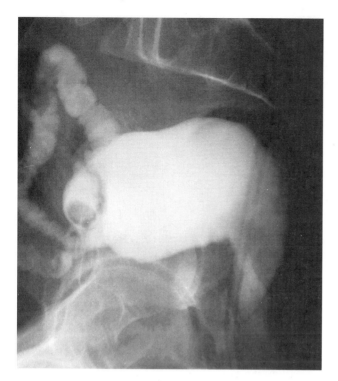

Figure 7-16. "W" pouch. No leak. Normal presacral space with free reflux into proximal small bowel.

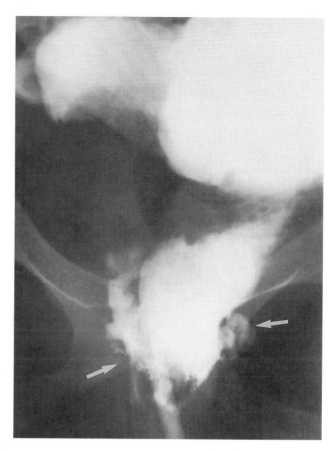

Figure 7-17. Bilateral extravasation from the ileoanal anastomosis (arrows) with some displacement of staples.

technique. Except in the immediate postoperative period, barium suspension is the preferred contrast agent to evaluate valve or pouch dysfunction. A Foley catheter should be inserted through the stoma, just into the valve (Fig. 7-18). Contrast is injected slowly during screening to ascertain the length of the valve, and exclude any fistula or stenosis. The catheter is then passed into the pouch, more contrast injected, gas insufflated, and the patient turned from side to side to obtain good double-contrast images of the pouch and distal small bowel.[32] The valve should lie within the pouch. A common problem is reduction of the valve so that it lies outside the pouch. The mucosal surface and any stricture in the distal small bowel or fistula should be noted.

Obstructive problems with long-standing pouches may relate to adhesion and stricture formation, often at the site of the covering ileostomy. These cases are best examined by a barium study of the small bowel. The distal small bowel often becomes quite dilated as it takes on an additional reservoir function,[33] which is a normal adaptive response.

FISTULOGRAPHY

Fistulography is an undervalued radiologic examination, as it is often crucial to patient management. Enterocutaneous fistulas are particularly complex,[34] and require careful investigation. There are several ground rules to follow radiologically. The first is that fistulography should be the initial examination. It should not be performed after barium studies, as these may obscure the fistula. Demonstrating the viscus involved in the abnormal communication may also help target the next most appropriate study. The cutaneous opening must be catheterized

gently, but the catheter inserted as far as possible into the track, otherwise contrast will reflux back up the track. Small (6 to 8 French) Foley catheters are useful[35] to seal the track by inflating the balloon just enough so that the catheter is held in place. This prevents contrast reflux during injection, and allows complete filling of the proximal extent of the track. A water-soluble contrast is always used, and spot films taken at right angles, (i.e., PA and either a very steep oblique, lateral, or horizontal shoot-through if the patient cannot be turned).

Fistulograms of anal fistulas (Fig. 7-19) may show the primary track, and any branching, abscess, or communication into the anal canal or rectum.[36] Fistulography has been reported to be only 16% accurate in demonstrating internal openings or extensions, with a 10% false-positive rate,[37] but may influence surgical management.[38] Fistulography has a limited role in the investigation of anal fistula, but is very useful in patients with chronic fistula, particularly where the cutaneous opening is distant from the anus. The entire track system may be clearly shown, probably because the track is epithelialized[39] and so open, rather than partially blocked by granulation tissue as is usual in a more acute fistula. Some fistulae have an intra-abdominal origin,[40] usually secondary to diverticular disease, which may be picked up on fistulography or cross-sectional imaging, and confirmed with a water-soluble contrast enema.

Enterovesical fistulae are demonstrated optimally by CT[41] by the presence of intravesical gas, passage of contrast from

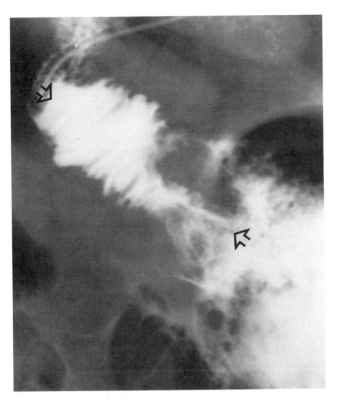

Figure 7-18. The valve (between arrows) of the Kock's pouch has been outlined, and lies outside the reservoir of the pouch due to detachment of the pouch and reduction of the intussuscepted valve.

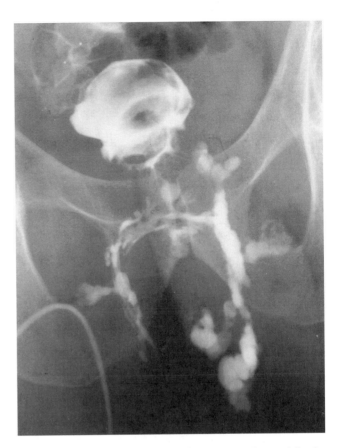

Figure 7-19. Fistulography of a chronic complex anal fistula, showing horseshoe extension with bilateral ischioanal fossa abscesses and internal opening into the midanal canal with retrograde filling of the rectum.

bowel into the bladder, localized thickening of the bladder wall, or an extraluminal gas-containing mass adjacent to the bladder.[42]

Colovaginal fistula should initially be investigated with an unprepared water-soluble contrast enema and transvaginal ultrasound to exclude any abscess mass related to the vagina or rectovaginal septum. If these are negative, vaginography[43] using the balloon of a large Foley catheter to occlude the vagina and distend it with contrast, may be helpful.

Entero-enteric fistulae are revealed by inappropriate filling of part of the gastrointestinal tract during a contrast study. The fistulous track and any intervening abscess cavity may be shown, providing these fill with sufficient contrast to be visible on the imaging modality used. CT is much more sensitive than standard films, as very small amounts of contrast are detectable. Fistulae may close intermittently, so are not completely excluded by negative radiology.

ILEOSTOMY ENEMA

An ileostomy enema is a useful technique to obtain double-contrast views of the distal small bowel and prestomal segment, either at the end of a standard small bowel examination, or as a separate study. The ileostomy is catheterized with a 16F Foley, the balloon inflated to a maximum of 10 ml of air, and withdrawn so that it abuts the abdominal wall. Atonia is induced with 20 mg of hyoscine butylbromide IV, and up to 150 ml of

barium suspension is injected, followed by gaseous insufflation[44] with spot films taken (Fig. 7-20).

EVACUATION PROCTOGRAPHY

Evacuation proctography (EP) is a radiologic study of the dynamics of rectal emptying. There are considerable variations in techniques used, although most are based on the original description by Mahieu.[45] The examination has variously been termed evacuation proctography,[46] defecography,[45] videoproctography,[47] cinedefecography,[48] and dynamic rectal examination.[49] The examination tests only voluntary rectal evacuation. "Defecography" is misleading in that physiologic defecation is not simulated, because the colonic contraction and reflex anorectal changes that accompany normal defecation are absent.[50] "Evacuation proctography" or a related term is therefore preferred.

Technique

Rectal cleansing, either with glycerine suppositories or enema, is recommended. This has been criticized as being unphysiologic,[50] but allows standardization of the procedure. Contrast consistency should approximate to feces. Suitable preparations can be made by mixing a barium suspension with potato starch

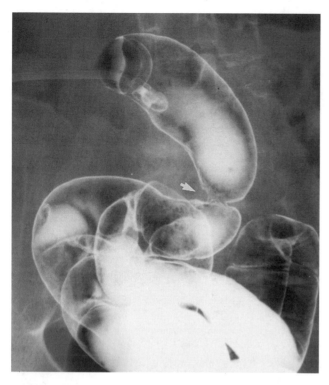

Figure 7-20. Ileostomy enema with a short stricture due to localized Crohn's disease (arrow) in the prestomal ileum.

or methylcellulose.[51] Commerical preparations are available (E-Z-Paste; E-Z-EM Ltd, London). The total volume used is variable. Contrast may be instilled until a strong urge to evacuate is provoked,[52] whereas most use a fixed volume of 120 to 200 ml. Because the contrast is of high viscosity, it must be syringed into the rectum.

Oral barium suspension should be given prior to the procedure, to opacify the small bowel and visualize enteroceles.[53] A vaginal marker may be helpful to indicate rectogenital prolapse from rectovaginal separation during evacuation. A viscous barium paste is preferable, as a tampon may inhibit prolapse by splinting the vagina.[54] Liquid barium can be instilled prior to rectal paste into the sigmoid colon to identify any sigmoidocele.[51] Recent reports have promoted bladder opacification in addition to the above modifications so that cystocele can be

diagnosed,[53,55,56] and some investigators have combined the examination with peritoneography to delineate the pelvic peritoneal recesses during evacuation.[57,58]

The commode that the patient sits on is placed sideways on the footstep of the table top. It must incorporate some added filtration, equivalent to 4 mm of copper,[46] to prevent screen flare. Where a commode is unavailable, the examination may be carried out with the patient lying on his or her left side.[59] Static values for pelvic floor position are higher in the left lateral than seated position.[60]

Evacuation is recorded either by a 105-mm ampliphotography camera, videofluoroscopy, or digital spot films at one frame per second. Patient dose is lowest with videofluoroscopy, but copy from spot films is easier to review.

THE NORMAL EXAMINATION

Mahieu[45] defined five stages of a normal examination: increase in anorectal angulation, obliteration of the puborectalis impression, wide opening of the anal canal, total evacuation of contrast, and normal pelvic floor descent. Subsequent studies of asymptomatic volunteers revealed a wide range of normal values, with some overlap into pathologic states.[46,61–64] Nevertheless, a consensus of opinion regarding normal EP findings[51] agrees broadly with Mahieu's original description.

It is convenient to consider the examination in three stages[46]: resting, evacuation, and recovery. The initial lateral view determines the resting anorectal configuration and pelvic floor position. The anorectal angle (ARA) was thought to be important for maintaining continence, and considerable attention has been devoted to its measurement. It may be measured between the anal canal axis and the posterior rectal wall, or the central axis of the rectum.[65] The junction between the rectal ampulla and anal canal, the anorectal junction (ARJ), is easy to appreciate at rest with the anal canal closed and rectum filled. The level of the pelvic floor is traditionally defined by the pubococcygeal line, but the fluoroscopic field of view is too limited to define this, and the inferior aspect of the ischial tuberosities is used instead. At rest the ARJ should be at, or just above, this plane, and the anal canal should be closed with no leakage of contrast. The ARA should be approximately 90°. ''Squeeze'' views may be used to evaluate pelvic floor contraction,[62] and cough views to stress the continence mechanism. The patient may also be asked to bear down without evacuating, to assess pelvic floor

Figure 7-21. Evacuation proctography. The film on the left shows pelvic floor descent, opening of the anal canal with a wide anorectal angle. Evacuation is rapid and completed within a few seconds.

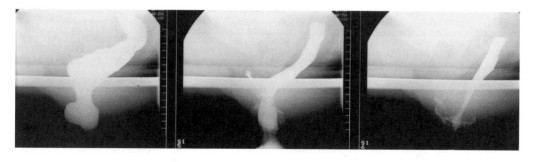

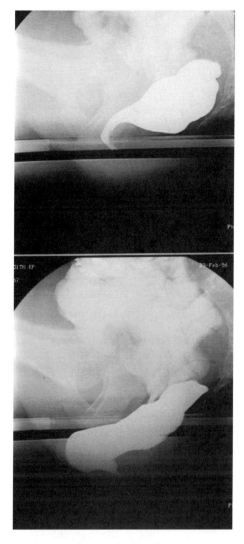

Figure 7-22. The upper view at rest shows a closed anal canal, acute anorectal angle, and normal pelvic floor position. The small bowel has been opacified. The lower view during attempted evacuation shows pelvic floor descent and a large anterior rectocele.

descent. Paradoxically the ARA may increase during this maneuver in 30% of normal individuals, suggesting pelvic floor contraction to ensure continence.[52] These supplementary maneuvers yield relatively little information for the additional radiation incurred, and are not essential.

The patient is then instructed to empty the rectum as rapidly and completely as possible. Evacuation should be initiated rapidly, first with pelvic floor descent (Fig. 7-21), then effacement of the puborectalis impression with the ARA widening by approximately 20°, as the anal canal opens. Evacuation should be rapid (less than 30 seconds) and complete, with almost total effacement of the anal canal. Only the distal rectum, below the main fold, is usually emptied. It is common for contrast to be retained in the rectosigmoid. When the patient stops straining, the anal canal closes and puborectalis tone returns, elevating the pelvic floor and restoring the ARJ and ARA to their resting positions and the recovery phase is complete.

It may be helpful to image the rectum in the PA plane after emptying, to reveal the coronal configuration of the rectum at rest and during straining,[66] as this improves the diagnostic accuracy of intussusception.

ABNORMAL FINDINGS

Structural abnormalities, such as rectocele, intussusception, pelvic floor prolapse, or abnormal pelvic floor descent are often observed only during or at the end of evacuation. Function assesses the patient's ability to evacuate. EP may reveal abnormalities of structure or function, or a combination of both.

Rectocele

Rectocele describes an anterior bulge of the rectal wall during evacuation,[62] and is considered a normal variant in females unless greater than 2 cm deep, as measured from the anterior anal canal to the most anterior point of the rectocele (Fig. 7-22). Large rectoceles may be associated with difficult evacuation.[67] Barium trapped within the rectocele at the end of evacuation[58] may lead to a sense of incomplete evacuation (Fig. 7-23), and is often associated with vaginal digitation[68] to complete rectal emptying.

Posterior rectoceles, more correctly termed *posterior perineal hernias*,[69,70] are due to defects in the levator ani.

Intussusception

Intussusception confined to the rectum is termed intrarectal, and intra-anal when the apex enters the anal canal. The EP appearances of intussusception have been graded on a seven-

Figure 7-23. There is a large residue of barium trapped in the anterior rectocele at the end of evacuation when the rectum has emptied.

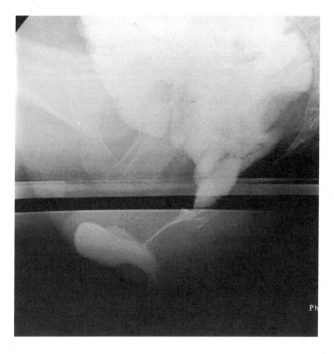

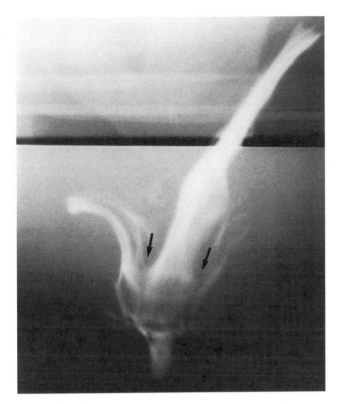

Figure 7-24. Intra-anal intussusception with infolding of the distal rectum (arrows) down to the anal canal.

point scale,[71] although a simpler division into high and low grades is possible.[49] Classification is based on rectal appearances at the end of evacuation. Generally, low-grade intussusception is defined as rectal wall infolding less than 3 mm thick, which does not enter the anal canal. Full thickness intussusception defines high-grade prolapse, which is assumed if the prolapsing folds are greater than 3 mm,[62] and the intussusception penetrates the anal canal (Fig. 7-24) or impedes evacuation.[46] The relationship of anterior mucosal prolapse[72] to proctographic intussusception has not been established.

Any rectal configuration during voiding, other than that of a symmetrically collapsing tube, has been considered abnormal. However, using this criterion some degree of intussusception has been reported[62] in 80% of asymptomatic subjects. Most interpretations are based solely on a lateral view of the rectum. The valves of Houston govern rectum collapse, and these are observed better in the PA than the lateral plane. Many so-called intussusceptions in the PA plane will then be seen to be no more than folding over of the rectum. Intra-anal intussusception is defined on PA views by the folded rectum entering the anal canal and widening this[66] during straining (Fig. 7-25).

Pelvic Floor Prolapse

Bladder or bowel may herniate into a deep rectogenital space, forming a cystocele, enterocele, or sigmoidocele (Fig. 7-26). This may be inferred during EP from widening of the rectovaginal distance (Fig. 7-27) or compression of the anterior rectal wall[53] during evacuation, but is demonstrated best by opacify-

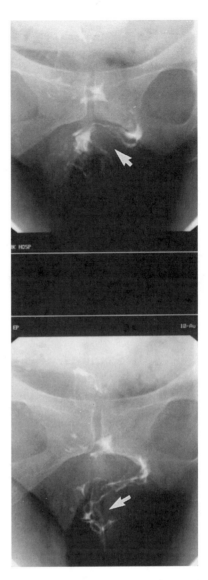

Figure 7-25. Posteroanterior view at rest (upper view) with the distal rectum folded over. On straining (lower view) the distal rectal fold prolapses down into the anus (arrow), confirming an intra-anal intussusception.

ing the bowel or bladder.[56,73] Peritoneography has shown that small pelvic floor hernias during evacuation may not fill with any particular structure.[57,58]

Pelvic Floor Descent

Normally the pelvic floor descends less than 3.0 cm during evacuation.[46,62] The significance of excessive pelvic floor descent is uncertain. A low resting position may be seen in incontinent patients[74] or the elderly,[75] with only minimal further descent on evacuation. Some studies show significant differences between constipated patients and controls,[75] whereas others have not found any difference between incontinent and constipated patients.[76] Although chronic straining is considered a cause of pudendal neuropathy, no correlation between neuropathy and pelvic floor descent on EP has been found.[77] Reduced

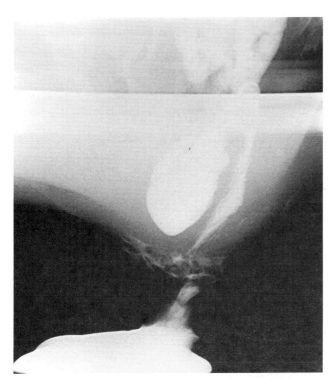

Figure 7-26. Sigmoidocele at the end of evacuation. The patient has had a rectopexy.

descent during evacuation suggests a poor increase in intrarectal pressure.[78]

FUNCTIONAL CHANGES

Changes in the ARA have been emphasized in the literature, despite proven intraobserver error in making this measurement.[79,80] Of greater clinical relevance may be the ability to demonstrate if a patient can evacuate normally or not. Failure of the anorectal angle to open and a prominent puborectalis impression are frequently cited as proctographic signs of anismus,[52,65,77,81] although no correlation between the anorectal angle and anorectal physiologic tests has been proved.[82]

Proctography provides an accurate estimate of the rate and degree of rectal emptying.[83] In a study of 24 patients with a diagnosis of anismus based on multiple criteria, only measurements of rectal emptying were able to distinguish patients from controls.[84] Normal values for evacuation time may depend on the volume and viscosity of contrast instilled. Using 100 ml of a commercial barium paste, voiding was completed within 30 seconds.[85] The relationship between a proctographic definition of anismus based on the time and completeness of evacuation, and paradoxical contraction on electromyography (EMG) studies is uncertain. In 42 patients with proctographic anismus, only 28 (67%) demonstrated changes on EMG.[48] Conversely, in 70 individuals with normal proctographic emptying, 12 (17%) had anismus by EMG criteria. Another study of 24 constipated patients demonstrated no correlation between EMG evidence of anismus and the ability to evacuate on EP.[86] Integrated proctography and EMG activity from the puborectalis[87,88] also failed to show a definite relationship between voiding and EMG activity. The situation is further confused by ambulatory studies sug-

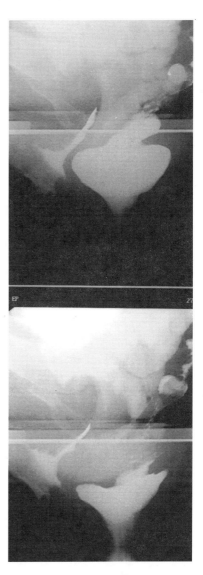

Figure 7-27. The vagina and small bowel have also been opacified in this study. At rest (upper view) small bowel is seen within the pouch of Douglas. The rectum is closely applied to the posterior wall of the vagina. During evacuation (lower view) there is separation of the rectum and vagina, with further prolapse of the small bowel forming a large enterocele.

gesting that some of the signs of anismus may be a laboratory phenomenon.[89]

Patients who can evacuate rapidly and completely are unlikely to have anismus. Those who are unable to evacuate properly may have anismus, but this could be artifactual due to inhibition. Failure to lower the pelvic floor during evacuation attempts may be considered a supplementary sign of anismus, related to reduced intrarectal pressure[78] or part of the spectrum of anismus as suggested by integrated studies.[90]

CONCLUSIONS

Difficult defecation is a complex symptom. Although proctography provides only a mechanistic viewpoint of the process, it does give some hard evidence as to functional or structural abnormality.

Proctography will show if there is a large rectocele, or an enterocele. The diagnosis of internal intussusception is more difficult, and reference to PA stress views is helpful. There are no absolute criteria for anismus, but the diagnosis should be considered when there is delayed and incomplete evacuation. Anismus will frequently coexist with structural abnormalities.

ULTRASOUND

TRANSABDOMINAL ULTRASOUND

Ultrasound (US) is undergoing continual technical development. The latest generation of scanners are capable of giving highly detailed images of the bowel from transabdominal scanning. Complete reflection of the US beam at a gas interface limits examination of gas-filled bowel. However, it is usually possible to compress bowel to obtain adequate views. Graded compression is an essential technique for transabdominal examination, not only for this reason, but also to show that bowel loops are mobile, and that there is no fixed loop or mass. Enlarged lymph nodes, thickened mesentery, peritoneal deposits, and ascites may be identified.

The "pseudokidney" sign of localized thickened hypoechoic bowel wall around echogenic bowel lumen may be seen in a wide variety of inflammatory or neoplastic lesions. Colonic cancer may be picked up on abdominal scanning,[91] especially in the right colon.[92] Limberg has pioneered the use of hydrocolonic sonography, filling the prepared colon with water.[93] This improved cancer detection from 31% to 97%. The sensitivity for detecting polyps larger than 7 mm was 91%, a figure that has been challenged in one study,[94] although supported by two others.[95,96]

Hydrocolonic sonography has also been used for the detection of colitis, with an accuracy of 91% for Crohn's disease and 89% for ulcerative colitis.[96,97] Differentiation of Crohn's from ulcerative colitis (Figs. 7-28 to 7-30) may be possible in 93% of cases by preservation of the five-layer pattern with only moderate wall thickening[98] in ulcerative colitis. Abdominal US with careful compression may also be quite accurate, and there are suggestions that this has a role in the primary detection of inflammatory bowel disease.[99–101]

US is useful in the diagnosis of acute diverticulitis, particularly in the early stages where there is typically a hypoechoic area (Fig. 7-31), tender to compression, the colonic wall and surrounded by rather echogenic mesenteric fat.[102,103] US may be helpful in the diagnosis of acute appendicitis (Fig. 7-32), and demonstrate abscess formation.[104]

ENDORECTAL ULTRASOUND

Rectal endosonography (RES) with rigid probes (Fig. 7-33) was developed to stage rectal cancer.[105] Endoscopic systems now allow complete colorectal examination,[106] but most published work relates to rectal disease.

Technique

The rectum must be prepared prior to examination. Enemas or suppositories are satisfactory. Blind insertion of a rigid probe allows examination of only the distal 12 cm of rectum. Some

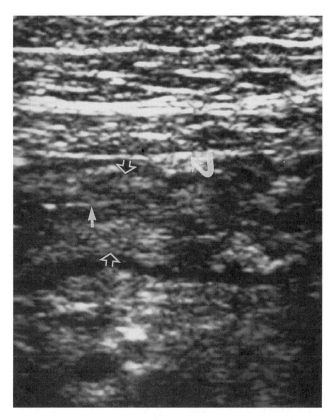

Figure 7-28. Longitudinal compression view of the descending colon in ulcerative colitis. The thickened bowel lies just under the peritoneal reflection on the inner border of the abdominal wall (curved arrow). The interface between the mucosal surfaces creates another interface (white arrow). The thickened submucosa (open arrows) is seen just deep to the muscularis propria layer.

transrectal probes can be passed through a short rectoscope. This allows proximal rectal lesions to be investigated, and is useful for localizing a small tumor. The probe should be inserted proximal to the lesion, the balloon distended with water, and the transducer then slowly withdrawn across the lesion. The degree of distension is important. Good contact with the rectal wall must be obtained, but overdistension should be avoided, because this squashes the second mucosal layer,[107] and forces an elevated lesion into the wall, which may distort the image of its base.

Rectal Wall Pattern

The rectal wall is less than 4 mm thick sonographically[108] with a five-layer pattern, composed of reflections from individual layers, and interfaces between layers of different acoustic impedance. Interface echoes extend into the deeper layer for a depth that equates to the axial resolution of the probe.[109] The layers are as follows (Fig. 7-34):

1. An interface with the superficial mucosa
2. A layer of poorly reflective deep mucosa
3. A composite layer and interface with increased reflectivity from the submucosa and the interface between the submucosa and the muscularis propria

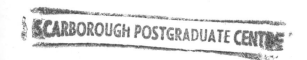

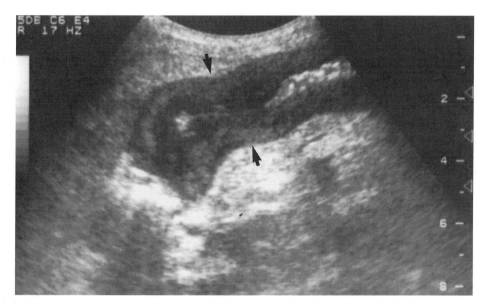

Figure 7-29. Thickened bowel loop (arrows) due to Crohn's disease. Note the bright fat inferiorly to this loop, indicating transmural inflammation with changes in the mesentery.

4. A layer of the muscularis propria of low reflectivity and reduced in thickness by the depth of the interface echo

5. An interface with the adventitia

With high-frequency probes (greater than 10 MHz) the (fourth) muscle layer may be seen to be divided by the fascial plane between the inner circular and outer longitudinal muscle. The muscularis mucosae is less than 0.1 mm thick[109] in the large bowel. Recent work suggests that the interface between the lamina propria and the muscularis mucosae summates with the echogenic third layer.[110] Unless the muscularis is abnormally thick, it is not visualized as a separate layer.

Figure 7-30. Oblique axial view of thickened bowel wall (arrowheads) in Crohn's disease, with color Doppler showing enhanced flow (arrow).

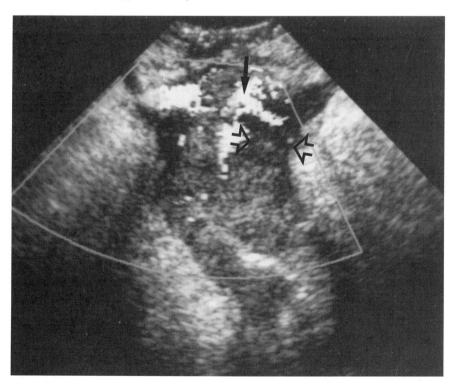

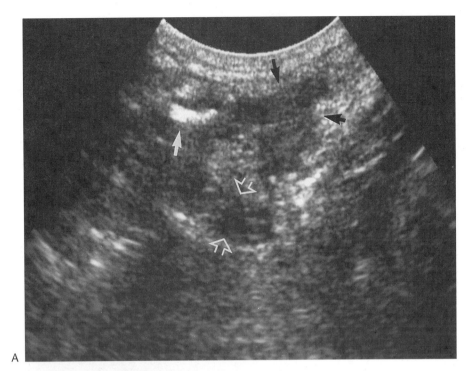

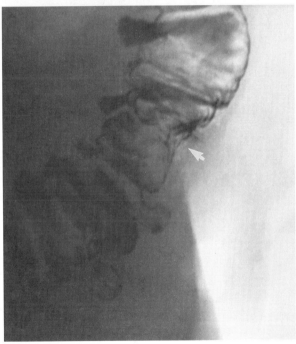

Figure 7-31. (**A**) Transverse view through a segment of diverticular disease with thickened wall (open white arrows) and localized pericolic inflammatory mass (black arrows) with adjacent rather bright fat. There is a bright reflection from gas within a diverticulum (white arrow). (**B**) Double-contrast barium enema performed 3 weeks later shows a residual deformity at the site of the diverticulitis.

Artifacts

Sonographic artifacts require recognition to avoid misinterpretation.[111] Gas bubbles, either within the water-filled balloon or between the balloon and rectal wall, cause a strong reverberation echo with complete loss of detail deep to the echo (Fig. 7-35). A large intraluminal mass will result in a discrepancy of US attenuation between the beam traveling through water with minimal attenuation, compared to attenuation by the mass. If the gain is set to show the wall adjacent to the mass, the base of the mass may suggest malignant infiltration because echoes from this level are not adequately amplified. This is simply rectified by increasing the gain, so that the base of the lesion will become visible, although the surrounding normal wall may then be too bright. Major reflections from air/fluid interfaces produce "mirror imaging," where part of the field of view is reflected onto the other side. This may seem to enlarge a mass or even form a pseudomass. The US beam has a certain thickness, and to register reflections from the very thin layers of the bowel wall, these must be scanned at right angles. An oblique

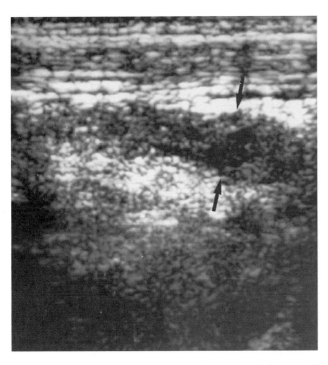

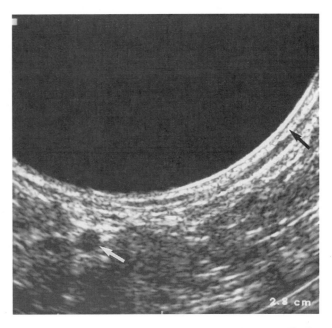

Figure 7-34. Endosonography of the normal rectal wall. The bright submucosa (black arrow) is well defined. The thin hypo-echoic deep mucosa is seen on the inside of this layer, with a bright reflection at the interface between this and the water/balloon. Outside the submucosa is the hypoechoic muscularis propria, with a bright interface between this and the perirectal fat. A small perirectal vein is present (white arrow).

Figure 7-32. Acute appendicitis with a distended appendix (arrows) surrounded by inflamed acoustically bright fat. There is no free fluid or abscess formation.

view may obliterate the layer pattern and thus the ability to "T" stage a tumor. This is a problem in the rectal ampulla, and by the folds of Houston.

Cancer Staging

Cancers are typically of low reflectivity. T1 tumors are confined to the submucosa, so that the bright third layer is involved but not breached. Once breached the lesion involves the echo-poor

fourth layer of the muscularis propria, and is a T2 stage (Fig. 7-36). When the rectal wall is breached, the lesion becomes a T3. An early T3 tumor is recognized by the presence of small tumorous pseudopodia that create peglike projections from the outer edge of the muscle layer, interrupting the fifth adventitial layer (Fig. 7-37). More extensive perirectal infiltration presents as a large extramural mass. With infiltration of an adjacent structure, such as the prostate, the tumor becomes a T4 stage.

Figure 7-33. B&K Medical rectal endoprobe with water-filled balloon. This may be inserted high into the rectum, via the short rectoscope.

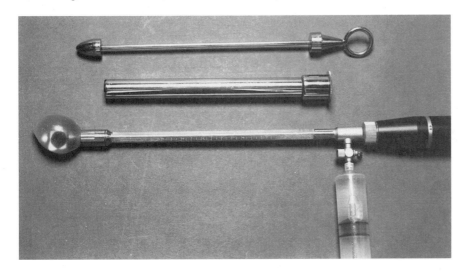

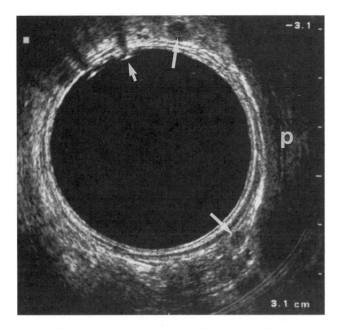

Figure 7-35. Small gas bubbles within the water-filled balloon (short arrow) causing acoustic shadowing. The prostate (p) and two small reactive nodes (long arrows) are noted.

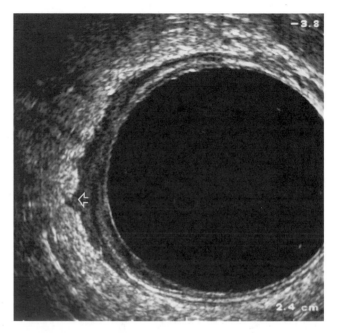

Figure 7-37. T3 cancer. Small projections of tumor (arrow-head) extend into the perirectal fat.

Reported comparisons of endosonographic compared to histologic ''T'' staging suggest an accuracy of 79% to 94.3%.[112–122] Solomon and McLeod[123] in a meta-analysis of 11 studies found a weighted kappa of 0.85 for all T stages, with sensitivities of 84%, 76%, 96%, and 76% for individual T1–4 stages, respectively. Accuracy improves with experience.[124] Errors are more frequent in the lower rectum (16.7%) compared to the mid- and upper rectum (6.3%)[125] due to the technical

Figure 7-36. T2 cancer. Note the break in the submucosa with involvement of the muscularis propria (arrow).

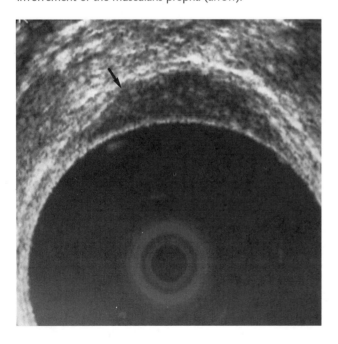

problems that result from not viewing a lesion at right angles (Figs. 7-38 and 7-39), as described above. T2 lesions are the most frequently overstaged. This is due to an inflammatory response around the tumor[117,126,127] that is indistinguishable sonographically from malignant infiltration. Stenotic lesions are difficult to examine, but may be staged with an 82% accuracy using a forward-viewing transducer.[128]

Lymph Node Involvement

Lymph node ''N'' staging is more controversial, with an unweighted kappa of only 0.58 reported for endosonographic detection of involved nodes.[123] Malignant nodes are typically large (greater than 5 mm), rounded rather than ovoid, and have a homogeneous echo-poor pattern (Figs. 7-40 and 7-41) without any internal reflectivity.[128–130] These features depend on the degree of node replacement. With complete replacement typical sonographic changes may be expected, but with micrometastases there may be no alteration in the echogenicity or configuration of the node. In vitro studies suggest a positive predictive value of only 59% for nodal involvement,[129] and because less than half the nodes in a surgical specimen will be visualized by endosonography,[131] node detection rate must be considered poor. If suspected nodal involvement requires preoperative confirmation, the node may be biopsied under ultrasound guidance.[132,133]

Indications

Staging—?local resection

Large villous adenomas—?malignant

Follow-up following resection—?recurrent disease

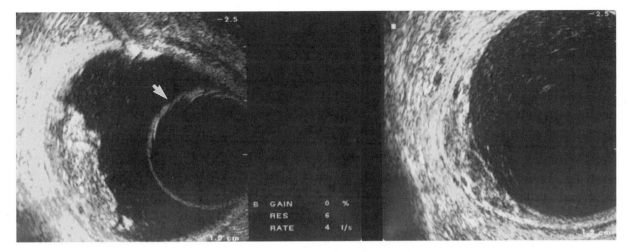

Figure 7-38. Collapse of the balloon (arrow) due to perforation with filling of the rectum shows how a tumor, in this case a benign villous adenoma, is pushed into the rectal wall by the balloon (see right-hand view). This may deform the lesion and prevent a correctly oriented view from being obtained.

Several studies have confirmed the value of RES staging in planning sphincter-saving surgery, and local resection.[118,134,135] It is also useful in detecting early malignant change in large villous tumors.[136,137] Following radiotherapy there is an increased reflectivity in the primary tumor as well as involved nodes,[138] and loss of wall definition makes "T" staging less accurate.[139,140] Early recurrent cancer may be detected by RES[141-143] before it is apparent on digital or sigmoidoscopic examination. The anastomosis is recognized as a narrow segment of loss or fusion of bowel wall layers.[144] Reflections from staples may be noted. Granulomas at the anastomosis must not be confused with recurrence. If the lesion cannot be biopsied intraluminally, transrectal biopsy under US guidance should be undertaken.[145,146]

ANAL ENDOSONOGRAPHY

The anal sphincters are circular structures, most clearly imaged in cross section. Balloon systems are unsuitable in the anal canal, as sphincter tone deforms the musculature around the

Figure 7-39. T2 carcinoma in the posterior wall of the distal rectum (arrow shows infiltration of muscularis propria) viewed with a linear probe in the longitudinal plane.

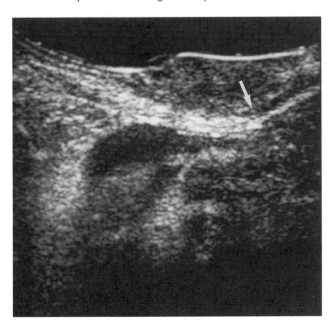

Figure 7-40. Small malignant lymph node (black arrow) with a T3 carcinoma. Fascia to the prostate is intact (white arrow). Gas outside the balloon has created an acoustic shadow (arrowhead).

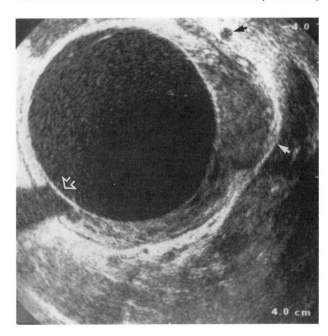

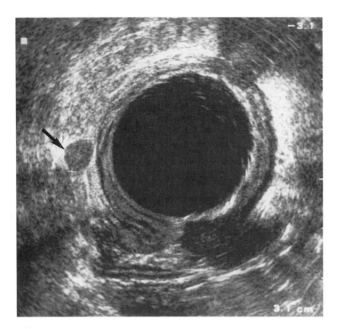

Figure 7-41. A 7-mm malignant node with slightly hyperechoic texture.

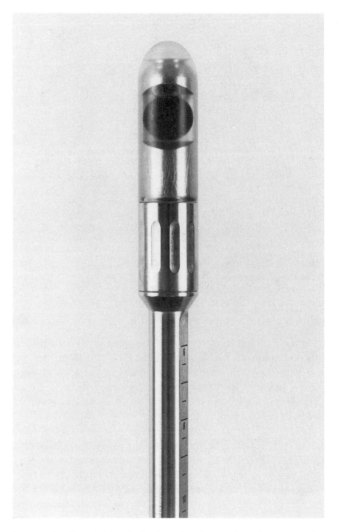

Figure 7-42. B&K Medical probe for anal endosonography with plastic cone filled with degassed water.

balloon. The probe should have parallel walls so that the anatomy of the canal is not altered as the probe is moved longitudinally within it. Systems that are suitable for anal endosonography include B&K Medical (Gentofte, Denmark) where a mechanically rotated 10 MHz probe with a water-filled plastic cone (Fig. 7-42) 1.7 cm in diameter gives a 360° image at right angles to the probe, and Kretz-technik (Zipf, Austria), which has a 7.5 MHz probe giving a 355° cross-sectional image.

Technique

The examination is simple and with practice takes only a few minutes. No patient preparation is needed. The patient is examined in the left lateral position. The probe, covered with a condom, is inserted gently into the canal. The probe should be cleaned with industrial spirit between cases, or soaked in glutaraldehyde if contaminated, or at the end of a session.

Normal Anatomy

A four-layer pattern is present in the anal canal: subepithelium, internal sphincter, longitudinal muscle, and external sphincter (Fig. 7-43).

The cone creates two bright interface echoes. The mucosa is not visible, as it is part of the strong outer echo, although with high-frequency catheter probes it may be seen.[147] The subepithelial tissues are moderately reflective. Low-reflective channels with this layer represent vascular spaces.

The internal sphincter is a well-defined hypoechoic ring. It increases in thickness with age, being about 1 mm thick in individuals younger than 20 years, 2 mm in individuals younger than 55 years, and 2 to 3 mm in the elderly.[148] The thickness is dependent on the size of the probe. The internal sphincter is stretched and thinned by a larger probe,[149] and is thicker with

smaller probes,[147] or when viewed transvaginally without any probe in the canal.[150] Immediately peripheral to the internal sphincter is the longitudinal muscle, a broad band of predominant fibroelastic tissue of moderate echogenicity. A wavy hypoechoic line at its outer edge demarcates the intersphincteric space.

The external sphincter is complex. Striated muscle has a characteristic sonographic appearance with thin parallel reflective striae of fibroadipose tissue separating the poorly reflective muscle fibers (Fig. 7-44). A trilaminar arrangement[151] with the deep part indistinguishable from the puborectalis with the same striated texture is seen sonographically. The superficial part is often hyporeflective in males relative to the longitudinal muscle, whereas in females it may be of the same reflectivity. The subcutaneous part, below the termination of the internal sphincter, shows increased reflectivity in both sexes (Fig. 7-45). Another difference between the sexes is that in males all three parts are roughly symmetric, but in females the deep and superficial parts slope downward as they travel forward around the canal, to join into an anterior muscle bundle in the lower canal. This starts just above the termination of the internal sphincter.

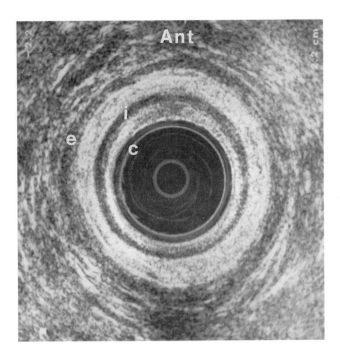

Figure 7-43. Normal endosonography in midanal canal in male. Anterior (Ant) is uppermost at 12 o'clock. Two interfaces form the cone (c), with echogenic subepithelium outside this. The internal sphincter (i) is a well-defined hypoechoic ring. Outside this is the echogenic longitudinal muscle, and then the hypoechoic, slightly striated external sphincter (e).

Figure 7-44. Deep external sphincter (between arrows) in a male demonstrating the typical striated pattern of voluntary muscle.

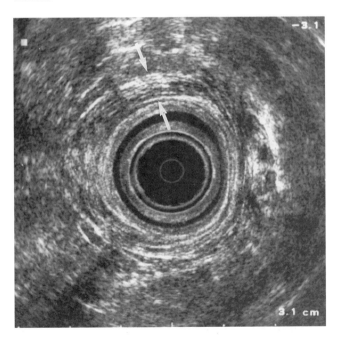

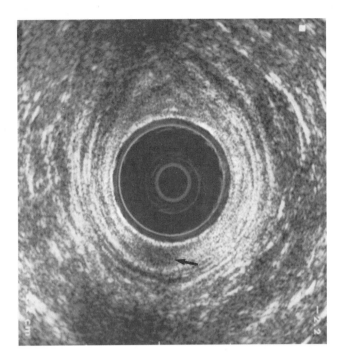

Figure 7-45. Normal subcutaneous external sphincter. Posteriorly a hypoechoic area in the subepithelium (arrow) is due to a vascular space. These are commonly seen at either 6 or 12 o'clock.

This creates the appearance of a defect high in the canal in females (Fig. 7-46), where the fibers of the external sphincter are cut across by the cross-sectional image as they run forward to downward to the anterior muscle bundle. As the probe is withdrawn, these ends can be seen joining together into the intact anterior muscle bundle.

A triangular acoustic shadow posteriorly is due to the anococcygeal ligament. Anteriorly the transverse perineii may be seen on either side of the bulbospongiosus. Bartholin's glands may be seen in the female. At the deep level the puborectalis can be seen attaching to the inner border of the pubic bones. Lateral to this is the ischiocavernosus. Fat in the ischioanal fossae creates an ill-defined striated texture. At the deep level the closely striated pattern of the levator ani may be seen.

Internal Sphincter

Abnormalities in thickness are age dependent. An internal sphincter of 3 mm is normal in an elderly patient, but abnormal in a 20-year-old individual. Using the B&K Medical probe, any sphincter greater than 3.5 mm thick is abnormal irrespective of age. Sphincters 4 to 5 mm in thickness (Fig. 7-47) may be associated with intussusception[152] or anal pain. Hereditary internal sphincter myopathies[153] are rare, but seem to have sphincters greater than 5 mm thick (Fig. 7-48). A moderate increase of internal sphincter thickness is common in solitary rectal ulcer syndrome.[152] Internal sphincter thickness is reduced following pouch formation,[154] and in some primary smooth muscle disorders.[155]

Any disruption in the intact ring is abnormal. The most common cause is obstetric trauma, where the internal sphincter disruption is associated with external sphincter damage.[156] Anal

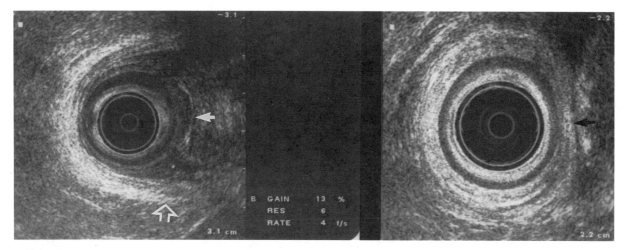

Figure 7-46. The lowermost view shows the puborectalis (arrowhead) running anteriorly toward the inner border of the pubic bone. There is no obvious circular sphincteric muscle anteriorly at this deep level. The vagina (white arrow) lies anterior to the internal sphincter. Lower down in the canal (upper view) the external sphincter has joined together anteriorly into the anterior muscle ring (black arrow).

dilatation or stretch procedures may cause single or multiple defects in the internal sphincter.[157,158] Fragmentation of the sphincter (Fig. 7-49) is pathognomonic of dilatation. Lateral internal sphincterotomy normally creates a well-defined defect in the lower third of the internal sphincter (Fig. 7-50). The ends are clearly defined and pull apart so that the remaining sphincter bunches up and looks thicker. In females the shorter anal canal may result in the sphincterotomy being more extensive (Fig. 7-51) than intended.[159] If the entire length of the sphincter is divided, incontinence may result. Sexual abuse with anal penetration may result in internal and sometimes external sphincter damage.[160]

External Sphincter

Muscle tears heal by fibrous tissue replacement, which is homogeneous and relatively poorly reflective compared to normal striated muscle. Endosonography has been proven operatively

Figure 7-47. A thick internal sphincter (4.4 mm) in a 43-year-old patient with solitary rectal ulcer syndrome and intra-anal intussusception on proctography.

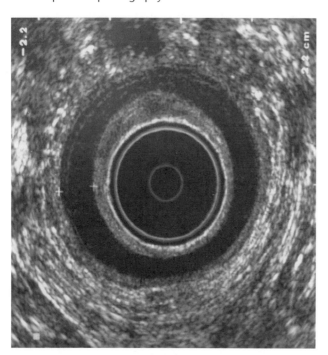

Figure 7-48. Internal sphincter 7.1 mm thick in a 70-year-old female with proctalgia fugax and family history of this affecting females only.

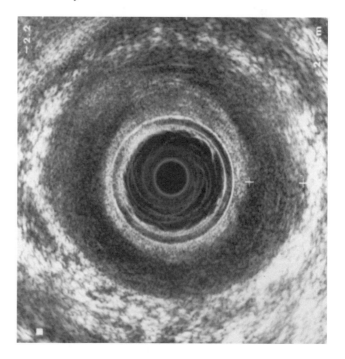

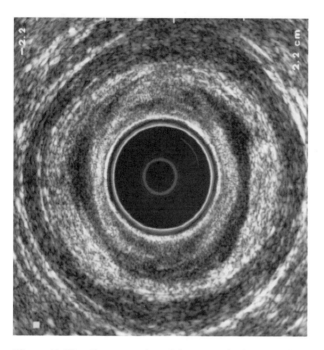

Figure 7-49. Fragmentation of the internal sphincter following anal dilatation.

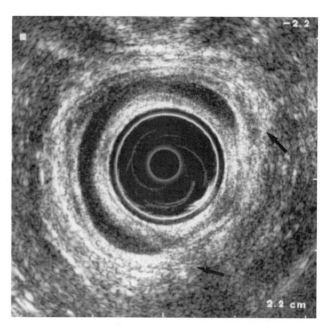

Figure 7-51. Lateral sphincterotomy that extended throughout the length of the canal, but also involved the longitudinal muscle and disrupted the external sphincter (arrows).

to be highly accurate in detecting external sphincter tears,[161,162] and more accurate than clinical assessment, EMG mapping, or manometry.[161] It is now preferred to EMG mapping[163,164] for the diagnosis of external sphincter tears.

Obstetric trauma is the most common cause of sphincter dam-

age,[165] with almost one-third of vaginal deliveries (Fig. 7-52) resulting in some degree of loss of sphincter continuity.[156] Forceps delivery is a high-risk factor.[166] Endosonography has shown that primary repair after a third-degree tear is frequently inadequate[167,168] (Fig. 7-53). Good function is associated with

Figure 7-50. Lateral internal anal sphincterotomy with well-defined edges to the sphincterotomy (arrows). Note that the longitudinal muscle and external sphincter are intact adjacent to the sphincterotomy.

Figure 7-52. Anterior defects in the internal and external sphincters between 10 and 2 (arrows) due to obstetric trauma.

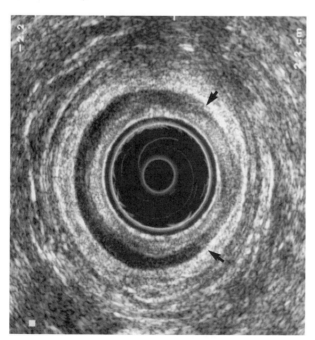

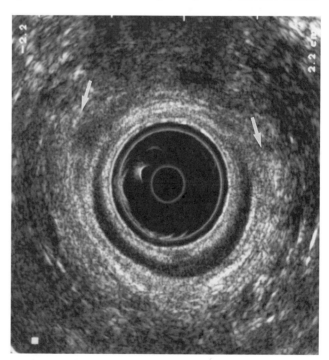

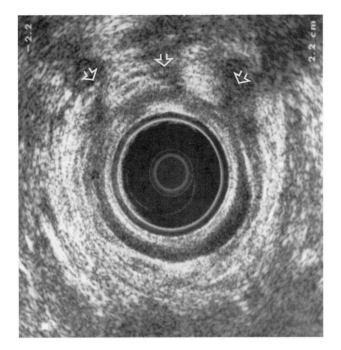

Figure 7-53. Defects (arrowheads) in the anterior part of the external sphincter remaining after a primary repair for a third-degree tear.

restoration of an intact anterior muscle ring by sphincter repair.[169,170]

Anal Sepsis

The primary track is seen as a rounded hypoechoic area within the longitudinal muscle (Fig. 7-54). The extent of the track and any secondary branching may be traced as the probe is moved along the canal. Internal openings are seldom recognized directly as tracks through the internal sphincter into the subepithelium, but are inferred by the point where the primary track fuses with the internal sphincter.[171] Transphincteric extension is present when tracks are seen penetrating through the external sphincter. Using these criterion, endosonographic accuracy has been shown to be comparable to digital examination under anesthesia.[171] Gas bubbles, easily seen as small bright spots, may be induced by injecting hydrogen peroxide into the primary track, to enhance imaging of complex tracks.[172] Gas bubbles are frequently spontaneously present in tracks. Foreign bodies may also cause a localized bright echo.[173] Fluid collections are clearly shown sonographically (Fig. 7-55), even when not palpable.[174]

Suprasphincteric extension will not be seen if only the hard cone is used, because there is loss of contact in the ampulla. With a water-filled balloon system, pararectal extensions may be visualized. Endosonography is not as accurate as MRI, which with fat suppression sequences to highlight inflammatory tissue is the gold standard for anal sepsis diagnosis.[175]

Anal Malignancy

Anal cancer is poorly reflective, and tumor penetration of the sphincters demonstrated by endosonography. This allows accurate staging and follow-up of irradiated tumors.[176]

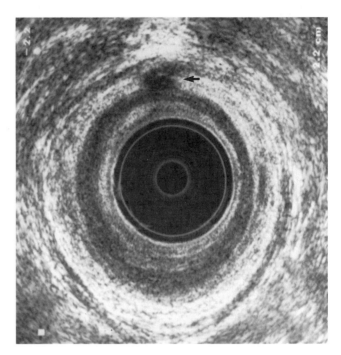

Figure 7-54. Primary track (arrow) of an anal fistula running within the longitudinal muscle.

Indications

Fecal incontinence—to show sphincter damage

Sepsis—fluid collections may not be palpable

Pain—?abnormal internal sphincter

Figure 7-55. Small superficial abscess (arrowhead).

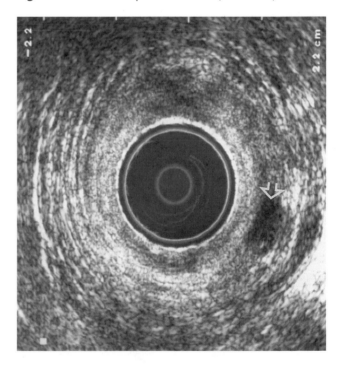

Solitary rectal ulcer syndrome/prolapse—?thick internal sphincter

Surgical followup—to confirm sphincter integrity

Anal malignancy—staging, follow-up

REFERENCES

1. Welin S (1967) Results of the Malmo technique of colon examination. JAMA 199:369–373
2. Bartram CI (1994) Bowel preparation—principles and practice. Clin Radiol 49:365–367
3. Fasano JJ (1985) Surgery for complications resulting from para-clinical colorectal examinations. Ann Gastroenterol Hepatol (Paris) 21:371–375
4. Martin CJ, Hunter S (1994) Reduction of patient doses from barium meal and barium enema examinations through changes in equipment factors. Br J Radiol 67:1196–1205
5. Elliott PR, Williams CB, Lennard-Jones JE et al (1982) Colonoscopic diagnosis of minimal change colitis in patients with a normal sigmoidoscopy and normal air-contrast barium enema. Lancet 1:650–651
6. Stevenson GW (1991) Medical imaging in the prevention, diagnosis, and management of colon cancer. pp. 1–20. In Herlinger H, Megibow AJ (eds): Advances in Gastrointestinal Radiology. Mosby Year Book, St Louis
7. Young AC (1963) The instant barium enema in proctocolitis. Proc R Soc Med 56:491–494
8. Thomas BM (1979) The instant enema in inflammatory disease of the colon. Clin Radiol 30:165–168
9. Patel U, Bartram CI (1993) Utility of the instant (unprepared) enema in Crohn's colitis. Clin Radiol 47:351–354
10. Bartram CI, Preston DM, Lennard-Jones JE (1983) The ''air enema'' in acute colitis. Gastrointest Radiol 8:61–65
11. Nelson JA, Daniels AU, Dodds WJ (1979) Rectal balloons: complications, causes, and recommendations. Invest Radiol 14:48–59
12. Reeders JW, Rosenbusch G (1994) Clinical Radiology and Endoscopy of the Colon. [Anonymous] George Thieme Verlag, New York
13. Sandikcioglu TG, Torp-Madsen S, Pedersen IK et al (1994) Contrast radiography in small bowel obstruction. A randomized trial of barium sulfate and a nonionic low-osmolar contrast medium. Acta Radiol 35:62–64
14. Saito Y, Slezak P, Rubio C (1989) The diagnostic value of combining flexible sigmoidoscopy and double-contrast barium enema as a one-stage procedure. Gastrointest Radiol 14:357–359
15. Glick SN, Teplick SK, Balfe DM (1989) Large colonic neoplasms missed by endoscopy. AJR 152:513–517
16. Jensen J, Kewenter J, Asztely M et al (1990) Double contrast barium enema and flexible rectosigmoidoscopy: a reliable diagnostic combination for detection of colorectal neoplasm. Br J Surg 77:270–277
17. Brewster NT, Grieve DC, Saunders JH (1994) Double-contrast barium enema and flexible sigmoidoscopy for routine colonic investigation. Br J Surg 81:445–447
18. Hough DM, Malone DE, Rawlinson J et al (1994) Colon cancer detection: an algorithm using endoscopy and barium enema. Clin Radiol 49:170–175
19. Gelfand DW (1980) Complications of gastrointestinal radiologic procedures:I. Complications of routine fluoroscopic studies. Gastrointest Radiol 5:293–315
20. Dorudi S, Berry AR, Kettlewell MGW (1992) Acute colonic pseudo-obstruction. Br J Surg 79:99–103
21. Barnes PRH, Lennard-Jones JE, Hawley PR, Todd IP (1986) Hirschsprung's disease and idiopathic megacolon in adults and adolescents. Gut 27:534–541
22. Chapman AH, McNamara M, Porter G (1992) The acute contrast enema in suspected large bowel obstruction: value and technique. Clin Radiol 46:273–278
23. Shorthouse AJ, Bartram CI, Eyers AA, Thomson JP (1982) The water soluble contrast enema after rectal anastomosis. Br J Surg 69:714–717
24. Akyol AM, McGregor JR, Galloway DJ, George WD (1992) Early postoperative contrast radiology in the assessment of colorectal anastomotic integrity. Int J Colorectal Dis 7:141–143
25. Pescatori M, Manhire A, Bartram CI (1983) Evacuation pouchography in the evaluation of ileoanal reservoir function. Dis Colon Rectum 26:365–368
26. Kmiot WA, Yoshioka K, Pinho M, Keighley MR (1990) Videoproctographic, assessment after restorative proctocolectomy. Dis Colon Rectum 33:566–572
27. Kelly IM, Bartram CI, Nicholls RJ (1994) Water-soluble contrast pouchography—technique and findings in 85 patients. Clin Radiol 49:612–616
28. Daly BD, Crowley BM (1989) Radiological appearances of colonic ring staple anastomosis. Br J Radiol 62:256–259
29. Jacquenod P, Hautefeuille P, Valleur P et al (1987) Contribution of radiology in the study of ileal reservoirs anastomosed to the anal canal. J Radiol 68:677–686
30. Tsao JI, Galandiuk S, Pemberton JH (1992) Pouchogram: predictor of clinical outcome following ileal pouch-anal anastomosis. Dis Colon Rectum 35:547–551
31. Thoeni RF, Fell SC, Engelstad B, Schrock TB (1990) Ileoanal pouches: comparison of CT, scintigraphy, and contrast enemas for diagnosing postsurgical complications. AJR Am J Roentgenol 154:73–78
32. Lycke KG, Gothlin JH, Jensen JK et al (1994) Radiology of the continent ileostomy reservoir: II. Findings in patients with late complications. Abdom Imaging 19:124–131
33. Hennild V, Kjaergard H, Kuld Hansen L (1986) Radiologic evaluation of the continent (S-pouch) ileal reservoir with anal anastomosis. Acta Radiol [Diagn] (Stockh) 27:301–304
34. McIntyre PB, Ritchie JK, Hawley PR et al (1984) Management of enterocutaneous fistulas: a review of 132 cases. Br J Surg 71:293–296
35. Alexander ES, Weinberg S, Clark RA, Belkin RD (1982) Fistulas and sinus tracts: radiographic evaluation, management, and outcome. Gastrointest Radiol 7:135–140
36. Ani AN, Lagundoye SB (1979) Radiological evaluation of anal fistulae: a prospective study of fistulograms. Clin Radiol 30:21–24

37. Kuijpers HC, Schulpen T (1985) Fistulography for fistula-in-ano. Is it useful? Dis Colon Rectum 28:103–104

38. Weisman RI, Orsay CP, Pearl RK, Abcarian H (1991) The role of fistulography in fistula-in-ano. Report of five cases. Dis Colon Rectum 34:181–184

39. Lunniss PJ, Sheffield JP, Talbot IC et al (1995) Persistence of idiopathic anal fistula may be related to epithelialization. Br J Surg 82:32–33

40. Parks AG, Gordon PH (1976) Fistula-in-ano: perineal fistula of intra-abdominal or intrapelvic origin simulating fistula-in-ano—report of seven cases. Dis Colon Rectum 19:500–506

41. Labs JD, Sarr MG, Fishman EK et al (1988) Complications of acute diverticulitis of the colon: improved early diagnosis with computerized tomography. Am J Surg 155:331–336

42. Goldman SM, Fishman EK, Gatewood OM et al (1985) CT in the diagnosis of enterovesical fistulae. AJR Am J Roentgenol 144:1229–1233

43. Arnold MW, Aguilar PS, Stewart WR (1990) Vaginography: an easy and safe technique for diagnosis of colovaginal fistulas. Dis Colon Rectum 33:344–345

44. White MM, Bartram CI (1987) Technique and evaluation of the double contrast ileostomy enema. Clin Radiol 38:621–624

45. Mahieu PH, Pringot J, Bodart P (1984) Defecography: 1. Description of a new procedure and results in normal patients. Gastrointest Radiol 9:247–251

46. Bartram CI, Turnbull GK, Lennard-Jones JE (1988) Evacuation proctography: an investigation of rectal expulsion in 20 subjects without defecatory disturbance. Gastrointest Radiol 13:72–80

47. Sunderland GT, Poon FW, Lauder JC, Finlay IG (1992) Videoproctography in selecting patients with constipation for colectomy. Dis Colon Rectum 35:235–237

48. Jorge JM, Wexner SD, Ger GC et al (1993) Cinedefecography and electromyography in the diagnosis of nonrelaxing puborectalis syndrome. Dis Colon Rectum 36:668–676

49. Wiersma TG, Mulder CJ, Reeders JW et al (1994) Dynamic rectal examination (defecography). Baillieres Clin Gastroenterol 8:729–741

50. Kamm MA, van der Sijp JR, Lennard-Jones JE (1992) Observations on the characteristics of stimulated defaecation in severe idiopathic constipation. Int J Colorectal Dis 7:197–201

51. Bartolo DC, Bartram CI, Ekberg O et al (1988) Symposium. Proctography. Int J Colorectal Dis 3:67–89

52. Kelvin FM, Stevenson GW (1994) Defecography: techniques and normal findings. pp. 840–851. In Freeny PC, Stevenson GW (eds): Margulis and Burhenne's Alimentary Tract Radiology. 5th eds Mosby, St. Louis

53. Kelvin FM, Maglinte DD, Hornback JA, Benson JT (1992) Pelvic prolapse: assessment with evacuation proctography (defecography). Radiology 184:547–551

54. Archer BD, Somers S, Stevenson GW (1992) Contrast medium gel for marking vaginal position during defecography. Radiology 182:278–279

55. Thorpe AC, Williams NS, Badenoch DF et al (1993) Simultaneous dynamic electromyographic proctography and cystometrography. Br J Surg 80:115–120

56. Hock D, Lombard R, Jehaes C et al (1993) Colpocystodefecography. Dis Colon Rectum 36:1015–1021

57. Bremmer S, Ahlback SO, Uden R, Mellgren A (1995) Simultaneous defecography and peritoneography in defecation disorders. Dis Colon Rectum 38:969–973

58. Halligan MS, Bartram CI (1995) Evacuation proctography combined with positive contrast peritoneography to demonstrate pelvic floor hernias. Abdom Imaging 20:442–445

59. Poon FW, Lauder JC, Finlay IG (1991) Technical report: evacuating proctography—a simplified technique. Clin Radiol 44:113–116

60. Jorge JM, Ger GC, Gonzalez L, Wexner SD (1994) Patient position during cinedefecography. Influence on perineal descent and other measurements. Dis Colon Rectum 37:927–931

61. Selvaggi F, Pesce G, Scotto Di Carlo E et al (1990) Evaluation of normal subjects by defecographic technique. Dis Colon Rectum 33:698–702

62. Shorvon PJ, McHugh S, Diamant NE et al (1989) Defecography in normal volunteers: results and implications. Gut 30:1737–1749

63. Freimanis MG, Wald A, Caruana B, Bauman DH (1991) Evacuation proctography in normal volunteers. Invest Radiol 26:581–585

64. Goei R, van Engelshoven J, Schouten H et al (1989) Anorectal function: defecographic measurement in asymptomatic subjects. Radiology 173:137–141

65. Bartolo DC, Roe AM, Virjee J et al (1988) An analysis of rectal morphology in obstructed defaecation. Int J Colorectal Dis 3:17–22

66. McGee SG, Bartram CI (1993) Intra-anal intussusception: diagnosis by posteroanterior stress proctography. Abdom Imaging 18:136–140

67. Siproudhis L, Ropert A, Vilotte J et al (1993) How accurate is clinical examination in diagnosing and quantifying pelvirectal disorders? A prospective study in a group of 50 patients complaining of defecatory difficulties. Dis Colon Rectum 36:430–438

68. Halligan MS, Bartram CI (1996) Is digitation associated with proctographic abnormality. Int J Colorect Dis (in press)

69. Kaasbol MA, Hauge C, Nielsen MB (1993) Case report:impaired rectal emptying caused by perineal herniation of the rectum: defaecographic demonstration using oblique projections. Br J Radiol 66:171–172

70. Poon FW, Lauder JC, Finlay IG (1993) Perineal herniation. Clin Radiol 47:49–51

70. Halligan S, Bartram CI (1995) Is barium trapping in rectoceles significant? Dis Colon Rectum 38:764–768

71. Ambrosetti P, Robert J, Witzig JA et al (1992) Prognostic factors from computed tomography in acute left colonic diverticulitis. Br J Surg 79:117–119

72. Allen-Mersh TG, Henry MM, Nicholls RJ (1987) Natural history of anterior mucosal prolapse. Br J Surg 74:679–682

73. Altringer WE, Saclarides TJ, Dominguez JM et al (1995) Four-contrast defecography: pelvic ''floor-oscopy.'' Dis Colon Rectum 38:695–699

74. Pinho M, Yoshioka K, Keighley MR (1991) Are pelvic floor movements abnormal in disordered defecation? Dis Colon Rectum 34:1117–1119

75. Pinho M, Yoshioka K, Ortiz J et al (1990) The effect of age on pelvic floor dynamics. Int J Colorectal Dis 5:207–208

76. Skomorowska E, Hegedus V, Christiansen J (1988) Evalua-

tion of perineal descent by defaecography. Int J Colorectal Dis 3:191–194

77. Jorge JM, Wexner SD, Ehrenpreis ED et al (1993) Does perineal descent correlate with pudendal neuropathy? Dis Colon Rectum 36:475–483

78. Halligan SH, Thomas J, Bartram CI (1995) Intrarectal pressures and balloon expulsion related to evacuation proctography. Gut 37:100–104

79. Penninckx F, Debruyne C, Lestar B, Kerremans R (1991) Intraobserver variation in the radiological measurement of the anorectal angle. Gastrointest Radiol 16:73–76

80. Jorgensen J, Stein P, King DW, Lubowski DZ (1993) The anorectal angle is not a reliable parameter on defaecating proctography. Aust N Z J Surg 63:105–108

81. Shorvon PJ, Henry MM (1994) Investigation of constipation and incontinence. pp. 852–872. In Freeny PC, Stevenson GW (eds): Margulis and Burhenne's Alimentary Tract Radiology. 5th ed Mosby, St Louis

82. Felt-Bersma RJ, Luth WJ, Janssen JJ, Meuwissen SG (1990) Defecography in patients with anorectal disorders. Which findings are clinically relevant? Dis Colon Rectum 33: 277–284

83. Halligan S, McGee S, Bartram CI (1994) Quantification of evacuation proctography. Dis Colon Rectum 37:1151–1154

84. Halligan MS, Bartram CI, Park HY, Kamm MA (1995) The proctographic features of anismus. Radiology (in press)

85. Kamm MA, Bartram CI, Lennard-Jones JE (1989) Rectodynamics—quantifying rectal evacuation. Int J Colorectal Dis 4:161–163

86. Borstad E, Skrede M, Rud T (1991) Failure to predict and attempts to explain urinary stress incontinence following vaginal repair in continent women by using a modified lateral urethrocystography, see comments. Acta Obstet Gynecol Scand 70:501–506

87. Johansson C, Ihre T, Holmstrom B et al (1990) A combined electromyographic and cineradiologic investigation in patients with defecation disorders. Dis Colon Rectum 33: 1009–1013

88. Womack NR, Williams NS, Holmfield JH et al (1985) New method for the dynamic assessment of anorectal function in constipation. Br J Surg 72:994–998

89. Bartolo DC, Duthie GS (1994) Pelvic floor incoordination. pp. 77–85. In Kamm MA, Lennard-Jones JE (eds): Constipation. Wrightson Biomedical Publishing Ltd, Petersfield, UK

90. Roberts JP, Womack NR, Hallan RI et al (1992) Evidence from dynamic integrated proctography to redefine anismus. Br J Surg 79:1213–1215

91. Shirahama M, Koga T, Ishibashi H et al (1994) Sonographic features of colon carcinoma seen with high-frequency transabdominal ultrasound. J Clin Ultrasound 22:359–365

92. Rutgeerts LJ, Verbanck JJ, Crape AW et al (1991) Detection of colorectal cancer by routine ultrasound. J Belge Radiol 74: 11–13

93. Limberg B (1992) Diagnosis and staging of colonic tumors by conventional abdominal sonography as compared with hydrocolonic sonography, see comments. N Engl J Med 327: 65–69

94. Chui DW, Gooding GA, McQuaid KR et al (1994) Hydrocolonic ultrasonography in the detection of colonic polyps and tumors. N Engl J Med 331:1685–1688

95. Hernandez-Socorro CR, Guerra C, Hernandez-Romero J et al (1995) Colorectal carcinomas: diagnosis and preoperative staging by hydrocolonic sonography. Surgery 117:609–615

96. Walter DF, Govil S, William RR et al (1993) Colonic sonography: preliminary observations. Clin Radiol 47:200–204

97. Limberg B (1989) Diagnosis of acute ulcerative colitis and colonic Crohn's disease by colonic sonography see comments. J Clin Ultrasound 17:25–31

98. Limberg B, Osswald B (1994) Diagnosis and differential diagnosis of ulcerative colitis and Crohn's disease by hydrocolonic sonography. Am J Gastroenterol 89:1051–1057

99. Sheridan MB, Nicholson DA, Martin DF (1993) Transabdominal ultrasonography as the primary investigation in patients with suspected Crohn's disease or recurrence: a prospective study. Clin Radiol 48:402–404

100. Hata J, Haruma K, Suenaga K et al (1992) Ultrasonographic assessment of inflammatory bowel disease, see comments. Am J Gastroenterol 87:443–447

101. Bozkurt T, Richter F, Lux G (1994) Ultrasonography as a primary diagnostic tool in patients with inflammatory disease and tumors of the small intestine and large bowel. J Clin Ultrasound 22:85–91

102. Schwerk WB, Schwarz S, Rothmund M (1992) Sonography in acute colonic diverticulitis. A prospective study. Dis Colon Rectum 35:1077–1084

103. Wilson SR, Toi A (1990) The value of sonography in the diagnosis of acute diverticulitis of the colon. AJR 154: 1199–1202

104. Pulyaert JBCM (1986) Acute appendicitis: US evaluation using graded compression. Radiology 158:355–358

105. Beynon J, Feifel G, Hildebrandt U, Mortensen NJ (1991) An atlas of rectal endosonography. [Anonymous] Springer-Verlag, Vienna, New York

106. Tio TL, Coene PP, van Delden OM, Tytgat GN (1991) Colorectal carcinoma: preoperative TNM classification with endosonography. Radiology 179:165–170

107. Odegaard S, Kimmey MB, Martin RW et al (1992) The effects of applied pressure on the thickness, layers, and echogenicity of gastrointestinal wall ultrasound images. Gastrointest Endosc 38:351–356

108. Van Outryve MJ, Pelckmans PA, Michielsen PP, Van Maercke YM (1991) Value of transrectal ultrasonography in Crohn's disease. Gastroenterology 101:1171–1177

109. Kimmey MB, Martin RW, Haggitt RC et al (1989) Histologic correlates of gastrointestinal ultrasound images. Gastroenterology 96(2 Pt 1): 433–441

110. Odegaard S, Kimmey MB (1994) Location of the muscularis mucosae on high frequency gastrointestinal ultrasound images. Eur J Ultrasound 1:39–50

111. Hulsmans FH, Castelijns JA, Reeders JW, Tytgat GN (1995) Review of artifacts associated with transrectal ultrasound: understanding, recognition, and prevention of misinterpretation. J Clin Ultrasound 23:483–494

112. Thaler W, Watzka S, Martin F et al (1994) Preoperative staging of rectal cancer by endoluminal ultrasound vs. magnetic resonance imaging. Preliminary results of a prospective, comparative study. Dis Colon Rectum 37:1189–1193

113. Sentovich SM, Blatchford GJ, Falk PM et al (1993) Transrectal ultrasound of rectal tumors. Am J Surg 166:638–641; discussion 641–642

114. Scialpi M, Andreatta R, Agugiaro S et al (1993) Rectal carcinoma: preoperative staging and detection of postoperative local recurrence with transrectal and transvaginal ultrasound. Abdom Imaging 18:381–389

115. Milsom JW, Graffner H (1990) Intrarectal ultrasonography in rectal cancer staging and in the evaluation of pelvic disease. Clinical uses of intrarectal ultrasound. Ann Surg 212:602–606

116. Lindmark G, Elvin A, Pahlman L, Glimelius B (1992) The value of endosonography in preoperative staging of rectal cancer. Int J Colorectal Dis 7:162–166

117. Katsura Y, Yamada K, Ishizawa T et al (1992) Endorectal ultrasonography for the assessment of wall invasion and lymph node metastasis in rectal cancer. Dis Colon Rectum 35:362–368

118. Hildebrandt U, Schuder G, Feifel G (1994) Preoperative staging of rectal and colonic cancer. Endoscopy 26:810–812

119. Goldman S, Arvidsson H, Norming U et al (1991) Transrectal ultrasound and computed tomography in preoperative staging of lower rectal adenocarcinoma. Gastrointest Radiol 16:259–263

120. Dershaw DD, Enker WE, Cohen AM, Sigurdson ER (1990) Transrectal ultrasonography of rectal carcinoma. Cancer 66:2336–2340

121. Derksen EJ, Cuesta MA, Meijer S (1992) Intraluminal ultrasound of rectal tumours: a prerequisite in decision making. Surg Oncol 1:193–198

122. Boyce GA, Sivak MV Jr, Lavery IC, et al (1992) Endoscopic ultrasound in the pre-operative staging of rectal carcinoma. Gastrointest Endosc 38:468–471

123. Solomon MJ, McLeod RS (1993) Endoluminal transrectal ultrasonography: accuracy, reliability, and validity. Dis Colon Rectum 36:200–205

124. Solomon MJ, McLeod RS, Cohen EK et al (1994) Reliability and validity studies of endoluminal ultrasonography for anorectal disorders. Dis Colon Rectum 37:546–551

125. Herzog U, von Flue M, Tondelli P, Schuppisser JP (1993) How accurate is endorectal ultrasound in the preoperative staging of rectal cancer? Dis Colon Rectum 36:127–134

126. Hawes RH (1993) New staging techniques. Endoscopic ultrasound. Cancer, 71 suppl 12:4207–4213

127. Hulsmans FJ, Tio TL, Fockens P, et al (1994) Assessment of tumor infiltration depth in rectal cancer with transrectal sonography: caution is necessary, see comments. Radiology 190:715–720

128. Nielsen MB, Pedersen JF, Christiansen J (1993) Rectal endosonography in the evaluation of stenotic rectal tumors. Dis Colon Rectum 36:275–279

129. Rafaelsen SR, Kronborg O, Fenger C (1992) Echo pattern of lymph nodes in colorectal cancer: an in vitro study. Br J Radiol 65:218–220

130. Hildebrandt U, Feifel G (1993) Endosonography in the diagnosis of lymph nodes, editorial. Endoscopy 25:243–245

131. Nielsen MB, Qvitzau S, Pedersen JF (1993) Detection of pericolonic lymph nodes in patients with colorectal cancer: an in vitro and in vivo study of the efficacy of endosonography. AJR Am J Roentgenol 161:57–60

132. Andersson R, Aus G (1990) Transrectal ultrasound-guided biopsy for verification of lymph-node metastasis in rectal cancer. Case report. Acta Chir Scand 156:659–660

133. Milsom JW, Czyrko C, Hull TL et al (1994) Preoperative biopsy of pararectal lymph nodes in rectal cancer using endoluminal ultrasonography. Dis Colon Rectum 37:364–368

134. Anderson BO, Hann LE, Enker WE et al (1994) Transrectal ultrasonography and operative selection for early carcinoma of the rectum. J Am Coll Surg 179:513–517

135. Detry RJ, Kartheuser A, Kestens PJ (1993) Endorectal ultrasonography for staging small rectal tumors: technique and contribution to treatment. World J Surg 17:271–275; discussion 275–276

136. Hulsmans FH, Tio TL, Mathus-Vliegen EM et al (1992) Colorectal villous adenoma: transrectal US in screening for invasive malignancy. Radiology 185:193–196

137. Mosnier H, Guivarch M, Meduri B et al (1990) Endorectal sonography in the management of rectal villous tumors. Int J Colorectal Dis 5:90–93

138. Glaser F, Kuntz C, Schlag P, Herfarth C (1993) Endorectal ultrasound for control of preoperative radiotherapy of rectal cancer. Ann Surg 217:64–71

139. Napoleon B, Pujol B, Berger F et al (1991) Accuracy of endosonography in the staging of rectal cancer treated by radiotherapy. Br J Surg 78:785–788

140. Fleshman JW, Myerson RJ, Fry RD, Kodner IJ (1992) Accuracy of transrectal ultrasound in predicting pathologic stage of rectal cancer before and after preoperative radiation therapy. Dis Colon Rectum 35:823–829

141. Dresing K, Stock W (1990) Ultrasonic endoluminal examination in the follow-up of colorectal cancer. Initial experience and results. Int J Colorectal Dis 5:188–194

142. Ramirez JM, Mortensen NJ, Takeuchi N, Humphreys MM (1994) Endoluminal ultrasonography in the follow-up of patients with rectal cancer. Br J Surg 81:692–694

143. Tschmelitsch J, Glaser K, Schwarz C et al (1992) Endosonography (ES) in the diagnosis of recurrent cancer of the rectum. J Ultrasound Med 11:149–153

144. Charnley RM, Heywood MF, Hardcastle JD (1990). Rectal endosonography for the visualisation of the anastomosis after anterior resection and its relevance to local recurrence. Int J Colorectal Dis 5:127–129

145. Milsom JW, Lavery IC, Stolfi VM et al (1992) The expanding utility of endoluminal ultrasonography in the management of rectal cancer. Surgery 112:832–840; discussion 840–841

146. Nielsen MB, Pedersen JF, Christiansen J (1992) Rectal endosonography and guided biopsy in the evaluation of recurrent rectal carcinoma. Br J Radiol 65:622

147. Alexander AA, Miller LS, Liu JB et al (1994) High-resolution endoluminal sonography of the anal sphincter complex. J Ultrasound Med 13:281–284

148. Burnett SJ, Bartram CI (1991) Endosonographic variations in the normal internal anal sphincter. Int J Colorectal Dis 6:2–4

149. Papachrysostomou M, Pye SD, Wild SR, Smith AN (1992) Anal endosonography: which endoprobe? Br J Radiol 65:715–717

150. Sultan AH, Loder PB, Bartram CI et al (1994) Vaginal endosonography. New approach to image the undisturbed anal sphincter. Dis Colon Rectum 37:1296–1299

151. Sultan AH, Kamm MA, Hudson CN et al (1994) Endosonography of the anal sphincters: normal anatomy and comparison with manometry. Clin Radiol 49:368–374

152. Halligan S, Sultan A, Rottenberg G, Bartram CI (1995) Endosonography of the anal sphincters in solitary rectal ulcer syndrome. Int J Colorectal Dis 10:79–82

153. Kamm MA, Hoyle CH, Burleigh DE et al (1991) Hereditary internal anal sphincter myopathy causing proctalgia fugax and constipation. A newly identified condition. Gastroenterology 100:805–810

154. Silvis R, van Eekelen JW, Delemarre JB, Gooszen HG (1995) Endosonography of the anal sphincter after ileal pouch-anal anastomosis. Relation with anal manometry and fecal continence. Dis Colon Rectum 38:383–388

155. Eckardt VF, Nix W (1991) The anal sphincter in patients with myotonic muscular dystrophy. Gastroenterology 100:424–430

156. Sultan AH, Kamm MA, Hudson CN et al (1993) Anal-sphincter disruption during vaginal delivery. N Engl J Med 329:1905–1911

157. Nielsen MB, Rasmussen OO, Pedersen JF, Christiansen J (1993) Risk of sphincter damage and anal incontinence after anal dilatation for fissure-in-ano. An endosonographic study. Dis Colon Rectum 36:677–680

158. Speakman CT, Burnett SJ, Kamm MA, Bartram CI (1991) Sphincter injury after anal dilatation demonstrated by anal endosonography. Br J Surg 78:1429–1430

159. Sultan AH, Kamm MA, Nicholls RJ, Bartram CI (1994) Prospective study of the extent of internal anal sphincter division during lateral sphincterotomy. Dis Colon Rectum 37:1031–1033

160. Engel AF, Kamm MA, Bartram CI (1995) Unwanted anal penetration as a physical cause of faecal incontinence. Eur J Gastroenterol Hepatol 7:65–67

161. Sultan AH, Kamm MA, Talbot IC et al (1994) Anal endosonography for identifying external sphincter defects confirmed histologically. Br J Surg 81:463–465

162. Deen KI, Kumar D, Williams JG et al (1993) Anal sphincter defects. Correlation between endoanal ultrasound and surgery. Ann Surg 218:201–205

163. Nielsen MB, Hauge C, Pedersen JF, Christiansen J (1993) Endosonographic evaluation of patients with anal incontinence: findings and influence on surgical management. AJR Am J Roentgenol 160:771–775

164. Tjandra JJ, Milsom JW, Schroeder T, Fazio VW (1993) Endoluminal ultrasound is preferable to electromyography in mapping anal sphincteric defects. Dis Colon Rectum 36:689–692

165. Kamm MA (1994) Obstetric damage and faecal incontinence, see comments. Lancet 344:730–733

166. Sultan AH, Kamm MA, Bartram CI, Hudson CN (1993) Anal sphincter trauma during instrumental delivery. Int J Gynaecol Obstet 43:263–270

167. Sultan AH, Kamm MA, Hudson CN, Bartram CI (1994) Third degree obstetric anal sphincter tears: risk factors and outcome of primary repair. BMJ 308:887–891

168. Nielsen MB, Hauge C, Rasmussen OO et al (1992) Anal endosonographic findings in the follow-up of primarily sutured sphincteric ruptures. Br J Surg 79:104–106

169. Nielsen MB, Dammegaard L, Pedersen JF (1994) Endosonographic assessment of the anal sphincter after surgical reconstruction. Dis Colon Rectum 37:434–438

170. Engel AF, Kamm MA, Sultan AH et al (1994) Anterior anal sphincter repair in patients with obstetric trauma. Br J Surg 81:1231–1234

171. Choen S, Burnett S, Bartram CI, Nicholls RJ (1991) Comparison between anal endosonography and digital examination in the evaluation of anal fistulae. Br J Surg 78:445–447

172. Cheong DM, Nogueras JJ, Wexner SD, Jagelman DG (1993) Anal endosonography for recurrent anal fistulas: image enhancement with hydrogen peroxide. Dis Colon Rectum 36:1158–1160

173. Law PJ, Talbot RW, Bartram CI, Northover JM (1989) Anal endosonography in the evaluation of perianal sepsis and fistula in ano. Br J Surg 76:752–755

174. Deen KI, Williams JG, Hutchinson R et al (1994) Fistulas in ano: endoanal ultrasonographic assessment assists decision making for surgery. Gut 35:391–394

175. Lunniss PJ, Barker PG, Sultan AH et al (1994) Magnetic resonance imaging of fistula-in-ano. Dis Colon Rectum 37:708–718

176. Herzog U, Boss M, Spichtin HP (1994) Endoanal ultrasonography in the follow-up of anal carcinoma. Surg Endosc 8:1186–1189

177. Schwander D, Zurbriggen S, Schwander A (1973) Peritonitis caused by barium and other complications of barium enema. Ann Radiol (Paris) 16:521–526

COMPUTED TOMOGRAPHY AND MAGNETIC RESONANCE IMAGING

W. Ross Stevens

C. Daniel Johnson

Computed tomography (CT) plays an important role in the evaluation of patients with colorectal diseases. CT does not have the resolution of colonoscopy or contrast enema for evaluation of the bowel mucosa, but its advantage is its ability to image the bowel wall in its entirety and the extraluminal extent of colorectal disease. CT has impact on the diagnosis, management, and follow-up of inflammatory and neoplastic conditions that affect the colon and rectum. Although magnetic resonance imaging (MRI) has not been utilized to directly image the colon, it has superior contrast resolution over CT and sonography and is having an increasing role in specific applications of abdominal imaging. Currently, evaluation of the liver for metastatic disease is the most common application of MRI in evaluation of colorectal diseases. This section discusses the use of CT and MRI in evaluation of colorectal diseases, including techniques of examination, the indications and limitations of cross-sectional imaging, and the imaging findings of common disease processes.

TECHNIQUES OF EXAMINATION

Computed Tomography

Current generation spiral CT scanners have become increasingly versatile as volumetric scanning and faster scan speeds expand the imaging options available. Thin sections for assessment of small anatomic structures or multiplanar image display is possible using volumetric data acquired during spiral CT scanning. More rapid scanning allows an area of interest to be imaged sequentially in order to demonstrate a lesion's enhancement pattern after intravenous contrast material is administered. The information provided by rapid, volumetric scanning techniques may improve the visualization or characterization of a lesion. CT examinations can be tailored to provide the most useful information when radiologists are provided pertinent clinical information and the questions to be answered by the study. In selected patients, the effectiveness of CT and MRI in evaluation of the colon can be optimized by using laxatives prior to the study for cleansing of the bowel and by ensuring

good distension of the bowel wall with air, water, or contrast material during the examination. Dilute oral contrast material can be given several hours before the study or a dilute contrast enema can be given at the time of the study for good opacification of the colon and rectum. For rectal lesions, prone positioning during CT scanning may provide better visualization of the primary tumor. Intravenous contrast material is especially helpful in the evaluation of the solid abdominal organs and in distinguishing vessels from enlarged lymph nodes.

For the detection of metastatic disease to the liver, intravenous iodinated contrast enhanced CT scans are more sensitive than unenhanced scans. Normally, 75% to 80% of the blood supply to the liver comes from the portal venous system, with the remainder coming from the hepatic arterial supply. The blood supply to hepatic neoplasms arises almost entirely from the arterial system. Because most colorectal metastases are hypovascular, enhanced CT scans of the liver obtained when portal venous opacification is at its peak will provide the best discrimination between the enhanced high-attenuation hepatic parenchyma and the relatively lower attenuation metastases. Metastases may appear hyperdense to liver when scans are obtained during the arterial phase of contrast enhancement. This appearance is most prominently seen in hypervascular metastases such as those from neuroendocrine, renal, and thyroid tumors. Using current generation spiral CT scanners, it is possible to obtain images of the liver during both the arterial and the portal venous phases of a single intravenous contrast injection. This dual-phase scanning may increase the sensitivity of CT for identification of hypervascular metastases.

CT arterial portography (CTAP) is another scanning method that capitalizes on the differential blood supply between the liver and hepatic tumors. For CTAP, CT scans are obtained after injection of iodinated contrast material into the portal venous system via a catheter positioned in the superior mesenteric artery. This results in a more selective portal phase scan than is available with the usual delivery of contrast material via peripheral veins (no contrast material in the hepatic arterial system). Hepatic metastases appear hypodense compared to the markedly enhanced hepatic parenchyma. The CTAP technique has been shown to be more sensitive than conventional CT and MRI in detection of hepatic metastases.[1] However, CTAP has the disadvantages of being more expensive and more invasive than conventional CT and is usually reserved for patients who do not have evidence of unresectable disease on conventional studies. Perfusion defects in the liver are commonly encountered with this technique and can simulate hepatic masses. Considerable experience is required for accurate interpretation of these images.

Magnetic Resonance Imaging

MRI, like CT, has many options available for individualizing the examination to address the clinical concerns. Effective communication between the radiologist and surgeon is necessary so that the appropriate study can be obtained in the optimal manner for each patient. Because MRI is usually a longer examination than CT, it is most useful for evaluating a specific area of interest. MRI is not well suited for survey examinations of the entire abdomen. With respect to colorectal disease, MRI is currently most often used in evaluation of the liver for metastases. Some investigators,[2-4] have found it useful for staging rectal tumors and for assessing recurrent tumor following abdominoperitoneal resections. The basis and theory of MRI pulse sequence selection is beyond the scope of this review. Typically, standard T_1- and T_2-weighted images are obtained in the axial plane. Coronal, sagittal, or oblique planes can be selected to optimally display anatomic findings. Gradient echo images may be used to increase lesion conspicuity or to depict flowing blood in order to exclude portal venous thrombosis. Fat saturation or chemical shift images can help to determine the fat content of a lesion. Gadolinium-based intravenous contrast agents can be used in MRI examinations to demonstrate the vascularity and enhancement patterns of lesions and provide information similar to that derived from contrast-enhanced CT scans. Gadolinium-enhanced MR images are sometimes more sensitive than unenhanced images in detection of small hepatic tumors.

Various radiofrequency coils are available to image different anatomic structures. The body coil is the standard coil used in MRI. It has a large field of view useful for coverage of large anatomic regions but provides the lowest signal to noise compared to other dedicated coils. Surface coils, such as the abdominal or pelvic phased array multicoils, have been shown to provide at least twice the signal to noise available for liver or pelvic imaging.[5] Endorectal coils have been developed that facilitate imaging of the rectum, prostate, or cervix. Using an endorectal coil, it may become possible to reliably image the rectal wall and depict the depth of invasion of rectal tumors.

MALIGNANT TUMORS

Colorectal Carcinoma

Detection and Staging of Primary Tumor

Conventional intraluminal contrast radiography and endoscopy are currently the best methods for the initial diagnosis and evaluation of primary tumors and mucosal lesions in the colon and rectum.[6] Although CT and MRI studies may incidentally identify a primary colorectal tumor, conventional cross-sectional imaging studies are insensitive for screening of intraluminal tumors. CT and MRI are most useful in the preoperative staging of colorectal carcinoma and in the postoperative surveillance for recurrent or metastatic disease. These techniques can demonstrate extracolonic tumor spread to adjacent structures and distant organs. The layers of the bowel wall and the depth of tumor invasion can be determined using endorectal ultrasound and MRI. MRI is less useful in evaluation of primary colonic tumors above the reach of the endorectal coil because of its lower spatial resolution (using the body coil) and bowel motion artifacts.

Compared with the normal colon (see Fig. 7-56), primary colorectal masses are often seen at CT as an area of circumferential bowel wall thickening and mass, corresponding to the typical "apple core" appearance of colorectal cancers on conventional barium enema studies.[7] Local invasion of the tumor may be suggested by the presence of soft tissue stranding in the pericolonic fat, obliteration of pericolonic fat planes, or by extension of the mass into adjacent structures such as muscle, bone, or solid organs (Fig. 7-57). The gastrocolic ligament is a natural pathway for tumor arising in the transverse colon to spread to the greater curvature of the stomach.[8] Lymph node metastases can be suggested by the finding of enlarged lymph nodes (greater than 1.0 cm diameter) in the pericolonic fat, mesentery, or retroperitoneum. Unfortunately, metastatic lymphadenopathy often occurs in microscopic quantities within normal-sized lymph nodes. Without nodal enlargement, this pathway of disease spread cannot be currently detected by imaging examinations.[9,10]

Although findings of colon wall thickening and pericolonic mass or soft tissue stranding are helpful in the staging of primary tumors, these findings are not specific.[7,11] Inflammatory conditions such as diverticulitis or colitis can have a similar appearance. Poor preparation of the colon results in residual colonic contents and incomplete distension of the colon and makes detection of intralumenal masses and wall thickening more difficult. Because of these limitations, the reported sensitivity of CT ranges from 53% to 77% in identification of local tumor extension and from 22% to 73% in detection of lymph node metastases.[7,10-12] MRI has similar limitations and has been shown to have sensitivities similar to those of CT in staging of primary lesions of the colon.[10]

Assessment of Metastases

Cross-sectional imaging has its greatest impact on the clinical management of colorectal cancer patients in the assessment for distant metastatic disease. Common sites for early metastases from colorectal cancer include the liver, adrenal, and retroperitoneal lymph nodes. Detection of metastatic disease indicates a poorer prognosis and may change the planned clinical and surgical management of these patients. Resection of localized metastases may prolong disease-free survival in colorectal cancer patients, but diffuse metastases may not be resectable. Palliative surgery, chemotherapy, and/or irradiation therapy may be indicated in these patients.

Because of the high prevalence of metastases to the liver, preoperative evaluation of the liver can be helpful in selected colorectal cancer patients.[12] Ultrasound and/or intravenous contrast-enhanced CT are typically obtained initially. Ultrasound

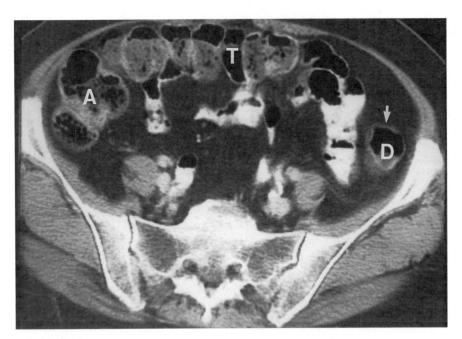

Figure 7-56. CT of normal colon. CT scan with oral contrast material shows the normal ascending (A), transverse (T), and descending (D) colon. The colon is normal in caliber and contains gas and fecal material. The colon wall is almost imperceptibly thin (arrow).

provides a less expensive examination of the liver, but CT has the advantage of providing better visualization of extrahepatic disease extent including the adrenal glands and retroperitoneum.[13] If diffuse, unresectable metastases are encountered on the initial studies, the imaging assessment is complete. If metastases amenable to resection are discovered, additional evaluation of the liver with MRI, CTAP, or intraoperative ultrasound is indicated to search for additional lesions.[9]

Indeterminate lesions may be detected on the initial CT or ultrasound studies and provide a diagnostic dilemma. If prior studies are not available for comparison, MRI may provide improved tissue characterization of the lesion in question. Benign lesions such as focal fatty infiltration, cysts, or cavernous hemangiomas can simulate metastases and are readily diagnosed at MRI examination. Alternatively, CT or ultrasound can provide guidance for percutaneous needle biopsy of an indeterminate lesion to obtain a pathologic diagnosis.

Hepatic metastases from colorectal carcinoma usually appear on CT as discrete low attenuation masses on unenhanced scans (Fig. 7-58). Calcification may be present and usually indicates a mucinous primary tumor. The hepatic calcifications within mucinous metastases are characteristically fine, punctate calcifications that may be diffuse. Similar calcifications can also be seen in other mucinous metastases, such as those from breast or ovarian primary tumors. Colorectal metastases are usually hypovascular and are therefore hypodense to liver on contrast-enhanced CT scans. Low-attenuation, unenhancing areas within metastatic lesions are often due to necrosis. Enhancing regions of the lesions and peripheral rims represent viable tumor. The reported sensitivity of CT for detection of hepatic metastases is in the range of 70% to 80%.[11,14] CT is least sensitive for detection of metastases less than 1 cm diameter. Spiral CT

should improve the sensitivity of CT because of its more rapid scan time. Rapid scanning allows for thinner sections and for completion of the study during the optimal phase of hepatic enhancement.

At MRI, hepatic metastases are generally discrete masses that are hypointense to liver on T_1-weighted (short TR/short TE) scans and moderately hyperintense on T_2-weighted (long TR/long TE) scans[15] (see Fig. 7-58). The sensitivity of MRI in detection of liver metastases is similar to or slightly greater than that of CT scans.[14,16] Like CT, MRI is least sensitive in detection of smaller lesions. Because the sensitivities of CT and MRI are similar and the cost of MRI is greater, CT is generally preferred for the initial screening of patients for hepatic metastases. In our practice MRI is used as an adjunct to CT and ultrasound for the characterization of indeterminate lesions and in the preoperative search for inoperable disease. In addition, flow-sensitive MR images can be used to define the vascular anatomy of the liver in order to localize resectable lesions with respect to the relevant surgical anatomy. Spiral CT angiography may prove to be of equal value in demonstrating the vascular anatomy of the liver.

Postoperative Surveillance

As many as 30% to 50% of colorectal cancers will recur after attempted curative resection of the primary lesion.[12] Eighty percent of recurrences are found within 2 years of the initial resection.[7,11] Metastatic lesions to the liver account for almost one-half of recurrences, local recurrence at the area of bowel resection for about one-third, and peritoneal seeding for 22%.[12] Early identification of recurrent or metastatic disease is important because treatment of early metastases can result in improved

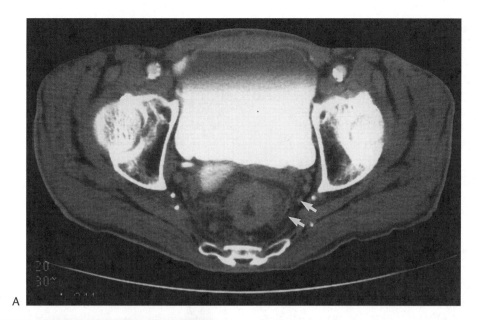

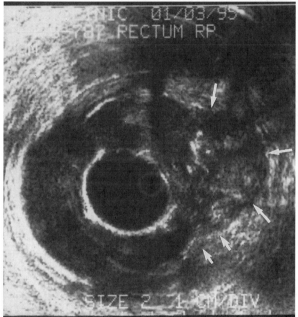

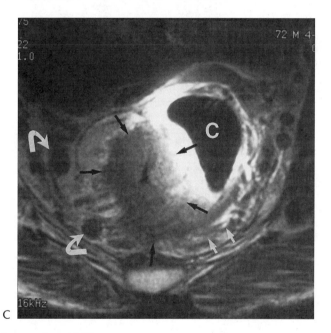

Figure 7-57. Rectal carcinoma evaluated with CT, transrectal ultrasound, and MRI using endorectal coil. (**A**) Intravenous contrast-enhanced CT shows circumferential thickening of the rectal wall by tumor. Soft tissue stranding in the perirectal fat indicates tumor extension (arrows). (**B**) Ultrasound of the rectum shows circumferential abnormal thickening of the rectal wall by tumor. The tumor extends through the echogenic muscularis propria into the perirectal fat (arrows). (**C**) T$_2$-weighted MRI using endorectal coil (C) shows the rectal tumor mass (black arrows) with perirectal invasion (white arrows), and enlarged lymph nodes (curved arrows).

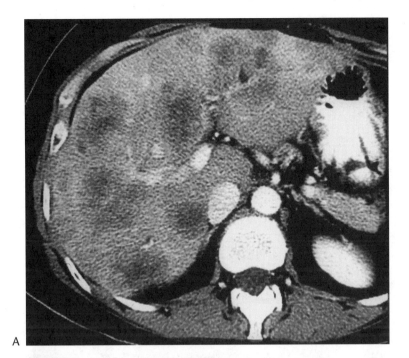

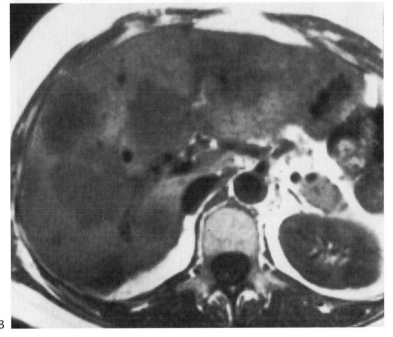

Figure 7-58. CT and MRI of metastatic colon carcinoma to the liver. (**A**) Intravenous contrast-enhanced CT shows multiple low-attenuation, hypovascular metastases throughout the liver. MRI examination of the same patient shows that compared to the normal liver, the metastases (**B**) are of low signal intensity on the T_1-weighted (short TR/TE) image. (*Figure continues.*)

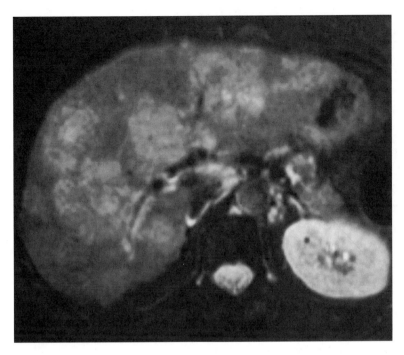

Figure 7-58 *(Continued).* (**C**) The metastases have higher signal intensity on the T_2-weighted (long TR/TE) image.

patient survival. The postoperative surveillance of patients with resected colorectal carcinomas often represents a multimodality approach in which cross-sectional imaging plays an important role.[17]

Appropriate strategies for postoperative imaging in patients with colorectal cancer are determined by the location and stage of the primary tumor and by the results of other postoperative evaluations. Tumor recurrence after attempted curative resection of colorectal carcinoma may involve the colonic anastamosis, local tissues, or distant sites. Imaging strategies for postoperative surveillance should include all of these areas. CT is the most useful imaging study for overall postoperative screening of the abdomen and pelvis in patients with resected colorectal cancer. CT can detect hepatic metastases, extraluminal recurrence, and lymphadenopathy or peritoneal implants. MRI is equivalent to CT in detection of hepatic metastases and is useful in distinguishing some benign lesions such as cavernous hemangiomas from metastases.[16] MRI has shown promise in the ability to differentiate locally recurrent carcinoma from postoperative fibrosis.[2–4] MRI is less sensitive than CT for evaluation of extraluminal tumor recurrence and peritoneal seeding. In patients who had higher staged tumors (Duke's B or C lesions) and are therefore more likely to develop metastases, routine interval follow-up CT scans may detect recurrent or metastatic lesions before they are large enough to produce clinical symptoms or abnormal laboratory values.[11,12] In patients with lower staged (Duke's A) primary lesions, a more conservative approach might be employed and imaging reserved for those patients with clinical symptoms, laboratory abnormalities, or barium enema or colonoscopic findings suggestive of recurrence.[17]

Anastomotic recurrence after partial colonic resection and ileocolic or colocolic anastomosis is the least common site of recurrence encountered. Barium enema and colonoscopy are best suited for evaluation of anastomotic recurrence.[14,18] On barium enema, anastomotic recurrence can be seen as an area of anastomotic narrowing and is usually asymmetric and irregular. Adjacent mass effect and obstruction may also be present.[18] CT is less sensitive than barium enema for detection of anastomotic recurrence and may miss smaller mucosal lesions. However, CT can often show more extensive extraluminal disease adjacent to the involved anastomotic segment.[18] On CT, the diagnosis of anastomotic recurrence requires the presence of a discrete mass or local invasion of adjacent structures or fat planes. This extraluminal tumor spread is not as well seen on barium enema or colonoscopic examinations and may be of importance to patient management. Therefore, CT can be considered complementary to barium enema or colonoscopy in the evaluation of anastomotic disease.

CT is of particular importance in the postoperative follow-up of patients who have had abdominoperineal resections for rectal carcinoma. The sensitivity of CT is significantly greater for the diagnosis of local recurrence after abdominoperineal resection than after anterior resection and reanastomosis.[19] Tumor recurrence in the pelvis is common, occurring in up to 50% of patients, and frequently is the cause of death in these patients.[12] Clinical symptoms suggesting recurrence are nonspecific and generally occur only in the advanced stages of local recurrence after direct invasion of adjacent structures.[12,20,21] Resection of the rectum precludes colonoscopy or barium enema examination for detection of locally recurrent disease. Local recurrence of rectal carcinoma after abdominoperitoneal resection most often is manifested as a mass in the presacral space. Recurrent tumor may also spread locally to involve the pelvic side walls or other pelvic organs such as bladder, prostate, uterus, or vagina. Secondary ureteral obstruction by tumor may also be observed.[22] On CT, pelvic recurrence generally appears as an irregular, heterogeneous, expanding, soft tissue-

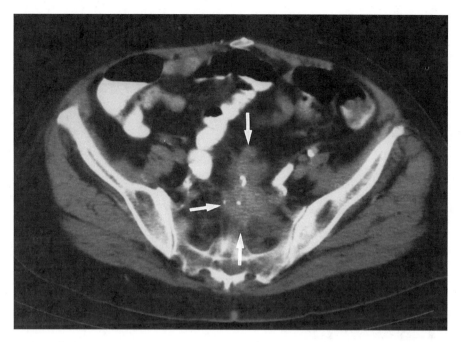

Figure 7-59. CT of recurrent rectal carcinoma. CT with oral contrast material shows irregular soft tissue mass arising in the presacral region (arrows) with standing of the adjacent fat. This lesion was not present on a prior postoperative baseline study and represents recurrence of rectal cancer at the rectal stump anastomosis. (From Johnson,[61] with permission.)

density presacral mass with indistinct margins (Fig. 7-59). However, these changes are not specific for recurrence. The differential diagnosis for a presacral mass includes, in addition to tumor recurrence, postoperative changes such as fibrosis, hematoma, or abscess.[19,22,23] Postoperative irradiation of the pelvis often incites the development of granulation or fibrous tissue that results in the CT findings of linear, streaky soft tissue density in the presacral and pelvic fat.[10,20] The appearance of these normal postoperative and postirradiation changes may be indistinguishable from that of tumor recurrence.[7,10–12] Displaced but otherwise normal pelvic structures such as small bowel, prostate, seminal vesicles, or uterus can simulate recurrent masses.[23] Ureteral stones causing hydronephrosis have been reportedly mistaken for malignant ureteral obstruction.[22] Invasive tumors may coincidentally arise in other pelvic organs and produce misleading imaging features.[19]

The most sensitive use of CT for accurate detection of an early recurrence and differentiation of recurrence from benign presacral changes is with a baseline study obtained early in the postoperative period for comparison with subsequent follow-up scans and biopsy of suspicious lesions.[22] On serial follow-up studies, postoperative changes may remain unchanged or may become smaller and better delineated. CT findings indicating tumor recurrence include new or enlarging soft tissue masses on consecutive examinations, development of invasion into adjacent tissues, or development of pelvic lymphadenopathy.[19] Masses with low attenuation centers may indicate central necrosis within a recurrent mass.[19,24] The recommended protocols[9–11,22] for postoperative surveillance after abdominoperineal resection includes a baseline CT scan obtained during the first 2 to 4 postoperative months. Serial follow-up scans are

then obtained every 6 to 8 months. After 2 to 3 years, the follow-up CT examinations can probably be obtained yearly if the patient remains disease free. Of course, studies can be obtained more frequently if the patient develops signs or symptoms that suggest recurrence.

CT-guided percutaneous needle biopsy is often necessary to supplement the diagnostic CT evaluation of recurrent tumor. Suspicious or equivocal CT findings of recurrence can be biopsied via percutaneous approach using CT guidance for a more definitive diagnosis of recurrence.[11,22] Biopsy may be indicated if there are clinical signs or laboratory studies suggesting recurrence but the CT findings indicate only postoperative changes.[19] CT is used to guide percutaneous placement of the biopsy needle, typically via a transgluteal approach with the patient in the prone position.[25] A thin needle (20 to 22 G) aspiration may be sufficient to obtain diagnostic tissue, but the presence of a desmoplastic fibrosis with infiltrating tumor cells may require tissue core biopsy with a larger bore needle (16 to 18 G).[19]

Successful differentiation of recurrent tumor from fibrosis using MRI has been reported.[3,4,20,23] On MRI, most malignant tumors have intermediate to high signal intensity on T_2-weighted (long TR/long TE) images, whereas fibrous tissue has low signal intensity.[3,4,24] The presence of high signal intensity on T_2-weighted images has been found to be accurate in predicting recurrent tumor in up to 80% of patients.[23] In addition, studies comparing MRI to CT indicate that without the benefit of baseline comparison examinations, MRI was more accurate than CT for diagnosis of recurrent tumor.[20,23] The sensitivity of MRI in detection of local recurrence is reportedly from 80% to 91% with a specificity of as high as 100%.[14,23] This compares with a reported 82% sensitivity and 50% specificity for CT.[23]

The greater sensitivity and specificity of MRI over CT can be attributed to better differentiation of displaced normal anatomic structures such as seminal vesicle or uterus as well as to discrimination of fibrosis from recurrent tumor.[20,23] MRI in some cases demonstrated sacral metastases or neural tumor involvement that was not apparent on CT.[23]

However, MRI examinations can be limited in the evaluation of some patients. Susceptibility artifacts produced by metallic suture material or surgical clips in the postoperative bed may obscure visualization of some areas.[20] Abscesses, fluid collections, or inflammatory changes may have high signal intensity on T_2-weighted images and may be difficult to distinguish from postoperative recurrence.[20,24] MRI is also sometimes limited in the differentiation between recurrence and fibrosis in some patients in whom recurrent tumor arises in an area of postoperative fibrosis.[2,10] In these cases, malignant cells may be interspersed within fibrous tissues or inflammatory changes and are not easily distinguished on the MR images because the tumor does not necessarily exhibit the characteristic high signal intensity on T_2-weighted images. In a study comparing histologic findings to MRI in patients with recurrent rectal carcinomas, de Lange et al.[24] found a variable histologic character to the recurrent tumor and the host response resulting in a broad distribution of signal intensities in malignant lesions on the T_2-weighted images. High signal intensity was found in areas consisting predominantly of carcinoma or tumor necrosis, low signal intensity in areas of predominant desmoplasia (fibrosis) and a paucity of malignant cells, and intermediate signal intensity in areas of fibrosis interspersed with larger amounts of tumor cells.[24] Therefore, the signal intensity of a suspicious presacral lesion may not reliably differentiate between benign and malignant histology.[24] Because of these imaging limitations, confirmatory CT-directed biopsy is usually performed at our institutions rather than MRI, with MRI examinations used to supplement information obtained at CT.

MRI is generally considered to be better than CT in evaluation of the cardiac, musculoskeletal, and nervous systems and has proven to be useful in evaluation of these organs for metastases from colorectal carcinoma.[26–28] Colorectal metastases to these organs are not as common as metastases to the liver or peritoneum and routine studies are not indicated. However, if metastases are clinically suspected, MRI would probably be the study of choice for visualization and characterization of potential metastatic lesions in the heart, brain, or bones. CT remains the most sensitive study for evaluation of the lungs for metastases.

The use of CT and MRI in detection and characterization of hepatic metastases was discussed previously with respect to tumor staging. Cross-sectional imaging can also aid in the treatment of some metastatic lesions in the liver. CT or ultrasound can be used to guide needle placement for percutaneous ablation of hepatic metastases with ethanol. Using CT or ultrasound for guidance, ethanol is injected into a hepatic lesion, resulting in cell death and tumor necrosis. Ethanol ablation is most successful when performed on single focal lesions of less than 5 cm diameter. It can be performed only if the lesion is accessible by needle with image guidance. Other ablative agents such as cryogenics, radiofrequency pulses, and immunotherapy can be delivered using CT or ultrasound guidance and are currently being investigated for treatment of primary and metastatic liver lesions.[29]

Complications of Colorectal Tumors

Intussusception

In adults, colonic intussusception usually occurs because of an underlying bowel abnormality, such as a primary or secondary malignancy, a benign tumor, or Meckel's diverticulum. Carcinoma of the colon is the most common cause of colonic intussusceptions.[12] Intussusception has a characteristic appearance on both contrast enema studies and on CT. Many patients with intussusception present with abdominal pain and a palpable mass, and CT is often the initial examination obtained in these patients.

On CT, intussusception is characterized by a shortened and thickened segment of bowel that results from the invagination of one segment, the intussusceptum, into the adjacent segment, the intussuscipiens[30] (Fig. 7-60). Mesenteric fat and vessels are pulled into the intussuscipiens along with the intussusceptum. Identification of these mesenteric contents within the mass is pathognomonic for intussusception on CT. The underlying mass responsible for the intussusception can occasionally be identified. In the absence of a mass on CT, further evaluation is recommended.[12] In most adults, urgent surgery will be required to reduce the intussusception and resect the underlying mass. Often, the findings of intussusception may be the first or only indication of a primary or metastatic tumor.[30] Secondary features and complications that may be seen include bowel obstruction proximal to the intussusception, bowel ischemia, and perforation due to vascular compromise of the intussuscepting segment.

Although MRI is not often used for evaluation of intussusception, it may be indicated in selected patients such as pregnant women in whom exposure to ionizing radiation is contraindicated.[31] The MRI findings of intussusception are identical to those at CT.

Perforation

Perforation in colon carcinoma is an uncommon complication that can present difficulty in the diagnosis of the underlying malignancy.[12] At CT, the features of perforated cancer include a soft tissue mass with inflammatory changes in the adjacent pericolonic fat, abscess, and/or extracolonic gas (Fig. 7-61). The appearance may be indistinguishable from colonic diverticulitis. Inflammatory disease of the colon with a significant masslike component should be regarded with suspicion and exclusion of underlying neoplasm is warranted.[32] The presence of perforation in colon cancer increases the likelihood of peritoneal tumor spread. Resection of these lesions may be more difficult and the operative mortality is increased.

Lymphoma

Lymphoma may involve the colon primarily or as a secondary manifestation of diffuse abdominal lymphoma. Lymphoma of the gastrointestinal tract is usually of the non-Hodgkin's type. CT is complementary to contrast enema studies for the evalua-

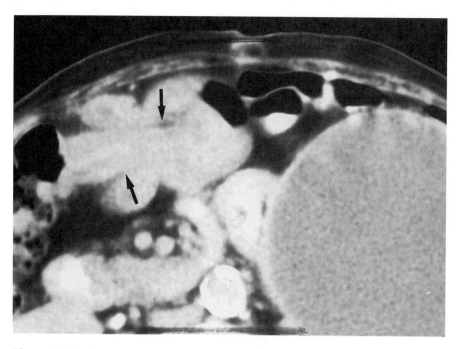

Figure 7-60. Intussuscepting colon cancer. An intussusception is present in the right transverse colon. The linear low density (fat) region (arrows) within the mass represents mesenteric fat. The lead point mass is not visible, but at contrast enema a polypoid carcinoma was discovered. A large cystic mass is also visible arising from the left kidney. (From Johnson,[61] with permission.)

tion of primary colorectal lymphoma. It is useful in the characterization and staging of lymphoma, and in its differentiation from adenocarcinoma.[33] Colonic lymphoma may appear on CT as a discrete bulky mass, a focal area of mural infiltration, or may involve the colon diffusely, either in its entirety or over a long segment[34] (Fig. 7-62). Lesions may be single or multiple and most commonly involve the cecum or rectum. CT findings can help in distinguishing primary colorectal lymphoma from adenocarcinoma. The diagnosis of lymphoma is suggested for cecal tumors that extend into the terminal ileum and for tumors that involve long segments of the colon. Adenocarcinomas are more likely than lymphomas to invade adjacent structures. Colorectal lymphoma is often associated with bulky mesenteric or retroperitoneal lymphadenopathy.[11,34] The bulky, conglomerate lymphadenopathy of lymphoma is usually distinguishable from the mildly enlarged, distinct inflammatory lymph nodes that can be seen in Crohn's disease.[35,36]

Metastatic Disease to the Colon

Metastatic disease to the colon is much less common than primary malignancy. Metastases to the colon can arise from intraperitoneal spread of tumor with colonic implants, from direct extension of tumor from other abdominal organs, and from hematogenous spread.[8] Common primary tumors that may metastasize to the colon include tumors of the ovary, uterus, prostate, breast, stomach, and pancreas. Diffuse intraperitoneal carcinomatosis is most often associated with ovarian carcinoma. CT will demonstrate heterogeneous soft tissue stranding and nodularity of the mesentery, omentum, and peritoneal wall. Ascites

and liver metastases may also be present. Ovarian, uterine, or prostatic carcinomas may invade directly into the adjacent rectum or sigmoid colon. A soft tissue mass deforming these organs is usually identified at CT. Direct extension may produce asymmetric mass effect on the bowel or thickening of the bowel wall in the involved region. The appearance can be difficult to differentiate from a primary colorectal lesion. Primary tumors of the stomach or pancreas can extend directly into the transverse colon by way of the gastrocolic ligament and transverse mesocolon. A soft tissue mass involving these organs and extending into the colon is usually seen at CT. Hematogenous metastases can occur from primary cancers such as breast carcinoma or melanoma. These would appear as soft tissue nodules in the bowel wall or as larger masses involving the bowel. As with any cause of colonic mass or wall thickening, dilation of bowel loops proximal to the area of pathology may indicate secondary obstruction.

BENIGN TUMORS OF THE COLON AND RECTUM

Polyps and Villous Tumors

CT and MRI, as they are currently available, are not sensitive for depiction of polypoid lesions in the colorectal lumen. Larger villous tumors can be seen on CT and may be suggested by the presence of contrast material within frondlike interstices of the tumors.[11] Villous tumors may have low attenuation levels on CT because of their high mucin content.[7] With good cleansing of the colon prior to examination and good distension of the colon during the examination, CT can sometimes identify colorectal pol-

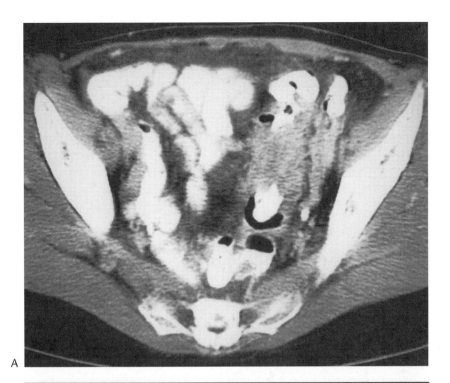

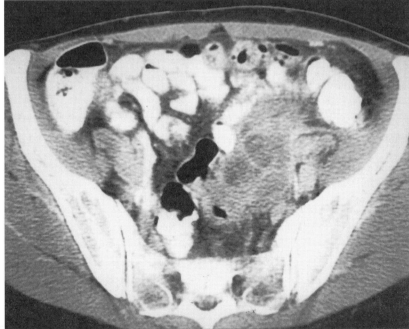

Figure 7-61.   Perforated colon cancer.
(**A**) Circumferential bowel wall thickening is present about the sigmoid colon (**B**), with a large heterogeneous density mass (arrows) on an adjacent section. Differential considerations include diverticulitis with a pericolonic abscess or a perforated colon cancer. At operation, a perforated cancer was removed. (From Johnson,[61] with permission.)

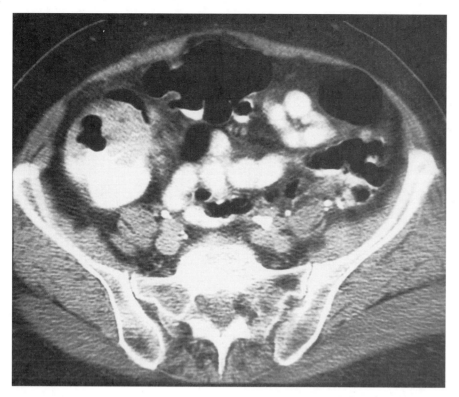

Figure 7-62.   Colonic lymphoma. Bowel wall thickening is present within the right colon and rectum. Several prominent lymph nodes are visible within the perirectal fat. The multifocal nature of this mass makes lymphoma an important consideration, although a synchronous adenocarcinoma could present in a similar fashion. Non-Hodgkin's lymphoma was confirmed histologically. (From Johnson,[61] with permission.)

yps. However, in the unprepared colon imaged with CT slice thickness of 5 mm or greater, generally only polyps larger than 2 cm in diameter will be seen with any degree of certainty.[11] The finding of polyps on routine CT scans should be considered incidental and conventional CT should not be used for screening of the colon for polyps. However, using current generation spiral CT scanners with thin sections and three-dimensional virtual reality computer reconstructions, it may be possible to detect polyps as small as 5 mm in diameter (see Fig. 7-63). If "CT colography" becomes routinely available, it may be a viable alternative to contrast enema and colonoscopy for screening and surveillance of the colon for polyps. Studies are now being conducted to evaluate the feasibility of detecting polyps in the unprepared colon using this new technology.[37]

Figure 7-63.   CT colography. CT colography with transaxial and longitudinal image reconstructions shows a 1-cm pedunculated polyp arising from the colonic wall (arrows point to polyp head).

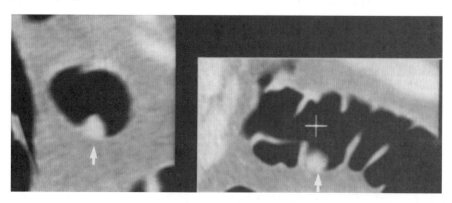

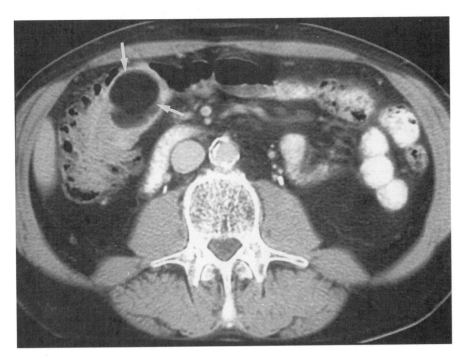

Figure 7-64. Lipoma. A uniformly fatty-density mass (arrows) is present within the lumen of the hepatic flexure of the colon. The fat density is pathognomonic of a lipoma. (From Johnson,[61] with permission.)

Lipoma

Colonic lipomas are benign tumors of the colonic submucosa that are usually small and asymptomatic and may be discovered during colonoscopy or contrast enema examinations. Up to 25% of large lipomas may be symptomatic. Symptomatic lipomas can present with features such as abdominal pain, rectal bleeding, and intussusception and thus can be confused clinically with malignant tumors.[38] CT and MRI can readily identify the presence of fat within the lipomas and distinguish them as benign fatty lesions. On CT, lipomas are homogeneous and are composed of negative attenuation, fat density tissue[39] (Fig. 7-64). Similarly, on MRI lipomas contain homogeneous tissue that has high signal intensity on T_1-weighted images and mirrors the appearance of subcutaneous fat on all imaging sequences.[38] The diagnosis of a lipoma can be made unequivocally if these typical features are present.[11] The preoperative diagnosis of a colonic lipoma can eliminate the need for surgery in asymptomatic patients and can result in a less aggressive procedure if surgery is required for symptomatic lesions.

TUMORS OF THE APPENDIX

Primary tumors of the appendix include carcinoid tumors, mucinous cystadenomas or cystadenocarcinomas, mucoceles, and adenocarcinoma. On CT, the tumors may be identified directly as mass lesions, as a fluid-distended appendix, or they may present with acute appendicitis or abscess due to obstruction of the appendix by the mass.

Carcinoid tumors are the most common type of primary appendiceal tumor, accounting for 85% of malignant primary tumors in the appendix.[40] Although they have malignant potential,

most carcinoid tumors of the appendix are discovered incidentally and have a benign behavior. Distant metastases may occur from appendiceal carcinoids that are greater than 2 cm diameter, but carcinoid tumors that metastasize are usually found to arise in the terminal ileum. An appendiceal soft tissue density mass of greater than 2 cm on CT should raise suspicion of a significant tumor and surgical intervention may be warranted.

An appendiceal mucocele represents a distended, mucous-filled appendix. The cause of the obstruction may be benign (fecalith, foreign body, or adhesion) or neoplastic (mucinous cystadenoma or cystadenocarcinoma). On CT, the mucocele is seen as a thin-walled cystic or tubular structure with internal water density[41] (Fig. 7-65). Curvilinear calcification can be seen in the wall of the appendix. Mucinous cystadenocarcinomas or cystadenomas are low-attenuation mass lesions on CT because of the abundant mucous material that they produce. They may contain calcification in their walls. At the time of discovery, about one-half of patients with mucinous cystadenocarcinomas will have diffuse peritoneal metastases, or pseudomyxoma peritonei.[40] Massive amounts of water density tumor can fill the peritoneal cavity. Diffuse tumoral calcification can be seen, especially in long-standing, well-differentiated tumors.

INFLAMMATORY DISEASES OF THE COLON AND RECTUM

Diverticulitis

Diverticulosis is a common condition, affecting over one-half of patients in the United States by the age of 85.[42] As many as one-fourth of these patients will develop diverticulitis.[42] The diagnosis of diverticulitis can be suggested by clinical features

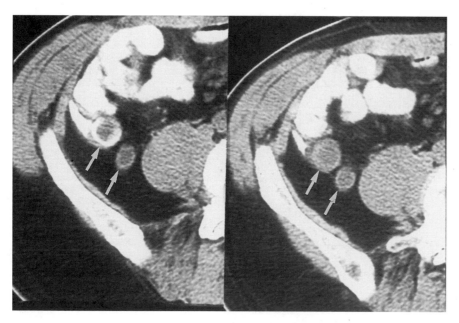

Figure 7-65. Mucocele. At the base of the cecum is a distended, fluid-filled, tubular mass (arrows). Linear calcification is visible within its wall. This is a characteristic appearance for a benign mucocele. CT is also helpful to assess for metastases in patients with cystadenocarcinoma of the appendix. (From Johnson,[61] with permission.)

of left lower quadrant pain and tenderness, fever, and leukocytosis. In the appropriate clinical setting, radiologic investigation may not be necessary and patients may be treated with antibiotics and followed clinically until resolution of symptoms. However, if the clinical features are not specific, radiologic studies may be needed to confirm the diagnosis of diverticulitis, to identify the extent of the inflammation, and to exclude complications such as abscess formation, perforation, or bowel obstruction.[43] CT and contrast enema studies remain the primary imaging modalities for imaging of patients with diverticulitis. The choice of CT or contrast enema as the initial study for diagnosis of diverticulitis remains controversial.[44–48] Contrast enema can demonstrate findings suggestive of diverticulitis in a majority of patients and it is better than CT in the demonstration of sinus tracts. However, CT is better than contrast enema in showing the pericolonic features of diverticulitis, defining the extent of inflammatory changes, and documenting complications of the disease. CT can identify distant changes (e.g., liver or psoas abscess) that may be associated with diverticulitis, and can better identify other abdominal or pelvic pathology (e.g., appendicitis or tubo-ovarian abscess) that may mimic diverticulitis clinically. CT can also guide percutaneous placement of catheters for drainage of diverticular abscesses. For these reasons, most authors recommend CT as the preferred modality for initial evaluation of diverticular disease.[32,42,43,45]

CT plays an important role in the diagnosis and management of patients with diverticulitis because of its ability to depict extraluminal disease. The CT findings of diverticulitis correspond to the severity of the disease and can be used to guide surgical management and provide prognostic information for patients.[49] Ultrasound has been used in the evaluation of diverticulitis and can demonstrate associated bowel wall thickening and pelvic abscesses. Ultrasound can also guide catheter place-

ment for percutaneous abscess drainage. However, compared to CT, ultrasound is limited by its smaller field of view that results in decreased sensitivity for evaluation of distant disease extent. Therefore, ultrasound is currently not preferred by most investigators for initial diagnostic imaging of diverticulitis. Although MRI can depict bowel wall thickening and pelvic abscesses, it is limited by motion artifacts and poorer spatial resolution than CT. At this time, MRI has no documented role in the evaluation of diverticulitis.

Computed Tomography Findings in Diverticulitis

The CT features used to diagnose diverticulitis were first described by Hulnick et al.[50] in 1984. They include presence of diverticula, colon wall thickening, pericolonic inflammation, extracolic abscess or gas collection, and fistula formation (Figs. 7-66 and 7-67). Pericolonic abscess formation is the most specific CT finding in the diagnosis of diverticulitis.[42] An abscess is represented on CT as a well-defined pericolic or distant collection of fluid and may also contain gas or contrast material if it is associated with either colonic perforation, fistulas, or gas-forming organisms. Colon wall thickening represents an early finding in diverticulitis and is almost always present in patients with diverticulitis. Intramural sinus tracts can sometimes be seen as linear fluid or contrast collections within the thickened bowel wall. Pericolonic inflammation is seen on CT as hazy, poorly defined strands of soft tissue density in the pericolonic fat or mesentery. Although colon wall thickening and pericolonic inflammation have a high positive predictive value for the diagnosis of diverticulitis,[42] they are not specific features. Other inflammatory conditions such as Crohn's disease, pseudomembranous colitis, and neutropenic colitis, as well as radiation enteritis, ischemia, or carcinoma can also have

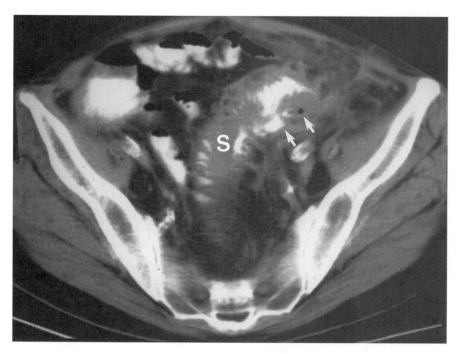

Figure 7-66. CT of sigmoid diverticulitis: CT with oral contrast material shows thickening of the wall of the sigmoid colon with soft tissue inflammatory stranding in the pelvic fat (S) and extraluminal air and contrast (arrows). These findings indicate stage 1 disease (see Table 7-1). (From Johnson,[61] with permission.)

a similar appearance.[11,32] In patients with atypical clinical or CT features, or in patients with a soft tissue mass–like component, a follow-up contrast enema or colonoscopy is recommended to exclude an underlying carcinoma.[11,32,43] Colonic diverticula are often seen on CT studies of asymptomatic patients and do not aid in the diagnosis of diverticulitis except to document the presence of the underlying condition that leads to the development of the disease.

Computed Tomographic Staging of Diverticulitis

Neff and vanSonnenberg[43] have proposed a CT staging system for diverticulitis that correlates with the surgical staging of the disease. This system is summarized in Table 7-1. In stage 0 diverticulitis, inflammation is confined within the serosa and may include pericolonic inflammatory changes. The CT signs of stage 0 disease are colon wall thickening, possibly with mild pericolonic infiltration. Stage 0 patients can be managed conservatively and usually respond to prompt antibiotic therapy without progression to more advanced stages. No follow-up imaging is routinely needed.

Formation of small (less than 3 cm diameter) pericolic abscesses that are confined to the adjacent mesentery characterizes stage 1 diverticulitis (Fig. 7-66). Stage 1 patients also usually respond to conservative therapy, but follow-up imaging is recommended after 7 to 10 days of antibiotics to ensure adequate therapeutic response.

Stage 2 diverticulitis occurs as the inflammatory changes extend outside the mesentery to form a larger pelvic abscess (usually 5 to 15 cm diameter) bounded by pelvic structures such as omentum, small bowel, or colon (Fig. 7-67). Treatment

usually involves percutaneous drainage of the abscess followed by surgical resection of the diseased portion of the colon.

Stage 3 diverticulitis is characterized by spread of the pelvic abscess into the retroperitoneum or peritoneal cavity. Surgical intervention is necessary for treatment of stage 3 patients. However, these patients may be critically ill at presentation and can be poor surgical candidates. Percutaneous drainage may be useful to evacuate as much of the abscess as possible. This temporizing measure can allow surgery to be delayed until the patient has stabilized clinically.[42,43]

Stage 4 diverticulitis occurs when a large diverticular perforation leads to free spillage of fecal material into the peritoneal cavity. These patients present with acute peritonitis, sepsis, and shock. The CT appearance is similar to that of stage 3 disease, but stage 4 patients require immediate surgical intervention and are easily recognized clinically without the need for radiologic confirmation.

Percutaneous Drainage of Diverticular Abscesses

CT-guided percutaneous abscess drainage has proven to be an effective adjunct to surgical sigmoidectomy in patients with stage 2 or stage 3 diverticulitis.[51] In these patients, the goal of the surgical treatment is to drain the abscess, resect the involved portion of colon, and re-anastomose the colonic segments. In many patients who have not been drained percutaneously, a two-stage procedure is indicated. In a two-stage procedure, the colon is resected and the abscess drained during the initial procedure and a diverting colostomy is left in place for re-anastomosis at a later time. Preoperative percutaneous CT-guided abscess drainage, when possible, decreases the amount of

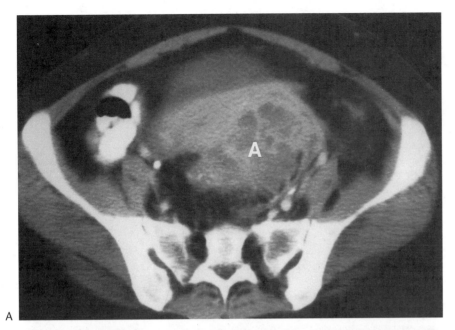

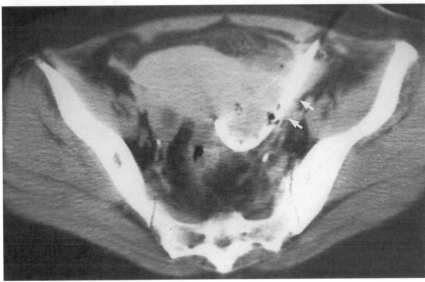

Figure 7-67. CT-guided drainage of diverticular abscess.
(**A**) CT scan shows a large, heterogeneous pelvic fluid collection (A) in a patient with
diverticulitis, indicating stage 2 disease. (**B**) CT scan obtained after percutaneous
abscess drainage shows the drainage catheter in place (arrows) after evacuation of the
contents of the abscess.

inflammation in the surgical field, reducing the surgical morbidity, and allows for performance of a single-stage surgical procedure in a majority of patients.[43,51,52] CT-guided drainage procedures can be performed at the time of the initial diagnostic scan (Fig. 7-67). A Seldinger or trochanter technique is used to place the drainage catheter into the abscess cavity. The approach may be anterior or transgluteal and is selected on an individual basis depending on the location of the abscess and its relationship to adjacent pelvic structures.[42,51] Catheter drainage is continued until the abscess closes and drainage is less than 10 ml in 24 hours. Drainage duration of 10 to 30 days is often required.[42] Sinograms, using fluoroscopy or CT, can be obtained periodi-

cally during drainage to assess the size of the remaining abscess cavity, to identify fistulas or sinus tracts, and to aid in catheter repositioning for optimal drainage. Sinograms are especially helpful if the patient develops recurrent fever or pain, or if the character or volume of drainage changes significantly.

CT is a valuable tool in the diagnosis and management of diverticulitis because of its ability to image the colonic, pericolic, and more distant extent of disease and to guide catheter placement for percutaneous abscess drainage. CT provides information that correlates to the surgical staging of diverticulitis and has prognostic value that is useful in the patients' clinical management. CT can also detect other abdominal and pelvic

Table 7-1. Computed Tomography (CT) of Colonic
Diverticulitis

	CT Signs	Treatment
Stage 0	Diverticula Pericolonic inflammation Thickening of the colon wall	Conservatively

Stage 1	Pericolonic abscess (up
	  to 3 cm, limited to
	  the mesentery)
		Conservatively

Stage 2	Pelvic abscess
	  (perforation through
	  the mesentery)
		Percutaneous
		  drainage, one-stage
		  sigmoid resection

Stage 3	Extrapelvic abscess	Surgery, or
		  percutaneous
		  drainage followed
		  by elective surgery

Stage 4	Large diverticular
	  penetration with
	  spread of fecal
	  material into
	  abdominal cavity
		Emergent surgery

(Adapted from Doringer,[42] with permission.)

processes that may mimic diverticulitis clinically. CT is limited by its inability to distinguish changes of diverticulitis from colon cancer in some cases. Follow-up contrast enema or colonoscopy is recommended in patients with atypical clinical features or equivocal CT findings to exclude underlying carcinoma.

Appendicitis

Appendicitis can usually be diagnosed using clinical and laboratory data without the need for radiologic confirmation. Imaging studies are useful in patients with atypical or nonspecific clinical features and may be of particular value in elderly patients or in young women in whom the diagnosis is difficult.[32,41] Both CT and ultrasound are considered to be the ''best'' methods for imaging of patients with suspected appendicitis. Contrast enema examination can be used to exclude the diagnosis of appendicitis if the appendix is completely filled, but this study has been largely replaced by CT and ultrasound that directly visualize the appendix and periappendiceal tissues. On ultrasound, appendicitis is diagnosed by the presence of a distended appendix measuring greater than 5 mm diameter and having circumferential wall thickening. The positive predictive value of ultrasound for appendicitis is very high if an abnormal appendix is identified. The sensitivity of ultrasound for appendicitis is about 85% and the specificity is 94% to 100%.[32,41] Patient pain and guarding can result in an inadequate examination if satisfactory compression cannot be maintained. Aberrant appendiceal location or retrocecal location can also be problematic and lead to a false-negative examination.

Pericecal inflammatory changes at CT are suggestive of appendicitis in the appropriate clinical setting, but are not specific and can also be seen in Crohn's disease, neutropenic colitis, cecal diverticulitis, or perforated carcinoma. A specific CT di-

agnosis of appendicitis can be made if the abnormal appendix is seen (Fig. 7-68) or if an appendicolith with pericecal inflammation is identified.[32,41] An inflamed appendix is distended more than 5 mm diameter and has a circumferentially thickened wall. A target appearance (alternating rings of high density serosa and mucosa with intramural water density changes) may be seen on intravenous contrast-enhanced scans. The intramural water density changes correspond to edema in the thickened appendiceal wall. Pericecal inflammation is commonly seen in association with the inflamed appendix (Fig. 7-68). Appendicoliths may be seen in asymptomatic patients and are only diagnostic of appendicitis in the presence of pericecal inflammation or an abnormal appendix. Birnbaum and Balthazar[32] found CT to have a higher sensitivity, accuracy, and negative predictive value for appendicitis than ultrasound. They reported that CT was superior to ultrasound in depiction of the extent of inflammatory changes and in exclusion of appendicitis by demonstrating a normal appendix. However, because of the lower cost of ultrasound, its lack of ionizing radiation, and its high positive predictive value, Birnbaum and Balthazar[32] recommended ultrasonography in children, young women, and pregnant women. CT is recommended in other patients.

CT or ultrasound can be used for guidance of percutaneous drainage of appendiceal abscesses. The techniques of appendiceal abscess drainage are similar to those employed for drainage of diverticular abscesses. In some cases, percutaneous drainage and antibiotic therapy have been successful in treatment of appendicitis without the need for surgical appendectomy or drainage.[41] In most cases, percutaneous drainage is used as a temporizing measure in patients who are unfit for immediate surgery or in order to decrease the amount of inflammation in the operative field during definitive surgical treatment.

Inflammatory Bowel Diseases

The appearance of inflammatory bowel diseases at CT is usually nonspecific. Bowel wall thickening is the hallmark finding and can be seen in all inflammatory bowel diseases. CT is useful for assessment of extraluminal disease in patients with inflammatory bowel diseases.[11,35,53] The diagnosis of an inflammatory bowel disease is usually based on clinical features and endoscopic or contrast enema findings. In indeterminate cases, CT features of extraluminal findings and the distribution of changes can be useful in narrowing the differential diagnosis. Although case reports suggest potential in the use of MRI in the evaluation of inflammatory bowel diseases,[2] at this time MRI has limited application in this patient group. Ultrasound has been used to demonstrate cecal and ileal wall thickening in inflammatory bowel disease, but its value is limited by its small field of view and susceptibility to artifact caused by bowel gas. Currently, CT is the most appropriate cross-sectional imaging modality for evaluation of inflammatory bowel disease.

Crohn's disease

CT is useful in the evaluation of patients with Crohn's disease to aid in the differential diagnosis from other inflammatory conditions such as ulcerative colitis, to define the extracolonic extent of disease, and to guide percutaneous placement of abscess drainage catheters. The classic CT features of Crohn's disease include bowel wall thickening, mesenteric soft tissue

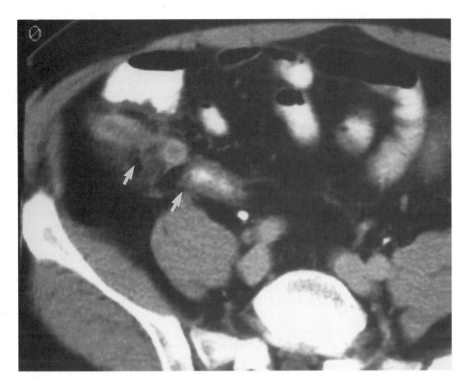

Figure 7-68. CT of appendicitis. CT scan after administration of oral and intravenous contrast material shows changes of acute appendicitis, including circumferential thickening of the appendix with inflammatory changes (soft tissue stranding) in the surrounding fat (arrows).

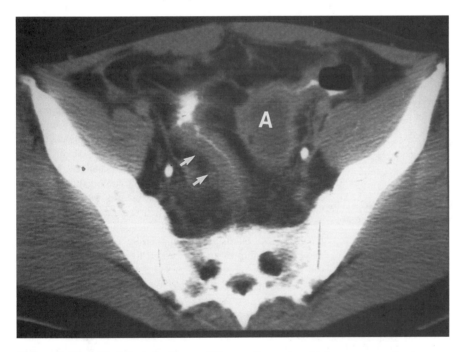

Figure 7-69. CT of Crohn's disease: CT scan after oral and intravenous contrast administration shows wall thickening, stricturing, and soft tissue stranding in the sigmoid and sigmoid mesocolon due to Crohn's disease (arrows). Soft tissue strands, possibly representing fistulas, extend to a pelvic abscess (A). (From Johnson,[61] with permission.)

stranding, abscess, fistulae or sinus tracts, and fibrofatty mesenteric proliferation. Bowel wall thickening, due to edema, fibrosis, and inflammation of the colon wall, is the most common CT finding in Crohn's disease (Fig. 7-69). Although this feature is not specific, Crohn's disease is associated with a greater degree of wall thickening than other inflammatory bowel diseases.[35,53] CT can detect colonic narrowing, stricture formation, and secondary obstruction of the bowel in patients with Crohn's disease. Early mucosal changes of Crohn's disease, such as aphthous ulcers, are not detectable by CT and are best evaluated by contrast enema or colonoscopy.

Extracolonic extension of Crohn's disease causes inflammation of the pericolonic fat or mesentery and results in CT findings of mesenteric soft tissue stranding and abscess (Fig. 7-69). Inflammatory bowel conglomerates, characterized by heterogeneous masses of thickened bowel loops matted together by inflammation or abscess, may occur.[36] Fistulae can be seen on CT as strands of soft tissue extending from a diseased segment of bowel to other bowel loops, abdominal or pelvic organs, inflammatory tissue or abscesses, or to the cutaneous surface. Extracolonic collections of fluid, contrast material, or gas suggest the presence of fistulas or sinus tracts. MRI of the pelvis can aid in the evaluation of fistulas and sinus tracts in patients with Crohn's disease, sometimes providing information not available on CT or clinical examinations.[54,55] On MR images, fistulae appear as linear structures with low intensity on T_1-weighted images and high intensity on T_2-weighted images.[55] MRI has proved useful in demonstrating the orifice of fistulae in the bowel wall and the connection of fistulae to muscles, viscera, and skin.[55] Coronal MR images provide good visualization of the levator ani muscles and can be particularly useful for surgical planning in the preoperative localization of fistulae and sinus tracts with respect to the anal sphincter and levator compartments.[54,55]

Mesenteric changes of Crohn's disease include fibrofatty proliferation of the mesentery. Fibrofatty proliferation is identified at CT by abnormal fatty tissue with increased attenuation and soft tissue stranding. The accumulation of fat in the mesentery produces the secondary sign of separation of bowel loops that is seen on small bowel studies as well as on CT. Mildly enlarged mesenteric lymph nodes are also commonly seen in patients with Crohn's disease.

The CT findings of Crohn disease can aid in the differential diagnosis with ulcerative colitis (see box). Discontinuous, asymmetric colonic involvement is associated with Crohn's disease and can help to exclude ulcerative colitis. Philpotts et al.[53] noted an even distribution between right-sided, left-sided, and bilateral involvement in Crohn's disease, whereas ulcerative colitis was found to have only left-sided or bilateral involvement. Coexisting disease in the small bowel, stomach, or esophagus is associated with Crohn's disease. The presence of mesenteric changes, abscesses, or fistulae favors the diagnosis of Crohn's disease.

CT-guided percutaneous drainage of abscesses in Crohn's patients can be used to evacuate abscess cavities prior to surgical treatment, or may lead to complete resolution of the abscess and serve as definitive therapy.[35] Although surgical resection of enteric fistulae is usually necessary, percutaneous abscess drainage is sometimes effective for treatment of patients with

---

CT Features of Ulcerative Colitis Versus Crohn's Disease

Ulcerative Colitis

> Mural thickening <1 cm
> Inhomogeneous CT density of wall
> Target appearance of rectum
> Increased perirectal fat

Crohn's Disease

> Mural thickening, often >1 cm
> Homogeneous CT density of wall
> Small bowel thickening
> Abscess, fistula, sinus tract
> Fibrofatty mesenteric proliferation

Common to Both Ulcerative Colitis and Crohn's Disease

> Mural thickening
> Narrowed lumen
> Increased lymph node size and number

(Adapted from Gore,[35] with permission.)

---

fistulae.[35] The techniques used for CT-guided abscess drainage are described previously in the discussion of diverticulitis.

Ulcerative Colitis

Bowel wall thickening in ulcerative colitis is usually less than 1 cm and involves the distal to proximal colon in a continuous fashion. Unilateral right-sided involvement is uncommon.[35,53] Occasionally, inflammatory polyps in ulcerative colitis may be detected, but usually mucosal changes are not depicted at CT. Toxic megacolon can produce colonic dilatation of an inflamed segment and is often associated with thinning or thickening of the bowel wall.[35] Pneumatosis coli can be identified and is a worrisome finding that indicates impending perforation or infarction. Fatty infiltration of the submucosa in ulcerative colitis can produce a targetlike appearance of the bowel wall on CT.[35,53] This change is associated with chronic or inactive disease and is often encountered in patients receiving steroid therapy. Enlargement of the presacral space by perirectal fatty proliferation can also be seen in patients with ulcerative colitis.

The incidence of colon cancer is higher in patients with ulcerative colitis than in the general population. Although CT is not a primary imaging modality for screening for colon cancer, focal regions of bowel wall thickening should be regarded with suspicion. Systemic complications associated with ulcerative colitis that can be identified on CT include hepatic steatosis, primary sclerosing cholangitis, renal lithiasis, pyelonephritis, and sacroiliitis.[35]

Acute Colitis

Pseudomembranous colitis, neutropenic colitis, ischemic colitis, and radiation-induced colitis are all characterized by colon wall thickening on CT[35,53] (Fig. 7-70). Although CT may be

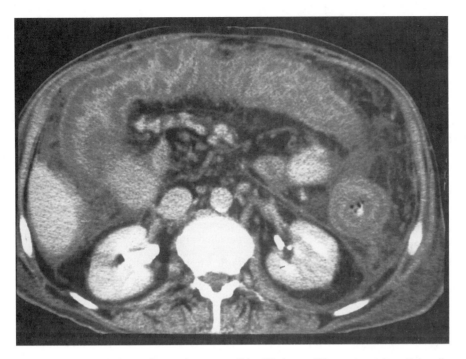

Figure 7-70.   CT of pseudomembranous colitis. CT shows diffuse, circumferential wall thickening and edema (water density changes in the colon wall) of the colon due to pseudomembranous colitis (arrows). Enhancement of the muscularis mucosa within the low-attenuation mural edema produces a "target" appearance (curved arrow).

used for detection of changes associated with these processes, the diagnosis is usually made on the basis of other clinical, laboratory, or radiographic data.

Pseudomembranous colitis is associated with marked bowel wall and haustral fold thickening.[56–58] Usually, the colon is diffusely involved, but segmental disease can occur. Often, edematous changes in the bowel wall and marked serosal and mucosal enhancement can be detected on CT scans obtained after administration of intravenous contrast material (Fig. 7-71). Ascites may also be present. Pseudomembranous colitis is generally suspected because of a history of antibiotic therapy and the diagnosis is confirmed by endoscopic examination and stool assay for *Clostridium difficile* endotoxin.

Neutropenic colitis, or typhlitis, is a necrotizing colitis found in neutropenic patients who are being treated with chemotherapy. Classically, neutropenic colitis involves the cecum and ascending colon, producing concentric bowel wall thickening. Neutropenic colitis may progress to produce necrosis and perforation of the colon. CT findings of this complication include pericolonic fluid and inflammation, pneumatosis coli, and pneumoperitoneum.[35,53]

Radiation colitis most commonly involves the rectosigmoid colon after pelvic irradiation when radiation doses in excess of 40 Gy have been administered. Often, pelvic loops of small bowel are also involved. Radiation injury produces an endarteritis of the bowel and leads to bowel ischemia. Early changes include bowel wall thickening and edema in the involved colonic segment and edema in the adjacent mesentery. Later chronic changes include wall thickening and luminal narrowing due to fibrosis. Changes are confined to the irradiated field.[35,53,59]

Bowel infarction may be diffuse or focal and conforms to the boundaries of the involved vascular supply. Abnormal CT findings include bowel wall thickening, edema, intramural pneumatosis, and portal venous gas. Portal venous gas is a late finding that indicates a poor prognosis. Peritoneal fluid can be seen in association with bowel perforation or peritonitis. Identification of a filling defect (thrombus) in the proximal superior mesenteric artery or vein can be a helpful finding to suggest the diagnosis of bowel infarction in patients with bowel wall thickening at CT.[59,60]

SUMMARY

The role of cross-sectional imaging studies is complementary to that of the contrast enema and endoscopy in the complete evaluation of diseases affecting the colon and rectum. Although endoscopy and enema studies are necessary to evaluate the colorectal mucosa, cross-sectional examinations are used to define the extraluminal extent of tumors and inflammatory conditions of the colon and rectum. The techniques used for CT and MRI examinations can be tailored to optimally address specific clinical questions. Of the cross-sectional imaging modalities, CT is the most versatile. CT is usually the initial cross-sectional imaging examination indicated for the preoperative and postoperative assessment of patients with colorectal cancer, and for the evaluation of inflammatory bowel diseases. CT may guide percutaneous biopsy of suspicious lesions or percutaneous placement of abscess drainage catheters. With respect to colorectal diseases, MRI is currently most often used for evaluation of metastatic liver disease. It may provide better anatomic detail than CT in selected areas such as the rectum. MRI may be

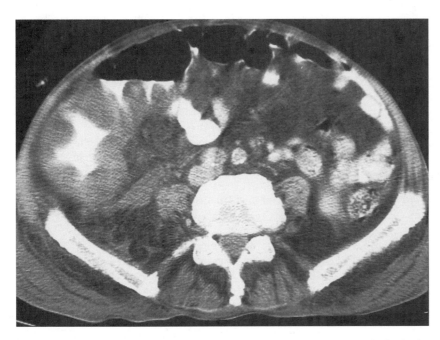

Figure 7-71. Acute ischemic colitis. The wall of the right colon is markedly thickened causing "thumbprinting" throughout the ascending colon. Soft tissue stranding is seen within the pericolonic fat. These findings are nonspecific, and could be due to ischemic, inflammatory, or even neoplastic disorders. Additional findings of pneumatosis coli and portal venous gas would be more suggestive of ischemia, but often angiography is required to confirm the diagnosis in patients with suspicious clinical findings. (From Johnson,[61] with permission.)

indicated in patients such as pregnant women, for whom irradiation is contraindicated. CT and MRI examinations have become an integral part of the overall assessment and treatment of patients with colorectal diseases.

REFERENCES

1. Soyer P, Levesque M, Caudron C et al (1993) MRI of liver metastases from colorectal cancer vs. CT during arterial porto-graphy. J Comput Assist Tomogr 17:67–74

2. Goldberg HI, Thoeni RF (1989) MRI of the gastrointestinal tract. Radiol Clin North Am 27:805–814

3. Gomberg JS, Freidman AC, Radecki PD et al (1986) MRI differentiation of recurrent colorectal carcinoma from postoperative fibrosis. Gastrointest Radiol 11:361–363

4. Rafto SE, Amendola MA, Gefter WB (1988) MR imaging of recurrent colorectal carcinoma versus fibrosis. J Comput Assist Tomogr 12:521–523

5. Campeau NG, Johnson CD, Felmlee JP et al (1995) MR imaging of the abdomen with a phased-array multicoil: prospective clinical evaluation. Radiology 195:769–776

6. Gelfand DW (1991) Imaging of the colon. Curr Opin Radiol 3:422–426

7. Thoeni RF (1989) CT evaluation of carcinomas of the colon and rectum. Radiol Clin North Am 27:731–741

8. Meyers MA (1988) Dynamic Radiology of the Abdomen: Normal and Pathologic Anatomy, 3rd Ed. Springer-Verlag, New York

9. Stevenson GW (1993) Radiology and endoscopy in the pretreatment diagnostic management of colorectal cancer. Cancer 71:4198–4206

10. Thoeni RF (1991) Colorectal carcinoma: cross-sectional imaging for staging of primary tumor and detection of local recurrence. Am J Roentgen 156:909–915

11. Johnson CD, Stephens DH (1989) Computed tomography of the large bowel and appendix. Mayo Clinic Proc 64:1276–1283

12. Kelvin FM, Maglinte DDT (1987) Colorectal carcinoma: a radiologic and clinical review. Radiology 164:1–8

13. Collier BD (1993) New radiographic techniques for colorectal cancer. Cancer 71:4214–4216

14. Charnsangavej C (1993) New imaging modalities for follow-up of colorectal carcinoma. Cancer 71:4236–4240

15. Outwater E, Tomaszewski JE, Daly JM, Kressel HY (1991) Hepatic colorectal metastases: correlation of MR imaging and pathologic appearance. Radiology 180:327–332

16. Stark DD, Wittenberg J, Butch RJ, Ferrucci JT (1987) Hepatic metastases: randomized, controlled comparison of detection with MR imaging and CT. Radiology 165:399–406

17. Fantini GA, DeCosse JJ (1990) Surveillance strategies after resection of carcinoma of the colon and rectum. Surg, Gynecol, Obstet 171:267–273

18. Chen YM, Ott DJ, Wolfman NT et al (1987) Recurrent colorectal carcinoma: evaluation with barium enema and CT. Radiology 163:307–310

19. Mendez RJ, Rodriguez R, Kovacevich T et al (1993) CT in local recurrence of rectal carcinoma. J Comput Assist Tomogr 17:741–744
20. Krestin GP, Steinbrich W, Friedmann G (1988) Recurrent rectal cancer: diagnosis with MR imaging versus CT. Radiology 168:307–311
21. DuBrow RA, David CL, Curley SA (1995) Anastomotic leaks after low anterior resection for rectal carcinoma: evaluation with CT and barium enema. Am J Roentgenol 165:567–571
22. Thompson WM, Halvorsen RA, Foster Jr WL et al (1986) Preoperative and postoperative CT staging of rectosigmoid carcinoma. Am J Roentgenol 146:703–710
23. Pema PJ, Bennett WF, Bova JG, Warman P (1994) J Comput Assist Tomogr 18:256–261
24. de Lange EE, Fechner RE, Wanebo HJ (1989) Suspected recurrent rectosigmoid carcinoma after abdominoperineal resection: MR imaging and histopathologic findings. Radiology 170:323–328
25. Butch RJ, Wittenberg J, Mueller PR et al (1985) Presacral masses after abdominoperineal resection for colorectal carcinoma: the need for biopsy. Am J Roentgenol 144:309–312
26. Schmidt RG, Cecchini AJ, Mayer DP, Kabbani Y (1994) Magnetic resonance diagnosis of an occult metastatic colon carcinoma of the calcaneous. Foot Ankle Int 15:334–339
27. Suzuki M, Takashima T, Kadoya M et al (1993) Signal intensity of brain metastases on T2-weighted images: specificity for metastases from colonic cancers. Neurochirurgia 16:151–155
28. Testempassi E, Takeuchi H, Fukuda Y et al (1994) Cardiac metastasis of colon adenocarcinoma diagnosed by magnetic resonance imaging. Acta Cardiol 49:191–196
29. Dawson SL, Lee MJ, Mueller PR (eds) (1993) Nonsurgical treatment of liver tumors. Semin Intervent Radiol Vol. 10
30. Lorigan JG, DuBrow RA (1990) The computed tomographic appearances and clinical significance of intussusception in adults with malignant neoplasms. Br J Radiol 63:257–262
31. Seidman DS, Heyman Z, Ben-Ari GY et al (1992) Use of magnetic resonance imaging in pregnancy to diagnose intussusception induced by colon cancer. Obstet Gynecol 79:822–823
32. Birnbaum BA, Balthazar EJ (1994) CT of appendicitis and diverticulitis. Radiol Clin North Am 32:885–898
33. Wyatt SH, Fishman EK, Jones B (1993) Primary lymphoma of the colon and rectum: CT and barium enema correlation. Abdom Imaging 18:376–380
34. Wyatt SH, Fishman EK, Hruban RH, Siegelman SS (1994) CT of primary colonic lymphoma. Clini Imaging 18:131–141
35. Gore RM (1989) CT of inflammatory bowel disease. Radiol Clin North Am 27:717–729
36. Kleinhaus U, Weich Y (1987) Computed tomography of Crohn's disease—reevaluation. Fortschr Rontgenstr 147:607–611
37. Hara AK, Johnson CD, Reed JE et al (1996) Colorectal polyp detection with CT colography: two- versus three-dimensional techniques. Work in progress. Radiology 200:49–54
38. Younathan CM, Ros PR, Burton SS (1991) MR imaging of colonic lipoma. J Comput Assist Tomogr 15:492–494
39. Kakitsuba Y, Kakitsuba S, Nagatomo H et al (1993) CT manifestations of lipomas of the small intestine and colon. Clin Imaging 17:179–182
40. Rutledge RH, Alexander JW (1992) Primary appendiceal malignancies: rare but important. Surgery 111:244–250
41. Shapiro MP, Gale ME, Gerzof SG (1989) CT of appendicitis: diagnosis and treatment. Radiol Clin North Am 27:753–762
42. Doringer E (1992) Computerized tomography of colonic diverticulitis. Criti Revi Diagno Imaging 33:421–435
43. Neff CC, vanSonnenberg E (1989) CT of diverticulitis: diagnosis and treatment. Radiol Clini North Am 27:743–754
44. Balthazar EJ, Megibow A, Schinella RA, Gordon R (1990) Limitations in the CT diagnosis of acute diverticulitis: comparison of CT, contrast enema, and pathologic findings in 16 patients. Am J Roentgen 154:281–285
45. Cho KC, Morehouse HT, Alterman DD, Thornhill BA (1990) Sigmoid diverticulitis: diagnostic role of CT—comparison with barium enema studies. Radiology 176:111–115
46. Johnson CD, Baker ME, Rice RP et al (1987) Diagnosis of acute colonic diverticulitis: comparison of barium enema and CT. Am J Roentgen 148:541–546
47. McKee RF, Deignan RW, Krukowski ZH (1993) Radiological investigation in acute diverticulitis. Br J Surg 80:560–565
48. Smith TR, Cho KC, Morehouse HT, Kratka PS (1990) Comparison of computed tomography and contrast enema evaluation of diverticulitis. Dis Colon Rectum 33:1–6
49. Ambrosetti P, Robert J, Witzig JA, et al (1992) Prognostic factors from computed tomography in acute left colonic diverticulitis. Br J Surg 79:117–119
50. Hulnick DH, Megibow AJ, Balthazar EJ et al (1984) Computed tomography in the evaluation of diverticulitis. Radiology 152:491–495
51. Mueller PR, Saini S, Wittenberg J et al (1987) Sigmoid diverticular abscesses: percutaneous drainage as an adjunct to surgical resection in 24 cases. Radiology 164:321–325
52. Saini S, Mueller PR, Wittenberg J et al (1986) Percutaneous drainage of diverticular abscess: an adjunct to surgical therapy. Arch Surg 121:475–478
53. Philpotts LE, Heiken JP, Westcott MA, Gore RM (1994) Colitis: use of CT findings in differential diagnosis. Radiology 190:445–449
54. Jenss H, Starlinger M, Skaleij M (1992) Magnetic resonance imaging in perianal Crohn's disease, letter. Lancet 340:1286
55. Koelbel G, Schmiedl U, Majer MC et al (1989) Diagnosis of fistulae and sinus tracts in patients with Crohn disease: value of MR imaging. Am J Roentgen 152:999–1003
56. Boland GW, Lee MJ, Cats AM (1994) Antibiotic-induced diarrhea: specificity of abdominal CT for the diagnosis of *Clostridium difficile* disease. Radiology 191:103–106
57. Fishman EK, Kavuru M, Jones B et al (1991) Pseudomembranous colitis: CT evaluation of 26 cases. Radiology 180:57–60
58. Merine D, Fishman EK, Jones B (1987) Pseudomembranous colitis: CT evaluation. J Comput Assist Tomogr 11:1017–1020
59. Scholz FJ (1993) Ischemic bowel disease. Radiolo Clin North Am 31:1197–1218
60. Clark RA (1987) Computed tomography of bowel infarction. J Comput Assist Tomogr 11:757–762
61. Johnson CD (1993) Alimentary Tract Imaging—A Teaching File. Mosby Year Book, St. Louis

ENDORECTAL MAGNETIC RESONANCE IMAGING

W.A. Kmiot   N.M. de Souza

A.P. Zbar

Traditionally, contrast radiology has been used in the assessment of malignant and functional disorders of the colon and rectum. More recently, computed tomography (CT) has been used in the preoperative assessment of patients with known colorectal carcinoma. Endorectal ultrasound has been advocated both for the preoperative determination of tumor depth in low rectal cancer and for the identification of patients with potentially repairable sphincter defects presenting with fecal incontinence.

Magnetic resonance imaging (MRI) is the latest modality used to study the colon, anorectum, and pelvic floor. Its superior soft tissue contrast and multiplanar imaging facility provides anatomic information about the relationship of disease to the pelvic floor. This is of importance in the delineation of complex fistulae and congenital anorectal deformities and their relationship to the levator plate. MRI is less operator dependent than endorectal ultrasonography but is more time consuming and expensive. Recently, dedicated internal coils have produced high-resolution images of the sphincter musculature in patients with fecal incontinence (Fig. 7-72) although comparative studies between these techniques are still awaited. The internal coil is immobilized by an external clamp to prevent movement artifact.

MRI using both external and internal coils is being used in the examination of patients with complex and recurrent anorectal sepsis, obstetric sphincter injury, low rectal cancer, and congenital anorectal malformations. It is anticipated that highly detailed preoperative imaging may define those cases with low rectal cancer who may benefit from local excision with early tumors or preoperative radiation and chemoradiation in advanced lesions as well as guide the surgeon in complex anorectal sepsis and perianal Crohn's disease, minimizing recurrence of fistula-in-ano and inadvertent sphincter injury.

TECHNICAL ASPECTS

Pelvic MRI requires adequate bowel preparation and may sometimes be improved in the prone position in order to reduce respiratory motion artifact. Cancer tissue shows moderate signal intensity and contrasts well with the high signal intensity of perirectal fat and intraluminal air (Fig. 7-73). The use of fast spin-echo sequences provides a substantial reduction in scan times and motion artifact at the expense of brightening the fat signal.[1,2] The STIR (short tau inversion recovery) sequence results in fat suppression while highlighting fistulous tracks, collections, and tumors (Fig. 7-74). MRI with external coils has been used to define the normal anatomy of the sphincter musculature as well as the dynamic behavior of the pelvic floor. Most studies have difficulty with sphincter muscle resolution as well as in differentiation of the mucosal/submucosal interface and the entirety of the levator plate. The differentiation of these layers is of considerable importance in patients with perirectal sepsis for the demonstration of the relationship of fistula tracks, abscess collections, and internal openings to the puborectalis sling.[3–5]

In perirectal sepsis, multiplanar images are well suited to outlining the anatomy of the tracks. Axial scans provide images of the intersphincteric plane, whereas coronal images define the point at which high tracks cross the pelvic floor. STIR imaging is of particular benefit in demonstrating complex fistulas. Epithelialization of tracks in long-standing cases will, however, be missed by MRI because of absence of granulation tissue. Further, MRI may miss tracks or abscess cavities that are relatively collapsed as well as misdiagnose neurovascular structures in the perineum as inflammatory fistulae if performed by an inexperienced practitioner (Fig. 7-75).

In malignant disease, MRI relies on differentiation between the rectum and adjacent organs by recognizing the integrity of perirectal fat planes. Inflammatory thickening may be difficult to separate from neoplastic infiltration and this may result in overstaging of tumor depth. In the case of adjacent malignant lymphadenopathy the use of size criteria alone to define malignancy will only improve specificity, because it has been shown that up to 10% of nodal metastases may be microscopic.[6]

An increased signal-to-noise ratio (SNR) may be obtained by placing the coil closer to the region of interest. Dedicated endorectal coils were first introduced for imaging the prostate gland in 1989 and then subsequently for the uterine cervix,[7–9] use of an endorectal receiver coil allows increased resolution of the rectal wall. Advanced tumors producing luminal stenosis may prevent optimal coil placement and peristalsis may degrade

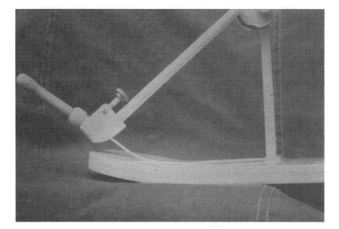

Figure 7-72. Endoanal coil as used at Hammersmith Hospital during MRI of the anorectum.

images as well as cause migration of the coil, necessitating repositioning.

In balloon-designed coil systems, overinflation of the balloon will flatten early mucosal lesions and prevent adequate definition of surface layers. The use of an endorectal coil awaits evaluation against standard modalities, but it may be of advantage when combined with surface pelvic phased array imaging to outline the presence of pelvic visceral infiltration (prostate, seminal vesicles, uterus) in bulky tumors as well as pelvic sidewall lymphadenopathy.[10-12]

The use of the internal coil for anorectal imaging was first reported by deSouza and co-workers[13] in 1994 after preliminary experiments correlating histology with imaging in cadaveric specimens. These coils have been designed to encompass the normal contours of the anal sphincter and are inserted in the

Figure 7-73. Pelvic MRI demonstrating adenocarcinoma of the rectum.

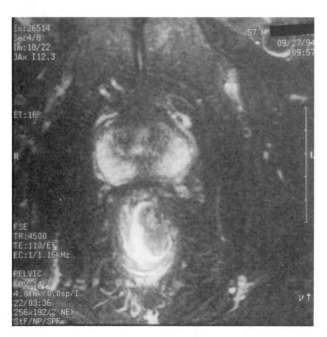

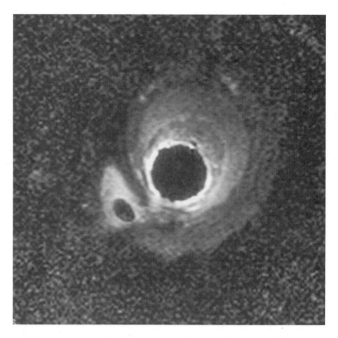

Figure 7-74. Endoanal coil MRI using the STIR sequence demonstrating an intersphincteric abscess at 7 o'clock with an associated fistula into the rectum.

left lateral position covered with a rubber sheath. Patients are scanned in the supine position without the need for sedation although some patients with perianal sepsis and chronic anal fissure have required local lignocaine anesthesia. Coils are sterilized between patient examinations by soaking in 1% glutaraldehyde solution.

Standard imaging using T_1-weighted spin-echo, T_2-weighted

Figure 7-75. Endoanal coil MRI demonstrating an intact internal sphincter (bright halo) surrounded by normal vascular markings (STIR) sequence.

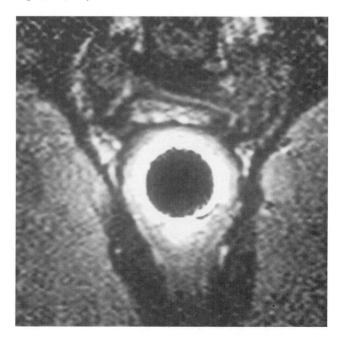

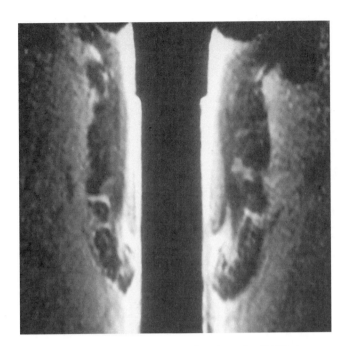

Figure 7-76. T_1-weighted coronal endoanal coil MRI demonstrating the normal anal sphincter configuration.

spin-echo, and STIR sequences is adequate. Standard imaging times range from 30 to 45 minutes. Phantom studies have shown a rapid falloff of signal from the surface of the coil radially, but with a gain in SNR when compared with standard phased array images up to 2 cm from the coil.

NORMAL APPEARANCES

The general configuration of the anal sphincter complex is shown in Figure 7-76. There is good separation of the deep, superficial, and subcutaneous external sphincter muscles, which is best seen in oblique coronal images. The deep external anal sphincter (EAS) is continuous with the puborectalis sling. The superficial EAS extends inferior to the internal anal sphincter (IAS). The subcutaneous EAS is well developed and forms a distal cap over the superficial sphincter, but in some it forms a more condensed bundle medially. Anteriorly the EAS is separable from the puborectalis muscle. The longitudinal muscle is best seen on transverse images where it has a typically beaded appearance surrounded by high signal fat and fibroelastic tissue (Fig. 7-77). This muscle is seen to merge in some cases with the subcutaneous EAS, a phenomenon noted in recent anatomic dissection.[14]

The IAS has a naturally high signal on all sequences, particularly on T_2-weighted and STIR images. This feature may be a function of its inherent smooth muscle content. It is seen to be continuous with the longitudinal rectal muscle layer above and is either circular or crescentic in cross section. It is well delineated laterally by high-signal intersphincteric fat and enhances strikingly after gadolinium-DTPA contrast. Relatively high vascularity, capillary permeability or innate metabolic activity consequent upon maintenance of basal resting tone may also account for the contrast enhancement.[15] The EAS also enhances but to a much lesser degree (Fig. 7-78). This phenomenon of normal enhancement needs to be recognized and not mistaken for infection.

The musculus submucosae is demonstrable running in the submucosa as a low signal intensity stripe. This type of layer definition is superior to body coil images where there is no capacity to separate the internal sphincter from the submucosa. The degree of sphincter distension is much greater with the larger diameter endoanal ultrasound probe, resulting in lower values for sphincter thickness when compared with endoanal MRI.

The main sex differences are visible anteriorly where in males the superficial EAS is elliptical with some anterior decussation. In females the superficial EAS is more circular and merges with the superficial transverse perineal muscles and with

Figure 7-77. Transverse endoanal coil MRI demonstrating intact, bright, internal anal sphincter surrounded by fragmented external anal sphincter interspersed with high signal fat and fibroelastic tissue (T_1-weighted).

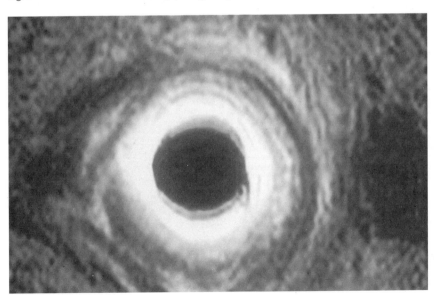

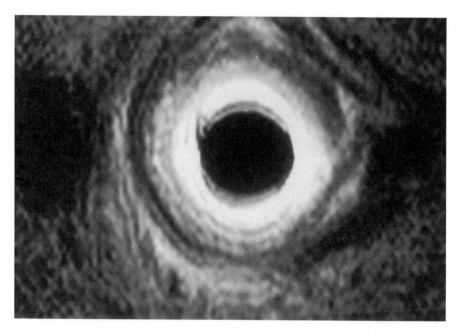

Figure 7-78. Endoanal coil MRI transverse section demonstrating high enhancement of the internal anal sphincter and patchy appearance of the external anal sphincter (T_2-weighted).

the homogeneous mass of the perineal body. Table 7-2 summarizes the dimensions of the muscle layers as recorded in normal patients of both sexes. The values obtained, although consistent with cadaveric measurements for the EAS, tend to vary for the IAS, possibly because of loss of tone. Specimen measurements of thickness are also inaccurate because of the change in signal intensity at postmortem or after tissue fixation.[16] Comparisons with endorectal ultrasound cannot readily be made because different echogenicity with increasing age occurs consequent upon fatty and fibrous tissue replacement of muscle.[17]

CONTRAST ENHANCEMENT

Contrast agents have been used selectively to alter the T_1 and T_2 relaxation times of pathologic tissue.[18,19] Paramagnetic substances such as gadolinium (Gd; a trivalent lanthanide heavy metal) have positive magnetic susceptibility (i.e., a positive effect on local magnetic fields). This results in increased signal intensity on T_1-weighted images. Thus Gd and related compounds are T_1 enhancers. The main contrast agent for clinical use is a Gd-DTPA chelate (''Magnevist'', Schering AG, Berlin, Germany). It functions as an extracellular space marker with the same pharmacokinetics as iodinated contrast agents. Chelation renders the compound nontoxic although it does compromise its effect on relaxation enhancement. Newer Gd chelates with different osmolality, ionization, and hepatic excretion (Gd-HP-DO3A, *gadoteridol*; Gd-DTPA-BMA, *gadodiamide*; Gd-DO-TA,*gadoterate*; Gd-BOPTA) have been developed. The side effects of these agents are minimal when compared with conventional iodinated contrast agents. In some patients transient increases in bilirubin and serum iron levels have been recorded.

Table 7-2. Thickness of Components of the Normal Anal Sphincter in Males and Females

	Musculus Submucosa, Mean ± SD (mm)	Internal Sphincter, Mean ± SD (mm)		External Sphincter, Mean ± SD (mm)		
		Anterior	Posterior	Subcutaneous	Superficial	Deep
Males (n = 8)	3.0 ± 1.7	5.4 ± 1.0	2.0 ± 1.3	3.6 ± 0.6	5.1 ± 1.3	6.5 ± 0.9
Females (n = 9)	2.5 ± 1.4	5.3 ± 1.9	2.2 ± 1.4	4.0 ± 0.9	5.4 ± 1.0	6.7 ± 1.2

Length of Components of the Normal Anal Sphincter in Males and Females in the Oblique Coronal Plane

	Internal Sphincter, Mean ± SD (mm)	External Sphincter, Mean ± SD (mm)		
		Subcutaneous	Superficial	Deep
Males (n = 7)	36 ± 6	8 ± 2	22 ± 8	26 ± 4
Females (n = 7)	37 ± 7	9 ± 2	26 ± 4	25 ± 5

(From de Souza et al.,[97] with permission.)

Headaches, nausea, rashes, and rarely transient hypotension have been reported.

The next section describes the clinical application of MRI in perirectal sepsis, obstetric sphincter injury and repair, low rectal cancer, functional evacuatory disorders, and congenital anorectal malformations.

MRI IN PERIRECTAL SEPSIS

Most anal fistulae and abscesses are simple in nature and easy to treat surgically. About 5% to 15% of patients with anorectal sepsis will have complex or recurrent disease and the accurate preoperative definition of the anatomy of primary and secondary tracks and associated collections with their relationship to the puborectalis sling is desirable in order to prevent recurrence and inadvertent sphincter injury. In long-term follow-up even simple fistulae are associated with a small but definable recurrence rate of about 6% with most recurrent or residual disease occurring because of missed primary tracks.[20]

A range of imaging techniques have been described for the delineation of primary and secondary tracks in fistulous anorectal disease. Traditionally fistulography has been used and although accurate at representing tracks, ramifications, and internal openings, the relationship of the disease to the anorectal sphincter complex and the levator plate can only be inferred and is frequently overestimated.[21–23] The technique is painful for the patient and has the potential for disseminating sepsis.

CT scanning of complex fistulae and sepsis has also been disappointing. In many cases the levator plate is poorly visualized and because of volume averaging effects in the ischiorectal fossae, lateral (and frequently extrasphincteric) fistulae are poorly visualized. The internal opening is not seen in most cases.[24,25]

Endorectal ultrasound has proved to be of only limited value in the preoperative assessment of perirectal sepsis and has been shown to be inferior to experienced clinical examination.[26] In this technique, primary tracks are identified as hypoechoic lines running either trans-sphincterically or in the intersphincteric space. Endoanal ultrasonography frequently fails to define the presence of suprasphincteric fistulae and supralevator/translevator abscesses because of poor acoustic coupling of the cone above the puborectalis. Further, because of limited focal range, lateral extensions are often not detected. Both situations are precisely the occasions when additional preoperative anatomic information is sought by the coloproctologist in the complex case. In some instances the presence of a substantial intersphincteric collection will create sufficient acoustic shadowing so as to overstage the collection as trans-sphincteric. This difficulty has not been improved by the use of image enhancement with hydrogen peroxide.[27,28] The indirect endosonographic sign of a mucosal layer break, that has been advocated for diagnosis of the internal opening site has proven inaccurate. Moreover, there is no facility for distinguishing scarred burnt-out tracks from recrudescent sepsis.[29]

MRI using an external coil has been advocated for the delineation of perirectal sepsis and has been shown to be highly accurate in outlining the course of the primary tracks, secondary extensions, and collections and the presence and plane of horseshoeing. The sensitivity of these parameters in concordance with operative findings is over 90%.[30,31] The MR images of a

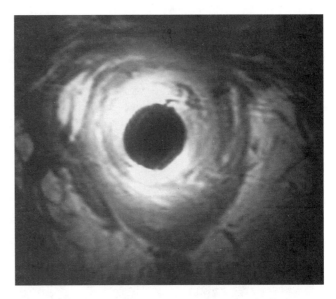

Figure 7-79. Transverse section of endoanal coil MRI showing the apex of a suprasphincteric fistula at 11 o'clock using a T_1-weighted sequence.

case of complex recurrent fistula-in-ano are shown in Figure 7-79.

MRI has failed to identify epithelialized long-standing tracks. Granulation tissue in the subepithelial layer may cause difficulty in identifying the site of the internal opening. The STIR sequence will usually show the inflammatory track well without the need for contrast, but the relationship to the main sphincter complex may be difficult to define. MRI with an external coil allows identification of distant tracks and supralevator or associated pelvic disease. This is of particular importance in patients with inflammatory bowel disease and in recurrent or residual cases where contrast enhancement will distinguish scar from recrudescent sepsis. Images in multiple planes provide an improved diagnosis of horseshoeing and relationship to the levator plate. The presence of pus is best depicted on T_2-weighted images and here contrast enhancement will differentiate active disease. Recently the use of saline instillation during MRI has been advocated to define tracks and to expand relatively collapsed collections, although there is no substantial improvement in imaging if the fistula is simple or short.[32] The use of MRI may also prove advantageous in the evaluation of children because of its relative accuracy and avoidance of ionizing radiation.[33]

Endoanal MRI has been recently assessed both in simple cryptogenic and complex perirectal sepsis. In adults with acute perianal infection the technique may be performed without the need for sedation. The concordance rate with operative findings in a small number of patients with simple cryptogenic infection (where the surgeon and radiologist were blinded to the results of each other's findings) has been 100% for abscesses and 80% for tracks and internal openings. The only track missed by MRI was located below the level of the dentate line.[34] Examples of the endoanal findings in simple perianal sepsis are shown in Figures 7-80 to 7-83.

Endoanal MRI has performed well in complex disease.[35] The definition in our study of a complex case included recurrent or residual sepsis following initial surgical management where the

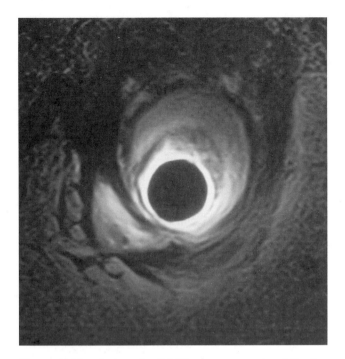

Figure 7-80. Endoanal coil MRI transverse section following administration of intravenous contrast showing an intersphincteric abscess and fistula-in-ano at 6 o'clock (T_1-weighted).

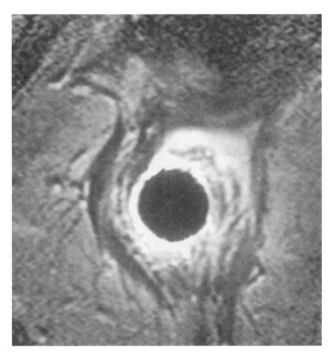

Figure 7-81. Transverse section T_2-weighted endoanal coil MRI image demonstrating a fistula secondary to Behçet's disease at 12 o-clock.

internal opening lay above the anorectal ring (mostly in patients with inflammatory bowel disease). In 11 cases recently reported where the surgeon was initially blinded to the MRI results and after surgical exploration was able to consult the MRI findings, the images provided relevant new information in one patient with Crohn's disease with an epithelialized extrasphincteric fistula who would have otherwise had the fistula missed at surgery. Unfortunately, MRI missed a supralevator abscess and extra-

sphincteric fistula in another patient with Crohn's disease as well as the internal openings of fistulae in three other patients found at surgery. Poor visualization above the levator plate remains an inherent problem of any endoanal imaging technique and it is likely that the presence of the endorectal probe obscures

Figure 7-82. A sagittal endoanal coil MR image prior to administration of intravenous contrast in a patient with Crohn's disease.

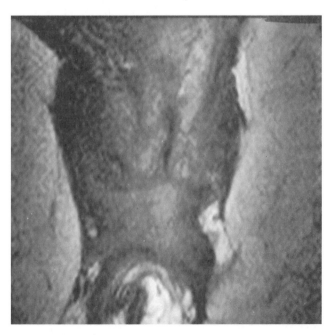

Table 7-3. Clinical and Radiologic Concordance of Patients With Complex Fistula-in-Ano[a]

Etiology of disease	6 Crohn's disease
	2 Behçet's disease
	3 Recurrent cryptogenic
Abscess (n = 7)	2 Intersphincteric
	5 Supralevator
Fistula-in-ano (n = 14)	5 Extrasphincteric
	5 Trans-sphincteric
	4 Rectovaginal
Surgery Versus Radiology: Concordance	
Abscess	
Presence	85.7%
Site	100%
Fistula-in-ano	
Presence	85.7%
Site	100%
Internal opening	
Position	78.5%
Horseshoeing	
Presence	100%

[a] n = 11 (7 males, 4 females); median age = 32 years (range 18–56).

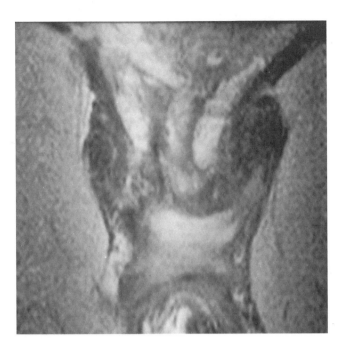

Figure 7-83. The same patient in Figure 7-81 following intravenous contrast administration demonstrating enhancement by an intersphincteric collection in front of the anal canal.

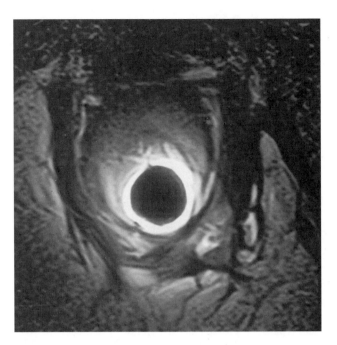

Figure 7-84. T_1-weighted endoanal coil MR image without intravenous contrast in a patient with intersphincteric sepsis.

the internal opening in some cases. The details of the cases are shown in Table 7-3 and depicted in Figures 7-81 to 7-83.

It has been shown that recurrent disease after primary fistula surgery, particularly in the complex or noncryptogenic case, occurs as a result of missed primary and secondary tracks and in attempts to preserve anal continence where the primary track traverses the external sphincter above the levator plate.[36] It is anticipated that MRI will help prevent these recurrences after primary surgery. It is recommended that the use of endoanal MRI in particular to outline complex disease may be of value for the specialist coloproctologist referred a patient with multiply recurrent sepsis where clinical examination in the presence of scarring may be unreliable. Further, the general surgeon with a proctologic interest may use the technology to decide which patients with high fistulae may be better referred to specialist centers. It remains to be seen how endoanal MRI will compare with external coil MRI (Fig. 7-84).

MRI IN LOW RECTAL CANCER

Accurate preoperative staging of rectal cancer assists in selection of appropriate surgery, the determination of prognosis, and in the identification of patients likely to benefit from adjuvant therapies.

The incidence of pelvic recurrence after radical surgery is dependent on the depth of rectal wall involvement by the tumor and the presence of adjacent malignant lymphadenopathy.[37–39] Preoperative tumor staging taken together with well-described histopathologic features such as degree of differentiation and microvascular or lymphatic invasion may define those patients suitable for local excision or ablation therapy as well as determine appropriate cases for this approach with more aggressive

histology who are poor candidates for major resectional surgery.[40,41]

Accurate imaging of patients with advanced but resectable rectal cancer before surgery will help determine patients who will benefit from preoperative adjuvant radiotherapy[42] as well as assist in detection of locally advanced cancers with extrarectal fixity and adjacent organ invasion where preoperative chemoradiation may enhance resection.[43]

The clinical examination of the patient with low rectal cancer is only moderately accurate, tending to overstage early lesions with an inability either to separate extensive from minimal perirectal spread or to distinguish inflammatory from neoplastic fixity.[44,45]

Endorectal ultrasonography (ERUS) has become the "gold standard" in the preoperative determination of tumor depth with a reported accuracy of 80%, but a tendency to overstage early lesions.[46,47] In four trials comparing transrectal ultrasound with external coil MRI, accuracy of assessment of tumor depth appears to be similar. The sensitivity of nodal detection by MRI is inferior to that of ultrasound (on average 60% compared with 80%) and comprehensive TN staging by MRI appears to be relatively poor. The delineation of advanced local disease by disruption of perirectal fat planes appears to be equivalent when comparing MRI with CT and is not enhanced by the availability of multiple planes afforded by MRI.[11,48–50]

MRI is inaccurate in the detection of nodes and mesorectal tumor deposits. The ultrasonographic features of involved nodes have been extensively described both in vitro and in vivo, although there is no evidence that an MRI classification based on recognized ultrasonographic features of neoplastic node replacement is valid. The changes noted by ultrasound to be associated with malignancy include hypoechoic appearance, inhomogeneity, altered shape, and reduced sonar attenuation coefficient.[51–53] Definition of the presence of a definable mass in the mesorectum larger than 0.5 cm in diameter has a 50% to 70% chance of malignancy whereas nodes smaller than 4 mm in diameter have less than a 20% chance of being neoplastic.[54]

Despite this, nodal size appears to be the predominant feature predicting malignant change in most MRI studies because it is nearly impossible to analyze the internal structure of very small nodes. It is likely that given size differences in resected specimens that up to 20% of patients will have involved but undetectable nodes preoperatively because their diameter is less than 3 mm.[55]

Comparative studies such as these must also take into account differences in nodal yield in part dependent on the diligence of the pathologist and the use of node clearance techniques.[56] MRI is accurate in the detection of locally recurrent disease with improved sensitivity, specificity, and accuracy when compared with CT.[57] In theory, fibrous tissue and postradiation reaction appears as a relatively low signal intensity on both T_1- and T_2-weighted images. Distinction between tumor and fibrosis has been shown in pulmonary and gynecologic malignancy and highlights the advantage of MRI over endoanal ultrasound particularly after radiotherapy.[58–61] This effect is not absolute if there is tumor necrosis, extensive desmoplastic reaction, or if the recurrence is hypocellular. In these situations, differentiation of the presacral mass early after surgery still remains difficult[62,63] (Fig. 7-85). Endorectal surface coils have been used

to stage rectal cancer with an overall accuracy of T status of 80%. Like endorectal ultrasound there is an inherent tendency to overstage early (T1) lesions. Overstaging of T2 tumors as T3, which may occur in cases where there is advanced desmoplasia or surrounding edema (occasionally secondary to recent biopsy) may, in the current climate of adjuvant therapy, result in unnecessary radiotherapy to the pelvis. Technical difficulties may prevent accurate positioning of the probe if the tumor is constrictive. In the advanced case, where the craniocaudal extent of the tumor exceeds the dimensions of the probe, supplementary images will complement the examination by showing potential prostatic or uterine invasion as well as involvement of the pelvic side wall. Where pelvic exenteration is being contemplated, the demonstration of lateral pelvic wall and para-aortic lymph nodes will preclude radical surgery.[10,64]

We have recently examined 15 patients with low rectal cancer, prospectively combining endoanal MRI with CT before operation. Discrete soft tissue masses of any size detected in the mesorectal fat were recorded as positive. All patients underwent surgery within 2 weeks of imaging, with two patients undergoing abdominoperineal resection and two patients proving inoperable by virtue of pelvic side-wall invasion. One patient was treated by transanal excision of a villous lesion. In the cases treated by major resection, the bowel was immediately pinned on cork and fixed in formalin with documentation of the extent

Figure 7-85. Pelvic MRI in a patient with an adenocarcinoma of the rectum. (T_1-weighted).

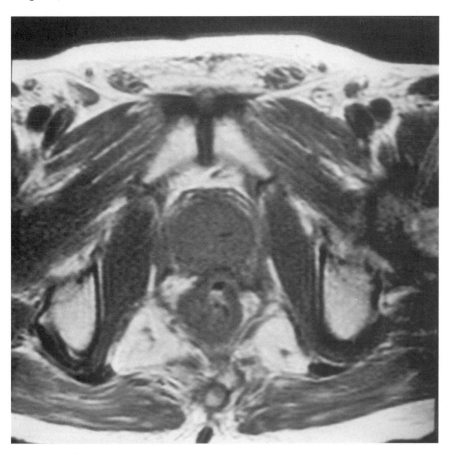

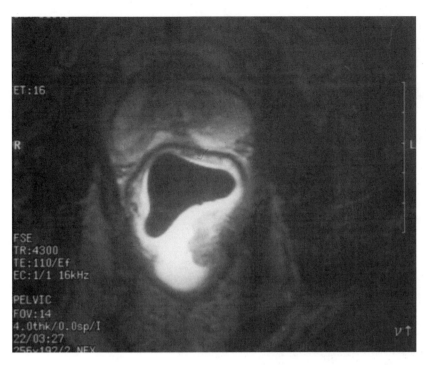

Figure 7-86. Transverse section of endoanal coil MRI (endoanal coil) as used at the Mayo Clinic, Rochester, Minnesota, demonstrating an adenocarcinoma of the rectum confined to the rectal wall.

of bowel wall invasion and the presence of either mesorectal nodal or extranodal deposits. Serial sectioning of the entire specimen was performed in the transverse plane with determination of the presence or absence of tumor involvement of the lateral resection margins in accordance with the technique of Quirke et al.[65] Anterior resections were carried out with total mesorectal excision as described by Heald et al.[66]

Of the 15 patients evaluated with endoanal MRI, 13 were able to be compared with resected histology. In two patients, MRI predicted extensive tumors invading the pelvic side wall; one showed malignant infiltration of the coccyx, prostate, and seminal vesicles and the other showed seminal vesicle infiltration with extensive pararectal and pelvic side-wall lymphadenopathy. Both patients proved to have disease at surgery that was irresectable for cure. In another patient, endoanal MRI, CT, and the clinical findings were complementary in successful transanal excision of a villous cancer with confirmed histologic clearance.

Of six patients with tumors limited to the bowel wall, five were correctly identified with a specificity of 83.3% (Figs. 7-86 and 7-87). Of the seven patients with T3/T4 lesions MRI correctly identified four with a sensitivity for tumor beyond the muscularis propria of 57.1% (Fig. 7-88). The sensitivity of nodal detection was only 50%. Of the 13 patients evaluable for T staging MRI correctly identified 9 (69.2%). Correct identification of N stage was made in only five patients (41.7%). Importantly, of 12 patients evaluable for lateral resection margins, MRI correctly predicted 91.7% (11 of 12) with a negative predictive value of 90.9% (10 of 11) and a specificity of 100%.

When MRI was compared with operative findings, there was good concordance with failure of agreement in only one case.

At operation, there was extension of an anterior rectal carcinoma into the prostatic capsule with confirmation of infiltration histologically. MRI failed to detect prostatic invasion because the tumor was stenotic and did not admit a larger endorectal coil for optimal examination of the prostate.

The results of this preliminary study show that MRI is disappointing in terms of detection both of T status and N status in low rectal cancer. The tendency to overstage early lesions is as much a feature of endoanal MRI as it is of endoanal ultrasound. The poor predictive capacity for detection of involved mesorectal nodes is disappointing although not unexpected. With increasing diligence by pathologists and the use of fat clearance techniques many nodes with micrometastases are found in the resection specimens and it is impossible for endorectal technologies to assess the internal structure of these small nodes. Furthermore, many nodes will be located beyond the field of view of the probe. The value of endorectal MRI in predicting the status of lateral resection margins is of importance for standard total mesorectal excision. Identification before operation of patients where pelvic residuum is likely despite radical surgery will permit the utilization of preoperative adjuvant strategies that might improve resectability and possibly outcome. It may also help to define those patients unsuitable for pelvic exenteration.

MRI IN THE ASSESSMENT OF THE PATIENT WITH FECAL INCONTINENCE

Endorectal ultrasound has become a "gold standard" in the definition of sphincter integrity in patients presenting with fecal incontinence. In vivo anatomy has proven to be concordant

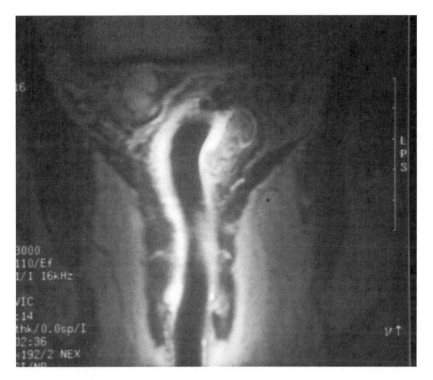

Figure 7-87. Longitudinal section of the adenocarcinoma of the rectum confined to the rectal wall as seen in longitudinal section (Mayo Clinic) coil.

with operative findings at the time of either sphincteroplasty or postanal repair and correlates with the known anatomic descriptions of the sphincter musculature in cadaveric dissection.[67–71]

The technique has effectively replaced concentric needle electromyography for the diagnosis of external sphincter defects.[72] More recently, it has become recognized that there is a higher incidence of occult sphincter defects than previously thought in the female population after normal vaginal delivery and that a high proportion of these patients have demonstrated loss of anterior sphincter integrity.[73,74] In these patients there is relatively poor correlation of symptoms with the presence of either an internal or external sphincter defect on endosonography.[75,76] The clinical importance of this finding has been based around the comparatively poor long-term outcome in patients without sphincter defects subjected to postanal repair when contrasted with the improved results at least in the short term in patients with demonstrable external sphincter defects undergoing overlapping sphincteroplasty.[77–83]

Endoanal MRI has recently been assessed in a group of patients operated on for fecal incontinence due to obstetric trauma.[84] In six patients with solid fecal incontinence immediately following vaginal delivery with forceps instrumentation, EAS disruption was noted on MRI in five (Fig. 7-89). The site and extent of each of these defects was subsequently confirmed at the time of surgery. EAS atrophy was universally demonstrable in another 16 patients with delayed fecal incontinence presenting at least 15 years after traumatic vaginal delivery. Statistically significant differences in muscle measurement are seen for both the superficial and deep EAS when compared with age-matched controls. Endoanal MRI has also shown two patients

presenting with delayed incontinence who had associated rectovaginal fistulae. An additional two patients had associated internal sphincter defects represented as a marked loss in the normally high signal intensity of the IAS ring. T_2 weighting appears to be the best sequence for establishing contrast between the EAS and the IAS. This degree of resolution showing the site and extent of the sphincter defect is not demonstrable with MRI using an external coil alone.

Endoanal MRI also provides excellent postoperative imaging after sphincteroplasty (Fig. 7-90) and complements anal manometry after postanal repair. Following hemorrhoidectomy, IAS injury has been shown using the endoanal coil, the morphologic appearances of which correlate with low resting maximal anal pressure and resting anal vector volume. This anatomic definition may be of value for medicolegal purposes in patients whose sphincter function is compromised postoperatively as well as for predicting the likely outcome after sphincter repair. In patients with recurrent or residual incontinence who have failed primary surgery, high-resolution imaging defines candidates for further attempts at anterior plication, levatorplasty, graciloplasty, or permanent colostomy.[85–87]

DYNAMIC MRI IN FUNCTIONAL DISORDERS

MRI is not well suited to the investigation of functional disorders of the anorectum; however, dynamic studies have been used to assess movement of the pelvic floor. The technique involves the use of an axial scout view at the sacrococcygeal junction with 10-mm sections obtained at rest using conventional spin-echo sequencing. Images are repeated during perineal squeeze and straining. Measurements include the anorectal

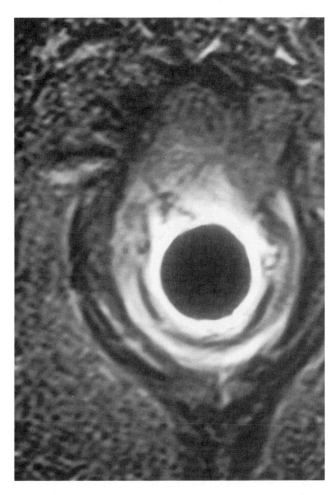

Figure 7-88. Endoanal coil MRI demonstrating invasion of anal carcinoma through the wall of the anal canal and into the surrounding external sphincter muscle (T$_2$-weighted).

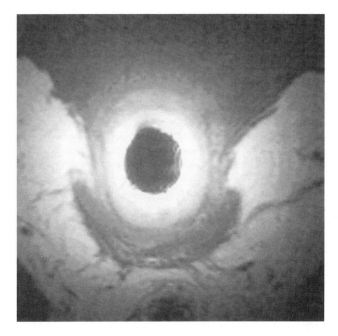

Figure 7-89. T$_1$-weighted endoanal coil MRI demonstrating disrupted external anal sphincter following obstetric injury.

MRI IN CONGENITAL ANORECTAL MALFORMATIONS

MRI has been used in the assessment of congenital anorectal abnormalities, cloacal anomalies, sacral agenesis, and in imaging of the pelvic floor after rectoplasty. It complements invertography of the infant, which may provide the false impression

Figure 7-90. T$_1$-weighted endoanal coil MRI in the same patient as in Figure 7-88 3 months later demonstrating an overlapped external anal sphincter repair.

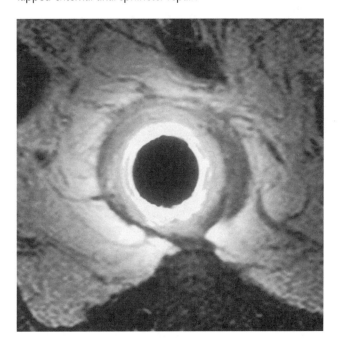

angle (between the posterior border of the rectum and the central axis of the anal canal), relative movement of the anorectal junction in relation to the symphysiosacral line, and determination of the retrorectal (presacral) distance. The anorectal angle is measured in exactly the same way as during defecography and cannot readily be performed if the rectum or bladder are not empty or if there is indentation of the rectum by an enterocele. Dynamic MRI may display pathologic mobility of the anorectum, which is implicated in intra-anal intussception and anterior mucosal rectal prolapse syndrome. Abnormal movement of the anorectal junction may imply anismus (paradoxical puborectalis contraction syndrome) and an excessive presacral space may be diagnostic of full-thickness prolapse as well as define the presence of a presacral mass.[88,89]

MRI of the pelvic floor is less physiologic than defecography and does not witness the actual act of defecation. However, it avoids unnecessary gonadal irradiation, opacification of the vagina and rectum is not required, and there appears to be less interobserver variation. Its exact role in the patient with functional disease remains to be determined although it may have a place in situations where patients either cannot retain or release rectal contrast during conventional proctography.[4,90,91]

of rectal atresia in cases where there is a high rectal fistula or meconium plugging of an atretic distal rectum. The approach with MRI uses transaxial and sagittal images because in many cases the funnel of the pelvic floor has a more sagittal orientation. In children, multiplanar imaging and the avoidance of ionizing radiation are distinct advantages. Where appropriate, it may be combined with peristomal contrast to outline high rectourethral fistulae. Differences between the measured puborectalis sphincter thickness and MRI nomograms confirm levator atrophy in cases of high anomaly.

Postoperative images sensitively depict the relation of the neorectum to the puborectalis sling and will define those cases that may benefit from neosphincter transplantation as well as predict the possible continence outcome after pull-through surgery.[92–94] Sagittal views display the distal development and attachment of the EAS to the coccyx, the anococcygeal raphe, and the blind rectal stump. Associated vertebral and sacrococcygeal anomalies (tethered spinal cord, coccygeal deviation, lateral sacral hypoplasia) may be demonstrated in 20% to 40% of cases as well as upper tract urinary anomalies (hydronephrosis, renal agenesis, renal ectopia) and lower genitourinary malformations (rectovesical/rectourethral fistulae, vaginal agenesis).[95]

MRI also demonstrates sacrococcygeal tumors, presacral teratomas, anterior myelomeningocele, or the Currarino triad[96] (anorectal malformation, presacral mass, and sacral anomaly).

SUMMARY

MRI has considerable advantages in cases of low rectal cancer and perirectal sepsis where examination of the pelvis, iliac, and para-aortic lymph nodes and liver is necessary in addition to the images of the primary pathology.

MRI utilizing an internal coil provides detailed images of the anal sphincter that correlate with in vitro and in vivo anatomy and that seem to be less operator dependent than endoanal ultrasound. Comparative studies using endoanal ultrasound and endoanal MRI in patients with fecal incontinence and rectal and anal cancer are awaited.

The practical advantages of endoanal MRI over ultrasound in perirectal sepsis are outlined in this chapter. MRI in the setting of complicated and recurrent infection where supralevator and extrasphincteric tracks and collections are suspected is advised as clinical examination is frequently unreliable.

In preliminary work, endoanal MRI appears to be an inferior modality for predicting TN status in low rectal malignancy, but it is highly predictive for pelvic side-wall involvement. This may have considerable bearing on the expected outcome after standard total mesorectal excision and should influence the choice of preoperative radiotherapy or chemoradiation.

The disadvantages of endoanal MRI compared with endoanal ultrasound include cost, lack of portability (particularly for use in the operating suite), and the present limited availability of the internal coils. The presence in some patients of ferromagnetic metallic implants (aneurysm clips, intravascular stents, otologic implants, and cardiac pacemakers) is a contraindication to the use of MRI technology where the magnetic forces used may impose dangerous torque and heating effects.

In patients with fecal incontinence secondary to obstetric trauma, endoanal MRI provides exquisite detail that has uniform concordance with operative findings and manometry. It also defines anatomy in those patients with continence impairment after routine anorectal surgery and it is hoped that it may select patients who will benefit from secondary surgery to restore continence after failed postanal or anterior sphincter repair.

The role of dynamic MRI in the assessment of the pelvic floor appears limited at present but may be complementary in cases where defecography proves difficult to interpret. MRI is superior when compared with CT in the assessment of congenital anorectal malformations because of its multiplanar capability and improved soft tissue resolution.

REFERENCES

1. Hesselink JR, Martin JF, Edelman RR (1990) Fast imaging. Neuroradiology 32:348
2. Frahm J, Gyngell ML, Hanicke W (1992) Rapid scan techniques. pp. 165–203. In Stark DD, Bradley WG (eds): Magnetic Resonance Imaging. 2nd Ed. Mosby Year Book, St. Louis
3. Plattner V, Leborgne J Heloury Y et al (1991) MRI evaluation of the levator ani muscle: anatomic correlations and practical implications. Surg Radiol Anat 13:129–131
4. Aronson MP, Lee RA, Berquist TH (1990) Anatomy of the anal sphincters and related structures in continent women studied with magnetic resonance imaging. Obstet Gynaecol 76: 846–851
5. Schafer A, Enck P, Furst G et al (1994) Anatomy of the anal sphincters: comparison of anal endosonography to magnetic resonance imaging. Dis Colon Rectum 37:777–781
6. Herrera-Ornelas L, Justiniano J, Castillo N et al (1987) Metastases in small lymph nodes from colon cancer. Arch Surg 122: 1253–1256
7. Schnall MD, Lenkinski RE, Pollack HM et al (1989) Prostate: MR imaging with an endorectal surface coil. Radiology 172: 570–574

8. Badouin CJ, Soutter WP, Gilderdale DJ, Coutts GA (1992) Magnetic resonance imaging of the uterine cervix using an intravaginal coil. Magnet Res Med 24:196–203
9. deSouza NM, Hawley IC, Schwieso JE et al (1994) The uterine cervix on in vitro and in vivo MR images: a study of zonal anatomy and vascularity using an enveloping cervical coil. Am J Roentgenol 163:607–612
10. Schnall MD, Furth EE, Rosato EF, Kressel HY (1994) Rectal tumour stage: correlation of endorectal MR imaging and pathologic findings. Radiology 190:709–714
11. Joosten FB, Jansen JBMJ, Joosten HJM, Rosenbusch G (1995) Staging of rectal carcinoma using MR double surface coil, MR endorectal coil and intraectal ultrasound: correlation with histopathologic findings. J Comput Assist Tomogr 19: 752–758
12. Meyenberger C, Huch-Boni RA, Bertschinger P et al (1995) Endoscopic ultrasound and endorectal magnetic resonance imaging: a prospective comparative study for preoperative staging and followup of rectal cancer. Endoscopy 27:469–479
13. Puni R, Hall AS, Coutts GA, deSouza NM (1994) Development of an insertable surface coil for MRI of the anal sphincter.

Proceedings of progress in Magnetic Resonance British Institute of Radiology. Radiology 68:679(A)

14. Lunniss PJ, Phillips RKS (1992) Anatomy and function of the anal longitudinal muscle. Br J Surg 79:882–884

15. Yamashita Y, Harada M, Sawada T et al (1993) Normal uterus and FIGO stage I endometrial carcinoma: dynamic gadolinium enhanced MR imaging. Radiology 186:495–501

16. Thickman DI, Kundel HL, Wolf G (1983) Nuclear magnetic resonance characteristics of fresh and fixed tissue: the effect of elapsed time. Radiology 148:183–185

17. Bartram CI, Burnett SJD (1991) Atlas of Anal Endosonography. Butterworth Heineman

18. Dawson P, Blomley M (1994) Gadolinium chelate MR contrast agents, editorial. Clin Radiol 49:439–442

19. Lauffer RB (1990) Magnetic resonance contrast media: principles and progress. Magn Reson Q 6:65–84

20. Sangwan YP, Rosen L, Riether R et al (1994) Is simple fistula-in-ano simple? Dis Colon Rectum 37:885–889

21. Kuijpers HC, Schulpen T (1985) Fistulography for fistula-in-ano: is it useful? Dis Colon Rectum 28:103–104

22. Ani AA, Langundoye SB (1979) Radiological evaluation of anal fistulae: a prospective study of fistulograms. Clin Radiol 30:21–24

23. Weisman RI, Orsay CP, Pearl RK, Abcarian H (1991) The role of fistulography in fistula-in-ano. Dis Colon Rectum 34:181–184

24. Guillaumin E, Jeffrey RB, Shea WJ et al (1986) Perirectal inflammatory disease: CT findings. Radiology 161:153–157

25. Yousem DM Fishman EK, Jones B (1988) Crohn's disease: perirectal and perianal findings at CT. Radiology 167:331–334

26. Choen S, Burnett S, Bartram CI, Nicholls RJ (1991) Comparison between anal endosonography and digital examination in the evaluation of anal fistulae. Br J Surg 78:445–447

27. Cheong DMO, Nogueras JJ, Wexner SD, Jagelman DG (1993) Anal endosonography for recurrent anal fistulas: image enhancement with hydrogen peroxide. Dis Colon Rectum 36:1158–1160

28. Tio TL, Mulder CJJ, Wijers OB et al (1990) Endosonography of perianal and pericolorectal fistulae and/or abscess in Crohn's disease. Gastrointest Endosc 36:331–336

29. Law PJ, Talbot RW, Bartram CL, Northover JMA (1989) Anal endosonography in the evaluation of perianal sepsis and fistula-in-ano. Br J Surg 76:752–757

30. Lunniss PJ, Barker PG, Sultan AH et al (1994) Magnetic resonance imaging of fistula-in-ano. Dis Colon Rectum 37:707–718

31. Barker PG, Lunniss PJ, Armstrong P et al (1994) Magnetic resonance imaging of fistula-in-ano: technique, interpretation and accuracy. Clin Radiol 49:7–13

32. Myrh GE, Myrvold HE, Nilsen G, et al (1994) Perianal fistulas: use of MR imaging for diagnosis. Radiology 191:545–549

33. Tjandra JJ, Sissons GRJ (1994) Magnetic resonance imaging facilitates assessment of perianal Crohn's disease. Aust N Z J Surg 64:470–474

34. Zbar AP, deSouza NM, Hall A et al (1996) Magnetic resonance imaging of anal sphincter sepsis using an endoanal coil: pilot studies. Br J Surg 83:694(A)

35. Zbar AP, deSouza NM, Puni R et al (1996) Magnetic resonance imaging (MRI) of anal sphincter sepsis with an internal coil. Proceedings Tripartite Colorectal Meeting July 1996 London. Int J Colorect Dis 11:135(A)

36. Seow-Choen F, Phillips RKS (1991) Insights gained from the management of problematical anal fistulae at St Mark's Hospital 1984–8. Br J Surg 78:539–541

37. Morson BC (1966) Factors influencing the prognosis of early carcinoma of the rectum. Proc R Soc Med 59:607–608

38. Pilipshen SJ, Hulweil M, Quan SHQ et al (1984) Patterns of pelvic recurrence following definitive resections of rectal carcinoma. Cancer 53:1351–1362

39. Duncan W, Smith AN, Freedman LF et al (1984) Clinicopathological features of prognostic significance in operable rectal cancer in 17 centres in the United Kingdom: third report of the MRC trial. Br J Cancer 50:435–442

40. Buess G, Mentgen B, Manncke et al (1991) Minimal invasive surgery in the local treatment of rectal carcinoma. Int J Colorect Dis 6:77–81

41. Morson B (1985) Histologic criteria for local excision. Br J Surg 72:S53–S54

42. Påhlman L, Glimelius B (1990) Pre and post-operative radiotherapy in rectal carcinoma: report from a randomized multicenter trial. Ann Surg 211:187–195

43. Chen E-T, Mohiuddin M, Brodovsky H et al (1994) Downstaging of advanced rectal cancer following combined preoperative chemotherapy and high-dose radiation. Int J Radiat Oncol Biol Phys 30:169–175

44. Nicholls RJ, York Mason A, Morson BC et al (1982) The clinical staging of rectal cancer. Br J Surg 69:404–409

45. Durdey P, Williams NS (1984) The effect of malignant and inflammatory fixation of rectal cancer on prognosis after rectal excision. Br J Surg 71:787–790

46. Hildebrandt U, Feifel G (1985) Preoperative staging of rectal cancer by intrarectal ultrasonography. Dis Colon Rectum 28:42–46

47. Orrom WJ, Wong WD, Rothenberger DA et al (1990) Endorectal ultrasonography in the preoperative staging of rectal tumours: a learning experience. Dis Colon Rectum 33:654–659

48. Guinet C, Buy J-N, Ghossain MA et al (1990) Comparison of magnetic resonance imaging and computed tomography in the preoperative staging of rectal cancer. Arch Surg 125:385–388

49. Waizer A, Powsner E, Russo I et al (1991) Prospective comparative study of magnetic resonance imaging versus transrectal ultrasound for preoperative staging and followup of rectal cancer—preliminary report. Dis Colon Rectum 34:1068–1072

50. Thaler W, Watzka S, Martin F et al (1994) Preoperative staging of rectal cancer by endoluminal ultrasound vs magnetic resonance imaging: preliminary results of a prospective comparative study. Dis Colon Rectum 37:1189–1193

51. Hildebrandt U, Klein T, Feifel G et al (1990) Endosonography of pararectal lymph nodes: in vitro and in vivo evaluation. Dis Colon Rectum 33:863–868

52. Bachmann-Nielsen M, Qvitzau S, Pedersen J-F (1993) Detection of pericolonic lymph nodes in patients with colorectal cancer: an in vitro and in vivo study of the efficacy of endosonography. Radiology 161:57–60

53. Hulsmans FH, Bosma A, Mulder PJJ et al (1992) Perirectal lymph nodes in rectal cancer: in vitro correlation of sonographic parameters and histopathologic findings. Radiology 184:553–560

54. Beynon J, Mortensen NJMcC, Foy DMA et al (1989) Preoperative assessment of mesorectal lymph node involvement in rectal cancer. Br J Surg 76:276–279

55. Dworak O (1989) Number and size of lymph nodes and node metastases in rectal carcinoma. Surg Endosc 3:96–99
56. Hyder JW, Talbott TM, Maycroft TC (1990) A critical review of chemical lymph node clearance and staging of colon and rectal cancer at Ferguson Hospital 1977–1982. Dis Colon Rectum 33:923–925
57. Pema PJ, Bennett WF, Bova JG, Warman P (1994) CT vs MRI in diagnosis of recurrent rectosigmoid carcinoma. J Comput Assist Tomogr 18:256–261
58. Glazer HS, Levitt RG, Lee JKT et al (1984) Differentiation of radiation fibrosis from recurrent pulmonary neoplasm by magnetic resonance imaging. Am J Roentgenol 143:729–730
59. Ebner F, Kressel HY, Mintz MC et al (1988) Tumour recurrence versus fibrosis in the female pelvis: differentiation with MR imaging at 1.5T. Radiology 166:333–340
60. Glazer HS, Lee JKT, Levitt RG et al (1985) Radiation fibrosis: differentiation from recurrent tumour by MR imaging. Radiology 156:721–726
61. Gomberg JS, Friedman AC, Radecki PD et al (1986) MRI differentiation of recurrent colorectal carcinoma from postoperative fibrosis. Gastrointest Radiol 11:361–363
62. Sundaram M, McGuire MH, Schajowicz F (1986) Soft-tissue masses: histologic basis for decreased signal (short T2) on T2-weighted MR images. Am J Roentgenol 148:1247–1250
63. deLange EE, Fechner RE, Wanebo HJ (1989) Suspected recurrent rectosigmoid carcinoma after abdominoperineal resection: MR imaging and histopathologic findings. Radiology 170:323–328
64. deLange EE (1994) Staging rectal carcinoma with endorectal imaging: how much detail do we really need? Editorial. Radiology 190:633–635
65. Quirke P, Durdey P, Dixon MF, Williams NS (1986) Local recurrence of rectal adenocarcinoma due to inadequate surgical resection: histopathological study of lateral tumour spread and surgical excision. Lancet 1:996–999
66. Heald RJ, Husband EM, Ryall RDH (1982) The mesorectum in rectal cancer surgery—the clue to pelvic recurrence? Br J Surg 69:613–616
67. Dalley AF (1987) The riddle of the sphincters: the morphophysiology of the anorectal mechanism reviewed. Am Surg 53:298–306
68. Gorsch RV (1955) Proctologic Anatomy. 2nd Ed. Williams & Wilkins, Baltimore
69. Sultan AH, Kamm MA, Talbot IC et al (1994) Anal endosonography for identifying external sphincter defects confirmed histologically. Br J Surg 81:463–465
70. Sultan AH, Nicholls RJ, Kamm MA et al (1993) Anal endosonography and correlation with in vitro and in vivo anatomy. Br J Surg 80:508–511
71. Law PJ, Bartram CI (1989) Anal endosonography: technique and normal anatomy. Gastrointest Radiol 14:349–353
72. Law PJ, Kamm MA, Bartram CI (1990) A comparison between electromyography and anal endosonography in mapping external anal sphincter defects. Dis Colon Rectum 33:370–373
73. Sultan AH, Kamm MA, Hudson CN et al (1993) Anal sphincter disruption during vaginal delivery. N Engl J Med 329:1905–1911
74. Burnett SJD, Spence-Jones C, Speakman CTM et al (1991) Unsuspected sphincter damage following childbirth revealed by endoanal ultrasonography. Br J Radiol 64:225–227
75. Engel AF, Kamm MA, Bartram CI, Nicholls RJ (1995) Relationship of symptoms in faecal incontinence to specific sphincter abnormalities. Int J Colorect Dis 10:152–155
76. Felt-Bersma RJF, Cuesta MA, Koorevaar M et al (1992) Anal endosonography: relationship with anal manometry and neurophysiologic tests. Dis Colon Rectum 35:944–949
77. Setti-Carraro P, Kamm MA, Nicholls RJ (1994) Long term followup of postanal repair for faecal incontinence. Br J Surg 81:140–144
78. Scheuer M, Kuijpers H, Jacobs PP (1989) Postanal repair restores anatomy rather than function. Dis Colon Rectum 32:960–963
79. Engel AF, Kamm MA, Sultan AH et al (1994) Anterior anal sphincter repair in patients with obstetric trauma. Br J Surg 81:1231–1234
80. Oliveria L, Pfeifer J, Wexner SD (1996) Physiological and clinical outcome of anterior sphincteroplasty. Br J Surg 83:502–505
81. Wexner SD, Marchetti F, Jagelman DG (1990) The role of sphincteroplasty for fecal incontinence reevaluated: a prospective physiologic and functional review. Dis Colon Rectum 34:22–30
82. Londono-Schimmer EE, Garcia-Duperly R, Nicholls RJ et al (1994) Overlapping anal sphincter repair for faecal incontinence due to sphincter trauma: five year functional followup results. Int J Colorect Dis 9:110–113
83. Engel AF, van Baal SJ, Brummelkamp WH (1994) Late results of anterior sphincter plication for traumatic faecal incontinence. Eur J Surg 160:633–636
84. deSouza NM, Puni R, Zbar A et al (1996) MR imaging of the anal sphincter in multiparous females using an endoanal coil: correlation with in vitro anatomy and appearances in faecal incontinence. Am J Roentgenol 167:1465–1471
85. Engel AF, Sultan AH, Kamm MA et al (1993) Outcome after sphincter repair is related to external sphincter function and ultrasound appearance. Gut 34:S40
86. Browning GGP, Henry MM, Motson RW (1988) Combined sphincter repair and postanal repair for the treatment of combined injuries to the anal sphincters. Ann R Coll Surg Engl 70:324–328
87. Miller R, Orrom WJ, Cornes H et al (1989) Anterior sphincter plication and levatorplasty in the treatment of faecal incontinence. Br J Surg 76:1058–1060
88. Yang A, Mostwin JL, Rosenshein NB, Zerhouni EA (1991) Pelvic floor descent in women: dynamic evaluation with fast MR imaging and cinematic display. Radiology 179:25–33
89. Chrispin AR, Fry IK (1963) The presacral space shown by barium enema. Br J Radiol 36:319–322
90. Kruyt RH, Delemarre JBVM, Doornbos J, Vogel HJ (1991) Normal anorectum: dynamic MR imaging anatomy. Radiology 179:159–163
91. Delemarre JBVM, Kruyt RH, Doornbos J et al (1994) Anterior rectocoele: assessment with radiographic defecography, dynamic magnetic resonance imaging and physical examination. Dis Colon Rectum 37:249–259
92. Vade A, Reyes H, Wilbur A, et al (1989) The anorectal sphincter after rectal pull through surgery for anorectal anomalies: MRI evaluation. Pediatr Radiol 19:179–183
93. Sato Y, Pringle KC, Bergman RA et al (1988) Congenital anorectal anomalies: MR imaging. Radiology 168:157–162

94. Mezzacappa PM, Price AP, Haller JO et al (1987) MR and CT demonstration of levator sling in congenital anorectal anomalies. J Comput Assist Tomogr 11:273–275
95. Denton JR (1982) Association of congenital spinal anomalies with imperforate anus. Clin Orthopaed Rel Res 162:91–98
96. Currarino G, Dale C, Votteler T (1981) Triad of anorectal, sacral and presacral anomalies. Am J Radiol 137:395–398
97. de Souza NM, Puni R, Gilderdale DJ, Bydder GM (1995) Magnetic resonance imaging of the anal sphincter using an internal coil. Magn Reson Q 11:45–56

NUCLEAR MEDICINE

Keith E. Britton
Marie Granowska

Nuclear medicine is an independent medical monospecialty that embraces all applications of radioactive materials in the diagnosis and treatment of patients and in medical research. The principal radionuclide from the 1940s was iodine-131 (^{131}I), used for thyroid imaging and the treatment of thyrotoxicosis and thyroid cancer. The present radionuclides for imaging are indium-111 (^{111}In) and technetium-99m (^{99m}Tc) and for therapy are ^{131}I and yttrium-90. ^{111}In has a half-life of 67 hours and gives off gamma rays of two energies, 171 and 243 MeV. It must be ordered for use and is expensive. ^{99m}Tc is available daily on site in the department as the daughter of the molybdenum-99 generator. ^{99m}Tc is the basis of most nuclear medicine imaging and is relatively inexpensive. It has a half-life of 6 hours and an energy of 140 MeV.

Imaging is undertaken with a gamma camera that is designed for the 140-MeV energy. It consists of a large crystal covered by a collimator, which is a lead sheet perforated with thousands of parallel holes so that the only gamma rays normal to the face of the crystal are received. Multiple photomultipliers behind the crystal turn the light flashes in the crystal into electrical impulses that, through special circuitry, record the site and strength of the received gamma rays to build up an image on a photographic plate or through buffers directly into minicomputers. Scattered radiation is of lower energy and is rejected by a pulse height analyzer window that allows in the primary gamma rays. The gamma camera might be rotated around the patient to collect data that are reformated into transverse, coronal, and/or sagittal sections (single photon emission tomography, SPET). Radiopharmaceuticals are produced under aseptic conditions in special cabinets using the eluted ^{99m}Tc from the molybdenum generator, which is combined with various kits such as methylenediphosphonate (MDP) for bone scanning and macroaggregated albumin for lung perfusion scans; or by special techniques such as the radiolabeling of monoclonal antibodies. The amount of activity injected is measured in megabequerels (MBq; 37 MBq equals 1 millicurie, mCi). Typically 600 MBq ^{99m}Tc MDP are used for a bone scan and 600 MBq ^{99m}Tc monoclonal antibodies for monoclonal antibody imaging. The energy received by the patient is measured in millisieverts (mSv). A typical absorbed effective dose from the above is 4 mSv. Normal annual background is about 2 mSv whereas a barium enema gives the patient about 9 mSv. The International Committee on Radiation Protection states that up to 5 mSv is of negligible risk to members of the public (World Health Organization [WHO] II classification).

Side effects from radiopharmaceuticals including monoclonal antibodies (1 mg injected) occur in about 1 in 1,000 as compared with 1 in 100 for x-ray contrast media and 1 in 10 for penicillin.

APPLICATIONS

This section considers the application of nuclear medicine techniques in the detection and management of primary and recurrent colorectal cancer including the use of the peroperative probe; the demonstration of inflammation and infection related to the large bowel; and the localization of gastrointestinal bleeding.

Cancer

The physical imaging techniques of conventional radiology, radiography, computed tomography (CT), ultrasound, and magnetic resonance imaging (MRI) demonstrate cancer as a mass distorting or invading normal structures. The conventional nuclear medicine techniques generally depend on the metabolic activity of the organ or tissue and are sensitive but not specific. The bone scan shows increased uptake focally as a result of the effect of a metastasis or any other disease on its metabolic mechanisms of repair. The liver colloid scan shows a defect due to replacement of Kupffer cells by a metastasis or any space-occupying lesion. Sensitive but not specific techniques include gallium-67 citrate imaging of lymphomas and inflammatory disorder, and fluorine-18 deoxyglucose (FDG), a glucose substitute taken up by many different active tissues including cancers and imaged using positron emission tomography (PET), which can be more sensitive than radiography CT, or MRI. The alternative approach is to develop and apply methods of tissue characterization.

The cancer cell differs subtly from the normal cell and the new techniques depend on the binder/bindee concept.[1] Binding sites on the cancer cell surface are selected that differ quantitatively and qualitatively from those on normal cells and are used to demonstrate the presence of cancer. The bindees that are applied are either appropriate radiolabeled monoclonal antibodies targeting surface antigens or radiolabeled peptides or other compounds targeting receptor sites. It should be noted that the size of the lesion is not a restriction per se because a pinhead with sufficient radioactive signal on it is detectable. Furthermore, plaque-like extensions of recurrent tumor in the peritoneum of a few cells in thickness are invisible to radiologic techniques but are not a restriction for radiolabeled tissue characterizing agents.

The detection of colorectal cancer depends on the history, clinical and digital rectal examination, barium enema, and/or endoscopy. Nuclear medicine techniques have no routine role in this phase of the patients' management. Although radioimmunoscintigraphy, the use of radiolabeled monoclonal antibodies in tissue characterization, has a place in staging primary colorectal cancer, its main applications are in the detection of para-aortic nodes and liver involvement, in the demonstration of recurrent cancer before serum markers are elevated, in the demonstration of the site of recurrent cancer when serum markers are elevated, in the evaluation of the success of chemotherapy and/or radiotherapy, in the demonstration of the distribution of the recurrence for radiotherapy planning and surgery, and in the demonstration of antibody uptake prior to consideration of radioimmunotherapy (i.e., the use of radiotherapy radionuclide labeled monoclonal antibodies in the treatment of cancer). Radiolabeled monoclonal antibodies may be injected prior to surgery to enable the use of the peroperative probe. This may aid in the detection of unsuspected disease, in the demonstration that a tumor bed is free of tumor after surgery, in the demonstration that a piece of bowel for anastomosis is free from tumor, and particularly in demonstrating that tissue removed at operation does or does not contain malignancy prior to its being sent for frozen section.

RADIOIMMUNOSCINTIGRAPHY

The requirements of radioimmunoscintigraphy include the selection of an antigen as specific as possible to the cancer and a monoclonal antibody directed against this antigen; the best radiolabel appropriate to the kinetics of uptake of the antibody by the cancer; a radiolabeling method that preserves immunoreactivity; a gamma camera imaging system optimized for the radiolabel and the site of the cancer; and an analysis system that makes best use of the image data.[2]

Tumor-associated antigens are of several types. First, the epithelial surface antigens are separated by biologic barriers from the blood by being in the inner surfaces of cells and do not react with a monoclonal antibody injected intravenously. However, with the architectural disruption that characterizes the malignant process such antigens may become exposed to the blood and thus colorectal tumors may be detected using radiolabeled monoclonal antibodies that react with these antigens. One such example is PR1A3 produced by the Imperial Cancer Research Fund.[3,4] A second well-used group are the oncofetal antigens such as carcinoembryonic antigen (CEA).[5,6] Antibodies such as B-72.3 against the tumor-associated antigen TAG 72 are available.[7,8] Antigens may either be fixed to the tumor or released from it. CEA is released from the tumor and therefore

is available as a serum marker for cancer. However, a tumor must reach a certain size to release sufficient CEA to overcome uptake by the liver and reticuloendothelial system and the normal biologic variations in the blood to make it useful as a serum marker. Both CEA and B-72.3 are released by the tumor into lymphatics and therefore detection of the antigen in lymph node does not mean that tumor cells are present. Conversely PR1A3 is fixed to the tumor. It is not found in lymph nodes draining a primary cancer and therefore detection of uptake in lymph nodes represents malignant involvement when PR1A3 is used. When the cancer cell dies the PR1A3 antigen is destroyed with it, whereas the CEA antigen may be still detectable in the environment of dead cancer cells.

It has been shown that the CEA molecule is very complex. It consists of a large structure with a tail buried in the surface membrane of the cell. The part known as CEA breaks off from this tail and diffuses into lymphatics and blood vessels, a process that causes a conformational change to conceal the antigen against which the monoclonal antibody PR1A3 is produced. PR1A3 only binds to the membrane-fixed antigen, a fact discovered only once the three-dimensional structure of this antigen had been described. The sites of the two negative charges that bind to the antigen have been identified in the structure of PR1A3. Such information will help to develop peptides derived from antibodies with even higher binding affinity to cancer antigens.[9]

The radionuclides used for labeling monoclonal antibodies include ^{111}In and ^{99m}Tc. The B-72.3 antibody labeled with ^{111}In is available commercially (Oncoscint). Its main problem is that up to 20% of colorectal cancers do not express the TAG-72 antigen so at best sensitivity is only 80%; in contrast, PR1A3 labeled with ^{111}In or ^{99m}Tc reacts with 97% of colorectal cancers as does the anti-CEA antibody.[5,6,10,11]

The choice of radiolabel is very important.[2] The shorter its half-life the greater the activity that may be administered and the higher the count rate obtained. The detection of tumor depends on achieving the highest possible count rate from the target by the imaging system. The need for this high count rate is to minimize the noise due to the signal. Noise is a term used generally from anything that degrades the signal and has many sources but the most important is the signal itself (Poisson noise). The weaker the signal the more the noise inherent in the signal and this is more important than the effect of any contribution from nontarget background. Poisson noise depends on the square route of the count rate, thus the lower the count rate the disproportionally higher the noise. At a count rate of 100 counts per minute (cpm) the noise is 10 cpm, that is, 10% of the counts recorded, whereas at a count of 10,000 cpm, the noise is 100 cpm, or 1% of the counts recorded. The lower the count rate the more noisy the image so that the target is less separable from the background. The high variability of the background itself may give rise to noise that may be falsely interpreted as tumor signals. A good signal enables detection however high the nonspecific tissue background activity. The higher the count rate achieved the smaller the tumor detectable. The count rate from ^{99m}Tc is about three times as good as that from ^{111}In given the usual permitted activities administered, hence the reason for preferring ^{99m}Tc as the radiolabel for monoclonal antibody imaging.

Once the signal has been maximized attention can be given

to reducing the amount of nonsignal activity due to that in the blood and tissue background. SPET allows one to separate activity in a normal structure, such as the bladder, from sites of specific uptake. This is particularly important for imaging the pelvis when recurrent colorectal cancer is suspected. Reconstruction of the data in transverse, coronal, and sagittal sections gives a three-dimensional view of tumor uptake in relation to its environment. For this a high standard of camera, preferably double headed, and good quality control and imaging technique are required.

Background subtraction techniques have been used in an attempt to reduce the tissue contribution. The conventional subtraction techniques only work for large tumors. Change detection algorithms can work for very small tumors whereby the early image taken at 5 to 10 minutes is used as a template with which to compare the later image, which has specific uptake of the monoclonal antibody. Such change detection algorithms, also called kinetic analysis with probability mapping,[12] have not been applied to colorectal cancer mainly because of the movement of activity in bowel giving false signals between the early and late image.

RADIOLABELING OF MONOCLONAL ANTIBODIES

[111]In is attached to a monoclonal antibody in two stages. First, the monoclonal antibody has a chelating group fixed to it or else a macrocycle that is a ring structure into which ^{111}In can fit snugly. The second stage is to add the ^{111}In to label the chelate or macrocycle. The system must be kept scrupulously free of metal ions because they can interfere or compete with the ^{111}In uptake into the chelate.

[99m]Tc was first attached to monoclonal antibodies using a method called pretinning, where it was reduced using tin and then bound to the monoclonal antibody.[13] This method, however, led to the attachment of some strongly bound ^{99m}Tc but also some weakly bound ^{99m}Tc that became detached in vivo. A significant advance came with the reduction method described by Schwarz and Steinstrasser[14] and modified by Mather and Ellison.[15] This provided a simple method for labeling whole antibodies that was applicable in every nuclear medicine department. The S-S bonds linking the heavy chains together in the stem of the Y of the gamma globulin are opened using 2-mercapto ethanol in a 1:1,000 molar ratio. In this state the gamma globulin can be stored deep frozen and taken out when an investigation is planned. The next stage is to use a bone imaging kit such as MDP, which provides some tin-reducing agent to help the technetium bind to the free sulfur groups and some phosphate compound to prevent the weak binding of the ^{99m}Tc to the antibody. The resulting ^{99m}Tc-labeled antibody is stable in vivo with no thyroid uptake of free ^{99m}Tc even after 24 hours, and thus the patient does not require any thyroid blockade.

Patient Protocol

The test is explained in detail to the patient. Because many of these studies are performed under ethical committee control, signed informed consent must be obtained. It is absolutely essential to ask the patient whether there is a history of allergy to foreign proteins and such patients should not be studied. Skin testing, which was used previously, is inappropriate and leads to

immunization of the patient so that human antimouse antibodies (HAMA) are produced that may interfere with the imaging procedure if a series of injections is given for imaging purposes or therapy. The injection consists of 600 MBq of ^{99m}Tc monoclonal antibody or 120 MBq of ^{111}In monoclonal antibody of the chosen type. The amount of protein injected is normally less than 1 mg and this reduces the chance of side effects or sensitization. Before the injection, the vital signs are observed and the patient is then set on the imaging couch with the camera over the pelvis.

[111]In Radiolabeled Antibody

For ^{111}In labeled antibody the camera is set up with a medium energy (up to 300 KeV) general purpose parallel hole collimator with windows of 15% around the 171 and 20% around the 247 KeV photo peaks of [111]In. The data are transferred automatically to the minicomputer for subsequent image analysis and presentation. The vial containing the ^{111}In anti-CEA is transferred to a weighed syringe and needle and the amount assayed in an ionizing chamber to ensure that the correct activity is to be injected. After injection the syringe and needle are reweighed and the residual activity reassessed so that the activity and the weight of the antibody injected are recorded. The injection is given intravenously into an anticubital vein slowly over 10 seconds. Vital signs are recorded before and after the injection.

A series of images is made over the anterior and posterior chest, upper abdomen, lower abdomen, and pelvis, starting about 10 minutes after the injection. Other images are taken at 24 hours and 72 hours with SPET around 24 hours (Fig. 7-91). The camera undergoes a 360° rotation with 64 projections and takes about 32 minutes. It is essential that the patient remains absolutely still during this period. Each planar image should contain at least 800, 000 counts. To aid repositioning a similar image to each of the planar images may be undertaken with radioactive markers over prominent bony landmarks such as the symphysis pubis, iliac spines, costal margins, and xiphisternum.[10,16] The planar and SPET images are analyzed in the absence of clinical and radiologic information and decisions are made as to whether an unequivocal site of abnormal antibody uptake is seen. Specific uptake of a monoclonal antibody by tumor increases with time and thus the 10-minute image should show no abnormality; subsequent images should show increasing uptake at the site of a specific abnormality. Nonspecific uptake decreases with time after the initial distribution.

[99m]Tc-Radiolabeled Monoclonal Antibody

For ^{99m}Tc the gamma camera is set up with a low-energy general purpose parallel hole collimator. The photopeak is set at 140 KeV with a 15% window and for data transfer on line to the minicomputer. The patient protocol is as above. A quantity of 600 MBq ^{99m}Tc-labeled monoclonal antibody either anti-CEA[6] or PR1A3[4] is injected intravenously over 10 seconds. Images are taken of the lower chest and upper abdomen, lower abdomen, and pelvis anteriorly and posteriorly at 10 minutes, 5 to 6 hours, and 18 to 24 hours (Fig. 7-92). Each planar image contains a minimum of 800,000 counts. Thyroid blockade is not required.[16]

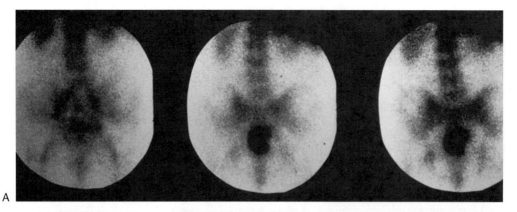

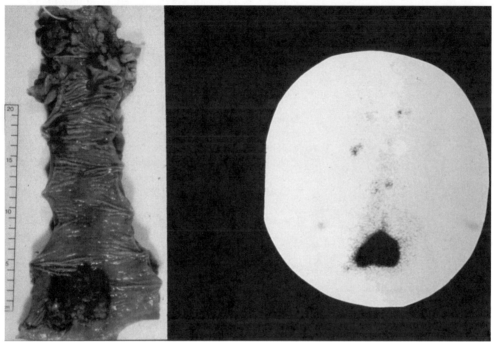

Figure 7-91. Rectal cancer. (**A**) [111]In PR1A3 monoclonal antibody images of the posterior pelvis at 10 minutes, left; 24 hours, center; and 48 hours, right. Focally increased uptake is seen on the 24- and 48-hour images in the region of the rectum consistent with rectal carcinoma. (**B**) Photograph of the pathologic specimen showing the rectal carcinoma inferiorly and several polyps on the left. An image of the specimen on the right showing tumor uptake and some uptake in the polyps but no abnormal uptake in the normal lymph glands draining the tumor.

Requirement for the Monoclonal Antibody
High uptake by tumor
Long residence time on tumor
Minimal metabolism
Blood clearance $T_{1/2}$ about 24 hours
High affinity
Easy and stable radiolabeling
High immunoreactivity

CLINICAL DIAGNOSIS

Primary Colorectal Cancer

The identification of primary colorectal cancer is straightforward using ^{99m}Tc anti-CEA or ^{99m}Tc PR1A3. The 10-minute image shows normal vascular, marrow, renal, urinary, and liver uptake. The 5-hour and 22-hour images show the focal area of increased uptake at the site of the cancer. Because the CEA antigen is released it may be possible to image normal lymph nodes and areas of inflammatory bowel disease such as Crohn's disease and ulcerative colitis. Through the series of images these areas of bowel show fixed uptake whereas some secretion into

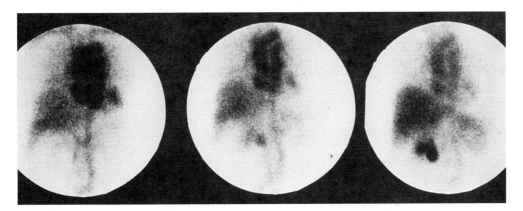

Figure 7-92. Transverse colon cancer. ^{99m}Tc PR1A3 images: anterior views of the upper abdomen and lower chest; at 10 minutes, left; 6 hours, center; 24 hours, right. The decreasing blood pool in the cardiac region is seen and the increasing uptake in the transverse colon cancer is noted to be maximal in the 24-hour image, which is greater than the liver uptake.

normal bowel contents will show movement between the 5- and 24-hour images. It is not unusual to see some diffuse uptake in the ascending colon particularly if the patient has undergone bowel preparation prior to colonoscopy or surgery, where the slightly inflamed bowel becomes somewhat leaky to protein such as the gamma globulin injected. In addition to identifying the primary colorectal cancer, on occasion a second site of focal uptake may be seen. This may represent a second cancer, for example, if the distal primary cancer has caused stricture of the large bowel so that a colonoscope cannot pass (Fig. 7-93).

The identification of a second cancer may be important. On one occasion in our experience a primary abnormality was noted in the region of the rectum both on imaging and sigmoidoscopy and an unsuspected second cancer was identified in the hepatic flexure only on imaging. The injection of the ^{99m}Tc-labeled monoclonal antibody 24 hours before surgery is indicated and allows the imaging to be combined with the use of the preoperative probe during surgery (see below).

If rectal cancer is suspected it is essential to take a series of squat views at the three time points because this may be the best indicator of a low-lying rectal cancer posterior to the bladder. The planar anterior and posterior views may not define it due to superimposition with the bladder or genitalia, which usually appear vascular. Some activity often persists in the genitalia, which is thought to be due to binding of the Fc portion of the whole antibody to gonadal tissue. SPET of the pelvis is always undertaken. This gives good definition of the position of the bladder in relation to any abnormality in the pelvis. The

Figure 7-93. Synchronous cancer with liver metastasis. (**A**) Anterior view of the abdomen and pelvis on the left at 24 hours after injection of ^{99m}Tc PR1A3: uptake in a sigmoid colon cancer is seen centrally between the iliac vessels. This caused a stricture and the second cancer in the descending colon could not be visualized by colonoscopy but is evident on the image. (**B**) Anterior view of the liver on the right at 24 hours in the same patient. A focal area of increased uptake is seen in the left lobe of the liver confirmed as a liver metastasis at surgery and not detected by ultrasound.

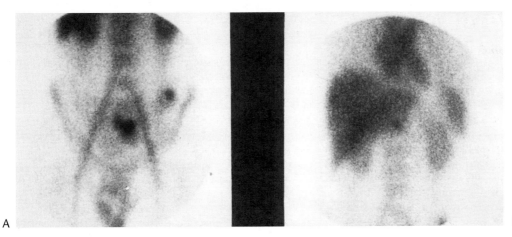

A   B

uterus may be seen as a vascular area on the early image but fades with time.

Liver Metastases

Liver metastases from colorectal cancer are mainly supplied by the hepatic artery rather than the portal vein. Measurement of the hepatic arterial to total blood flow has been used as a predictor of liver metastases before any focal abnormality is seen and has found favor in some centers.[17,18] Because hepatic arterial supply is less than the portal venous supply per unit volume of liver, a metastasis will appear as a defect in uptake on the 10-minute image against the background of normal liver uptake.

Four patterns of liver metastases are seen on radioimmunoscintigraphy. The first is that of a defect in uptake seen on the 10-minute image, which persists in the 5-hour and 24-hour images. This is usually large and may represent a space-occupying lesion due to causes other than liver metastasis. A more typical pattern is a defect on the 10-minute image that becomes slightly smaller in size on the 5-hour image and even smaller in size on the 24-hour image, often with a halo of increased uptake around its periphery. This is typical of a moderate-sized liver metastasis. A small liver metastasis may show a defect on the 10-minute image but appear undetectable on the 5-hour and 24-hour images because its uptake is balanced by the normal uptake in the liver. Without the 10-minute image this type of liver metastasis, which is not uncommon, would not be detectable. The last pattern is a normal 10-minute image and 5-hour image with a focal area of increased uptake seen on the 24-hour image. This is usually found in very small metastases (Fig. 7-93).

SPET of the liver may help to confirm the presence of a metastasis when interpreted in conjunction with the planar images. Very small focal metastases with increased uptake may be detected when the planar image is normal. It should be confirmed on all the orthogonal sections (coronal, transverse, and sagittal) before being called a metastasis. SPET is not as helpful in large metastases where a defect may be difficult to distinguish from the normal variation of the liver lobes. Focal areas of increased uptake in the periaortic region should be interpreted with caution when anti-CEA is used but indicates positive involvement with an antibody against a fixed antigen such as PR1A3. Rarely lung metastases are identified but these usually occur only when the liver has become extensively invaded. They are, however, not uncommon once liver metastases have been treated.

Recurrent Colorectal Cancer

Recurrent colorectal cancer is the main application of radioimmunoscintigraphy because recurrences may be plaquelike, a few cells thick, distributed over a wide area, and not detectable by radiography, CT, MRI, or ultrasound. They may be detectable by scintigraphy before any change in serum markers or symptoms occur. A Dukes' C cancer has a chance of recurrence at 1 year approaching 50% in some studies. The authors have undertaken imaging of such patients at 1 year after primary surgery at a time when they may have no symptoms and a normal CEA and have shown in approximately 30% of patients evidence of recurrence that is subsequently confirmed. The im-

aging technique is by its nature more sensitive than the use of serum markers because a tumor must be of a certain size to shed sufficient antigen to raise the serum marker in the blood, whereas with a good signal such as ^{99m}Tc, focal recurrences having the pattern of increasing uptake with time can be seen. Indeed radioimmunoscintigraphy may be the only modality able to detect such recurrences. As surgeons became confident with this technique, surgery, with the help of the radiodetection probe, or radiotherapy, may be undertaken on the basis of a positive radioimmunoscintigraphic image alone.

When serum markers are elevated radioimmunoscintigraphy can identify the sites of recurrence in the pelvis, abdomen, or liver, even when other radiologic modalities are negative. Radiography, CT, and MRI are able to demonstrate an abnormal mass in the pelvis or abdomen in a patient who has had surgery for primary colorectal cancer. It is often not possible, however, to identify whether such a mass represents postsurgical or postradiotherapy fibrosis, an inflammatory mass, or recurrence. The monoclonal antibody uptake will be absent if the mass is due to fibrosis. Uptake will be early and fade with time if the mass is due to an inflammatory process and it will show no uptake on the early image with progressively increasing uptake with time if the mass is due to viable recurrent tumor. The greater extent of a recurrence in the abdomen may be seen by radioimmunoscintigraphy to be due to the plaquelike spread of the tumor over the abdomen, whereas only the more masslike part of the tumor recurrence may be appreciated by CT. Para-aortic lymph node involvement may be well visualized (Fig. 7-94).

PEROPERATIVE RADIOIMMUNODETECTION

The history of localization of cancer with radiodetection probes goes back to 1949 when P-32 phosphate was used for localizing brain tumors.

Osteomas in the bone have been identified with probes for many years surgically. The work of Martin and his group using ^{125}I-labeled antibodies[19-21] has applied this approach to large bowel cancer as others have subsequently done.[22] ^{111}In-labeled antibodies[23,24] and ^{99m}Tc-labeled antibodies[25,26] are available.[27]

How does peroperative radioimmunodetection (PROD) aid surgery? It is used to identify tumor sites particularly in lymph nodes, in peritoneal plaques, in adhesions, and in the omentum at the time of surgery. It is also used to monitor the tumor bed after excision of tumor and to show whether the edges of an anastomosis are free of tumor before it is completed.

Some probes are designed to have the whole range of sensitivity from ^{125}I to ^{99m}Tc; others are suitable just for ^{111}In and ^{99m}Tc. It would be best if the probe were optimized just for one radionuclide, because the requirements for ^{125}I, ^{111}In, and ^{99m}Tc are quite different with respect to collimation, depth of resolution, and sensitivity. ^{125}I emissions are very soft, thus only very superficial lesions will be detected.

The count rate is crucial. The higher the count rate, the less the noise in the signal by the square root relationship. For ^{125}I this is about 25% whereas for ^{111}In (10%) and ^{99m}Tc (5%) it is considerably less. The delay between injection and surgery is important. Typically with ^{125}I, one must wait up to 30 days from the injection for the background activity to fall. For ^{111}In this period lies between 1 and 10 days and for ^{99m}Tc between 18 and 24 hours (Table 7-4). Surgery must therefore be planned

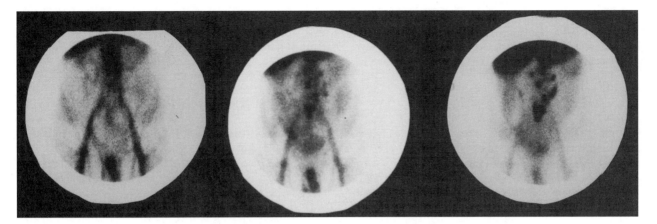

Figure 7-94. Recurrent colorectal cancer. ^{99m}Tc PR1A3 monoclonal antibody image. At 10 minutes, left; 6 hours, center; 24 hours, right. Anterior views of the abdomen and pelvis. There is intense uptake in the pelvis and para-aortic regions increasing with time, typical of pelvic and abdominal recurrences of colorectal cancer.

an appropriate time in advance. The absorbed dose to the patient is lowest with ^{99m}Tc compared with the other radionuclides. A dose of 5 mCi (185 MBq) of ^{125}I, which has been used in the United States, would not be allowed in Europe.

Probes differ in type and it is sometimes difficult to obtain adequate information from the manufacturer. The following are important: the type of crystal, its diameter and length and whether angled or straight; the material of the collimator; weight; shielding; and spatial resolution. Clearly these properties need to be determined for the particular radionuclide. It is also essential to know the sensitivity and how this was measured, the precision (i.e., the minimal detectable count rate), the depth of resolution, and the linearity of the response. It is also necessary to know how to sterilize the probe and how to keep it sterile during surgery. Usually this is with some sort of sheath as used for intraoperative ultrasound. Linearity needs to be tested up to 1,000 counts per second. The spectrum of response of the probe in air or in a patient-equivalent material demonstrates its sensitivity and resolution.[28,29]

Having decided which of three radionuclides and which of the five probes presently available to use, it is then necessary to choose the antigen. Clearly it should be expressed in all tumors and most important it should be fixed to the tumor and not released. There should be a high antigen density and it should be reasonably homogeneous. A little heterogeneity is

not a problem because only the surface of the tumor is sampled by the counting. The three most common types of monoclonal antibodies that are used include those directed against fixed antigens such as PR1A3, antigens that are released such as CEA, and antigens that are partly released such as B72.3 (Table 7-5). A high uptake of the antibody is necessary. There should be minimal metabolism, or if metabolism occurs, the label should be fixed or internalized into the tumor so it is still marking the tumor cell. The required blood clearance rate should have a half-life of about 24 hours to guarantee a reasonable amount of uptake by the tumor. High affinity, stable radiolabeling, and high immunoreactivity of the antibody after labeling are all important (Table 7-6).

Table 7-5. Monoclonal Antibodies Used for Peroperative Probe Work

	CEA	B72.3	PR1A3
Fixation	Released	Partly fixed	Fixed
Specificity	Low	Moderate	High
Antigen expression	Very high	80%	Very high

Table 7-4. Nuclides Suitable for Peroperative Probe Work

	Long Half-Life	Short Half-Life	
	^{125}I	^{111}In	^{99m}Tc
Preoperative wait (days)	10–30	1–10	1
Signal	Very low	High	Very high
Background	Very low	High	Very high
Retention of labeled antibody	Long	Short	Short
Imaging presurgery	No	Yes	Yes
Depth of penetration	Poor	Fair	Fair

Table 7-6. Radionuclides Suitable for Tissue Characterization in Inflammatory Diseases

Nonspecific	Bone scan
	Gallium-67 citrate
Inflammation specific	^{111}In oxine white cells
	^{99m}Tc HMPAO white cells
	^{99m}Tc monoclonal antibody to label white cells in vivo
	^{111}In human immunoglobulin
	^{99m}Tc human immunoglobulin
Disease specific	^{123}I serum amyloid protein for amyloid
	^{123}I and ^{99m}Tc interleukin-2 for autoimmune disorders
	^{99m}Tc infecton for bacterial infection

Kuhn et al.[23] showed that by using labeled antibody to a nonfixed antigen with a probe placed at the porta hepatis area, positive readings may occur when there is no tumor. It is now recognized that in the drainage region of primary tumors, a nonfixed antigen may give false-positive readings in nodes particularly in the porta hepatis. Using a fixed antigen, only nodes that are involved are detected.

Perhaps the most important variable is the surgeon. Clearly he or she needs to be trained in the principles of probe usage. There are surgeons who adapt to this very easily and like the approach and there are surgeons who do not. Using the probe lengthens the operation time by about 20 minutes but this may be longer depending on the surgeon. There may be difficulties in using the probe intra-abdominally owing to awkward angles and inaccessible recesses. Readings may be made with the probe over suspicious excised tissue and compared with a piece of normal tissue. The difference in counts is usually dramatic and allows selection of tissue for frozen section.

To what extent the probe alters surgical management is at present difficult to judge. Using ^{99m}Tc-labeled monoclonal antibody, imaging is performed the day before surgery and on the morning of the operation. Surgery thus follows the injection by about 24 hours, giving sufficient time for tissue activity to be established and blood activity to fall.

Most researchers recommend recording counts three times each for 5 or 10 seconds with the probe stationary over the tumor. If the normal tissue activity is taken as 1, a ratio of 1.5:1 would indicate significant uptake, and over 2.3:1 would be highly significant. From the authors' data from 35 patients, there is a gradient of ratios from normal tissue to abnormal with no real cutoff point defining the presence of tumor. If 1.5 is taken as the ratio of significance this will give a sensitivity of about 70%. If 2.3:1 is used sensitivity will fall to under 50%.

The choice of normal bowel during the operation for reference counting must be made. Sigmoid or descending colon well away from any tumor gives the most consistent results. The transverse colon may be affected by liver scatter although a tungsten shield in a surgical glove may be used to shield the liver if one is probing in its vicinity. ^{99m}Tc may show a small amount of biliary excretion and there may be some activity in the normal ascending colon at 24 hours, and therefore the right colon is not a good site for reference counting.

The ^{125}I B72.3 neoprobe data have shown a sensitivity for primary colorectal cancer of about 77%, for recurrent colorectal cancer about 72%, and for ovarian cancer 63%.[21]

The results of Stella et al.[30,31] using ^{125}I B72.3 showed sensitivity of only 50% but 20% of excised specimens were found to be antigen negative. The demonstration of tumor tissue was found to be of definite value to the surgeon in 10% to 20% of cases. Using an anti-CEA, sensitivity increased to 67% but the combination of both antibodies did not enhance this further although the numbers were small. Useful clinical information was obtained in about 16% of patients. Kuhn et al.[23] using the oncoprobe with ^{111}In B72.3 reported similar results in 21 patients with a sensitivity of 67% for monoclonal antibody external imaging and 86% for the probe.

Using the arithmetic average of three 5-second counts over the tumor, a ''normal'' reference point (sigmoid or descending colon), and the tumor bed, a ratio of about 1.5 to 2.0:1 was obtained. The excised tumor, however, gave a ratio of 18:1

(Table 7-6). The identification of liver metastases is not effective, with counts usually being not significantly different from those of the normal liver. Involved lymph nodes can, however, be identified.

In a series of 19 patients the probe was correct in 17 (89%) in identifying tumor using a ratio of 1.5:1.[25,27] When this study was expanded to include five surgeons, not all were able to take the time necessary and the sensitivity fell to 65%[26] using the same ratio. The reduction in sensitivity appears to be surgeon related and surgeons who are interested in probe work will achieve good results. In the same study counting the excised specimen gave 100% discrimination between malignant and nonmalignant tissue.

Ovarian cancer tends to spread throughout the peritoneal cavity and it is often difficult to detect and excise all tumor. Using the ^{99m}Tc-SM3 monoclonal antibody[32] ovarian tumor in the pelvis with PROD gave similar ratios of around 1.5 to 1. One patient who had a ratio of 1:1 was subsequently found to have a disseminated mucinous adenocarcinoma of the bowel with which the ovarian antibody does not react.

There are many other agents that localize to tumor. These include radiolabeled peptides and ^{111}In-octreotide, the latter having affinity for carcinoid,[33] as well as insulinoma, gastrinoma, glucagonoma, and vipoma.[34] Vasoactive intestinal peptide labeled with ^{123}I may also show small tumors.[35] Radiolabeled peptides give intraoperative tissue ratios normal/abnormal of 1:10, higher than achieved with monoclonal antibodies.

Paganelli et al.,[36,37] have used a two-stage approach with an initial PROD with an ^{125}I antibody tagged with biotin. Avidin, which binds to biotin, is then given and the antibody level falls as the biotinylated antibody is taken to the liver. However, tumor uptake remains. Using this technique it was possible to reduce the delay between injection of ^{125}I-labeled antibody and surgery from 24 days to 6 days. Reduction of background noise is important as it interferes with the signal. A similar two-stage approach can be applied to ^{99m}Tc-labeled monoclonal antibody.

Summary

There are advantages and disadvantages to probe work. It can confirm the surgical impression of malignancy in tissue during surgery and can examine suspicious areas. It can show that the tumor bed is clear after removal and demonstrate that anastomotic margins are free from tumor. Intraoperative scintigraphy can, however, be time consuming and is operator dependent. Small nodal involvement can be missed.

A ^{99m}Tc-labeled antibody is preferable to using a low-count rate label such as ^{125}I. The radiation dose is negligible.[38] Results will be improved by better training of staff and through taking more time and more readings as well as the development of new markers.

IDENTIFICATION OF BLEEDING IN THE COLON

Hemorrhage into the gastrointestinal tract is occasionally difficult to localize. Over 80% of cases occur in the upper tract. Bleeding from the small intestine, including Meckel's diverticulum, is rare. Massive colorectal bleeding requiring admission and transfusion is not common. It is, however, an important medical emergency. The subject has been reviewed by Robinson.[39]

The differential diagnosis of lesions that can cause bleeding from the lower gastrointestinal tract are fully discussed in Chapter 19. There has been some controversy as to the importance of diverticular disease in this regard[40–42] as well as anal lesions such as hemorrhoids and degenerative vascular disease, for example, angiodysplasia.[41,43] Identification of the source of bleeding and its cause can be difficult in an emergency situation. Blood may obscure the lumen making colonoscopy difficult, and contrast intestinal radiology is not helpful. Angiography will not identify the site of bleeding unless it is active (0.5 to 1 ml/min) at the time of examination. Under these circumstances labeled red cell scintigraphy is indicated and can be expected to localize the bleeding in about one-third of cases.[44,45]

Scintigraphy

There are two approaches. In the first an injection of ^{99m}Tc-DTPA[46] (diethylenetriamine penta-acetic acid) or ^{99m}Tc colloid is given.[47] The former is excreted rapidly through the kidneys and the latter taken up by the liver. The technique is useful only if bleeding is occurring at the time of injection. Focal accumulation at the bleeding site will then be evident on serial imaging. Positivity depends on the rate of bleeding and a minimum of 1 ml/min is thought to be required. In this respect it is as limited as angiography. Both compounds are readily available in any nuclear medicine department.

The usual technique is to label autologous red cells in vivo with ^{99m}Tc. Pyrophosphate from a bone-scanning kit that contains tin is injected first. Blood is taken at 20 minutes into a large syringe containing the ^{99m}Tc, mixed, and reinjected. Most of the red cells become labeled but there is a small amount of free pertechnetate. Over the next 24 hours the level of blood activity will slowly decline. Provided bleeding is occurring at around 70 ml/24 h, it should be identifiable. Serial scans at 1, 2, 4, 6, and 18 hours are taken.

There are several pitfalls in interpretation of blood pool images partly due to background activity. For example, abnormal vascularity in an aneurysm or an ischemic bowel loop might be interpreted as a site of bleeding. Other sites of increased vascularity such as a horseshoe or pelvic kidney, varices or bleeding into the abdominal wall or into a renal or pancreatic cyst, or else vascular bone disease such as Paget's disease of

---

Minor Symptomatic Bleeding

Outlet Bleeding

Bright red blood on the toilet paper or in the bowl
Bleeding associated with defecation
No change in bowel habits
No familial or personal history of colorectal neoplasm

Suspicious Bleeding

Dark blood, blood mixed with or streaked on stool
Change in bowel habits or passage of mucus
Positive personal or familial history of colorectal neoplasm

---

the ilium may give a false-positive picture. A positive result is defined by an intensity of the blood pool more than that of the liver blood pool.[48]

Meckel's Diverticulum

The occurrence of ectopic gastric mucosa in a Meckel's diverticulum can cause local ulceration and bleeding. This is rare but is more common in babies and children than adults. ^{99m}Tc pertechnetate is taken up by gastric mucosa and therefore the test must be undertaken without any thyroid blockage, iodine, perchlorate, periodate, or recent iodine-containing contrast media, etc. The ^{99m}Tc pertechnetate 40 MBq is injected intravenously. Anterior and posterior images of the abdomen, with lateral views if appropriate, are taken at 10, 20, 40, and 60 minutes after injection. A focal area of increased activity in the right side of the abdomen is compatible with a Meckel's diverticulum (Fig. 7-95).

Cimetidine has been used to enhance uptake by blocking gastric secretions,[49] and gastric stimulants such as pentagastrin or glucagon have been recommended although there is no proof that these maneuvers help. Pertechnetate is distributed in the blood pool and slowly excreted through the kidneys. Many anomalies can be misinterpreted as a Meckel's diverticulum. These are the result of accumulation of pertechnetate in blood pool of the kidneys or urinary tract particularly if anomalous, and sites of inflammation, infection, or tumor particularly if vascular. False-negative results may be due to the inadvertent administration of a thyroid-blocking agent.[50,51]

INFLAMMATORY BOWEL DISEASE

Inflammation is a general response to tissue damage whether traumatic, infective, autoimmune, or toxic. Nuclear medicine can offer several techniques for evaluating inflammation, some general and some specific (Table 7-7).

Nonspecific Agents

The first approach was to label white blood cells with ^{111}In.[52] This is a difficult technique in which the white cells are separated from plasma and labeled with ^{111}In in a metal-free environment. Because the white cells are separated from plasma, their phagocytic properties deteriorate to some extent. This problem has been overcome by the use of ^{111}In tropolone,[53] but this product is not yet commercially available. ^{111}In-labeled white cells require imaging at 1, 4, and 24 hours. The technique successfully identifies inflamed segments of bowel[54–58] and the 67-hour half-life of In means that excreted white cells can be detected in the feces by counting of ^{111}In.[55,59]

^{99m}Tc HMPAO (hexamethyl propylene amine oxime) used initially as a brain-scanning agent is highly lipophilic and can bind to white cells.[60,61] These are separated from red cells but are maintained in plasma and labeled with ^{99m}Tc HMPAO. Imaging is undertaken at 1 and 4 hours and usually a 24-hour image is not necessary. Because of the short life of ^{99m}Tc (6 hours), collection of feces for quantitative estimate of cell loss cannot be undertaken. Both these techniques require the taking of blood from the patient, and an in vitro labeling procedure. Imaging with ^{99m}Tc HMPAO white cells is now the usual technique used for detecting inflammatory bowel disease.[58,60,62–67]

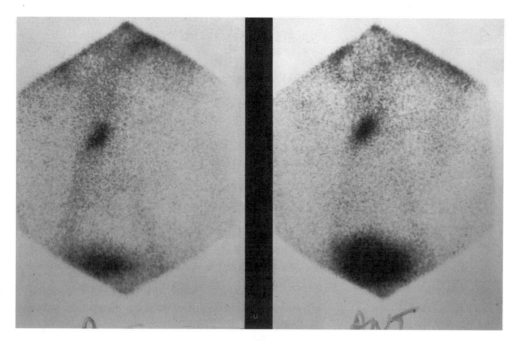

Figure 7-95. Meckel's diverticulum. Anterior views of the abdomen at 10 minutes, left, and 20 minutes, right, showing focally increased uptake just to the right of the midline, typical of a Meckel's diverticulum with ectopic gastric mucosa. Stomach activity superiorly and bladder activity inferiorly are evident.

In vivo labeling of white cells may be undertaken using an antibody against the NCA antigen on white cells. The monoclonal antibody is labeled with ^{99m}Tc and injected intravenously.[68,69] About 10% to 20% of white cells are labeled in the circulation and images are taken at 1, 4, and 24 hours.

^{111}In human immunoglobulin (HIG)[70] is a commercially available nonspecific agent injected intravenously. It pools at sites of inflammation where it is deposited. ^{99m}Tc HIG is also available,[71] but not recommended.[72] Gallium-67 imaging is not recommended for abdominal imaging due to considerable uptake in the normal large bowel.[73]

White cell scans will demonstrate uptake in areas of inflammation due to any cause. They will not distinguish inflammatory bowel disease due to infection from ulcerative colitis or Crohn's disease.

Specific Agents for Inflammation

Serum Amyloid Protein

Serum amyloid protein was labeled with ^{123}I and showed specific uptake in most forms of amyloid.[74] Its usual sites of uptake are the kidneys, liver, and adrenals but rarely in the gut. The compound is not commercially available and must be extracted from the patient's blood and labeled with ^{123}I. Nevertheless, it is a well-established technique.

Interleukin-2

Interleukin-2 is one of many cytokines that are bound to activated T cells that form an important cellular component of autoimmune disease, many allergic responses, and tissue rejection. It has been labeled with ^{123}I and used to detect insulitis in the prediabetic state,[75] in celiac disease,[76] and Crohn's disease.[77] It has been labeled with ^{99m}Tc.[78] and used in autoimmune thyroiditis and thyrotoxicosis.[79] It is likely to be a marker of activity of autoimmune disease but this has yet to be established.

Infecton

^{99m}Tc Infecton has been developed as a bacterial-specific imaging agent.[80,81] It is based on the 4-fluoroquinolone group of antibiotics and ciprofloxacin is used as the starting material. The final injection of ^{99m}Tc Infecton contains only about a milligram of ciprofloxacin (compared with the normal single tablet of 250 mg used therapeutically). A kit formulation has made the labeling procedure straightforward and no blood needs to be taken. It is patented but not yet commercially available. Imaging is taken 1 and 4 hours after injection. There is a high concordance with white cell scans in bacterial causes of inflammation. There are, however, true positives when white cell scans are negative, particularly in patients who have had chronic antibiotic treatment. Similarly, there are many true negatives when white cell scans are positive as, for example, in Crohn's disease[82,83] (Fig. 7-96). There is

Table 7-7. Small Bowel and Colon Transit Times (TT) (Mean and Range) in Normal Individuals and in Severe Idiopathic Constipation

	Normal	Constipated
Small bowel TT in minutes	55	75
	30–70	50–115
Colon TT in hours	31	96
	24–48	46–168

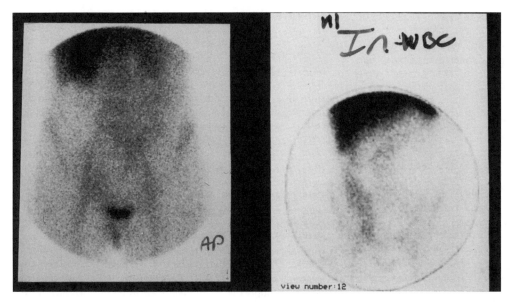

Figure 7-96. Crohn's disease. On the left ^{99m}Tc-Infecton image at 4 hours shows some renal and urinary activity but no abnormality in the right iliac fossa or right flank. On the right ^{111}In white cell scan at 4 hours showing increased uptake in the ascending colon confirmed subsequently to be the site of Crohn's disease. High liver uptake is also evident. The white cell study shows inflammation of Crohn's disease and the negative Infecton study indicates the absence of bacterial infection.

evidence that successful antibiotic therapy will cause loss of uptake of ^{99m}Tc infecton. Thus imaging after antibiotic therapy has commenced may give a false-negative result for bacterial infection if the treatment is effective. A study is being initiated whereby ^{99m}Tc Infecton imaging is undertaken before, during, and after a course of antibiotics to see if responsiveness to treatment can be predicted by conversion of a positive to a negative image at the site of the infection.

Infected diarrhea will be positive, both with ^{99m}Tc Infecton and ^{99m}Tc HMPAO white cells (Fig. 7-97). The clinical place

Figure 7-97. Infective diarrhea. Anterior views of the abdomen; left ^{99m}Tc Infecton showing uptake in the ascending colon; right ^{111}In white cell scan at 4 hours showing uptake in the ascending colon. The concordant pattern indicates the findings are due to bacterial infection and not sterile inflammation of the bowel.

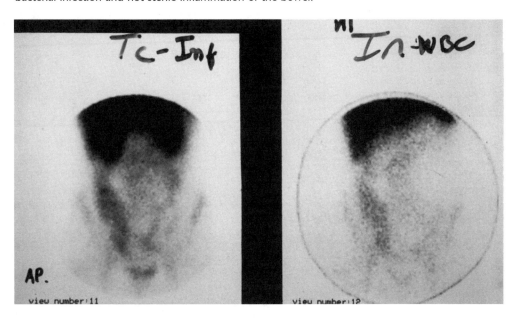

of this technique in inflammatory bowel disease has yet to be established.

The normal features of a white cell image show the following. Immediately after injection there is some lung activity that should clear rapidly. Failure to clear suggests damage to the white cells during preparation or focal uptake seen with any form of pneumonia. Next the spleen shows very high uptake, much more than the liver; a roughly equal uptake by liver and spleen is also a feature of damaged white cells. In such situations the reliability of a negative white cell scan in excluding inflammation is reduced. By 4 hours there may be some uptake related to the small intestine and ascending colon. It is not entirely clear why this happens but it may be related to biliary excretion of the technetium ligand coupled with relative stasis in the cecum.

Image interpretation may be aided by scoring as suggested by Li et al.[58]: grade 0 for no abnormal uptake; I, II, and III where bowel uptake is less than, equal to, or greater than the bone marrow uptake, respectively; and IV where bowel uptake is greater than splenic uptake. In a study comparing 152 patients imaged with ^{99m}Tc-HMPAO white cells and 88 patients with ^{111}In leukocytes the sensitivities, specificities, and accuracies were the same at 96%, 97%, and 97%, respectively.

Clinical Applications

Intra-Abdominal Abscess

All the general agents will image abdominal abscess formation. The most widely used at present is ^{99m}Tc HMPAO WBC. Positive uptake before 4 hours indicates the site of abscess. [99m]Tc Infecton will also be positive. At the center of an abscess where bacteria are dead the white cell uptake is focal, but the [99m]Tc Infecton being taken up by living bacteria may show a halo of activity around an abscess and uptake is often greater than by the labeled white cells.

Specific Abscess Formation

Paracolic abscess as in diverticulitis may not be evident on the barium enema but easily detected using labeled white cells.

Liver abscess should be first investigated with ultrasound but confirmation of the inflammatory nature by labeled white cells or [99m]Tc Infecton may be helpful. Acute pancreatitis, acute appendicitis, appendix abscess, pelvic abscess, subphrenic abscess, infection in the lesser sac, and wound infection all may be demonstrated using labeled white cells. In the frozen pelvis, labeled white cells and [99m]Tc Infecton are both able to localize sites of infection.

[99m]Tc Infecton shows no lung or bone marrow uptake, it has a roughly equal low uptake by spleen and liver but its main site of uptake are the kidneys because it is excreted into the urine. Distorted renal or ureteric anatomy may thus lead to diagnostic error. Occasionally the gallbladder is visualized early in the scan and some cecal activity may be seen at about 4 hours in normal individuals. Normal gut bacteria are not seen because of the biologic barriers preventing the intravenously injected [99m]Tc Infecton from entering the lumen. It is the inflammatory response to an infective diarrhea that allows the [99m]Tc Infecton to localize in bacteria in the bowel wall.

Noninfective

It is now recognized that the extent of inflammatory bowel disease can be well demonstrated using radiolabeled white cells. There is often some discordance with the extent of ulcerative colitis or Crohn's disease as determined by barium enema examination. Quiescent disease may, however, show distortion that may not be sufficiently inflamed to cause white cell uptake. Only ^{111}In-labeled white cells may be directly quantitative in inflammatory bowel disease by fecal collection.[59] Skip lesions of Crohn's disease in the small intestine as well as colon are well demonstrated using labeled white cells.[56,57]

CONCLUSION

Radiolabeled white cell studies have a definite place for the localization of pus in the evaluation of postoperative patients who develop fever and in the assessment of inflammatory bowel disease. [99m]Tc Infecton scanning has a place in demonstrating bacterial abscesses. It can also detect bacterial infection, for example, salmonella as the cause of inflammatory bowel disease. [123]I and ^{99m}Tc-labeled interleukin-2 shows uptake in celiac disease and Crohn's disease but their use in these conditions still needs to be evaluated. Radiolabeled HIG and ^{99m}Tc nanocolloids are not recommended for the investigation of inflammatory bowel disease or abdominal abscess.

COLONIC TRANSIT TIMES

Colonic transit is lengthened in cases of constipation. The movement of colonic contents can be demonstrated from one part of the colon to another using a radiolabeled nonabsorbable

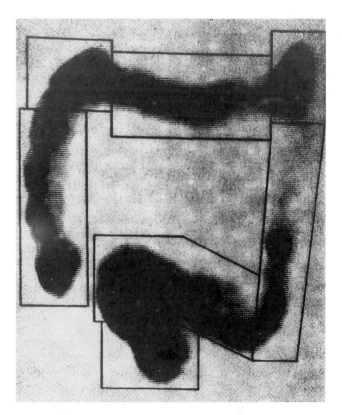

Figure 7-98.   Regions of interest set over the colon.

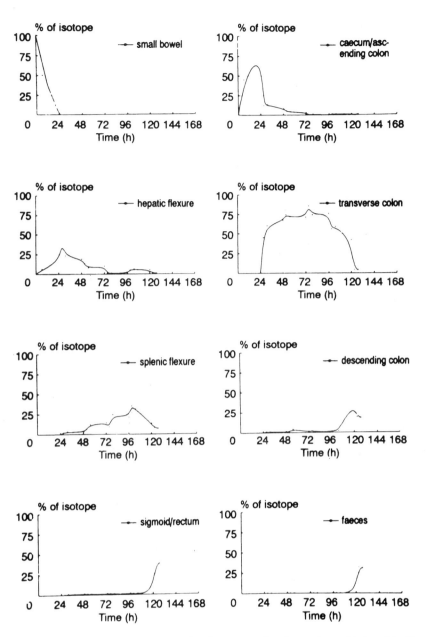

Figure 7-99. Colonic transit activity time curves for the regions of interest in Figure 7-97 as well as small bowel and feces.

marker in solid food. Rare forms of constipation where stasis occurs in a particular segment of the colon can be identified. The measurement of colonic transit follows those of gastric emptying and small bowel transit.

Methods

A pancake approximating to normal food in its bulk, total calorie content, and proportion of fat, protein, and carbohydrate has been developed. It is easy to prepare, and to label with [111]In (weight 492 g, fat 27 g, protein 18 g, calories 625).[84] Five grams of an anion exchange resin (Amberlite 1R-120) are washed five times with 10 ml 0.04 M hydrochloric acid. The supernatant is then decanted. Fifty mg of thick slurry is weighed out. Then

18 MBq ^{111}In chloride (Amersham International) is added. The resin is incubated for at least 30 minutes on a roller mixer and then washed twice with 500 μl of 0.04 M hydrochloric acid. The labeled resin is set aside. A browning dish is preheated in an industrial microwave oven for 8 minutes. To a blending bowl the following are added and blended until well mixed: 57 g flour, 142 g milk, 14 g oil, and an egg. Then 50 ml of the mixture is poured into a 50-ml polypropylene tube (Falcon). The labeled resin is pipetted into the pancake mixture in this tube and it is mixed by vortex.

These contents are then well mixed with the pancake in the blending bowl. The mixture is poured onto the browning dish and cooked in the microwave for 4 minutes and then turned over and heated for another 3 minutes. The ^{111}In gives good

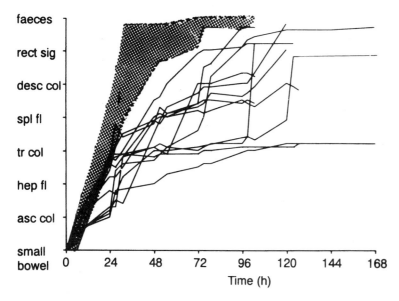

Figure 7-100. Normal range (shaded area) for colonic transit of the center of mass of the solid radionuclide marker. Patients with idiopathic constipation are shown as single lines outside the envelope of normal ranges. (From Van der Sijp et al.,[86] with permission.)

representation of the solid phase.[84] Note ^{99m}Tc DTPA should not be used for the liquid phase as it can leach out the Indium; ^{99m}Tc-labeled rhenium or tin colloid in orange juice is preferred. A ^{111}In-labeled methacrylate polymer (Eudragit S) is an alternative.[85]

Colonic Imaging

Six regions of interest are created on the images of the colon, obtained from the gamma camera that is set up for ^{111}In with a medium-energy parallel collimator.[86] These include cecum and ascending colon, hepatic flexure, transverse colon, splenic flexure, descending colon, and rectosigmoid (Fig. 7-98). Stool is taken as the seventh region.

The counts from each region of interest are determined by the geometric mean of immediately consecutive anterior and posterior views of the abdomen to reduce the effects of tissue attenuation. (The geometric mean is given by the square root of the product of the anterior and posterior counts for each region.) The counts are corrected for the decay of ^{111}In, half-life 67 hours. Time activity curves may also be obtained from each region of interest. These help to evaluate the proportion of time that the ^{111}In spends in each ROI during the imaging period to indicate possible sites of colonic delay (Fig. 7-99).

The center of mass of radionuclide may be derived from the following formula:

$$\text{Center of mass} = F_{ROI1}X1 + F_{ROI2}X2 + \ldots F_{ROIn}XN)$$

where F denotes the fraction of counts per ROI and n the number of the region according to the predefined sequence, from cecum (region 1) to stool (region 7).[87]

An alternative expression is:

$$\text{Center of mass}_n = [\text{Sum}^7 Ci.i] / [\text{Sum}^7 Ci]n$$
$$i = 1 \qquad i = 1$$

where n is the frame number, i is the number of the ROI in order, and Ci is the counts in region i. This number represents the point in the colon related to the predefined ROIs that lies ahead of 50% of the radionuclide mass and thus gives a guide to the effectiveness of colon transport.

A related graphic approach is to represent the percentage of activity for each region on the y-axis and the time or frame number on the x-axis to show the dispersion and progression of activity—a "condensed image."[85]

Normal results and the findings in severe idiopathic constipation are given in Table 7-7 and Figure 7-100.

CONCLUSION

Colonic transit assessment contributes to an understanding of colonic motility in health and disease,[87,88] idiopathic constipation,[85,86] fecal incontinence,[88] and mega rectum.[89]

REFERENCES

1. Britton KE, Granowska M (1993) The present and future of radiolabelled antibodies in oncology. Ann Nucl Med 7: 127–132
2. Britton KE, Granowska M (1988) Radioimmunoscintigraphy in tumour identification. Cancer Surveys 6:247–267
3. Richman PI, Bodmer WF (1987) Monoclonal antibodies to human colorectal epithelium: markers for differentiation and tumour characterisation. Br J Cancer 39:317–328
4. Granowska M, Britton KE, Mather SJ et al (1993) Radioimmunoscintigraphy with Technetium-99m labelled monoclonal antibody, IA3, in colorectal cancer. Eur J Nucl Med 20: 690–698

5. Baum RP, Hertel A, Lorenz M et al (1989) Tc-99m anti CEA monoclonal antibody for tumour immunoscintigraphy: first clinical results. Nucl Med Commun 10:345–348

6. Lind P, Lechner P, Arian-Schad K et al (1991) Anti carcino embryonic antigen immunoscintigraphy (technetium-99m monoclonal antibody BW 431/26) and serum CEA levels in patients with suspected primary and recurrent colorectal carcinoma. J Nucl Med 32:1319–1325

7. Doerr RJ, Andel-Nabi H, Krag D, Mitchell E (1991) Radiolabelled antibody imaging in the management of colorectal cancer. Arch Surg 214:118–124

8. Maguire RJ, Van Nostrand DV (1992) Diagnosis of Colorectal and Ovarian Cancer. Marcel Dekker, New York

9. Durbin H, Young S, Stewart LM et al (1994) An epitope on carcinoembryonic antigen defined by the clinically revelant antibody PR1A3. Proc Natl Acad Sci 91:4314–4317

10. Granowska M, Jass JR, Britton KE, Northover JMA (1989) A prospective study of the use of ^{111}In-labelled monoclonal antibody against carcinoembryonic antigen in colorectal cancer and of some biological factors affecting its uptake. Int J Colorect Dis 4:97–108

11. Granowska M, Mather SJ, Britton KE (1991) Diagnostic evaluation of 111-In and 99mTc radiolabelled monoclonal antibodies in ovarian and colorectal cancer: correlations with surgery. Nucl Med Biol 18:413–424

12. Granowska M, Nimmon CC, Britton KE et al (1988) Kinetic analysis and probability mapping applied to the detection of ovarian cancer by radioimmunoscintigraphy. J Nucl Med 29:599–607

13. Rhodes BA, Burchiel SW (1983) Radiolabeling of antibodies with technetium-99m. pp. 207–222. In Burchiel SW, Rhodes BA (eds): Radioimmunoimaging. Elsevier Science, New York

14. Schwartz A, Steinstrasser A (1987) A novel approach to Tc-99m-labelled monoclonal antibodies. J Nucl Med 28:721

15. Mather SJ, Ellison D (1990) Reduction-mediated technetium-99m labelling of monoclonal antibodies. J Nucl Med 31:692–697

16. Britton KE, Granowska M, Mather SJ (1991) Radiolabelled monoclonal antibodies in oncology, I. Technical aspects. Nucl Med Commun 12:65–76

17. Parkin A, Robinson PJ, Baxter P et al (1983) Liver perfusion scintigraphy—method, normal range and laparotomy correlation in 100 patients. Nucl Med Commun 4:395–402

18. Cooke DA, Parkin A, Wiggins P et al (1987) Hepatic perfusion index and the evolution of liver metastases. Nucl Med Commun 8:128–130

19. Martin TM, Hinkle GH, Tuttle S et al (1985) Intraoperative radioimmunodetection of colorectal tumours with a handheld radiation detector. Am J Surg 150:672–675

20. Martin EW, Mojzisik C, Hinkle GH et al (1988) Radioimmunoguided surgery using monoclonal antibody. Am J Surg 156:386–392

21. Petty LR, Mojzisik C, Hinkle GH et al (1991) Radioimmunoguided surgery: a phase I/II study using Iodine-125 labelled 17-1A 1gG^{2A} in patients with colorectal cancer. Antibod Immunoconj Radiopharm 4:603–611

22. Aprile C (1993) Interoperative radioimmunolocalisation of colorectal cancer: a review. Int J Biol Markers 8:166–171

23. Kuhn JA, Corbisiero RM, Buras RR et al (1991) Intraoperative gamma detection with presurgical imaging in colon cancer. Arch Surg 126:1398–1403

24. Curtet C, Vuillez JP, Daniel G et al (1990) Feasibility study of radioimmunoguided surgery of colorectal carcinomas using Indium-111 CEA-specific monoclonal antibody. Eur J Nucl Med 17:299–304

25. Granowska M, Britton KE, Morris G et al (1992) Intraoperative probe with 99mTc-labelled monoclonal antibodies in colorectal and gynaecological surgery. Eur J Nucl Med 19:599

26. Howell R, Hawley PR, Granowska M et al (1995) Peroperative radioimmunodetection, PROD, of colorectal cancer using Tc-99m PR1A3 monoclonal antibody. Tumori, suppl. 81:107–108

27. Granowska M, Britton KE, Morris G et al (1993) Probe peroperative radioimmunodetection (PROD) with monoclonal antibody (Moab) labelled with $^{99m}Tc^m$. Nucl Med Commun 14:259

28. Waddington WA, Davidson BR, Todd Pokropek A et al (1991) Evaluation of a technique for the intraoperative detection of a radiolabelled monoclonal antibody against colorectal cancer. Eur J Nucl Med 18:964–972

29. Roncari G, Benevento A, Bianchi L et al (1993) Performance evaluation of a hand held gamma detector probe used for radioimmunoguided surgery. J Nucl Biol Med 37:21–25

30. Stella M, De Nardi P, Paganelli G et al (1994) Radioimmunoguided surgery: clinical experience with I-125 radiolabelled monoclonal antibodies B72.3 and F023C5. p. 21. In Epenetos AA (ed): Advances in the Applications of Monoclonal Antibodies in Clinical Oncology. 11th International Hammersmith Conference Molyvos, Lesvos

31. Stella M, De Nardi P, Paganelli G et al (1991) Surgery of colorectal cancer guided by radiodetecting probe: clinical evaluation using monoclonal antibody B72.3. Eur J Surg 157:485–488

32. Ind TEJ, Granowska M, Britton KE et al (1994) Peroperative radioimmunodetection of ovarian carcinoma using a hand held gamma detection probe. Br J Cancer 70:1263–1266

33. Wangberg B, Forssell-Aronsson E, Tisell L-E et al (1996) Intraoperative detection of somatostatin-receptor positive neuroendocrine tumours using 111-In-DTPA-Phe I-octreotide. Br J Cancer 73:770–775

34. Krenning EP, Keboom DJ, Bakker WH et al (1993) Somatostatin receptor scintigraphy with 111-In-DTPA-D-PheI- and 123-I-Tyr 3-octreotide: the Rotterdam experience with more than 1000 patients. Eur J Nucl Med 20:716–731

35. Virgolini I, Raderer M, Kurtaran A et al (1994) Vasoactive intestinal peptide receptor imaging for the localisation of intestinal adenocarcinomas and endocrine tumours. N Engl J Med 331:1116–1121

36. Paganelli G, Stella M, De Nardi P et al (1991) A new method for faster blood clearance in radioimmunoguided surgery. J Nucl Med Allied Sci 35:88–89

37. Stella N, De Nardi P, Paganelli G et al (1994) Avidin-Biotin system in radioimmunoguided surgery for colorectal cancer: advantages and limits. Dis Colon Rectum 37:355–343

38. Bares R, Muller B, Fass J et al (1992) The radiation dose to surgical personnel during intraoperative radioimmunoscintigraphy. Eur J Nucl Med 19:110–112

39. Robinson P (1993) The role of nuclear medicine in acute gastrointestinal bleeding. Nucl Med Commun 14:849–855

40. Myers MA, Alonson DR, Gray GF et al (1976) Pathogenesis of bleeding colonic diverticulosis. Gastroenterology 91:577–583
41. Jaramillo E, Slezak P (1992) Comparison between double contrast barium enema and colonoscopy to investigate lower gastrointestinal bleeding. Gastrointest Radiol 17:81–83
42. Stevenson GW, Hunt RH (1988) Prospective comparison of double contrast barium enema plus flexible sigmoidoscopy v colonoscopy in rectal bleeding. Gut 29:1188–1193
43. Jenson DN, Machicado GA (1988) Diagnosis and treatment of severe haematochezia. Gastroenterology 95:1569–1574
44. Hunt PS, Hansky J, Korman MG (1979) Mortality in patients with haematemesis and melaena: a prospective study. BMJ 1:1238–1240
45. Bearn P, Persad R, Wilson N et al (1992) 99m Technetium labelled red blood cell scintigraphy as an alternative to angiography in the investigation of gastrointestinal bleeding: clinical experience in a district general hospital. Ann R Coll Surg 74:192–199
46. Abdel-Dayem HM, Ziada G, Owunewanne A et al (1984) Scintigraphic detection of acute gastrointestinal bleeding using 99mTc DTPA. Nucl Med Commun 5:633–639
47. Alavi A, Dann RW, Baum S, Biery D (1977) Scintigraphic detection of acute gastrointestinal bleeding. Radiology 124:753–756
48. Gupta SN, Spencer RP, Chak SP (1991) Significance of intensity of delayed activity during technetium 99m RBC gastrointestinal bleeding study. J Nucl Med 32:249–252
49. Petrokubi RJ, Baum S, Rohrer GV (1978) Cimetidine administration resulting in improved imaging of Meckel's diverticulum. Clin Nucl Med 3:385–388
50. Gordon I (1980) Gastrointestinal haemorrhage unrelated to gastric mucosa diagnosed on 99mTc pertechnetate scans. Br J Radiol 53:322–324
51. Conway JJ (1980) Radionuclide diagnosis of Meckel's diverticulum. Gastrointest Radiol 5:209–213
52. Thakur ML, Lavender JP, Arnold RW et al (1977) 111-In labelled autologous leukocytes in man. J Nucl Med 18:1014–1021
53. Danpure HJ, Osman S, Brady F (1982) The labelling of blood cells in plasma with In-111 tropolonate. Br J Radiol 55:247–249
54. Saverymuttu SH, Lavender JP, Hodgson HFJ et al (1983) Assessment of disease activity in inflammatory bowel disease. A new approach using 111-Indium-granulocyte scanning. BMJ 287:1751–1753
55. Saverymuttu SH, Peters AM, Lavender JP et al (1983) Quantitative fecal Indium-111 labelled leukocyte excretion in the assessment of disease in Crohn's disease. Gastroenterology 85:1333–1339
56. Poitras P, Carrier L, Chartrand R et al (1987) 111-In leukocyte scanning of the abdomen. Analysis of its value for diagnosis and management of inflammatory bowel disease. J Clin Gastroenterol 9:418–423
57. Froehlich JW, Field SA (1988) The role of 111-In white blood cells in inflammatory bowel disease. Semin Nucl Med 18:300–307
58. Li DJ, Middleton SJ, Wraight EP (1992) 99mTc and 111-In leucocyte scintigraphy in inflammatory bowel disease. Nucl Med Commun 13:867–870
59. Saverymuttu SH, Camilieri M, Reese M et al (1986) 111-In granulocyte scanning in the assessment of disease extent and disease activity in inflammatory bowel disease. Gastroenterology 90:1121–1128
60. Peters AM, Osman S, Henderson BL et al (1986) Clinical experience with Tc-99m HMPAO for labelling leukocytes and imaging inflammation. Lancet 2:966–969
61. Solanki KK, Mather SJ, Janabi M Al- et al (1988) A rapid method for the preparation of Tc-99m hexametazine labelled leukocytes. Nucl Med Commun 9:753–761
62. Schumichen C, Scholmerich J (1986) 99Tcm-HMPAO labelling of leucocytes for detection of inflammatory bowel disease. NucCompact 17:274–276
63. Roddie ME, Peters AM, Danpure HJ et al (1988) Inflammation: imaging with 99Tcm-HMPAO-labelled leukocytes. Radiology 166:767–772
64. Peters AM (1994) The utility of 99Tcm-HMPAO leukocytes for imaging infection. Semin Nucl Med 24:110–127
65. Allan RA, Sladen GE, Bassingham S et al (1993) Comparison of simultaneous 99Tcm-HMPAO and 111In oxine labelled white cell scans in the assessment of inflammatory bowel disease. Eur J Nucl Med 20:195–200
66. Arndt JW, Veer A vd S, Blok D et al (1993) Prospective comparative study of Technetium-99m-WBC and Indium-111 granulocytes for the examination of patients with inflammatory bowel disease. J Nucl Med 34:1052–1057
67. Chanon M, Orenstein SR, Bhargara S (1994) Detection of inflammatory bowel disease in paediatric patients with Technetium-99m-HMPAO labelled leukocytes. J Nucl Med 33:4451–4455
68. Becker W, Borst U, Fischbach W et al (1989) Kinetic data of in-vivo labelled granulocytes in humans with a murine Tc-99m labelled monoclonal antibody. Eur J Nucl Med 15:361–366
69. Joseph K, Hoffken H, Bosslet K, Schorlemmer HU (1988) In vivo labelling of granulocytes with Tc-99m-anti-NCA monoclonal antibodies for imaging inflammation. Eur J Nucl Med 14:367–373, 1988
70. Rubin RH, Fischman AJ, Callahan RJ et al (1989) 111-In labelled nonspecific immunoglobulin scanning in the detection of focal infection. N Engl J Med 321:935–950
71. Buscombe JR, Lin D, Ensing G et al (1990) 99mTc human immunoglobulin (hIgG): first result of a new agent for localisation of infection and inflammation. Eur J Nucl Med 16:649–655
72. Hebbard GS, Salehi N, Gibson PR et al (1992) 99Tcm-labelled 1gG scanning does not predict the distribution of intestinal inflammation in patients with inflammatory bowel disease. Nucl Med Commun 13:336–341
73. Palestro CJ (1994) The current role of gallium imaging in infection. Semin Nucl Med 24:128–141
74. Hawkins PN, Lavender JP, Myers MJ, Pepys MB (1988) Diagnostic radionuclide imaging of amyloidosis: biological targetting by circulating human serum amyloid P component. Lancet 25:1413–1418
75. Signore A, Chianelli M, Ferretti E et al (1994) A new approach for in vivo detection of insulitis: activated lymphocyte targetting with 123-I labelled interleukin-2. Eur J Endocrinol 131:431–437
76. Signore A, Chianelli M, Ferretti E et al (1993) Use of 123I-interleukin-2 for in vivo detection of activated lymphocytes in chronic inflammatory diseases. Eur J Nucl Med 20:834

77. Signore A, Chianelli M, Picarelli A et al (in press) ^{123}I-IL2 for in vivo detection of activated lymphocytes in organ specific autoimmune diseases. J Endocrinol Invest

78. Chianelli M, Signore A, Ronga G et al (1994) Labelling, purification and biodistribution of ^{99m}Tc-interleukin-2: a new radiopharmaceutical for in vivo detection of activated lymphocytes. Eur J Nucl Med 21:807

79. Chianelli M, Signore A, Biassoni L et al (1995) In vivo imaging of autoimmunity by ^{99m}Tc interleukin-2. Eur J Nucl Med 22: 781

80. Solanki KK, Bomanji J, Mather SJ et al (1993) [99]Tc[m]-Infecton: development of a new radiopharmaceutical for imaging infection. Nucl Med Commun 14:925

81. Solanki KK, Bomanji J, Siraj Q et al (1993) Tc-99m 'Infecton' a new class of radiopharmaceutical for imaging infection. J Nucl Med 34:119P

82. Vinjamuri S, Hall AV, Solanki KK et al (1995) Tc-99m Infecton, Tc-I, a bacterial specific infection imaging agent. Eur J Nucl Med 22:916

83. Vinjamuri S, Hall AV, Solanki KK et al (1996) Comparison of Tc-99m infecton imaging with radiolabelled white cell imaging in the evaluation of bacterial infection. Lancet 347: 233–235

84. Mather SJ, Ellison D, Nightingale JMD et al (1991) The design of a two phase radiolabelled meal for gastric emptying studies. Nucl Med Commun 12:409–416

85. Notghi A, Kumar D, Panagamuwa B et al (1993) Measurement of colonic transit time using radionuclide imaging: analysis by condensed images. Nucl Med Commun 14:204–211

86. Van der Sijp JRM, Kamm MA, Nightingale JMD et al (1993) Radioisotope determination of regional colonic transit in severe constipation: comparison with radio opaque markers. Gut 34:402–408

87. Krevsky B, Malmud LS, D'Ercole F et al (1986) Colonic transit scintigraphy: a physiological approach to the quantitative measurement of colonic transit in humans. Gastroenterology 91: 1102–1112

88. Herbst F, Kamm MA, Morris GP et al (submitted) Gastrointestinal transit and prolonged ambulatory colonic motility in health and faecal incontinence. Gastroenterology

89. Gattuso JM, Kamm MA, Morris G, Britton KE (1996) Gastrointestinal transit in patients with idiopathic mega rectum. 39: 1046–1050

8

PHYSIOLOGIC INVESTIGATIONS

David Z. Lubowski
Michael L. Kennedy

ANORECTAL MANOMETRY

The anal sphincter produces a high-pressure zone around the anal canal. Although the mechanisms of continence and defecation are highly complex, involving integrated visceral and somatic motor and sensory function as well as higher centers, a simple pressure zone provides an important contribution to normal anorectal function. The pressure increases in response to rises in abdominal pressure and decreases during defecation. Manometry is a simple, noninvasive method of studying the anal sphincter pressure zone. It has an important role in the assessment of anal sphincter and rectal function and has become a standard test in clinical laboratories.

Technique of Anal Manometry

For the purpose of clinical investigation, minor pressure differences that are found with different recording techniques are not important. All recording systems allow assessment of basal and squeeze pressures, and functional anal canal length. Whichever system is used, three principles must be observed: the recording catheter must not be of large diameter, the system must be standardized to zero before each recording, and adequate time must be allowed for the pressure to equilibrate at each recording site. A large diameter (greater than 8 mm) recording catheter should not be used because it artifically raises both resting and squeeze pressure.[1-4]

Balloon Recording Systems

The use of a balloon connected to a pressure transducer via a thin, nondistensible tube is a simple and inexpensive method of recording anal pressure. The system devised by Schuster[5] was popular but the large diameter balloons raise the anal pressure. Even when this is taken into account by establishing pressures with this system in normal subjects, the variation of anal sphincter stretch by the balloons renders the technique unreliable. In addition, the outer and inner balloons do not selectively record external and internal sphincter pressures as they were intended to do. If a balloon system is used, then a small diameter (0.4 cm) "microballoon" is better than the older 1.0- to 1.5-cm diameter balloon. Air-filled and water-filled systems produce similar results[6] although some have found the pressure with an air-filled system to be slightly lower.[7]

A station pull-through technique is used. The balloon is inserted into the rectum and then slowly withdrawn into the anal canal. Once within the high pressure zone in the upper anal canal, the resting pressure is allowed to stablize. The catheter should have markings 1 cm apart, and the mark at the anal verge allows the observer to determine the position of the balloon in the anus. The patient is then asked to maximally contract the anal sphincter for 3 seconds, and this is done three times. The catheter is then withdrawn at 1 cm intervals and the procedure is repeated at each interval. Thus the maximal resting pressure, maximal voluntary contraction pressure, and anal canal length are recorded.

Perfusion Systems

A perfusion system consists of a multichannel catheter containing narrow diameter low-compliance tubes that are perfused with water via sideholes at a constant rate. The water is pumped from a container that is pressurized by a high-pressure air cylinder, and passes via resistance capillary tubing to the multichannel catheter. The diameter of the resistance tube is varied and controls the rate of flow of water. Flow rates of 0.4 to 0.6 ml/min are optimal. The perfusion catheter contains six to eight channels. The channel opening at the tip is used for inflation of a rectal balloon. The first sidehole is 2 cm proximal to the tip and records rectal pressure. Three centimeters proximal to this is the first of a series of sideholes 1 cm apart for recording anal pressure. Recordings can be made on a standard paper chart recorder, but collection and storage of data on a computerized

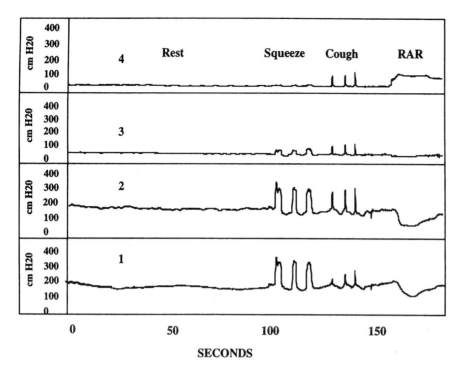

Figure 8-1. Anorectal manometry recorded with a four-channel perfusion system. Channel 4 records rectal pressure, and channels 1, 2, and 3 are lower, mid-, and upper anal canal, respectively. Pressures are recorded at rest, and then during a voluntary squeeze and cough. Rectal pressure increases during coughing but not during squeezing. The rectoanal reflex (RAR) is shown at the right—pressure increases in the rectum as the rectal balloon is inflated, and this is accompanied by a fall in anal pressure followed by spontaneous recovery.

system has considerable advantages. The catheter should be positioned and the basal resting pressure is allowed to stabilize. The maximal resting pressure will be observed at one of the recording sites. The patient is then asked to maximally contract the sphincter three times at 10-second intervals. Then the basal pressure is again allowed to stabilize for 1 to 3 minutes, after which the patient is asked to cough as forcefully as possible three times at 10-second intervals. Hence the maximal squeeze and cough pressures are recorded (Fig. 8-1).

Strain Gauge Transducers

Early forms of strain gauge transducers involved a cantilever that incorporated a semiconductor strain gauge that was set in a resistance bridge.[8] Modern microtransducers are more accurate and employ the principle of a Wheatstone bridge, containing resistors that are placed on a metal diaphragm within a vacuum. Pressure on the sensing diaphragm changes the resistance on the bridge, and this change is converted to pressure.[9] A single transducer is used with a station pull-through technique, or a catheter with multiple transducers may be used for simultaneous recording at more than one site. Although these transducers are easy to use,[10,11] they are expensive and in most centers have been used only for ambulatory manometry.

Clinical Relevance of Manometry

Anorectal manometry provides a direct measure of internal and external sphincter tone. Digital examination by an experienced clinician undoubtedly gives an accurate assessment of the

sphincter in most cases, and a significant overall correlation between clinical and manometric assessment of resting and squeeze pressure has been demonstrated.[12,13] However in a small number of patients the manometric measurement shows the clinical examination to be incorrect. In a patient with fecal incontinence this may have an important influence on the decision to carry out surgical treatment. It is more difficult to clinically assess the functional length of the anal sphincter than to assess the tone, and although there is also a significant overall correlation with manometric assessment of sphincter length marked differences are seen in individual cases (Lubowski DZ, Nicholls RJ, unpublished observations; Fig. 8-2). Thus manometry may have an important bearing in assessing the length of sphincter enclosed by a seton when making a decision about laying open an anal fistula. Several aspects of resting and squeeze pressure should be considered.

Resting Anal Pressure

Frenckner and von Euler[14] carried out pudendal nerve blocks to eliminate external sphincter contraction, and showed that 85% of the resting pressure was due to tonic contraction of the internal anal sphincter. Other studies have shown a larger contribution by the external sphincter[15,16] but the figure of 15% from the external sphincter is generally accepted to be correct. In practice, a reduction in resting pressure implies loss of internal sphincter tone. The internal sphincter is in a state of spontaneous intrinsic contraction.[14,17] Electrical activity may be

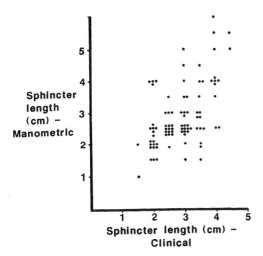

Figure 8-2. Sphincter length assessed manometrically, and then with digital examination by observers blinded to the manometric recording. There is an overall significant correlation between the two measures ($P < .001$) but in several patients digital assessment differs widely from manometric measurement.

recorded in internal sphincter smooth muscle cells, showing phasic activity at a rate of 6 to 26 cycles/min known as basic electrical rhythm (BER).[8,18] This is accompanied by phasic pressure waves recorded manometrically called slow waves, usually occurring at a frequency of 6 to 20 per minute[19,20] and amplitude 10 to 25 cm H_2O, although sometimes of higher frequency.[21,22] In addition, there are ultra-slow waves of frequency 1 to 3 per minute and amplitude up to 200 cm H_2O.

The internal sphincter relaxes in response to rectal distension. This occurs spontaneously on average seven times per hour.[23–25] Duthie and Bennet[26] originally proposed that this was a "sampling" reflex that was important in the continence mechanism, allowing discrimination of flatus and stool. Spontaneous internal sphincter relaxation is usually accompanied by rectal distension or contraction[27,28] although it may also occur without changes in rectal pressure[29,30] and is observed during routine manometric recordings.[30]

Slow wave frequency is higher in the lower anal canal than the upper canal[31,32] and it has been postulated that this may produce a distal to proximal pressure gradient to prevent incontinence during the sampling events. This theory is supported by the observation that the lowest part of the external sphincter contracts during rectal distension, the "inflation reflex".[15,33,34] Ultra-slow waves are observed in 3% to 5% of normal subjects[32,35] although Haynes and Read[21] recorded them in 40% when resting pressure was greater than 100 cm H_2O (Fig. 8-3). They are present in conditions known to be associated with high resting pressure due to internal sphincter spasm, namely hemorrhoids[32,35–37] and anal fissure.[38–40]

Resting pressures are lower in women than men.[41,42] They have also been found to be lower in elderly subjects in some studies[43,44] but not in others.[45]

The length of the internal sphincter high-pressure zone is slightly longer in men (mean 2.5 cm) than women (mean 2.0 cm).[42] Other studies have reported a high-pressure zone 2.5 to 5.0 cm in length[46] but this was using a continuous pull-through technique that probably includes a variable amount of reflex external sphincter contraction.

Radial variation in anal pressure is observed, usually in the upper anal canal where the resting and squeeze pressures are usually lower anteriorly than posteriorly.[47,48] This is thought to be due to the absence anteriorly of the puborectalis muscle. Radial variation is measured using a perfusion system with four sideholes placed at one level (Fig. 8-4) and is not detected when using a standard multichannel perfusion catheter, nor with a microballoon system. Radial variation is usually not of clinical importance because the chief parameters of interest, the maximum resting and squeeze pressures, are most commonly found in the mid- or lower anal canal.

Resting anal pressures are reduced in patients with neurogenic fecal incontinence[49–51] and rectal prolapse[49] (Fig. 8-5). Internal sphincter function recovers in some patients after abdominal rectopexy.[52] In neurogenic incontinence reduced resting anal pressure is associated with histologic[53] and electromyographic[22] evidence of internal sphincter muscle damage, although the condition is thought to predominantly affect the somatic external sphincter muscle. Incontinence in patients with ulcerative colitis has not been found to be associated with low anal pressure.[54] Resting pressure is reduced with sacral nerve damage,[55] but not in patients with paraplegia.[56,57]

Rectoanal Inhibitory Reflex

Internal sphincter relaxation in response to rectal distension is mediated via an intrinsic neural pathway in the wall of the anorectum.[27,58] It has long been known that this reflex can be tested by distending the rectum with air.[27,59,60] Sphincter relaxation is defined as a fall in basal pressure of 20%, but this should also be accompanied by spontaneous pressure recovery. With progressive distension of the rectum, the sphincter tone does not recover.[61] The threshold and amplitude of the rectoanal reflex is not affected by age or sex.[41] The reflex is absent in Hirschsprung's disease[62] and manometry is a useful screening test for this condition. The reflex is, however, also absent when the resting pressure is very low, either due to a weak internal anal sphincter or due to sphincter relaxation resulting from fecal impaction. A negative reflex is also sometimes found with megarectum despite inflation with a very large volume, and also with fecal impaction when the internal sphincter is normally contracted but stool in the rectum prevents inflation of the rectal balloon. Following excision of the rectum with anastomosis, the coloanal inhibition reflex returns in some subjects,[63,64] presumably due to regrowth of intramural nerve fibers across the anastomosis.[65]

Technique of Testing the Rectoanal Inhibitory Reflex

If a balloon manometric system is used, a separate firm catheter with a party balloon at the tip is initially inserted into the rectum. The microballoon is then inserted into the anal canal for pressure recording. If a perfusion system is used, then the catheter contains a rectal balloon at its tip. The resting pressure must be allowed to stabilize completely. The rectal balloon is then inflated with 20 ml air over 5 to 10 seconds, ensuring that there is no movement of the pressure recording catheter. The anal

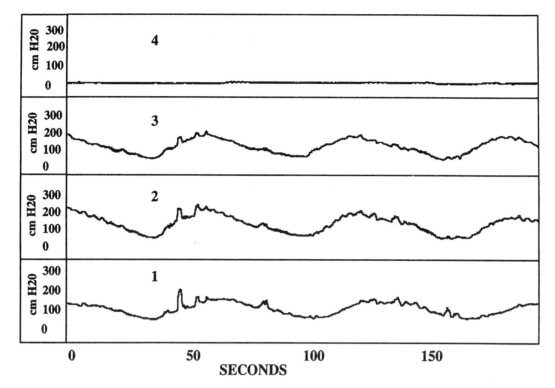

Figure 8-3. Resting anal pressure showing ultra-slow waves at 50-sec cycles. Channels 1 to 3 represent lower, mid-, and upper anal canal. Channel 4 is rectal pressure.

pressure is observed to fall and recover. If the pressure does not fall then 20-ml boluses of air are instilled until the reflex is observed. If megarectum is present then up to 800 ml may be needed. A false-positive reflex may be obtained if the anal pressure recording catheter is drawn upward into the rectum as the rectal balloon is inflated. If the pressure does not recover spontaneously but does so after the rectal balloon is deflated, then this is also considered a positive reflex, as long as there is certainty that the position of the pressure catheter has been perfectly maintained.

Figure 8-4. Radial variation in anal pressures. Pressure recording in the upper anal canal, channel 4 = posterior, 3 = left side, 2 = anterior, 1 = right side. Posteriorly the resting pressure is reduced and the squeeze pressure is higher than in the other positions. The most common pattern of reduced resting and squeeze pressure anteriorly is not present in this patient, illustrating the variations that are sometimes found.

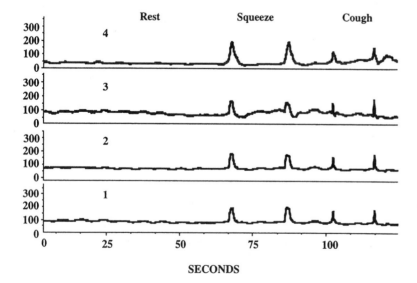

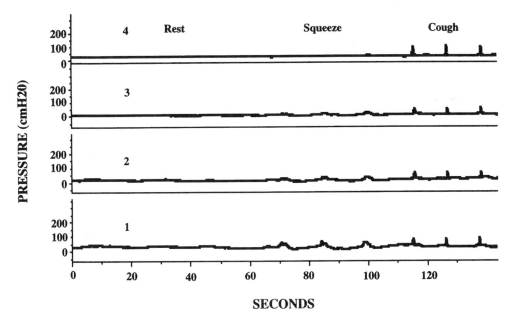

Figure 8-5. Anal manometry in a patient with neurogenic incontinence. Resting pressures are reduced, and squeeze and cough pressures are markedly reduced along the length of the anal canal. Channels 1, 2, 3 = lower, mid-, upper anal canal, channel 4 = rectum.

Voluntary Contraction Pressure

Voluntary contraction (squeeze) pressure is produced by the external sphincter muscle, and is defined as the highest pressure recorded during a maximum sphincter contraction[66] (Fig. 8-2). It is higher in men than women[41,42] and reduces with age.[43,44] The squeeze pressure is reduced in patients with neurogenic incontinence or incontinence due to sphincter injury.[22,43,43a,49,67] The squeeze pressure is dependent on the ability of the patient to cooperate and maximally contract the sphincter while lying in the lateral position, a maneuver that some patients find difficult in the laboratory setting. In a study comparing squeeze pressure and cough pressure, although we observed a significant linear relationship between squeeze and cough pressure, the true correlation was relatively poor with wide scatter of data ($r = 0.67$)[68] (Fig. 8-6). Therefore measurement of cough pressure provides additional information about external sphincter strength in some subjects.

Ambulatory Anorectal Manometry

The continence mechanism is complex and incontinence may occur in the presence of anal pressures that are within normal limits when measured with a conventional static recording system. Conversely, some subjects with a weak anal sphincter may have normal continence. The presence of a rectoanal pressure gradient produced when abdominal pressure is raised only has a 43% sensitivity in predicting incontinence[68] and it is clear that factors other than sphincter pressure and stool consistency are contributory. Attempts have been made to devise methods that study patients under conditions that are more physiologic than those in an investigative laboratory.

Ambulatory anorectal manometry was developed as a modifi-

cation of ambulatory esophageal manometry and was first reported by Miller et al.[23] and Kumar et al.[25] Improvement in data collection and storage has increased continuous multichannel recording time to over 24 hours. Although ambulatory perfusion systems have recently become available, all systems currently commercially available employ strain gauge pressure transducers. The transducers are mounted on a narrow-diameter probe that is flexible but firm, and is connected to a small portable data recording box (Fig. 8-7). It is advantageous to have a three-channel probe with two transducers 2 cm apart for recording anal pressure and a third transducer at the tip for rectal pressure. Each transducer adds considerable cost to the probe, and if only one transducer is available for recording anal pressure then particular care must be taken to record from the midanal canal in order to compensate for any upward or downward catheter movement (Fig. 8-8). After calibrating the transducers, the catheter is inserted and its position is maintained by adhesive strapping that secures the catheter at the anal verge and then in the natal cleft. Real-time pressure readings are taken to confirm the correct position of the transducers. The subject carries the recording box using a shoulder strap, and uses the event button while documenting events in a diary. The events of interest are passage of flatus, urge to defecate, defecation, incontinence, and movements such as running.

When the recording has been completed, the data are downloaded into the computer for analysis. The data are analyzed in two ways: analysis of individual marked events; and quantitative analysis, for example of mean pressure over a given length of time, number of designated waveforms, or number of pressure spikes using software packages. There are two particular problems in interpretation: (1) catheter movement—even a small movement of the transducer in the anal canal—can result in an artifactual pressure change if the transducer is displaced

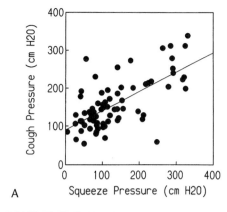

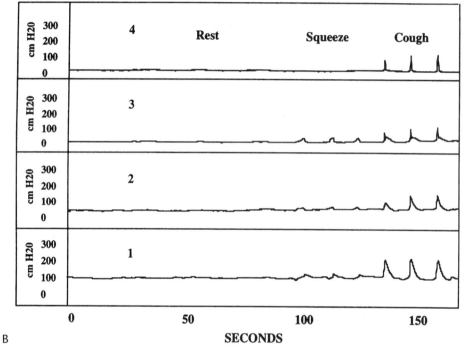

Figure 8-6. Cough pressure. (**A**) Relationship between cough pressure and squeeze pressure, $r = 0.67$, $P < .001$. Note wide scatter of data around the line of best fit. (From Meagher et al,[68] with permission). (**B**) Anal manometry to illustrate cough pressure. The tracing shows poor squeeze pressures but strong cough pressures. Inability to voluntarily contract the external sphincter does not reflect sphincter weakness in this patient because the sphincter is able to contract normally during coughing.

cranially or caudally from the anal canal (Fig. 8-9); (2) subject movement may produce severe artifacts that may completely obscure normal pressure waves. This occurs particularly during rapid movements or when abdominal pressure is suddenly raised.

Clinical Relevance of Ambulatory Manometry

Miller et al.[23] demonstrated spontaneous relaxation of the internal sphincter, which seemed to confirm the rectoanal sampling reflex theory put forward by Duthie and Bennett.[26] A rectal pressure rise does not always accompany anal relaxation,[23] so that the classic rectoanal neural pathway may not always be causal, and relaxation may be spontaneous and intrinsic, or controlled by extrinsic autonomic nerves. When resting anal pressure is high, sampling occurs more frequently than normal.[69] Patients with long-standing constipation have lower than normal sampling rates.[69]

In patients with incontinence, standard static recordings may show normal anal sphincter pressures in some patients but using

ambulatory manometry Roberts and Williams[9] have shown rectal high-pressure waves that coincide with a feeling of urgency. Similar proximal pressure waves may be associated with incontinence after proctocolectomy with ileoanal reservoir,[70] and we have observed them after rectal excision with coloanal anastomosis (Fig. 8-9). Patients with pruritus ani have abnormal transient internal sphincter relaxation, with more frequent episodes that are also of longer duration than in normal subjects.[52] This may be associated with minor soiling, causing pruritus.

Obstructed defecation has been investigated with ambulatory manometry. This common clinical entity, called anismus,[71] has been said to be due to paradoxic contraction of the puborectalis and levator muscles.[71–73] A variety of treatments have been attempted including puborectalis division,[74] *Botulinum* toxin,[75] and biofeedback.[76–78] Some have questioned whether the observations made in the physiology laboratory using electromyography (EMG) and evacuation proctography leading to the diagnosis may be due to the unphysiologic nature of laboratory tests.[79–81] Using combined ambulatory manometry and EMG Duthie et al.[82] showed that 8 of 11 patients who had been diag-

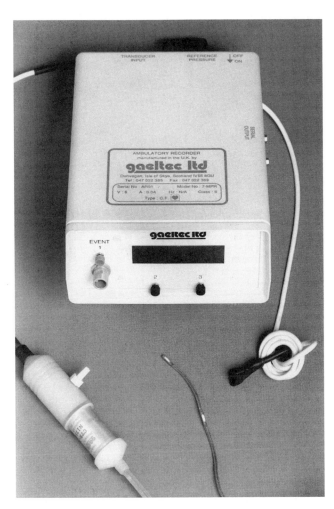

Figure 8-7. Ambulatory recording system (Gaeltec, Isle of Skye, Scotland). The recording box is shown with connection lines to recording catheters.

Figure 8-8. Ambulatory recording catheter with two strain gauge microtransducers.

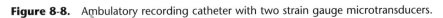

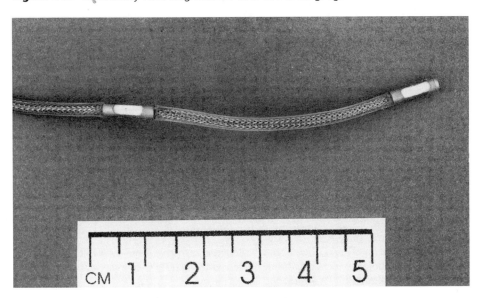

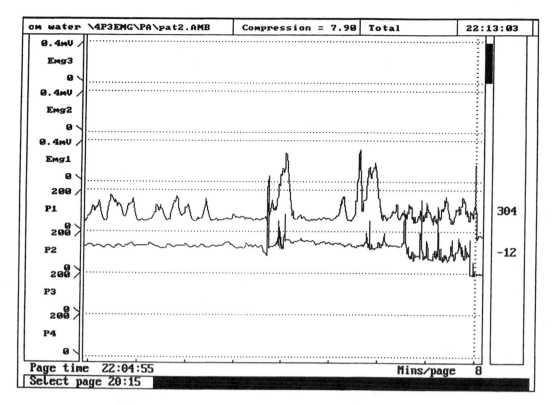

| cm water | \4P3EMG\PA\pat2.AMB | Compression = 7.90 | Total | 22:13:03 |

Page time 22:04:55   Mins/page   8

Select page 20:15

Figure 8-9. A 24-hour ambulatory manometric recording in a patient after rectal excision with coloanal anastomosis. Upper trace is the neorectal pressure, lower trace is anal canal pressure. Recording from an 8-minute segment shown. The two high-pressure colonic waves were associated with an episode of soiling. In minute 7 there is a spontaneous reduction in anal pressure. At the end of the trace the cursor indicates the point at which the anal transducer has become displaced from the anal canal, thus registering a negative pressure.

nosed with anismus in the laboratory demonstrated normal muscle relaxation when studied under physiologic conditions using ambulatory techniques and this has provided a new insight into this condition. It is likely that ambulatory studies will provide further important information in this difficult group of patients.

ELECTROPHYSIOLOGY

In patients with fecal incontinence, once the anal sphincter has been shown manometrically to be weak, it is then necessary to further investigate sphincter function in order to determine the cause for the muscle weakness. The impetus to develop electrophysiologic techniques for this purpose came from the work of Parks and Swash who identified histologic changes in the anal sphincter in patients with fecal incontinence, showing evidence of denervation of the muscle.[83,84] Standard electromyographic and nerve conduction studies used elsewhere in the body were adapted to study the anal sphincter and other pelvic floor muscles. These tests have provided a detailed understanding of the pathophysiology of incontinence and several other conditions affecting the pelvic floor muscles, and a large literature has grown around the subject. The tests are now used routinely in the clinical investigation of patients. In the United States and Britain surgeons practicing in coloproctology are using anorectal physiology studies with increasing frequency,[85] although

some still find difficulty obtaining easy access to a laboratory carrying out physiology studies.

Motor Nerve Conduction Studies

Pudendal Nerve Motor Latency

In 1984 Kiff and Swash[36] reported a novel test to assess motor conduction in the pudendal nerves.[86] This involves transrectal stimulation of the pudendal nerves, and was based on a technique of nerve stimulation to induce ejaculation in patients with paraplegia.[87] Electrical stimulation of the pudendal nerves allows assessment of conduction time along the distal part of the nerve. This is the section of the nerve that is most vulnerable to injury. Weakness of the external anal sphincter due to pudendal nerve damage may occur in two ways. A direct stretch-induced injury during vaginal delivery and chronic straining at stool has been well established, and in addition, damage to the pelvic nerves causing perineal descent in turn leads to pudendal nerve stretch.[88,89]

Anatomy of the Pudendal Nerves

The pudendal nerve derives fibers from the ventral rami of the second, third, and fourth sacral nerves. The sacral nerves join to form the sacral plexus, which lies on the medial aspect of the piriformis muscle. The pudendal nerve arises from the sacral plexus, passes out of the pelvis through the greater sciatic foramen below the piriformis, and comes to lie on the posterior surface of the ischial spine. From here it passes forward below the ischial spine through the lesser sciatic foramen to enter the perineum, where it lies in the lateral part of the ischiorectal fossa in the pudendal (Alcock's) canal. It passes forward on the perineal surface of the levator ani and divides into the inferior rectal nerve (to the external sphincter), perineal nerve (to the anterior parts of the external sphincter, puborectalis, and pubococcygeus), and dorsal nerve of the penis/clitoris. There is some disagreement about the origin of the nerve to the urethral sphincter, some authors describing it arising from the proximal part of the dorsal nerve of the penis[90] whereas others believe it arises from the perineal nerve,[91] and the latter is believed to be correct.[92]

Nerve Supply to the Levator Ani

The *nerves to levator ani*, which arise from the sacral plexus deriving fibers from S3 and S4, and the *perineal branch of S4* all supply the puborectalis and pubococcygeus muscle from the superior surface. Anatomic texts describe the main nerve supply to the levator ani, particularly the puborectalis, being mainly from the pudendal nerves. However Percy et al[93] showed that

the pubococcygeus and puborectalis muscles are mainly supplied by the S3, S4 nerves to levator ani, and that each nerve supplied only the ipsilateral muscle. The perineal branch of S4 is said to also supply the external sphincter[90] but Percy et al.[93] found that this muscle was supplied only by the pudendal nerves.

Technique of Pudendal Nerve Stimulation

The patient is placed in the left lateral position with the hips flexed. A ground electrode soaked in normal saline is placed around the thigh. A disposable St. Mark's electrode (Dantec 13L40, Skoulunde, Denmark) is attached to the gloved right index finger (Fig. 8-10). The stimulating anode/cathode electrodes should be positioned just proximal to the tip of the finger. The disposable electrode has replaced the original nondisposable finger-stall device[86] because the latter cannot be sterilized. Pudendal stimulation tests using the disposable electrode have been validated.[94] The finger is inserted into the rectum and then curved around the puborectalis, usually first on the left side where it is easier to record. The nerve is stimulated near the ischial spine. Contrary to many reports, it is usually *not* possible to accurately palpate the ischial spine and the optimal point to stimulate is determined by the wave form on the EMG machine. Repeated stimuli are delivered at 1-second intervals, and the tip

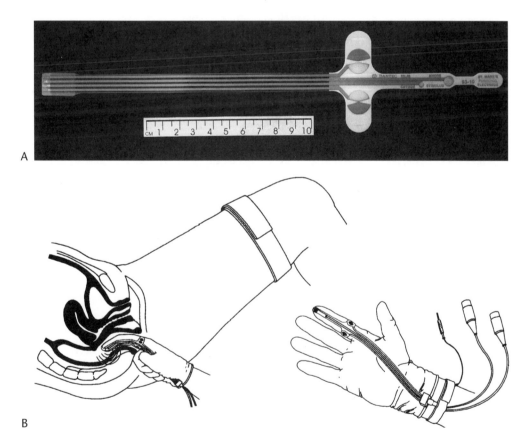

Figure 8-10. (**A**) Disposable pudendal stimulating device (Dantec, Denmark). The stimulating anode and cathode electrodes are at the tip, and the recording electrodes are at the base. (**B**) Disposable pudendal stimulating device mounted on gloved index finger. (Courtesy of Dantec, Denmark.)

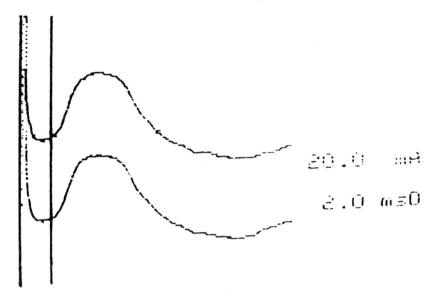

Figure 8-11. Pudendal nerve terminal motor latency. Two identical traces with short latency confirms that the stimulating electrode is in correct position. Cursors placed at onset of stimulus (time zero) and onset of contraction (latency 2 msec).

of the finger is moved until a tracing with precisely reproducible shape and latency is achieved (Fig. 8-11). When the stimulus is being delivered at some distance from the pudendal nerve, the latency is prolonged and it shortens progressively as the stimulating electrode is moved closer to the nerve. The image is stored on the screen and the procedure is repeated on the right side. The latency represents the time taken for the impulse to pass along the pudendal nerve to the external sphincter and is measured on the screen by placing the cursors at the point of stimulation and at the beginning of the deflection. In patients with a long or tight internal sphincter it can occasionally be difficult to adequately reach over the edge of the puborectalis, particularly on the right side, and if a reproducible tracing cannot be recorded then the latency should be disregarded.

Equipment and Filter Settings

Most standard EMG machines are suitable for pudendal nerve studies. Recently developed software packages used for recording anorectal manometry have the facility for recording needle EMG and nerve conduction studies so that a dedicated EMG machine is no longer needed (Neomedix, Sydney, Australia). Square-wave stimuli, duration 0.1 msec are delivered at 1-second intervals. A constant current stimulator, which corrects for tissue resistance, should be used. A stimulus of 20 mA is always supramaximal. It is best to progressively increase the stimulus strength from about 10 mA until 20 mA is reached in order not to produce a sudden, strong muscle contraction. If a voltage stimulator is used then a 50-V stimulus is required. Filter settings are low frequency 20 Hz, high frequency 5 KHz. Sweep speed is 2 msec/div.

Clinical Relevance

The underlying pathology affecting the pudendal nerves, and forming the basis for pudendal nerve motor studies, is a stretch-induced injury. The position of the nerves is fixed as they pass behind the ischial spine. Distal to this point the nerves are able to move freely and may be damaged if there is excessive pelvic floor descent. In normal subjects the pelvic floor descends up to 2 cm during straining down.[88,95–97] Descent of more than 2 to 3 cm is abnormal.[79,95,96,98] It has been estimated that perineal descent of this magnitude will produce a stretch of the pudendal nerves of 20% above their usual length[83] and because a stretch of only 12% produces nerve damage[99] it is postulated that abnormal perineal descent causes pudendal nerve damage. Jones et al.[79] found a linear correlation between amount of perineal descent and degree of pudendal nerve damage, and other studies have also shown a significant relationship between descent and pudendal latency.[100–103] Abnormal perineal descent and nerve damage are caused by chronic straining at stool[104,105] and difficult vaginal delivery.[106–109] Acute change in nerve conduction has been demonstrated during straining down in patients with abnormal perineal descent[110,111] (Fig. 8-12). Although nerve conduction returns to normal at the end of straining, repeated neuropraxia occurring over a long period of time leads to permanent nerve damage. Thus abnormal pudendal nerve motor latency occurs in patients with neurogenic fecal incontinence[22,79,102,112–117] Tetzschner et al.[118] found that women with prolonged pudendal nerve terminal motor latency after vaginal delivery had an increased risk of developing fecal incontinence compared with women who had normal latencies (odds ratio 2.2). Long-term follow-up of patients with fecal incontinence has shown progression of nerve damage over time[119] and this was also seen in paients who had undergone postanal repair.[120]

Abnormal pudendal latency is also found in patients with combined fecal and urinary incontinence,[89,121,122] patients with incontinence persisting after rectopexy for prolapse,[123] and in patients with chronic constipation,[105,124] hemorrhoids,[125] symptomatic uterovaginal prolapse,[97,126,127] and solitary rectal ulcer syndrome.[128,129] Vaccaro et al[124] found evidence of pudendal neuropathy in 24% of constipated patients. They found no difference in the incidence of pudendal neuropathy in constipated

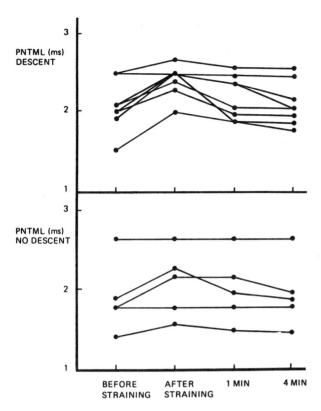

Figure 8-12. Change in pudendal nerve terminal motor latency before and after straining, and 1 and 4 minutes later. Top, patients with abnormal perineal descent; bottom, patients without abnormal descent (From Lubowski et al.,[110] with permission.)

patients with or without evidence of obstructed defecation on proctography.[130] The same group also found no correlation between perineal descent and pudendal nerve damage in a large group of patients with constipation, incontinence, or chronic pelvic pain.[131]

Rogers et al.[113] found normal pudendal latencies in patients with diabetes and normal continence. However Pinna Pintor et al.[132] found prolonged pudendal latencies in diabetic patients with or without incontinence.

Pudendal latencies should always be measured bilaterally because nerve damage is sometimes asymmetric.[109,133,134] Pudendal latency increases with age[101,135] and in normal subjects is higher in men than women.[101] In patients with constipation no sex differences were found.[136] Mean pudendal latencies in normal subjects are shown in Table 8-1.

Table 8-1. Mean Pudendal Nerve Motor Latencies in Normal Subjects. Standard Deviation or Range Is Shown in Brackets

No.	Mean Age (yr)	Motor Latency (msec)	Reference
40	50	2.1 (0.2)	86
11	58	1.95 (1.7–2.25)	113
15	51	Right 1.9 (0.2) Left 2.0 (0.2)	97

Practical Application of Pudendal Nerve Studies

In the clinical assessment of individual patients, pudendal nerve studies are of particular value in patients with fecal incontinence. In other conditions such as solitary rectal ulcer syndrome and hemorrhoids pudendal nerve studies have established the link between straining at stool and nerve damage, but measurement of pudendal latency usually does not directly influence the management of an individual patient. For example, a patient with solitary rectal ulcer syndrome, normal continence, and perineal descent would be advised to avoid straining at stool whether the pudendal latencies were prolonged or normal. However, in patients with fecal incontinence the pudendal latencies, taken in conjunction with the results of other tests, may determine whether surgical treatment is required, and which procedure is most suitable. The results of postanal repair for incontinence have varied in the literature and this may be accounted for in part by patient selection. Evidence of pudendal neuropathy is essential if a patient is to be considered for this procedure. In a large study pudendal nerve terminal motor latency was the only preoperative variable that correlated with long-term outcome of postanal repair.[120]

Perineal Nerve Motor Latency

The perineal branch of the pudendal nerve innervates the striated urethral sphincter muscle. The course of the perineal nerve to the urethral sphincter is longer than that of the inferior rectal

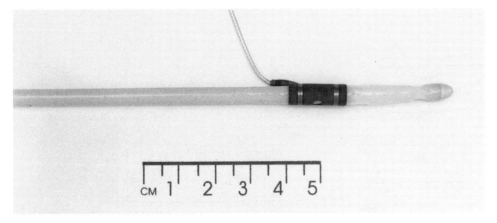

Figure 8-13. Bipolar ring electrode (Dantec, Denmark) for recording perineal nerve latency, and for mucosal electrosensitivity testing.

nerve to the external anal sphincter and hence the perineal motor latency is longer than pudendal latency. The perineal nerve latency is measured in the same way as pudendal latency using the intrarectal nerve-stimulating device but the muscle response is recorded in the urethral sphincter, using a bipolar ring electrode mounted on a urethral Foley catheter (Fig. 8-13). It is preferable to use the smaller diameter electrode (Dantec 21L 10, Skoulunde, Denmark) which fits a correspondingly smaller Foley catheter. The electrode is positioned just proximal to the catheter balloon, and when inserted into the bladder, the catheter with inflated balloon should be drawn down and held in this position so that the recording electrodes remain correctly positioned.

The mean perineal latency in normal control female subjects is shown in Table 8-2. The perineal motor latency is increased in patients with neurogenic fecal incontinence[121] and patients with urinary stress incontinence.[121,137,138] The latency is greater in those patients with double incontinence than those with fecal or urinary incontinence alone. There is a significant correlation between perineal latency and pudendal latency in patients with fecal incontinence and double incontinence.[121]

Clinical Application of Tests of Perineal Latency

Perineal nerve latency is a useful measure of denervation in patients with urinary stress incontinence. However, clinicians investigating and treating patients with this condition have not

Table 8-2. Mean Perineal Nerve Motor Latency in Normal Subjects and Patients With Fecal or Urinary Incontinence. Standard Deviation in Brackets.

	No.	Motor Latency (msec)	Reference
Normal controls	20	2.4 (0.2)	223
Normal controls	40	2.1 (0.3)	138
Fecal incontinence	20	3.2 (0.6)	223
Double incontinence	20	4.3 (1.6)	223
Stress urinary incontinence	34	2.8 (0.4)	138
Urinary incontinence plus genital prolapse	42	3.0 (0.5)	138

widely embraced the test, relying mainly on the results of urodynamic studies. Similarly, perineal latency has not been a popular test in most laboratories investigating patients with anorectal incontinence. It is more difficult and time consuming to measure perineal latency than pudendal latency and there is also the theoretical risk of introducing urinary sepsis despite aseptic techniques. Perineal latency has therefore remained a research tool in most laboratories.

Spinal Stimulation

The majority of patients with neurogenic incontinence and other pelvic floor conditions associated with straining at stool have damage to the pudendal nerves distal to the ischial spine. The nerves proximal to the ischial spines may also be subject to injury, from a variety of causes. It has been established that in patients with neurogenic fecal and urinary incontinence there is damage to the external anal sphincter and also the puborectalis and levator ani muscles.[138,139] Because the nerve supply to the puborectalis and levators is almost entirely from direct pelvic nerves, it follows that these nerves have been injured. The mechanism of this nerve injury has not been clearly identified. It has been assumed that they are not subject to the same stretch injury as the pudendal nerves distal to the ischial spines. In parous women direct pressure of the fetal head on the nerves during the second stage of labor may cause nerve damage.[107] Other proximal nerve lesions are considered as supranuclear or infranuclear, depending on their relation to the Onuf nucleus.[140] Infranuclear (lower motor neurone) lesions result from damage to the sacral nerve roots in the pelvis or within the cauda equina.

Conditions in the pelvis are primary tumors or cysts. Cauda equina disease results from sacral spondylosis, disc prolapse, trauma, or intraspinal neoplasms.

Transcutaneous stimulation of the cauda equina over the lumbar spine measures conduction along the cauda equina, the sacral plexus, and the branches arising from the plexus (Fig. 8-14). Damage to the nerves at any of these points will result in slowing of conduction. The injury may be regarded as occurring in: (1) the cauda equina; (2) the pelvis, affecting the sacral plexus and the direct branches innervating the levator ani; or (3) the pudendal nerves distal to the ischial spines.

The evoked response can be measured at three sites: the pu-

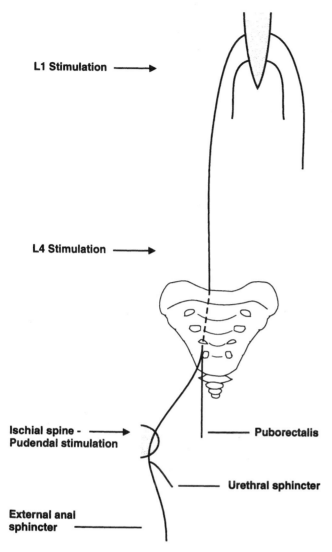

L1 Stimulation →

L4 Stimulation →

Ischial spine - →
Pudendal stimulation

Puborectalis

Urethral sphincter

External anal
sphincter

Figure 8-14. Position of spinal stimulation, showing L1 and L4 stimulation at the proximal and distal ends of the cauda equina. (Adapted from Swash,[92] with permission.)

borectalis muscle, external sphincter, or urethral sphincter (Fig. 8-15). If there is a stretch-induced injury to the pudendal nerves then conduction time from the spinal cord to the external sphincter (spinal latency) will be prolonged, as will pudendal nerve terminal motor latency. If the injury is above the ischial spine level then the spinal latency will be prolonged and the pudendal latency will be normal. A spinal latency ratio (SLR) is calculated to determine whether the abnormality lies within the cauda equina or beyond that site:

$$ \text{SLR} = \frac{\text{Latency when stimulating at L1 level}}{\text{Latency when stimulating at L4 level}} $$

If the abnormality lies distal to the cauda equina then the latency from both sites will be prolonged and SLR is constant. If the abnormality is within the cauda equina then only the L1 latency will be prolonged as the SLR will be increased. Normal values of spinal latency and SLR are given in Table 8-3.

Technique of Spinal Stimulation

The test is based on the technique of Merton et al.[141] for transcutaneous cortical stimulation, using a high-voltage low-impedance stimulator (Digitimer, Hertfordshire, UK). The patient is placed in the left lateral position and is connected to a ground electrode. Markings are placed on the skin at the L1 and L4 levels in the midline of the lower back, and these areas are shaved and cleaned. A single impulse of 1500 V, 0.5-msec duration, decaying with a precise time constant of 50 μsec is delivered through two small pad electrodes soaked in saline (Fig. 8-16). The cathode is positioned for stimulation at the L1 mark, with the anode placed cranially. An initial stimulus of about 200 V is delivered after warning the patient about a ''thump'' on the back. The stimulus is then increased to 1500 V. The evoked response may be recorded in the puborectalis muscle using two electrode plates mounted on the tip of a finger stall. However, because of difficulties sterilizing this device, it

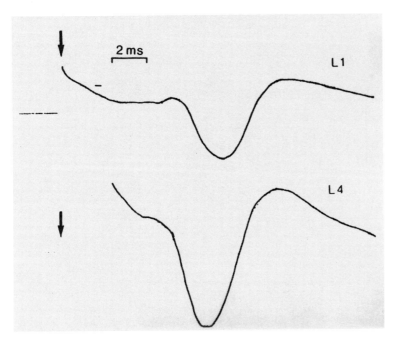

Figure 8-15. Spinal stimulation latencies. Arrows indicate onset of stimulus. Top, L1 stimulation; bottom, L4 stimulation showing shorter latency than L1. (From Lubowski et al.,[140] with permission.)

is preferable to record from the external anal sphincter using the recording electrodes of the St. Mark's pudendal stimulator (Fig. 8-10).

Practical Application of Spinal Stimulation

Spinal latencies are increased in patients with fecal incontinence.[139] In the majority of patients this is due to slowed conduction in the distal part of the pudendal nerves but in a small number of patients it is due to a cauda equina abnormality. Therefore spinal stimulation should be carried out in patients with incontinence when there is no obvious predisposing cause. These patients include men or nulliparous women with incontinence without rectal prolapse or evidence of direct sphincter injury on EMG or endoanal ultrasound. Spinal stimulation is also indicated in patients with suspected spinal disease causing other symptoms such as perineal pain. An abnormal spinal latency provides supportive evidence for a diagnosis of spinal disease, particularly when computed tomography (CT) myelography shows equivocal evidence of spinal stenosis or arachnoiditis.[142]

Table 8-3. Transcutaneous Spinal Stimulation Latencies in Normal Subjects

Recording Site	L1 Latency (msec)	L4 Latency (msec)	SLR
External anal sphincter	5.5 (0.4)	4.4 (0.4)	1.33 (0.1)
Puborectalis	4.8 (0.4)	3.7 (0.4)	1.3 (0.1)

Abbreviation: SLR, spinal latency ratio.
(From Snooks et al.,[114,139] with permission.)

Electromyography

History of Electromyography

EMG has been used for over half a century in the study of peripheral skeletal muscle activity. Although electrical impulses were recorded in contracting muscle in the early part of the

Figure 8-16. Transcutaneous electrode for spinal stimulation (Digitimer, Hertfordshire, UK).

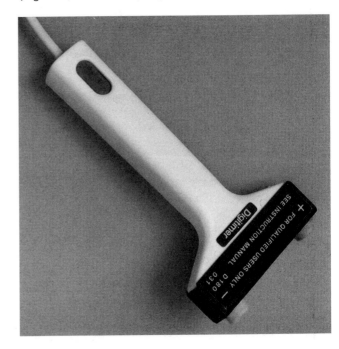

century, it was not until Adrian and Bronk[143] developed the concentric needle electrode that the technique was applied to clinical investigation. The motor unit was studied in animals[144–146] and concentric needle EMG was then used widely in the investigation of muscle disorders.[147] Difficulties in the investigation of muscle fatigue when using conventional concentric needle electrodes led to the development of an electrode with a much smaller recording surface, and hence the technique of single-fiber EMG was established.[148–151] Floyd and Walls[152] and Kawakami[153] recorded electromyographic activity in the external anal sphincter, but only more recently has EMG been applied in the investigation of disorders affecting the pelvic floor muscles, using single-fiber EMG[49,154] and concentric needle EMG techniques.[155]

The Motor Unit

Depolarization of the muscle fiber membrane leads to the muscle action potential, which passes along the length of the muscle fiber. This depolarization is initiated by a nerve impulse that arrives at the motor end plate and releases acetylcholine. The resting membrane potential of the muscle fiber is of the order of 80 mV, and the action potential of the changing electrical field during depolarization of the muscle is recorded outside the muscle fiber.

The motor unit consists of the axon, its branches, and the muscle fibers innervated by these branches. The number of muscle fibers in a motor unit varies enormously, depending on the size and complexity of function of the muscle; for example, the extraocular muscle has 9 to 10 fibers, the small muscles of the hand have 200 to 350 fibers, while the gastrocnemius has 1,900 fibers.[156–159] The precise number of fibers in the external anal sphincter is still uncertain. In human muscle there are two types of fibers, type I and type II. Peripheral limb muscles contain predominantly type II fibers, whereas the external anal sphincter and pelvic floor muscles have a predominance of type I fibers. All muscle fibers in a motor unit belong to one or the other type. The muscle fibers of an individual unit are scattered randomly through an area of the muscle.[92,160–162] Electrical activity generated by contraction of the muscle fibers of a motor unit is recorded as the motor unit action potential (MUP).

Electromyographic Recording

EMG of the external anal sphincter (EAS), puborectalis, and pubococcygeus is carried out for two basic purposes: overall qualitative activity of the whole muscle or part of the muscle may be recorded; or denervation and reinnervation of the muscle may be tested. The former is carried out using surface electrodes or a concentric needle electrode, and the latter using either concentric or single-fiber EMG electrodes.

Concentric Needle Electromyography

The concentric needle electrode is a bipolar electrode, consisting of a platinum wire 0.1 mm in diameter insulated in resin within a stainless steel cannula. The recording surface is 0.5 × 0.15 mm in size at the bare tip of the wire (Fig. 8-17).

Motor Unit Potential Duration

The normal motor unit action potentials are biphasic (one negative peak, one positive peak) with a recovery period. Action potentials become polyphasic when the muscle is denervated, and hence the MUP duration is prolonged. The mean motor unit potential duration (MUPD) in normal subjects in the anal and urinary sphincter muscle is 5 to 7.5 msec.[163] Bartolo et al.[155] found that the MUPD in the external anal sphincter increases with age. In neurogenic incontinence with denervation of the puborectalis muscle MUPD is increased.[156]

Technique of Recording Motor Unit Potential Duration

The mean of 10 separate motor unit potentials is calculated, using at least two passes of the needle into the external sphincter muscle, one on each side. Filter settings on the EMG machine are low frequency 20 Hz, high frequency 5 KHz. The sweep speed of the trace is set at 2 msec/div in order to separate the individual motor units for analysis.

Sphincter Mapping

Assessment of muscle activity using a concentric needle provides accurate information about the presence of functional muscle in a patient with a suspected sphincter defect. The amount of muscle activity can be quantified using rectified EMG activity[92] but this has not been shown to be superior to nonquantitative assessment when determining the need for surgical repair of an anal sphincter defect. EMG localizes a

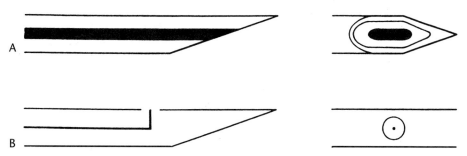

Figure 8-17. Electromyography needle electrodes. (**A**) Concentric electrode with insulated wire recording from the tip of the needle. (**B**) Single-fiber electrode with wire terminating on side of needle. (Adapted from Stalberg and Trontelj,[223] with permission.)

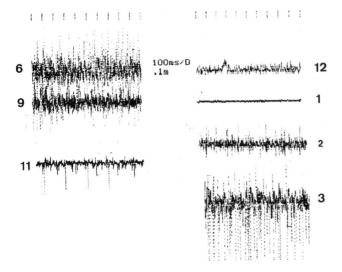

Figure 8-18. Concentric electromyography sphincter mapping in the external anal sphincter. The numbers represent the position in the sphincter, 12 o'clock anterior. Absence of action potentials between 12 o'clock and 1 o'clock demonstrates an anterior sphincter defect.

sphincter defect accurately in the majority of cases.[164] An operator with experience in the technique is essential.

Technique of Sphincter Mapping

The patient is placed in the supine left lateral position. It is sometimes necessary to have an assistant to adequately retract the upper buttock. A digital examination is carried out to determine the site of a suspected sphincter defect. Needle EMG is sometimes a painful test, and the number of passes of the needle should be minimized. The first pass should be into apparently healthy muscle at the edge of the sphincter defect. The next is into the defect adjacent to the healthy muscle, and then subsequent passes map the extent of the defect until healthy muscle is recorded on the opposite side of the defect (Fig. 8-18). In some cases it may be necessary to map the sphincter circumferentially to locate the sphincter defect. Local anesthetic is not used because it may interfere with recording. On rare occasions it is necessary to carry out the test under general anesthesia. Because overall muscle activity is being assessed, it is not necessary to separate individual motor unit potentials. Instead, the sweep of the trace is set at a slow rate of 100 msec/div in order to gain a picture of global muscle contraction. Filter settings are 20 Hz, 5 KHz.

Concentric Electromyography in Obstructed Defecation

The EAS and puborectalis are in a state of slight continuous activity at rest and even during sleep.[152,153,165–166] Activity increases as intra-abdominal pressure is increased, under control of a spinal reflex through the Onuf nucleus. During defecation, activity in the puborectalis muscle is inhibited.[167] Increased EMG activity during defecation straining has been found in a variety of conditions that have in common the symptom of chronic excessive straining at stool.[128,168–170] A similar finding

is made using surface EMG electrodes mounted on an anal plug[76] or with fine wire electrodes.[73] However, the validity of this technique has been questioned because the test is carried out under somewhat unphysiologic conditions and it has been suggested that the finding of increased EMG activity may be a laboratory artifact.[171] Using a similar technique to that of Womack et al.,[73] Miller et al.[172] showed evacuation of the rectum in some patients with muscle contraction and also failed evacuation in other patients who had muscle relaxation. Increased muscle activity is observed in patients with conditions not associated with straining at stool[171] and is also found in normal subjects[173,174] (Fig. 8-19). Simultaneous ambulatory EMG and manometry carried out in patients with obstructed defecation under more physiologic conditions shows that the majority of subjects do not demonstrate the same increased muscle activity, and the incidence of paradoxic EMG activity and anismus has been overestimated.[82]

Single-Fiber Electromyography

In order to obtain more accurate information about muscle injury, it is possible to measure action potentials from individual muscle fibers. The single-fiber EMG electrode is a modification of the concentric needle electrode, consisting of a platinum wire 25 μm in diameter, insulated within a stainless steel cannula, and terminating on the side of the cannula 5 mm before the tip (Fig. 8-17). The recording surface is 25 μm in diameter.

Technique of Recording Single-Fiber Electromyography

Action potentials from distant muscle fibers have a larger proportion of low-frequency components than those from fibers nearby. Thus by reducing the low-frequency response with the appropriate filter settings, interference is reduced, allowing analysis of individual muscle action potentials. The signals are

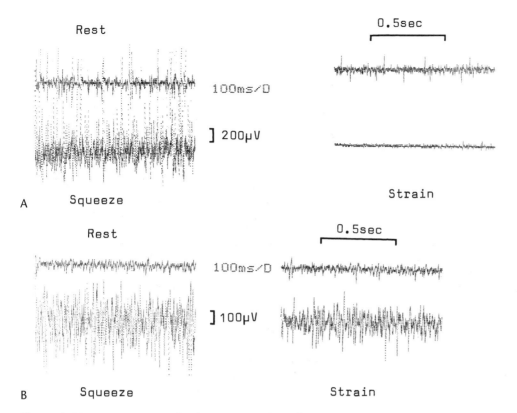

Figure 8-19. Concentric needle electromyography with tracings at rest, voluntary squeeze, and straining down. (**A**) The two top traces are taken at rest, the bottom traces during squeezing and straining. Absence of action potentials in the muscle during straining indicates muscle relaxation. (**B**) Increased activity in the muscle during straining indicates muscle contraction.

amplified by the EMG machine and a trigger-delay line is used, with sweep speed 2 msec/div. Most of the spectral energy of single action potentials is found between 100 Hz and 10 KHz with a peak value of 1.61 (SD 0.3) KHz.[175] Filter settings used are therefore low frequency 500 Hz, high frequency 2 KHz. All action potentials greater than 100 μV are accepted, and the trigger on the EMG machine is set to record only action potentials of at least this magnitude. Two to four passes of the EMG needle are made into the external sphincter muscle and 20 consecutive action potentials are recorded for analysis. If there is insufficient muscle activity at rest then the sphincter can be stimulated by gentle downward traction on an inflated rectal balloon. Various aspects of single-fiber recording can be analyzed, including jitter and fiber density.[176] The latter has been applied in the study of pelvic floor disorders.

Fiber Density

Axonal damage resulting in denervation of the external anal sphincter and puborectalis muscle fibers is followed by reinnervation by neighboring healthy axons. This leads to a change in the arrangement of muscle fibers, with type I and type II grouping.[83,84] These histologic changes can be quantified with single-fiber EMG by measuring muscle fiber density. The mean fiber density is calculated by counting the number of muscle fibers in a motor unit within the uptake area of the single-fiber electrode, measured at several positions.[177] This is done by finding the mean number of action potentials recorded at 20 sites. With reinnervation and fiber type grouping action potentials become polyphasic and there is therefore an increase in the mean number of spikes, leading to an increase in the fiber density (Fig. 8-20).

Clinical Relevance of Single-Fiber Electromyography

Normal fiber density in the external sphincter muscle is 1.5 (SD 0.16),[154] and fiber density greater than 2.0 indicates denervation and reinnervation of the muscle. Single-fiber EMG has been shown to be repeatable with interobserver studies.[178] Fiber density increases with age.[135] In neurogenic incontinence fiber density is increased.[22,49,116,121,154,179] It is also increased in patients with rectal prolapse and incontinence,[49] and in patients with urinary stress incontinence.[138] Fiber density is increased in other conditions in which straining at stool produces pudendal nerve damage, including solitary rectal ulcer syndrome,[128] hemorrhoids,[125] and symptomatic uterovaginal prolapse.[97] Diabetic patients with normal continence have raised fiber density in the external anal sphincter,[113] possibly reflecting a generalized metabolic change affecting all muscle because similar abnormalities on single-fiber EMG have been shown in other muscles.[180]

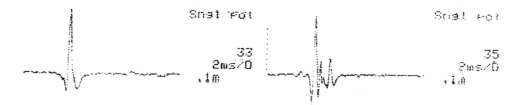

Figure 8-20. Single-fiber electromyography in the external anal sphincter, in a patient with sphincter denervation. Left, normal monophasic action potential; right, prolonged polyphasic action potential.

The most sensitive measure of limb muscle denervation (and reinnervation) is single-fibre EMG and it is often stated that this also applies to the anal sphincter. The degree of nerve and muscle damage has, however, not been correlated quantitatively with severity of symptoms such as fecal incontinence. Some studies have shown raised fiber density but normal mean pudendal latencies in patients with pelvic floor abnormalities.[181] In these same patients a significant relationship between fiber density and pudendal latency was present, and these observations taken together may suggest that single-fiber EMG is a more sensitive test.

In clinical investigation we do not use single-fiber EMG in every patient with fecal incontinence. If a patient is thought to have neurogenic incontinence and this is confirmed with pudendal nerve terminal motor latency studies and supported by findings on anal mucosal electrosensitivity, then single-fiber EMG is not done. If pudendal nerve studies (motor and sensory) are equivocal then single-fiber EMG is carried out.

Internal Sphincter Electromyography

Electrical activity in the internal sphincter can be recorded using a concentric needle or a small surface electrode.[22] Specific filter settings are needed to detect internal sphincter slow wave activity and exclude external sphincter artifact: 0.05 Hz and 2 KHz, with sweep speed 500 msec/cm. Slow wave electrical activity corresponding to slow pressure waves is observed. The electrical activity is absent in patients with severe neurogenic incontinence.[22]

The best method of recording internal sphincter EMG is using an ambulatory technique with fine wire electrodes. Using this technique in patients following abdominal rectopexy for rectal prolapse, Farouk et al.[52] showed a return of internal sphincter EMG corresponding with an improvement in resting anal pressure. This technique promises to provide useful information about internal anal sphincter function, but is unlikely to become a routine clinical test.

ANAL AND RECTAL SENSATION

Anal Sensation

The anal mucosa is sensitive to pain, touch, temperature, and movement. The upper level of pain sensation varies between 0.5 and 1.5 cm above the dentate line and usually extends slightly higher than sensation to light touch and temperature.[182] The perianal skin is innervated by free nerve endings, and the anal mucosa contains an abundance of free and organized nerve endings including Meissner's corpuscles, genital and pacinian corpuscles, Golgi bodies, and Krause end bulbs.

Anal sensation is mediated via the pudendal nerves to the S2–S4 sacral nerves. Sensory fibers also pass from the anal mucosa in the nerves to the levator ani, which arise directly from S3 and S4. Quantitative assessment of anal sensation may be carried out by testing mucosal electrosensitivity or temperature sensation. Testing for temperature involves the use of a somewhat complex system, consisting of a probe through which water of three different controlled temperatures is pumped.[183] The temperature in the probe can be rapidly increased or decreased and this change is detected by the anal mucosa. The magnitude of the temperature change reported by the patient gives a quantitative measure of mucosal sensitivity. The complexity of the technique makes it unsuitable for use in clinical studies. In 1986 Roe and colleagues[184] reported the technique of measuring anal mucosal electrosensitivity, based on the methods of measuring urethral sensation.[185,186] This test is performed quickly and easily, and is readily applied in clinical investigation.

Technique of Mucosal Electrosensitivity

The original technique involved a custom-built electrode containing two platinum wires 1 cm apart. A ring electrode is now commercially available (Dantec, Skoulunde, Denmark). The electrode is the same as that used for perineal motor latency tests although the larger diameter electrode (Dantec 21L11) is applicable. The electrode is connected to a constant current stimulator, which should have a rheostat for increments of 0.1 mA. The stimulator in most modern EMG machines is suitable for this technique. The stimulus is set at 0.1 msec and rate of 5 Hz. The test should be done following anorectal manometry, during which the functional length of the anal canal has been measured in order to place the electrosensitivity electrode correctly in the anal canal. The lubricated electrode is inserted and the current is increased from zero until a buzzing or tingling sensation is reported. This is carried out three times at each position in the upper, mid-, and lower anal canal and the mean value determined at each site.

Clinical Relevance of Anal Mucosal Electrosensitivity

Mucosal electrosensitivity testing is a useful test, taken in conjunction with pudendal nerve terminal motor latency tests in the assessment of patients with fecal incontinence. The test is reproducible.[178,184] Normal median and range of values in 20 control subjects[184] were:

Lower anal canal (mA): 4.8 (3.0–7.0)
Mid-anal canal (mA): 4.2 (2.0–6.0)
Upper anal canal (mA): 5.7 (3.3–7.3)

Patients with hemorrhoids have normal sensation in the lower canal but reduced sensation in the mid- and upper anal canal, and Roe et al.[184] postulated that this was due to prolapse of the anal cushions with accompanying prolapse of insensitive mucosa into the upper anal canal. Another explanation is that the raised sensory threshold is in keeping with the pudendal nerve damage that is known to occur in patients with hemorrhoids.[125]

Anal sensation is abnormal in patients with neurogenic fecal incontinence.[67,184] This may simply reflect the pudendal neuropathy in this condition and may not be a factor contributing independently to the incontinence. The role of anal sensation in the continence mechanism is still not clear. Although sampling of rectal contents has been said to be important,[26] anesthetizing the anal mucosa was not found to impair continence in normal subjects.[187] After restorative proctocolectomy for ulcerative colitis, although anal sensation is impaired when the anal transitional zone has been removed,[188,189] this was not found to be accompanied by impairment of continence.[189]

Rectal Sensation

The rectum is insensitive to painful stimuli but is sensitive to distension. The site for the receptors producing the sensation of rectal distension is debated. The mucosa of the anal canal is richly innervated with nerve endings, which are not found in the rectal mucosa.[182] In particular, there are no organized nerve endings in the rectum. Balloon distension of the rectum produces a "pelvic" sensation, whereas distension of the sigmoid colon produces a different visceral sensation[190] and it was suggested that "rectal" sensation was due to distension of receptors in the pelvic floor muscles.[191] This is supported by the observation that rectal-type sensation is felt after rectal excision when a balloon is distended in the colon that has been anastomosed to the anus.[63,64] Stretch receptors[192,193] and muscle spindles[92] have been identified in the pelvic floor muscles.

Technique of Testing Rectal Sensation

Rectal Balloon Distension

The patient is placed in the left lateral position. A firm catheter with a fully deflated pear-shaped party balloon is inserted so that the lower end of the balloon lies above the anorectal ring. The balloon is inflated with 10-ml volumes of air until the inflated balloon is first perceived by the patient. This is called the *rectal sensitivity threshold* (RST). The inflation is continued until the *urge to defecate* is felt. This urge becomes increasingly intense as distension continues, until pain is felt. The volume at which this becomes intolerable is called the *maximum tolerable volume* (MTV).

There is considerable variation in RST and MTV depending on the technique used. Distension with water and air are felt at similar volumes.[194] Threshold of sensation is lower with inflation of smaller incremental amounts, or with slower inflation. It is also lower with intermittent inflation compared with continuous inflation using a pump.[194] The height of the balloon in the rectum influences the sensory threshold.[45] Normal values are given in Table 8-4.

Rectal Mucosal Electrosensitivity

Electrosensitivity testing in the rectal mucosa was described by Kamm and Lennard-Jones[195] and is carried out using a similar technique to that used for testing anal mucosal electrosensitivity. A ring electrode is mounted on a Foley catheter and inserted 6 cm above the anorectal junction. A constant current stimulus of 500 μsec and 10 Hz is delivered, slowly increasing from zero in 0.5-mA increments. A sensation, described as tapping or buzzing, is reported by the patient. The procedure is performed three times and the lowest of the readings represents the sensory threshold.

Clinical Relevance of Rectal Sensation

Patients with severe slow transit constipation have reduced rectal sensation on balloon testing. Several studies have demonstrated an elevated rectal sensory threshold,[195,196] although other studies did not confirm this.[197,198] Most studies, however, have shown an elevated volume required for the sensation of call to stool.[195–198]

Patients with fecal incontinence have normal rectal sensation

Table 8-4. Rectal Sensation. Balloon Distension Volumes in Normal Subjects. Standard Deviation in Brackets

Reference		No.	M:F	Mean age (yr)	RST (ml)	Urge to Defecate (ml)	MTV (ml)
195		13	0:13	13	16.9 (4.4)	61.6 (9.1)	231.9 (17)
41		18	9:9	29	17 (8)	173 (64)	
41		18	9:9	72	17 (9)	151 (61)	
37	Bolus	12	12:0	22	12 (1)	75 (10)	110 (10)
	Continuous 20 ml/min				20 (5)	128 (10)	178 (20)
	Continuous 100 ml/min				43 (10)	167 (7)	230 (21)

Abbreviations: RST, rectal sensitivity threshold; MTV, maximum tolerable volume.

on balloon testing.[67] A small subgroup of men with incontinence and normal anal sphincter function have reduced rectal sensation on balloon distension testing and incontinence seems to result from internal sphincter relaxation at a volume of rectal distension less than the rectal sensory threshold.[199]

Kamm and Lennard-Jones[195] found reduced rectal mucosal electrosensitivity in patients with idiopathic constipation and concluded that a rectal sensory neuropathy was present. They also found reduced rectal mucosal electrosensitivity after abdominal rectopexy when the lateral ligaments had been divided but not when the ligaments were intact,[129] and this supported the hypothesis that denervation of the rectum might be the cause of abnormal defecation after rectopexy. The interpretation of rectal mucosal electrosensitivity tests have, however, been questioned, because marked circumferential variation in sensitivity threshold, as well as the presence of a normal ''rectal'' sensation observed in patients after rectal excision and coloanal or ileoanal anastomosis, suggests that the test may be measuring sensation in the somatic pelvic floor muscles rather than the rectal mucosa.[200] This test may prove to be useful but needs further evaluation.

RECTAL BALLOON EXPULSION

Expulsion of an inflated balloon from the rectum has been used as a means of testing rectal evacuation. Preston and Lennard-Jones[71] suggested that constipation may be due to a disorder of defecation in addition to an abnormality of colon transit and showed that some patients with chronic constipation were unable to expel a rectal balloon while normal subjects were able to do so. They used the term *anismus* to describe an apparent disorder caused by failure of the pelvic floor muscles to relax during defecation. There have been many subsequent reports of patients with symptoms of obstructed defecation being unable to expel a rectal balloon.[224,225] The test should be interpreted with caution since it is unphysiologic, particularly when carried out with the patient in the lateral position. A recent study found that both normal subjects and patients with anismus were unable to expel a rectal balloon.[226] Unlike other static tests of anorectal function such as manometry or electromyography that measure intrinsic muscle strength or neuromuscular function, balloon expulsion attempts to simulate defecation, which is a complex dynamic process.

The test is carried out with the patient in the left lateral position. A pear-shaped party balloon attached to a firm plastic tube is inserted into the rectum and inflated with 50 ml water. Slight traction may be applied to draw the balloon down to the pelvic floor and the subject is asked to bear down to expel the balloon. Variations of the technique include inflating the balloon to the volume first felt or to that producing the urge to defecate; applying weights over a pulley[71]; or carrying out the test with the patient in the seated position.

MEASUREMENT OF COLONIC TRANSIT

Disorders of colonic transit are frequently encountered in clinical practice. Diarrhea of colonic origin is usually associated with a condition affecting the colonic mucosa and is diagnosed colonoscopically. However, constipation that is not due to mechanical obstruction of the lumen and does not have an extracolonic cause may be associated with an abnormality of colonic motility. Over the past two decades there has been an increasing interest in the pathophysiology of severe constipation, and the importance of evaluation of colonic transit in these patients has become apparent, particularly if surgical treatment is being considered.

Colonic transit was initially investigated using barium[201,202] but this does not provide a quantitative measure of colonic activity because only the position of the head of barium can be accurately recorded. In addition, barium itself can alter colonic transit.[203] The two methods that are currently used for assessment of colonic transit are radiopaque markers, and radioisotopes.

Radiopaque Marker Studies

Whole Gut Transit Time

Hinton et al.[204] described a method for measuring whole gut transit. Twenty markers are taken orally, and Hinton et al. found that 14 (80%) have passed by day 5. This may be assessed by collecting the stool for radiography, but a single abdominal radiograph taken on day 5 is a much simpler method.

If whole gut transit is normal then colonic transit time can assumed to be normal in the majority of cases because colonic transit time forms a large percentage of whole gut transit time. This is therefore a useful screening test of colonic transit. An abnormal test does not differentiate abnormal gastric emptying or slow small bowel transit from slow colonic transit, and to do so requires multiple radiographs to be taken, which is undesirable. A more detailed analysis of colonic transit is obtained by measuring segmental transit.

Segmental Colonic Transit

Segmental colonic transit can be measured by taking serial radiographs for several days after ingestion of 20 markers.[205,206] The colon is arbitrarily divided into sections on the abdominal

Table 8-5. Mean Segmental Colonic Transit Time in Hours, in Healthy Subjects. Standard Deviation in Brackets.

	Right Colon	Left Colon	Rectosigmoid	Total Colon
Male (n = 34)	8.9 (1.1)	8.7 (1.5)	13.0 (1.7)	30.7 (3.0)
Female (n = 39)	13.3 (1.6)	13.7 (2.1)	11.8 (1.6)	38.8 (2.9)

(From Metcalf et al.,[207] with permission.)

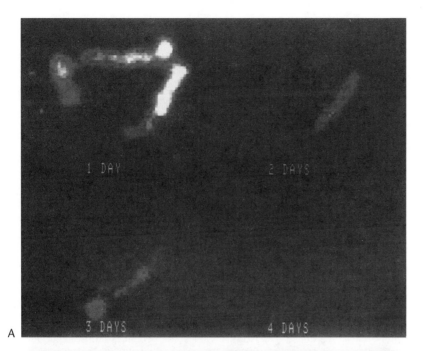

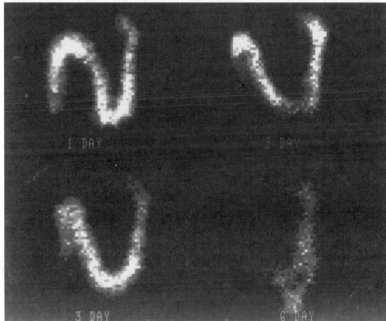

Figure 8-21. Radioisotope colon transit study.
(**A**) Normal subject showing transit to the rectum by day 1, and minimal retention of isotope in the left colon on day 2. (**B**) Patient with severe idiopathic constipation showing retention of isotope throughout the colon on day 3, and retention in the left colon up to day 6. The position of the transverse colon in the lower abdomen in this patient illustrates the difficulty that may occur with interpreting the site of radiopaque markers in the colon.

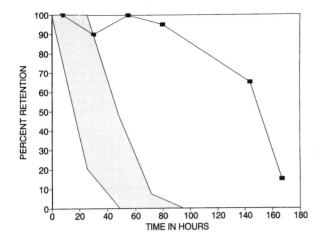

Figure 8-22. Plot of total percent isotope retention against time in a patient with constipation. There is markedly increased retention of isotope. Normal values[216] are represented in the shaded area.

radiograph: right colon (to the right of the vertebral column and above a line joining L5 vertebra to the pelvic brim), left colon (to the left and above a line joining L5 to the left anterior superior iliac spine), and sigmoid/rectum (below the latter line). Radiation exposure is substantially reduced by taking 20 markers per day on three successive days and obtaining a single abdominal radiograph on day 4.[207] The test assumes that colon transit is similar on each of the days, and although colon transit measured in this way correlates with the sequential radiograph technique, the test can be further refined by assessing daily transit after ingesting markers of different shape on the 3 days. Segmental colonic transit times are shown in Table 8-5.

Radioisotope Scintigraphy

An alternative to radiopaque markers is an isotope that emits gamma radiation. With this technique the colon can be imaged as frequently as necessary without excessive exposure to radiation. Initial techniques of delivery of isotope involved intuba-

tion of the cecum to instill isotope directly.[208–210] An alternative method that avoided nasocecal or colonoscopic intubation used isotope placed within capsules that dissolved in the terminal ileum.[211] These techniques are not readily used in the routine clinical investigation of patients.

Malagelada et al.[212] developed a technique to study small intestinal transit in a dog model using orally ingested ^{131}I bound to cellulose, and because it was difficult to define the precise position of isotope in the small bowel, they used entry into the cecum as a measure of small bowel exit time. The colon is well visualized with this technique, and we adapted this to study colon transit, initially using orally ingested ^{131}I bound to cellulose[213] and later with In-III-DTPA,[214] which is less expensive and easier to prepare. Using this technique the colon can be accurately divided into segments for analysis (Fig. 8-21). Segmental transit is calculated by measuring percent isotope retained in the right colon (arbitrarily defined to midtransverse colon), left colon, and sigmoid/rectum, or by calculating the position of the midpoint of the isotope column (mean activity position).[214,215] The percent isotope retention is a particularly simple measure to use and is readily applied in clinical practice (Fig. 8-22) Normal values for percent isotope retention are shown in Table 8-6. The test is reproducible.[216] Transit time is significantly faster in males than females but does not change significantly with age.[216]

Clinical Relevance

In clinical practice radioisotope studies are more time consuming for the patient than radiopaque marker studies because it is necessary to visit the nuclear medicine department on successive days for scanning. Nevertheless, we find the study is readily accepted by patients with severe constipation and it is used routinely in our department.

Patients with severe constipation should be fully assessed with anorectal physiologic studies and colon transit studies in order to plan management.[217,218] It is important to distinguish normal transit constipation (i.e., constipation-predominant irritable bowel syndrome) from slow transit constipation. An appro-

Table 8-6. Mean Total and Segmental Percent Colonic Retention of [131]I. Standard Deviation in Brackets.

	Right Colon	Left Colon	Rectosigmoid	Total Colon
Normal Subjects				
24 hr	16 (7)	26 (17)	15 (9)	48 (28)
48 hr	3 (3)	5 (5)	6 (7)	11 (11)
72 hr	0.8 (1)	1 (2)	0.5 (0.5)	2 (4)
96 hr	0.2 (0.6)	0.1 (0.3)	0	0.3 (0.9)
Patients With Severe Idiopathic Constipation				
24 hr	37 (19)	37 (16)	18 (13)	84 (23)
48 hr	18 (10)	33 (24)	22 (20)	63 (28)
72 hr	9 (5)	18 (20)	19 (18)	43 (28)
96 hr	4 (3)	13 (15)	16 (15)	30 (25)

(From Smart et al.,[214] with permission.)

priate laxative regimen can be given, and patients can be selected for biofeedback. It is essential to have accurate information about colonic transit before considering surgery in a patient with severe constipation, and it is satisfactory to use radiopaque markers[217,219–221] or radioisotopes[222] for this purpose. Outcome of subtotal colectomy is dependent on careful patient selection.

REFERENCES

1. Gibbons CP, Bannister JJ, Trowbridge GA, Read NW (1986) An analysis of anal sphincter pressure and anal compliance in normal subjects. Int J Colorectal Dis 1:231–237
2. Duthie HL, Watts JM (1965) Contribution of the external anal sphincter to the pressure zone in the anal canal. Gut 6: 64–68
3. Gutierrez JG, Oliai A, Chey WY (1975) Manometric profile of the internal anal sphincter in man. Gastroenterology 68: 907
4. Akervall S, Fasth S, Nordgren S et al (1988) Manovolumetry—a new method for investigation of anorectal function. Gut 29:614–623
5. Schuster MM, Hookman P, Hendrix TR, Mendeloff AI (1965) Simultaneous manometric recording of internal and external anal sphincter reflexes. Bull Johns Hopkins Hosp 116:79–88
6. Orrom WJ, Wong WD, Rothenberger DA, Jensen LL (1990) Evaluation of an air-filled microballoon and mini-transducer in the clinical practice of anorectal manometry. Dis Colon Rectum 33:594–597
7. Miller R, Bartolo DCC, James D, Mortensen NJMcC (1989) Air-filled microballoon manometry for use in anorectal physiology. Br J Surg 76:72–75
8. Wankling WJ, Brown BH, Collins CD, Duthie HL (1968) Basal electrical activity in the anal canal in man. Gut 9: 457–460
9. Roberts JP, Williams NS (1992) The role and technique of ambulatory manometry. Bailliere's Clin Gastroenterol 6: 163–178
10. Schouten WR, van Vroonhoven TJ (1983) A simple method of anorectal manometry. Dis Colon Rectum 26:721–724
11. Miller R, Bartolo DCC, Roe AM, Mortensen NJ (1988) Assessment of microtransducers in anorectal manometry. Br J Surg 75:40–43
12. Felt-Bersma RJF, Klinkenberg-Knol EC, Meuwissen SGM (1988) Investigation of anorectal function. Br J Surg 75: 53–55
13. Hallan RI, Marzouk DEMM, Waldron DJ et al (1989) Comparison of digital and manometric assessment of anal sphincter function. Br J Surg 76:973–976
14. Frenckner B, von Euler C (1975) Influence of pudendal block on the function of the anal sphincters. Gut 16:482–489
15. Bannister JJ, Read NW, Donnelly C, Sun WM (1989) External and internal anal sphincter responses to rectal distension in normal subjects and in patients with idiopathic faecal incontinence. Br J Surg 76:617–621
16. Lestar B, Penninckx F, Kerremans R (1989) The composition of anal basal pressure. An in vivo and in vitro study in man. Int J Colorectal Dis 4:118–122
17. Gutierrez JG, Shah AN (1975) Autonomic control of the internal anal sphincter in man. pp. 363–373. In von Trappen G (ed): International Symposium of Gastrointestinal Motility. Typoff Press, Leuven, Belgium
18. Monges HO, Salducci J, Naudy B et al (1980) The electrical activity of the internal anal sphincter: a comparative study in man and in cats. pp. 495–501. In Christensen J (ed): Gastrointestinal Motility. Lippincott-Raven, Philadelphia
19. Kerremans R (1969) Morphological and Physiological Aspects of Anal Continence and Defaecation. Editions Arscia, Brussels
20. Hancock BD, Smith K (1975) The internal sphincter and Lord's procedure for haemorrhoids. Br J Surg 62:833–866
21. Haynes WG, Read NW (1982) Anorectal activity in man during rectal infusion of saline: a dynamic assessment of the anal continence mechanism. J Physiol 330:45–46
22. Lubowski DZ, Nicholls RJ, Burleigh DE, Swash M (1988) Internal anal sphincter in neurogenic fecal incontinence. Gastroenterology 95:997–1002
23. Miller R, Lewis GT, Bartolo DCC et al (1988) Sensory discrimination and dynamic activity in the anorectum: evidence using a new ambulatory technique. Br J Surg 75:1003–1007
24. Miller R, Bartolo DCC, Cervero F, Mortensen NJMcC (1988) Anorectal sampling: a comparison of normal and incontinent patients. Br J Surg 75:44–47
25. Kumar D, Williams NS, Waldron D, Wingate DL (1989) Prolonged manometric recording of anorectal motor activity in ambulant human subjects: evidence of periodic activity. Gut 30:1007–1011
26. Duthie HL, Bennett RC (1963) The relations of sensation in the anal canal to the functional anal sphincter: a possible factor in anal continence. Gut 4:179–182
27. Denny-Brown D, Robertson EG (1935) An investigation of the nervous control of defaecation. Brain 58:256–310
28. Callaghan RP, Nixon HH (1984) Megarectum physiology observation. Arch Dis Childhood 39:153–157
29. Naudy B, Planche D, Monges B, Salducci J (1984) Relaxations of the internal anal sphincter, elicited by rectal and extrarectal distensions in man. pp. 451–458. In Roman C (ed): Gastrointestinal Motility MTP Press, London
30. Sun WM, Read NW, Miner PB et al (1990) The role of transient internal sphincter relaxation in faecal incontinence? Int J Colorectal Dis 5:31–36
31. Penninckx F, Kerremans R, Beckers J (1973) Pharmacological characteristics of the non-striated anorectal musculature in cats. Gut 14:393–398
32. Hancock BD (1976) Measurement of anal pressure and motility. Gut 17:645–651
33. Ihre T (1974) Studies on anal function in continent and incontinent patients. Scand J Gastroenterol, suppl. 9:25
34. Whitehead WE, Orr WC, Engel BT, Schuster MM (1982) External anal sphincter response to rectal distension: learned response or reflex? Psychophysiology 19:57–72
35. Hancock BD (1977) Internal sphincter and the nature of haemorrhoids. Gut 18: 651–656
36. Deutsch AA, Moshkovitz M, Nudelman I et al (1987) Anal pressure measurements in the study of hemorrhoid etiology and their relation to treatment. Dis Colon Rectum 30:855–857

37. Sun WM, Donnelly TC, Read NW, Johnson AG (1990) The hypertensive anal cushion as a cause of the high anal pressures in patients with haemorrhoids. Br J Surg 77:458–462

38. Hancock BD (1977) The internal anal sphincter and anal fissure. Br J Surg 64:92–95

39. Gibbons CP, Read NW (1986) Anal hypertonia in fissures: cause or effect? Br J Surg 73:443–445

40. McNamara MJ, Percy JP, Fielding IR (1990) A manometric study of anal fissure treated by subcutaneous lateral internal sphincterotomy. Ann Surg 211:235–238

41. Loening-Baucke V, Anuras S (1985) Effects of age and sex on anorectal manometry. Am J Gastroenterol 80:50–53

42. Sun WM, Read NW (1989) Anorectal function in normal subjects: the effect of gender. Int J Colorectal Dis 4:188–196

43. Read NW, Harford WV, Schmulen AC et al (1979) A clinical study of patients with fecal incontinence and diarhea. Gastroenterology 76:747–756

43a. Read NW, Bartolo DCC, Read MG (1984) Differences in anal function in patients with incontinence to solids and in patients with incontinence to liquids. Br J Surg 71:39–42

44. Matheson DM, Keighley M (1981) Manometric evaluation of rectal prolapse and faecal incontinence. Gut 22:126–129

45. Loening-Baucke V, Anuras S (1985) Anorectal manometry in healthy elderly subjects. J Am Geriatr Soc 32:636–639

46. Nivatvongs S, Stern HS, Fryd DS (1981) The length of the anal canal. Dis Colon Rectum 24:600–601

47. Collins CD, Brown BH, Whittaker GE, Duthie HL (1969) New method of measuring forces in the anal canal. Gut 10:160–163

48. Taylor BM, Beart RW, Phillips SF (1984) Longitudinal and radial variations of pressure in the human anal sphincter. Gastroenterology 86:693–697

49. Neill ME, Parks AG, Swash M (1981) Physiological studies of the pelvic floor in idiopathic faecal incontinence and rectal prolapse. Br J Surg 68:531–536

50. Womack NR, Morrison JFB, Williams NS (1986) The role of pelvic floor denervation in the aetiology of idiopathic faecal incontinence. Br J Surg 73:404–407

51. Deen KI, Kumar D, Williams JG et al (1993) The prevalence of anal sphincter defects in faecal incontinence: a prospective endosonic study. Gut 34:685–688

52. Farouk R, Duthie GS, Bartolo DC, MacGregor AB (1992) Restoration of continence following rectopexy for rectal prolapse and recovery of the internal anal sphincter electromyogram. Br J Surg 79:439–440

53. Swash M, Gray A, Lubowski DZ, Nicholls RJ (1988) Ultrastructural changes in internal anal sphincter in neurogenic faecal incontinence. Gut 29:1692–1698

54. Loening-Baucke V, Metcalf AM, Shirazi S (1989) Anorectal manometry in active and quiescent ulcerative colitis. Am J Gastroenterol 84:892–897

55. Gunterberg B, Kewenter J, Petersen I, Stenar B (1976) Anorectal function after major resection of the sacrum with bilateral or unilateral sacrifice of sacral nerves. Br J Surg 63:546–554

56. Frenckner B (1975) Function of the anal sphincters in spinal man. Gut 16:638–644

57. Meunier P, Mollard P (1977) Control of the internal anal sphincter (manometric study with human subjects). Pflugers Arch 370:233–239

58. Lubowski DZ, Nicholls RI, Swash M, Jordan MJ (1987) Neural control of internal anal sphincter function. Br J Surg 74:668–670

59. Gowers WR (1877) The autonomic action of the sphincter ani. Proc R Soc Med 26:77–84

60. Gaston EA (1948) The physiology of faecal incontinence. Surg Gynecol Obstet 87:280–290

61. Schuster MM, Hendrix TR, Mendeloff AI (1963) The internal anal sphincter response: manometric studies on its normal physiology, neural pathways and alteration in bowel disorders. J Clin Invest 42:196–207

62. Lawson JON, Nixon HH (1967) Anal canal pressure in the diagnosis of Hirschsprung's disease. J Pediatr Surg 2:544–552

63. Lane RHS, Parks AG (1977) Function of the anal sphincters following coloanal anastomosis. Br J Surg 64:596–599

64. Nicholls RJ, Lubowski DZ, Donaldson DR (1988) Comparison of colonic reservoir and straight coloanal reconstruction following rectal excision. Br J Surg 75:318–320

65. Brookes SJH, Lam TCF, Lubowski DZ et al (1996) Regeneration of nerves across a colonic anastomosis in the guinea-pig. J Gastroenterol Hepatol 11:29–33

66. Keighley MRB, Henry MM, Bartolo DCC, Mortensen NJMcC (1989) Anorectal physiology measurement: report of a working party. Br J Surg 76:356–357

67. Rogers J, Henry MM, Misiewicz JJ (1988) Combined sensory and motor deficit in primary neuropathic faecal incontinence. Gut 29:5–9

68. Meagher AP, Lubowski DZ, King DW (1993) The cough response of the anal sphincter. Int J Colorectal Dis 8:217–219

69. Waldron D, Kumar D, Hallan RI, Williams NS (1989) Prolonged ambulant assessment of anorectal function in patients with prolapsing hemorrhoids. Dis Colon Rectum 32:968–974

70. Miller R, Orrom WJ, Duthie G et al (1990) Ambulatory anorectal physiology in patients following restorative proctocolectomy for ulcerative colitis: comparison with normal controls. Br J Surg 77:895–897

71. Preston DM, Lennard-Jones JE (1985) Anismus in chronic constipation. Dig Dis Sci 30:413–418

72. Kuijpers HC, Bleijenberg G (1985) The spastic pelvic floor syndrome. Dis Colon Rectum 28:669–672

73. Womack NR, Williams NS, Holmfield JHM et al (1985) New method for the dynamic assessment of anorectal function in constipation. Br J Surg 69:470–472

74. Kamm MA, Hawley PR, Lennard-Jones JE (1988) Lateral puborectalis division in the management of severe constipation. Br J Surg 75:661–663

75. Hallan RI, Williams NS, Melling J (1988) Treatment of anismus in intractable constipation with Botulinum A toxin. Lancet 2:714–717

76. Bleijenberg G, Kuijpers HC (1987) Treatment of the spastic pelvic floor syndrome with biofeedback. Dis Colon Rectum 30:108–111

77. Kawimbe BM, Papachrysostomou M, Binnie NR et al (1991) Outlet obstruction constipation (anismus) managed by biofeedback. Gut 32:1175–1179

78. Fleshman JW, Dreznik Z, Meyer K et al (1992) Outpatient protocol for biofeedback therapy of pelvic floor outlet obstruction. Dis Colon Rectum 35:1–7

79. Jones PN, Lubowski DZ, Swash M, Henry MM (1987) Rela-

tion between perineal descent and pudendal nerve damage in idiopathic faecal incontinence. Int J Colorectal Dis 2:93–95

80. Duthie HL, Bartolo DCC (1992) Anismus: the cause of constipation? Results of investigation and treatment. World J Surg 16:831–835

81. Lubowski DZ, King DW (1995) Obstructed defaecation—current status of pathophysiology and management. Aust N Z J Surg 65:87–92

82. Duthie HL, Bartolo DCC, Miller R (1991) Estimation of the incidence of anismus by laboratory tests. Br J Surg 78:747

83. Beersiek F, Parks AG, Swash M (1979) Pathogenesis of anorectal incontinence: a histometric study of the anal sphincter musculature. J Neurol Sci 42:111–127

84. Parks AG, Swash M, Urich H (1977) Sphincter denervation in ano-rectal incontinence and rectal prolapse. Gut 18:656–665

85. Karulf RE, Coller JA, Bartolo DC et al (1991) Anorectal physiology testing. A survey of availability and use. Dis Colon Rectum 34:464–468

86. Kiff ES, Swash M (1984) Slowed conduction in the pudendal nerves in idiopathic (neurogenic) faecal incontinence. Br J Surg 71:614–616

87. Brindley GA (1981) Electrojaculation: its technique, neurological implications and uses. J Neurol Neurosurg Psychiatry 44:9–18

88. Henry MM, Parks AG, Swash M (1982) The pelvic floor musculature in the descending perineum syndrome. Br J Surg 69:470–472

89. Swash M, Snooks SJ, Henry MM (1985) Unifying concept of pelvic floor disorders and incontinence. J R Soc Med 78:906–911

90. Gardner E, Gray DJ, O'Rahilly R (1975) Anatomy. pp. 454–455. 4th Ed. WB Saunders, Philadelphia

91. Williams PL, Warwick R (1980) Grays Anatomy. pp. 1115–1116, 36th Ed. Churchill Livingstone, New York

92. Swash M (1992) Histopathology of pelvic floor muscles in pelvic floor disorders. pp. 176–181, 185. In Henry MM, Swash M (eds): Electromyography in Pelvic Floor Disorders. 2nd Ed. Butterworth-Heinemann, Oxford

93. Percy JP, Neill ME, Swash M, Parks AG (1981) Electrophysiological study of motor nerve supply of pelvic floor. Lancet 1:16–17 (see also Lancet, 1981, 1:999–1000)

94. Rogers J, Henry MM, Misiewicz JJ (1988) Disposable pudendal nerve stimulator: evaluation of the standard instrument and new device. Gut 29:1131–1133

95. Oettle GJ, Roe AM, Bartolo DCC, Mortensen NJMcC (1985) What is the best way of measuring perineal descent? A comparison of radiographic and clinical methods. Br J Surg 72:999–1001

96. Ambrose WL, Keighley MRB (1986) Outpatient measurement of perineal descent. Ann R Coll Surg Eng 67:306–308

97. Beevors MA, Lubowski DZ, King DW, Carlton MA (1991) Pudendal nerve damage in women with symptomatic uterovaginal prolapse. Int J Colorectal Dis 6:24–28

98. Bartolo DCC, Roe AM, Mortensen NJMcC (1986) The relationship between perineal descent and denervation of the puborectalis in continent patients. Int J Colorectal Dis 1:91–95

99. Sunderland S (1978) Nerves and Nerve Injuries. 2nd Ed. pp. 82–86. Churchill Livingstone, Edinburgh

100. Laurberg S, Swash M, Snooks SJ, Henry MM (1988) Neuro-

101. logic cause of idiopathic incontinence. Arch Neurol 45:1250–1253

101. Jameson JS, Chia YW, Kamm MA et al (1994) Effect of age, sex and parity on anorectal function. Br J Surg 81:1689–1692

102. Roig JV, Villoslada C, Lledo S et al (1995) Prevalence of pudendal neuropathy in faecal incontinence. Results of a prospective study. Dis Colon Rectum 38:952–958

103. Ho YH, Goh HS (1995) The neurophysiological significance of perineal descent. Int J Colorectal Dis 10:107–111

104. Kiff ES, Barnes P, Swash M (1984) Evidence of pudendal neuropathy in patients with perineal descent and chronic straining at stool. Gut 25:1279–1282

105. Snooks SJ, Barnes PRH, Swash M, Henry MM (1985) Damage to the innervation of the pelvic floor musculature in chronic constipation. Gastroenterology 89:977–981

106. Snooks SJ, Setchell M, Swash M, Henry MM (1984) Injury to the innervation of the pelvic floor musculature in childbirth. Lancet 2:546–550

107. Snooks SJ, Swash M, Henry MM, Setchell M (1986) Risk factors in childbirth causing damage to the pelvic floor innervation: a precursor of stress incontinence. Int J Colorectal Dis 1:20–24

108. Snooks SJ, Swash M, Mathers SE, Henry MM (1990) Effect of vaginal delivery on the pelvic floor: a 5 year follow-up. Br J Surg 77:1358–1360

109. Sultan AH, Kamm MA, Hudson CN (1994) Pudendal nerve damage during labour: prospective study before and after childbirth. Br J Obstet Gynaecol 101:22–28

110. Lubowski DZ, Swash M, Nicholls RJ, Henry MM (1988) Increase in pudendal nerve terminal motor latency with defaecation straining. Br J Surg 75:1095–1097

111. Engel AF, Kamm MA (1994) The acute effect of straining on pelvic floor neurological function. Int J Colorectal Dis 9:8–12

112. Kiff ES, Swash M (1984) Normal proximal and delayed distal conduction in the pudendal nerves of patients with idiopathic (neurogenic) faecal incontinence. J Neurol Neurosurg Psychiatry 47:820–823

113. Rogers J, Levy DM, Henry MM, Misiewicz JJ (1988) Pelvic floor neuropathy: a comparative study of diabetes mellitus and idiopathic faecal incontinence. Gut 29:756–761

114. Snooks SJ, Henry MM, Swash M (1985) Faecal incontinence due to urethral anal sphincter division in childbirth is associated with damage to the innervation of the pelvic floor musculature: a double pathology. Br J Obstet Gynaecol 92:824–828

115. Vernava AM, Longo WE, Daniel GL (1993) Pudendal neuropathy and the importance of EMG evaluation of faecal incontinence. Dis Colon Rectum 36:23–27

116. Emblem R, Dhaenens G, Stein R et al (1994) The importance of anal endosonography in the evaluation of idiopathic faecal incontinence. Dis Colon Rectum 37:42–48

117. Tjandra JJ, Sharma ER, McKirdy HC et al (1994) Anorectal physiological testing in defecatory disorders: a prospective study. Aust N Z J Surg 64:322–326

118. Tetzschner T, Sorensen M, Rasmussen OO et al (1995) Pudendal nerve damage increases the risk of faecal incontinence in women with anal sphincter rupture after childbirth. Acta Obstet Gynecol Scand 74:434–440

119. Hill J, Mumtaz A, Kiff ES (1994) Pudendal neuropathy in

patients with idiopathic faecal incontinence progresses with time. Br J Surg 81:1492–1494

120. Setti Carraro P, Kamm MA, Nicholls RJ (1994) Long-term results of postanal repair for neurogenic faecal incontinence. Br J Surg 81:140–144

121. Snooks SJ, Barnes RPH, Swash M (1984) Damage to the innervation of the voluntary anal and periurethral sphincter musculature in incontinence: an electrophysiological study. J Neurol Neurosurg Psychiatry 47:1269–1273

122. Snooks SJ, Henry MM, Swash M (1985) Abnormalities in central and peripheral nerve conduction in anorectal incontinence. J R Soc Med 78:294–300

123. Setti Carraro P, Nicholls RJ (1994) Postanal repair for faecal incontinence persisting after rectopexy. Br J Surg 81: 305–307

124. Vaccaro CA, Wexner SD, Teoh TA et al (1995) Pudendal neuropathy is not related to physiologic pelvic outlet obstruction. Dis Colon Rectum 38:630–634

125. Bruck CE, Lubowski DZ, King DW (1988) Do patients with haemorrhoids have pelvic floor denervation? Int J Colorectal Dis 3:210–214

126. Benson JT, McClellan E (1993) The effect of vaginal dissection on the pudendal nerve. Obstet Gynecol 82:387–389

127. Spence-Jones C, Kamm MA, Henry MM, Hudson CN (1994) Bowel dysfunction: a pathogenic factor in uterovaginal prolapse and urinary stress incontinence. Br J Obstet Gynaecol 101:147–152

128. Snooks SJ, Nicholls RJ, Henry MM, Swash M (1985) Electrophysiological and manometric assessment of the pelvic floor in the solitary rectal ulcer syndrome. Br J Surg 72:131–133

129. Speakman CTM, Madden MV, Nicholls RJ, Kamm MA (1991) Lateral ligament division during rectopexy causes constipation but prevents recurrence: results of a prospective randomized study. Br J Surg 78:1431–1433

130. Vaccaro CA, Cheong DM, Wexner SD et al (1995) Pudendal neuropathy in evacuatory disorders. Dis Colon Rectum 38: 166–171

131. Jorge JM, Wexner SD, Ehrempreis ED et al (1993) Does perineal descent correlate with pudendal neuropathy? Dis Colon Rectum 36:475–483

132. Pinna Pintor M, Zara GP, Falletto E et al (1994) Pudendal neuropathy in diabetic patients with faecal incontinence. Int J Colorectal Dis 9:105–109

133. Lubowski DZ, Jones PN, Swash M, Henry MM (1988) Asymmetrical pudendal nerve damage in pelvic floor disorders. Int J Colorectal Dis 3:158–160

134. Cheong DM, Vaccaro CA, Salanga VD et al (1995) Electrodiagnostic evaluation of faecal incontinence. Muscle Nerve 18: 612–619

135. Laurberg S, Swash M (1989) Effects of ageing on the anorectal sphincters and their innervation. Dis Colon Rectum 32: 734–742

136. Vaccaro CA, Cheong DM, Wexner SD et al (1994) Role of pudendal nerve terminal motor latency assessment in constipated patients. Dis Colon Rectum 37:1250–1254

137. Snooks SJ, Badenoch D, Tiptaft R, Swash M (1985) Perineal nerve damage in genuine stress urinary incontinence: an electrophysiological study. Br J Urol 57:422–426

138. Smith ARB, Hosker GL, Warrell DW (1989) The role of partial denervation of the pelvic floor in the aetiology of genitourinary prolapse and stress incontinence of urine: a neurophysiological study. Br J Obstet Gynaecol 96:24–28

139. Snooks SJ, Henry MM, Swash M (1985) Anorectal incontinence and rectal prolapse: differential assessment of the innervation to puborectalis and external anal sphincter muscles. Gut 26:470–476

140. Lubowski DZ, Swash M, Henry MM (1988) Neural mechanisms in disorders of defaecation. pp. 201–223. In Grundy D, Read NW (eds): Clinical Gastroenterology. Gastrointestinal Neurophysiology. Bailliere Tindall, WB Saunders, London

141. Merton PA, Hill DK, Morton HB, Marsden CD (1982) Scope of a technique for electrical stimulation of human brain, spinal cord, and muscle. Lancet 2:597–600

142. Swash M, Snooks SJ (1986) Slowed motor conduction in lumbosacral nerve roots in cauda equina lesions: a new diagnostic technique. J Neurol Neurosurg Psychiatry 49:808–816

143. Adrian ED, Bronk DV (1929) Discharge of impulses in motor nerve fibres. J Physio 67:119–151

144. Edds MV (1950) Collateral reinnervation of residual motor axons in partially denervated muscles. J Exp Zool 113: 517–552

145. Buchthal F, Guld CH, Rosenfalck P (1957) Multielectrode study of the territory of a motor unit. Acta Physiol Scand 39: 83–103

146. Krnjevic K, Miledi R (1958) Motor units in the rat diaphragm. J Physiol 140:427–439

147. Goodgold J, Eberstein A (1972) Electrodiagnosis of Neuromuscular Diseases. Williams & Wilkins, Baltimore

148. Ekstedt J (1964) Human single muscle fibre action potentials. Acta Physiol Scand, 61 suppl. 226:1–96

149. Ekstedt J, Haggqvist P, Stalberg E (1969) The construction of needle multi-electrodes for single fibre electromyography. Electroenceph Clin Neurophysiol 27:540–543

150. Stalberg E, Trontelj J, Schwartz MS (1976) Single muscle fibre recording of the jitter phenomenon in patients with myasthenia gravis and in members of their families. Ann NY Acad Sci 274:189–262

151. Thiele B, Stalberg E (1974) The bimodal jitter: A single fibre electromyographic finding. J Neurol Neurosurg Psychiatry 37:403–411

152. Floyd WF, Walls EW (1953) Electromyography of the sphincter ani externus in man. J Physiol 122:599–609

153. Kawakami M (1954) Electromyographic investigation of the human external sphincter muscle of anus. Jpn J Physiol 4: 1961

154. Neill ME, Swash M (1980) Increases motor unit fibre density in the external sphincter muscle in anorectal incontinence: a single fibre EMG study. J Neurol Neurosurg Psychiatry 43: 343–347

155. Bartolo DCC, Jarrett JA, Read NW (1983) The use of conventional electromyography to assess external sphincter neuropathy in man. J Neurol Neurosurg Psychiatry 46:1115–1118

156. Bartolo DCC, Jarratt JA, Read MG et al (1983) The role of partial denervation of the puborectalis in idiopathic faecal incontinence. Br J Surg 70:664–667

156a. Feinstein BB, Lindegard EN, Wohlfart G (1955) Morphological studies of motor units in normal human muscles. Acta Anat 23:127–142

157. McComas AJ, Fawcett PRW, Campbell MJ, Sica REP (1971) Electrophysiological estimation of the number of motor units

within a human muscle. J Neurol Neurosurg Psychiatry 34: 121–131

158. Ballantyne JP, Hansen S (1974) A new method for the estimation of the number of motor units in a muscle. 1. Control subjects and patients with myasthenia gravis. J Neurol Neurosurg Psychiatry 37:907–915

159. Brown WF (1972) A method for estimating the number of motor units in thenar muscles and the changes in motor unit counting with ageing. J Neurol Neurosurg Psychiatry 35: 845–852

160. Stalberg E, Ekstedt J (1973) Single fibre EMG and microphysiology of the motor unit in normal and diseased human muscle. pp. 113–129. In Desmedt JE (ed): New Developments in Electromyography and Clinical Neurophysiology. Vol. 1. Karger, Basel

161. Stalberg E, Schiller HH, Schwatrz MS (1975) Safety factor in single human motor end-plates studied in vivo with single fibre electromyography. J Neurol Neurosurg Psychiatry 38: 799–804

162. Stalberg E, Schwartz B, Thiele B, Schiller HH (1976) The normal motor unit in man. J Neurol Sci 27:291–301

163. Petersen I, Franksson EE (1955) Electromyographic study of the striated muscles of the male urethra. Br J Urol 27:148–153

164. Sultan AH, Kamm MA, Talbot IC et al (1994) Anal endosonography for identifying external sphincter defects confirmed histologically. Br J Surg 81:463–465

165. Taverner D, Smiddy FG (1959) An electromyographic study of the normal function of the external anal sphincter and pelvic diaphragm. Dis Colon Rectum 2:153–160

166. Ruskin AP, Davis JE (1969) Anal sphincter electromyography. Electroencephalog Clin Neurophysiol 27:713

167. Porter NH (1961) Physiological study of the pelvic floor in rectal prolapse. Ann R Soc Med 286:379–404

168. Lane RHS (1974) Clinical application of anorectal physiology. Proc R Soc Med 68:28–30

169. Rutter KPR (1974) Electromyographic changes in certain pelvic floor abnormalities. Proc R Soc Med 67:53–56

170. Rutter KPR, Riddell RH (1975) Solitary ulcer syndrome of the rectum. Clin Gastroenterol 4:503–530

171. Jones PN, Lubowski DZ, Swash M, Henry MM (1987) Is paradoxical contraction of puborectalis muscle of functional importance? Dis Colon Rectum 30:667–670

172. Miller R, Duthie GS, Bartolo DCC et al (1991) Anismus in patients with normal and slow transit constipation. Br J Surg 78:690–692

173. Ambrose WL, Pemberton JH, Litchy WJ, Hanson RB (1990) The myoelectric activity of the pubococcygeus muscle. Dis Colon Rectum 33:29

174. Lubowski DZ, King DW, Finlay IG (1992) Electromyography of the pubococcygeus muscles in patients with obstructed defaecation. Int J Colorectal Dis 7:184–187

175. Gath I, Stalberg E (1975) Frequency and time domain characteristics of single muscle fibre action potential. Electroencephalogr Clin Neurophysiol 39:371–376

176. Trontelj JV, Stalberg E (1995) Single fiber electromyography in studies of neuromuscular function. Adv Exp Med Biol 384: 109–119

177. Stalberg E, Thiele B (1975) Motor unit fibre density in the extensor digitorum communis muscle. J Neurol Neurosurg Psychiatry 38:874–880

178. Rogers J, Laurberg S, Misiewicz JJ et al (1989) Anorectal physiology validated: a repeatability study of the motor and sensory tests of anorectal function. Br J Surg 76:607–609

179. Fink RL, Roberts LJ, Scott M (1992) The role of manometry, electromyography and radiology in the assessment of faecal incontinence. Aust N Z J Surg 62:951–958

180. Aanestad O, Flink R (1994) Interference pattern in perineal muscles. A quantitative electromyographic study in patients with faecal incontinence. Eur J Surg 160:111–118

180a. Bril V, Werb MR, Greene DA, Sima AA (1996) Single-fiber electromyography in diabetic peripheral polyneuropathy. Muscle Nerve 19:2–9

181. Strijers RL, Felt-Bersma RJ, Visser SL, Meuwissen SG (1989) Anal sphincter EMG in anorectal disorders. Electromyogr Clin Neurophysiol 29:405–408

182. Duthie HL, Gairns FW (1960) Sensory nerve endings and sensation in the anal region of man. Br J Surg 47:585–595

183. Miller R, Bartolo DCC, Cervero F, Mortensen NJMcC (1987) Anorectal temperature sensation: a comparison of normal and incontinent patients. Br J Surg 74:511–515

184. Roe AM, Bartolo DCC, Mortensen NJMcC (1986) New method for assessment of anal sensation in various anorectal disorders. Br J Surg 73:310–312

185. Kiesewetter H (1977) Mucosal sensory threshold of urinary bladder and urethra measured electrically. Urol Int 32: 437–448

186. Powell PH, Feneley RCL (1980) The role of urethral sensation in clinical urology. Br J Urol 52:539–541

187. Read MG, Read NW (1982) Role of anorectal sensation in preserving continence. Gut 23:345–347

188. Holdsworth PJ, Johnston D (1988) Anal sensation after restorative proctocolectomy for ulcerative colitis. Br J Surg 75: 993–996

189. Keighley MRB, Winslet MC, Yoshioka K, Lightwood R (1987) Discrimination is not impaired by excision of the anal transitional zone after restorative proctocolectomy. Br J Surg 74:1118–1121

190. Goligher J, Hughes F (1951) Sensibility of the rectum and colon: its role in the mechanism of anal continence. Lancet 1:543–548

191. Scharli AF, Kiesewetter WB (1970) Defaecation and continence: some new concepts. Dis Colon Rectum 13:81–107

192. Winckler G (1958) Remarques sur la morphologie et l'innervation du muscle releveur de l'anus. Arch Anat Histol Embryol 41:77–95

193. Walls EW (1959) Recent observations on the anatomy of the anal canal. Proc R Soc Med 52:85–87

194. Sun WM, Prior A, Daly J et al (1990) Sensory and motor responses to rectal distension vary according to rate and pattern of balloon inflation. Gastroenterology 99:1008–1015

195. Kamm MA, Lennard-Jones JE (1990) Rectal mucosal electrosensitivity testing—evidence for a rectal sensory neuropathy in idiopathic constipation. Dis Colon Rectum 33:419–423

196. Baldi F, Ferrarini F, Corinaldesi R et al (1982) Function of the internal anal sphincter and rectal sensitivity in idiopathic constipation. Digestion 24:14–22

197. Keighley MRB, Shouler P (1984) Outlet syndrome: is there a surgical option. J R Soc Med 77:559–563

198. Read NW, Timms JM, Barfield LJ et al (1986) Impairment

of defaecation in young women with severe constipation. Gastroenterology 90:53–60

199. Lubowski DZ, Nicholls RJ (1988) Faecal incontinence associated with reduced pelvic sensation. Br J Surg 75:1086–1088

200. Meagher AP, Kennedy ML, Lubowski DZ (1996) Rectal mucosal electrosensitivity—what is being tested? Int J Colorectal Dis 11:29–33

201. Manousos ON, Truelove SC, Lumsden K (1967) Transit times of food in patients with diverticulosis or irritable colon syndrome and normal subjects. BMJ 760–762

202. Ritchie JA, Truelove SC, Ardran GM, Tuckey MS (1971) Propulsion and retropulsion of normal colonic contents. Dig Dis 16:697–704

203. Alvarez WC, Freedlander BL (1924) The rate of progress of food residues through the bowel. JAMA 83:576–580

204. Hinton JM, Lennard-Jones JE, Young AC (1969) A new method for studying gut transit times using radio-opaque markers. Gut 10:842–847

205. Arhan P, Devroede G, Jehannin B et al (1981) Segmental colonic transit time. Dis Colon Rectum 24:625–629

206. Martelli H, Devroede G, Arhan P et al (1978) Some parameters of large bowel motility in normal man. Gastroenterology 75:612–618

207. Metcalf AM, Phillips SF, Zinsmeister AR et al (1987) Simplified assessment of segmental colonic transit. Gastroenterology 92:40–47

208. Krevsky B, Malmund LS, D'Ercole F et al (1986) Colonic transit scintigraphy: a physiologic approach to the quantitative measurement of colonic transit in humans. Gastroenterology 91:1002–1012

209. Spiller RC, Brown ML, Phillips SF (1986) Decreased fluid intolerance, accelerated transit and abnormal motility of the human colon induced by oleic acid. Gastroenterology 91:100–107

210. Kamm MA, Lennard-Jones JE, Thompson DG et al (1988) Dynamic scanning defines a colonic defect in severe idiopathic constipation. Gut 29:1085–1092

211. Proano M, Camilleri M, Phillips SF et al (1990) Transit of solids through the human colon: regional quantification in the unprepared bowel. Am J Physiol 258:G856–862

212. Malagelada JR, Robertson JS, Brown ML et al (1984) Intestinal transit of solid and liquid components of a meal in health. Gastroenterology 87:1255–1263

213. McLean RG, Smart RC, Gaston-Parry D et al (1990) Colon transit scintigraphy in health and constipation using I-131-cellulose. J Nucl Med 31:985–989

214. Smart RC, McLean RG, Gaston-Parry D et al (1991) Comparison of oral iodine-131-cellulose and Indium-III DTPA as tracers for colon transit scintigraphy: analysis by colon activity profiles. J Nucl Med 32:1668–1674

215. van der Sijp JR, Kamm MA, Nightingale JM et al (1993) Radioisotope determination of regional colonic transit in severe constipation: comparison with radio opaque markers. Gut 34:402–408

216. McLean RG, Smart RC, Lubowski DZ et al (1992) Oral colon transit scintigraphy using indium-III DTPA: variability in healthy subjects. Int J Colorectal Dis 7:173–176

217. Pemberton JH, Rath DM, Illstrup DM (1991) Evaluation and surgical treatment of severe chronic constipation. Ann Surg 214:403–413

218. Kamm MA (1989) Constipation. Br J Hosp Med 41:244–250

219. Kamm MA, Hawley PR, Lennard-Jones JE (1988) Outcome of colectomy for severe idiopathic constipation. Gut 29:969–973

220. Wexner SD, Daniel N, Jagelman DG (1991) Colectomy for constipation: physiological investigation is the key to success. Dis Colon Rectum 34:851–856

221. Yoshioka K, Keighley MR (1989) Clinical results of colectomy for severe constipation. Br J Surg 76:600–604

222. Lubowski DZ, Chen FC, Kennedy ML, King DW (1996) Results of colectomy for severe slow transit constipation. Dis Colon Rectum 39:23–29

223. Stalberg E, Trontelj J (1979) Single Fibre Electromyography. pp. 33–86. Mirvalle Press, Surry

224. Barnes PRH, Lennard-Jones JE (1985) Balloon expulsion from the rectum in constipation of different types. Gut 26:1049–1052

225. Fleshman JW, Dreznick Z, Cohen E et al (1992) Balloon expulsion test facilitates diagnosis of pelvic floor outlet obstruction due to nonrelaxing puborectalis muscle. Dis Colon Rectum 35:1019–1025

226. Schoutten WR, Gosselink M, Briel JW et al (1995) Anismus: Fact or Fiction? Presented American Soc Colon and Rectal Surgeons Meeting, Montreal, May 9

9

MICROBIOLOGY

Douglas W. Burdon

The microbial flora of the colon and rectum is complex; it is composed predominantly of bacteria, of which 99% are anaerobic. About 60% of the fecal material within the colon consists of viable organisms that reach counts in excess of 10^{12} organisms per gram. Yeastlike fungi are also present in up to 30% of persons, and nonpathogenic parasites are sometimes found in individuals exposed to poor hygienic living conditions. Viruses occur transiently as infections and are normally absent, but the presence of bacteriophage is more common. In terms of the bacterial species present, the composition of the flora throughout the colon and rectum of an individual is essentially uniform, and qualitatively can be treated as one as far as the luminal contents are concerned. Less is known about the mucosal flora, which may vary at different sites within the large bowel. Quantitatively, however, there are significant differences between the flora of the right colon and that of the left colon and rectum, reflecting differences in the amount and type of nutrients available for bacterial growth and metabolism. The right colon is rich in undigested nutrients, enzymes, cellular debris, and mucin from the small intestine. Carbohydrate breakdown is predominant, resulting in maximal bacterial growth, with high levels of short chain fatty acids and ethanol. In the left colon the environment is more proteolytic with production of high levels of branched chain fatty acids, ammonia, and phenols, and low levels of volatile fatty acids.[1,2]

During the last decade, research into the influence of the microbial flora on health and disease has shifted from study of the composition of the flora to investigation of the metabolism and especially the end products of metabolism of individual bacterial species that are found within the colonic flora.

IMPORTANCE OF THE INTESTINAL FLORA

A knowledge of the composition of the intestinal flora is an essential prerequisite for gaining an insight into the effect of bacterial growth and metabolism on human health and any possible involvement in the pathogenesis of disease.

There are various ways in which the flora might influence host health. Although colonic digestion is not essential as an energy source in well-nourished humans, it is likely to be important for many who live in poor areas of the Third World on an inadequate diet.[1] Besides their overall nutritional value, the products of bacterial fermentation in the colon may influence the host in other ways. Short chain fatty acids produced by anaerobic bacteria provide an energy source that is utilized by colonic mucosal cells,[3] and some products of fermentation such as hydrogen, methane, and ammonia are absorbed from the colon and influence host metabolism and homeostasis. Most noninfective large bowel diseases, including cancer, diverticulosis, ulcerative colitis, and possibly irritable bowel syndrome, affect the left colon and rectosigmoid region. Differences between the left and right sides of the colon in the metabolic activity of the bacterial flora may play an important role in the pathogenesis of these disorders and explain their distribution. One of the ways in which the bacterial flora may be related to disease is the induction of carcinoma of the colon. Metabolism by particular species of bacteria might generate carcinogenic substances from dietary fats or from host secretions such as bile steroids.[4,5]

If bacteria do have a role in the etiology of large bowel disorders, this is likely to be mediated by the products of bacterial metabolism. Because unrelated bacteria can have common metabolic pathways, the occurrence of particular disorders will not necessarily correlate with the presence of increased numbers of a single bacterial species or even genus. This underlies the present emphasis on investigation of possible associations of disease with specific bacterial metabolites rather than with individual bacterial components of the flora.

LIMITATIONS TO STUDY OF THE COLONIC FLORA

There are several limitations to investigation of the colonic bacterial flora. First, it is difficult to obtain suitable samples because of the inaccessibility of the colonic contents. Second, the complexity of the flora, which is composed of an estimated 400 species, of which only about 60% have been identified, necessitates the use of a large number of selective media incubated under differing atmospheric conditions. Investigation of the flora is therefore time consuming and costly. No single investigation can realistically expect to analyze the total flora in large numbers of subjects, so that it is desirable to define the objectives of any investigation, and target selected species or types of organism. Third, many intestinal bacteria are sensitive to oxygen, and the chosen method must protect the sample from air, and ensure that the organisms of interest are unaffected by the method used. Moore et al.[6] tested the effects of freezing, transporting, or storing fecal specimens prior to culture including the method of Aries et al.[7] In each instance they detected changes in the composition of the flora of stored specimens as compared with results obtained from immediate processing of specimens. Lastly, the enumeration of bacteria from the feces is not highly reproducible, and generally requires at least a 10-fold difference between samples for significance. Differences in counts of 10-fold or less are therefore unlikely to be detected.

SAMPLING AND STORAGE METHODS

A variety of methods for sampling the colon contents have been utilized, all of which have disadvantages. These include examination of freshly collected feces,[8] which have similar bacteriologic counts of those species that can be regarded as potential human soft tissue pathogens, as the right colonic contents. Intestinal intubation has been used by some investigators,[9,10] but it is difficult to locate the tube at the desired site and aspiration of the semisolid contents of the colon is difficult. Aspiration during surgery[11,12] provides good samples, but the flora may be modified by the underlying pathology for which the surgery is being undertaken, and by preoperative bowel preparation. Sampling of colostomy effluents[13] is convenient, but the presence of the colostomy is likely to alter the ecology of the site. Examination of necropsy samples[2] may only provide valid data if samples are obtained immediately after death in previously healthy subjects such as trauma victims. The use of swallowed sampling capsules containing a mechanism allowing for remote control of sampling provides a good method for obtaining material from the proximal colon.[14,15] This method can be criticized for allowing time for organisms to multiply during the period between sampling and recovery of the capsule. This is less likely to be a significant problem in colonic sampling than in intestinal sampling and Pochart et al.[15] found that counts in control samples were little changed.

Whichever method of collection is adopted, samples should preferably be cultured immediately. Delays will cause significant losses of some bacterial species even if the samples are transported under anaerobic conditions or are frozen during storage and transport.[6]

CULTURAL METHODS

To investigate the total colonic flora, which includes many organisms with fastidious growth requirements, it is important to use a large selection of media providing for different nutritional requirements. Selective media must also be used to recover organisms present in small numbers that would otherwise be masked by more numerous species. For anaerobic culture, pre-reduced media are essential, and strictly anaerobic conditions must be provided. Anaerobic cultures must remain in an anaerobic atmosphere during inspection and subculture. Whereas some of the most important of the earlier studies utilized the roll-tube technique, in which the tubes containing the cultures had a self-contained oxygen-free atmosphere,[16] modern anaerobic cabinets provide a more convenient means of fulfilling all of the requirements for successful culture of the colonic flora. However, when samples are collected from locations that are distant from the laboratory, the roll-tube technique has the advantage that pre-prepared tubes can be taken to the place of sample collection for immediate inoculation. Microaerophilic and aerobic incubation should also be provided for a full analysis of the flora.

QUANTITATIVE FINDINGS ON THE LUMINAL FLORA AND FECES

The average bacterial count of cultivable organisms in colonic feces is 10^{12} per gram (dry weight). When compared to microscopic counts, the cultivable organisms represent 63% to 93% of the total count.[16,17] The complexity of the colonic flora is well illustrated by the study of Moore and Holdeman,[16] who isolated over 100 species from fecal specimens. On the basis of statistical analysis of their findings they concluded that there were probably more than 400 or 500 species present at any one time, but that most of these are represented by less than 10^8 cells per gram of feces or less than one ten-thousandth of the total bacterial population. A notable finding was that there is greater person-to-person variation in the composition of the flora than there is between samples taken from the same individual over a period of several months.

The highest bacterial counts are found in stool specimens and Bentley et al.[11] found counts were 2 to 3 $\log_{10}$ higher than in samples from the transverse colon. A similar but smaller difference in total counts was found by Arabi et al.,[12] who compared counts in stools sampled by aspiration from the right, transverse, and left colon in six subjects undergoing abdominal surgery. However, the finding of higher counts in the left than in the right colon was not true for individual species. They found higher counts of *Bacteroides* spp. in the left colon but for *Escherichia coli* and *Klebsiella* spp. counts were higher on the right side. Counts of clostridia were highest in the transverse colon, and for *Streptococcus faecalis* and lactobacilli counts were higher in the left and right colon than in the transverse colon. Apart from the difference in counts there does not appear to be any variation in the major groups of bacterial species present in different areas of colon. It is not known whether this also applies to the less numerous species, but it is likely that it does.

MUCOSAL FLORA

A substantial part of the flora of the large intestine is closely associated with the epithelial lining of the intestinal wall, and forms layers within the glycoprotein-rich mucus material. These organisms may be important in protecting the host from invasion by pathogenic organisms by providing a barrier between the gut lumen and the intestinal epithelial surface. They appear also to contribute to maintenance of the stability of the colonic luminal flora by replenishing the organisms in the fecal stream, and in effect providing colonization resistance to new bacterial species, which unless they can establish themselves on the mucosa will most likely be removed in the fecal stream. New organisms entering the colon will not find a niche in the mucosal flora except by chance, and this is unlikely unless they are introduced in very large numbers.

Some organisms adhere by means of surface macromolecules that attach to specific cell surface binding sites. Others do not attach to the epithelium but colonize the mucus layer, the most frequent being gram-positive bacilli and cocci with smaller numbers of gram-negative bacilli. Bacteria associated with the mucosal surface in this way are present at levels of 10^7 to 10^8 organisms per gram of tissue homogenate of which anaerobic species occur in counts of at least 10^7 per gram and aerobes at 10^6 per gram. The genera present are the same as those found in the lumen, and it is likely that the species are also the same. Nelson and Mata[18] observed mucosa-associated gram-positive and negative bacilli and gram-positive cocci. The most prevalent bacteria that they cultured from colonic mucosa were anaerobic and microaerophilic streptococci, but lactobacilli, bifidobacteria, bacteroides, clostridia, veillonella, and enterobacteriaceae were also isolated. Peach et al.[19] cultured similar organisms and found counts in colonic mucosal biopsies of 3.8 to 6.3 $\log_{10}$ per gram of tissue. Their isolates were mostly facultative anaerobes and they suggested that the mucosal flora was not dominated by anaerobes in the way that the luminal flora is. However, their findings probably reflect insufficiently long incubation for isolation of fastidious anaerobes. They also noted wide variations in total counts present at different sites but these did not correlate with particular areas of the colon.

Edmiston et al.[20] observed bacilli and cocci by scanning and transmission electron microscopy, and cultured bacteroides, fusobacteria, clostridia, eubacteria, peptostreptococci, and peptococci. Other genera such as megasphaera, veillonella, acidaminacocci, and lactobacilli were also found but their presence did not contribute significantly to the overall quantitation. There were no differences for the total number of species and recovery of species between samples from the ascending colon and transverse colon, but in the descending colon and sigmoid colon total counts were significantly reduced, although there were no differences in the genera present. They suggested that this may have been due to precolonoscopic preparation of the patients.

CONTROL OF THE FECAL FLORA

The major mechanism controlling the intestinal flora is believed to be substrate competition, with each limiting nutrient supporting the bacterial species best adapted to utilize it. Taking into consideration the large number of dietary and host-derived substances in the gut, and the many metabolic end products arising from their fermentation, which in turn provide further substrates for bacterial metabolism, the total number of nutrients available to competing species is very great. Such diversity in the range of nutrients may be the principal determinant of the large number of bacterial species that constitute the colonic flora. Bacterial metabolic waste products may be inhibitory to the bacteria that produce them and to other bacteria but may also be a source of nutrient to other species. The success of any particular bacter-

ium to maintain its presence in the intestine will depend on its ability to utilize competitively a particular substrate in the presence of the prevailing inhibitory substances.

Apart from these mechanisms determined by substrate availability, bacteria interact in other ways to promote or inhibit growth and maintain the balance between competing species. One method is the rapid removal of oxygen, which diffuses into the intestinal lumen, by facultative anaerobes. This maintains the low redox potential required by the predominantly anaerobic flora. Some species produce inhibitory substances or bacteriocins usually with activity directed against different strains of the same species or closely related species, for example the colicins of *E. coli*. Lactic acid bacteria, which include lactobacillus and other genera, are thought to have an important role in maintaining the fecal flora. Their antagonistic effects against other organisms have been attributed to production of lactic acid and hydrogen peroxide as well as the secretion of bacteriocins. Bifidobacteria are also thought to exert beneficial effects by inhibiting bacterial colonization by newly ingested organisms and especially by pathogenic species. The mechanism has also been attributed to lactate production and a lowering of pH. However eight species of bifidobacteria have been shown to produce substances that inhibit *E. coli*, *Clostridium perfringens*, *Bacteroides fragilis*, and intestinal pathogenic bacteria, independent of pH.[21]

NOMENCLATURE OF FECAL FLORA

During the past 25 years, in which much of our current knowledge of the large bowel flora has been obtained, many new species of bacteria have been discovered. As a result of detailed study of these organisms and greater knowledge of their physical and biochemical characteristics, new genera have been created and the definitions of others have been revised. Consequently, the names of many anaerobic bacteria have changed. The most numerous changes in classification and nomenclature apply to the nonsporing gram-negative bacilli, and the reader should be especially careful when comparing data from publications that span this period of change. In particular many species formerly classified within the genus *Bacteroides* are now classified in new genera named *Prevotella* and *Porphyromonas*. Changes of nomenclature have also occurred among gram-positive cocci, and there is now only one species of *Peptococcus*, *Peptococcus niger*, others having been reclassified as peptostreptococci. In this chapter, when citing published work, the nomenclature used by the authors has been retained.

ANAEROBIC NONSPORING GRAM-NEGATIVE FLORA

Moore and Holdeman[16] found *Bacteroides* and *Fusobacterium* in stools from 20 healthy Japanese-Americans with mean counts of more than 10^{10}. Finegold et al.[22-24] investigated feces from healthy individuals on different diets and with different disease states, and found little difference between the groups. *Bacteroides* spp. were found in 100% of all groups on a Western diet and in 93% on a Japanese diet in total counts of $10^{9.2}$ to $10^{13.5}$. The most frequently found species were *Bacteroides thetaiotaomicron*, *B. vulgatus*, *B. distasonis*, and *B. fragilis*. Duerden[25] studied the stools of 20 healthy adults and also found *B. vulga-*

Table 9-1. Bacteria Isolated From Feces of 10% or More of 62 Subjects Taking a Western Diet

	Percent Positive	Range ($\log_{10}/g$ dry weight)
Anaerobic bacteria		
Bacteroides spp.	100	9.2–13.5
Fusobacterium spp.	24	5.1–11.0
Acidaminococcus spp.	27	3.7–11.6
Anaerobic streptococci	32	8.6–12.6
Peptococcus spp.	37	5.1–12.9
Peptostreptococcus spp.	35	5.4–12.6
Ruminococcus spp.	45	4.6–12.7
Veillonella spp.	34	3.5–13.4
Bifidobacterium spp.	79	5.7–13.4
Eubacterium spp.	95	5.9–13.3
Lactobacillus spp.	73	3.6–12.5
Clostridium spp.	100	6.5–13.1
Facultative bacteria		
Streptococcus spp.	100	5.1–12.9
Citrobacter spp.	10	6.3–9.7
Escherichia coli	94	4.4–12.3
Klebsiella spp.	24	3.5–10.1
Bacillus spp.	82	0.6–9.9
Micrococcus spp.	11	3.7–9.3
Staphylococcus aureus	11	3.6–6.4
Staphylococcus epidermidis	27	3.9–12.7

(From Finegold et al.,[26] with permission.)

tus, *B. thetaiotaomicron*, and *B. distasonis* to be the most common. *B. fragilis* accounted for only 9%. Fusobacterium was found in 18.4% of subjects in counts of $10^{5.1}$ to $10^{11.0}$ [26] (Table 9-1). Some of the gram-negative bacilli previously classified as *Bacteroides* spp., especially pigment-producing strains such as *B. melaninogenicus* and *B. asaccharolyticus*, have as a result of taxonomic changes been renamed in new genera as *Prevotella melaninogenica* and *Porphyromonas asaccharolytica*, respectively.

ANAEROBIC COCCI

The most frequently isolated anaerobic gram-positive cocci are *Streptococcus intermedius*, *Peptococcus* (now *Peptostreptococcus*) *prevotii*, *Peptostreptococcus productus*, and *Ruminococcus albus*. Other genera of gram-positive cocci found in feces are *Coprococcus* and *Sarcina*. The gram-negative cocci that inhabit the colon are classified in the genera *Veillonella*, *Acidaminococcus*, and *Megasphaera*.

ANAEROBIC NONSPORING GRAM-POSITIVE BACILLI

These are represented predominantly by species of *Bifidobacterium*, *Eubacterium*, and *Lactobacillus*. *Actinomyces* were found in only 2% of subjects eating a typical Western diet,[22] but occurred in 29% to 31% of vegetarians.[24] Similar differences were seen with *Propionibacterium acnes*.

CLOSTRIDIA

Clostridia are found in the feces of all subjects except vegetarians in whom they are present in 92%[26] (Table 9-1). The most frequently isolated clostridium is *C. ramosum* in 60% of subjects with *C. perfringens* occurring in 55%. The latter was found more commonly in subjects on a Japanese diet (73%), and was absent from the feces of strict vegetarians.[26] Drasar et al.[27] found *C. perfringens* to be more common in a study of clostridia from diverse populations. Other clostridia isolated from more than 10% of persons are *C. bifermentans*, *C. paraputrificum*, *C. inocuum*, and *C. aminovalericum*. *C. difficile* was found in 2% of subjects on a Western diet,[26] an incidence consistent with more recent studies.

FACULTATIVE ANAEROBES

Streptococci are found in almost all subjects,[26] the most common being *S. faecalis* in 82%. *S. faecium*, *S. mitis*, *S. lactis*, *S. bovis*, *S. sanguis*, *S. durans*, *S. mutans*, and *S. salivarius* are present in more than 10% of subjects. Of the facultative gram-negative bacteria, *E. coli* is by far the most common in over 90% of individuals,[9,26] with *Klebsiella* and *Citrobacter* next in frequency (Table 9-1).

AEROBIC BACTERIA

Pseudomonas aeruginosa, a strictly aerobic bacterium, was found in only 5% of subjects eating a Western diet, but in 20% of Japanese subjects and 23% of strict vegetarians.[26]

METHANOGENIC FLORA

Methanogenic bacteria are found in the right and left colon and in feces, with the highest counts in the left colon and feces. In respiratory excretors of methane, counts of methanogens in the feces are significantly higher than in nonexcretors, and methanogens accounted for 12% of the anaerobic flora compared with 0.003% in nonexcretors.[15] The sole source of energy for methanogens is hydrogen, which is produced in considerable volumes by intestinal bacteria. The predominant methanogenic bacterium in humans is *Methanibrevibacter smithii*, an anaerobic gram-positive coccobacillus that uses hydrogen to convert carbon dioxide to methane, a reaction that greatly reduces the volume of gas that would otherwise be present in the colon. A less numerous methanogen, *Methanosphaera stadtmaniae*, forms methane by reducing methanol with hydrogen.[28] Methane production was found to be the main method of hydrogen disposal in 23 of 30 subjects.[29] The methanogens compete for hydrogen with sulfate-reducing bacteria and appear to predominate, but the conditions that favor methanogens are unknown.[30]

SULFATE-REDUCING BACTERIA

The sulfate-reducing bacteria belong to several morphologically and nutritionally distinct genera of which *Desulfovibrio*, *Desulfobacter*, *Desulfobulbus*, and *Desulfotomaculum* are predominant. Counts of more than 10^7 sulfate-reducing bacteria per gram dry weight are only found in fecal samples from individuals whose breath methane excretion is low or undetectable.

Methane-producing fecal flora usually contains less than 10^7 sulfate-reducing bacteria per gram dry weight, suggesting that sulfate reduction and methanogenesis are mutually exclusive in the colon.[29,31] Unlike methanogens, sulfate-reducing bacteria can utilize substrates other than hydrogen, but are dependent on the availability of sulfate.

SPIROCHETELIKE ORGANISMS

Intestinal spirochetes were first described in 1884 by Escherich who observed them in feces by microscopy. Further observations reviewed by Jones et al.[32] were made during the subsequent 40 years, but significant progress was hindered by inability to culture spirochetes. Interest in them was renewed by their rediscovery by Harland and Lee[33] using electron microscopy, who described them as short and borrelia like. Histologic examination of the same specimens revealed a blue haze about 3 μm in thickness along the surface of epithelial cells. This was due to a dense forest of spiral organisms attached end-on to the surface epithelium, and was seen in 9 out of 100 rectal biopsies reviewed retrospectively. Spirochetes were also found in sections of appendiceal, colonic, and rectal biopsies reviewed retrospectively in mucosal specimens obtained up to 6 years previously.[33,34] Successful isolation of spirochetes from feces or rectal mucosa[35,36] allowed detailed characterization of isolates and led to the recognition that intestinal spirochetes form a heterogeneous group,[32,37] some of which are presently classified as *Treponema* and others placed in the genus *Brachyspira* of which *B. aalborgi*[36] is the species associated with intestinal spirochetosis.

YEASTS AND YEASTLIKE FUNGI

Candida albicans is found in 14% of feces, other *Candida* spp. in 8%, and various yeastlike fungi in 31%.[26] The yeastlike fungi found in feces include *Torulopsis glabrata*. Filamentous fungi are uncommonly isolated from feces.

BACTERIAL FERMENTATION IN THE COLON

Fermentation is the process of breakdown by anaerobic bacteria of residual undigested food remnants, of host-derived substrates such as glycoproteins in mucin and pancreatic secretions, and of exfoliated cells that reach the cecum. The end products include the short chain fatty acids, acetate, propionate and butyrate, hydrogen and carbon dioxide gas, ammonia, amines, and phenols. The diverse flora in the colon include saccharolytic species such as bacteroides, eubacteria, bifidobacteria, lactobacilli, ruminococci, peptostreptococci, and clostridia.[38,39] Proteins, peptides, and amino acids are utilized by bacteroides, eubacteria, peptococci, peptostreptococci, and clostridia.[40] Other bacteria such as methanogens and sulfur-reducing bacteria utilize intermediate products of fermentation that include hydrogen, lactate, and ethanol.[31] In a study of 14 subjects, 5 consumed hydrogen by methanogenesis, 4 via sulfate reduction, and 5 by an unidentified route,[41] which was possibly acetogenesis. Densities of methanogenic bacteria increase distally through the large intestine and are 10,000-fold greater in the rectosigmoid region than in the cecum, and methanogenesis is higher in the left than the right colon. In contrast, sulfate-reducing bacteria are more uniformly distributed throughout the colon but sulfate reduction is greater in the ascending and transverse colons. Acetogenesis provides an alternative route for hydrogen utilization in which carbon dioxide is reduced to acetate by hydrogen, a process that appears to be active in humans who are not high methane excretors.[42]

The cecum is the richest part of the colon in nutrients, and consequently bacterial growth and metabolism is greatest in the right colon. Carbohydrate fermentation is maximal in this area and volatile fatty acids, lactate, and ethanol concentrations are higher and pH is lower in the cecum and ascending colon than in other areas of the large intestine. In contrast, products of protein fermentation such as ammonia, branched chain fatty acids, and phenols progressively increase from the right to the left colon and pH rises.[2] It has also been inferred from data in animals that the right colon is the main site of breakdown of dietary fiber.

EFFECT OF DIET AND GEOGRAPHIC LOCATION ON COLONIC FLORA

Investigations into the effects of diet on fecal flora have provided conflicting data and are difficult to interpret. Most studies have compared the fecal flora of subjects from different ethnic groups taking their customary diet, and have not shown significant variation between the groups in the composition of their flora.

Investigation of individuals who have undergone drastic changes of diet have similarly not shown significant changes in the fecal flora.[6] Among native populations of African and Japanese subjects, most individuals maintain high concentrations of a few species, whereas subjects on a Western diet usually have a more heterogeneous flora. This may reflect a more uniform intestinal physiology in the former group and a more routine existence and diet.[43] Hill et al.[4] compared specimens from British and American subjects representing a group with a high risk for colon cancer, with Ugandans, Indians, and Japanese subjects from a population with a low risk for colon cancer. They found that the British and Americans had more bacteroides, whereas the Africans and Asians had more aerobic streptococci and enterobacteria. A further study by the same group noted that subjects taking a Western-type diet had a large proportion of gram-negative anaerobes comprising bacteroides and fusobacteria and also large numbers of clostridia belonging to the *C. paraputrificum* group. In contrast, in subjects consuming a high carbohydrate diet from India, Uganda, and Japan, there was a higher proportion of gram-positive organisms and a statistically significant increase in eubacteria.[44] Similarly Aries et al.[7] found a higher incidence of bacteroides and bifidobacteria in English and North American subjects compared with Ugandans. However, a rural Japanese population had a higher incidence of bacteroides and bifidobacteria than North Americans.[6] Drasar et al.[27] also noted that the *C. paraputrificum* group was common in American and British subjects and rare in subjects from Uganda and Japan.[41] In a comparison of two groups of Japanese-Americans, one of which took a traditional Japanese diet and the other took a Western diet, there were some differences in counts of individual species, but considering the large number of species tested, the authors concluded that these differences might have occurred by chance.[22] They found no differences for the *C. paraputrificum* group. In another study comparing vegetarian and nonvegetarian Seventh Day Adventists with non-Adventists, they again found some differences including significantly fewer *C. septicum* and *C. tertium*, and again concluded that these might have arisen by chance. Among the paraputrificum group, the only differences noted were for *C. septicum* and *C. tertium*. Some of the differences reported in fecal flora from early studies may have occurred as a result of selective loss of some bacterial species as a result of the procedures used for transport and storage of the specimens. Investigators using the roll-tube technique were able to initiate their cultures within a few minutes of sample collection in each geographic location and avoid this problem.[17,45]

FECAL FLORA AND COLON CANCER

Feces from subjects on a Western diet were found to contain higher concentrations of steroids than those from African and Eastern countries and the steroids were more degraded. However, the major correlation with colon cancer is the Western high-fat and low-fiber diet.[4] Studies of the colonic flora have found significant differences in the counts of a few species of fecal bacteria in populations with differing dietary habits, but considering the large number of species tested, the authors con-

cluded that these differences might have occurred by chance.[22,43,46] Moore al.[6] found a positive correlation between the incidence of colon cancer and *Bacteroides vulgatus*, *B. distasonis*, and *Peptostreptococcus productus* and an inverse relationship with *Eubacterium aureofaciens*, *B. fragilis*, and *E. coli*, but were also uncertain what significance to attach to these observations. Interpretation of these data is also difficult because identification of organisms to the species level has not always been complete and within genera there are often large numbers of species with differing metabolic activities. This highlights the difficulty in establishing whether bacteria play a role in the etiology of cancer.

Nevertheless, it is possible that some bacterial species among those that are normally resident in the fecal microflora might be capable of producing carcinogenic substances, in which case it will probably be necessary to identify the carcinogens before the responsible organisms can be identified. An example of a potential carcinogen is a mutagen found in the feces of 15% to 20% of the population, which is produced by many strains of five species of *Bacteroides*, from an unidentified precursor substance in the presence of bile.[5] The five species that included *Bacteroides fragilis* are all commonly found in the colonic microflora, so that if this particular mutagen is important in colonic disease, factors other than the presence of the organisms must play a part.

REFERENCES

1. Cummings JH, MacFarlane GT (1991) The control and consequences of bacterial fermentation in the human colon. J Appl Bacteriol 70:443–459
2. MacFarlane GT, Gibson GR, Cummings JH (1992) Comparison of fermentation reactions in different regions of the human colon. J Appl Bacteriol 72:57–64
3. Roediger WEW (1980) Role of anaerobic bacteria in the metabolic welfare of the colonic mucosa in man. Gut 21:793–798
4. Hill MJ, Drasar BS, Aries V et al (1971) Bacteria and aetiology of cancer of large bowel. Lancet 1:95–100
5. Van Tassell RL, MacDonald DK, Wilkins TD (1982) Production of a faecal mutagen in human feces by Bacteroides spp. Infect Immun 37:975–980
6. Moore WEC, Cato EP, Holdeman LV (1978) Some current concepts in intestinal bacteriology. Am J Clin Nutr 31:S33–42
7. Aries V, Crowther JS, Drasar BS et al (1969) Bacteria and the aetiology of cancer of the large bowel. Gut 10:334–335
8. Arabi Y, Dimock D, Burdon DW et al (1979) Influence of neomycin and metronidazole on colonic microflora of volunteers. J Antimicrob Chemother 5:531–537
9. Gorbach SL, Plaut AG, Nahas L, Weinstein L (1967) Studies of intestinal flora. II. Microorganisms of the small intestine and their relations to oral and fecal flora. Gastroenterology 53:856–867
10. Flourie B, Etanchaud F, Florent C et al (1990) Comparative study of hydrogen and methane production in the human colon by means of cecal and fecal homogenates. Gut 31:684–685
11. Bentley DW, Nichols R, Condon RE, Gorbach S (1972) The microflora of the human ileum and intra-abdominal colon: results of direct needle aspiration at surgery and evaluation of the technique. J Lab Clin Med 79:421–429

12. Arabi Y, Dimock D, Burdon DW et al (1978) Influence of bowel preparation and antimicrobials on colonic microflora. Br J Surg 65:555–559
13. Finegold SM, Sutter VL, Boyle JD, Shimada K (1970) The normal flora of ileostomy and transverse colostomy effluents. J Infect Dis 122:376–381
14. Drasar BS, Hill MJ (1974) Human Intestinal Flora. Academic Press, New York
15. Pochart P, Lemann F, Flourie B et al (1993) Pyxigraphic sampling to enumerate methanogens and anaerobes in the right colon of healthy humans. Gastroenterology 105:1281–1285
16. Moore WEC, Holdeman LV (1974) Human fecal flora: the normal flora of 20 Japanese-Hawaiians. Appl Microbiol 27:961–979
17. Holdeman LV, Good IJ, Moore WEC (1976) Human fecal flora: a variation in bacterial composition within individuals and a possible effect of emotional stress. Appl Environ Microbiol 31:359–375
18. Nelson DP, Mata LJ (1970) Bacterial flora associated with human gastrointestinal mucosa. Gastroenterology 58:56–61
19. Peach S, Lock MR, Katz D et al (1978) Mucosal-associated bacterial flora of the intestine in patients with Crohn's disease and a control group. Gut 19:1034–1042
20. Edmiston CE, Avant GR, Wilson FA (1982) Anaerobic bacterial populations on normal and diseased human biopsy tissue obtained at colonoscopy. Appl Environ Microbiol 43:1173–1181
21. Gibson GR, Wang X (1994) Regulatory effects of bifidobacteria on the growth of other colonic bacteria. J Appl Bacteriol 77:12–20
22. Finegold SM, Attebery HR, Sutter VL (1974) Effect of diet

on human fecal flora: comparison of Japanese and American diets. Am J Clin Nutr 27:1456–1469

23. Finegold SM, Flora DJ, Attebery HR, Sutter VL (1975) Fecal bacteriology of colonic polyp patients and control patients. Cancer Res 35:3407–3417

24. Finegold SM, Sutter VL, Sugihar PT et al (1977) Fecal microbial flora in Seventh Day Adventist populations and control subjects. Am J Clin Nutr 30:1781–1792

25. Duerden BI (1980) The isolation and identification of *Bacteroides* spp. from the normal human faecal flora. J Med Microbiol 13:69–78

26. Finegold SM, Sutter VL, Mathisen GE (1983) Normal indigenous intestinal flora. pp. 3–31. In Hentges DJ (ed): Human Intestinal Microflora in Health and Disease. Academic Press, New York

27. Drasar BS, Goddard P, Heaton S et al (1976) Clostridia isolated from faeces. J Med Microbiol 9:63–71

28. Miller TL, Wolin MJ (1985) *Methanosphaera stadtmaniae* gen. nov., sp. nov.: a species that forms methane by reducing methanol with hydrogen. Arch Microbiol 141:116–122

29. Gibson GR, Cummings JH, Macfarlane GT et al (1990) Alternative pathways for hydrogen disposal during fermentation in the human colon. Gut 31:679–683

30. Strocchi A, Furne JK, Ellis CJ, Levitt MD (1991) Competition for hydrogen by human faecal bacteria: evidence for the predominance of methane producing bacteria. Gut 32:1498–1501

31. Gibson GR, Macfarlane GT, Cummings JH (1988) Occurrence of sulphate-reducing bacteria in human faeces and the relationship of dissimilatory sulphate reduction to methanogenesis in the large gut. J Appl Bacteriol 65:103–111

32. Jones MJ, Miller JN, George WL (1986) Microbiological and biochemical characterization of spirochetes isolated from the feces of homosexual males. J Clin Microbiol 24:1071–1074

33. Harland WA, Lee FD (1967) Intestinal spirochaetosis. BMJ 3: 718–719

34. Lee FD, Kraszewski A, Gordon J et al (1971) Intestinal spirochaetosis. Gut 12:126–133

35. Tompkins DS, Waugh MA, Cooke EM (1981) Isolation of intestinal spirochaetes from homosexuals. J Clin Pathol 34: 1385–1387

36. Hovind-Hougen K, Birch-Andergon A, Heurik-Nielson R et al (1982) Intestinal spirochetosis: morphological characterization and cultivation of the spirochete *Brachyspira aalborgi* gen. nov., sp. nov. J Clin Microbiol

37. Tompkins DS, Foulkes SJ, Godwin PGR, West AP et al (1986) Isolation and characterisation of intestinal spirochaetes. J Clin Pathol 39:535–541

38. Vercelotti JR, Salyers AA, Bullard WS, Wilkins TD (1977) Breakdown of mucin and plant polysaccharides in the human colon. Can J Biochem 55:1190–1196

39. Salyers AA, Leedle JAZ (1983) Carbohydrate utilization in the human colon. pp. 129–146. In Hentges DJ (ed): Human Intestinal Microflora in Health and Disease. Academic Press, New York

40. MacFarlane, Allison C, Gibson SAW, Cummings JH et al (1988) Contribution of the microflora to proteolysis in the human colon. J Appl Bacteriol 64:37–46

41. Strocchi A, Ellis CJ, Levitt MD (1993) Use of metabolic inhibitors to study H_2 consumption by human feces: evidence for a pathway other than methanogenesis and sulphate reduction. J Lab Clin Med 121:320–327

42. Lajoie SF, Bank S, Miller TL, Wolin MJ (1988) Acetate production from hydrogen and [^{13}C] carbon dioxide by the microflora of human feces. Appl Environ Microbiol 54: 2723–2727

43. Moore WEC, Holdemann LV (1975) Discussion of current bacteriological investigations of the relationships between intestinal flora, diet and colon cancer. Cancer Res 35:3418–3420

44. Peach S, Fernandez F, Johnson K, Drasar BS (1974) The nonsporing anaerobic bacteria in human faeces. J Med Microbiol 7:213–221

45. Holdeman LV, Moore WEC (1974) New genus, *Coprococcus*, twelve new species, and emended description of four previously described species of bacteria from human feces. Int J Syst Bacteriol 24:260–277

46. Finegold SM, Sutter VL (1978) Fecal flora in different populations with special reference to diet. Am J Clin Nutr 31: S116–122

10

PRESENTING SYMPTOMS

Jacques Heppell

This chapter deals with the presenting symptoms of anorectal diseases including bleeding, pain, discharge, and pruritus. This limited number of symptoms represents the complaints of the great majority of patients seen in the Proctology Clinic at the Mayo Clinic, Scottsdale.

A carefully taken medical history will often lead to a diagnosis of anorectal disease that can be confirmed by physical examination. However, the clinical history is sometimes limited, because patients are reluctant or uncomfortable to describe their anorectal symptoms in detail, as fear and embarrassment associated with this part of the anatomy are common. Patients often need help in order to describe the periodicity of symptoms, their frequency, the nature of exacerbating and relieving factors, the associations with other symptoms, and the predisposing causes. A direct physical or endoscopic examination of the anorectal area will most often give an ''instant'' diagnosis, thus minimizing the importance of a detailed questionnaire. Certainly, an accurate description of anal symptoms is important preoperatively, and realistic expectations should be given regarding the correction of such symptoms by surgical procedures.

Benign and malignant anorectal disorders have similar presenting features. Unfortunately, patients can delay consultation because their symptoms are commonly attributed to hemorrhoids or other benign anorectal conditions. Commercial preparations, which are readily available, make self-treatment easy. The reported prevalence rates of anal diseases have varied widely, depending on the method of evaluation and definition. A recent survey[1] of benign anal disease symptoms in a randomly selective American population showed that history of hemorrhoids and recurrent anal symptomatology were highly prevalent, and yet 80% of subjects with anal symptoms had not consulted a physician. Data analyzed from a number of governmental services concluded that the prevalence is 4.4% in the United States (11 million people).[2] The significance of such a high prevalence of anal symptoms in the general population is unknown. Certainly, the economic aspects are substantial. It was estimated that in 1989, total wholesale sales for pharmaceutical preparations used for anorectal symptoms reached $22.5 million in Canada and $151.3 million in the

United States.[3] These numbers are probably an underestimation of the actual amount expended. The efficacy of these drugs to relieve anorectal symptoms has not been well documented. On a lighter note, the presence of severe anal symptoms may have serious consequences in a head of state. If a great man has an itch, millions of others might be forced to scratch.[4,5]

PAST MEDICAL HISTORY

In patients presenting with anorectal symptoms, the previous medical history often helps to make the correct diagnosis. It is important to learn the obstetric history, and the history of previous abdominal, anorectal, urologic, or gynecologic operations. Obstetric trauma or prior anal operation may leave a muscle defect or dysfunction. Patients who have had previous radiotherapy for prostate or cervical neoplasia may have proctitis or fibrosis of the anal sphincter. A family history of inflammatory bowel disease or colorectal neoplasia among first degree relatives should lead to a suspicion of a similar problem. A detailed interrogation about the characteristics of any accompanying abdominal complaint such as pain, vomiting, or altered bowel habits is important. Anal diseases may precede intestinal manifestations of Crohn's disease.[6] A high degree of suspicion is necessary in patients with associated gastrointestinal symptoms or in whom there are unusual features to the perianal lesions (for example, a wide-based, eccentrically placed fissure with large skin tags or a fistula with multiple tracts or opening).[7] Also, a history of a previous dysentery or travel to tropical or subtropical countries should be investigated. The presence of concomitant medical disease, including cardiac valvular disease or prosthetic implants, which may necessitate the use of prophylactic antibiotics before surgical procedures, should be sought. An immunosuppressed patient may also need prophylactic antibiotics. It is important to know what medication the patients is taking, such as warfarin or aspirin. A history of bleeding tendencies may make anorectal procedures hazardous. Drugs and special diets that can affect bowel function should be identified. All pertinent letters, reports of examinations, and operative and pathologic reports from referring physicians should be reviewed.

A sexual history is important in all patients but particularly in men presenting with anorectal complaints. Information regarding previous sexually transmitted diseases and sexual activities may be helpful. Reticence is common about asking or answering such personal questions. Some patients will deny homosexuality or taking part in high risk activities.[8] The anal-receptive males have an increased risk for various infectious,[9] neoplastic,[10] and traumatic[11] lesions of the anorectum. In addition, men who test positive for the human immunodeficiency virus (HIV) have a high prevalence (33%) of anorectal pathologic symptoms.[12]

BLEEDING

The passage of blood from the anus is always abnormal, and although the most common cause are benign, the possibility of an underlying colorectal neoplasm should always be considered. Any assessment of bleeding requires a review of both the quality and quantity of blood. Blood may be pink, bright red, dark red, black, or occult. It may be noticed on the toilet paper, in the toilet bowl, or both. It may also be present on the clothing, on the stool, or mixed within the stool. Anal sources of bleeding usually result in bright red blood on the toilet paper, on the clothing, or within the toilet bowl. Bleeding from a site in the colon or upper rectum is suggested by the passage of dark blood and clots, especially if the blood is mixed with the stool.

Anal bleeding is usually not an isolated symptom. The duration, quantity, and relationship of bleeding to defecation is important to elicit. In women, an anorectal source should be distinguished from urinary or vaginal sources. When associated with a painful lump and when unrelated to defecation, it is usually due to a thrombosed external hemorrhoid. Bright red blood that drips into the bowl, streaks the stool, and appears on toilet tissue is frequently caused by internal hemorrhoids. Occasionally, chronic blood loss may be severe enough to cause a profound symptomatic anemia. Blood escaping from hemorrhoids is bright red in color and therefore arterial rather than venous in character, because of the presence of arteriovenous communications in corpus cavernosum recti.[13] When related to painful defecation, it is often caused by an anal fissure or abrasion. Small amounts of blood on toilet tissue are also seen in patients with pruritus ani.[14] When bleeding accompanies diarrhea, inflammatory bowel disease must be considered. Bleeding accompanied by a large amount of mucus suggests the presence of a villous adenoma. It should be remembered that ingestion of certain pigmented foods, such as beets, may mimic the appearance of blood in the stool.[15]

Minor symptomatic bleeding is common and occurs in about 10% of the normal population between 25 and 65 years.[16–20] Few of these individuals seek medical attention, presumably because the bleeding resolves and does not recur. It would appear, therefore, that rectal bleeding is common in healthy adults and that the prevalence may vary from population to population. This variation will depend on the type of population studied, the way in which the question is asked, the perception of the question by the interviewee, and on how often the stool or toilet paper is inspected. In evaluating these patients with chronic rectal bleeding, a careful history should provide enough information to make a provisional diagnosis and to classify the bleeding as typical outlet bleeding or as suspicious.[21,22] In patients with outlet bleeding, most lesions are within reach of the ano-scope and flexible sigmoidoscope. However, colonoscopy is the investigation of choice in patients with suspicious, occult, or severe rectal bleeding. When treatment of the anal lesion does not lead to resolution of bleeding, a full colonic investigation is mandatory. In high-risk patients, colonic investigation should precede surgical treatment. Bleeding was the presenting symptom in 70% (308) of a series of 440 consecutive new patients seen at the rectal clinic of the St. Mark's Hospital, London.[17] The final diagnosis were hemorrhoids (54%), perianal lesion (7%), anal fissure (18%), neoplastic disease (benign 2.5%, malignant 4%), inflammatory bowel disease (ulcerative colitis 4%, Crohn's disease 1%), others 6.5%, and no diagnosis was made in 3%. Most diagnoses were made with simple means (rigid proctosigmoidoscopy 85%, barium enema and/or flexible sigmoidoscopy 10%, and colonoscopy 2%).

A large amount of bleeding raises concern about the patient's hemodynamic stability and leads to a suspicion of diverticular disease, angiodysplasia, or Crohn's disease of the colon.[14] Severe bleeding can also occur in patients with portal hypertension and coagulation disorders or exacerbated by diarrhea during the treatment of encephalopathy.[23] However, the incidence of hemorrhoidal disease in patients with portal hypertension is not greater than in the general population. Bleeding from hemorrhoids in these patients must be distinguished from anorectal varices, a true consequence of portal hypertension, which can lead to massive bleeding.[24]

Public education programs designed to encourage adults to inspect their stools for blood, and medical education to highlight adequate investigation of this symptom, may lead to earlier diagnosis of colorectal cancer. Rectal bleeding is considered a symptom of early rather than late colorectal cancer.[25,26] A common source of physician delay in diagnosis of colorectal cancer occurs when rectal bleeding is wrongly attributed to hemorrhoids or other anal pathology.[27] Public education should discourage the self-diagnosis and self-treatment of hemorrhoids, and should advise general practitioner consultation for all rectal bleeding. However, this recommendation may lead to unnecessary procedures that may not be cost-effective.[28]

PAIN

Anorectal pain can be most disabling to the patient. It is important to distinguish true pain from the sensation of burning and irritation of the skin caused by perianal skin disorders. Pain may be acute or chronic. Traumatic laceration of the anorectal region is painful and should be recognized from the patient's acute history. Most commonly, an acute anorectal pain is caused by a fissure, an abscess, a thrombosed external hemorrhoid, or a strangulated internal hemorrhoid. The patient's description should help differentiate these causes. In some cases the anorectal pain is so severe that an examination under general or regional anesthesia is necessary to fully assess the extent of involvement of anorectal disease and find the exact cause. Sometimes reexamination when symptoms are maximal or after an interval of time may be helpful.

Anal fissure often results from the trauma of a hard stool. The pain is worsened by having a bowel movement, and may persist as a stinging or burning for a period of time varying from a few seconds to several hours. The pain can be so agonizing that the patient is afraid to have a bowel movement. Bleeding associated with pain is often caused by a fissure. The bleeding is often manifest as streaking on the outside of the fecal bolus or spotting on the toilet tissue.

Severe pain is usually not due to hemorrhoids unless the hemorrhoid is thrombosed, ulcerated, or gangrenous. If the pain is continuous, not related to defecation, and associated with a purplish tender mass, a thrombosed external hemorrhoid (perianal hematoma) is the probable diagnosis. It is often of sudden onset after straining or heavy lifting, but some patients give no history of straining or physical exertion. The natural history of a thrombosed external hemorrhoid is one of resolution with decreasing pain after 2 to 3 days. Thrombosis of an internal hemorrhoid is associated with its prolapse through a spastic anus tending to produce edema, strangulation, and necrosis. The pain is intense and may be associated with urinary retention. The mass is very tender and ranges in color from red to black depending upon the degree of strangulation.

A perianal abscess is another cause of acute anal pain. In such case, the pain is associated with the presence of a tender, diffuse swelling, usually located unilaterally. It is a continuous throbbing pain and the patient may complain of a fever. In severe cases the infection can be bilateral (horseshoe abscess) and be associated with urinary retention. Severe pain, especially in the posterior aspect of the anus, in the absence of external signs, is typical of an abscess in the post anal space.[29] Pain increases in intensity when the patient coughs or sneezes. More virulent necrotizing infections can present with severe pain and intense toxemia.[30] Contrary to popular belief, syphilitic lesions in the anal region are not always painless, and occur approximately 3 weeks after anal intercourse. Very few pains in the anal region are so severe as that of herpes. A history of sacral paresthesias suggests an acute herpetic infection.[9]

Tenesmus, which is a symptom complex of straining and the urge to defecate, frequently is associated with inflammatory or neoplastic conditions of the rectum. Anorectal pain is rarely associated with a tumor unless the lesion invades the internal sphincter to produce tenesmus. Inflammatory and neoplastic involvement of the anal canal by condyloma acuminatum or epidermoid carcinoma may cause pain.[14] Carcinoma of the rectum extending into the sacral region also causes a severe, deep, aching kind of pain. Referred pain to the rectum may occur from aneurysmal dilatations in the pelvic vessels. The pain associated with retrorectal neoplasms is frequently postural.[31] The pain is worse while sitting and better with walking or standing. It is generally poorly localized as low back or perianal pain, rectal ache, or deep rectal pain. In the later stages, if the sacral plexus is involved, patients experience referred pain to the legs and buttocks. The presence of a painful mass in an old episiotomy scar noticeable at the time of menstruation and subsiding several days after the termination of menses suggests a diagnosis of perineal endometriosis.[32,33]

Strictures of the anal canal are rare but manifest as progressive obstruction with constipation. Patients have to strain vigorously, with painful sensation and incomplete evacuation. These strictures most commonly follow anal surgery. Inflammatory causes include lymphogranuloma venereum, tuberculosis, and Crohn's disease. Strictures may also result from previous radiation therapy.

Anal or perianal pain can be chronic without any evidence of a cause. The management of these patients is difficult. Patients are often referred from one physician to another and a variety of different but ineffective treatments are tried. Several syndromes of chronic perianal pain have been described.[34] A *coccygodynia* consists of a vague tenderness or ache in the region of the sacrum and coccyx, and in the adjacent muscles and soft tissues. It is associated with similar rectal and perianal discomfort. Sometimes the pain radiates to the back of the thighs and buttocks. It occurs more frequently in women in their 50s and 60s. Symptoms often persist for many years. Sitting induces or exacerbates the pain. An association between coccygodynia and depression was described.[35] *Proctalgia fugax*[36] is a well-defined syndrome of obscure causation. The pain is deep seated and unrelated to defecation. It often begins in young adult males and occurs spontaneously in late middle life. It occurs at any time, but is particularly common at night and awakens the patient. It begins suddenly and progresses to a cramp-like pain that may be excruciating, but that usually resolves within 30 minutes. The duration and location usually remain constant in a given patient. The pain is felt at a constant site above the level of the external anal sphincter. It is not accompanied by an acute bowel disturbance. Between attacks, no consistent physical abnormality is evident. The pain is sometimes relieved by passing flatus, having a bowel movement, or sitting in a warm tub of water. Subjectively, pain is considerably ameliorated by the application of heat. Understandably, a significant decrease in anal resting pressure was observed after immersion in warm water.[37] Because patients with certain anal conditions often have elevated pressures, the lowering of resting anal canal pressures may result in improvement.

The *descending perineum syndrome*[38] is a dull aching pain in the posterior perineum associated with abnormal descent of the perineum during straining at defecation, and sometimes with prolapse of the anterior rectal mucosa. A vague, dull, aching pain in the perineum and sacral region may follow defecation, and a sensation of incomplete evacuation ensues. The pain sometimes improves by lying down or when the abnormal defecation habit is modified. *Chronic idiopathic perianal pain*[34] is an ill-defined and perhaps heterogenous clinical syndrome. In many cases there are strong indications that psychiatric disturbances are present. The pain may be precipitated by sitting and is often described as "like sitting on a ball." It is usually relieved, if only partially, by standing or lying on one side. This group of patients presents both a diagnostic and therapeutic challenge. It is of paramount importance to exclude all organic causes for the pain prior to relegation of the patient into the frustrating group labeled as having "chronic" intractable rectal pain.[39]

ANAL DISCHARGE

Patients often complain of a discharge or moisture in the perianal region, which may be due to a pathologic condition, dietary indiscretion, or poor hygiene. Discharge may produce an offensive odor, which is often a reason to consult.

Mucus is secreted by the colonic mucosa and may be seen in the stool under many circumstances. It may be the result of normal production of mucus, the early sign of a villous adenoma of the rectum, the indication of an early inflammatory process, or caused by chemical irritants. The packaged buffered phosphate enema can elicit a tremendous response from the bowel.[15] If the mucus is associated with bleeding, it may be the sign of a neoplasm or an inflammatory process. Normally, mucus should not leak through the anus unless the patient is incontinent. Soiling of underclothes with mucus may be a sign of rectal mucosal prolapse, ectropion from a previous hemorrhoidectomy, or overproduction of mucus such as occurs with a villous adenoma. The mucoid discharge is most severe in patients with internal hemorrhoids that are in permanently prolapsed condition.

A purulent discharge is indicative of an infectious process. A history of purulent discharge and pain is suggestive of an anorectal abscess, whereas a painless purulent discharge more likely is due to fistula-in-ano. Passing pus per rectum is suspicious for a gonococcal proctitis or a spontaneously drained high intermuscular abscess.[15] Patients presenting with an anal fistula may have had one or more operations to treat the original abscess or fistula. On rare occasions when patients with long-standing chronic anal fistula see a change in the nature of fistulous drainage with increasing pain or mass, a carcinoma should be suspected.[40,41] Watery pus draining from multiple openings of superficial and deep sinus tracts and pitted scars are characteristic of patient with hidradenitis suppurativa.[42] Occasionally, a sinus tract from pilonidal disease will run caudad and may be the cause of purulent perianal discharge.[43] A rectovaginal fistula can lead to development of a discharge with fecal odor or recurrent vaginitis. Spontaneous passage of urine via the rectum as a consequence of rectoprostatic fistula is a rare complication of prostatic operations.[44]

In patients with *fecal soiling*, the history is of key importance to establish the degree of disability and to identify etiologic factors. An underlying neurologic cause should be considered if patients complain of perineal or low back pain or if motor or sensory symptoms in the legs or buttocks are present. Incontinence may be partial or major.[45] Partial incontinence is defined as a loss of control of flatus and minor soiling of the underwear. Major incontinence is defined as frequent and regular deficiency in ability to control stools of normal consistency. Fecal soiling of the underwear can be asymptomatic and occurs frequently in the general population. It can be an early consequence of anorectal procedures, and a common problem in the elderly and in patients with neurologic diseases. Fecal impaction and laxative abuses should be excluded. Major incontinence is a most disabling problem. Afflicted individuals frequently become socially and professionally isolated. Patients are confined to the house and may be rejected by family and friends. In the elderly, it often results in admission to nursing homes.[46] Patients in their fourth and fifth decades can also develop denervation

of pelvic floor musculature. History of difficult and prolonged labor,[47] prolonged straining with pelvic floor descent,[48] complete rectal prolapse,[49] or solitary rectal ulcer syndrome[50] may be a contributing factor. Traumatic damage, tumor, and infection can lead to destruction of pelvic floor muscle and cause incontinence. Peripheral neuropathies associated with alcohol or diabetes mellitus are rare causes. Laxity of the anal sphincter and saddle anesthesia of the perineum support involvement of coccygeal nerves.

PRURITUS

Pruritus ani is a common complaint. It is associated with a variety of anorectal conditions producing increased local moisture.[51] The questionnaire should define if present day or night, or both, and if it is associated with discharge or not. Varying degrees of pruritus may occur in the perianal area in patients with systemic skin conditions, such as psoriasis. Skin irritation or eruption elsewhere in the body should be excluded. Skin diseases such as fungal infections, candidiasis, and scabies may produce pruritus ani as may systemic illness such as diabetes mellitus, jaundice, or lymphoma. In rare cases, pruritus ani in adults may be caused by *Enterobius vermicularis* (pinworms),[15] which often affect other members of the family. Contact dermatitis is often due to local anesthetic application. The long-term use of topical steroids may produce an itchy atrophic dermatosis. Itching is associated with Bowen's disease and Paget's disease. Pruritus is associated with healing of anal conditions such as a healing anal fissure or hemorrhoidectomy incision. Shaving of perianal hairs aggravates itching postoperatively and should be omitted. Patients with anal discharge or seepage of stools may experience pruritus if they are unable to properly cleanse the anal area. Adequate hygiene may be difficult in hirsute or sweaty individuals or if skin tags or prolapsed hemorrhoids are present. Severe pruritus ani usually is associated with a mucoid discharge, which may be blood tinged due to open ulceration of the perianal skin. Any lesion that produces a discharge can cause pruritus. A mucosal ectropion or Whitehead deformity must be excluded.

Pruritus ani is often attributed to hemorrhoids, but frequently the examination fails to reveal significant hemorrhoidal disease. That is also why, unfortunately, many patients who undergo hemorrhoidectomy discover that the pruritic symptoms persist.[52]

References

1. Nelson RL, Abcarian H, Davis FG et al (1995) Prevalence of benign anorectal disease in a randomly selected population. Dis Colon Rectum 38:34–41

2. Johanson JF, Sonnenberg A (1990) The prevalence of hemorrhoids and constipation: an epidemiological study. Gastroenterology 98:380

3. Gordon PH (1992) Pharmacology of anorectal preparations. pp. 149–155. In Principles and Practice of Surgery for the Colon, Rectum, and Anus. Quality Medical Publishing, St. Louis

4. Welling DR, Wolff BG, Dozois RR (1988) Piles of defeat: Napoleon at Waterloo. Dis Colon Rectum 31:303–305

5. Karlen A (1984) pp. 7–34. In Napoleon's Glands and Other Ventures in Biohistory. Little Brown, Boston

6. Lockhart-Mummery HE (1975) Crohn's disease: anal lesions. Dis Colon Rectum 18:200–202

7. Cohen Z, McLeod RS (1987) Perianal Crohn's disease. Gastroenterol Clin North Am 16:175–189

8. Quinn TC, Glasser D, Cannon RO et al (1988) Human immunodeficiency virus infection among patients attending clinics for sexually transmitted diseases. N Engl J Med 318:197–203

9. Gottesman L (1991) Treatment of anorectal ulcers in the HIV-positive patient. pp. 19–33. In Perspectives in Colon and Rectal Surgery. Vol. 4. Quality Medical Publishing, St. Louis.

10. Daling JR, Weiss NS, Hislop TG et al (1987) Sexual practices, sexually transmitted diseases, and the incidence of anal cancer. N Engl J Med 317:973–977

11. Elam AL, Ray VG (1986) Sexually related trauma: a review. Ann Emerg Med 15:576–584

12. Edwards P, Wodak A, Cooper DA et al (1990) The gastrointestinal manifestations of AIDS. Aus N Z J Med 20:141–148

13. Stelzner F (1958) Uber die Haemorrhoiden. Dtsch Med Wochenschr 83:569

14. Veidenheimer MC (1992) Clinical evaluation of the anorectum, perineum, and pelvic floor. In Henry MM, Swash M (eds): Coloproctology and the Pelvic Floor. 2nd Ed. Butterworth-Heineman, Oxford, England

15. Nivatvongs S (1992) Diagnosis. pp. 81–114. In Gordon PH, Nivatvongs S (eds): Principles and Practice of Surgery for the Colon, Rectum and Anus. Quality Medical Publishing, St. Louis

16. Dent OF, Goulston KJ, Zubrzycki J et al (1986) Bowel symptoms in an apparently well population. Dis Colon Rectum 29:243–247

17. Nicholls J, Glass R (1986) Clinical presentations in coloproctology. pp. 243–247. In Diagnosis and Outpatient Management. Springer-Verlag, Berlin

18. Silman AJ, Mitchell P, Nicholls RJ et al (1983) Self-reported dark red bleeding as a marker comparable to occult blood testing in screening for large bowel neoplasms. Br J Surg 70:721–724

19. Farrands PA, Hardcastle JD (1984) Colorectal screening by self-completion questionnaire. Gut 25:445–447

20. Drossman DA, Sandler ES, McKee DC et al (1982) Bowel patterns among subjects not seeking health care: use of a questionnaire to identify a population with bowel dysfunction. Gastroenterology 83:529–534

21. Church JM (1995) Chronic rectal bleeding. pp. 71–74. In Wexner SD, Vernara AM (eds): Clinical Decision Making in Colorectal Surgery. Igaku-Shoin, New York

22. Church JM (1991) Analysis of the colonoscopic findings in patients presenting with rectal bleeding according to the pattern of their presenting symptoms. Dis Colon Rectum 34:391–395

23. Bernstein WC (1983) What are hemorrhoids and what is their relationship to portal venous system? Dis Colon Rectum 26:829–834

24. Johansen K, Bacdin J, Orloff MJ (1980) Massive bleeding from hemorrhoidal varices in portal hypertension. JAMA 244:2084–2085

25. Goulston KJ, Cook I, Dent OF (1986) How important is rectal bleeding in the diagnosis of bowel cancer and polyps? Lancet 2:261–264

26. Raftery TL, Sanison N (1980) Carcinoma of the colon: a clinical correlation between presenting symptoms and survival. Am J Surg 46:600–606

27. Funch DP (1985) Diagnostic delay in symptomatic colorectal cancer. Cancer 56:2120–2124

28. Chapuis PH, Goulston KJ, Dent OF et al (1985) Predictive value of rectal bleeding in screening for rectal and sigmoid polyp. Br Med J 290:1546–1548

29. Roberts PG (1992) Patient evaluation. pp. 25–35. In Beck DE, Wexner SD (eds): Fundamentals of Anorectal Surgery. McGraw-Hill, New York

30. Heppell J, Benard F (1991) Life-threatening perineal sepsis. Perspect Colon Rectal Surg 4:1–18

31. Dozois RR (1990) Retro rectal tumors: spectrum of disease, diagnosis, and surgical management. Perspec Colon Rectal Surg 3:241–255

32. Pollack R, Gordon PH, Ferency A et al (1990) Perineal endometriosis: a case report and review of the literature. J Reprod Med 2:109–112

33. Gordon PH, Schottler JL, Baccos EG et al (1976) Perianal endometrioma: report of five cases. Dis Colon Rectum 19:260–265

34. Swash M, Foster JMG (1992) Chronic perianal pain syndromes. pp. 449–454. In Henry MM, Swash M (eds): Coloproctology and the Pelvic Floor. 2nd Ed. Butterworth-Heineman, Oxford, England

35. Maroy R (1988) Spontaneous and evoked coccygeal pain in depression. Dis Colon Rectum 31:210–215

36. Thaysen TH EH (1935) Proctalgia fugax: a little known form of pain in the rectum. Lancet 2:243–246

37. Dodi G, Bogoni F, Infantino A et al (1986) Hot or cold in anal pain? A study of the changes in internal anal sphincter pressure profiles. Dis Colon Rectum 29:248

38. Parks AG, Porter NH, Hardcastle JD (1966) The syndrome of descending perineum. Proc R Soc Lon 59:477–482

39. Ger GC, Wexner SD, Jorge JMN et al (1993) Evaluation and treatment of chronic intractable rectal pain—a frustrating endeavor. Dis Colon Rectum 36:139–145

40. Kline RJ, Spencer RJ, Harrison EG Jr (1964) Carcinoma associated with fistula-in-ano. Arch Surg 89:989–994

41. Getz SB, Ovgit YD, Patterson RB et al (1981) Mucinous adenocarcinoma developing in a chronic anal fistula: report of 2 cases and review of the literature. Dis Colon Rectum 24:562–566

42. Culp CE (1983) Chronic hidradenitis suppurativa of the anal canal: a surgical skin disease. Dis Colon Rectum 26:669–676

43. Notaras MJ (1970) A review of three popular methods of post-anal (pilonidal) sinus disease. Br J Surg 57:886–890

44. Bauer AW, Sturm W, Schmiedt E (1984) Surgical correction of rectoprostatic fistula. Urology 24:452–455

45. Henry MM (1987) Pathogenesis and management of fecal incontinence in the adult. Gastroenterol Clin North Am 16:35–45

46. McCormick KA, Burgio KL (1984) Incontinence: an update on nursing care measures. J Gerontol Nurs 10:16–23

47. Snooks SJ, Swash M, Henry MM et al (1986) Risk factors in childbirth causing damage to the pelvic floor innervation. Int J Colorectal Dis 1:20–24

48. Henry MM, Parks AG, Swash M (1982) The pelvic floor musculature in the descending perineum syndrome. Br J Surg 69/0–472

49. Neil ME, Parks AG, Swash M (1981) Physiological studies of the anal sphincter musculature in fecal incontinence and rectal prolapse. Br J Surg 68:531–536

50. Snooks SJ, Swash M, Henry MM et al (1985) Electrophysiological and manometric assessment of the pelvic floor in the solitary rectal ulcer syndrome. Br J Surg 72:131–133

51. Daniel GL, Longo WE, Vernava AM (1994) Pruritus ani, causes and concerns. Dis Colon Rectum 37:670–674

52. Corman ML (1993) pp. 54–115. In Corman MC (ed): Hemorrhoids in Colon and Rectal Surgery. 3rd Ed. J.B. Lippincott, Philadelphia

11

HEMORRHOIDS

Neil Mortensen
John Romanos

It used to be said that the successful physician needed to have gray hair to give an air of seniority and wisdom, and hemorrhoids to give a look of constant anxiety that patients would think was a natural concern for their well-being. Hemorrhoids are, of course, important to the colorectal surgeon because they form a major part of his or her work. They have been described and treated since the very beginnings of medical practice. Although many patients present with symptomatic disease, the same vascular cushions are present in normal individuals and in those who present with a hemorrhoidal problem. The word "hemorrhoid" is derived from the Greek haemorrhoids, meaning flowing of blood (haema = blood, rhoos = flowing). The word "pile" comes from the Latin pila, meaning a ball or a pill. Perhaps the term pile should be reserved for anal cushions that enlarge but then bleed, and the term hemorrhoids for those that actually present with bleeding. The causes of hemorrhoidal disease are unknown. Constipation and an abnormal bowel habit are commonly blamed, but there is very little evidence to support this.

NORMAL ANAL LINING

The anal canal is lined in its upper two thirds by a columnar epithelium and in the lower third by squamous epithelium, which meet at the dentate line. The junctional area between these two epithelial surfaces is called the anal transitional zone, which may vary in extent from a few millimeters to several centimeters, and circumferentially can be patchy or a complete ring of specialized epithelium. In the upper anal canal beneath this epithelium there are vascular cushions continuous with the rectal columns above (Fig. 11-1), which when distended give a stellate cross-section to the anal lumen. Classically, three are described, two on the right and one on the left, but their arrangement varies greatly. Thomson[1] found that only 19% of normal subjects had the classical arrangement at 3, 7, and 11 o'clock.

The anal cushions receive a rich intercommunicating blood supply from the superior, middle, and inferior rectal arteries. Up to eight branches of the superior rectal artery pass from the mesorectum through the rectal wall, descending into the anal subepithelial space and anastomosizing circumferentially to then communicate with the venous system, not only through the capillaries but by direct arterial venous shunts.[1]

Specialized veins running beneath the anoderm, particularly below the dentate line, have discrete dilatations along their core. They drain mainly into the superior rectal vein but also downwards into the systemic circulation. Thin- and thick-walled vascular spaces have been described, and some 19th century authors noted a resemblance to erectile tissue, but this is tenuous.[2] The venous dilations are supported by smooth muscle and fibroelastic tissue. Specialized sensory nerve endings and many nerve fibers in and around the vascular spaces have led to the suggestion that this represents a specialized regulatory system controlling anal pressure.

The anal cushions are supported against the extruding and shearing forces of defecation by smooth muscle. This was first described by Treitz in 1853, and is probably best termed the musculus submucosae ani. Slips of smooth muscle emerge from the inner surface of the internal anal sphincter at varying levels to pass into the subepithelial space. Hansen[3] demonstrated continuity of fibers between the conjoined longitudinal muscle layer and the musculus submucosae ani that pass through the upper internal anal sphincter (Figs. 11-2 and 11-3). They are most concentrated at the area of the dentate line, and this probably corresponds to the mucosal suspensory ligament described by Parks.[4] The physiology and pharmacology of these muscle fibers is not known, but it has been suggested that their contraction during defecation flattens the cushions and holds them up against the internal sphincter.

FUNCTION OF THE NORMAL ANAL CUSHIONS

There is good evidence to suggest that the anal cushions provide the final watertight seal to the anal canal. The internal anal sphincter cannot completely close the anal canal on its own.

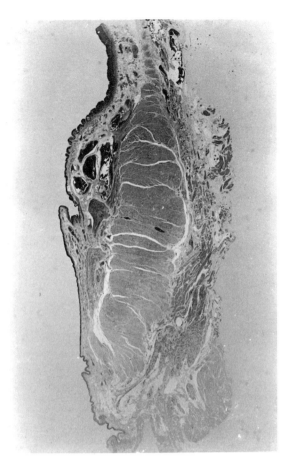

Figure 11-1.   Longitudinal section through anal canal showing the internal anal sphincter with vascular cushions below the columnar and transitional epithelium in the upper anal canal.

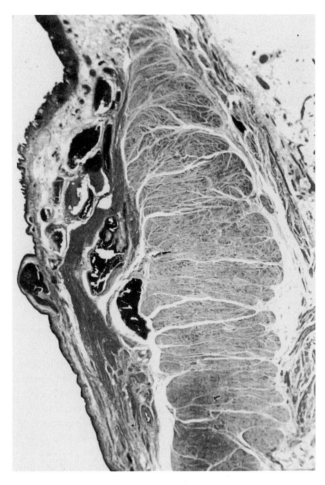

Figure 11-2.   Higher-power longitudinal section of anal canal showing the vascular cushions with enveloping slips of smooth muscle. Note the separate arrangement of the internal anal sphincter allowing fibers of the anal longitudinal muscle to pass through and join the musculus mucosae ani.

Vascular filling probably contributes 15% to 20% of resting anal pressure. The sacculated venous plexus of the anal cushions provides a spongy plug of infinitely variable volume, which, together with the tougher subepithelial space in the lower part of the anal canal, provides the final seal for perfect continence (Fig 11-4). Conversely, they can also be emptied to permit greater anal distension and therefore easier defecation.[1]

Emptying of the anal cushions may occur by passive compression due to the passage of a solid stool, and due to the action of contracted subepithelial muscle fibers from the conjoined longitudinal muscle, which act to compress the anal cushion complex under its arching fibers.[2]

THE PATHOPHYSIOLOGY OF HEMORRHOIDS

Varicose dilatation of anal veins was generally described and accepted until recently, but Thomson[1] was unable to show any difference between the histology of hemorrhoidectomy specimens and those of normal cadavers. Both aging and hemorrhoids lead to disordered connective tissue in the subepithelial space. Enlarged lamina propria capillaries can bleed in the absence of clinical hemorrhoids. There is hypertrophy of the subepithelial muscle together with squamous metaplasia of prolapsing hemorrhoids and edema.

The "pecten band" described by Miles is probably the free edge of the internal sphincter, and histologic studies have failed to show any fibrous rings or bands.[2] Fibrosis of the internal anal sphincter has been described in patients with symptomatic hemorrhoids, although anal endosonography does not show any increase in thickness in the internal anal sphincter. Changes in external sphincter striated muscle composition have been described but their significance is uncertain.

FUNCTIONAL ABNORMALITIES IN HEMORRHOIDS

Anal Pressure

The most widely and consistently reported change is a high maximum resting pressure in the anal canal, an indicator of increased resting internal anal sphincter tone.[2,5–7] Symptoms and pressure may be related since prolapsing hemorrhoids are associated with a lower resting pressure than nonprolapsing hemorrhoids.[8] Increased external sphincter tone and pressure within the vascular spaces could also account for the increased resting pressure.

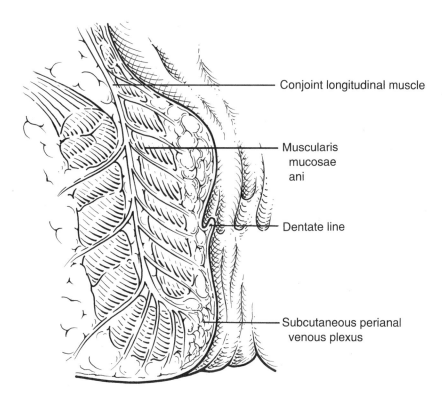

Conjoint longitudinal muscle

Muscularis mucosae ani

Dentate line

Subcutaneous perianal venous plexus

Figure 11-3.   Line drawing to show the relationship between the fibers of the musculus mucosae ani and the vascular cushions, and their relationship with the internal and external anal sphincter.

Figure 11-4.   Colonoscopic view of the upper anal canal and normal anal cushions seen on retroversion.

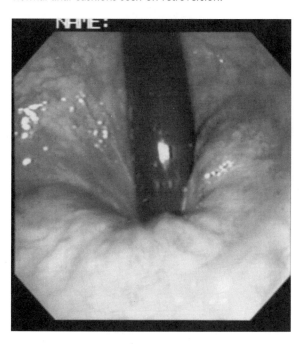

Abnormalities in rectoanal inhibition have been described, as have abnormalities in slow waves arising in the internal sphincter, particularly in its upper part. Ultraslow waves are also more common in patients with hemorrhoids.

Electrophysiology

Changes in external sphincter EMG are inconsistent and no clear changes in electrical activity in the internal anal sphincter have been confirmed in patients with hemorrhoids.

Anal Sensation

Anal electrosensitivity and temperature sensation are reduced in patients with hemorrhoids, particularly in the proximal and midanal canal, probably as a result of prolapse of less sensitive rectal mucosa contributing to decreased continence.[9]

EPIDEMIOLOGY

Accurate prevalence figures are impossible to ascertain. Personal, cultural, social, and economic differences can explain wide variations in hospital admission and operation rates, as well as self-reporting and medical practitioner attendances for hemorrhoidal disease.

Much has been made of dietary differences between developed countries and those, for example, in rural Africa. The observation that hemorrhoidal disease was uncommon in rural

Africa may not just be due to Burkitt's dietary fiber hypothesis[10] but to variations in availability and acceptance of medical care.

Hemorrhoids are common in the West. In the United States, 1177 physician visits for hemorrhoids are reported annually per 100,000 population compared with 1123 visits for England and Wales. Annual hospital discharge rates for hemorrhoids per 100,000 population are 47.65 in the United States and 40.69 in England and Wales. Hemorrhoidectomy rates in the United States have been estimated annually at 60.24 and 48.65 per 100,000 population. In France, the figure is 46 per 100,000 annually.[2]

There is some evidence that treatment rates are decreasing, but it is not known whether this is a true change in prevalence or a change in health behavior.[11]

SEX

Although the prevalence of hemorrhoids in the general population seems to be equal between the sexes, men are hospitalized for hemorrhoids more than women. Symptoms occurring during pregnancy and coinciding with the menstrual cycle can be explained by the high estrogen receptor content of hemorrhoids. Mechanical events during pregnancy may, of course, be just as important as hormone levels.

SOCIAL FACTORS

Hemorrhoids increase in prevalence with age. People in higher socioeconomic groups report hemorrhoids more frequently. There is an association with hernia, genitourinary prolapse, and prostatism, which may be a reflection of abdominal straining. There is no association with varicose veins or any other vascular disease. Despite Burkitt's hypothesis it has been difficult to prove a relationship between fiber intake and the prevalence of hemorrhoids.[12]

A positive family history is common, but this is more likely to be due to dietary, cultural, or behavioral causes rather than a genetic one. Constipation and straining at stool have been the most commonly described association with hemorrhoids, but many patients have a normal bowel frequency, and hemorrhoids do occur in vegetarians. Thomson et al.[13] found that the time spent in the lavatory was significantly longer in patients with hemorrhoids rather than straining at stool itself. They felt that sitting with a relaxed perineum and unsupported anal cushions was a potential cause of hemorrhoids.

A THEORY OF PATHOGENESIS

The notion of varicose veins of the anal canal has largely been discounted, and there is no relationship between hemorrhoidal disease and portal hypertension. Rectal varices are a clinically separate entity. Constipation and straining were once generally accepted as the major cause of hemorrhoidal disease, but this is now considered to be a gross oversimplification.[2]

Disruption of Anal Cushions

The anal cushions are disrupted by the forces of defecation and displaced distally. The delicate subepithelial connective tissue, with its slips of muscle fibers from the conjoined longitudinal

muscle, becomes loose and fragmented. The effect of raised intra-abdominal pressure engorges the cushions, and the shearing force of hard stool increases the damage. It is probably an over simplification to think of a common single etiology. Some patients claim a lifetime of regular easy bowel action, and perhaps from the effects of aging and a deficiency in the supporting tissues of the anal cushions, develop hemorrhoids as an effect of aging and a decrease in anal canal pressure. Many women date their hemorrhoids not to pregnancy itself but to parturition, when supporting tissues to the anal cushions can be stretched and torn. The terms internal and external hemorrhoids should probably be abandoned. It is simpler to describe the degree of disruption of the anal cushions and whether or not there is in addition a superimposed skin tag.

Classification of Hemorrhoids

It has been traditional to grade hemorrhoidal disease into four degrees depending on the extent of prolapse. This has limited value because it refers to only one aspect of the disease, the severity of blood loss or degree of discomfort being as important to some patients as the degree of prolapse. Many elderly patients can have third- or fourth-degree hemorrhoids with few symptoms. Some form of classification is, however, helpful in assessing different therapies, but keep in mind that the degree of prolapse may vary from day to day and, as mentioned, the different times in the menstrual cycle for women.

1. *First-degree piles.* These are anal cushions that do not descend below the dentate line on straining. By this definition all normal subjects have first-degree piles but only have hemorrhoidal disease when they develop symptoms.

2. *Second-degree piles.* These are anal cushions that protrude below the dentate line on straining. They can be seen at the anal verge only to disappear when straining ceases.

3. *Third-degree piles.* These anal cushions descend to the anal verge on straining or defecation and remain prolapsed until they are digitally replaced (Fig. 11-5).

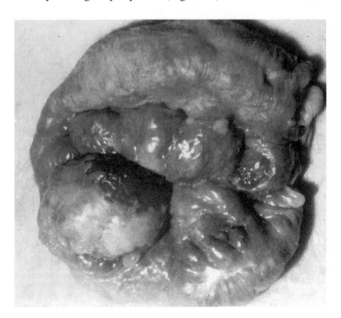

Figure 11-5. Third-degree hemorrhoids.

4. *Fourth-degree piles*. This is a term used by some to describe rectal mucosal covered internal cushions permanently outside the anal verge, which immediately prolapse on replacement.

Perhaps a more useful classification is that described by Nicholls and Glass.[14] In this the emphasis is on choice of treatment. They propose four stages as follows:

1. *Occasional symptoms*. Reassurance after exclusion of colorectal disease is all that is required.

2. *Bleeding with no prolapse*. Treatment with suppositories or injection is likely to be helpful.

3. *Prolapse*. Rubber band ligation may be indicated.

4. *Prolapse with large symptomatic external component*. Conservative measures are unlikely to help, and hemorrhoidectomy is the treatment of choice.

SYMPTOMS

Hemorrhoidal disease can give rise to varying degrees of bleeding, anal swelling, pain, discomfort, discharge, and puritis. The larger the cushions and the more they prolapse, the more troublesome the symptoms; but this is not invariable. Young men with a tight anal canal can have severe discomfort and profuse bleeding with minimal prolapse, while some elderly patients with huge cushions and major degrees of prolapse may have no complaints.

Bleeding

Bleeding is the most common complaint and the earliest in the development of the problem. The capillaries of the lamina propria are protected by only a single layer of epithelial cells, which is fragile and easily broken. The blood is often bright red and is first noticed on the lavatory paper after passing a non-blood stained firm stool. Repeated trauma due to wiping or contact with clothes to the extroverted prolapsed cushion produces a chronic inflammatory response, making the damaged mucosa a brighter red and granular and so more friable and likely to bleed.

As the problem becomes more protracted, the bright red rectal bleeding may be profuse, dripping into the pan or splattering the sides at the end of defecation. This is characteristic of hemorrhoidal bleeding but occasionally can be mimicked by a prolapsing rectal polyp on a long stalk.

Bleeding unrelated to defecation tends to occur in elderly patients with marked prolapse and can be described as a bright red mucousy discharge or occasionally spontaneous bleeding staining underclothing. Blood smeared on the stool in the pan is unlikely to be coming from piles and suggests a higher lesion.

The passage of clotted blood can occasionally occur due to a large pile bleeding back into the rectum, but this is unusual. Dark rectal bleeding usually indicates a higher lesion. Profuse bleeding can occasionally be of such a degree as to cause anemia.

Prolapse

It is unusual for patients to report for treatment for prolapse alone, but on questioning, patients may describe the symptom of protrusion of a lump or prolapse occurring during defecation and requiring self-digital reduction back into the anal canal. Some patients experience prolapse on exertion causing perianal discomfort, often due to exuding mucous and restricting their work and leisure activity. Hypertrophied anal papillae and low rectal polyps are often erroneously diagnosed as prolapsing piles.

Pain

Although pain is often described as a symptom of hemorrhoids, disrupted anal cushions in otherwise uncomplicated hemorrhoidal disease are unlikely to cause pain. The presence of severe pain would indicate a serious complication of hemorrhoidal disease such as thrombosed hemorrhoids resulting from obstruction of venous drainage and consecutive clotting in the sacculated venous complex. However, when trapped outside the closed anus, distortion together with edema and congestion from lymphatic and venous impairment may well cause discomfort. It is usually relieved by reduction of the prolapse. Prolapsed cushions in those with low anal canal tone is usually painless.

Itching and Discharge

When disrupted anal cushions are constantly prolapsed beyond the anal verge, a mucous discharge from the anus, with or without blood staining, is characteristic. This may soil the underclothing or cause excoriation of the perianal skin with secondary fungal infection. True fecal seepage is unusual in hemorrhoidal disease, and an intractable pruritis is usually due to a perianal skin condition. Perianal skin tags may result from a local derangement of lymphatic drainage consequent upon repeated eversion of the anal canal or perhaps the result of past episodes of complications such as thrombosis. They become increasingly common with the passage of time and can also give rise to problems with hygiene and pruritis.

NATURAL HISTORY AND COMPLICATIONS

It is not known what percentage of patients who suffer from uncomplicated hemorrhoids subsequently develop severe complications or have no further problems. The natural history of untreated hemorrhoidal disease is not known.

Thrombosis of Prolapsed Internal Anal Cushions

Thrombosis of prolapsed internal anal cushions is the most dramatic complication of hemorrhoidal disease and usually the most painful. It can occasionally occur as the first manifestation of the disease but is usually present in those with large piles who previously have been able to reduce them. Once thrombosis has occurred, the anal cushions are usually so swollen that they remain outside. There is often accompanying edema of the perianal skin, pressure rises in the anal canal, and there is pain and

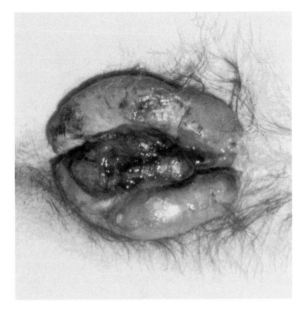

Figure 11-6. Thrombosed hemorrhoids. Note the marked swelling at the anal margin and necrosis of mucosa. The most marked features of thrombosis will be within the anal canal.

edema. Thrombosis can occur in one or more of the primary cushions, with pain such as to prevent sitting, walking, or defecation.

On parting the edematous perianal skin, a dark dense mucous membrane overlying the thrombosis can be seen, and on gentle rectal examination, a hard thrombosed cord-like cushion can be palpated (Fig. 11-6). The patient is in severe pain and digital examination is not justified. Further examination needs to be accomplished under sedation or anesthesia.

Without treatment by excision or dilatation, the internal cushion thrombosis will slowly and naturally resolve. Between 1 and 4 days after the initial thrombosis, edema and inflammation are at their greatest. Within 10 days resolution begins to occur, and may not be complete by as much as 6 to 8 weeks. An enlarged of fibrous skin tag may be a lasting reminder of the event.

True necrosis of the mucosa over the thrombosis is rare. Occasionally spontaneous extrusion of a clot can give symptomatic relief, but it is unusual for all of them to be extruded because they are present in a number of noncommunicating venous spaces. Very rarely the ischemic epithelium allows bacterial superinfection and may need to be treated with antibiotics.

Thrombosis of a Perianal Vascular Channel: Perianal Hematoma or Thrombosed Pericanal Vazgx

The term *perianal hematoma* is a misnomer, and thrombosis seems to be intravascular.[15] The clot has an endothelial lining. Tense swelling within the confines of this vascular space gives a hard, smooth swelling that causes extreme perianal pain. It usually occurs in patients who do not have symptomatic or hypertrophied internal anal cushions. Careful parting of the perianal skin shows that it is outside and not within the anal

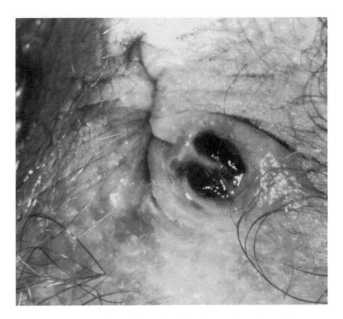

Figure 11-7. A thrombosed perianal vascular channel.

canal. A tender lump has a bluish appearance, and the hard clot does not extend up into the anal canal (Fig. 11-7).

Without treatment, it causes a few days of acute discomfort followed by gradual resolution over 5 to 7 days.

PATIENT ASSESSMENT AND EXAMINATION

History

Although a careful history may be very suggestive of the diagnosis of hemorrhoids, with particular attention to the color and character of rectal bleeding and the relief of discomfort on reduction of any prolapsing hemorrhoid, the diagnosis still must always be confirmed by endoscopy.

Examination

With the patient in either the left lateral position or the modified knee elbow position, the anal margin is inspected and the patient asked to bear down. The anal margin is gently parted and a careful rectal examination carried out. In the absence of an acute thrombosis, pain is rarely a feature of uncomplicated hemorrhoidal disease. Pain on digital examination would more commonly suggest a fissure in ano, an abscess, or perhaps an anal carcinoma; these are likely to be evident on inspection.

Sigmoidoscopy

Sigmoidoscopic exclusion of rectal disease is essential in establishing the diagnosis. In patients with bright red rectal bleeding, flexible sigmoidoscopy to 60 cm is the method of choice to rule out sigmoid neoplasms, and it is mandatory whenever there is blood mixed with the stool. In those patients with bright red blood on the toilet paper or with the characteristic blood splattering, it may be permissible to confine examination to the rectum, provided any symptoms are cured by hemorrhoidal treatment. In patients with any other colorectal symptoms or when there is any further doubt, either barium enema or colonoscopy will be required.

Proctoscopy

Because anal cushions are normal structures, their distinction from piles is one of degree. Bright red granularity of the mucosa over an anal cushion is evidence of recent disruption, and the extent to which the cushions bulge into the instrument on straining and follow it out on withdrawal, are also helpful signs. It is important to emphasize, however, that the presence of congested anal cushions does not necessarily mean that they have been the cause of bleeding. Inflamed mucosa in the upper anal canal may be due to proctitis. If there is doubt, a biopsy should be taken.

Anal manometry and anal ultrasound

The routine use of manometry and anal ultrasound is unnecessary. Some elderly patients or younger multiparous females with large prolapsing hemorrhoids have a low-pressure anal canal, and excisional surgery for hemorrhoids could result in a degree of anorectal incontinence. Here such specialized tests may be helpful in planning treatment, and this is especially so in patients who have recurrent hemorrhoidal problems following previous surgery.

TREATMENT

A Brief History of Hemorrhoidal Therapy

No area in coloproctology has been more subject to the vagaries of fad and fashion than the treatment of hemorrhoidal disease. So-called new treatments are often rediscoveries or modifications of older therapies. Variations on the theme of heating, freezing, ligating, or excising have followed each other in quick succession, sometimes making or breaking the careers of their advocates.

In the 19th century controversy raged over the relative advantages and disadvantages of ligation or excision. A form of submucosal hemorrhoidectomy had been described by Samuel Cooper in 1809. Dupuytren the 1820s used simple excision without ligation, sometimes with disastrous results. Von Langenbeck, in Berlin in 1870, popularized ligation of the hemorrhoids and tissue coagulation with a hot iron.[16]

Dr Mitchell of Illinois was the pioneer of injection therapy in the United States using 30% phenol in olive oil. He sold his formula secretly, giving rise to large numbers of unqualified itinerant commercial "pile doctors" but by 1900 the method had been accepted and recorded in legitimate medical literature. Injections were usually placed low in the anal canal and the high concentration of phenol acted as an anesthetic.

Anal spasm was also a popular theory of hemorrhoidal disease in the 19th century. Therapy was directed towards gentle stretching with bougies or by division of the anal sphincter. A comparison between anal dilatation and internal sphincterotomy was reported by Bodenheimer in the United States as early as 1868.

The most radical operation was described by Whitehead,[17] in which total excision of the pile bearing area with primary suture was advocated. The breakdown rate of this primary suture was considerable, however, and subsequent slow healing of the granulating wound often lead to a severe stenosis with mucosal ectropion, which became known as Whitehead's deformity. The operation was, however, logical, and Whitehead himself emphasized the need to ensure a mucocutaneous suture proximal to the anal verge to avoid ectropion with the consequent mucous leakage. It still has a place today.

The most common procedure was ligation of the whole prolapsed hemorrhoid including the skin and mucous membrane. This was usually a very painful procedure, and Salmon in 1836 introduced the first modification of this technique in Britain in which a cut was made with scissors at the mucocutaneous junction so that the base of the hemorrhoid could be ligated in the insensitive area of the mucosa, decreasing postoperative pain.

During the early part of the 20th century the most important descriptions of hemorrhoidal surgery came from the surgeons at St Mark's Hospital, London. Miles[18] had described a wide V-shaped excision of the perianal skin, and Milligan[19] described the low ligation technique. Together with Naunton Morgan, their technique *he described what* became known as the Milligan-Morgan hemorrhoidectomy. The closed hemorrhoidectomy technique was popularised by Ferguson and Heaton[20] at Grand Rapids, Michigan, and is still the operation most commonly used in the United States and Australia.

While operative hemorrhoidectomy became widely used, it was still seen as a very painful procedure, and this lead to the widespread interest in more conservative methods. Fixation by submucosal injection was revived and developed, and the technique of the injection of a weak solution of phenol (5% in arachis oil) was introduced by Blanchard.[21]

Rubber band ligation was rediscovered by Blaisdel in 1954, and Barron[22] modified his technique, producing a robust instrument for placing a strong rubber band to strangulate the base of a vascular cushion.[16]

Although cooling with ice had been used for many years to give local relief to thrombosed prolapsed hemorrhoids, the development of cryosurgical techniques allowed the clinical application of tissue destruction by freezing with liquid nitrogen. The method was popularized in the United States by Lewis[23] and in the United Kingdom by Lloyd Williams.[24] Infrared photocoagulation is the most recent addition, developed by Nath.[25]

Although there is considerable controversy over the exact nature of the pecten band, spasm or narrowing of the anal canal in association with hemorrhoids has been the focus of a further rediscovery. Lord[26] reintroduced the earlier French procedure of anal dilatation and stressed the importance of destroying the pecten band. Now at the end of the 20th century, things have again turned full circle, and Lord's anal dilatation procedure is once more out of favor.

MEDICAL MANAGEMENT

Advice

Most patients who only have minor symptoms, or an incorrect diet or personal hygiene, will often respond to advice in the first instance. A description of the degree of the severity of the problem, the simple pathophysiology of hemorrhoids and a discussion about diet, together with reassurance that there is no serious underlying abnormality, will often be effective. Advice about a high-fiber diet, avoiding foods or drink that cause diarrhea, and careful personal perianal hygiene are important elements. It is reassuring for patients to know that hemorrhoids have no malignant potential.

Defecatory Habits

Excessive straining at stool and prolonged periods of sitting on the lavatory are discouraged, while the adoption of a more squatting position is encouraged.

Dietary Manipulation

The aim is to achieve a bulky stool that is easy to pass, and the simplest way of achieving this is to ask the patient to change to a high-fiber diet. This is often best accomplished by advice cards and charts. A simple prescription of bran is often not tolerated, and many doctors prescribe simple bulk-forming agents such as sterculia, ispaghula husk, or psilium seed extract.

In a controlled trial, comparing the use of sterculia (Normacol) over a starch placebo in 40 patients with hemorrhoidal disease, Broader et al.[27] were unable to demonstrate a significant advantage. Compliance was poor and over 50% of patients stopped taking the sterculia at the end of the trial. Similar studies looking at Fybogel and psilium seed as bulking agents have been unable to demonstrate a clear effect between high fiber and the control of first- and second-degree hemorrhoidal disease.

Senapati and Nicholls[28] reported a prospective randomized trial of 43 patients with bleeding hemorrhoids who were allocated to receive either a bulk laxative together with injection sclerotherapy, or a bulk laxative alone. No significant difference in bleeding at 6 months was detected.

Although some proctologists argue that injection or photocoagulation therapies are very safe and more effective and that they should be the treatment of first choice, it would seem commonsense in the majority of cases to commence with dietary manipulation before invasive therapy.[29]

Topical Applications

There are a host of preparations available for hemorrhoidal disease and although patients often report that they give symptomatic relief, there is no clear evidence that they are effective. Most contain several ingredients including steroids, topical anesthetics, and antiseptics. Although topical anesthetics can give temporary relief for discomfort, they can provoke skin hypersensitivity. Hemorrhoidal symptoms, especially bleeding, go.[27] This aspect of natural history has no doubt been an important reason for the apparent success of local preparation.

MUCOSAL FIXATION

The aim of these mucosal fixation methods is to fix the mucosa and submucosal vascular cushions to the underlying muscle by creating submucosal fibrosis or full-thickness ulceration. Before carrying this out, the patient should be given a careful explanation of hemorrhoids and the technique to be advised. Success in abolishing symptoms can be expected in about 50% of cases, and this may be of only a few months duration.

Injection Sclerotherapy

The most commonly used equipment for injection sclerotherapy has been the Gabriel syringe and needle. Although the traditional glass syringe and needle were easy to use, they have been largely superseded by the disposable version made of phenol-resistant plastic and the luer lock device to prevent the needle becoming forced off (Fig. 11-8). Five percent phenol in almond or arachis oil is drawn up from individual 10-ml phials to allow for about 3 ml of injection into the base of each vascular cushion. Although 5% phenol in oil is the most common injection agent used in the United Kingdom, 5% quinine and urea hydrochloride is commonly used in the United States.

Technique

Although it is usually quite possible to accomplish hemorrhoidal sclerotherapy in an unprepared rectum, a small disposable microenema taken by the patient, either before the clinic

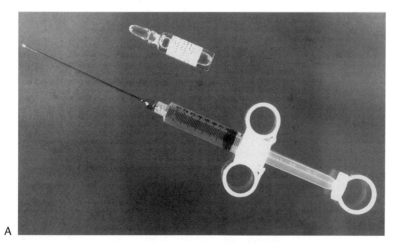
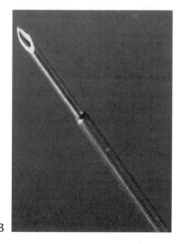

A   B

Figure 11-8. A disposable Gabriel syringe (**A**) and needle (**B**) for injection sclerotherapy.

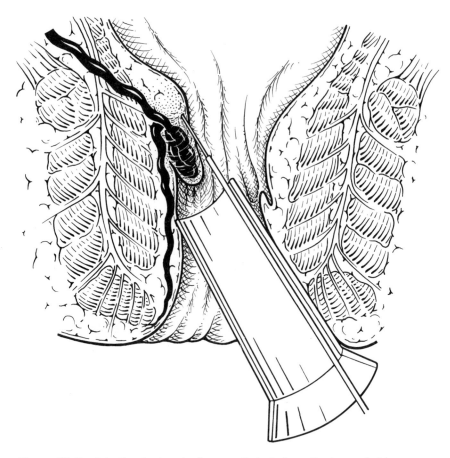

Figure 11-9. Injection is placed submucosally just above the hemorrhoid.

or at the clinic itself, ensures that the rectum is empty and good views of the anal canal are obtained. Treatment can take place in the left lateral position, the knee chest position, or on a special proctology table. After a preliminary sigmoidoscopy, the proctoscope is passed into the rectum, the obturator withdrawn, and the proctoscope gradually moved down the anal canal, and at the point where the reddish mucosa changes to the purplish mucosa, indicating engorged underlying vascular cushions, the sclerosant is injected immediately under the mucosa (Fig. 11-9). The procedure should be entirely painless. Pain or discomfort indicates either too deep an injection or positioning of the needle too near the anal verge. Three to five milliliters are injected into each vascular cushion.

Complications

1. Pain from an inappropriate injection site or submucosal extravasation.
2. Hemorrhage from a puncture point, which can, on occasion, be controlled by application of a band. More useful is application of a gauze swab soaked in topical adrenaline (1/1,000).
3. Prostatitis, lower urinary tract sepsis, or hematospermia from a grossly misplaced injection.
4. A fibrous band in the upper anal canal due to radial extravasation.

5. Pronounced inflammatory response associated with an oleogranuloma.

After Treatment

An advice sheet about the technique and any likely complications is usually given. If there has been any discomfort it is advisable that the patient rests for a while afterwards. A dull perianal ache may result several hours after the injection and a mild analgesic is usually sufficient. Most patients can return to work almost immediately. Those who are constipated should be advised to use a laxative and as usual, general advice should be given about diet and straining.

Results

There are disappointingly few large published series with reasonable length of follow-up after injection sclerotherapy. Khoury et al.[30] performed a randomized trial comparing single with multiple injection treatments. One hundred and two patients treated initially with conservative medical treatment and who had first- or second-degree hemorrhoids were randomized. At 3 months, 89.9% were either cured or improved of their symptoms, and this was maintained for 12 months after injection. There was, however, no difference in the degree of improvement between the two treatment regimes. Senapati and Nicholls[28] have reported a small study in which 43 patients were randomized to receive either bulk laxatives and injection therapy or bulk laxatives alone. After 6 months no significant difference in symptoms could be demonstrated.

Although injection sclerotherapy is very safe and probably upward of 70% of patients are satisfied with the results of treatment, it would seem sensible to start with conservative measures initially. Thereafter injection sclerotherapy is the first line of treatment for minor degrees of hemorrhoidal disease, particularly causing bleeding without prolapse. One course of injection seems to be sufficient. There is no evidence that repeated injections at monthly intervals are any better. In most patients a single outpatient visit with advice to return if the bleeding persists, should be sufficient.

RUBBER BAND LIGATION

Rubber band ligation probably works by causing some tissue loss and ulceration, and therefore fixation of the mucosa. A small rubber band, or O ring, is applied tightly around the neck of a tongue of mucosa, pulled into the barrel of an applicator. There is then ischemic sloughing of the mucosa and ulceration over the next few days. There is no evidence that using more than one band for each hemorrhoid is more effective, although this is widely practiced.

The original Barron ligator is the most widely used. A simpler version by McGiveny is also popular (Fig. 11-10).

Modifications of the device to allow a one-handed procedure have been described by Van Hoorn and more recently by Thomson (Fig. 11-11).[31] Another one-handed ligator uses suction to pull the mucosa into the cylinder for ligation.

Technique

Banding is more easily achieved if the patient has used a small microenema before attending the clinic so that the rectum is empty. Any of the positions described for injection sclerotherapy can be used. A straight oblique-ended or grooved procto-

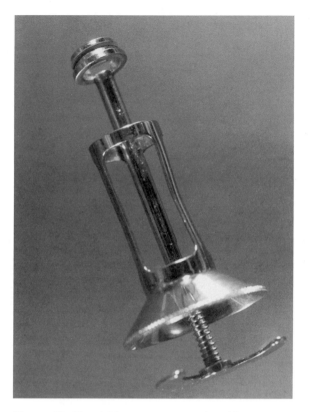

Figure 11-11.   A Thomson one-man band ligator.

scope, depending on personal preference, can be passed into the rectum and then gradually withdrawn. The whole of the internal cushion is then allowed to prolapse into the lumen so that its apex can be clearly seen. The proctoscope is passed back up into the upper anal canal, and while an assistant holds the proctoscope in position, the apex of the hemorrhoidal cushion is grasped and a rubber band applied to its base (Fig. 11-12). The principal problem and complication of the technique

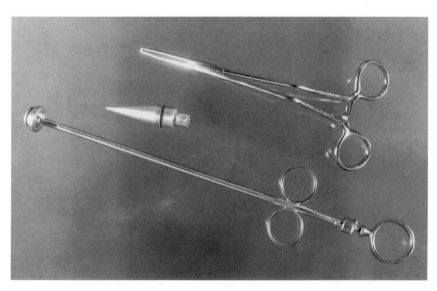

Figure 11-10.   A McGiveney simplified band ligator.

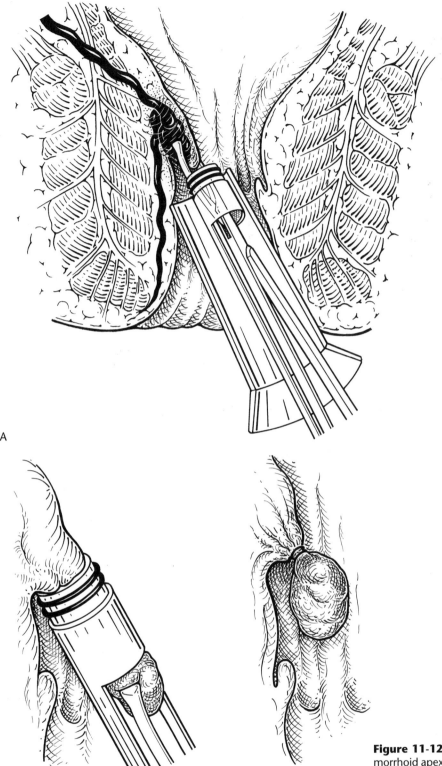

A

B

Figure 11-12. (**A & B**) Rubber band ligation. The hemorrhoid apex is grasped at least 6 mm above the dentate line. Here 2 bands are shown, but 1 is probably sufficient.

relates to the exact placing of the rubber band. If this is too near the dentate line, it may result in considerable pain and discomfort. The area of acute sensation can sometimes extend a centimeter or more above the dentate line and the apex of the cushions usually lies 1.5 to 2 cm above the dentate line. An indication that the band is being placed too low may be discomfort when the apex of the hemorrhoidal cushion is grasped with the grasping forceps. Severe pain immediately on banding is also an important sign that the band should be removed immediately. To do so it is easiest to use a small scalpel (#15) or fine scissors.

In the original description by Barron,[22] one ligation was performed at each session and repeated at three weekly intervals. It is however, perfectly feasible to perform two or three ligations at one session.

Some advocate the further injection of local anesthetic or phenol into the strangulated tissue, but there is no evidence that this improves either comfort or long-term results.

Complications

Pain is the most common complication of rubber band ligation. It is usually mild (20%), but on occasion can be severe (around 5%). If the pain is severe, the band must be removed. Patients are usually given an advice sheet warning them to take some mild analgesia and bed rest if the pain persists after the first 24 hours.

Some patients experience a vasovagal fainting episode on standing up after banding, but this usually passes if they lie back down on the couch for a while and mild analgesics are prescribed.

Since rubber band ligation causes tissue necrosis, secondary hemorrhage can occur when the tissue included in the rubber band separates. Patients should be warned that a show of blood may occur between days 5 and 7 after banding. This is generally not severe enough to require consultation or hospitalization.

The first case of fatal *Clostridium* infection resulting from banding of hemorrhoids was reported by O'Hara.[32] The most alarming report by Russell and Donohue[33] described 4 men between 34 and 54 years of age who developed pelvic cellulitis and died. Early recognition of this complication and aggressive antibiotic treatment can prevent a serious outcome. Although this is exceptionally rare, it emphasises the importance of meticulous technique and the signs and symptoms of fever, malaise, urinary hesitancy or retention, and increasing local discomfort should be taken very seriously.

Results

Here again the assessment of the effectiveness of rubber band ligation is hampered by reported series being small with only short-term follow up. In a randomized prospective trial, Murie et al.[34] assessed the results in 43 patients at 1 year. Most patients had an excellent result and only 12% had no improvement. In patients with third-degree hemorrhoids, 70% had no prolapse at 1 year. Pain, however, was a significant problem. Fifteen patients had pain for more than 48 hours. They concluded that rubber band ligation was the treatment of choice for first- and second-degree hemorrhoids. The largest series was reported by Bartizal and Slosberger,[35] who carried out a retrospective re-

view, 670 patients having had 3208 rubber band ligations. Mild to moderate discomfort was reported in 4.8% and pain, severe enough to limit activity, occurred in 0.6%. One percent of patients had severe bleeding. Two patients required readmission to hospital.

Khubchandani[36] randomly allocated 100 patients to one, two, or three ligations at a single session. No differences were found in the morbidity comparing multiple with single ligations. Mild discomfort occurred in 28, 32, and 35%, respectively, and pain severe enough to require an analgesic occurred in 28, 5 and 23%.

Long-term outcomes have been reported by Wrobleski et al.[37] Two hundred sixty-six patients with a minimum of 36 months and a mean of 60 months follow-up were reviewed. Eighty percent considered themselves improved and 69% were totally free of symptoms. Hemorrhoidectomy had been required in 7.5%. Steinberg et al.[38] used a questionnaire follow up in 147 patients at a mean of 4.8 years after rubber band ligation. Eighty-nine percent of patients were either cured or satisfied with the results, but only 44% were totally symptom free. Further conservative measures such as rubber band ligation or dilatation had been required in 12%, but only 2% required a hemorrhoidectomy.

Rubber band ligation was compared with hemorrhoidectomy, anal dilatation, and cryotherapy by Lewis et al.[39] One hundred twelve patients were randomly divided into 4 groups. They all had prolapsing hemorrhoids failing to respond to injection sclerotherapy. Of the 30 patients treated by rubber band ligation, 24 had required further treatment, including hemorrhoidectomy in 12, anal dilatation in 3, and injection in 9. These disappointing results may be a reflection of severe degrees of hemorrhoidal disease being selected, those patients usually requiring hemorrhoidectomy. When rubber band ligation is compared with injection therapy as first-line treatment, however, both therapies seem to be equally effective.[40]

CRYOTHERAPY

Cryodestruction of skin lesions using liquid carbon dioxide or liquid nitrogen is well established. The freezing of tissue below $-22°C$ causes permanent destruction by infarction and thrombosis, which occurs within 24 hours. The tissue then becomes necrotic, and sloughing and separation of the frozen from the undamaged tissue takes 10 to 14 days. Although freezing destroys nerve endings and induces anesthesia, on rewarming the edema and inflammatory response cause pain.

Liquid nitrous oxide cryoprobes are the most widely used. The principal disadvantage of the technique is that patients may be frightened by the cold sensation and adequate freezing may take 20 to 25 minutes. In the office or outpatient setting this is clearly too time consuming and the use of anaesthesia or sedation makes the technique less attractive as an ambulatory procedure.

The tip of the probe is applied to the anal cushion to produce an ice ball over 2 or 3 minutes. Most proponents of the technique advise a second application to the same cushion after a period of 5 to 10 minutes of thawing.

Complications

Although early enthusiasts described cryotherapy as a painless technique, it can only be used for tissue destruction of hemorrhoidal cushions above the dentate line without additional analgesia or general anesthesia.

The major problem is a profuse serous discharge occurring between the 2nd and 10th day after treatment. Bleeding, on the other hand, is extremely uncommon. The effects of cryotherapy take some time to subside, in some cases up to 8 weeks.

Results

In an interesting study, Smith et al.[41] compared hemorrhoidectomy with cryodestruction on opposite sides of the anal canal in the same patient. In 26 patients they concluded that the site of excision and primary suture after hemorrhoidectomy healed faster than the site of cryodestruction. There were also more frequent residual hemorrhoid, adjacent thrombosis, and skin tags after cryotreatment.

In treating large prolapsing third-degree hemorrhoids, which would otherwise have required hemorrhoidectomy, Lewis et al.[39] reported that 5 (20%) of 25 patients subsequently required conventional hemorrhoidectomy for residual piles and that cryosurgery was unsuitable for this group of patients. O'Callaghan et al.,[42] in a similar group of 97 patients, compared cryosurgery with hemorrhoidectomy in a group of 99 patients. Cryodestruction gave equally good results with fewer complications, and less time in hospital or off work. Goligher,[43] however, was less enthusiastic. In 68 patients who were on the waiting list for hemorrhoidectomy, adequate cryodestruction was obtained in 50 patients and 50 were able to return immediately to normal activity. Only 38 considered that they were pleased with the result and 12 were disappointed owing to continuing symptoms.

Although enjoying a brief period en vogue in the late 1970s and early 1980s, most proctology clinics have now abandoned the technique on the grounds of pain and profuse discharge. Hemorrhoidectomy would still appear to be the best treatment for third degree prolapsing hemorrhoids.

PHOTOCOAGULATION

Neiger[44] first adapted infrared photocoagulation for the treatment of hemorrhoidal disease. The infrared pulse causes a circumscribed area of tissue destruction by heating to 100°C. The burnt tissue reacts in a similar way to that treated by cryotherapy or rubber band ligation.

Technique

Infrared coagulation is applied in pulses to the base of the hemorrhoidal cushion. The tip must be in complete contact with the mucosa, and three to six coagulations are performed at the base of each hemorrhoid.

Complications

This technique has the fewest complications of any of the conservative methods described, because the depth of tissue destruction is limited to 3 mm. Pain is unusual, and the incidence and severity of secondary hemorrhage is negligible. Urinary retention and infection are very unusual.

Results

Leicester et al.[45] reported cessation of bleeding at 12 months in 17 (49%) of 35 patients treated by injection and 20 (53%) of 38 by infrared coagulation. For prolapse, photocoagulation was successful in 17 (39%) of 43 patients compared with 12 (35%) of 34 having rubber band ligation. Photocoagulation has been compared with rubber band ligation. Ambrose et al.[47] found that photocoagulation was associated with significantly fewer side effects than rubber band ligation but the clinical results were similar. Templeton et al.[46] found a satisfactory outcome in 85% of patients after infrared coagulation. There were fewer complications and better patient acceptability. Ambrose et al.[47] compared photocoagulation with injection therapy and found that fewer patients needed further treatment after injections than after photocoagulation. Photocoagulation is most useful in dealing with first-degree hemorrhoids and is less effective for third-degree piles. It has, however, declined in use.

OTHER TECHNIQUES

Bipolar diathermy[48,49] and Nd:YAG laser[50] have been used for the treatment of hemorrhoids. As yet there is no evidence that they confer any advantage over established techniques.

OPERATIVE TREATMENT

The Anal Stretch Procedure

Anal dilatation is an age-old remedy described and popularized in 19th century France by Recamier and Maisonneuve. The rationale lies in the questionable anatomic structure known as the pecten band, first described by Miles. Eisenhammer[51] of South Africa in the 1950s described a constricting band in the anal canal that he felt it was important to stretch, and Lord, on introducing the technique of forcible anal dilatation, stressed the importance of dividing or stretching constricting bands, both at the position of the pecten band and higher in the anal canal.

There has not, however, been any firm histologic evidence for fibrotic bands encircling the anorectum. It is more likely that the anal canal tightness found in hemorrhoidal disease is caused by muscle spasm and not by any anatomic fibrous structure.

The eight finger dilatation procedure popularized by Lord[52] has largely been abandoned owing to the incidence of incontinence in as many as 10% of patients postoperatively. A more judicious digital dilatation, by only four fingers, may be justifiable in some patients with thrombosed hemorrhoids, or anal pain. It should never be used in multiparous or aged females and should not be repeated even in males.

Results

Lord[53] reported results in over 300 patients, and claimed that only a tiny minority subsequently needed a hemorrhoidectomy and that the vast majority were rendered asymptomatic.

Randomized controlled trials comparing dilatation with rubber band ligation and hemorrhoidectomy failed to show any advantage of the anal dilatation technique. Vellacot and Hardcastle[54] were unable to confirm any benefit from the use of an anal dilator after maximal anal dilatation, and they and Hancock[55] showed that after anal dilatation there was a persisting reduction in resting pressures in the anal canal by as much as 50%, which persisted 5 years after the procedure.

Lord himself admitted that transient incontinence to flatus or mucous was common in the first few days after the procedure but stated that this resolved in time. This cannot always be the case, however, because a small number of patients persist with incapacitating incontinence in the longer term. There is now anal ultrasound evidence that anal dilatation can disrupt the internal anal sphincter. At a conservative estimate, up to 10% of patients may have a degree of persisting incontinence after the procedure, which is clearly unacceptable and a major reason for the decline in popularity of the procedure.

Bruising or bleeding after anal dilatation are unusual but sometimes the skin of the anal canal can split. Mucosal and even rectal prolapse have been described after the procedure.

Internal Anal Sphincterotomy

In patients who have a high resting anal pressure, the concept of a more controlled reduction in pressure is attractive, and internal sphincterotomy has been described in these patients. No clear benefit has been demonstrated over other treatments including anal dilatation, and indeed postoperative incontinence is a major concern.[56]

Suture

Simple suture rather than excision of hemorrhoids has been described, but there does not seem to be any clear advantage over rubber band ligation or sclerotherapy.

Hemorrhoidectomy

There are essentially two varieties of hemorrhoidectomy, open and closed. The former is the most popular in the United Kingdom, and the latter is widely used in North America.

Closed Hemorrhoidectomy

Closed hemorrhoidectomy was popularized by Ferguson et al.[57] Its aim was to remove as much internal hemorrhoid as possible without sacrificing anoderm, to prevent stenosis that he thought resulted from large raw wounds. Closure was also considered to be an important part of the technique to minimize postoperative serous discharge.

Indications

Some 10% of patients managed conservatively will eventually require a hemorrhoidectomy for excessive bleeding, severe prolapse or pain, or in those requiring surgery for other anorectal diseases. Contraindications to hemorrhoidectomy include the presence of Crohn's disease,[58] portal hypertension, leukaemia, lymphoma, or bleeding diathesis. Patients who have a symptomatic external hemorrhoidal component comprise the most common indication. Those who continue to have bleeding or prolapse after conservative or minimally invasive treatments should also be considered. Hemorrhoidectomy for pruritus is not usually effective and should be undertaken with great caution.

Preparation and Operation

The patient's bowel is prepared with a microenema, and in selected cases, day surgery may well be possible. The preferred position is the prone jackknife position. The perianal area is blocked with local anaesthesia (bupivacaine with adrenaline 1/300,000). Regional anaesthesia including causal or spinal, block may also be employed. With the buttocks strapped apart, the anal canal is examined with a Pratt bivalve anoscope or a Fansler anoscope. Although a three-quadrant hemorrhoidectomy is common, this is by no means the rule. In addition to a search for excessive hemorrhoidal tissue in other positions, the presence of rectal mucosa or prolapse is noted. The hemorrhoid is grasped with the forceps and excised. Bleeding from the submucosal vessels is controlled with diathermy. Undermining of the anoderm on either side allows complete removal of any vascular tissue. The wound is then closed using a running adsorbable suture (gauge 30) and small bites of the internal anal sphincter may be included to fix the endoderm to the anal canal (Fig. 11-13). The other hemorrhoidal sites are then selected and treated in the same way. Skin tags should be excised wherever possible with the hemorrhoid but occasionally they may have to be excised separately if they are displaced from the surgical wound. At the end of the procedure, the excision sites and suture lines are inspected using the anoscope and any persisting bleeding point is underrun.

Submucosal Hemorrhoidectomy

Parks described submucosal hemorrhoidectomy in 1956.[4] It is a plastic operation, removing the hemorrhoid while leaving the epithelial layer largely intact. This is then sutured to constitute the anal canal without tissue loss. A Parks self-retaining bivalve speculum exposes the anal canal throughout its length. A longitudinal incision is made along the mucosa over each hemorrhoid and the anoderm undermined on either side to create flaps to expose the underlying hemorrhoidal tissue, which is then removed. At the apex of each wound, the pedicle is transfixed and ligated. The mucosa is closed taking the suture through the internal sphincter to fix it. An open wound is left at the most distal lower end of the incision to allow drainage of blood and serum (Fig. 11-14).

Postoperative Care

Intravenous fluid administration during surgery is kept to a minimum to reduce the incidence of acute retention of urine. Patients are started on a combination of high-fiber diet and mild laxatives and appropriate analgesia are given. The systematic arrangements for counseling, preoperative preparation, aggressive analgesia, and careful hemostasis will allow increasing numbers of patients to have hemorrhoidectomy as a day care procedure. Complications include wound dehiscence, bleeding, fecal impaction, and persistent soiling or mild incontinence. Comparative studies between open and closed hemorrhoidectomy are few. In Goldberg's series of 500 consecutive closed hemorrhoidectomies, 10% had urinary retention, 4% had bleed-

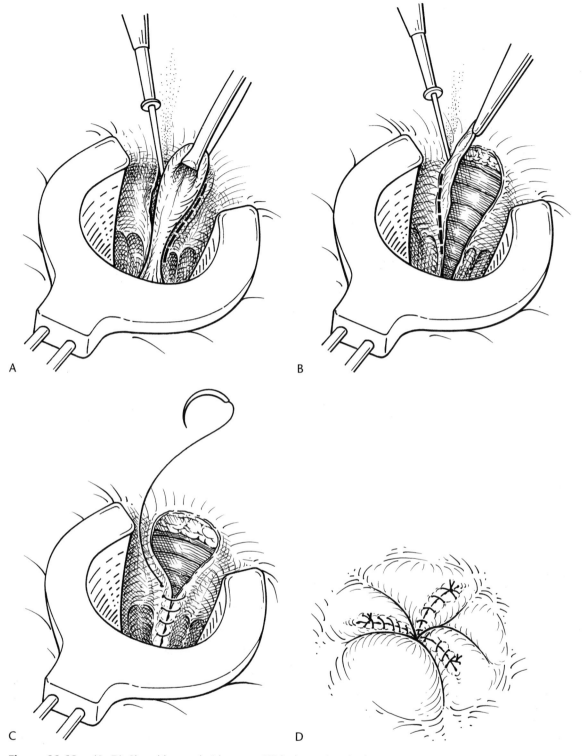

Figure 11-13. (**A–D**) Closed hemorrhoidectomy. With the patient in the prone jackknife position, the pile is excised, the mucosa edges diathermized and undermined, and finally the mucosal edges are approximated with a running absorbable suture.

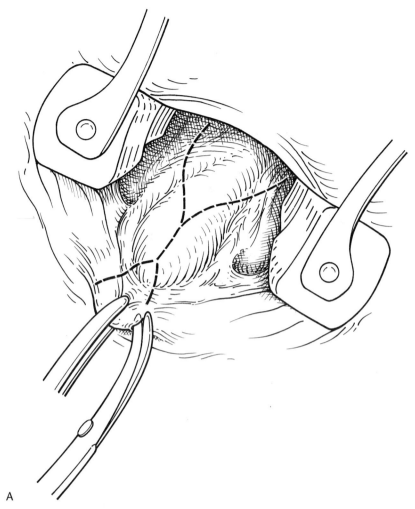

A

Figure 11-14. (**A–E**) Submucosal hemorrhoidectomy. The hemorrhoid is filletted from beneath the mucosa and the mucosa partly closed. (*Figure continues.*)

ing, 6% had skin tags, fistula-in-ano occurred in 0.4%, anal stenosis in 1%, and incontinence in 0.4%.[59]

Although those surgeons who use the closed technique are convinced of its efficacy, particularly in reduction in postoperative pain, there are no objective data to confirm this.

Open Hemorrhoidectomy

Open hemorrhoidectomy is the operation most widely used in the United Kingdom and is based on the technique originally described by Milligan in 1937[19] and now generally referred to as the Milligan-Morgan operation. General or regional anaesthesia can be used. Either the lithotomy or prone jackknife position can be used. Infiltration with 1 in 300,000 adrenaline assists in hemostasis. Although in the original description an anal retractor was not used, a Parks, Eisenhammer, or Pratt speculum allows the technique to be carried out under direct vision and aids hemostasis, even if a closed technique is not being used. The skin over each of the main hemorrhoids is grasped with artery forceps and retracted outwards (Fig. 11-15). The more proximal mucosa is then retracted distally with a second artery

forceps. With one finger in the anal canal supporting the hemorrhoid stretched under tension by retraction on the artery forceps, a V-shaped incision is made at the skin base of each hemorrhoid. The incision is developed laterally to circumvent the perianal venous plexus, which is then displaced medially until the lower border of the internal sphincter is identified. This is the key to safe hemorrhoidecomty. It enables easy access to the submucosal plane without damage to the muscle. Any slips of the longitudinal muscle (musculus submucosae ani) are divided by blunt resection or diathermy during this part of the dissection. Having identified the lower border of the internal sphincter, longitudinal incisions are extended up the anal canal on each side of the hemorrhoidal pedicle, converging them to a point about a centimeter above the dentate line. The submucosal plane is entered dissecting laterally fibers of the internal sphincter to the level of the upper anal canal. This dissection will create a pedicle that is transfixed by absorbable suture material and the isolated hemorrhoid is then excised. The area is carefully checked for hemostasis. An alternative technique is to use electrocoagulation to dissect the hemorrhoid. With this procedure ligation of the pedicle is not necessary, since individual vessels are usually easily identified for coagulation.

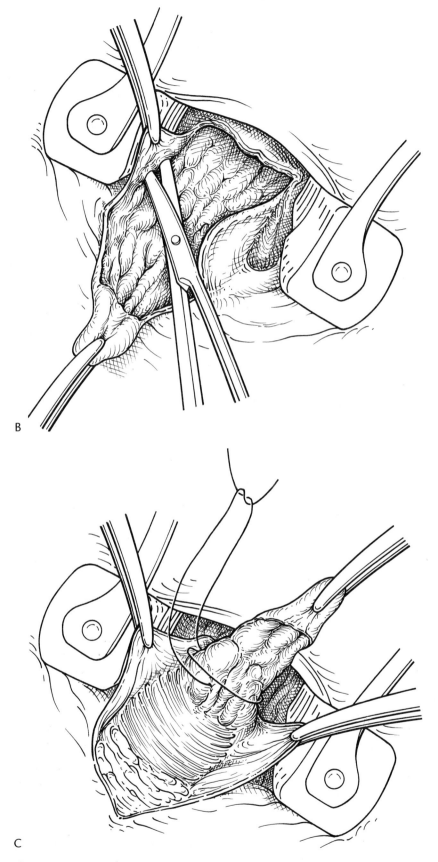

B

C

Figure 11-14. *(Continued)*

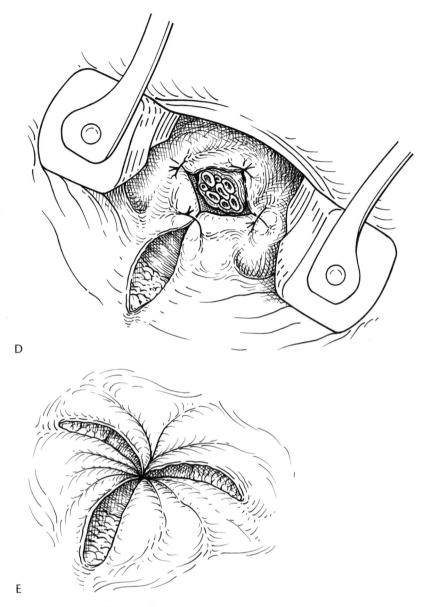

D

E

Figure 11-14. *(Continued)*

It is generally best to tackle the left lateral and right posterior hemorrhoid first since bleeding from the right anterior hemorrhoid can impair the view of any subsequent hemorrhoidectomy. When making the skin incisions in the anal canal, it is important to ensure that there is an intact bridge of anoderm between each excised hemorrhoid.[60] It is usually not necessary to pack the anal canal, which is simply dressed with paraffin gauze and a dry pad. Commercially available sponge plugs and pads do not seem to have any advantage. There is no evidence that the addition of either a sphincterotomy or anal stretch improves the incidence of postoperative pain or healing.

Postoperative Care and Complications

Patients are usually started on a fiber preparation and a mild laxative, together with nonnarcotic analgesics. Pain is very variable after open hemorrhoidectomy. Relief can be obtained by immersion in a hot bath. The area should be kept scrupulously clean after defecation, and a detachable shower head can be useful to wash the area. Patients are usually confined in hospital until their first bowel action 2 or 3 days after the procedure. A phosphate enema can be used if the patient becomes constipated. There is no evidence that the routine use of antibiotics reduces postoperative pain. However, in exceptional circumstances of severe pain, metronidazole can undoubtedly produce relief. Daycare hemorrhoidectomy is commonly used, particularly in the United States. This requires adequate home facilities, full access to the surgeon and hospital, and a degree of understanding on the part of the patient.

Results

There are few long-term published results of the Milligan-Morgan hemorrhoidectomy. Up to 10% of patients have treatment failure, but around 90%, when questioned, are satisfied with

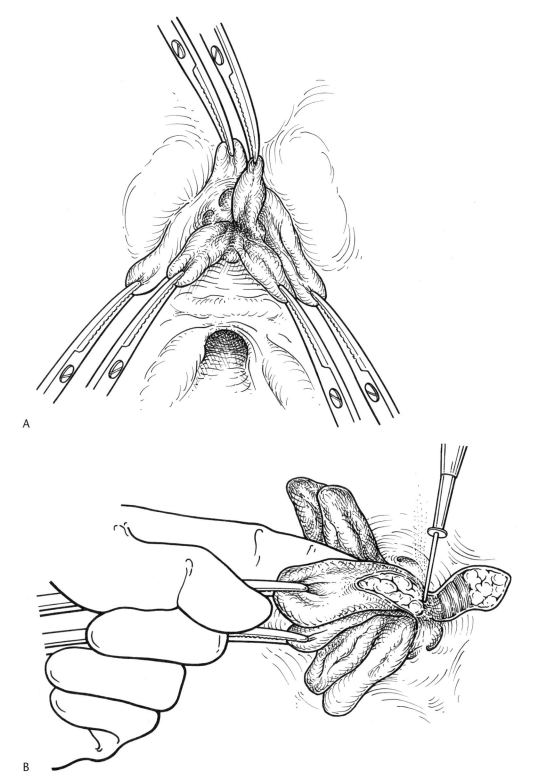

A

B

Figure 11-15.   (**A–E**) The classical Milligan-Morgan hemorrhoidectomy. (*Figure continues.*)

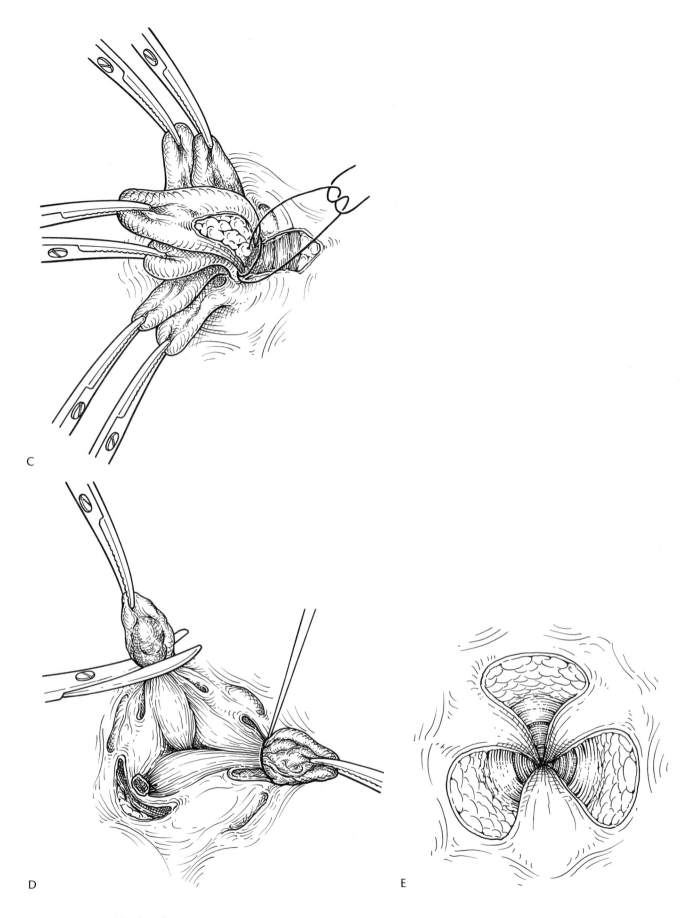

C

D

E

Figure 11-15. *(Continued)*

their operation. Roe et al.[61] compared submucosal excision with the Milligan-Morgan operation and found no difference in postoperative pain as measured by linear analog scores. True closed hemorrhoidectomy has never been compared in this way with the Milligan-Morgan operation and it would be interesting to see the results.

Reactionary hemorrhage is usually due to a slipped ligature or small bleeding point in one of the anal wounds. Gentle oozing can be stopped by external pressure but it is important to remember that bleeding from a pedicle can pass up into the rectum and remain undetected. Patients who are hemodynamically unstable, or in whom there is any doubt as to the source of the bleeding, should be returned to the operating room for an examination under anesthesia. After irrigation the bleeding point can be detected and underrun, but balloon tamponade and packing have also been used. Usually bleeding arises from the edge of the external wound. Local application of gauze-soaked adrenaline may stop it but if this is not successful an examination under anesthesia should be carried out. The incidence of secondary hemorrhage ranges from 1.2 to 4% and occurs between the 7th and 10th postoperative days. It is often described by the patient as an urge to evacuate followed by the passage of large amounts of fluid and clotted blood. Readmission to hospital may be necessary. Before an examination under anesthetic, the passage of a wide-bore rubber drain with paraffin gauze wrapped around it or a Foley catheter inserted into the rectum should be attempted.

Failure of one of the hemorrhoidectomy sites to heal adequately may result in anal fissure. This is usually only apparent weeks to months postoperatively, and should be treated by a lateral sphincterotomy. Abscess and fistula formation have been described but are rare. Edema in the perianal skin following a hemorrhoidectomy indicates that skin tags are likely to result.

The most feared complication of hemorrhoidectomy is the development of an anal stenosis. Provided skin bridges are retained, the complication is unlikely. Its true incidence is not known. If there is any evidence of anal narrowing, patients can use an anal dilator, take bulk laxatives, or have an examination under anesthesia and a judicious anal stretch, or even in some cases, an anoplasty. The Whitehead operation may result in this complication, but like Delorme's procedure (with which it has close similarity) this is usually manageable by dilation in the rare case where it occurs.

Minor disturbances of continence are quite common after any form of hemorrhoidectomy. Roe et al.[61] found that in both submucosal hemorrhoidectomy and excision ligation patients, some 50% equally divided between the two groups complained of soiling in the early postoperative period, but this settled uneventfully. It is important to remember that in elderly patients with a weak anal sphincter, enlarged anal cushions may be an important contributory factor in their continence, and hemorrhoidectomy should be offered in these circumstances only rarely.

Comparison of Treatments

Table 11-1 shows the results of comparative trials. It can be seen that subgroup analysis is necessary. In correctly selected cases, hemorrhoidectomy performs well. The outcome for other treatments is similar to the conclusion drawn from a meta-analysis reported by MacRae and McLeod.[62] These authors have presented a superb comparison of the various methods. Eighteen trials were rigorously selected and analyzed. Hemorrhoidectomy was found to be more effective than manual dilatation of the anus, with less need for further treatment, no difference in complications, but more pain. Hemorrhoidectomy was also

Table 11-1. Results of Comparative Trials of Treatments of Hemorrhoids

	Follow-up (Months)	Symptom	No. of Asymptomatic Patients/No. of Patients Followed						
			Injection	RBL	MDA	IR	C	LS	H
Keighley et al.[56]	12	Not specified	—	16/35	11/37	—	4/36	6/34	—
Cheng et al.[64]	12	Bleeding	14/21	15/20	19/22	—	—	—	18/19
		Prolapse	4/9	10/10	5/8	—	—	—	11/11
Sim et al.[65]	12	Bleeding	14/24	15/22	—	—	—	—	—
		Prolapse	0/7	5/7	—	—	—	—	—
Greca et al.[40]	12	Not specified	13/33	15/28	—	—	—	—	—
Murie et al.[34]	42	Bleeding	—	27/38	—	—	—	—	32/38
		Prolapse	—	17/25	—	—	—	—	27/29
O'Callaghan et al.[42]	48	Not specified	—	—	—	—	65/89	—	64/88
Hancock[55]	60	1st, 2nd degree	—	—	19/22	—	—	—	—
		3rd degree	—	—	12/26	—	—	—	—
Leicester et al.[45]	12	Bleeding	17/35	—	—	20/38	—	—	—
		Prolapse	—	12/34	—	17/43	—	—	—
Templeton et al.[46]	3–12	Not specified	—	33/62	—	34/60	—	—	—
Ambrose et al.[66]	12	1st degree	—	6/17	—	8/22	—	—	—
		2nd degree	—	20/62	—	26/68	—	—	—

RBL, rubber band ligation; MDA, maximal dilatation of the anus; IR, infrared coagulation; C, cryotherapy; LS, lateral sphincterotomy; H, hemorrhoidectomy.
[a] Noncontrolled trial.

more effective than rubber band ligation, but patients had more complications and pain. Rubber band ligation was more effective than injection sclerotherapy and infrared coagulation, but was associated with more pain.

Thrombosed Perianal Varyx or Perianal Hematoma

Thrombosed perianal varyx is a characteristic pea-sized subcutaneous swelling that may be hard, tender, and have a purplish appearance. There is no internal component and minimal perianal swelling. The condition is a thrombosis in the subcutaneous venous plexus. It may occur after an episode of vigorous exercise, for example on the sports field, in the home on lifting heavy weights, or straining in the lavatory. If the patient presents early in the history of the condition, it is best treated by the use of topical anesthesia and evacuation of a clot by making a small incision in the most distended area, with immediate and dramatic relief of symptoms. This rarely occurs in practice and

patients usually present a few days later with the acute symptoms, which are already subsiding. Subsequently they will settle on conservative management.

Examination will show a tender tense anal nodule, usually with a blue coloration. Treatment at this stage includes analgesics, a mild laxative, hot baths, and a suitable cream such as a local anesthetic steroid preparation. There is no place for "reduction" of a prolapsed hemorrhoid since the lesion is external. Following resolution, which occurs over a few days to several weeks, a full anorectal examination should be carried out. If normal (as it almost always is), the patient can be discharged.

Fibrosed Anal Polyp

Fibrous anal polyp is an interesting condition. It is a prolongation of one of the anal papillae, which then may prolapse. The cause is unknown. Taking origin from the innervated part of the anal canal, rubber band ligation is not indicated. Excision under local anesthetic with under-running of the pedicle by a suture is the correct treatment.

REFERENCES

1. Thomson WHF (1975) The nature of haemorrhoids. Br J Surg 62:542
2. Loder PB, Kamm MA, Nicholls RJ, Phillips RKS (1994) Haemorrhoids: pathology, pathophysiology and aetiology. Br J Surg 81:946–954
3. Hansen HH (1976) Die Bedeutung des Musculus canalis ani fur die Kontinenz und anorectale Erkrankungen. Langenbecks Arch Chir 341:23–37
4. Parks AG (1956) The surgical treatment of haemorrhoids. Br J Surg 43:337–351
5. Hancock BD, Smith K (1975) The internal sphincter and Lord's procedure for haemorrhoids. Br J Surg 62:833–836
6. Sun WM, Read NW, Shorthouse AJ (1990) Hypertensive anal cushions as a cause of the high anal canal pressures in patients with haemorrhoids. Br J Surg 77:458–462
7. Sun WM, Peck RJ, Shorthouse AJ, Read NW (1992) Haemorrhoids are associated not with hypertrophy of the internal anal sphincter but with hypertension of the anal cushions. Br J Surg 79:592–594
8. Arabi Y, Alexander-Williams J, Keighley MRB (1977) Anal pressures in haemorrhoids and anal fissure. Am J Surg 134:608–610
9. Roe AM, Bartolo DCC, Mortensen NJM (1986) New method for assessment of anal sensation in various anorectal disorders. Br J Surg 73:310–312
10. Burkitt DP (1972) Varicose veins, deep vein thrombosis, and haemorrhoids: epidemiology and suggested aetiology. Br Med J 2:556–561
11. Nelson RL (1991) Temporal changes in the occurrence of haemorrhoids in the United States and England. Dis Colon Rectum 34:591–599. Editorial comment
12. Johanson JF, Sonnenberg A (1991) Temporal changes in the occurrence of haemorrhoids in the United States and England. Dis Colon Rectum 34:585–591
13. Thomson JPS, Leicester RJ, Smith LE (1992) Haemorrhoids. pp. 373–393. In Coloproctology and the Pelvic Floor. 2nd Ed. Butterworth-Heinemann, Oxford
14. Nicholls RJ, Glass RE (1985) p. 84. In Coloproctology: Diagnosis and Outpatient Management. Springer Verlag, Berlin
15. Thomson WHF (1982) The nature of perianal haematoma. Lancet 2:467
16. Keighley MRB, Williams NS (eds) (1993) Surgery of the Anus, Rectum and Colon. WB Saunders, London
17. Whitehead W (1882) Surgical treatment of haemorrhoids. Br Med J 1:149
18. Miles WE (1919) Observations upon internal piles. Surg Gynecol Obstet 29:496
19. Milligan ETC, Morgan C, Naughton Jones LF, Officer R (1937) Surgical anatomy of the anal canal and the operative treatment of haemorrhoids. Lancet 2:1119
20. Ferguson JA, Heaton JR (1959) Closed hemorrhoidectomy. Dis Colon Rectum 2:176
21. Blanchard CE (1928) p. 134. In Textbook of Ambulant Proctology.
22. Barron J (1963) Office ligation of internal hemorrhoids. Am J Surg 195:563
23. Lewis MI (1973) Diverse methods of managing hemorrhoids: cryohemorrhoidectomy. Dis Colon Rectum 16:175
24. Williams KL, Haq IU, Elem B (1973) Cryodestruction of haemorrhoids. Br Med J 1(854):666–668
25. Nath G, Kreitmaier A, Kiefhaber P et al (1977) Neue Infrarotkoagulationsmethode. Verhandlungsband des 3 Kongresses der Deutscher Gesellschaft fur Gastroenterologie, Munich
26. Lord PH (1968) A new regime for the treatment of haemorrhoids. Proc R Soc Med 61:935
27. Broader JH, Gunn IF, Alexander-Williams J (1974) Evaluation of a bulk forming evacuant in the management of haemorrhoids. Br J Surg 61:142
28. Senapati A, Nicholls RJ (1988) A randomised trial to compare the results of injection sclerotherapy with a bulk laxative alone in the treatment of bleeding haemorrhoids. Int J Colorectal Dis 3:124–126
29. Standards Task Force, American Society of Colon and Rectal

Surgeons (1993) Practice parameters for the treatment of hemorrhoids. Dis Colon Rectum 36:1118–1120

30. Khoury GA, Lake SP, Lewis MCA, Lewis AAM (1985) A randomised trial to compare single with multiple phenol injection treatment for haemorrhoids. Br J Surg 72:741–742

31. Thomson WHF (1980) The one-man bander: a new instrument for elastic ligation of piles. Lancet 2:1006

32. O'Hara VS (1980) Fatal clostridial infection following haemorrhoidal banding. Dis Colon Rectum 23:570–571

33. Russell TR, Donohue JH (1985) Hemorrhoidal banding: a warning. Dis Colon Rectum 28:291–293

34. Murie JA, Mackenzie I, Sim AJW (1980) Comparison of rubber band ligation and haemorrhoidectomy for second and third-degree haemorrhoids: a prospective clinical trial. Br J Surg 67: 786

35. Bartizal J, Slosberger PA (1977) An alternative to haemorrhoidectomy. Arch Surg 112:534

36. Khubchandani IT (1983) A randomised comparison of single and multiple rubber band ligations. Dis Colon Rectum 26: 705–708

37. Wrobleski DE, Corman ML, Veidenheimer MC et al (1980) Long-term evaluation of rubber band ligation in hemorrhoidal disease. Dis Colon Rectum 23:478

38. Steinberg DM, Liegois H, Alexander-Williams J (1975) Long-term review of the results of rubber band ligation of haemorrhoids. Br J Surg 62:144

39. Lewis AAM, Rogers HS, Leighton M (1983) Trial of maximal anal dilatation and elastic band ligation as alternatives to haemorrhoidectomy in the treatment of large prolapsing haemorrhoids. Br J Surg 70:54–56

40. Greca F, Hares MM, Nevah E et al (1981) A randomised trial to compare rubber band ligation with phenol injection for treatment of haemorrhoids. Br J Surg 68:250

41. Smith LE, Goodreau JJ, Fouty WJ (1979) Operative hemorrhoidectomy versus cryodestruction. Dis Colon Rectum 22:10

42. O'Callaghan JD, Matheson TS, Hall R (1982) In-patient treatment of prolapsing piles: cryosurgery versus Milligan-Morgan haemorrhoidectomy. Br J Surg 69:157–159

43. Goligher JC (1976) Cryosurgery for haemorrhoids. Dis Colon Rectum 19:223

44. Neiger A (1979) Haemorrhoids in everyday practice. Proctology 2:22

45. Leicester RJ, Nicholls RJ, Mann CV (1981) Infrared coagulation: a new treatment for haemorrhoids. Dis Colon Rectum 24: 602–605

46. Templeton JL, Spence RAJ, Kennedy TL et al (1983) Comparison of infrared coagulation and rubber band ligation for first and second degree haemorrhoids: a randomised prospective clinical trial. Br Med J 286:1387–1389

47. Ambrose NS, Morris D, Alexander-Williams J, Keighley MRB (1983) A randomised trial of photocoagulation or injection sclerotherapy for the treatment of first and second-degree haemorrhoids. Dis Colon Rectum 28:238–240

48. Griffith CD, Morris DL, Wherry DC, Hardcastle JD (1987) Out-patient treatment of haemorrhoids: a randomised trial comparing contact bipolar diathermy with rubber band ligation. Coloproctology 6:322–334

49. Dennison A, Whiston BM, Rooney S et al (1990) A randomised comparison of infrared photocoagulation with bipolar diathermy for the out-patient treatment of haemorrhoids. Dis Colon Rectum 33:32–35

50. Senagore A, Mazier PW, Luchtefeld MA et al (1993) Treatment of advanced hemorrhoidal disease: a prospective, randomised comparison of cold scalpel vs contact Nd: YAG laser. Dis Colon Rectum 36:1042–1049

51. Eisenhammer S (1951) The surgical correction of internal anal (sphincteric) contracture. South Afr Med J 25:486–487

52. Lord PH (1969) A day-case procedure for the cure of third degree haemorrhoids. Br J Surg 56:747

53. Lord PH (1977) Approach to the treatment of anorectal disease, with special reference to haemorrhoids. Surg Ann 9:195–211

54. Vellacott KD, Hardcastle JD (1980) Is continued dilatation necessary after a Lord's procedure for haemorrhoids? Br J Surg 67:658–659

55. Hancock BD (1981) Lord's procedure for haemorrhoids: a prospective anal pressure study. Br J Surg 68:729–730

56. Keighley MRB, Buchemann P et al (1979) Prospective trials of minor surgical procedures and high fibre diet for haemorrhoids. Br Med J 11:967–969

57. Ferguson JA, Mazier WP, Ganchrow MI, Friend WG (1971) The closed technique of hemorrhoidectomy. Surgery 70: 480–484

58. Jeffrey PJ, Ritchie JK, Parks AG (1977) Treatment of haemorrhoids in patients with inflammatory bowel disease. Lancet 1: 1084–1088

59. Goldberg SM, Gordon PH, Nivatvongs S (1980) Hemorrhoids. In Essentials of Anorectal Surgery. Lippincott, Philadelphia

60. Seow-Choen F, Low HC (1995) Prospective, randomised study of radical versus four piles haemorrhoidectomy for symptomatic large circumferential prolapsed piles. Br J Surg 82: 188–189

61. Roe AM, Bartolo DCC, Vellacott KD et al (1987) Submucosal versus ligation excision haemorrhoidectomy: a comparison of anal sensation, and sphincter manometry and post-operative pain and function. Br J Surg 74:948–951

62. MacRae HM, McLeod RS (1995) Comparison of hemorrhoidal treatment modalities. A meta-analysis. Dis Colon Rectum 38: 687–694

63. Heald RJ, Gudgeon AM (1986) Limited haemorrhoidectomy in the treatment of acute strangulated haemorrhoids. Br J Surg 73:1002

64. Cheng FCY, Shum DWP, Ong GB (1981) The treatment of second degree haemorrhoids by injection, rubber band ligation, MDA and haemorrhoidectomy—a prospective clinical tracal. Aust NZ J Surg 51:458–462

65. Sim AJW, Murli JA, Mackenzie I (1981) Comparison of rubber band ligation and sclerosant injection for 1st and 2nd degree haemorrhoids: a prospective clinical trial. Acta Clin Scand 147: 717

66. Ambrose NS, Hares MM, Alexander J, Keighley MRB (1983) Prospective randomised comparison of photocoagulation and rubber band ligation in treatment of haemorrhoids. Br Med J 1:1389–1391

12

ANAL FISSURE

Donald G. Kim
W. Douglas Wong

Anal fissure (fissure-in-ano) is one of the most common causes of severe anal pain. The patient's symptoms can be highly distressing, often out of proportion to the findings on physical examination.

An anal fissure is a linear longitudinal tear or ulcer, situated in the anal canal, and extending from just below the dentate line to the margin of the anus. Fissures can be classified as either acute or chronic, and may be either primary idiopathic or secondary. In the acute phase, it is often a mere cut or crack in the anal epithelium, but nevertheless may cause severe pain and spasm. Chronic fissures are distinguished from their acute precursor by several features including a sentinel pile, an indurated anal ulcer, and a hypertrophied anal papilla. The vast majority of fissures encountered in clinical practice are of primary idiopathic origin. The lesion is usually encountered in younger and middle-aged adults but may occur at the extremes of age. Anal fissure is the most common cause of rectal bleeding in infants. Men and women are affected equally, but women are more likely to develop an anterior fissure. Anterior fissures account for 10% of all fissures in women versus only 1% of fissures in men.[1] Clearly, the majority of fissures in both men and women are located posteriorly.

HISTORICAL PERSPECTIVE

Much of the classic literature associated with anal fissure focuses on operative management. Anal dilatation remains a popular technique for treatment of anal fissure, especially in the United Kingdom. The first description of anal dilatation by Récamier in 1838[2] has since been translated into English.[3] Récamier detailed his observations in a variety of abnormal contractile states of voluntary and involuntary muscles, including several patients with anal fissure and associated sphincter spasm on whom he performed anal dilatation resulting in immediate pain relief and subsequent cure of the fissure. The procedure was reintroduced and popularized by Goligher.[4] Lord[5] applied the procedure to the treatment of hemorrhoids, a technique that still bears his name.

Anal sphincterotomy for the treatment of anal fissure was first described by Brodie in 1835.[6] He advocated the procedure for "preternatural contraction of the sphincter ani" and rectal ulcer (anal fissure).[6] His description advised lateral division rather than the posterior or anterior location. Miles is usually credited as the surgeon who gave the procedure real credence; however, internal sphincterotomy was performed for treating anal fissure under a complete misapprehension. Miles[7] treated anal fissure by pectenotomy, by dividing what he called the "pecten band." In 1951, Eisenhammer[8] advocated internal sphincterotomy as a treatment for anal fissure, with a true understanding of which muscle he was dividing. He initially described an incision along the "left lateral line of the anal canal axis" with division of at least four-fifths of the internal sphincter. Eisenhammer[9] later advocated dividing one-half of the sphincter in the lateral position in an open fashion. With lateral placement of the sphincterotomy, Eisenhammer noted less functional disturbance and prompt healing as compared to posteriorly placed wounds.

Despite this information, posterior internal sphincterotomy was probably the most popular surgical technique used in the treatment of chronic anal fissure at that time. This technique was not without significant morbidity. Bennett and Goligher[10] reported a 93% cure rate using a posterior internal sphincterotomy, but observed incontinence to flatus and feces in 34% and 15% of patients, respectively. In 1969, Notaras[11] introduced a new minimally invasive, closed technique using a narrow-bladed cataract scalpel to perform an internal sphincterotomy in the lateral position. His technique introduced a narrow blade through the perianal skin submucosally between the internal sphincter and the anoderm of the anal canal, followed by division of the internal sphincter by cutting outwards. The lateral internal sphincterotomy continues to be a popular treatment for

233

anal fissure with several variations from the originally described technique.

ETIOLOGY AND PATHOGENESIS

Despite what seems to be a rather common, straightforward malady, much is unknown about the etiology and pathogenesis of this disorder. Generally, anal fissure has been associated with the passage of a hard, constipated stool that theoretically traumatizes the anal canal leading to the onset of symptoms. Yet many questions remain poorly understood, such as why fissures are most commonly located in the posterior midline, and why some heal spontaneously while others become chronic. More recent studies have suggested that ischemia may play a role in the etiology of anal fissure and may explain some of the questions that have baffled clinicians managing this disease.

The etiology of anal fissure is largely speculative but it is generally agreed that the initiating factor is the passage of a large, hard stool that tears the anoderm, resulting in a linear tear that manifests as a fissure. Alternatively an anal fissure can be instigated by passage of an explosive diarrheal stool. In both instances, trauma to the anal canal seems to be the causative factor. Constipation has been incriminated in perpetuating an anal fissure through repetitive trauma to the injured anoderm. In a prospective case control study Jensen[12] identified risk factors associated with anal fissure by comparing 174 chronic anal fissure patients to matched controls. Significantly decreased risk was associated with frequent intake of raw fruits, vegetables, and whole grain breads, whereas significantly increased risk was associated with frequent intake of white bread, sauces thickened with roux, and bacon or sausages. No differences in risk ratios were noted for coffee, tea, or alcohol intake. No statistical associations were identified with particular occupational exposures. However, a history of previous anal surgery was reported more often for fissure patients than for controls. Previous anal surgery may be a predisposing factor, as the resultant scar is inelastic, tethered, and susceptible to traumatic injury resulting in fissure formation.

Although the initiating factor in fissure development may be traumatic, its perpetuation may be due to an abnormality of internal sphincter function leading to chronicity. Several investigators have studied anorectal pressures in anal fissure patients. Using an open-tipped catheter, Duthie and Bennet[13] found no differences in resting pressures between patients with and without anal fissures. However, several investigators have demonstrated high resting pressures in fissure patients.[14–18] Schuster[19] suggested that the discrepancy in these findings may be explained by the differences in the measurement techniques. The first group of authors[13] used open-tipped catheters while the second group used balloon manometry[14,16,18] or perfusion catheters.[15,17] This difference has been suggested by Schuster.[19]

Nothman and Schuster[18] demonstrated a normal reflex relaxation of the internal sphincter in response to rectal distention in patients without anal disease. However, anal fissure patients demonstrated an initial relaxation followed by an abnormal "overshoot" contraction. When a rectoanal inhibitory reflex is elicited, there is a marked and prolonged contraction above normal resting pressure following the reflex relaxation (Fig. 12-

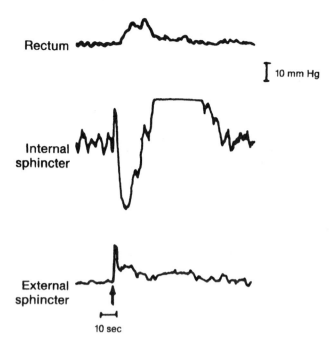

Figure 12-1. "Overshoot" contraction. (From Gordon,[76] with permission.)

1). All 7 fissure patients studied demonstrated this phenomenon. Five demonstrated an overshoot response 100% of the time with suprathreshold distension, and the other 2 patients 66% of the time. This "overshoot" phenomenon may explain the sphincter spasm and pain that results after anorectal stimulation during defecation. They also studied 3 patients after successful treatment of the fissures demonstrating disappearance of the "overshoot" phenomenon with return of normal reflex responses. Increased ultraslow-wave activity has also been identified in patients with anal fissure. Ultraslow waves in the anal canal are discrete pressure fluctuations with a low frequency (1 to 2/ min) and high amplitude (10% above or below basal resting pressure).[20] They have been demonstrated to occur in 50 to 80% of fissure patients compared to 5 to 10% of controls.[16,20] Recently, Keck et al.[21] demonstrated ultraslow waves in 91% of anal fissure patients and 73% of controls. Furthermore, ultraslow wave amplitudes were significantly higher, with mean amplitude of 31 mmHg in fissure patients and 15 mmHg in controls. Ultraslow waves have been reported to disappear after adequate internal sphincterotomy once resting pressures are reduced to a normal level.[16,20] Based on these findings it can be concluded that ultraslow waves are a manifestation of increased activity of an abnormal internal anal sphincter, which can be corrected by dilatation or lateral internal sphincterotomy. Other authors have demonstrated reduction of internal anal sphincter resting pressures after dilatation or sphincterotomy.[14,17,22,23]

One of the most recent and interesting hypotheses suggests that ischemia is the underlying pathophysiology for fissure development. Gibbons and Read,[15] using perfusion probes of varying diameters, demonstrated elevated resting pressures in all fissure patients when compared with controls, regardless of probe diameter. They suggest that the high resting pressures recorded in chronic anal fissure patients even when using small probes are unlikely to be due to spasm, but probably represent a true increase in basal sphincter tone. Thus the elevated resting pressure is a primary event rather than a consequence of the fissure. They further proposed that elevated sphincter pressures may cause ischemia of the anoderm resulting in the pain of anal fissures and their inability to heal. Excessive resting pressure could potentially reduce vascular perfusion pressure to the anoderm to levels that in other body areas would result in ischemic ulceration. The resultant fissure would then persist due to chronic ischemia.

Klosterhalfen et al.[24] studied the topography of the inferior rectal artery and suggested a causal relationship with chronic primary anal fissure. Postmortem angiography showed that in 85% of nonselected autopsy cases the posterior commissure was considered the end of the capillary system for the inferior rectal artery. In this case, the posterior commissure is less perfused than other sections of the anal canal. Anastomoses of rectal arteries at this site of the anal canal are rare; hence an anatomic basis for hypoperfusion in the posterior midline exists. In 15% of autopsy specimens, the posterior commissure was adequately vascularized by the inferior rectal artery to a similar extent as other areas of the anal canal. They have also demonstrated that the major arterial vessels pass perpendicular to the fiber course of the internal anal sphincter within the intermuscular septa and may be susceptible to strong ''contusion'' during increased sphincter tone. This may result in diminished blood supply leading to ischemia and resultant fissure.

Schouten et al.[25] demonstrated that anodermal blood flow at the posterior midline is less than in the other anal canal segments, and that the perfusion of the anoderm at the posterior commissure is strongly correlated to anal pressure. Using combined Doppler laser flowmetry and anal manometry in 31 controls and 9 patients with anal fissure, they demonstrated that anodermal blood flow at the base of an anal fissure was significantly lower than the blood flow at the posterior midline in control patients. The influence of anesthesia was studied in 10 patients. During the administration of anesthesia, anal pressure dropped significantly, with a concomitant increase in anodermal blood flow in the posterior midline. The higher the pressure, the lower the flow. These findings further support the hypothesis that anal fissures are ischemic ulcers.

PRESENTATION

Symptoms

Patients commonly present to the physician's office complaining of problems with their ''hemorrhoids.'' A careful history alone will direct the experienced clinician to the correct diagnosis in most cases. Classically the patient will complain of severe, sharp, or searing pain associated with defecation, often of a hard constipated stool. The pain can last only a few minutes or for several hours after a bowel movement.

Bleeding commonly occurs with the passage of stool. The blood is bright red and is usually a small amount. It is frequently noted on the toilet paper but may occasionally drip into the toilet bowl. However, it is not uncommon for a patient to report no associated bleeding.

Patients who present with chronic anal fissure present with different symptoms associated with chronicity. A palpable large sentinel tag may be present, drawing attention to the anus. Discharge or drainage from the open wound may lead to soiling of the undergarments and to increased perianal moisture with resultant pruritis. Pruritis may occur independent of any discharge. Pain is usually mild and frequently absent in patients with chronic anal fissure.

Constipation is a frequent complaint and is often described as the initiating event. Patients may also recall an episode of diarrhea triggering their symptoms.

Occasionally patients with a painful fissure may develop micturition problems, including dysuria, retention, urgency, or frequency. Dyspareunia may also be caused by an anal fissure.

Diagnosis

Acute Fissure

As mentioned, the diagnosis of anal fissure can usually be made by history alone. The physical examination confirms the diagnosis and rules out any associated diseases.

The diagnosis can usually be confirmed by placing the patient on the examining table in the left lateral position and gently separating the buttocks while inspecting the anal verge for signs of a tear in the epithelium. It is understandable that patients are reluctant to be examined in the presence of a painful anal fissure and special care must be taken to make the examination as gentle as possible. Local application of an anesthetic jelly may be helpful during the examination, although it may only anesthetize the fissure itself, and not affect the spasm that keeps the anal orifice closed. The finding of sphincter spasm itself is suggestive of a fissure. Digital examination will confirm the presence of the sphincter spasm, although the pain and spasm may be so intense that a complete digital examination cannot be performed. The acute fissure is superficial without fibrosis and may not be noticed by the examining finger.

Occasionally a patient is so tender that no pathology can be demonstrated. External inspection may be helpful in ruling out an obvious abscess or thrombosed external hemorrhoid, but it may be most prudent to examine the patient under anesthesia in the operating room. An intersphincteric abscess may mimic an acute fissure, presenting as severe anal pain with minimal physical findings, requiring an exam under anesthesia for diagnosis.

Once a fissure is identified, any attempts at instrumentation of the anus or anorectum should be deferred until treatment can be initiated, with the expectation that the patient can later be comfortably examined to rule out any associated pathology. Ideally, anoscopy and sigmoidoscopy should be performed. With an acute fissure, anoscopic exam is usually impossible secondary to the severe pain. Sigmoidoscopy is likewise impossible to perform at the initial visit, but both should be performed at a subsequent visit to rule out any associated conditions such as hemorrhoids, proctitis, carcinoma, or inflammatory bowel disease.

As discussed previously, the vast majority of fissures present posteriorly and anteriorly. A fissure located in the lateral position should increase one's suspicion of another cause (Fig. 12-2). If the suspicion of infection, neoplasm, or inflammatory bowel disease is raised, appropriate biopsies, cultures, endoscopy, or radiologic studies should be performed.

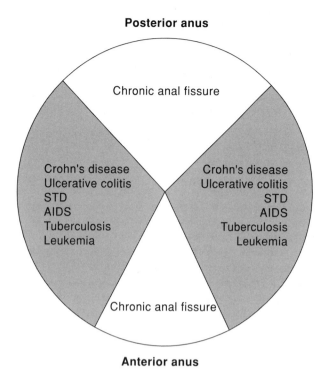

Posterior anus

Chronic anal fissure

Crohn's disease
Ulcerative colitis
STD
AIDS
Tuberculosis
Leukemia

Crohn's disease
Ulcerative colitis
STD
AIDS
Tuberculosis
Leukemia

Chronic anal fissure

Anterior anus

Figure 12-2. Common locations of chronic anal fissures and other anal conditions.

Chronic Fissure

Several features distinguish a chronic fissure from its acute precursor. The triad of a chronic fissure includes a sentinel pile, an indurated anal ulcer, and a hypertrophied anal papilla. The fissure edges become indurated and undermined, the circular fibers of the internal sphincter are visible in the depths of the ulcer, and a sentinel pile develops distally as does a hypertrophied anal papilla at the ulcer's apex. Once this stage is reached it is very unlikely that spontaneous healing will occur, and surgical intervention is usually necessary. A chronic fissure may be associated with anal stenosis, especially as a result of previous anal surgery (hemorrhoidectomy).

Digital examination of a chronic fissure reveals an open wound with an indurated and fibrotic base. A hypertrophied anal papilla may be palpable at the apex of the fissure.

Anoscopy can frequently be performed without difficulty because the pain of a chronic fissure is usually not severe. Sigmoidoscopy should also be performed to rule out an associated carcinoma or inflammatory bowel disease.

As with an acute fissure, any suspicion of infection, neoplasm, or inflammatory bowel disease warrants pursuit of the appropriate diagnostic tests. Any atypical fissure that fails to heal after treatment should be biopsied. A nonhealing fissure may represent unsuspected Crohn's disease or a neoplastic process.

TREATMENT

Conservative Management

The mainstay of treating an acute anal fissure is avoidance of constipation. The repetitive cycle of hard stool, pain, and spasm perpetuates the anal fissure and must be broken to allow the fissure to heal. A bulk-forming agent should be initiated and the dosage adjusted to maintain a formed but soft stool that is atraumatic to the anoderm during passage. Warm sitz baths are beneficial in relieving the spasm associated with a fissure. Dodi et al.[26] provided the first objective evidence for this recommendation. They measured the resting anal canal pressures of normal patients and patients with anorectal complaints including hemorrhoidal disease, anal fissure, and proctalgia fugax at room temperature (23°C). Subsequently, measurements were obtained while the anus was submerged in water at varying temperatures (5, 23, and 40°C). All patients demonstrated diminished resting anal canal pressures from baseline after immersion at 40°C but remained unchanged after immersion at 5° and 23°C.

Local application of anesthetic ointment may provide some symptomatic relief, but must be applied into the anal canal directly to the fissure. Recent data suggest that this may not be an effective means of treatment. In the only reported prospective, randomized trial, Jensen[27] studied 103 patients with a first episode of acute posterior anal fissure. Patients were randomized to three treatment categories: lignocaine (lidocaine hydrochloride) ointment, hydrocortisone ointment, or warm sitz baths combined with intake of unprocessed bran. After 1 and 2 weeks of treatment symptomatic relief was significantly better among patients treated with sitz baths and bran than among patients treated with lignocaine or hydrocortisone ointment. After 3 weeks there was no difference in symptomatic relief among the three groups, but patients treated with lignocaine had significantly fewer healed fissures (60%) than patients treated with hydrocortisone (82.4%) or warm sitz baths and bran (87%). Jensen advocated warm sitz baths and bran as the treatment of choice for an acute fissure and showed no particular advantage to using proprietary medications.

Topical nitroglycerine has recently been used in the treatment of anal fissures. Nitric oxide has emerged as one of the most important neurotransmitters mediating internal anal sphincter relaxation. Recent studies suggest that nitric oxide is probably the most important inhibitory neurotransmitter in the internal anal sphincter.[28–31] Neural stimulation of these nitric oxide-containing nerves releases nitric oxide, causing the internal anal sphincter to relax. Nitroglycerin is a readily available nitric oxide donor predominantly used to treat coronary heart disease. The drug is available as an ointment for topical systemic administration. Recent clinical studies have examined the effect of topical nitroglycerine on the anal sphincter. Loder et al.[32] studied the effects of glyceryl trinitrate on anal pressure in patients presenting for physiologic assessment of anal disorders. They demonstrated that application of 0.2% glyceryl trinitrate ointment to the anus resulted in a significant decrease in maximum resting anal pressure from pretreatment baseline values, which was not observed in the control patients receiving a placebo ointment. Guillemot et al.[33] studied two groups of constipated patients who differed in upper anal sphincter pressure measurements and a third group of asymptomatic controls. The first group demonstrated hypertonicity of the upper anal sphincter (> 70 mmHg) while the second group was without hypertonicity. Each patient acted as his own control and received a placebo followed by the nitroglycerine. No pressure decreases were noted with the placebo, but all groups experienced a significant decrease of upper anal sphincter pressure in response to nitroglycerine. Gorfine[34] has recently reported the use of topical nitroglycerin in benign anal disease. He reported the application of 0.5% nitroglycerin ointment in 5 thrombosed external hemorrhoid patients and 15 anal fissure patients. All patients reported dramatic relief of anal pain within 2 to 4 minutes following application of nitroglycerin, and the effect lasted 2 to 6 hours. Patients applied approximately 500 to 1000 mg of 0.5% NTG ointment to the external anus and distal anal canal four or more times daily and after bowel movement. Side effects were limited to transient self-limited headaches in 35% of the patients. The author's comments at the end of the article updated the series reporting on 43 fissure/ulcer patients. Forty-one (93%) reported pain relief within 5 minutes of application. Complete healing occurred in 30 patients (70%) within 4 weeks.

Solcoderm has also been used topically to treat anal fissure.[35] Solcoderm, an aqueous solution of organic and inorganic acids, copper ions, and nitrates has been used to treat various skin diseases since 1976. Patients were randomized to either a treatment or control group with 25 patients analyzed in each group. After 1 month, complete healing of the fissure was observed in 84% of the treated group while only 28% healed in the control group. Follow-up at 1 year showed complete healing in 84% of the treated group and 44% in the control group, with recurrence rates of 12% and 36%, respectively.

Other local therapies have been reported with some success. Antebi et al.[36] reported treatment of anal fissures with 1 ml of 2% lidocaine followed by an injection of 0.05 ml of sodium tetradecyl sulfate (Sotradecol). In the 96 patients treated, 80% were symptom free at 1 year follow-up.

Most recently, botulinum toxin has been utilized in Europe as a treatment for anal fissure.[37,38] Jost and Schimrigk, who first reported this in 1993,[39] have recently updated their series reporting on 26 patients treated with botulinum toxin injection.[40] Two doses of 0.1 ml diluted toxin are injected into the external sphincter on both sides lateral to the fissure. On the first day after injection, 19 of the 26 patients were free from pain. After 3 months, the fissure was completely healed in 21 (81%) of patients. No permanent incontinence was reported and only 1 patient had a recurrence. Botulinum toxin produces temporary chemical denervation of the internal sphincter, allowing fissures to heal, with minimal side effects reported to date. Future studies seem warranted.

With proper and timely administration of medical treatment, about 50 to 75% of acute anal fissures can be expected to heal. Measures as simple as bulk-forming agents can have a significant impact. This was supported by Jensen[41] in a prospective, double-blind, placebo-controlled study that demonstrated that unprocessed bran (5 g three times daily) resulted in a diminished recurrence rate. Patients taking 15 g of bran a day had a 16% recurrence rate, while those on 7.5 g per day (2.5 g three times daily) or placebo had recurrence rates of 60 and 68%, respectively. These data would suggest that those patients who heal with medical management should be maintained on bulk agents for life. Other conservative measures—such as the use of anal dilators, local injection of long-acting anesthetic agents, the usage of sclerosants such as Sotradecal, and injection of botulinum toxin as discussed—have not gained widespread usage. Preliminary data appear to support the use of topical nitroglycerine, especially to relieve the pain of an acute fissure. Further conclusions await a prospective, randomized trial.

Surgical Management

A variety of options for the surgical treatment of an anal fissure have been described. Lateral internal sphincterotomy continues to be the procedure of choice in this country, with anal dilatation popular in the United Kingdom. Surgical indications include persistent pain and bleeding unresponsive to medical management. Lock and Thomson[42] reported that the presence of a large sentinel tag and hypertrophied anal papilla indicated that spontaneous healing was unlikely.

Anal Dilatation

Anal dilatation requires forceful disruption of the internal sphincter fibers in a relatively uncontrolled manner. There is risk of significant incontinence, particularly in the older population, and recurrence rates are reported in the range of 10 to 30%.

Anal dilatation may be performed under local anesthesia in the office setting, but a general or regional anesthesia in a day surgery facility is preferred by many surgeons.

Technique

The technique as advocated by Lord for the treatment of hemorrhoids involved a forceful eight-finger maximal dilatation of the anus and was associated with a significant risk of incontinence. A more conservative dilatation has been advocated by gentle and progressive introduction of four fingers, maintaining this degree of sphincter stretch for 4 minutes.[43]

A standardized method of anorectal sphincter dilatation has been described for the treatment of anal fissure.[44] This precise method of anal dilatation is performed with a Parks retractor opened to 4.8 cm or with a 40-mm rectosigmoid balloon. Using this controlled technique, successful cure was achieved in 93 and 94% of patients, respectively. Twenty-two patients with acute or severely painful fissures all had pain relief within 12 hours of the procedure. Temporary incontinence to flatus, which resolved within 3 weeks, was noted in 2 patients. Late recurrence was noted in 2 patients, but substantial long term follow-up data are not available.

Results

Results in the literature are variable. Some authors report similar results for lateral internal sphincterotomy and anal dilatation.[43] MacDonald et al.[45] published a retrospective review of 100 consecutive patients undergoing anal dilatation and assessed morbidity with a follow-up questionnaire. Manual anal dilatation failed to relieve symptoms in 26 of the 46 patients with anal fissure, a persistence rate of 57%. These comparatively poorer results may be explained by the longer 90-month median follow-up in this study (range, 76 to 100 months) or may be related to the more specific questions asked via follow-up questionnaire.

Utilizing anorectal physiology and anal endosonography, Speakman et al.[46] studied 12 men presenting with fecal incontinence following anal dilatation. Resting anal pressures were low normal and pudendal nerve latencies were normal. Eleven men had disrupted internal anal sphincters, with a mean loss of 153 degrees of the circumference. Ten demonstrated fragmentation of the internal anal sphincter. Three also had external anal sphincter defects. Nielsen et al.[47] followed up 32 consecutive patients who had not undergone any additional anal surgery 2 to 6 years after anal dilatation for anal fissure. Minor anal incontinence was noted in 12.5%. Endoanal ultrasound documented internal anal sphincter defect in 13 of 20 patients evaluated. Two patients with anal incontinence were studied, demonstrating internal sphincter defects in both. Sphincteric defects were identified in 11 of 18 continent patients studied, 3 of these represented by internal sphincter fragmentation. Although anal dilatation results in sphincter damage in more than half of patients, few of them manifest anal incontinence.

An interesting study by Goldman et al.[48] demonstrated bacteremia in 8% of 100 patients undergoing anal dilatation for anal fissure. Based on these findings, prophylactic antibiotics were recommended for selected groups of patients such as those with valvular heart disease, those under steroid or immunosuppressive treatment, and those who are known to be immunosuppressed.

Lateral Internal Sphincterotomy

Initial experience with internal sphincterotomy was with the *posterior* sphincterotomy, commonly combined with fissurectomy. Unfortunately this technique was accompanied by prolonged healing and a significant incidence of anal incontinence.[10,49] Much of this incontinence was felt to be due to a keyhole deformity created after posterior sphincterotomy. Although this technique still has some proponents, it has largely

been abandoned in favor of *lateral* internal sphincterotomy. In North America the standard of care for the surgical treatment of chronic anal fissure is lateral internal sphincterotomy.

Technique

There are several variations to the technique of lateral sphincterotomy. The procedure may be performed under local, regional, or general anesthesia in the office or day surgery facility depending on the surgeon's preference. The patient may be placed in the lithotomy, left lateral, or prone jackknife position. The procedure can be performed using an open or closed (subcutaneous) technique. The muscle may be divided medially to laterally or laterally to medially.

At the University of Minnesota, we prefer the prone jackknife position. If local anesthesia is used, a 50/50 mixture of 1% lidocaine with 1:200,000 epinephrine and 0.5% bupicacaine is infiltrated to establish perianal anesthesia. The injection should start in the quadrant that has the fissure and be completed in the remaining three quadrants circumferentially. For an open sphincterotomy, the anal canal is exposed with a Pratt bivalve speculum and the anal canal is examined for any pathology. The speculum is then rotated to the lateral position, and a longitudinal incision is made in the anoderm (Fig. 12-3). The internal anal sphincter is identified by its pearly white appearance, which differentiates it from the redder external sphincter. The distal one-third of the internal anal sphincter is divided under direct vision using a 15 blade scalpel or Metzenbaum scissors followed by closure of the incision with a running 4–0 chromic suture.

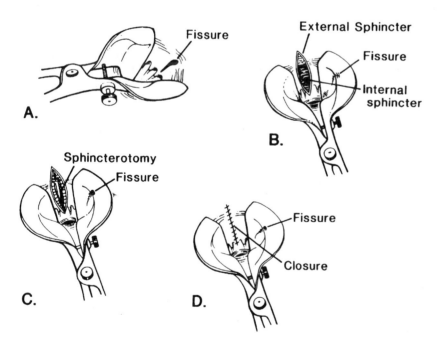

Figure 12-3. Internal sphincterotomy using an open technique. (**A**) The anal fissure is identified using a bivalve anal speculum. (**B**) A lateral anal quadrant is exposed and a longitudinal incision made in the anoderm and the internal sphincter identified. (**C**) The distal one-third of the internal sphincter is divided. (**D**) The incision is closed with an absorbable suture.

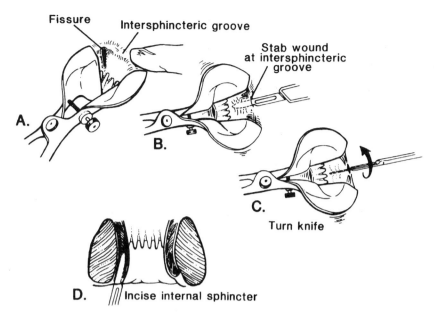

Figure 12-4. Internal sphincterotomy using a closed technique. (**A**) The anal fissure is identified using a bivalve anal speculum, and the intersphincteric groove is palpated. (**B**) A knife blade is inserted in the intersphincteric groove in a lateral quadrant. (**C**) The knife is rotated. (**D**) The distal one-third of the internal sphincter is divided.

Closed internal sphincterotomy is also performed in the lateral anal canal (Fig. 12-4). With gentle retraction of the anus using a bivalve speculum, the intersphincteric groove is easily accentuated and palpated. A knife blade is inserted into the lateral aspect of the anus with the blade oriented with the flat side parallel to the intersphincteric groove. The knife blade is then rotated medially and the distal one-third of the internal sphincter is divided. As the sphincter is divided, a "give" of the sphincter is noted, and the defect can be palpated. Alternatively, the blade can be introduced into the submucosal plane, rotating the sharp edge toward the internal sphincter and completing the sphincterotomy. The preferred knife blade is a Beaver #5100 blade used for cataract surgery, although a #11 blade can be used. The Beaver blade is optimal because the thin, narrow blade creates a very small wound.

The fissure needs no specific treatment, but large sentinel tags or prolapsing, hypertrophied anal papillae may be removed for anal hygiene purposes. Concomitant procedures including hemorrhoidectomy and fistulotomy have been performed without increasing the risk of postoperative complications.[50] Because prolapsing hemorrhoids are a recognized complication after lateral internal sphincterotomy, it would be reasonable to consider a concomitant hemorrhoidectomy in those patients presenting with large hemorrhoids.

Patients are discharged on the day of surgery with instruction for warm sitz baths and a prescription for a mild analgesic. Patients are continued on a bulk-forming laxative such as Metamucil. Postoperative pain is mild and is usually less than preoperative levels. Most patients resume their normal activities within 48 hours.

Results

The lateral internal sphincterotomy has become the procedure of choice for the management of chronic anal fissure. Comparison to the technique of posterior sphincterotomy demonstrated superiority of the lateral internal sphincterotomy.[51,52] Abacarian[53] retrospectively compared 150 lateral internal sphincterotomies to 150 fissurectomy-midline sphincterotomies. Lateral internal sphincterotomy tended towards shorter hospital stays, faster pain relief, and more rapid wound healing, but no statistical significance was assigned. Early loss of continence to flatus was common and noted in 30% of lateral internal sphincterotomies and 40% of fissurectomy-midline sphincterotomies. After the first or second postoperative week there was no incontinence to flatus or fecal soilage in the lateral internal sphincterotomy group. A "keyhole" deformity resulting in occasional loss of flatus and fecal soilage was identified in 5% of those undergoing fissurectomy-midline sphincterotomy. There were 2 recurrences in each group, for an incidence of 1.3%.

In a prospective study reported by Marby et al.[54] lateral subcutaneous sphincterotomy performed with local anesthesia was compared to manual dilatation of the anus performed under general anesthesia. The results indicated that manual dilatation was superior to sphincterotomy, with a surprising 29% recurrence rate for lateral subcutaneous sphincterotomy. Keighley et al.[55] subsequently advocated that lateral subcutaneous sphincterotomy be performed under general anesthesia, reporting a 50% (17 out of 34) recurrence rate versus 3% (1 out of 37) rate. Keighley's group[43] undertook another prospective randomized trial comparing the two procedures performed under general anesthesia, revealing no significant difference between the two techniques. Recurrence rates for both techniques were 5.1%. Other authors have failed to demonstrate similar high recurrence rates when lateral internal sphincterotomy is performed under local anesthesia.[56–58] Other authors have compared lateral sphincterotomy to anal dilatation. Jensen et al.[57] studied 58 patients in a randomized prospective trial comparing the two techniques. No differences were noted between groups for immediate pain relief, time to healing, complications, or time off work. One recurrence (3.3%) was noted in the sphincterotomy group, whereas 8 (28.6%) recurrences occurred in the dilatation group (p<0.05).

Immediate or early complications of lateral internal sphincterotomy include ecchymoses or hematoma, perianal abscess, fistula-in-ano, hemorrhage, and prolapsed thrombosed hemorrhoids. The overall immediate or early complication rate is approximately 5%, with ecchymosis occurring most frequently approximately 2% of the time. Each of the remaining complications occur in 1% or less of patients undergoing a lateral internal sphincterotomy.

Success of the procedure can be measured by the absence of unhealed or recurrent fissures. Reported recurrence rates have ranged from zero to 29%, with the majority in the 1 to 3% range (Table 12-1). Variations in recurrence rates probably reflect differences in the extent of sphincterotomy, the definition of recurrence, and the length and type of follow-up. The extent of the division of the internal sphincter is difficult to predict. Sultan et al.[59] assessed the anal sphincters in 15 patients with anal fissure (10 females and 5 males). Endoanal ultrasound was performed preoperatively and 2 months after open lateral internal sphincterotomy. All but 1 male, in whom no defect could be identified, had internal anal sphincter defects corresponding with the surgical site. In 9 of the 10 females, the defect involved

the full length of the sphincter, while in the remaining 4 males, the defect was noted distally only. The division of the females' internal sphincters tended to be more extensive than intended, probably related to a shorter canal. All were continent preoperatively, but 3 females were incontinent to flatus postoperatively. Two of 3 were noted to have external sphincter defects preoperatively presumably due to obstetrical trauma. These results emphasize that care should be exercised in performing sphincterotomy, especially in females with a prior history of obstetric trauma.

Problems with anal incontinence undoubtedly represent the most significant long-term complication of lateral internal sphincterotomy. Incontinence can take the form of incontinence to flatus, fecal soiling, or accidental bowel movements. A wide variation in results is reported in the literature. The reported incidence of incontinence varies from 0 to 38% of patients after lateral internal sphincterotomy. Factors that account for this variation include retrospective analysis, the method by which follow-up results were obtained, the unspecified duration of follow-up, and the lack of a precise definition of incontinence. Those series reporting higher incidences of incontinence[60,61] in the literature used patient questionnaires for patient follow-up. In the University of Minnesota series reviewed by Garcia-Aguilar et al.[60] comparison was made between open and closed lateral internal sphincterotomy. A total of 549 patients, 324 with open sphincterotomy and 225 with closed sphincterotomy, returned their questionnaires. The average follow-up was 36 months (range, 12 to 72 months). No statistical differences were noted for persistence of symptoms (3.4% open versus 5.3% closed), fissure recurrence (10.9% open versus 11.7% closed), or need for reoperation (3.4% open versus 4.0% closed). More than one-third of patients (37.8%) complained of some change

Table 12-1.   Results of Anal Fissure Procedures

Author	Procedure	No. Patients	Impaired Control Flatus (%)	Impaired Control Feces (%)	Fecal Soiling (%)	Unhealed or Recurrence (%)
Marby et al[54]	Dilatation	78	0	0	0	10
	Closed	78	0	0	0	29
Rosenthal[73]	Open	125	0	0	0	1.6
Abcarian[53]	Open	150	0	0	0	1.3
Marya et al[74]	Closed	100	0	0	0	2
Jensen et al[57]	Closed	30	0	0	3.3	
	Dilatation	28	28.6	7.1	39.3	
Gordon and Vasilevsky[5]	Open	133	0.8	0	0	2.3
Weaver et al[43]	Dilatation	59	0	0	0	5.1
	Closed	39	0	0	2.6	5.1
Lewis et al[58]	Open/closed	350	6.6[a]		2.6	6
Khubchandani and Reed[61]	Multiple	1057	35.1	5.3	22	2.3
Kortbeek et al[63]	Open	54	0	0	0	5.6
	Closed	58	0	0	0	3.4
Sohn et al[44]	Dil (Pratt)	105	1.9	0	0	1.9
	Dil (balloon)	66	0	0	0	0
Pernikoff et al[62]	Open/closed	500	2.8	4.4	0.4	1
Oh et al[75]	Open/closed	1313	0	0	0	1.4
Garcia-Aguilar et al[60]	Total	549	27.5	8.2	22.3	15
	Open	349	30.3	11.8	26.7	14.3
	Closed	225	23.6	3.1	16.1	17

[a] Impaired control for flatus and feces combined, 17% short-term (temporary) and 6.6% with long-term problems.

in anal continence after internal sphincterotomy. A statistically significant difference was noted for soiling of underwear (26.7% open versus 16.1% closed, $P < 0.001$) and stool incontinence (11.8% open versus 3.1% closed, $P < 0.001$); flatus incontinence trended towards significance (30.3% open versus 23.6% closed, $P < 0.062$). Unhealed or recurrent fissures were identified in 15% of patients. Despite reportedly high complication rates, patient satisfaction was 91%. Khubchandani and Reed[61] showed similar results for incontinence, but did not show differences between groups undergoing lateral, bilateral or posterior midline sphincterotomy. Recurrence rates were noted to be lower at 2.3%. Other authors have compared open sphincterotomy to the closed technique demonstrating similar statistically significant differences in complication rates.[62] Still others have shown no differences between the two groups.[58,63]

Lateral internal sphincterotomy is an effective treatment for anal fissure, with data suggesting that the subcutaneous technique may reduce complications related to incontinence. This may be due to a more limited sphincter division related to the ''blind'' nature of the technique. Certainly functional results are related to the method and duration of follow-up. Use of very strict criteria for morbidity evaluation has resulted in higher complication rates than previously reported. This information should be used to properly select and adequately counsel anal fissure patients prior to performing a lateral internal sphincterotomy. Lateral internal sphincterotomy is highly successful in the properly selected patient, and the minor morbidity is well accepted by grateful patients.

Anoplasty

Chronic anal fissure is often associated with some degree of anal stenosis. Complaints include difficulty with defecation associated with the narrowing of the anal canal. This problem is more common in the posthemorrhoidectomy patient, when too much anal canal mucosa has been removed, resulting in anal stenosis and fissure. Conservative medical management includes bulk-forming laxatives, lubricants, and dilators, but an anoplasty can be particularly useful in these patients.[64–66] The technique of a V-Y anoplasty will be described below.

Use in the chronic fissure patient combines excision of the fissure with an advancement flap of anoderm fashioned as a V-Y anoplasty (Fig. 12-5). Preoperative preparation includes a full bowel prep including intravenous antibiotics. The procedure can be performed under regional or general anesthesia. The patient is placed in the prone jackknife position. The fissure is excised, and an internal sphincterotomy is performed posteriorly. A triangular skin flap based outside of the anal canal is elevated in continuity with the excised fissure, keeping the base broad to ensure adequate blood supply. Adequate mobilization avoids tension on the suture line. Meticulous hemostasis is obtained to prevent a hematoma beneath the flap. The flap is then advanced proximally, approximating the apex of the flap to the rectal mucosa and closing the defect with a 3–0 chromic suture. The repair should be under no tension. The diameter of the anus is increased using this technique, and good results with minimal morbidity can be achieved.[66] The patient is started on a regular diet the evening of surgery and sitz baths are begun on the first postoperative day.

SPECIAL PROBLEMS

Anal Fissure in Crohn's Disease

Anal fissures, often in atypical locations (Fig. 12-2), may be associated with Crohn's disease. Perianal Crohn's disease may be the only manifestation of Crohn's disease without other intestinal or extraintestinal manifestations, but up to 97% of these

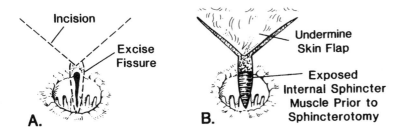

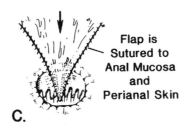

Figure 12-5. V-Y Anoplasty. (**A**) The anal fissure and stenotic area is excised. A V flap of posterior perianal skin is outlined ensuring a broad base. (**B**) The flap is raised and a partial internal sphincterotomy is performed. (**C**) The mobilized flap is advanced to the dentate line and sutured with absorbable suture. (From Zuidema,[77] with permission.)

patients will eventually develop Crohn's disease elsewhere.[67] Perianal Crohn's disease is more often associated with colonic Crohn's disease.[68] Traditionally Crohn's fissures are described as asymptomatic and painless occurring laterally, frequently, and multiple.

Sweeney et al.[69] reviewed the natural history of anal fissures in Crohn's disease. Sixty-one patients reportedly had a fissure as the only manifestation. Medical treatment of intestinal Crohn's disease healed 69% of the fissures. However, in 11 patients, fissure activity did not reflect disease activity elsewhere, because the fissure healed despite progressive intestinal disease. Contrary to popular belief the majority of the reported fissures were located anteriorly and posteriorly with 45% of the patients reporting associated pain not attributable to any other anal pathology. The authors concluded that Crohn's-related anal fissures should be managed conservatively, with anal surgery reserved for managing other anal disease. Metronidazole or azathioprine may be of benefit in managing symptomatic fissures in Crohn's patients. There is no role for lateral internal sphincterotomy in these patients.

Anal Fissure and Ulcerative Disease in HIV-Positive Patients

Anal ulcerative processes can be the most disabling of anal diseases in the HIV-positive patient. The spectrum ranges from typical "benign" fissure to AIDS-specific idiopathic anal ulcer and may be the presenting manifestation of HIV disease. Al-though these ulcers may be confused with the classic anal fissure, HIV ulcers usually have a unique appearance that differentiates them from the usual fissure. Benign fissures and idiopathic AIDS ulcers are distinct processes and a high index of suspicion is necessary for diagnosis. An appropriate workup including culture and biopsy of the fissure or ulcer should be obtained. Those fissures that appear to be typical uncomplicated anal fissures can be treated by sphincterotomy if medical management has been unsuccessful.[70] HIV-associated ulcers can be secondary to syphilis, chancroid, chlamydia, *Haemophilus ducreyi*, tuberculosis, herpes simplex virus, cytomegalovirus, squamous cell carcinoma, Kaposi's sarcoma, and B-cell lymphoma. In these cases, examination under anesthesia should include appropriate biopsy, culture, debridement, and therapy directed at the specific causative agent found. Those patients without an identifiable cause may benefit by aggressive debridement or intralesional steroid therapy.[70]

Anal Fissure and Tuberculosis

Tuberculosis of the anorectal region is rare. Sporadic case reports occur.[71,72] An anal fissure in an unusual location that is slow to heal should be biopsied with the appropriate stains and cultures obtained. Differentiating these lesions from Crohn's disease can be difficult, though they are usually associated with pulmonary tuberculosis. Antituberculous chemotherapy is highly effective in the treatment of ulcerative perianal tuberculosis. A high index of suspicion and appropriate histopathologic and microbiologic testing are required to exclude tuberculosis.

References

1. Goligher JC (1984) Anal fissure. In: Surgery of the Anus, Rectum, and Colon. 4th Ed. Tindall, London
2. Récamier JCA (1838) Extension, massage et percussion cadencee dans le traitement des contracture musculaires. Rev Med 1:74
3. Anonymous (1980) Classic articles in colonic and rectal surgery. Stretching, massage and rhythmic percussion in the treatment of muscular contractions: Joseph-Claude-Anthelme Récamier (1774–1852). Dis Colon Rectum 23:362–367
4. Watts JMK, Bennet RC, Goligher JC (1964) Stretching of the anal sphincters in the treatment of fissure-in-ano. Br Med J 342–343
5. Lord PH (1968) A new regime for the treatment of haemorrhoids. Proc R Soc Med 61:935–936
6. Brodie BC (1835) Lectures on diseases of the rectum, III. Preternatural contraction of the sphincter ani. London Med Gazette 16:26–31
7. Miles (1944) Rectal Surgery. 2nd Ed. Cassell, London
8. Eisenhammer S (1951) The surgical correction of chronic anal (sphincteric) contracture. S Afr Med J 25:486–489
9. Eisenhammer S (1959) The evaluation of the internal anal sphincterotomy operation with special reference to anal fissure. Surg Gynecol Obstet 109:583–590
10. Bennett RC, Goligher JC (1962) Results of internal sphincterotomy for anal fissure. Br J Surg 2:1500–1503
11. Notaras (1969) Lateral subcutaneous sphincterectomy for anal fissure—a new technique. Proc R Soc Med 62:713
12. Jensen SL (1988) Diet and other risk factors for fissure-in-ano. Prospective case control study. Dis Colon Rectum 31:770–773
13. Duthie HI, Bennett RC (1964) Anal sphincter pressure in fissure-in-ano. Surg Gynecol Obstet 119:19–21
14. Chowcat NL, Araujo JG, Boulos PB (1986) Internal sphincterotomy for chronic anal fissure: long term effects on anal pressure. Br J Surg 73:915–916
15. Gibbons CP, Read NW (1986) Anal hypertonia in fissures: cause or effect? Br J Surg 73:443–445
16. Hancock BD (1977) The internal sphincter and anal fissure. Br J Surg 64:92–95
17. Hiltunen KM, Matikainen M (1986) Anal manometric evaluation in anal fissure. Effect of anal dilation and lateral subcutaneous sphincterotomy. Acta Chir Scand 152:65–68
18. Nothmann BJ, Schuster MM (1974) Internal anal sphincter derangement with anal fissures. Gastroenterology 67:216–220
19. Schuster MM (1975) The riddle of the sphincters. Gastroenterology 69:249–262
20. Schouten WR, Blankensteijn JD (1992) Ultra slow wave pressure variations in the anal canal before and after lateral internal sphincterotomy. Int J Colorectal Dis 7:115–118
21. Keck JO, Staniunas RJ, Coller JA et al (1995) Computer-generated profiles of the anal canal in patients with anal fissure. Dis Colon Rectum 38:72–79
22. McNamara MJ, Percy JP, Fielding IR (1990) A manometric study of anal fissure treated by subcutaneous lateral internal sphincterotomy. Ann Surg 211:235–238
23. Xynos E, Tzortzinis A, Chrysos E et al (1993) Anal manometry

in patients with fissure-in-ano before and after internal sphincterotomy. Int J Colorectal Dis 8:125–128

24. Klosterhalfen B, Vogel P, Rixen H, Mittermayer C (1989) Topography of the inferior rectal artery: a possible cause of chronic, primary anal fissure. Dis Colon Rectum 32:43–52

25. Schouten WR, Briel JW, Auwerda JJ (1994) Relationship between anal pressure and anodermal blood flow. The vascular pathogenesis of anal fissures. Dis Colon Rectum 37:664–669

26. Dodi G, Bogoni F, Infantino A et al (1986) Hot or cold in anal pain? A study of the changes in internal anal sphincter pressure profiles. Dis Colon Rectum 29:248–251

27. Jensen SL (1986) Treatment of first episodes of acute anal fissure: prospective randomised study of lignocaine ointment versus hydrocortisone ointment or warm sitz baths plus bran. BMJ 292:1167–1169

28. O'Kelly T, Brading A, Mortensen N (1993) Nerve mediated relaxation of the human internal anal sphincter: the role of nitric oxide. Gut 34:689–693

29. Rattan S, Chakder S (1992) Role of nitric oxide as a mediator of internal anal sphincter relaxation. Am J Physiol 262: G107–G112

30. Rattan S, Sarkar A, Chakder S (1992) Nitric oxide pathway in rectoanal inhibitory reflex of opossum internal anal sphincter. Gastroenterology 103:43–50

31. Tottrup A, Glavind EB, Svane D (1992) Involvement of the L-arginine-nitric oxide pathway in internal anal sphincter relaxation. Gastroenterology 102:409–415

32. Loder PB, Kamm MA, Nicholls RJ, Phillips RK (1994) Reversible chemical sphincterotomy by local application of glyceryl trinitrate. Br J Surg 81:1386–1389

33. Guillemot F, Leroi H, Lone YC et al (1993) Action of in situ nitroglycerin on upper anal canal pressure of patients with terminal constipation. A pilot study. Dis Colon Rectum 36: 372–376

34. Gorfine SR (1995) Treatment of benign anal disease with topical nitroglycerin. Dis Colon Rectum 38:453–457

35. Chen J, Michowitz M, Bawnik JB (1992) Solcoderm as alternative conservative treatment for acute anal fissure: a controlled clinical study. Am Surg 58:705–709

36. Antebi E, Schwartz P, Gilon E (1985) Sclerotherapy for the treatment of fissure in ano. Surg Gynecol Obstet 160:204–206

37. Gui D, Cassetta E, Anastasio G et al (1994) Botulinum toxin for chronic anal fissure. Lancet 344:1127–1128

38. Jost WH, Schimrigk K (1994) Therapy of anal fissure using botulin toxin. Dis Colon Rectum 37:1321–1324

39. Jost WH, Schimrigk K (1993) Use of botulinum toxin in anal fissure. Dis Colon Rectum 36:974. Letter

40. Jost WH, Schimrigk K (1995) Botulinum toxin in therapy of anal fissure. Lancet 345:188–189. Letter

41. Jensen SL (1987) Maintenance therapy with unprocessed bran in the prevention of acute anal fissure recurrence. J R Soc Med 80:296–298

42. Lock MR, Thomson JP (1977) Fissure-in-ano: the initial management and prognosis. Br J Surg 64:355–358

43. Weaver RM, Ambrose NS, Alexander-Williams J, Keighley MR (1987) Manual dilatation of the anus vs. lateral subcutaneous sphincterotomy in the treatment of chronic fissure-in-ano. Results of a prospective, randomized, clinical trial. Dis Colon Rectum 30:420–423

44. Sohn N, Eisenberg MM, Weinstein MA et al (1992) Precise anorectal sphincter dilatation—its role in the therapy of anal fissures. Dis Colon Rectum 35:322–327

45. MacDonald A, Smith A, McNeill AD, Finlay IG (1992) Manual dilatation of the anus. Br J Surg 79:1381–1382

46. Speakman CT, Burnett SJ, Kamm MA, Bartram CI (1991) Sphincter injury after anal dilatation demonstrated by anal endosonography. Br J Surg 78:1429–1430

47. Nielsen MB, Rasmussen OO, Pedersen JF, Christiansen J (1993) Risk of sphincter damage and anal incontinence after anal dilatation for fissure-in-ano. An endosonographic study. Dis Colon Rectum 36:677–680

48. Goldman G, Zilberman M, Werbin N (1986) Bacteremia in anal dilatation. Dis Colon Rectum 29:304–305

49. Magee HR, Thompson HR (1966) Internal anal sphincterotomy as an out-patient operation. Gut 7:190–193

50. Leong AF, Husain MJ, Seow-Choen F, Goh HS (1994) Performing internal sphincterotomy with other anorectal procedures. Dis Colon Rectum 37:1130–1132

51. Hawley PR (1969) The treatment of chronic fissure-in-ano. A trial of methods. Br J Surg 56:915–918

52. Hoffmann DC, Goligher JC (1970) Lateral subcutaneous internal sphincterotomy in treatment of anal fissure. Br Med J 3: 673–675

53. Abcarian H (1980) Surgical correction of chronic anal fissure: results of lateral internal sphincterotomy vs. fissurectomy-midline sphincterotomy. Dis Colon Rectum 23:31–36

54. Marby M, Alexander-Williams J, Buchmann P et al (1979) A randomized controlled trial to compare anal dilatation with lateral subcutaneous sphincterotomy for anal fissure. Dis Colon Rectum 22:308–311

55. Keighley MR, Greca F, Nevah E et al (1981) Treatment of anal fissure by lateral subcutaneous sphincterotomy should be under general anaesthesia. Br J Surg 68:400–401

56. Gordon PH, Vasilevsky CA (1985) Symposium on outpatient anorectal procedures. Lateral internal sphincterotomy: rationale, technique and anesthesia. Can J Surg 28:228–230

57. Jensen SL, Lund F, Nielsen OV, Tange G (1984) Lateral subcutaneous sphincterotomy versus anal dilatation in the treatment of fissure in ano in outpatients: a prospective randomised study. BMJ 289:528–530

58. Lewis TH, Corman ML, Prager ED, Robertson WG (1988) Long-term results of open and closed sphincterotomy for anal fissure. Dis Colon Rectum 31:368–371

59. Sultan AH, Kamm MA, Nicholls RJ, Bartram CI (1994) Prospective study of the extent of internal anal sphincter division during lateral sphincterotomy. Dis Colon Rectum 37: 1031–1033

60. Garcia-Aguilar J, Belmonte C, Wong WD et al (1996) Open vs. closed sphincterotomy for chronic anal fissure: long-term results. Dis Colon Rectum 39:440–443

61. Khubchandani IT, Reed JF (1989) Sequelae of internal sphincterotomy for chronic fissure in ano. Br J Surg 76:431–434

62. Pernikoff BJ, Eisenstat TE, Rubin RJ et al (1994) Reappraisal of partial lateral internal sphincterotomy. Dis Colon Rectum 37:1291–1295

63. Kortbeek JB, Langevin JM, Khoo RE, Heine JA (1992) Chronic fissure-in-ano: a randomized study comparing open and subcutaneous lateral internal sphincterotomy. Dis Colon Rectum 35:835–837

64. Corman ML, Veidenheimer MC, Coller JA (1976) Anoplasty for anal stricture. Surg Clin North Am 56:727–731

65. Gonzalez AR, de Oliveira O Jr, Verzaro R et al (1995) Anoplasty for stenosis and other anorectal defects. Am Surg 61: 526–529

66. Samson RB, Stewart WR (1970) Sliding skin grafts in the treatment of anal fissures. Dis Colon Rectum 13:372–375

67. Williams DR, Coller JA, Corman ML, et al (1981) Anal complications in Crohn's disease. Dis Colon Rectum 24:22–24

68. Rankin GB, Watts HD, Melnyk CS, Kelley ML Jr (1979) National Cooperative Crohn's Disease Study: extraintestinal manifestations and perianal complications. Gastroenterology 77: 914–920

69. Sweeney JL, Ritchie JK, Nicholls RJ (1988) Anal fissure in Crohn's disease. Br J Surg 75:56–57

70. Viamonte M, Dailey TH, Gottesman L (1993) Ulcerative disease of the anorectum in the HIV + patient. Dis Colon Rectum 36:801–805. Published erratum appears in Dis Colon Rectum (1993) 36:990

71. Myers SR (1994) Tuberculous fissure-in ano. J R Soc Med 87:46

72. Whalen TV Jr Kovalcik PJ, Old WL Jr (1980) Tuberculous anal ulcer. Dis Colon Rectum 23:54–55

73. Rosenthal D (1979) Fissure-in-ano management in the military community. Mil Med 144:505–508

74. Marya SK, Mittal SS, Singla S (1980) Lateral subcutaneous internal sphincterotomy for acute fissure in ano. Br J Surg 67: 299

75. Oh C, Divino CM, Steinhagen RM (1995) Anal fissure. 20-year experience. Dis Colon Rectum 38:378–382

76. Gordon PH (1992) Fissure-in-ano. In Gordon PH, Nivatvongs S (eds): Principles and Practice of Surgery for the Colon, Rectum and Anus. Quality Medical Publishing, St. Louis

77. Zuidema GD (1990): Shackelford's Surgery of the Alimentary Tract. 3rd Ed. Vol. 4. WB Saunders, Philadelphia

13

PILONIDAL DISEASE

Santhat Nivatvongs

The first documented case of pilonidal sinus is believed to be from A. W. Anderson in a letter to the Boston Medical and Surgical Journal in 1847.[1] He described a young man of 21 years old with pain in his back. He found a "fistula opening" near the coccyx on the left side that was so small that he could not introduce a probe. Upon opening the cavity, he found a large amount of "very fine, closely matted hairs about two inches in length," with a very offensive smell. The wound healed in 3 weeks. In 1880, Hodges[2] coined the term "pilonidal sinus" (*pilus*, meaning hair, and *nidus*, meaning nest) to describe the chronic sinus containing hair and found between the buttocks. He believed the condition was congenital in origin, representing an imperfect union of the lateral halves of the body and involving the integument only. Buie[3] called it "jeep disease" because of the frequent reactivation of the quiescent sacrococcygeal sinuses among military personnel who entered training for combat duty, with rugged life and stresses of driving trucks, tanks, and jeeps. The time loss among patients with pilonidal disease in the military was tremendous. "A mild ailment, . . . it represents one of the most important surgical causes of lost time."[3] Pilonidal sinus is a chronic subcutaneous abscess in the natal cleft that spontaneously drains through the openings. It is not a "cyst" as frequently referred to in many textbooks and articles.

ETIOLOGY AND PATHOGENESIS

The origin of pilonidal sinus has been a subject of interest and debate for many years. The congenital theory, the remnant of the medullary canal and the infolding of the surface epithelium, or a faulty coalescence of the cutaneous covering in early embryonic life, was once popular.[4] In the modern era, the congenital theory still has its proponents. Lord[5] reasoned that hairs in the pilonidal sinuses are identical in length, diameter, color, and orientation. He said "it is hard to conceive any other theories that explain how hair can get into the pilonidal sinus from outside, which could possibly explain how 23 hairs should fol-

low each other into a pilonidal sinus and each hair be identical in every respect to the last."

The acquired theory is now widely accepted. Its mechanism, however, is speculative and varied. Bascom[6] believes the affected hair follicles become distended with keratin and subsequently infected, leading to folliculitis and an abscess which extends down into the subcutaneous fat (Fig. 13-1). Once the abscess cavity is formed, hairs can enter through the tiny pit and lodge into the abscess cavity from the suction created by movement of the gluteal area. Karydakis,[7] on the other hand, believes the loose hair, due to its scales with chisel-like root end, inserts into the depth of the natal cleft (Fig. 13-2). Once one hair inserts successfully, other hairs can insert more easily. A foreign body tissue reaction and infection follow and the primary sinus of pilonidal disease forms. Secondary openings often occur due to the self-propelling ability of hair and the opening of the abscess that often forms.

SURGICAL PATHOLOGY

The main feature of a pilonidal sinus is the subcutaneous fibrous track lined by gelatinous granulation tissue. The primary opening is in the midline, tiny, and usually noninfected (Fig. 13-3). It may be lined with squamous epithelium. The subcutaneous track extends for a variable distance, usually 2 to 5 cm. A small abscess cavity and branching tracks may come off the primary track. The secondary openings have a different appearance from the primary ones in that they are marked by elevation of granulation tissue and discharge of seropurulent material. Hairs, if seen sticking out of the secondary opening, are the hairs in the abscess cavity that the body tries to spit out (Fig. 13-3). Most sinus tracks (93%) run cephalad; the rest (7%) run caudad and may be confused with fistula-in-ano or hidradenitis suppurativa.[8]

NATURAL HISTORY

Pilonidal sinus is a chronic disease with a natural regression.[9] Usually the disease does not manifest until at puberty and seldom occurs after the third decade of life. However, pilonidal

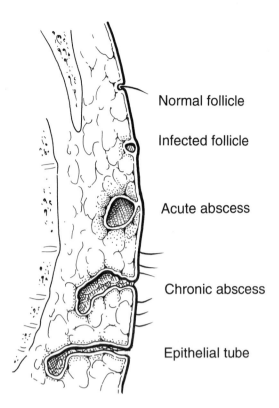

Figure 13-1. Pathogenesis of pilonidal abscess and sinus: hair follicle infection theory. (Modified from Bascom,[6] with permission.)

Figure 13-2. Pathogenesis of pilonidal abscess and sinus: hair penetration theory insertion of loose hair by primary sinus and exit by secondary sinus. (From Karydakis,[7] with permission.)

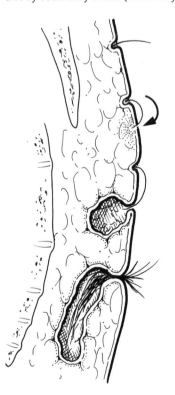

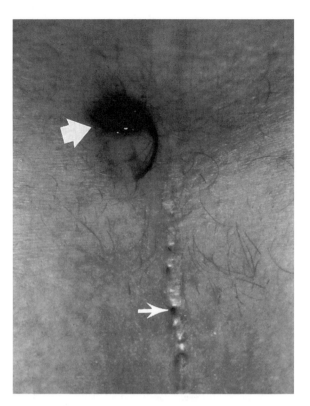

Figure 13-3. Typical pilonidal disease. The primary midline pit is uninflamed (small arrow). Extruding hairs in the secondary sinsus, which is much larger (larger arrow).

sinus may occur at any age. Sagi et al.[10] reported a patient with pilonidal sinus at 7 years of age that progressed to a squamous cell carcinoma at age 54. Karydakis[7] has seen an increased incidence of pilonidal sinus in Greece in the very young, down to 11 years of age, especially in girls. The average age of patients with pilonidal sinus is 32 years in men and 24 years in women in Sola and Rothenberger's series.[11]

Clothier and Haywood[9] studied 42 military personnel who had pilonidal disease; only 5 of 42 (12%) had duration of the disease less than 3 weeks and presented as an acute abscess. In only 2 patients (5%), in whom the disease commenced in their third decade, did it continue into the fourth decade, suggesting that there tends to be a natural tendency to ''burn out'' at about 30 years of age. However, there is also a small group of patients who develop the disease for the first time in their fourth decade.

PREDISPOSING FACTORS

Tiny skin dimples in the sacrococcygeal area are common in the normal population (9%), but almost never become a problem.[12] Because of the common problems of infected pilonidal sinuses among Army and Navy officers, it was speculated that a trauma to the sacrococcygeal area was the primary predisposing factor. However, the acquired theory of folliculitis[6] and spontaneous insertion of hair in the natal cleft[7] refute this theory. Most pilonidal abscesses and sinuses occur without known predisposing factors. More likely, the motion of the natal cleft creating vacuum and pulling forces on sitting down at work appears to be a significant factor in etiology.[9] The rarity of the disease in older people further complicates the issue.

CLINICAL MANIFESTATIONS

The average patient with pilonidal disease is a hirsute, moderately obese man in his second or third decade. However, people of both sexes and any age above puberty can be affected. Pilonidal disease initially may be seen as an acute abscess in the sacrococcygeal area. It frequently ruptures spontaneously, leaving unhealed sinuses with chronic drainage. Once the sinus develops, pain is usually minimal. In 71 to 85% of cases of pilonidal infection, men are affected.[4,11]

DIAGNOSIS

The diagnosis of this condition is usually made quite easily. The patients' history suggests the problem. A painful and fluctuant mass is the most common presentation of the acute process. In its earliest stage, only cellulitis may be present. In the chronic state, the diagnosis is confirmed by the sinus opening in the intergluteal fold approximately 5 cm above the anus. On careful examination, a tiny pit or pits in the midline, which are the main source of the disease, almost always can be found (Fig. 13-3).

The differential diagnosis that must be considered include any furuncle in the skin, an anal fistula, hidradenitis, specific granulomas such as syphilitic or tuberculous ones, and osteomyelitis with multiple draining sinuses in the skin. Actinomycosis in the sacral region has been described as virtually indistinguishable from pilonidal disease. When a fungus is suspected, the diagnosis should be confirmed by finding a ray fungus in the smear of the discharge or in a culture.

TREATMENT

Pilonidal Abscess

Although the infected epithelial sinus is in the midline, the abscess is usually lateral on either side and cephalad. It is well-known that the midline wound in the intergluteal cleft heals slowly and poorly. An attempt should be made to avoid the midline wound and, if necessary, to make it small. Drainage of a pilonidal abscess almost always can be done with the patient under local anesthesia in the clinic, office, or emergency room. A longitudinal incision is made lateral to the midline in the coccygeal area (Fig. 13-4). The incision is deepened into the subcutaneous tissue entering the abscess cavity. Hair in the abscess cavity, if present, must be completely removed. The patient is instructed to irrigate the abscess cavity with diluted hydrogen peroxide (dilution 1:4) twice a day followed by washing with soap and water or a bath. The wound is also swabbed with a Cytette brush, which is very effective in catching any hairs in the abscess cavity and the sinus tracks (Fig. 13-5). Complete healing is a rule. The most important aspect is to prevent and remove hairs from the abscess cavity.

Pilonidal Sinus

Treatment of pilonidal sinus can be done in one of several ways: nonoperative treatment, conservative excision, incision and marsupialization, wide local excision with or without primary closure, excision and Z-plasty, or advancing flap operation (Karydakis procedure).

Nonoperative Treatment

Klass[12] believes that the immediate cause of the infection in a pilonidal sinus is a collection of loose hairs and fecal residue in the internatal cleft, and that when an abscess has developed, incision and drainage is all that is required. He does treat his patients with strict hygiene by washing with soap and water in the perineal and sacrococcygeal area. An abscess is drained, the sinus is kept open, and the area is cleaned. In his series of 15 patients with chronic discharge from sinuses, 11 were cured with follow-up of 3 years or longer. In another group of 12 patients who required incision and drainage of the abscess, 10 patients healed and 2 patients required a second incision and drainage. The follow-up was at least 3 years. At the Tripler Army Medical Center, Hawaii, Armstrong and Barcia[13] treat

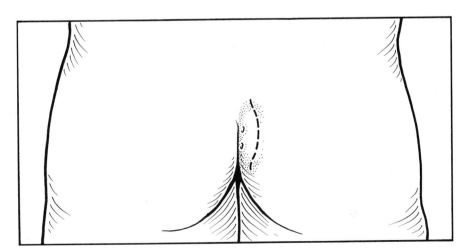

Figure 13-4. Drainage of pilonidal abscess. The incision is made off the midline. (Modified from Nivatvongs[30] with permission.)

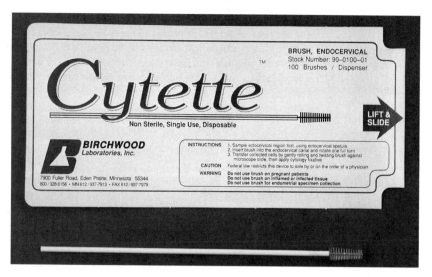

Figure 13-5. Cytette brush for removal of hair from the pilonidal abscess cavity and sinus track.

pilonidal disease mainly by shaving all hairs within the natal cleft, 5 cm from the anus to the sacrum. Visible hairs within the sinus are removed, but no attempt is made to probe for hairs within the sinus. If there is an abscess, a lateral incision for drainage is made. This conservative method was applied to 101 consecutive patients during a 1 year period. The wound healed in all patients. Unfortunately, the length of follow-up and the recurrence rate are not stated.

Injecting phenol into the sinus track has been advocated by some authors who obtained excellent results with its use.[14] The phenol serves to destroy epithelium, sterilize the track, and remove the embedded hair. An injection of 1 to 2 ml of 80%

phenol is given, with great care taken to protect the patient's skin. The injection can be repeated every 4 to 6 weeks as necessary. This technique, however, has never become popular.

Incisional Drainage and Excision of Midline Pits

Although Lord[5] believes in the congenital theory, in contrast to Bascom's strong advocacy of acquired etiology,[6] their concept of treatment is remarkably similar. Both advocate excision of the midline pits or sinuses and thorough cleansing of hair and debris from the abscess or sinus cavity. Bascom emphasizes

Figure 13-6. Bascom operation: midline pits excised and closed. Lateral incision to cavity. Granulating tissue curetted. (Modified from Bascom,[6] with permission.)

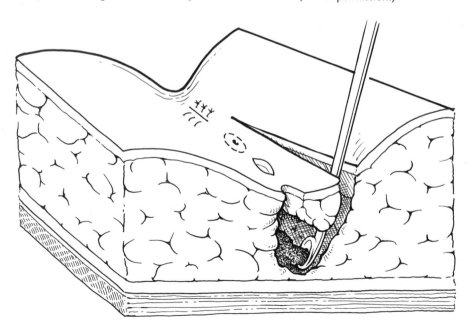

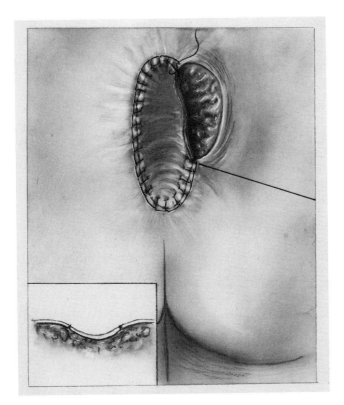

Figure 13-7. Marsupialization. Sinus laid open. Fibrotic wall at the base of the wound is sutured to the edges of the skin with continuous absorbable suture.

avoiding midline wounds by using a longitudinal incision off the midline to enter the abscess or sinus cavity (Fig. 13-6).[6] In a follow-up of 149 patients with a mean follow-up of 3 1/2 years (longest, 9 years), the cure rate was 84%.[15] Advantages of this technique are minimal surgery and small wounds. It can be done on an outpatient basis and the healing is rapid, usually complete within 3 weeks, with the majority within 1 to 2 weeks.

This is a technique of choice for most primary pilonidal sinuses with or without abscess. One should keep in mind that to be successful, the patient will have to make sure that hairs will not get into the wound. This is best performed by irrigating the wound with diluted hydrogen peroxide (dilution 1:4) and swabbing the wound with a Cytette brush once or twice a day, in addition to washing the area with soap and water.

Incision and Marsupialization

An open type of operation with marsupialization of the wound was advocated by Buie[3] and later by Culp.[16] The technique consists of opening the sinus track in the midline. The debris and granulation tissues are scraped with a curette. The fibrous tissue in the track is saved and is sutured to the edges of the wound. This technique not only minimizes the size and depth of the wound, but also prevents the wound from premature closure. In addition, it is easy to pack and clean the wound (Fig. 13-7). In so doing, the size of the wound is reduced 50 to 60%. Sola and Rothenberger[11] reported 125 patients treated with incision and marsupialization. The average age was 32 years. The average healing time was 4 weeks, with prolonged healing (12 to 20 weeks) in 2 to 4% of the patients. Although this technique is simple, it is still far more extensive than the incisional drainage and excision of the midline pits as described earlier.

Wide Local Excision with or Without Primary Closure

The sinus tracks and a 5-mm margin of normal tissue are excised en bloc. The dissection is carried down to the sacrococcygeal fascia, and the pilonidal abscess or sinuses are removed without entering the gluteal fascia laterally.[17] Some authors advocate performing a wide local excision with primary closure of the wound to minimize the healing time. In a randomized trial with 3-year follow-up, Kronborg et al.[18] found that excision with primary closure of the wound had a shorter healing time than

Figure 13-8. Z-plasty. **(A)** The pilonidal sinus is excised. The limbs of the Z are made as in diagram. **(B)** Full-thickness flaps are raised and **(C)** skin is closed. (Modified from Monroe,[31] with permission.)

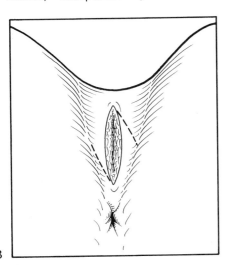
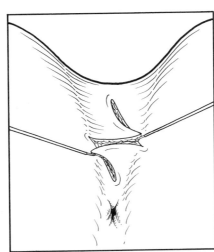
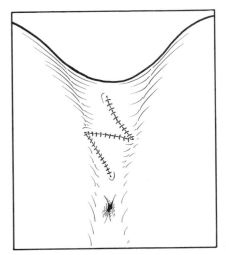

A,B   C

excision with an open wound. The recurrence rate varied from 0 to 38%.[19] This radical technique has no advantage over the simpler incisional drainage and excision of the midline pits.

Excision and Z-Plasty

Excision of pilonidal sinuses with primary closure of the wound is simple but has a high recurrence rate. The use of primary closure, however, is appealing because successful wound healing can be accomplished within 7 to 10 days. To avoid recurrence or breakdown of the midline wound, the anatomy of the natal crease must be altered. Z-plasty can be done to achieve this goal. Excision of pilonidal sinuses with primary Z-plasty fills out and flattens the natal crease, directs the hair points away from the midline, largely prevents maceration, reduces suction effects in the soft tissues of the buttock, and minimizes friction between their adjacent surfaces.[17] The excision is carried down to the subcutaneous tissue. The limbs of the Z are cut to form a 30-degree angle with the long axis of the wound. Full-thickness flaps are raised, and the flaps are transposed and sutured (Fig. 13-8). A closed suction drain is placed under the full-thickness flaps. Z-plasty thus avoids the midline wound, which is the main cause of slow healing and recurrences. In a series of 110 patients treated with Z-plasty by Toubanakis,[20] there were no recurrences. Mansoory and Dickson[21] reported similar good results. The main disadvantage of this procedure is that it is a rather extensive one for a noncomplicated pilonidal sinus and is not suitable for performance on an outpatient basis.

Advancing Flap Operation (Karydakis Procedure)

Karydakis[7] believes that recurrent pilonidal sinuses occur because of the entry of hair into the intergluteal fold from various parts of the body; the hairs are then forced by friction to the depth of the fold. He designed an operative technique to avoid this problem. A "semilateral" excision is made over the sinuses all the way down to presacral fascia (Fig. 13-9). Mobilization is carried to the opposite side so that the entire flap can be advanced toward the other side of closure. A closed suction drain is placed. This technique avoids midline wound. In the series of 7,471 patients who received the advancing flap procedure, the recurrence rate was 1%. In each recurrence, reinsertion of hair was observed. Follow-up ranged from 2 to 20 years. The complication rate was 8.5%, mainly infection and fluid collection. The mean hospital stay was 3 days, with many patients requiring 1 day of hospitalization or the procedure being performed on an outpatient basis. The Karydakis procedure has been proved to be effective[7,22] but is a moderately extensive procedure.

POSTOPERATIVE CARE

In the management of patients with pilonidal disease, the postoperative care is as important as the operation itself. The open wound should be irrigated with diluted peroxide and swabbed with a Cytette brush to get rid of the hairs, in addition to bathtub or shower twice a day. The open wound, if large, should be packed with fine gauze. Hairs around the wound must be shaved or plucked every 10 to 14 days for at least a few months after complete healing of the wound. The person responsible for taking care of the wound at home is instructed in proper care. The patient should return for a follow-up at 1- to 2-week intervals until the wound is completely healed.

Role of Hairs

During the initial operation, all hair present in the pilonidal sinus must be removed. The wound will not heal if even one hair is present in or enters the wound. There are three ways that the hair can enter the wound.

Ingrown Hair

Hairs from edges of the wound often are crooked and grow into the wound. The best way to avoid this problem is to pluck them out every 10 to 14 days until the wound is healed completely.

Local Hair

Hairs in the adjacent area, particularly from the perianal area, can grow to considerable length, with tips of hairs getting into the wound. Shaving or trimming with scissors is required.

Other Hair

Motion in the intergluteal cleft has been shown to attract loose hairs toward it. Irrigating the open wound with diluted hydrogen peroxide and swabbing with Cytette brush will get rid of those hairs. For closed wounds, washing the area with soap and water will get rid of those hairs.

RECURRENT DISEASE

The length of time needed for the pilonidal wound to heal depends on the type of operation and the extent of the disease. The recurrence rate varies widely from series to series (0 to 40%).[19,20,23] Karydakis believes insertion of hair into the intergluteal cleft is the main cause of recurrences.[7] The treatment of recurrent pilonidal sinus is the same as for the primary disease.

UNHEALED WOUNDS

It is common for the wound not to heal after treatment of pilonidal sinuses. Most commonly, the base is filled with gelatinous granulation tissue, which is usually the result of improper postoperative wound care. Hair is often found growing into the edge of the wound. With even a single hair in it, the wound will not heal completely, and therefore proper management is indicated.

Curettage, Reexcision, and Saucerization

The hairs around the unhealed wound must be shaved and plucked, after which a complete curettage of the granulation tissue is done. If the shape of the wound appears to fold together, causing "pocketing," it should be refashioned and saucerization performed to avoid accumulation of discharge. If the wound is infected with anaerobe bacteria, administering metronidazole (Flagyl) can improve healing.[24] Using a water-pulsating device (such as WaterPik) offers a simple method for irrigation of the

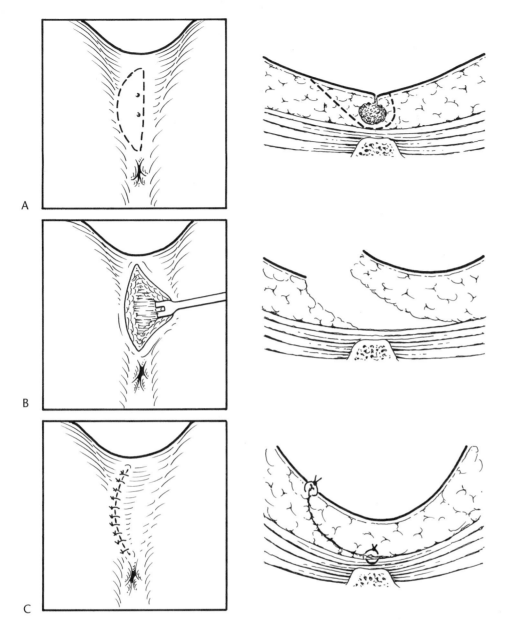

Figure 13-9.   Karydakis operation. **(A)** Semilateral excision. **(B)** Mobilization of the flap. **(C)** Suturing to the sacrococcygeal fascia and to the lateral edge of the wound. (From Karydakis,[7] with permission.)

wound, requires little inconvenience and time, and involves a simple instrument that is familiar to many people.[25] However, a simple packing of the wound with fine mesh gauze is the key to success.

Reverse Bandaging

Some pilonidal wounds heal well initially but fail to form epithelium. The problem is mainly mechanical, because most of the patients involved are obese and have a narrow intergluteal cleft. The motion of the buttocks traumatizes the wound constantly. Rosenberg[26] has used reverse bandaging with success. A wide piece of adhesive tape is placed on each side of the wound, stretching it outward. The tapes are tied in front of the abdomen. The net effect is to flatten the wound and remove most of the angle of the intergluteal cleft.

Gluteus Maximus Myocutaneous Flap

If the wound is extensive and conservative management fails, the wound should be excised. In this situation, use of gluteus maximus myocutaneous flap offers a secure repair. Although the procedure appears extensive, it is not complicated.

Under general anesthesia, the patient is placed in the prone position. The unhealed wound, along with scar and granulation tissue, is excised to reach normal surrounding fat and presacral fascia. A rotational buttock flap is raised, incorporating skin and the underlying superior portion of the gluteus maximus

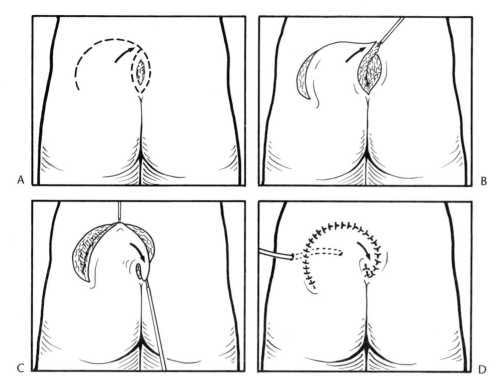

Figure 13-10. Gluteus maximus myocutaneous flap. **(A)** Incision. **(B)** Lesion is excised to sacrum, and the flap created. The flap is raised, incorporating superior portion of the gluteus maximus muscle, protecting gluteal vessels and nerve. **(C)** Myocutaneous flap is rotated to cover the presacral defect; apex rotated to inferior part of the wound. **(D)** Wound is closed and suction drain placed. Arrow indicates apex of flap. (Modified from Perez-Gurri,[27] with permission.)

muscle (Fig. 13-10). After the skin and subcutaneous tissue of the buttock have been traversed, the upper portion of gluteus maximus is transected to the level of gluteus medius and piriformis muscle, with care taken to protect the sciatic nerve. The myocutaneous flap is then rotated into place, a closed suction drain is inserted, and the wound is closed in layers.[27] The patient is not allowed to lie on the flap for 1 week. Z-plasty has been used successfully for treating recurrent pilonidal sinus.[20]

Figure 13-11. Cleft closure. **(A)** Buttocks pressed together, approximated edges marked on each side. (*Figure continues.*)

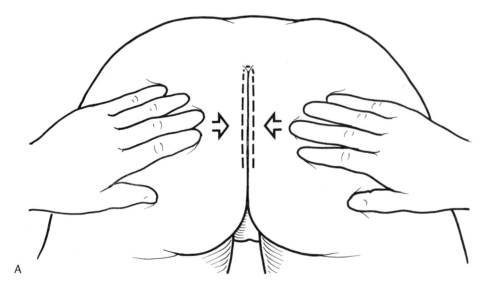

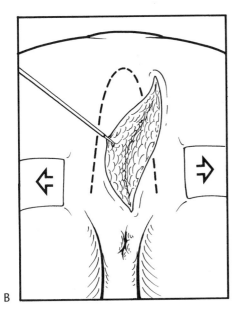
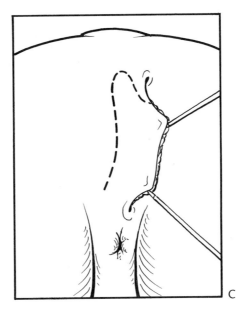

Figure 13-11. (*Continued*) **(B)** Lesion excised. **(C)** Skin flap positioned to overlap edges of wound on opposite side. Excess skin is excised. The skin is closed. (Modified from Bascom,[28] with permission.)

Cleft Closure

Cleft closure, a unique method for treating the unhealed wound, was devised by Bascom.[28] The basic concept is to excise the unhealed skin and the underlying subcutaneous tissue. The natal cleft is eliminated by replacing the defect at the depth of the cleft with a skin flap over a thick pad of fat.

The procedure is performed with the patient under general or spinal anesthesia. Cefazolin (Ancef) and metronidazole (Flagyl), 500 mg each, are given intravenously preoperatively and two doses every 6 hours thereafter. The patient is placed in the prone jackknife position.

With the patient's buttocks pressed together, the lines of contact of the cheeks of the buttocks are marked with a felt-tipped pen (Fig. 13-11A). The cheeks of the buttocks are then taped apart and the skin is prepared and draped. The skin in this region is infiltrated with 0.25% bupivacaine (Marcaine) containing 1:200,000 epinephrine to decrease bleeding. A triangle-shaped section of skin overlying the unhealed wound is excised, extending above and lateral to the apex of the cleft. The lower apex of excision is ''comma shaped'' and points toward the anus (Fig. 13-11B). The granulation tissues and hairs are removed. No mobilization of fat or muscle is done.

After the skin flap (dissected only into the dermis) is raised out to the previously marked line, the tapes are released. The skin flap is positioned to overlap the edges of the wound on the opposite side. The excess skin is excised. A closed suction drain is placed in the subcutaneous tissue. The subcutaneous tissue is closed with 3-0 chromic catgut and the skin is closed with subcuticular 4-0 polydioxanone suture (PDS) (Fig. 13-11C).

The drain is removed in about 4 days. We usually keep the patient in the hospital for a few days. Most patients are able to resume normal activities on the fourth day.[28] Because of its simplicity, cleft closure is the procedure of choice for the unhealed midline pilonidal wound.

PILONIDAL SINUS AND CARCINOMA

Carcinoma arising in a chronic pilonidal sinus is rare. Review of the world literature from 1900 to 1994 yields only 44 patients.[29] Thirty-nine of the cases were squamous cell carcinoma. There were also three basal cell carcinomas, one adenocarcinoma (sweat gland type), and one unspecified type. The etiology of pilonidal carcinoma appears to be the same as that by which other chronic inflamed wounds such as scars, skin ulcers, and

Table 13-1. World Literature on Pilonidal Carcinoma

Total patients	44
Male:female ratio	35:9
Age at presentation (yr.)	50
Mean duration of symptoms (yr.)	23
Inguinal adenopathy	5 (11%)
Treatment	
Excision	35
Chemotherapy only	1
Radiation only	0
No treatment	2
Excision and radiation	4
Excision and chemotherapy	1
Excision, chemotherapy, and radiation	1
Follow-up (mean)	29 months
Recurrence	34%
Time to recurrence	16 months
Total dead	12 (27%)
Total dead with disease	8 (18%)

(From Davis et al.,[29] with permission.)

fistulas undergo malignant degeneration. The average duration of pilonidal disease in these patients was 23 years. Pilonidal carcinoma has a distinctive appearance, and the diagnosis can frequently be made on inspection. A central ulceration is often present with a friable, indurated, erythematous, and fungating margin. It is usually a well-differentiated squamous cell carcinoma, frequently with focal areas of keratinization and rare mitotic figures. The carcinoma grows locally before metastasizing to inguinal lymph nodes. Preoperative evaluation of patients with pilonidal carcinoma should include examination of the inguinal areas, perineum, and the anorectum. The treatment is wide local excision to include the presacral fascia. The features of world literature on pilonidal carcinoma are shown in Table 13-1).

REFERENCES

1. Anderson AW (1847) Hair extracted from an ulcer. Boston Med Surg J 36:74

2. Hodges RM (1880) Pilonidal sinus. Boston Med Surg J 103:485–486

3. Buie LA (1944) Jeep disease. South Med J 37:103–109

4. Kooistra HP (1942) Pilonidal sinuses. Review of the literature and report of three hundred fifty cases. Am J Surg 55:3–17

5. Lord PH (1975) Etiology of pilonidal sinus. Dis Colon Rectum 18:661–664

6. Bascom J (1980) Pilonidal disease: origin from follicles of hairs and results of follicle removal as treatment. Surgery 87:567–572

7. Karydakis GE (1992) Easy and successful treatment of pilonidal sinus after explanation of its causative process. Aust NZ J Surg 62:385–389

8. Notaras MJ (1970) A review of three popular methods of post-anal (pilonidal) sinus disease. Br J Surg 57:886–890

9. Clothier PR, Haywood IR (1984) The natural history of post anal (pilonidal) sinus. Ann R Coll Surg Eng 66:201–203

10. Sagi A, Rosenberg L, Greiff M et al (1984) Squamous cell carcinoma arising in a pilonidal sinus: a case report and review of the literature. J Dermatol Surg Oncol 10:210–212

11. Sola JA, Rothenberger DA (1990) Chronic pilonidal disease. An assessment of 150 cases. Dis Colon Rectum 33:758–761

12. Klass AA (1956) The so-called pilonidal sinus. Can Med Assoc J 75:737–742

13. Armstrong JH, Barcia PJ (1994) Pilonidal sinus disease. The conservative approach. Arch Surg 129:914–918

14. Hegge HGJ, Vos GA, Patka P, Hoitsma HFW (1987) Treatment of complicated or infected pilonidal sinus disease by local application of phenol. Surgery 102:52–54

15. Bascom J (1983) Pilonidal disease: long-term results of follicle removal. Dis Colon Rectum 26:800–807

16. Culp CE (1967) Pilonidal disease and its treatment. Surg Clin North Am 47:1007–1014

17. Eftaiha M, Abcarian H (1977) The dilemma of pilonidal disease: surgical treatment. Dis Colon Rectum 20:279–286

18. Kronborg O, Christensen K, Zimmermann-Nielsen C (1985) Chronic pilonidal disease: a randomized trial with a complete three-year follow-up. Br J Surg 72:303–304

19. Duchateau J, De Mol J, Bostoen H, Allegaert W (1985) Pilonidal sinus. Excision–marsupialization–phenolization? Acta Chir Belg 85:325–328

20. Toubanakis G (1986) Treatment of pilonidal sinus disease with the Z-plasty procedure (modified). Am Surg 52:611–612

21. Mansoory A, Dickson D (1982) Z-plasty for treatment of disease of the pilonidal sinus. Surg Gynecol Obstet 155:409–411

22. Kitchen PRB (1982) Pilonidal sinus: excision and primary closure with a lateralized wound—the Karydakis operation. Aust NZ J Surg 52:302–305

23. Jensen SL, Harling H (1988) Prognosis after simple incision and drainage for a first-episode acute pilonidal abscess. Br J Surg 75:60–61

24. Marks J, Harding KG, Hughes LE, Ribeiro CD (1985) Pilonidal sinus excision—healing by open granulation. Br J Surg 72:637–640

25. Hoexter B (1976) Use of WaterPik lavage in pilonidal wound care. Dis Colon Rectum 19:470–471

26. Rosenberg I (1977) Reverse bandaging for cure of the reluctant pilonidal wound. Dis Colon Rectum 20:290–291

27. Perez-Gurri JA, Temple-Walley J, Ketcham AS (1984) Gluteus maximus myocutaneous flap for the treatment of recalcitrant pilonidal disease. Dis Colon Rectum 27:262–264

28. Bascom JW (1987) Repeat pilonidal operations. Am J Surg 154:118–122

29. Davis KA, Mock CN, Armand V et al (1994) Malignant degeneration of pilonidal cysts. Am Surg 60:200–204

30. Nivatvongs S (1987) p. 339. In Basic Surgical Practice. Hanley and Belfus, Philadelphia

31. Monro RS, McDermott FT (1965) The elimination of casual factors in pilonidal sinus treated by Z-plasty. Br J Surg 52:177–181

14

ANORECTAL SEPSIS

Robin K.S. Phillips
Peter J. Lunniss

Anorectal sepsis, whether presenting acutely as an abscess or chronically as an anal fistula, is common. Fortunately the majority of cases can be dealt with easily, but every experienced surgeon will have encountered more difficult cases that require a deeper understanding if recurrence or incontinence are to be avoided. St. Mark's Hospital was founded as the hospital ''for fistulae etc.,'' yet over 150 years later, certain fistulae may be just as challenging as they were in Frederick Salmon's day.

Most anal fistulae are preceded by an episode of acute anorectal sepsis. The converse is however not true: only about 60% of acute abscesses will go on to form a chronic anal fistula.

Epidemiology

Anal fistulae may be found in association with a variety of specific conditions. Most, however, are nonspecific (idiopathic, cryptoglandular), and in this group infection of an anal gland in the intersphincteric space may be the initiating pathology.[1] Fistulae occur in Crohn's disease,[2,3] tuberculosis,[4] malignancy[5] (which itself may arise in the track of a long-standing fistula), lymphogranuloma venereum,[6] presacral dermoid,[7] rectal duplication,[8] actinomycosis,[9] trauma, and foreign bodies.[10]

Information on incidence in the general population is scarce. Most comes from hospital analysis, often from tertiary referral centers, which attract more difficult cases. Buie[11] reported that approximately 5% of patients admitted to the Mayo Clinic with anorectal disease had an anal fistula. At St. Mark's between 1968 and 1973, about 4% of all new outpatients and 10% of all new inpatients had an anal fistula.[12] More accurate information about incidence comes from Scandinavia. In the County of Stockholm (population 1.5 million), about 170 patients with anal fistulae are operated upon annually, giving an approximate incidence of 1 in 10,000.[13] Sainio[14] similarly reported a mean incidence of 8.6 in 100,000 among the population of Helsinki.

Gender

All series have a male predominance. Most report a male-female ratio of between 2 to 1 and 4 to 1. The highest ratios come from the Indian subcontinent,[15–17] although this may reflect underreporting in women. The gender difference in incidence is unexplained. Lilius[18] showed that males have slightly more intramuscular anal glands than women, and that the anal glands tend to be more ramifying and cystic. However, McColl[19] found no sex difference in histology or distribution of the anal glands in 50 normal human anal canals.

The sex difference is not limited to humans. German shepherd dogs are particularly prone to develop anal fistulae compared with other breeds, and this is not due to any differences in anal crypt or gland anatomy.[20] Vasseur[21] has reported a 3 to 1 male-female ratio for canine fistulae, compared with a 1 to 1 sex ratio for the whole dog population. The incidence of fistulae is much lower in neutered dogs and bitches compared with those sexually intact.[22]

These findings suggest a possible role for sex hormones in fistula development and maintenance, and this factor might explain the observation that in babies only boys are affected.[23,24] A recent study from St. Mark's Hospital failed to demonstrate any significant difference in circulating sex hormone levels between patients with idiopathic anal fistulae and age- and sex-matched normal controls.[25] It is however possible that tissue sensitivity to endogenous hormones is more important rather than the levels of circulating hormones.

Other Factors

Anal fistulae most commonly afflict people in the third, fourth, or fifth decades of life.[12,18,26] There is little information on racial differences, although the peak incidence has been reported to be at a lower age in Nigerians[27] and in black Americans.[28] Lockhart-Mummery[10] wrote that members of mounted cavalry units developed anal fistulae twice as often as those of un-mounted units, although this was a retrospective revelation. More modern sedentary occupations, however, cannot be implicated.[14,18] It is not clear whether bowel habit is influential. Some authors take the view that diarrhea may allow easier access of bacteria to the anal glands, especially in infants.[29] Others feel that hard stools are at fault through the abrasive passage along the anal canal.[30] Any form of useful epidemiologic data are lacking in this respect.

Etiology

Anal glands were mentioned in the literature as far back as 1751 by van Haller.[19] Most writers today, however, attribute their demonstration and the link with anal fistulae to Chiari[31] and Herrmann & Desfosses.[32] The function of anal glands is uncertain; they secrete mucin,[1] but this is of a different type to that secreted by rectal mucosa.[33] McColl[19] showed that the anal glands were not vestigial remnants of sexual scent glands; and Shafik's[34] suggestion that they are not true glands at all, but rather vestigial epithelial remnants left after proctodeal invagination into the hindgut, has not been substantiated by a more scientific approach.[35]

Lockhart-Mummery[10] in 1929 rekindled the idea that anal glands are central to anorectal sepsis. Anal glands may be found in the submucous and intermuscular spaces; they have also been described lying outside the external sphincter,[36] although Parks[1] thought it unlikely that such visceral structures could penetrate somatic musculature. The number of glands within the anal canal is variable, ranging from more than 10 rarely,[36] to none.[18] Not all anal sinuses have gland ducts draining into them, but occasionally more than one gland can discharge into the same sinus.[1,37] The distribution of glands around the circumference of the anal canal is probably fairly even,[18,19] despite reports of a preponderance posteriorly.[38,39] Shropshear[40] felt that only glands lying in the submucosa were implicated in anorectal sepsis, infection spreading through the components of the anal sphincter along the ramifications of the conjoined longitudinal muscle.[41] This, however, was not supported by any objective evidence.

Modern thinkers blame intersphincteric anal glands as the source of sepsis. These constitute between one-third and two-thirds of all anal canal glands,[19,38] which might contribute to the cryptoglandular hypothesis.[1,42] Eisenhammer considered all nonspecific abscesses and fistulae to be the result of extension of sepsis from an intramuscular anal gland, the sepsis being unable to drain spontaneously into the anal lumen because of infective obstruction of the connecting duct across the internal sphincter into the crypt. Parks[1] proposed that when any initial abscess had subsided, the remaining diseased anal gland might become the seat of chronic infection with subsequent fistula formation. A fistula was thus regarded as a granulation tissue-lined track kept open by an abscess around a diseased anal gland deep to the internal sphincter.

Gordon-Watson and Dodd[43] provided histologic evidence that anal glands were implicated when they demonstrated anal glandular epithelium lining three anal fistula tracks. Parks[1] studied 30 consecutive cases of anal fistulae and found cystic dilatation of anal glands (Fig. 14-1) in 8, which he attributed to acquired duct dilatation or more probably a congenital abnormality, a precursor to infection within a mucin-filled cavity.

Goligher et al.[44] questioned the cryptoglandular hypothesis, reasoning that if abscess and fistula were acute and chronic manifestations of the same disease, then one would expect to find an intersphincteric abscess in (almost) all cases. In fact

Figure 14-1. Photomicrograph showing cystic dilatation of an intersphincteric anal gland, situated between the striated external anal sphincter and the conjoined longitudinal muscle fibers. The internal anal sphincter lies medial to the longitudinal muscle layer (H & E × 40).

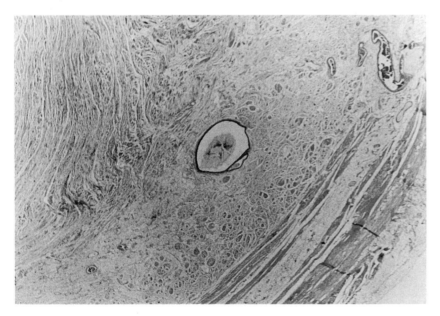

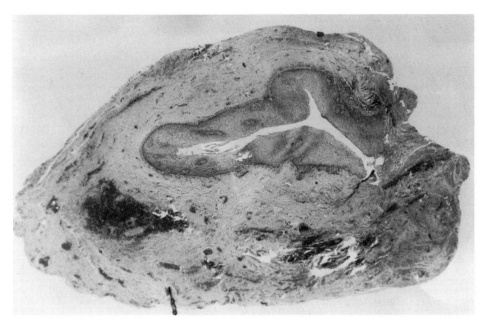

Figure 14-2.   Photomicrograph showing in cross-section the intersphincteric component of a chronic intersphincteric fistula. The fistula is lined by stratified squamous epithelium, and surrounded by dense fibrous tissue (H & E × 40). (From Lunniss et al.,[47] with permission.)

intersphincteric space sepsis was found in only 8 of 28 cases of acute anorectal sepsis. Of 32 cases of anal fistulae, only 14 had evidence of either intersphincteric sepsis or the track traveling within (rather than simply across) the intersphincteric space. Clearly not all anorectal sepsis has a cryptoglandular origin, some simply being skin boils that happen to be on the anus. It must be said, however, that surgical assessment during the acute phase of the disease is unlikely to be accurate in every case.

Microbiologic studies of anal fistula tissue also question the contribution of sepsis to the persistence of fistulae. Although acute infection and its effective drainage are primary problems, the possibility that anal glands are the seat of chronic infection in established fistulae is not wholly supported by the evidence.[45,46] An alternative theory as to why idiopathic fistulae persist is that they become epithelialized, at least partly. This factor is responsible for the persistence of fistulae at other sites in the body. A histologic study of the intersphincteric component of 18 consecutive idiopathic anal fistulae showed an association between anal gland and fistula in only a minority of cases (3), whereas epithelialization from either or both ends of the fistula track was much commoner (10 cases; Fig. 14-2).[47]

Shafik[48] considers the cryptoglandular hypothesis to be untenable, favoring instead infection developing beneath the intersphincteric space by abrasion of the overlying anoderm. He supports this theory by the fact that this region of the anal canal is inelastic and therefore more susceptible to trauma by hard stool. He named the central area deep to this susceptible anoderm the "central space" (probably synonymous with the "anal intermuscular interstices" described by Shropshear[40]). Infection here between the terminal fibers of the conjoined longitudinal muscle and the base loop of the external anal sphincter might spread along any of many named septa derived from the con-

joined longitudinal muscle to any anatomic space around the anal sphincter complex (Fig. 14-3). It must be said, however, that there is no evidence to support this theory. Whether the cryptoglandular hypothesis is true in most cases or not, it has allowed the creation of the classification of Parks, which has the merit of enabling clinical decisions to be made.[45]

ACUTE ANORECTAL SEPSIS

Acute anorectal sepsis may either arise as a simple area of cutaneous sepsis that happens to be close to the anus or as a result of cryptoglandular infection. This distinction is fundamental. The overall incidence of acute anorectal sepsis is higher in males than females, but this is not caused by an increased chance of infection by skin organisms (unrelated to fistulae). Infections of this sort are evenly distributed between men and women.[49]

The link between acute abscess and chronic fistula was stressed by Eisenhammer,[50] who considered the two to be manifestations of the same condition. Thus they were combined under the same title of ''fistulous-abscess.'' The cryptoglandular theory of intersphincteric anal gland infection allowed the concept of the spread of sepsis in the vertical, horizontal, or circumferential planes within the anorectal anatomy. Caudal spread[51] presents acutely as a perianal abscess or chronically as an intersphincteric fistula. Cephalad extension in the intersphincteric space will result in a high intermuscular abscess[52] or a supralevator abscess, depending on the relation of the sepsis to the longitudinal muscle layer. This situation is rare. More common is lateral spread across the external sphincter to enter the ischiorectal fossa. This will lead to an ischiorectal abscess and subsequently a trans-sphincteric fistula. Upward spread may penetrate the levators to form a supralevator abscess. At

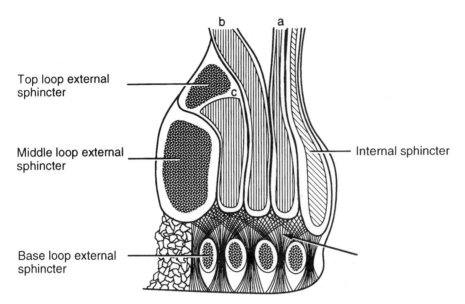

Figure 14-3. Diagram illustrating the arrangement of the muscle components of the anal sphincters according to Shafik.[48] Shafik recognizes three components of the conjoined longitudinal muscle, each bordered by named septa. (*a*) The medial longitudinal muscle, a direct continuation of the outer muscle coat of the rectum. (*b*) The intermediate layer, a direct prolongation of pubococcygeus (which therefore does not present anteriorly). (*c*) The lateral layer, an extension of the top loop of the external anal sphincter, again deficient anteriorly. The central space (arrowed) lies immediately below the intersphincteric space, from where sepsis can spread along the longitudinal muscle septa. (Adapted from Phillips and Lunniss,[146] with permission.)

any level, namely intermuscular (synonymous with intramuscular and equivalent to intersphincteric but with no restriction to a level beneath the anorectal ring), ischiorectal or supralevator, circumferential spread may occur, causing varieties of horseshoe extensions. Not all sepsis was considered cryptoglandular in origin by Eisenhammer,[53] who wrote of acute anorectal noncryptoglandular nonfistulous abscesses. Such lesions included submucous abscess, mucocutaneous or marginal abscess, perianal abscess caused by follicular skin infection, ischiorectal abscess caused by primary infection or foreign body, and pelvirectal supralevator abscess originating from pelvic disease (Fig. 14-4).

SURGICAL MANAGEMENT OF ACUTE ANORECTAL SEPSIS

Acute anorectal sepsis is the most common acute surgical emergency, accounting for between 5,000 and 6,000 admissions per year to hospitals in England and Wales.[54]

Presentation

Perianal sepsis usually presents with a short history of a few days pain and a palpable tender lump at the anal margin. Usually there are no systemic symptoms, but occasionally the patient may be severely septic. Examination usually reveals swelling to the side of the anus with induration. A tender enlarged inguinal node may be palpable. If sepsis is high, rectal pain and occasionally disturbance of micturition may be the only symptoms. In this circumstance, the diagnosis should be suspected,

and an examination under anesthetic with identification of the abscess and drainage should be carried out.

Management

Management is by drainage by an external skin incision over the most fluctuant part of the abscess. Recurrence of abscess or development of fistula following simple incision and drainage has been variously reported as 17%,[55] 25%,[56] 41%,[57] 62%,[58] 66%,[59] and 87%.[60] Vasilevsky and Gordon[61] reported a recurrence rate of 48% despite those with an intersphincteric abscess (18% of the study group) undergoing internal sphincterotomy to drain the abscess. Not one of the patients reported by Ramstead[56] was thought to have had an intersphincteric abscess, yet 60% of the subsequent fistulae were intersphincteric. Schouten and van Vroonhoven[62] reported a prospective randomized study of incision and drainage versus primary fistulotomy. There was a 40% recurrence rate following incision and drainage, with the same authors having earlier reported a recurrence rate of 85%.[63] Their explanation for the difference was inclusion in the first study of patients with recurrent abscesses.

Drainage With Primary Suture

Shorter healing time, shorter hospital stay, and less postoperative pain have been demonstrated after incision, curettage, and primary suture under antibiotic cover when compared with simple incision and drainage.[64–66] This method was first described in the management of anorectal sepsis by Ellis.[67] Only 22% of cases overall recur after such treatment, but 50% do so when

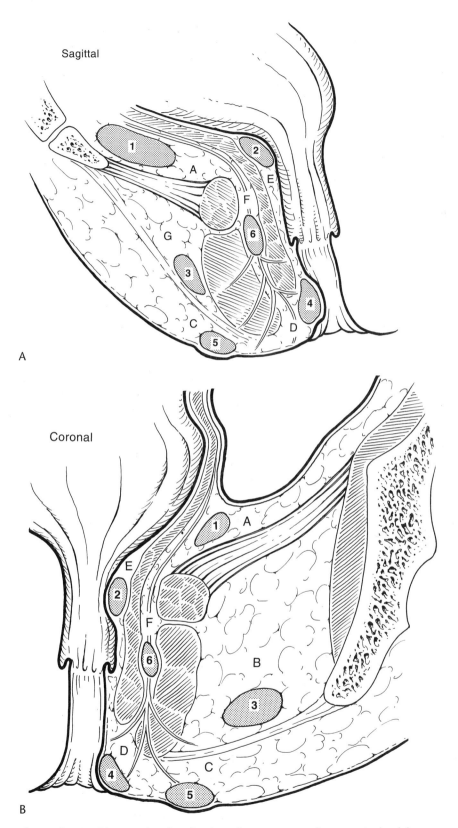

Sagittal

A

Coronal

B

Figure 14-4.   Diagram showing the sites of acute anorectal noncryptoglandular nonfistulous abscesses, according to Eisenhammer.[53] *A*, Pelvirectal supralevator space; *B* ischiorectal space; *C*, perianal or superficial ischiorectal space; *D*, marginal or mucocutaneous space; *E*, submucous space; *F*, anorectal intermuscular space; *G*, deep postanal space. *1*, Pelvirectal supralevator abscess; *2*, submucous abscess (infected hemorrhoid injection, trauma); *3*, ischiorectal foreign body abscess; *4*, mucocutaneous or marginal abscess (infected hematoma); *5*, subcutaneous or perianal abscess (follicular skin infection).

the causative organism is a coliform (described later).[64] A prospective randomized trial confirmed shorter healing times with primary closure.[66] Nevertheless, despite adequate treatment of any concomitant fistula, recurrence was common, occurring in 22% of the incision and drainage group and 39% of the primary suture group.

The Role of Microbiology

In spite of the obvious bacterial origin of anorectal sepsis, the significance of microbiologic findings has been largely ignored until the last decade. Grace et al.[49] prospectively studied 162 patients presenting with either a perianal (125 patients) or ischiorectal (37 patients) abscess, of whom 56 presented with recurrent sepsis at the site of a previous abscess. In 63 patients a fistula was found, and pus grew gut organisms in all but one. In 34 patients no fistula was found, and pus grew skin-derived organisms in all cases. There were another 52 patients in whom the pus grew gut organisms but who did not have a fistula at presentation. Ten of these patients later presented with recurrent sepsis at the same site, 5 of whom had a fistula. There were no cases of recurrence where pus had grown skin organisms.

Subsequent studies have supported the view that growth of skin organisms from an anorectal abscess means that the abscess has nothing to do with fistula, whereas there is a high probability of an underlying fistula if gut organisms are cultured.

The Operation

Protocol of Examination

The surgical management should be as follows:

1. Examine carefully under anesthesia (EUA) to determine the site of the abscess.
2. Apply external pressure on the abscess while examining the anal lumen with a proctoscope to demonstrate pus discharging into the anal canal at the site of any internal opening.
3. Drain the abscess at the most fluctuant point, and send the pus for culture.
4. Curette the cavity while placing a finger in the anus to avoid the creation of a false opening.
5. Look for the internal opening of a fistula.

If no fistula is found, the abscess is simply drained and the patient allowed home with instructions for dressings. Although some would await the results of microbiology, most surgeons would not, having not been convinced that microbiology has a useful part to play in practice. If the abscess does not heal over the next few weeks, then further assessment by EUA is indicated, and any fistula can then be treated.

The bacteriologic approach is rendered not useful by the fact that cutaneous infection may also be caused by gut organisms. Approximately 40% of anorectal abscesses with pus positive for enteric bacteria do not develop a fistula.[49,68,69] Secondly, the results of microbiology are not often available to be of practical use.

Primary or Delayed Fistulotomy?

According to Eisenhammer,[53] external incision and drainage alone can only work if the acute lesion is of noncryptoglandular origin; if the origin was cryptoglandular, the source of the sepsis in the intersphincteric space would not be adequately treated by this method. Eisenhammer further stated that a fistulous abscess follows a constant and predetermined anatomic path, which if not dealt with adequately in the early stages leads to a more complex form of fistula. He reasoned that because abscess and fistula are the same entity, initial treatment at the acute stage should include primary fistulotomy, so obviating the need for further surgery for any subsequent fistula. Proponents of primary fistulotomy, or primary partial internal sphincterectomy, report a recurrence rate of 0 to 7%,[53,58,60,63,70,71] much lower than that after simple external incision and drainage alone.

There are drawbacks to this aggressive approach. Internal openings may only be demonstrable in one-third of cases,[28,53,71] and false tracks may be created by overzealous probing. Eisenhammer[53] recommended injecting methylene blue (hydrogen peroxide could also be used) through the external wound to identify the internal opening, or passing forceps from the intersphincteric space into the anal lumen. Others have recommended Goodsall's rule to predict the correct site for internal sphincterotomy.[63] Laying open of an identified primary track may divide an uncertain amount of sphincter. Furthermore, a significant proportion of patients with acute abscesses do not develop recurrent sepsis or fistulae (even including many of those later shown by culture to contain gut-derived organisms). These patients will not be well served by unnecessary division of the internal sphincter or primary fistulotomy. Both procedures can result in flatus incontinence[55] and soiling.[62] This is even more aposite as a prospective randomized trial has shown no statistically significant difference in recurrence rates between incision and drainage and incision with early fistulotomy.[55] Perhaps performing an incision alone in those cases where no internal opening is evident, and primary fistulotomy when one is evident and low, is most sensible; it yields a recurrence rate of less than 1%.[71]

Intersphincteric Space Infection

A recent prospective study[72] has confirmed the importance of intersphincteric space infection in the pathogenesis of anal fistulae. Twenty-two consecutive patients presenting with either acute perianal or ischiorectal sepsis had a radial incision made over the abscess and pus taken for microbiologic culture. The incision was then extended medially as necessary to allow dissection of the intersphincteric space. Simple abscesses or those with intersphincteric space involvement but no obvious fistula were incised and drained. Any simple fistula was managed by primary fistulotomy, and more complex ones with a loose seton.

Of 22 abscesses, 10 had no internal opening or intersphincteric space involvement. Eleven fistulae were treated immediately by laying open (10 patients) or loose seton (1 patient). One patient had intersphincteric sepsis, but no internal opening could be identified. Treatment was therfore by simple drainage. Recurrent sepsis developed 28 weeks later when an internal opening was found and an intersphincteric fistula laid open.

Gut organisms were always cultured when there was intersphincteric space sepsis, as well as in 3 patients with simple cutaneous abscesses but no fistula. Skin and gut organisms were never cultured together.

There still remains the possibility that some anorectal abscesses of cryptoglandular origin might be cured by simple drainage without fistulotomy. A trial would be required resolve this issue. Current best practice must allow for the skills and experience of the surgeon.

Acute Supralevator Sepsis

Supralevator sepsis presenting acutely is uncommon. Correct and safe management depends upon diagnosis of the exact location of the sepsis.[1] The origin of supralevator sepsis may be (1) pelvic disease (appendiceal, diverticular, Crohn's disease, gynecologic, or malignant); (2) cephalad extension of an intersphincteric fistula; or (3) cephalad extension of a trans-sphincteric fistula. Of these, the third possibility is most likely. Inappropriate drainage through the perineum of a pelvic abscess may result in an extrasphincteric fistula, which would result in incontinence of rectal contents. In such a case, intrarectal drainage of a pelvic abscess would be the best course of action. Drainage of a supralevator extension of an intersphincteric fistula into the rectum would be safe, whereas drainage through the perineum would create a suprasphincteric or extrasphincteric fistula. In contrast, drainage of a supralevator extension of a trans-sphincteric fistula should be through the perineum, as drainage into the rectum would similarly create an extrasphincteric fistula (Fig. 14-5).

In practice it can be very difficult if not impossible to separate these two forms of suprasphincteric abscess. Furthermore, drainage of a supralevator abscess into the rectum leaves a closed sphincter below, which may inhibit free drainage. In the rare case of an intersphincteric supralevator abscess penetrating the levators to reach the ischiorectal fossa, drainage through the buttock will be needed. The resulting suprasphincteric fistula will then have to be treated on its merits. Such occasions are fortunately very rare, but when they occur, a colostomy may be necessary, especially in any patient who is immunocompromised or diabetic.

ANAL FISTULA

Classification

Historical Classification

Successful surgical management of anal fistula depends upon accurate knowledge of anal sphincter topography and the surgical anatomy of the fistula. Failure to understand either may result in recurrence or incontinence. Classification should provide accurate information that permits simple, comprehensible, and comparable usage.

At the beginning of the century, fistulae were divided simply into two main groups, those in which the track did not pass through the sphincters, and those in which it did.

Goodsall and Miles[73] noted three types of fistulae including complete, blind external, and blind internal, the latter regarded as the precursor of the majority of fistulae. Blind internal fistu-

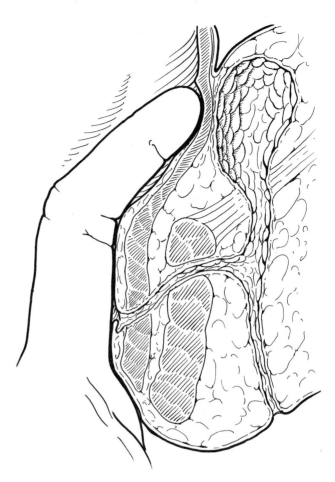

Figure 14-5. Palpation for deep induration, depicting a supralevator pelvirectal extension of a trans-sphincteric fistula. Drainage of this extension into the rectum would create an extrasphincteric fistula. (Adapted from Phillips and Lunniss,[146] with permission.)

lae were further subdivided into subcutaneous, submuscular, and submucous varieties according to the relations of the track to the anal sphincter; but appreciation of anal anatomy at that time was substantially different from the present view.

Milligan and Morgan[74] emphasized the importance of the anorectal ring (anatomically the puborectalis muscle) in maintaining continence, and accordingly classified fistulae as either anal or anorectal. *Anal* fistulae were further subdivided into low and high varieties according to the level of the internal opening, which in both types was below the anorectal ring and therefore safe to lay open. *Anorectal* fistulae were split into three groups: those with an internal opening below the anorectal ring but with a secondary track running above the ring; those without an internal opening; and those with an internal opening into the rectum. Goligher[75] modified this classification by dividing anorectal fistulae into ischiorectal and pararectal, both with extensions above the level of puborectalis but with the former confined by the roof of the ischiorectal fossa and the latter terminating in the pararectal space.

The classification of Stelzner[76] is closer to the system used today. He acknowledged three main fistula groups: intermuscular, in which the track ran in the plane between internal and external sphincters; trans-sphincteric, in which it extended across the external sphincter into the ischiorectal fossa; and extrasphincteric, where the track ran completely outside the sphincters communicating the rectum with the perineum. Thompson[77] emphasized the practical importance of classification and divided fistulae into simple, forming 95% of those encountered, and complex. A complex fistula was defined as one in which the internal opening lay above the anorectal ring, or one that, being laid open, would result in division of at least three-fourths of the sphincter musculature, irrespective of the site of the internal opening. These were the precursors of the Parks classification.

Parks Classification

The most comprehensive and practical classification and most widely used today is that devised by Parks.[78] It is derived from the cryptoglandular hypothesis, which holds that the majority of fistulae arise from an abscess in the intersphincteric plane that results in a primary track whose relations to the external sphincter dictates the type of fistula and therefore management. The classification is divided into four groups: intersphincteric, trans-sphincteric, suprasphincteric, and extrasphincteric fistulae. These groups may or may not be associated with the presence of secondary tracks.

Intersphincteric fistulae (Fig. 14-6) comprise 45% of fistulae.

Figure 14-6. Diagram showing the possible tracks of an intersphincteric fistula. Most pass caudally to present at the perianal skin, but some may track cephalad and even have a secondary opening into the rectum. (Adapted from Phillips and Lunniss,[146] with permission.)

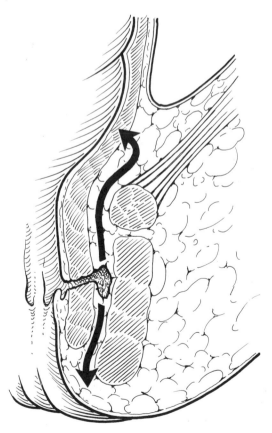

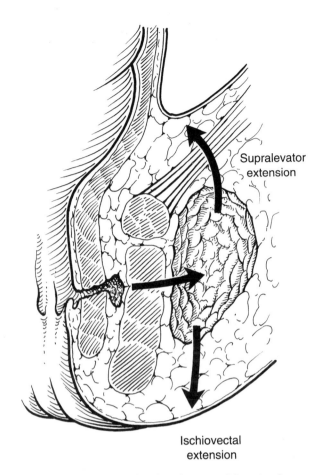

Figure 14-7. Diagram showing the potential tracks of a trans-sphincteric fistula, originating in disease in the intersphincteric space. The primary track may ascend in the intersphincteric plane to cross the external sphincter at a higher level than the dentate line and internal opening. (Adapted from Phillips and Lunniss,[146] with permission)

The majority are simple, but they occasionally deviate from this pattern, including having a high blind track, a high opening into the rectum, no perineal opening, or a pelvic extension.

Trans-sphincteric fistulae (Fig. 14-7) comprise 30% to 40% of cases. The primary track passes through the external sphincter into the ischiorectal fossa. The fistula may be uncomplicated, consisting simply of the primary track, or it may have associated secondary tracks terminating above or below the levator ani muscles. These usually extend to the apex of the ischiorectal fossa, and may undergo horseshoe formation at this level. Occasionally the secondary track may penetrate the levator plate to enter the supralevator space.

Suprasphincteric fistula is rare (Fig. 14-8). Although reported common in Parks' series, this probably reflected case selection through referral pattern. It is very rare to encounter a suprasphincteric fistula that has not been previously operated on. The inference is that most of these cases are likely to be iatrogenic. They are difficult to identify, and some are probably erroneously classified as suprasphincteric when in reality the lesion is high trans-sphincteric.

Extrasphincteric fistulae (1% to 2%) (Fig. 14-9) run directly from the viscera to the perineum or vagina lying outside the

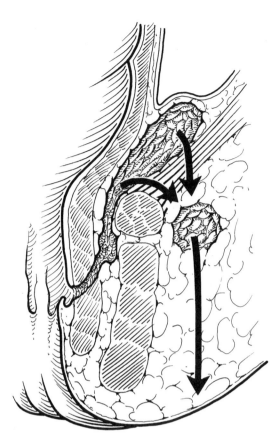

Figure 14-8. Diagram showing the course and associated extensions of a suprasphincteric fistula. (Adapted from Phillips and Lunniss,[146] with permission.)

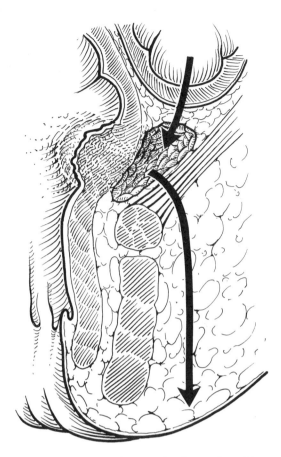

Figure 14-9. The extrasphincteric fistula, running without relation to the sphincters, and classified and managed according to specific etiology. (Adapted from Phillips and Lunniss,[146] with permission.)

Figure 14-10. Diagram showing the three planes in which circumferential spread may occur. Supralevator spread may be outside the rectal wall in the pararectal space, or between the circular and longitudinal muscle layers of the rectum in the inter- (or intra-) muscular space. (From ......,* with permission.)

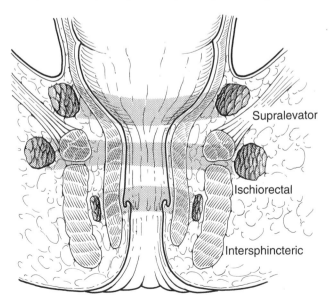

sphincter complex. These are not cryptoglandular in origin. They are usually associated with pathology including trauma, tumor, or infection.

Besides horizontal and vertical spread, sepsis may spread circumferentially in any of the three spaces—intersphincteric, ischiorectal, and pararectal (Fig. 14-10).

The Parks classification has certain minor defects,[79] which are of little clinical significance. Superficial fistulae, often associated with bridged fissures, are not included. Many, if not all, intersphincteric fistulae actually cross the lowermost fibers of the subcutaneous portion of the external sphincter, and although they strictly ought to be classified as trans-sphincteric, they are better regarded as intersphincteric for the purposes of treatment. Suprasphincteric fistulae are rare and difficult to distinguish from high trans-sphincteric tracks. Management is the same as for high trans-sphincteric fistulae. They may not have a cryptoglandular origin. Extrasphincteric fistulae are likewise noncryptoglandular.

Assessment

Clinical Assessment

Surgical success depends upon accurate assessment including a full medical history and proctosigmoidoscopy. It is necessary to exclude associated conditions. Nearly 100 years ago Goodsall

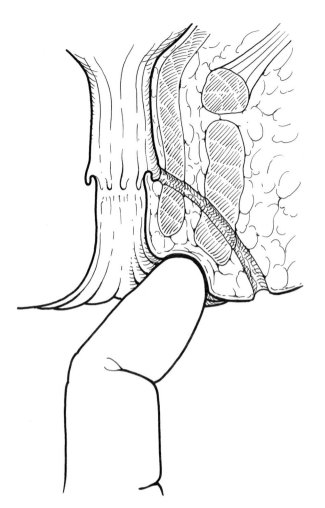

Figure 14-11. Superficial palpation to assess the primary track.

and Miles[73] defined the five essentials of clinical assessment. These include identification of the internal opening, the external opening, the course of the primary track, the presence of secondary extensions, and the presence of other diseases complicating the fistula. The internal opening is the key to the assessment. The relative positions of external and internal openings indicate the likely course of the primary track. Palpable superficial induration suggests a relatively superficial track (Fig. 14-11), whereas supralevator induration suggests a track high in the ischiorectal fossa or more likely a secondary extension (see Fig. 14-5). The distance of the external opening from the anal verge may help differentiate an intersphincteric from a trans-sphincteric fistula; the greater the distance, the greater the likelihood of a complex cephalad extension.[18,80] Goodsall's rule generally applies (Fig. 14-12). Exceptions include anterior openings more than 3 cm from the anal verge, which may be anterior extensions of posterior horseshoe fistulae, or fistulae associated with other diseases, especially Crohn's disease and cancer.

Preoperative Assessment

The first component of preoperative assessment is to identify the site and level of the primary track. The second component is to determine the presence or absence of any secondary track.

Primary Track

1. Identify any external openings.
2. Feel on the skin for the direction of the track using a well-lubricated finger between the external opening and the anal orifice. An indurated track suggests a fairly superficial course; its direction will give a hint to the circumferential location of the internal opening.
3. Identify the internal opening. This is the key to the surgical anatomy. Feel for induration within the anal canal using the index finger applying counterpressure on the perianal skin with the thumb. The internal opening is likely to be located at the level of the dentate line. There is often an enlarged papilla in the region of the internal opening and with experience, the opening itself can be felt in most cases. Seow Choen et al.[8] have shown that trainees can acquire this skill in a few months.
4. The level of the internal opening in relation to the puborectalis is then determined by asking the patient to contract the anal sphincter; it is possible to feel how much functioning muscle would remain were the primary track to be laid open.

Secondary Tracks

The presence of secondary track formation is detected by the sign of supralevator induration. It may be difficult to appreciate, but there is often a difference on each side that will help to reveal its presence. A secondary track most usually arises from a trans-sphincteric primary track, extending upwards to the apex of the ischiorectal fossa, or even through the levators. Alternatively supralevator induration may arise from upward extension from an intersphincteric track. Digital examination cannot distinguish between these two possibilities.

Examination Under Anesthesia

Anal examination should also be routinely carried out under general anesthetic immediately before proceeding with surgery. This may identify features not easy to determine with the patient awake. Examination in this way by the experienced surgeon is about 85% accurate when compared with the surgical findings following dissection of the fistula.[81] Probes should rarely be used in the awake patient.

Downward retraction of the dentate line helps expose concealed openings,[82] while retraction away from the anticipated site of an internal opening may reveal dimpling at the site of inflammatory tethering. Massage may release a bead of pus. Various agents injected along the track via the external opening have been used to locate the internal opening. These include saline,[83] hydrogen peroxide,[84] and dyes such as methylene blue and indigo carmine.[53,82] Although dyes may demonstrate both track and internal opening, they cause staining of the tissue obscuring the track if the internal opening is initially missed or if the track is transected.[85] In most cases with an anterior external opening, the internal opening will be located at the same circumferential point.

Careful probing can delineate primary and secondary tracks. If the internal and external openings are easily detected but the probe cannot easily traverse the path of the track, there may be

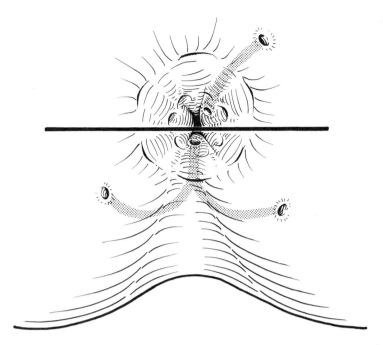

Figure 14-12. Diagram illustrating Goodsall's rule. The likely position of the internal opening of a fistula may be determined by the site of the external opening in relation to the (imaginary) transverse anal line.

a high extension. In this circumstance, a probe passed via each opening may then delineate the primary track. Persistence of granulation tissue after curettage indicates a continuing track.[85]

Assessment of a Difficult Fistula

Previous surgery leads to scarring and deformity and may result in unusual primary tracks, making assessment extremely difficult. Extensive track formation resulting from severe acute spsis will often result in a similar situation. Until recently imaging techniques had proved disappointing.

Fistulography

The accuracy and usefulness of fistulography has been variously reported. Kuypers[86] showed that preoperative fistulography correctly identified a patent internal opening in only 25% of cases, compared with a success rate for clinical explanation of 98% in detecting the site of the obliterated or patent opening. In a retrospective study from the same unit, comparing fistulographic and operative findings in 25 patients, Kuijpers and Schulpen[87] reported that the internal opening into the anal canal was accurately identified by fistulography in only 24% of cases and/or opening into the rectum in only 17%. High extensions were missed by fistulography in 44% of cases where they existed. Perhaps of more concern was a false-positive rate of 11% for high extensions that could not be demonstrated operatively. False rectal openings and high extensions were suggested in 12%.

Fistulography may be uncomfortable, and the introduction of radio-opaque contrast medium under high pressure (in order to demonstrate all tracks) risks dissemination of sepsis.[88]

Weisman et al.[89] found fistulography useful, revealing unsuspected pathology or altering surgical management in 48% of cases, and recommended it in patients with recurrent sepsis where perineal anatomy had been distorted by sepsis or surgery. Radio-opaque markers placed at either end of the anal canal used in conjunction with fistulography may assist interpretation.[90]

Fistulography is the essential investigation when an extrasphincteric fistula is suspected. Such cases are rare, but should be suspected where an external opening is present in the perineum in the presence of a completely normal anal canal. A sinogram using a water-soluble contrast medium may show a communication with the rectum, or the sigmoid, or the small bowel affected by primary pathology such as carcinoma, diverticular disease, or Crohn's disease.

CT Scanning

Computed tomography (CT) has also proved disappointing. The exact site of pathology in relation to the levators on axial CT scans can only be inferred indirectly through the relation of any abnormality to the piriformis and coccygeus muscles. The levators are not well identified,[91] and sphincter resolution is poor. Coronal imaging is rarely possible and there are many pitfalls in interpretation of the images.[92] CT also involves ionizing radiation and the need for contrast media.

Ultrasound

The endorectal probe was modified by Bartram for use in the anal canal by encasing the 7-MHz rotating tip with a hard sonolucent cone. The results in the evaluation of intersphincteric

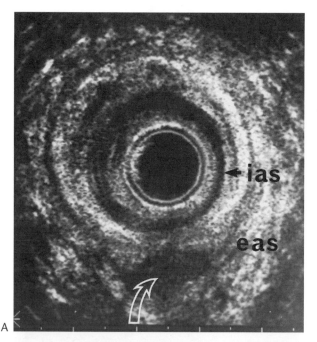

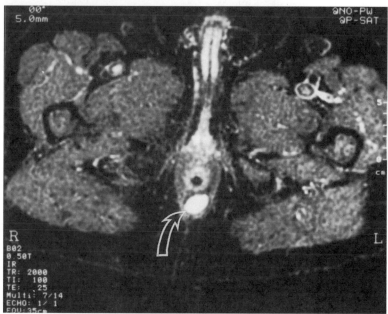

Figure 14-13. (**A**) Anal endosonographic image of a posterior intersphincteric abscess (arrow) lying between the internal (ias) and external (eas) anal sphincter; (**B**) The same pathology demonstrated by MRI using STIR sequencing. Anterior is to the top. (From Phillips and Lunniss,[146] with permission.)

and trans-sphincteric tracks were initially promising (Fig. 14-13).[93]

Unfortunately the limited focal range of the probe makes evaluation of the tissues lateral to or above the sphincters difficult to assess, in the very areas that difficulty in clinical assessment is encountered. Ultrasound probes of greater focal length might overcome this problem but this will be at the expense of reduced resolution of the sphincters themselves. Supralevator sepsis is not well seen owing to the difficulty in establishing

acoustic contact, but may be more accurately determined by using a rectal balloon attachment over the rigid endoprobe.

Although improvements in ultrasound will occur, to date the technique has not been shown to be any more accurate than digital examination. In a prospective comparison of ultrasound with digital examination in 36 patients, Seow Choen et al.[81] found the latter to be slightly more accurate in identifying the internal opening and much more so in detecting secondary track formation. Sepsis and scarring can confuse assessment in patients who have undergone previous surgery.[94] Although ultrasound is cheap and gives excellent images of the sphincters, its low positive predictive value in fistula-in-ano renders it of little value.[94]

Tio et al.[88] have assessed patients with perianal Crohn's disease by a combination of flexible and rigid nonoptical echoprobes, and by flexible echoendoscopy. Above the anal sphincters, reasonable images are obtained provided acoustic contact is established either by filling the rectal lumen with water, or by using a water-filled balloon placed around the probe. In another study, transrectal ultrasound has been shown to be superior to CT in determining the presence of abscesses and fistulae in patients with perianal Crohn's disease.[95]

Magnetic Resonance Imaging

The advantages of magnetic resonance imaging (MRI), which include lack of ionizing radiation, the ability to image in any plane, and the high soft-tissue resolution, became apparent in initial studies in patients with fistulae in Crohn's disease.[96,97] These studies were small, however, and did not compare results of imaging with the operative findings. The incorporation of "STIR" sequencing to highlight the presence of pus and granulation tissue without the need for any contrast medium (Fig. 14-14)[41] meant for the first time that there was the real possibility of an imaging technique useful in the assessment of difficult fistulae. A prospective study involving 35 patients comparing MRI scan interpretations with the operative findings independently documented by the surgeon[94] showed MRI to be as accurate. In five cases, pathology that was missed at operation and that was the cause of failure to heal had been demonstrated by MRI. In two cases the primary track was incorrectly assessed at surgery, and in 3 cases secondary extensions were missed.

The technique therefore gives the most accurate assessment possible at present. Owing to its expense, it should be reserved for difficult cases, but in these it is likely to be cost effective. The accuracy of MRI also means that we now have a method of monitoring fistula healing by nonsurgical methods, as well as being able to refute or confirm the presence of sepsis in patients with symptoms where clinical examination is unrevealing.

CONTINENCE AFTER FISTULA SURGERY

Fistula surgery aims to cure the fistula while maintaining continence. Continence may be regarded as a balance between rectal pressure and the power of the sphincters to withstand this. It also depends on intact sensory feedback. Most of the time the anus is closed by the involuntary action of the internal sphincter. At times stool descends to the sensitive transitional zone of the upper anal canal, where it is sampled[98–100] and a distinction made between solid matter and flatus.[100,101] The external sphincter then contracts and returns the stool to the rectum to await defecation at a socially convenient time. Thus perfect continence may theoretically be achieved through an intact internal sphincter and distensible compliant mucosa leading to a closed anus at rest, enough external sphincter to overcome rises in intrarectal pressure, and good sensation.

Milligan and Morgan[74] stressed the importance of the anorectal ring in fistula surgery: "If this ring be cut, loss of control surely results, yet as long as the narrowest complete ring of muscle remains, control is preserved. All the anal sphincter muscles below this ring may be divided in any manner without harmful loss of control." Most clinicians today might doubt the last sentence, but all would agree that complete division of the puborectalis sling will result in total incontinence to all rectal

Figure 14-14. Conventional axial MRI scan of the same patient as in Figure 14-13 at the same level of the perineum. Although T1-weighted spin echo sequences provide excellent soft tissue resolution, inflammatory changes are difficult to see. On the fat suppressing STIR sequence, however (**B**), a fistula track (arrow) is easily seen, running from the intersphincteric space in the posterior midline across the external sphincter to enter the fat of the left ischiorectal fossa. (From Phillips and Lunniss,[146] with permission.)

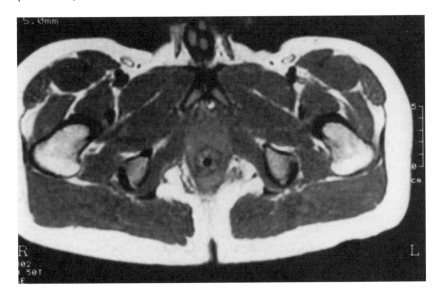

contents. Below this level the term incontinence becomes relative, dependent more upon the perception of the patient than measurements in the physiology laboratory. It is the case that the higher the fistula the greater the possibility of impaired function after fistulotomy.[102] Fistulotomy, however, is a sure way to cure a fistula, whereas the many sphincter-conserving operations have high failure rates.

We should be cautious when interpreting published results of function after fistula surgery because of the following factors:

1. The complexity of fisulae reported may be markedly different.
2. Classification of fistulae may be variable.
3. Follow-up may be inadequate.
4. Reports of successes may be preferred to the reporting of failures (publication bias).
5. Fistula variability and individual surgeon preference and skill make randomized trials practically impossible.

Traditionally, surgeons have attempted to preserve the external anal sphincter while being prepared to sacrifice the internal sphincter. Parks[1] advocated internal sphincterectomy in order to eradicate the presumed etiologic source lying in a diseased anal gland in the intersphincteric space. Most surgeons today divide the internal sphincter rather than excise it, but the concept of removing the intersphincteric source remains popular.

What, then, are the consequences of sphincter division in fistula surgery? There are no standard questionnaires to assess continence.[103] Those that exist tend to focus on gross changes and do not consider the finer aspects of continence, including minor disturbances that occur in a high proportion of patients after anal surgery for hemorrhoids[99] and fissure.[104] Functional disturbances short of actual fecal incontinence are generally labeled as "minor," although they may be distressing to the patient. The aim of fistula surgery is to cure the lesion with no functional disturbance. This ideal cannot be achieved in all cases, and a balance must be struck between effectiveness of cure and functional disturbance. Preservation of the sphincter, using, for example, a seton technique has a higher incidence of failure to cure compared with laying open. The gain is better function in those in whom the treatment is successful.

For example, Thomson and Ross[105] reported 34 patients with high trans-sphincteric fistulae managed with a loose seton. The treatment was successful in 18 cases (57%) and unsuccessful in 16 (46%). This latter group underwent subsequent division of the external sphincter. Continence was normal in 15 (83%) of those successfully treated without external sphincter division and in 5 (32%) in the unsuccessful group, who needed external sphincter division. Of the 16 patients in whom the external sphincter was divided, 9 reported some degree of incontinence to formed stool. In another study in which 25 patients were successfully treated by the loose seton technique, normal continence was however less frequent, occurring in 16 cases (64%).[106] Interestingly, Sainio[26] found the highest incidence of incontinence where a high intersphincteric track had been laid open (and in whom the external sphincter had not been divided).

In order to obtain an accurate comparison of continence before and after surgery, a prospective study was conducted in 37 patients successfully treated for either an intersphincteric (15 patients) or trans-sphincteric (22 patients) fistula. Patients

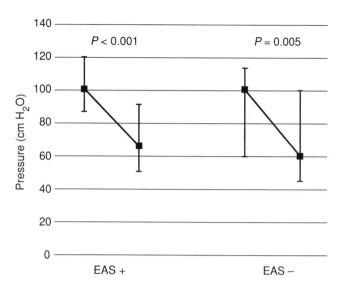

Figure 14-15. Diagram showing the pre- and postoperative maximum resting pressures (cm H_2O), median, interquartile range) in 22 patients with inter- and trans-sphincteric fistulae in whom the internal sphincter was divided but the external sphincter preserved (EAS +), and in 15 patients with trans-sphincteric fistulae in whom both internal and external sphincters were divided (EAS −). In both groups, surgery led to a significant reduction in maximum resting pressure, but there was no difference between the two groups. (From Phillips and Lunniss,[146] with permission.)

were assessed by physical and physiologic examination.[107] They were divided into two groups, those having internal sphincter division only and those who had division of internal and external sphincters. They were compared with a group of control patients who had had anal surgery without any sphincter division.

Controls showed no change in continence or anal pressures. As might be expected, both test groups had a similar fall in postoperative resting pressure (Fig. 14-15) and only those having external sphincter division had a significant fall postoperatively in squeeze pressure (Fig. 14-16). A disturbance of continence occurred in 53% and 50% of the two test groups and was not related to division of the external sphincter. Moreover the severity of disturbance was no different in the two groups, being evidently more related to loss of internal sphincter function and to mucosal scarring than to loss of external sphincter function.

This study demonstrated the importance of all the sphincter components and indicated that total sphincter conservation should ideally be the best form of treatment. Patients, however, want to be rid of the symptoms due to recurring anal sepsis, and many are prepared to accept a minor reduction in continence to achieve this. Nevertheless, techniques are available to eradicate the fistula without any sphincter division. The outcome of these procedures in achieving cure will be compared with laying open operations in the next section.

TREATMENT

Principles

The treatment is surgical with the aim of abolishing the primary track and draining any secondary tracks. The surgical anatomy should be known to the surgeon preoperatively in most cases,

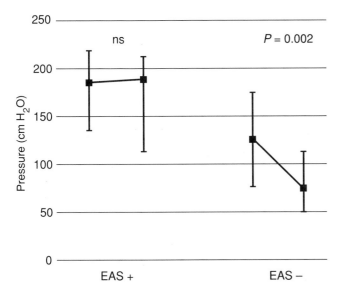

Figure 14-16. The pre- and postoperative maximum squeeze pressures (cm H_2O, median, interquartile range) in patients undergoing fistula surgery in whom the external sphincter was either preserved (EAS +) or divided (EAS −). Division of the external sphincter led to a significant reduction in squeeze pressures, but this was not associated with any greater detriment to continence than internal sphincter and anoderm division alone. (From Phillips and Lunniss,[146] with permission.)

but in some this will only become clear during the dissection. Accurate preoperative assessment, already outlined, is essential.

Most fistula operations are simple and can be performed without special preparation. Low fistulae can be operated upon under local anesthetic but more complicated ones require regional or general anesthesia. Surgical approaches to preserve the sphincters (advancement flap, "core-out" fistulectomy, and other approaches) require bowel preparation and perioperative antibiotics. The operation can be done with the patient in the lithotomy position or the prone jackknife position. A fistula operation sheet is useful in complex cases (Fig. 14-17) as the most accurate means of recording the surgical anatomy.

In general, sphincter-preserving operations should not be done in the presence of acute sepsis or when the surgical anatomy is complex with extensive secondary tracks. Such complexity should be simplified by an initial procedure to drain all secondary tracks, leaving a loose seton through the primary track. A second-stage operation can then be carried out 2 to 3 months later after the acute sepsis has resolved. The simple primary track can then be dealt with.

Fistulotomy

Fistulotomy is the classic operation for anal fistulae. Several instruments unearthed at Pompeii destroyed by the great eruption of Vesuvius in AD 79 were probably used for laying open anal fistula.[10] John of Arderne issued his treatise on the cure of fistula-in-ano in 1376, gaining his experience as a military surgeon in France during the earlier part of the Hundred Years War.[108,109]

The fistula was defined with a probe, ligature, and grooved director, and then the track was divided cleanly along its whole length in a single movement, while the opposite wall of the anorectum was protected with a spoon-shaped shield passed transanally.[108]

Technique

Fistulotomy is suitable for most straightforward fistulae. An appropriately shaped fistula probe is passed via the external opening along the length of the primary track (Fig. 14-18A) to emerge through the internal opening. The track is then laid open (Fig. 14-18B). Granulation tissue is curetted away and sent for histologic examination (Fig. 14-18C). Any adherent granulations indicating a possible secondary extension are carefully looked for. The wound is then trimmed (Fig. 14-18D) and in simple cases marsupialized (Fig. 14-18E). Any secondary extensions need full and adequate drainage, either by direct widening of the wound or by the use of drains.[110,111]

In certain types of fistulae fistulotomy should not be used, at least as the first intervention. These include all high trans-sphincteric tracks, anterior trans-sphincteric fistulae in females, and most trans-sphincteric fistulae in Crohn's disease. In these there is a high chance of incontinence following simple laying open. It is more prudent to place a seton through the primary track with drainage of secondary tracks and to reassess some weeks later.

Fistulectomy

In fistulectomy the track is excised rather than laid open. This is best done using the diathermy cautery to minimize bleeding and usually allows an excellent definition of the surgical anatomy of the fistula.[112] False tracks caused by injudicious probing are avoided, and granulation tissue leading from the primary to any secondary track is usually obvious. Healing after fistulectomy is slower than after fistulotomy, as demonstrated by Kronborg[113] in a randomized trial. Fistulectomy is often used as part of a sphincter-preserving technique (discussed later). Otherwise it can be useful in any case where the relation of the primary and secondary tracks to the anal sphincter mechanism is uncertain, as it supplies a clearer demonstration of anatomy. Such an approach is well worth adopting in cases where the anatomy has not been defined preoperatively, because it keeps open the options for a sphincter-preserving technique should the dissection show such an approach to be indicated.

Setons

The term *seton* is derived from the latin word *seta*, meaning a bristle. It is used in fistula surgery in various ways. Setons may be classified as loose, tight, or chemical according to their different properties and modes of action.

The Loose Seton

A seton thread, loosely tied, may be used to mark a fistula track when its exact position and level in relation to the external sphincter is unclear at the time of surgery. Scarring from previous surgery or the degree of relaxation of the external sphincter under anesthesia can make it impossible to determine the level

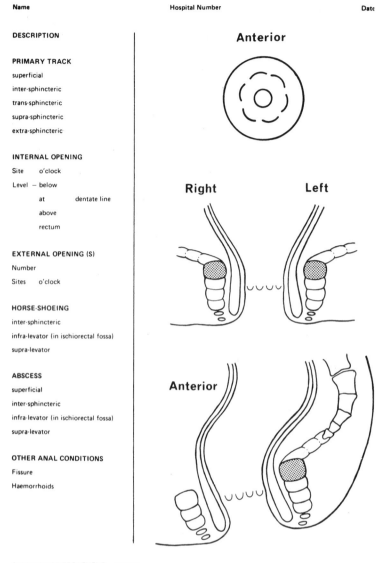

Name   Hospital Number   Date

DESCRIPTION

PRIMARY TRACK

superficial

inter-sphincteric

trans-sphincteric

supra-sphincteric

extra-sphincteric

INTERNAL OPENING

Site   o'clock

Level   – below

          at   dentate line

          above

          rectum

EXTERNAL OPENING (S)

Number

Sites   o'clock

HORSE-SHOEING

inter-sphincteric

infra-levator (in ischiorectal fossa)

supra-levator

ABSCESS

superficial

inter-sphincteric

infra-levator (in ischiorectal fossa)

supra-levator

OTHER ANAL CONDITIONS

Fissure

Haemorrhoids

Anterior

Right   **Left**

Anterior

SUMMARY OF TREATMENT – see over

Figure 14-17.   The St. Mark's Hospital fistula operation sheet.

of the track. In such circumstances it is prudent to insert a seton and to determine the proportion of muscle above and below the track when the patient is awake and with the track palpably delineated by the seton. Similarly, a loosely tied seton can facilitate drainage of acute sepsis, allow acute inflammation to subside, and permit safer subsequent fistula surgery.

A seton may be part of a surgical strategy aimed to preserve sphincter muscle by avoiding fistulotomy, and is therefore chiefly applicable to a trans-sphincteric fistula. It can be used in three ways: to preserve the entire external sphincter, to preserve the upper half of the voluntary muscle, or as part of a staged fistulotomy to reduce the degree of retraction of sphincter following division of large amounts of muscle. It has been suggested that a loose seton promotes fibrosis, but most modern seton materials are relatively inert, and it is hard to imagine how a thread in the fistula lumen might usefully increase the

degree of fibrosis already present around a chronic fistula track. Furthermore, the incidence of incontinence seen after division of external sphincter following failure of the loose seton method[102] demonstrates that any fibrosis that might result from the presence of the seton is insufficient to protect against incontinence.

Technique

A circumferential incision centered around the external opening is made outside the sphincter complex. The wound is deepened through the ischiorectal fossa, and any secondary tracks and chronic abscess cavities are laid open. The primary track across the external anal sphincter is then identified and a seton is passed through it and loosely tied. Various materials are suitable, including a braided or monofilament nonabsorbable suture,

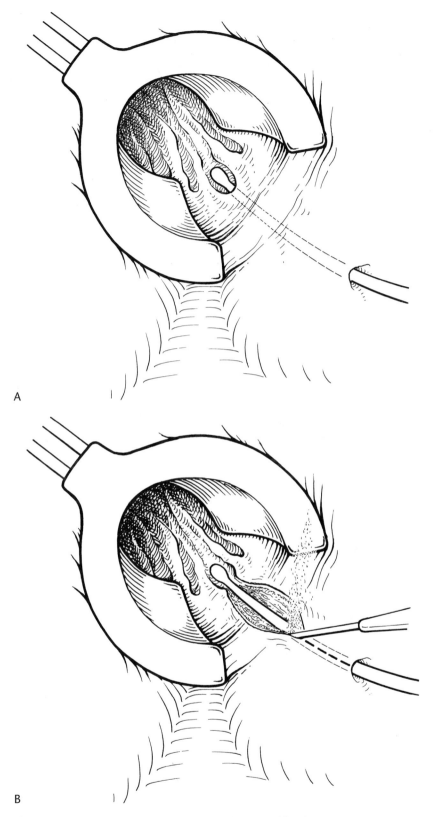

A

B

Figure 14-18. Diagram illustrating the technique of fistulotomy (**A & B**) incorporating marsupialization (**D & E**) (*Figure continues.*)

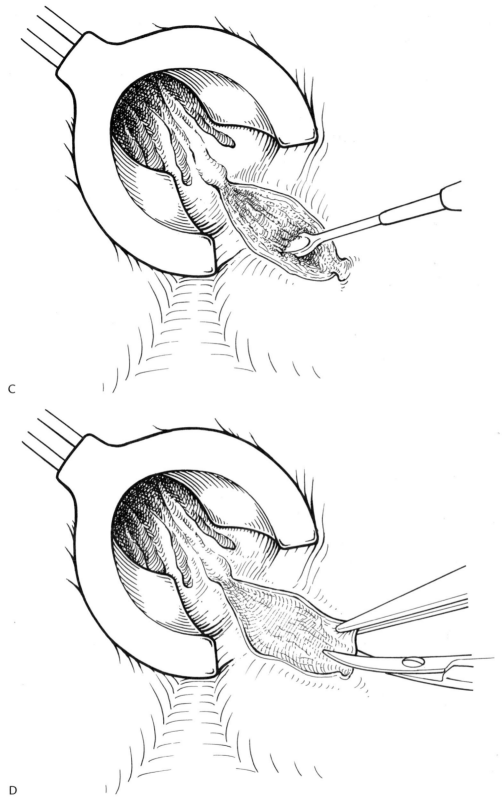

C

D

Figure 14-18 *(continued).*

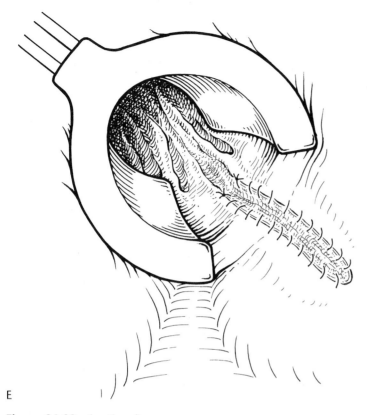

E

Figure 14-18   *(continued).*

or silastic. A malleable probe with an eye at its tip or a bodkin are useful instruments to draw the seton through the track, although Lockhart-Mummery probes are so designed that a thread can be negotiated along its groove. The wound is dressed over the subsequent weeks, when secondary tracks should gradually heal. Various options are then available, described in the next sections.

Staged Fistulotomy

Staged fistulotomy is the simplest option, but should be used only if there appears to be sufficient muscle above the level of the seton. After an interval of a few weeks, the primary track is laid open by division of muscle within the seton. At the same time the wound should be shaped if necessary to allow any residual secondary tracks to heal. Ramanujan et al.[114] reported a series of 45 patients with suprasphincteric fistulae in whom the first stage involved laying open the puborectalis while preserving the distal sphincter within a seton. This was divided about 2 months later. There was 1 recurrence, and 1 patient only suffered any disturbance of continence (to flatus). Others have preserved the upper sphincter within a seton in the first stage (divided at a later stage) while laying open the lower portion. Kuypers[115] described this technique in 10 patients with trans-sphincteric fistulae with supralevator extensions opening into the rectum. The seton-enclosed muscle was divided 3 months after the first stage; there were no recurrences, 1 patient was incontinent, and 6 reported minor soiling.

Parks and Stitz[116] reported a series of 80 patients with trans-

and suprasphincteric fistulae, in whom the lower one-third to one-half of the sphincter was divided at the first stage, with placement of a seton around the primary track crossing the upper sphincter. The second stage was carried out a few months later. Either the seton was removed if all extensions had healed or the muscle enclosed by the seton was divided in cases with a persisting high track or cavity. Thirty (38%) of patients required division to achieve healing; unfortunately the functional results were not described in this report.

Loose Seton Used Curatively

Technique. Secondary tracks and extensions outside the sphincters are widely laid open and the internal sphincter is divided to the level of the internal opening (or higher if a cephalad intersphincteric extension exists). In some cases with a high posterior trans-sphincteric track, its identification across the sphincter can only be made by dividing the anococcygeal ligaments. This maneuver dislocates the posterior sphincter attachments but allows access to the deep postanal space.[102] The seton is passed along the primary track across the external sphincter and then tied loosely (Fig. 14-19). Postoperatively the wounds are managed by daily dressing rather than by tight packing; irrigation of the wound helps keep it clean and occasional digitation may be necessary. After 7 to 10 days, under general anesthesia, the wounds are carefully examined to ensure that all tracks had been dealt with and that healing is progressing satisfactorily. The seton is left in situ for 2 to 3 months. If there is evidence of good healing it is removed.

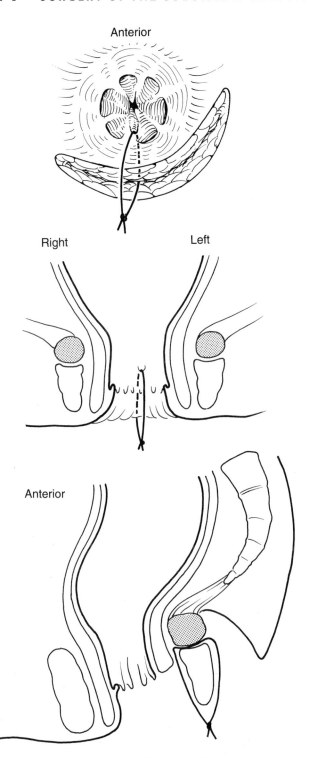

Anterior

Right   Left

Anterior

Figure 14-19. The operative details of a high posterior trans-sphincteric fistula with ischiorectal horseshoe extension treated by the loose seton technique. The internal sphincter has been divided to the level of the internal opening, and a loose seton passed along the primary track across the denuded external sphincter. The extensions in the ischiorectal fossae have been widely laid open. (Adapted from Phillips and Lunniss,[146] with permission.)

Results. In a series of 34 consecutive patients with trans-sphincteric fistulae[105] healing of the fistula without recourse to external sphincter division occurred in 16 (44%) cases. The functional outcome was better when the external sphincter was preserved. A later report achieved a success rate of 67% in 24 patients.[102] Kennedy and Zegarra[106] similarly used a loose silk seton to treat 32 patients with high trans-sphincteric and supra-sphincteric anal fistulae, reporting a success rate of 78%, higher with anterior (88%) than posterior (66%) fistulae.

Fistulectomy With Closure of Internal Opening

The residual primary track is cored out and the internal opening closed either by an advancement flap or by direct suture (described later).

Long-Standing Loose Seton

In certain cases (for example selected patients with a high fistula associated with Crohn's disease) it may be prudent to leave the seton indefinitely. This may be successful in achieving long-standing relief of symptoms of recurrent abscess formation.

The Tight Seton

A tight or cutting seton achieves a staged fistulotomy by slow division of the muscle below the track. The method was described by Hippocrates, who used a horse hair,[117] and has its present-day advocates mainly in the French school of proctologists.

Technique

Goldberg has recommended using a tight seton whenever more than 30% of the sphincter lies below the level of the primary track, or where local sepsis or fibrosis preclude an advancement flap.[118] The portion of the track outside the sphincters is opened or drained with Penrose drains,[119,120] and the anoderm and perianal skin covering the sphincter lying below the primary track are incised. The intersphincteric space is drained by internal sphincterotomy, which is extended proximally as necessary to drain any cephalad intersphincteric extension. The seton is then placed. When suppuration has resolved, usually at 3 weeks postoperatively, the seton is tightened at two weekly intervals using a silk tie or Barron band until it has cut through the muscle. An alternative is to use an elastic seton strapped to the thigh to maintain tension.

Results

Goldberg used a cutting seton in 13 patients with trans-sphincteric fistulae treated over a 5-year period. The average time for the seton to cut through was 16 weeks (range, 8 to 36 weeks). There were no recurrences at a median follow-up of 24 months (range, 4 to 60 months). There was however a relatively high incidence of functional morbidity, major in 1 patient and minor in a further 7 patients (54%) with incontinence of flatus or episodic loss of liquid stool.[118]

It seems that if the seton is tightened too quickly incontinence is more likely. Christensen et al.[121] tightened the seton every second day in a series of 24 patients with high trans-sphincteric fistulae. Fifteen (62%) patients reported some degree of incontinence, including 7 (29%) who wore a pad constantly. These high rates of disturbance of continence may however have been a reflection of the complex type of fistula treated rather than a defect of the method employed.

Misra and Kapur[122] reported the outpatient treatment of 56 anal fistulae using a braided stainless steel tight seton, tightened weekly, with pain used as an indicator of too much tension. Two recurrences were successfully treated by rewiring. No patient reported any functional disturbances, but 3 patients expressed a desire for some form of anesthesia while the wire was being tightened. All but 8 patients had fistulae classified as simple (that is, low trans-sphincteric, intersphincteric, or superficial), but the avoidance of inpatient treatment, time off work, and a large wound were advantages.

The Chemical Seton

In India the Kshara sutra, chemical seton technique has been used for centuries. It was probably first described by Sushruta, a surgeon who lived around 800 BC.

Technique

A specially prepared thread is passed through the fistula and changed weekly. Slow division of the track is achieved, about 1 cm of track every 6 days,[123,124] probably because of the caustic nature of the thread (pH 9.5). The herbally prepared thread also has antibacterial and anti-inflammatory properties.

Results

A prospective randomized trial involving 502 patients[125] showed this outpatient treatment to have comparable results to fistulotomy (incontinence rate 5 vs. 9%; recurrence rate at 1 year 4 vs. 11%), but with a longer healing time (8 vs. 4 weeks). Another series of 80 patients from Columbo reported no recurrences.[126] It would appear that the method can work only if the track is relatively straight and if there are no associated secondary tracks.

TECHNIQUES TO CLOSE THE INTERNAL OPENING

Advancement Flaps

Advancement flaps were first proposed by Noble[127] to repair rectovaginal fistulae. Elting described their use in managing anal fistulae 10 years later.[128] He stated two principles for their use, including the separation of the track from the anal lumen and the closure of the internal opening. The modern technique has added the creation of a flap of adequate vascularity and its anastomosis to the anoderm well distal to the internal opening.[129–133] Modifications include the use of flaps of different thickness, different incisions, curved or rhomboid, and the importance or otherwise of closing the external defect.[134]

Technique

Most surgeons would agree that an advancement flap should not be attempted in the presence of active sepsis. Furthermore the track should ideally be direct from internal to external open-

ing. Adequate access to the anal canal is essential. If there is much induration, the operation may not be possible. An Eisenhammer or Fansler retractor gives excellent exposure. A fistulectomy from external to internal opening is carried out. The anal retractor is then inserted and a flap of the lower rectum including mucosa and the underlying circular muscle is raised (Fig. 14-20). The distal portion of the flap including the internal opening is excised and the flap is advanced distally and sutured at a level below the internal opening. Fine PDS sutures are satisfactory. The external wound is then either left open or closed depending on the prejudice of the surgeon.

Results

Excellent results have been reported in several studies. Cure rates have ranged from between 90% and 100% with little functional disturbance. Information regarding the type of fistula has been incomplete in some reports,[135] making comparison of series impossible. These authors, however, had a remarkably high success rate of over 90% in a large series of patients. Kodner et al.[136] reported a 10-year experience of 107 patients, 24 of whom had Crohn's disease. The overall initial success rate was 84%. This rose to 94% with revisional surgery in 9 initial failures, including 4 patients who underwent successful repeat flap procedures. Finan[134] achieved healing in 10 of 11 patients with infralevator trans-sphincteric fistulae and provided prospective physiologic data to confirm the functional preservation of the sphincter and anoderm sensation. Despite these reported successes many surgeons still find the technique has a significant failure rate, but the problems encountered are not reported in the literature. Certainly there is a concern about further compromising the internal sphincter if the technique does fail.

Fistulectomy and Repair

Technique

Fistulectomy is a variant employing the same surgical principles. Instead of a flap, the internal opening is closed by direct suture. The external opening is circumcised using electrocoagulation and the primary track is dissected from the surrounding tissues. Initially the ischiorectal fat is encountered followed by the external and then the internal sphincter. Having completed the fistulectomy, the internal opening is closed by sutures through the mucosa and internal sphincter. The remaining external wound is either left open or closed according to the practice of the surgeon.

Results

Lewis[137] treated 32 high trans-sphincteric or suprasphincteric fistulae over a 20-year period by this technique; in 4 cases a temporary colostomy was performed, and there have been 3 recurrences to date.

Fistulotomy and Repair

Technique

The fistula is laid open and then immediately repaired with primary closure of the wound. This has been reported either as a one-[138] or two-staged[139] procedure. In the staged approach

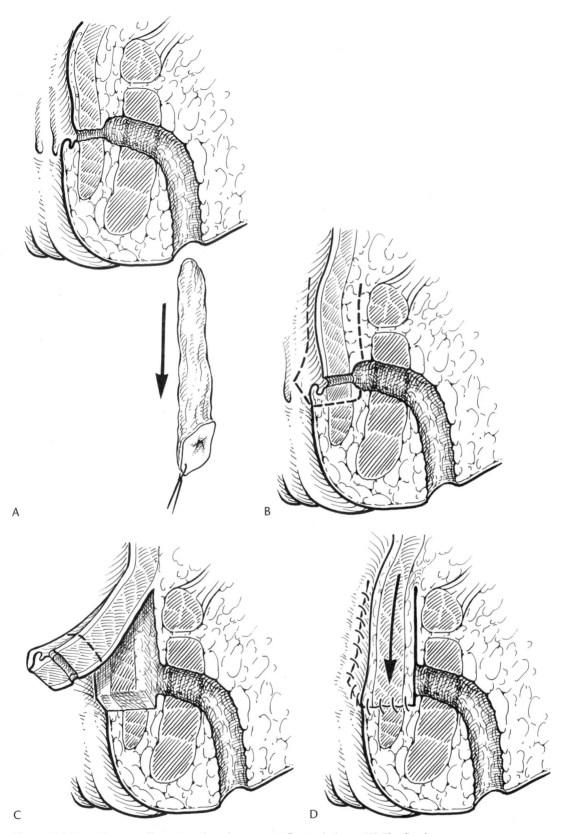

Figure 14-20.   Diagrams illustrating the advancement flap technique. (**A**) The fistula track is excised from the external opening to the intersphincteric plane. (**B**) The flap, incorporating the internal opening is raised, along with full-thickness internal sphincter. (**C**) The raised flap, with line marking level of division to excise the internal opening. (**D**) The advancement flap sutured to a site distal to the excised internal opening. (Adapted from Phillips and Lunniss,[146] with permission.)

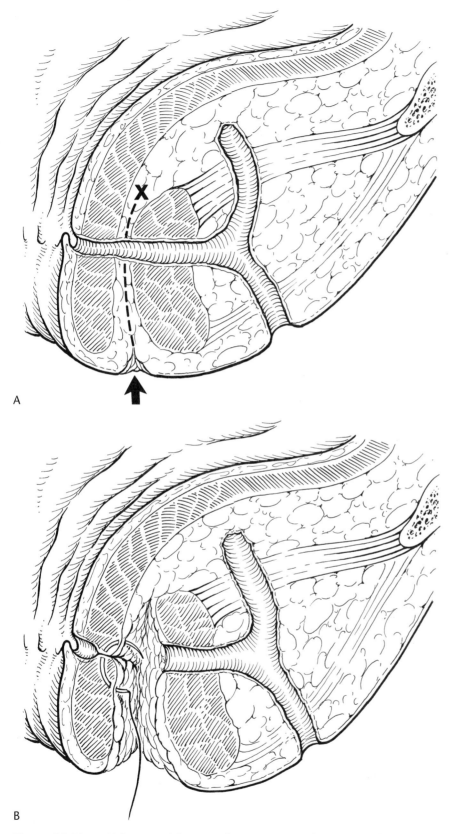

Figure 14-21. Initial stages of the intersphincteric approach to a transsphincteric fistula with blind supralevator pararectal extension. (**A**) A curvilinear incision is made over the intersphincteric groove between the external opening and the anus; the incision is deepened in the intersphincteric space (arrowed) and continued for 1 to 2 cm beyond the primary track (x marks the cephalad limit of the dissection). (**B**)

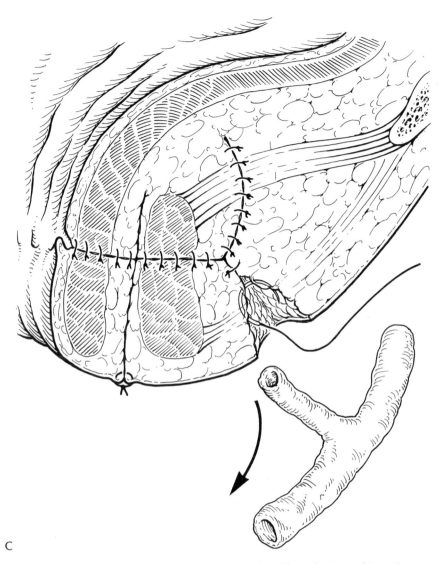

C

Figure 14-21 *(continued)*. The internal opening is closed from the intersphincteric space with an absorbable suture followed by fistulectomy and primary wound closure (**C**).

the trans-sphincteric track is cored out until the intersphincteric space is reached. The external sphincter is then divided and repaired immediately to create an intersphincteric fistula. Following healing of the wound, the transposed track, now lying intersphincterically, is laid open at a second stage. It is hard to see how the transposed fistula track maintains its blood supply, and the technique is rarely used.

Results

Parkash et al.[138] reported a series of 120 patients. Wound healing occurred at 2 weeks in 106 cases (88%). Only 5 patients (4%) developed recurrence. It is noteworthy, however, that all but two of the fistulae were intersphincteric or low trans-sphincteric in type, cases therefore in which functional disturbance after simple fistulotomy would be uncommon. Sood[140] achieved similar results in 136 patients with low fistulae.

Mann and Clifton[139] described 5 cases only. All had good results with no recurrence and satisfactory function. The technique requires two operations, however, and has not become generally popular owing to its complexity.

Kupferberg et al.[141] have advocated the use of gentamicin beads inserted into the wound after fistulectomy. They described 5 patients with a high fistula with no recurrence at 2 years.

The Intersphincteric Approach

Technique

The intersphincteric approach is a variant on fistulectomy with closure in which the track is arrived at via an intersphincteric dissection. A circumferential (Fig. 14-21A) incision is made and the intersphincteric space is entered (Fig. 14-21B). The fistula track is encountered and disconnected from the internal opening, which is then closed (Fig. 14-21C). Fistulectomy with primary closure of the external wound is then performed (Fig. 14-21D).

Results

Matos et al.[142] described 13 patients, all with complex fistulae, 5 of whom had inflammatory bowel disease. Sphincter preservation with wound healing and no functional disturbance was achieved in 7 (46%) cases. In 2 further patients the internal sphincter had to be laid open at a second stage to achieve cure, and in 4 the fistula ultimately required conventional laying open to achieve healing. As might be expected, functional disturbance correlated with the amount of sphincter finally divided.

Fibrin Glue

Two centers have reported the successful use of fibrin glue in sealing off fistula tracks in small numbers of patients.[143,144] Both stressed the importance of thorough curettage to remove as much granulation tissue and debris as possible, as well as generous antibiotic administration, either parenterally or along the fistula track itself.

APPROACH TO A DIFFICULT FISTULA

Fistulae may be difficult to treat for two main reasons. First, they may be complex, with secondary track formation or crossing the sphincters at a high level. Second, they may recur despite adequate management at the first attempt.[145] An algorithm suggesting a management plan is shown in Figure 14-22. Complexity due to secondary tracks can usually be reduced by drainage of these. Only later should the primary track be dealt with. Preoperative physiologic assessment comes a poor second to careful clinical assessment but may help identify patients at risk of impaired continence after fistulotomy. If the primary track is high, then an appropriate sphincter-preserving procedure should initially be undertaken; rarely a temporary diverting stoma will be needed.

Failure of sphincter-preserving methods and persistent symptoms will then make laying open or a long-term loose seton the only choices. After extensive fistulotomy some patients are able to lead normal lives with the narrowest of (often fibrotic) anorectal rings,[74] but others may need sphincter repair. MRI scanning is a useful way of making sure that there is no covert pathology before embarking on repair. Of the 20 patients over a 3-year period at St. Mark's Hospital who underwent sphincteroplasty for incontinence after previous surgery for idiopathic fistulae, a good outcome (Parks' grades 1 or 2 continence scores) was obtained in 13 (65%) (Engel et al., unpublished observations).

It is important to consider the possibility of an extrasphincteric fistula when a high "blind" track is encountered, arising from pelvic or abdominal disease or from a presacral dermoid cyst (Fig. 14-23). Failure to consider such a cause leads to delay in imaging by fistulography, barium studies, or MRI and is a major reason for delayed diagnosis. If a track is truly high and blind, this might be because the internal opening has closed, or that surgery has dealt with the primary track and recurrence is because of an overlooked secondary extension.[145] In such cases the component of the track outside the sphincters should

Figure 14-22. Algorithm for a patient with a difficult fistula. (From Phillips and Lunniss,[146] with permission.)

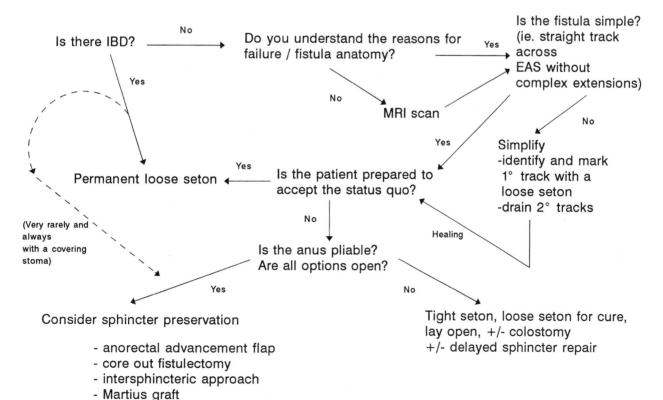

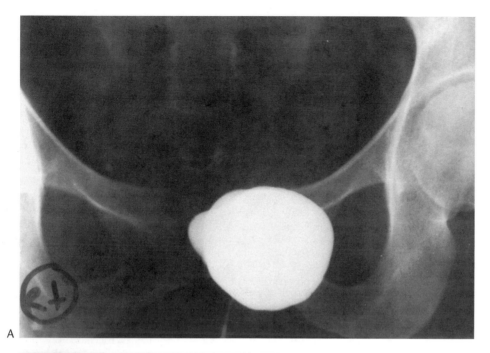

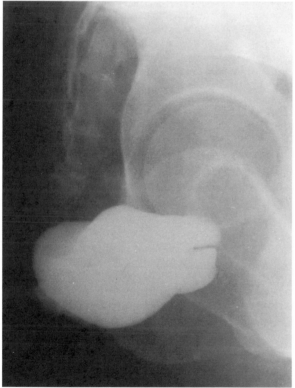

Figure 14-23. Sinogram demonstrating a postrectal dermoid cyst. (**A**) Anteroposterior view. (**B**) Lateral view. (From Phillips and Lunniss,[146] with permission.)

be laid open and curetted; as the resulting wound may be large, it is often wise to make a circular rather than a radial incision to avoid sphincter damage. Following granulation tissue with curette and probe should be carried out carefully to avoid false tracks. If the track peters out before reaching the intersphincteric space, it is safest to stop and come back another day. If the track enters the intersphincteric space but no internal opening can be identified, it is reasonable to assume that the opening

has healed or is extremely small; internal sphincterotomy is then justified to obviate recurrence.

CONCLUSION

Most fistulae are simple and can be cured by fistulotomy. The more difficult fistulae from time to time will require the application of more sophisticated techniques of imaging, such as MRI, and many of the alternative surgical techniques described in this chapter.

Almost all fistulae can be cured in expert hands. The residual functional defect is often slight and is seen by many patients to be a fair price to pay to be rid of persisting, painful, and debilitating bouts of anal sepsis.

REFERENCES

1. Parks AG (1961) The pathogenesis and treatment of fistula-in-ano. Br Med J 1:463–469

2. Lockhart-Mummery HE (1972) Anal Lesions of Crohn's disease. Clin Gastroenterol 1:377

3. Marks CG, Ritchie JK, Lockhart-Mummery HE (1981) Anal fistulae in Crohn's disease. Br J Surg 68:525–527

4. Shukla HS, Gupta SC, Singh G, Singh PA (1988) Tubercular fistula-in-ano. Br J Surg 75:38–39

5. Nelson RL, Prasad ML, Abcarian H (1985) Anal carcinoma presenting as perirectal abscess or fistula. Arch Surg 120: 632–635

6. Miles RPM (1957) Rectal lymphogranuloma venereum. Br J Surg 45:180–188

7. Pye G, Blundell JW (1987) Sacrococcygeal teratome masquerading as a fistula-in-ano. J R S Med 80:251–252

8. Narashimharao KL, Patel RV, Malik AK, Mitra SK (1987) Chronic perianal fistula: beware of rectal duplication. Postgrad Med J 63:213–214

9. Harris GJ, Metcalf AM (1988) Primary perianal actinomycosis. Report of a case and review of the literature. Dis Colon Rectum 31:311–312

10. Lockhart-Mummery JP (1929) Discussion on fistula-in-ano. Proc R Soc Med 22:1331–1341

11. Buie LA (1960) Practical Proctology. 2nd Ed. Charles C Thomas, Springfield, IL

12. Marks CG, Ritchie JK (1977) Anal fistulae at St. Mark's Hospital. Br J Surg 64:1003–1007

13. Ewerth S, Ahlberg J, Collste G, Holmstrom B (1978) Fistula-in-ano. A six year follow up study of 143 operated patients. Acta Chir Scand 482 (suppl):53–55

14. Sainio P (1984) Fistula-in-ano in a defined population. Incidence and epidemiological aspects. Ann Chir Gynaecol 73: 219–224

15. Deshpande PJ, Sharma KR, Sharma SK, Singh LM (1975) Ambulatory treatment of fistula-in-ano: results in 400 cases. Indian J Surg 37:85–89

16. Raghavaiah NV (1976) Anal fistula in India. Int J Surg 61: 243–245

17. Kesarwani RC (1984) Fistula-in-ano. J Indian Med Assoc 82: 113–115

18. Lilius HG (1968) Fistula-in-ano: a clinical study of 150 patients. Acta Chir Scand 383 (suppl):3–88

19. McColl I (1967) The comparative anatomy and pathology of anal glands. Ann R Coll Surg Engl 40:36–67

20. Budsberg C, Spurgeon TL, Liggitt HD (1985) Anatomic predisposition to perianal fistulae formation in the German shepherd dog. Am J Vet Res 46:1468–1472

21. Vasseur PB (1984) Results of surgical excision of perianal fistulae in dogs. J Am Vet Med Assoc 185:60–62

22. Killingsworth CR, Walshaw R, Dunstan RW, Rosser EJ (1988) Bacterial population and histologic changes in dogs with perianal fistula. Am J Vet Res 49:1736–1741

23. Duhamel J (1975) Anal fistulae in childhood. Am J Proctol 26:40–43

24. Longo WE, Touloukian RJ, Seashore JN (1991) Fistula in ano in infants and children: implications and management. Paediatrics 87:737–739

25. Lunniss PJ, Jenkins PJ, Besser GM et al (1995) Gender differences in incidence of idiopathic fistula-in-ano are not explained by circulating sex hormones. Int J Colorectal Dis 10: 25–28

26. Sainio P (1985) A manometric study of anorectal function after surgery for anal fistula, with special reference to incontinence. Acta Chir Scand 151:695–700

27. Ani AN, Solanke TF (1976) Anal fistula: a review of 82 cases. Dis Colon Rectum 19:51–55

28. Read DR, Abcarian H (1979) A prospective study of 474 patients with anorectal abscess. Dis Colon Rectum 22: 566–568

29. Matt JG (1960) Anal fistula in infants and children. Dis Colon Rectum 3:258–261

30. Eisenhammer S (1964) Long-tract anteroposterior intermuscular fistula. Dis Colon Rectum 7:438–440

31. Chiari H (1880) Uber die analen Divertikel der Rektumschleimhaut und ihre Beziehung zu den Analfisteln. Med Jahrbucher Wien 8:419–427

32. Herrmann G, Desfosses L (1880) Sur la Muquese de la region cloacale du rectum. Comptes Renditions Acadamie de Science Paris (III) 90:1301–1302

33. Fenger C, Filipe MI (1977) Pathology of the anal glands with special reference to their mucin histochemistry. Acta Pathol Microbiol Scand 85:273–285

34. Shafik A (1980) A new concept of the anatomy of the anal sphincter mechanism and the physiology of defaecation, X. Anorectal sinus and band: anatomic nature and surgical significance. Dis Colon Rectum 23:170–179

35. Klosterhalfen B, Offner O, Vogel P, Kirkpatrick CJ (1991) Anatomic nature and surgical siginficance of anal sinus and anal intramuscular glands. Dis Colon Rectum 34:156–160

36. Johnson FP (1914) The development of the rectum in the human embryo. Am J Anat 16:1–57

37. Kuster GG (1965) Relationship of anal glands to lymphatics. Dis Colon Rectum 8:329–333

38. Kratzer GL, Dockerty MB (1947) Histopathology of the anal ducts. Surg, Gynecol Obstet 84:333–338

39. Parks AG, Morson BC (1962) The pathogenesis of fistula-in-ano. Proc R Soc Med 55:751–754

40. Shropshear G (1960) Surgical anatomic aspects of the anorectal sphincter mechanism and its clinical significance. J Int Coll Surg 33:267–287

41. Lunniss PJ, Phillips RKS (1992) Anatomy and function of the anal longitudinal muscle. Br J Surg 79:882–884

42. Eisenhammer S (1956) The internal anal sphincter and the anorectal abscess. Surg Gynecol Obstet 103:501–506

43. Gordon-Watson C, Dodd H (1935) Observations on fistula

in ano in relation to perianal intermuscular glands. Br J Surg 22:703–709

44. Goligher JC, Ellis M, Pissides AG (1967) A critique of anal glandular infection in the aetiology and treatment of idiopathic anorectal abscesses and fistulae. Br J Surg 54:977–983

45. Seow-Choen F, Nicholls RJ (1992) Anal fistula. Br J Surg 79:197–205

46. Lunniss PJ, Faris B, Rees H et al (1993) Histological and microbiological assessment of the role of microorganisms in chronic anal fistulae. Br J Surg 80:1072

47. Lunniss PJ, Sheffield JP, Talbot IC et al (1995) Persistence of anal fistula may be related to epithelialization. Br J Surg 82:32–33

48. Shafik A (1979) A new concept of the anatomy of the anal sphincter mechanism and the physiology of defaecation, VI. The central abscess: a new clinicopathologic entity in the genesis of anorectal suppuration. Dis Colon Rectum 22:336–341

49. Grace RH, Harper IA, Thompson RG (1982) Anorectal sepsis: microbiology in relation to fistula-in-ano. Br J Surg 69:401–403

50. Eisenhammer S (1954) Advance of anorectal surgery with special reference to ambulatory treatment. S Afr Med J 28:264–266

51. Thomson JPS, Parks AG (1979) Anorectal abscesses and fistulae. Br J Hosp Med 417–424

52. Eisenhammer S (1958) A new approach to the anorectal fistulous abscess based on the high intermuscular lesion. Surg Gynecol Obstet 106:595–599

53. Eisenhammer S (1978) The final evaluation and classification of the surgical treatment of the primary anorectal, cryptoglandular intermuscular (intersphincteric) fistulous abscess and fistula. Dis Colon Rectum 21:237–254

54. Buchan R, Grace RH (1973) Anorectal suppuration: the results of treatment and the factors influencing the recurrence rate. Br J Surg 60:537–540

55. Hebjorn M, Olsen O, Haakansson T, Andersen B (1987) A randomized trial of fistulotomy in perianal abscesses. Scand J Gastroenterol 22:174–176

56. Ramstead KD (1983) Do anal abscesses lead to fistulae-in-ano? Br J Clin Pract 37:58–60

57. Lai CK, Wong J, Ong GB (1983) Anorectal suppuration: a review of 606 patients. Southeast Asian J Surg 6:22–26

58. Waggener HU (1969) Immediate fistulotomy in the treatment of perianal abscess. Surg Clin North Am 49:1227–1233

59. Scoma JA, Salvati EP, Rubin RO (1974) Incidence of fistulae subsequent to anal abscesses. Dis Colon Rectum 17:357–359

60. Fucini C (1991) One stage treatment of anal abscesses and fistulae. Int J Colorectal Dis 6:12–16

61. Vasilevsky CA, Gordon PH (1984) The incidence of recurrent abscesses or fistula-in-ano following anorectal suppuration. Dis Colon Rectum 27:126–130

62. Schouten WR, van Vroonhoven TJMV (1991) Treatment of anorectal abscess with or without primary fistulectomy: results of a prospective randomized trial. Dis Colon Rectum 34:60–63

63. Schouten WR, van Vroonhoven TJMV, van Berlo CLJ (1987) Primary partial internal sphincterotomy in the treatment of anorectal abscess. Neth J Surg 39:43–45

64. Wilson DH (1964) The late results of anorectal abscess treated by incision, curettage and primary suture under antibiotic cover. Br J Surg 51:828–831

65. Leaper DJ, Page RE, Rosenberg IL et al (1976) A controlled study comparing the conventional treatment of idiopathic anorectal abscess with that of incision, curettage and primary suture under antibiotic cover. Dis Colon Rectum 19:46–50

66. Kronborg O, Olsen H (1984) Incision and drainage v. incision, curettage and suture under antibiotic cover in anorectal abscess. Acta Chir Scand 150:689–692

67. Ellis M (1960) Incision and primary suture of abscesses in the anal region. Proc R Soc Med 53:652–654

68. Whitehead SM, Leach RD, Eykyn SJ, Phillips I (1982) The aetiology of perirectal sepsis. Br J Surg 69:166–168

69. Henrichsen S, Christiansen J (1986) Incidence of fistula-in-ano complicating anorectal sepsis: a prospective study. British J Surg 73:371–372

70. McElwain JW, Maclean D, Alexander RM et al (1975) Anorectal problems: experience with primary fistulectomy for anorectal abscess. A report of 1000 cases. Dis Colon Rectum 18:646–649

71. Ramanujan PS, Prasad ML, Abcarian H, Tan AB (1984) Perianal abscesses and fistulae. A report of 1023 cases. Dis Colon Rectum 27:593–597

72. Lunniss PJ, Phillips RKS (1994) Surgical assessment of acute anorectal sepsis is a better predictor of fistula than microbiological analysis. Br J Surg 81:368–369

73. Goodsall DH, Miles WE (1900) p. 92. In Diseases of the Anus and Rectum. Longmans, Green, London

74. Milligan ETC, Morgan CN (1934) Surgical anatomy of the anal canal with special reference to anorectal fistulae. Lancet 2:1150–1156, 1213–1217

75. Goligher JC (1967) Surgery of the Anus, Rectum and Colon. 4th Ed. Bailliere, Tindall & Cassell, London

76. Stelzner F (1959) Die Anorectalen Fisteln. Springer-Verlag, Berlin

77. Thompson H (1962) The orthodox conception of fistula-in-ano and its treatment. Proc R Soc Med 55:754–756

78. Parks AG, Gordon PH, Hardcastle JD (1976) A classification of fistula-in-ano. Br J Surg 63:1–12

79. Marks CG (1996) Classification. pp. 33–46. In Phillips RKS, Lunniss PJ (eds): Anal Fistula: Surgical Evaluation and Management. Chapman & Hall, London

80. Hawley PR (1975) Anorectal fistula. Clin Gastroenterol 4:635–649

81. Seow Choen F, Burnett S Bartram CI, Nicholls RJ (1991) A comparison between anal endosonography and digital examination in the evaluation of anal fistulae. Br J Surg 78:445–447

82. Fazio V (1987) Complex anal fistulae. Gastroenterol Clin North Am 16:93–114

83. Gingold BS (1983) Reducing the recurrence risk of fistula-in-ano. Surg Gynecol Obstet 156:661–662

84. Glen DC (1986) Use of hydrogen peroxide to identify internal opening of anal fistula and perianal abscess. Aust NZ J Surg 56:433–435

85. Seow-Choen F, Phillips RKS (1991) Insights gained from the management of problematical anal fistulae at St. Mark's Hospital, 1984–88. Br J Surg 78:539–541

86. Kuypers HC (1982) Diagnosis and treatment of fistula-in-ano. Neth J Surg 34:147–152

87. Kuijpers HC, Schulpen T (1985) Fistulography for fistula-in-ano. Dis Colon Rectum 28:103–104

88. Tio TL, Mulder CJJ, Wijers OB (1990) Endosonography of perianal and pericolorectal fistula and/or abscess in Crohn's disease. Gastrointest Endosc 36:331–336

89. Weisman RI, Orsay CP, Pearl RK, Abcarian H (1991) The role of fistulography in fistula-in-ano. Report of 5 cases. Dis Colon Rectum 34:181–184

90. Pommeri F, Pittarello F, Dodi G et al (1988) Diagnosi radiologica delle fistole anali con reperi radiopachi. Radiol Med (Torino) 75:632–637

91. Guillamin E, Jeffrey RB, Shea WJ et al (1986) Perirectal inflammatory disease: CT findings. Radiology 161:153–157

92. Youssem DM, Fishman EK, Jones B (1988) Crohn's disease: perirectal and perianal findings at CT. Radiology 167: 331–334

93. Law PJ, Talbot RW, Bartram CI, Northover JMA (1989) Anal endosonography in the evaluation of perianal sepsis and fistula-in-ano. Br J Surg 76:752–755

94. Lunniss PJ, Barker PG, Sultan AH (1994) Magnetic resonance imaging of fistula-in-ano. Dis Colon Rectum 37: 708–718

95. Schratter-Sehn AU, Lochs H, Vogelsang H et al (1992) Comparison of trans-rectal ultrsonography and computed tomography in the diagnosis of periano-rectal fistulae in patients with Crohn's disease. Gastroenterology 102:A691

96. Heiken JP, Lee JKT (1988) MR imaging of the pelvis. Radiology 166:11–16

97. Koelbel G, Schmiedl U, Majer MC et al (1989) Diagnosis of fistulae and sinus tracts in patients with Crohn disease: value of MR imaging. Am J Radiol 152:999–1003

98. Duthie HL, Bennett RC (1963) The relation of sensation in the anal canal to the functional anal sphincter: a possible factor in continence. Gut 4:179–183

99. Bennett RC, Friedman MHW, Goligher JC (1963) Late results of haemorrhoidectomy by ligature and excision. Br Med J 2: 216–219

100. Miller R, Lewis GT, Bartolo DCC, Mortensen NJM (1988) Sensory discrimination and dynamic activity in the anorectum: evidence using an ambulatory technique. Br J Surg 75: 1003–1007

101. Miller R, Bartolo DCC, Cervero F, Mortensen NJM (1988) Anorectal sampling: a comparison of normal and incontinent patients. Br J Surg 75:44–47

102. Lunniss PJ, Thomson JPS (1996) The loose seton. pp. 87–94. In Phillips RKS, Lunniss PJ (eds): Anal Fistula: Surgical Evaluation and Management. Chapman & Hall, London

103. Pescatori M, Anastasio G, Bottini C, Mentasti A (1992) New grading and scoring for anal incontinence: evaluation of 335 patients. Dis Colon Rectum 35:482–487

104. Khubchandani IT, Read JF (1989) Sequelae of internal sphincterotomy for chronic fissure in ano. Br J Surg 76: 431–434

105. Thomson JPS, Ross AH McL (1989) Can the external sphincter be preserved in the treatment of trans-sphincteric fistula-in-ano? Int J Colorectal Dis 4:247–250

106. Kennedy HL, Zegarra JP (1990) Fistulotomy without external sphincter division for high anal fistula. Br J Surg 77:898–901

107. Lunniss PJ, Kamm MA, Phillips RKS (1994) Factors affect-

ing continence after surgery for anal fistula. Br J Surg 81: 1382–1385

108. D'Arcy Power (1910) Arderne J. Treatise of Fistula in Ano, Haemorrhoid and Clysters from an Early Fifteenth Century Manuscript Translation. Kegan Paul, Trench, Trubner, London

109. Beynon J, Carr N (1988) Master John of Arderne—surgeon of Newark. J R Soc Med 81:43–44

110. Friend WG (1975) Anorectal problems: surgical incisions for complicated anal fistula. Dis Colon Rectum 18:652–656

111. Hanley (1978) Rubber band seton in the management of abscess-anal fistula. Ann Surg 187:435–437

112. Lewis A (1986) Excision of fistula in ano. Int J Colorectal Dis 1:265–267

113. Kronborg O (1985) To lay open or excise a fistula-in-ano. A randomized trial. Br J Surg 72:970

114. Ramanujan PS, Prasad ML, Abcarian H (1983) The role of seton in fistulotomy of the anus. Surg, Gynecol Obstet 157: 419–422

115. Kuypers HC (1984) Use of the seton in the treatment of extrasphincteric anal fistula. Dis Colon Rectum 27:109–110

116. Parks AG, Stitz RW (1976) The treatment of high fistula-in-ano. Dis Colon Rectum 19:487–499

117. Adams F (1849) p. 816. In the genuine works of Hippocrates translated from the Greek and with a preliminary discourse and annotations. Sydenham Society, London

118. Goldberg SM, Garcia-Aquilar J (1996) The cutting seton. pp. 95–102. In Phillips RKS, Lunniss PJ (eds): Anal Fistula: Surgical Evaluation and Management. Chapman & Hall, London

119. Held D, Khubchandani I, Sheets J et al (1986) Management of anorectal horseshoe abscess and fistula. Dis Colon Rectum 29:793–797

120. Ustynovsky K, Rosen L, Stasik J et al. (1990) Horseshoe abscess fistula. Dis Colon Rectum 33:602–605

121. Christensen A, Nilas L, Christiansen J (1986) Treatment of trans-sphincteric anal fistulae by the seton technique. Dis Colon Rectum 29:454–455

122. Misra MC, Kapur BML (1988) A new non-operative approach to fistula-in-ano. Br J Surg 75:1093–1094

123. Deshpande PJ, Sharma KR (1973) Treatment of fistula in ano by a new technique—review and follow-up of 200 cases. Am J Proctol 24:49–60

124. Deshpande PJ, Sharma KR (1976) Successful non-operative treatment of high rectal fistula. Am J Proctol February:39–47

125. Shukla NK, Narang R, Nair NG (1991) Multicentric randomized controlled clinical trial of Kshaarasootra (Ayurvedic medicated thread) in the management of fistula-in-ano. Indian J Med Res 94:177–185

126. Wolffers I (1986) Ayurvedic treatment for fistula-in-ano. Trop Doct 16:44

127. Noble GH (1902) A new operation for complete laceration of the perineum designed for the purpose of eliminating danger of infection from the rectum. Trans Am Gynecol Soc 27: 357–363

128. Elting AW (1912) The treatment of fistula in ano. *Ann* Surg 56:744–752

129. Jones IT, Fazio VW, Jagelman DG (1987) The use of transanal rectal advancement flaps in the management of fis-

tulae involving the anorectum. Dis Colon Rectum 30: 919–923

130. Wedell J, Meier zu Eissen P, Banzhaf G, Kleine L (1987) Sliding flap advancement for the treatment of high level fistulae. Br J Surg 74:390–391

131. Shemash EI, Kodner IJ, Fry RD, Neufeld DM (1988) Endorectal sliding flap repair of complicated anterior anoperineal fistulae. Dis Colon Rectum 31:22–24

132. Lewis P, Bartolo DCC (1990) Treatment of trans-sphincteric fistulae by full thickness anorectal advancement flaps. Br J Surg 77:1187–1189

133. Stone JM, Goldberg SM (1980) The endorectal advancement flap procedure. Int J Colorectal Dis 4:188–196

134. Finan PJ (1996) Management by advancement flap technique. pp. 107–114. In Phillips RKS, Lunniss PJ (eds). Anal Fistula: Surgical Evaluation and Management. Chapman & Hall, London

135. Aquilar PS, Plasencia G, Hardy TG et al (1985) Mucosal advancement in the treatment of anal fistula. Dis Colon Rectum 28:496–498

136. Kodner IJ, Mazor A, Shemesh EL et al (1993) Endorectal advancement flap repair of rectovaginal and other complicated anorectal fistulae. Surgery 114:682–690

137. Lewis A (1996) Core out. pp. 81–86. In Phillips RKS, Lunniss PJ (eds): Anal Fistula: Surgical Evaluation and Management. Chapman & Hall, London

138. Parkash S, Lakshmiratan V, Gajendran V (1985) Fistula-in-ano: treatment by fistulectomy, primary closure and reconstitiution. Aust NZ J Surg 55:23–27

139. Mann CV, Clifton MA (1985) Re-routing of the track for the treatment of high anal and anorectal fistulae. Br J Surg 72: 134–137

140. Sood ID (1968) Treatment of fistulae-in-ano and primary closure. In Menda RK (ed): Advances in Proctology. ISDCRA, Bombay

141. Kupferberg A, Zer M, Rabinson S (1984) The use of PMMA beads in recurrent high anal fistulae: a preliminary report. World J Surg 8:970–974

142. Matos D, Lunniss PJ, Phillips RKS (1993) Total sphincter conservation in high fistula in ano: results of a new approach. Br J Surg 80:802–804

143. Hjortrup A, Moesgaard F, Kjaegard J (1991) Fibrin adhesive in the treatment of perineal fistulae. Dis Colon Rectum 34: 752–754

144. Abel ME, Chiu YSY, Russell TR, Volpe PA (1993) Autologous fibrin glue in the treatment of rectovaginal and complex fistulae. Dis Colon Rectum 36:447–449

145. Phillips RKS, Lunniss PJ (1995) Approach to the difficult fistula. pp. 177–182. In: Phillips RKS, Lunniss PJ (eds): Anal Fistula: Surgical Evaluation and Management. Chapman & Hall, London

146. Phillips RKS, Lunniss PJ (eds) (1996) Anal Fistula: Surgical Evaluation and Management. Chapman & Hall, London

15

SEXUALLY TRANSMITTED DISEASES

Robert Gilliland
Steven D. Wexner

The anorectum has been used as a vehicle for obtaining sexual satisfaction for thousands of years.[1] However, the percentage of the population regularly performing anogenital, oroanal and other anal based erotic practices appears to be increasing. Wilcox[2] estimated that 2 to 2.5 million persons in the United Kingdom had regular anal intercourse. In the United States, 4 to 13% of the adult male population is predominately homosexual or bisexual for a significant proportion of their lives.[3] Promiscuity often plays a prominent role in homosexual behavior, with only an estimated 10% of the population having a "close-coupled" or monogamous relationship.[4] It has been estimated that the average homosexual has 1,000 sexual partners in a lifetime.[5,6] Other studies suggest that a "moderately active" homosexual man will have 100 partners per year,[7] and some may have as many as 200.[8] As a result, sexually transmitted diseases of the colorectum are rampant within this community, and have been grouped together under the umbrella of the "gay bowel syndrome."[9]

Anal intercourse however, is not confined to men. Bolling[10] reported that 25% of women attending a gynecologic clinic in the United States had had anal intercourse and 8% used that portal regularly. In the United Kingdom, figures from a genitourinary clinic estimated that 31% of women had had anal intercourse.[8]

Contrary to popular belief, the sexual proclivity of an individual cannot be determined by appearance or mannerisms.[4,11] Thus no colorectal consultation is complete without a thorough sexual history being obtained. Furthermore, the ever-widening scope of sexually transmitted diseases affecting the colorectum (Tables 15-1 to 15-3), plus the global epidemic of the human immunodeficiency virus (HIV), demands that all colorectal physicians have a working familiarity with these disorders.

GONORRHEA

Incidence

Up to 55% of homosexual men attending screening clinics have been found to harbor *Neisseria gonorrhoeae*, with the rectum being the only site infected in 40 to 50% of these patients.[12,13] In the United Kingdom, 13 to 45% of homosexual men attending genitourinary medicine clinics have rectal gonorrhea.[14] The rectal mucosa is infected in 35 to 50% of women with gonococcal cervicitis.[15–17] In the absence of cervical or urethral infection, rectal gonorrhea ocurs in 4 to 6%.[18,19]

From 1983 onwards, the incidence of rectal gonorrhea decreased significantly among homosexual men, probably in response to behavioural changes made to reduce the risk of infection with HIV.[20,21] However, the incidence has been increasing again since 1989.[22,23]

Transmission and Incubation

Gonococcal proctitis in men occurs as a result of anal receptive intercourse with a partner who has urethral gonorrhea. The incubation period is typically 5 to 7 days before symptoms commence. The method of inoculation in women is the subject of some debate. Some feel that rectal gonorrhea is only due to direct penile penetration while others suggest that infection is due to local spread of contaminated cervical secretions. This latter postulate is supported by the findings that rectal gonorrhea is uncommon in the absence of cervical or urethral involvement[19] and that its incidence is positively correlated with the duration of endocervical infection.[24]

Clinical Features

Many patients with rectal gonorrhea are asymptomatic and are only detected during the search for contacts of men with gonococcal urethritis. When local symptoms present they are usually

Table 15-1. Sexually Transmitted Bacterial Diseases

Organism	Symptoms	Proctoscopy and Sigmoidoscopy Findings	Laboratory Tests	Treatment
N. gonorrhoeae	Often asymptomatic, mucopurulent rectal discharge, pruritis, tenesmus	Anal sparing, proctitis, discharge	Gram-negative diplococci, Thayer-Martin culture	Ceftriaxone 250 mg IM for 1 day + doxycycline 100 mg PO bd for 7 days
T. pallidum	Often asymptomatic, rectal pain, mucoid discharge	Painful anal ulcer, occasional proctitis	Dark field microscopy of fresh scrapings	Benzathine penicillin 2.4 megaunits IM
H. ducreyii	Perineal pain	Perianal abscess, ulcers	Gram-negative bacillus, aerobic culture	Erythromycin 500 mg PO qid for 7 days
Chlamydia	Tenesmus, bloody discharge, lymphadenopathy	Proctitis, anal verge ulcer	Biopsy for tissue culture, microimmunofluorescent antibody titer	Tetracycline 500 mg PO qid for 14 days (Chlamydia) 21 days (LGV)
S. flexneri	Abdominal cramps, fever, bloody diarrhea	Proctitis, grayish-white ulceration of rectal mucosa	Stool culture	Co-trimoxazole (double strength) PO bd for 7 days
Campylobacter	Abdominal bloating, diarrhea, mucopurulent discharge	Proctitis, grayish-white ulceration of rectal mucosa	Stool culture	Supportive, erythromycin 500 mg PO qid for 7 days

(Adapted from Wexner and Beck,[201] with permission.)

mild, although Robbins et al.[25] have reported severe anal pain in some patients due to cryptitis and intersphincteric abscesses. Pruritis ani, tenesmus, and a bloody or mucoid discharge are the most common symptoms of gonococcal proctitis. In advanced disease, systemic infection can occur, most commonly causing a unilateral migratory suppurative arthritis of the large joints. Systemic spread may also result in perihepatitis, pericarditis, endocarditis, and meningitis.

Diagnosis

A mucopurulent discharge is the most common sign of infection with *N. gonorrheae*, and if present in conjunction with a nonspecific proctitis, is almost pathognomonic of rectal gonorrhea. The anal canal is typically spared and the area of inflammatory change is usually confined to the lower 8 cm of the rectum. The rectal mucosa may be erythematous, friable, and swollen but ulceration is rare. Avoidance of enemas prior to endoscopy

is recommended, as their use results in much of the discharge being evacuated. Furthermore, as many lubricants contain antibacterial agents, lubrication of the anoscope or sigmoidoscope with anything other than water prior to insertion is not advisable. It may be possible to express mucopus from the anal glands by applying gentle external pressure with the anoscope in place.

The diagnosis of rectal gonorrhea is confirmed by a swab culture and a Gram stain. Blind swabbing of the anus can be performed by inserting a pledget into the anal canal to a distance of 2 to 2.5 cm and rotating it from side to side. However, swabs taken blindly have only a 34 to 55% positive yield in culture-positive patients. This figure can be improved to 79% by swabbing under direct vision.[26-28]

Swabs should be Gram stained and cultured on Thayer-Martin or Stuart's (anaerobic) medium. Gram-negative diplococci may occasionally be seen within neutrophils or colonic mucosal cells, and positive identification allows therapy to be commenced immediately.

Table 15-2. Sexually Transmitted Viral Diseases

Organism	Symptoms	Proctoscopy and Sigmoidoscopy Findings	Laboratory Tests	Treatment
Herpes simplex virus	Anorectal pain, pruritis, mucoid/bloody discharge	Perianal erythema, vesicles, ulcers, diffusely inflamed friable rectal mucosa	Immunofluorescent staining or culture of vesicular fluid or scrapings	Acyclovir 400–800 mg 5 times daily for 7 days, prophylaxis
Human papilloma virus	Pruritis, discharge, bleeding, pain	Perianal/intra-anal warts	Excision biopsy	See Table 15-3
Molluscum contagiosum	Painless dermal lesions	Flattened, round, umbilicated lesions	Excision biopsy	Excision, cryotherapy

(Adapted from Wexner and Beck,[201] with permission.)

Table 15-3. Sexually Transmitted Parasitic Diseases

Organism	Symptoms	Proctoscopy and Sigmoidoscopy Findings	Laboratory Tests	Treatment
E. histolytica	Abdominal pain, bloody diarrhea, tenesmus, pyrexia	Proctitis, hourglass ulcers	Stool culture for cysts	Metronidazole 750 mg PO tid for 10 days
G. lamblia	Abdominal cramps, bloating, foul loose stools	Often normal, diffuse ulceration	Microscopic identification of trophozites in stool or scrapings	Metronidazole 750 mg PO tid for 7 days
Cryptococcus	Bloody diarrhea, usually self-limiting	Proctitis	Microscopic identification of oocytes in biopsy, Kinyoun stain	Supportive
I. belli	Bloody diarrhea	Proctitis	Microscopic identification of oocytes in biopsy, Kinyoun stain	Co-trimoxazole (double strength) PO bd for 7 days

(Adapted from Wexner and Beck,[201] with permission.)

Rectal biopsy is often unhelpful as histology is nonspecific and impossible to differentiate from other enteric infections such as *Shigella, Salmonella*, or *Yersinia*. These changes include crypt edema, infiltration of polymorphs and histiocytes within the lamina propria, and a reduction in the number of plasma cells and lymphocytes. More severe inflammation may result in exudates containing polymorphs being present in the crypts and on the mucosal surface. The crypt epithelium may be depleted of mucous and degenerative changes can occur.

Treatment

Rectal gonorrhea is more resistant to treatment than infection at other sites. This may be due to the presence of antibiotic inactivating enzymes, such as penicillinases, in the normal flora of the rectum.[29] As a result, the Centers for Disease Control (CDC) have recommended that the traditionally preferred treatment of procaine penicillin, 4.8 megaunits IM (or 3 g oral amoxicillin) in conjunction with 1 g of oral probenicid, be replaced by a single dose of cethtriaxone 250 mg IM followed by doxycycline 100 mg orally twice a day for 7 days.[30]

SYPHILIS

Venereal syphilis has been defined as an infective disease due to *Treponema pallidum*, which is systemic from the outset and is capable of involving practically every structure of the body in its course.[31]

Incidence

The rise in the incidence of syphilis seen during World War II in both the United Kingdom and United States was followed by a dramatic decrease during the next decade.[31] From 1971 to 1980 there was a further rise in the overall incidence, mainly due to a substantial increase within the homosexual male population.[32] The onset of the AIDS epidemic was mirrored by a fall in the incidence due to reduced partner changing within this group. However, the incidence has been rising again since 1989.[22] Currently 80% of cases of primary anal syphilis occur in homosexual men.[32]

Transmission

Primary syphilitic infections in the anorectum occur in both sexes as a result of direct penetration. Anal ulcers usually appear 2 to 6 weeks after exposure but may occur up to 3 months later.[33,34]

Clinical Features

The primary lesion of syphilis is the chancre. This starts as a dull red macule that rapidly becomes papular and ulcerates. The chancre is rounded with a well-defined margin and a rubbery, indurated base. Although usually painless at other sites, the anal chancre may cause extreme pain and may therefore be mistaken for an anal fissure.[35] The majority of ulcers are single but they may be multiple, eccentrically placed, or situated opposite each other in a "mirror image" or "kissing" configuration (Fig. 15-1). If the ulcers are painless, patients may not seek medical advice, and the lesions will heal in 3 to 4 weeks.[36] Occasionally the primary chancre presents as an anorectal ulcer, usually on the anterior wall of the rectum, where it mimics a rectal carcinoma or solitary rectal ulcer.[37] Proctitis in the absence of anal or rectal ulceration may occur causing tenesmus, rectal pain, and a mucoid discharge.[38] Any of these lesions may be associated with rubbery inguinal lymphadenopathy.

The secondary manifestations of anorectal syphilis begin to appear 6 to 8 weeks after the chancre has healed. *T. pallidum* organisms disseminate widely throughout the body and cause malaise, headaches, weight loss, fever, and musculoskeletal pains. This is usually accompanied by a dull red maculopapular rash that involves the entire body including the palms of the hands and soles of the feet. In intertriginous areas papules may become large and raised or may coalesce to form broad pale-brown or pink verrucous lesions called condylomata lata. These lesions, often found around the anus and genital areas, secrete mucous and may be associated with pruritis and an unpleasant odor. They are teeming with spirochetes and are highly infec-

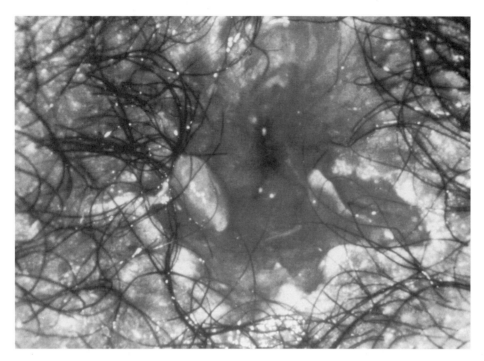

Figure 15-1. Irregular perianal syphilitic chancre. In this situation, chancres are often painful, eccentrically located, and occasionally in mirror-image configuration. (From Wexner,[69] with permission.)

tious. Secondary rectal syphilis may also present as rectal polyps, which are smooth, lobulated, and submucosal; or as mucosal ulceration.

Tertiary syphilis is rarely seen in the Western world but rectal gummata have been reported.[35] Tabes dorsalis can cause anal sphincter paralysis and severe perineal pain.

Diagnosis

Dark-field microscopy is the investigation of choice as early primary and secondary lesions are teeming with organisms. After cleaning the area with saline, the lesion should be squeezed and scrapings taken so as to collect serum rather than blood. Dark-field microscopy identifies treponemes as corkscrew-shaped motile, fluorescent yellowish-green organisms. Considerable expertise is required to make the diagnosis accurately.[39]

A number of serologic tests are available to aid in the diagnosis. Approximately 4 to 6 weeks after infection the fluorescent treponemal antibody (FTA) absorption test becomes positive.[34] The Venereal Disease Research Laboratory (VDRL) assay is positive in 75% of cases with untreated primary syphilis and in the secondary stage 100% should react. Biopsy of the lesions reveals an intense lymphocytic infiltrate in the submucosa and lamina propria with destruction of the muscularis mucosa. Organisms can be demonstrated throughout the infected tissue by immunofluorescent antibody staining.

Treatment

Patients with primary, secondary, or early tertiary syphilis are effectively treated by a single IM injection of 2.4 megaunits of penicillin G. Patients with long-standing disease may require up to 3 injections at weekly intervals. Patients allergic to penicillin may be treated with erythromycin or tetracycline, 500 mg orally four times a day for 2 to 4 weeks. All sexual contacts of patients within the previous 12 months should be treated prophylactically, and both patients and contacts should abstain from sexual activity until proven noninfective by low VDRL titers.

CHANCROID

Chancroid or "soft sore" is caused by *Haemophilus ducreyi*, a short, aerobic, gram-negative bacillus usually found in chains or groups. Infection is uncommon in temperate climates; most cases occur in patients who have traveled abroad. In the United States, the incidence fell dramatically between 1950 and 1978 but has been slowly rising since 1985. Males are affected about 10 times as often as females.[40] However, as females with the disease may be asymptomatic, prostitutes are the main reservoir of infection. Hence, the disease is not well characterized within homosexual males.

The incubation period is usually 4 to 7 days; no prodromal symptoms are recognized.[40] Infection is typified by painful genital ulcers and/or multiple perineal abscesses accompanied by suppuration of the regional lymph nodes.[33] The condition usually responds to erythromycin, 500 mg four times a day for 1 week. Alternatively, cotrimoxazole, one tablet (trimethoprim 80 mg/sulfamethoxazole 400 mg) twice a day for 1 week, is also curative.

CHLAMYDIA

Chlamydial species are obligate intracellular parasites and the cause of the most common sexually transmitted disease in the United States. These organisms cannot penetrate intact skin or mucous membranes and therefore entry is probably gained by minute lacerations and abrasions. There are 15 known immunotypes; serotypes D to K are responsible for most of the cases of proctitis and an increasing cause of this condition amongst homosexual men and anal-receptive women.[41,42] Serotypes L-1, L-2, and L-3 cause lymphogranuloma venereum (LGV).

Incidence

Chlamydial rectal infections are currently present in 15% of asymptomatic homosexual men.[43] The incidence in women has not yet been evaluated.

Transmission

Both anal-receptive and oroanal sex have been incriminated in the etiology of proctitis. The incubation period is 2 to 35 days in women and approximately 6 weeks in homosexual men.

Clinical Features

Infection is usually heralded by the formation of small vesicles, often unnoticed by the patient. These lesions progress over several weeks to form an ulcer at the anal verge. There is usually considerable inflammation of the inguinal nodes, which enlarge and become adherent to each other and the overlying skin. At this time they can be confused with the lymphadenopathy associated with syphilis. Untreated, the nodes may discharge resulting in purulent sinuses to the skin reminiscent of lymphogranuloma inguinale.

Proctitis may present with tenesmus, rectal pain, and the passage of blood per rectum. Sigmoidoscopy may reveal a range of findings from mild inflammation with occasional vesicles to severe proctitis with boggy, friable, ulcerated mucosa. Late findings may include an intraluminal stricture or mass, although these occur more commonly in those infected with LGV serovars.

Diagnosis

Rectal biopsy may demonstrate the presence of crypt abscesses, infectious granulomata, and giant cells.[43,44] A biopsy of inflamed rectal mucosa taken for culture must be transported in sucrose medium on ice for immediate tissue culture inoculation.

As the organism is an obligate intracellular pathogen, rectal swab culture is unhelpful. Furthermore, the complement fixation test is often negative, as titer elevation does not usually occur for 1 month after infection. Thus low antichlamydial antibody titers (greater than 1:64 is considered diagnostic)[34] should not be taken to indicate absence of the disease without either tissue culture testing or a microimmunofluorescent antibody titer. The latter procedure is the most sensitive seretyping test[45] but is not as yet universally available.

Treatment

These infections usually respond to tetracycline or erythromycin, 500 mg four times a day for 1 to 2 weeks.[46] Oral doxycycline, 100 mg twice daily for 1 week, is an acceptable alternative.

LYMPHOGRANULOMA VENEREUM

Incidence

Lymphogranuloma venereum (LGV) is a systemic disease predominately affecting lymphatic tissue. It is sporadic in Western communities, with cases usually occurring in patients who have traveled in Africa, India, Southeast Asia, South America, and the Caribbean where the condition is endemic. In these countries the incidence is 2 to 6% of patients attending genitourinary medicine clinics.[47]

Clinical Features

Features are similar to those of chlamydial proctitis, but gross inguinal lymphadenopathy is a prominent feature. Anorectal strictures occur more commonly in response to the L1 to L3 serovars and are a later manifestation. They occur about 3 to 10 cm from the anal verge. Other less common manifestations of LGV proctitis include fistula-in-ano, rectovaginal fistula, and perirectal abscesses. The diagnosis is again made by tissue culture of rectal biopsies or by the complement fixation test.

Treatment

Treatment with erythromycin and tetracycline is again effective but should be administered for 3 weeks.[46] The proctocolitis responds rapidly and the rectal mucosa is often healed within a few weeks after treatment.[43] A few treatment failures have been reported with tetracycline.[44]

HERPES SIMPLEX VIRUS

Herpes simplex virus (HSV) is a large enveloped DNA virus that may lie dormant after the initial infection but may be reactivated at any time in response to various stimuli including infection and malignancy. This chronic relapsing course is common and occurs in up to 40% of patients.[48] Two types are implicated in sexually transmitted coloanal disease; type II is responsible for 90% of infections, with type I responsible for almost all of the remainder.[49] The varicella-zoster strain is occasionally encountered.

Incidence

HSV has been identified on rectal culture from 6 to 30% of homosexual men with symptomatic rectal disease and in one third of these cases other pathogenic organisms coexist.[50–52] However, serologic testing reveals that over 95% of homosexual males have been infected with HSV type II.[53]

Transmission

HSV type II is spread by direct penile implantation. Type I is presumably spread by oroanal contact. The disease is highly contagious from the appearance of the vesicles until they completely reepithelialize.

Clinical Features

Clinical symptoms usually occur 4 to 21 days following infection.[13] Almost all patients have anorectal pain or burning exacerbated by defecation or intercourse,[54] and tenesmus is universal.[52] Pruritis afflicts 50 to 85% of patients.[55] Other symptoms include constipation and a mucoid or bloody rectal discharge. Approximately half the patients will have symptoms of a systemic viraemia at least during the first prodrome.[52] Bilateral tender inguinal lymphadenopathy is present in up to 57% of patients.[52]

HSV infection of the lumbosacral ganglia can result in urinary dysfunction, sacral paresthesia, impotence, and pain in the lower abdomen, thighs, and buttocks.[33] This radiculopathy is found in up to 50% of homosexual men[56] and often antedates the physical findings. Neurologic signs may persist long after the acute infection has subsided.[48,57]

During an acute episode the anus may be exquisitely tender, and internal examination may be impossible without the aid of local anesthetic gel. Initially small vesicles with surrounding erythema appear, but often rupture to form aphthous ulcers that may coalesce (Fig. 15-2). The vesicles may occur on the perianal skin and/or in the anal canal. They eventually crust over and heal within 2 weeks.

The proctitis induced by HSV is usually limited to the lower 10 cm of the rectum. The sigmoidoscopic findings include friable erythematous mucosa, diffuse ulceration, and occasional vesicles and pustules. Ulcerations within the anal canal may become secondarily infected and appear as grayish crypts with erythematous edges.

Diagnosis

Scrapings taken from the bed of the ulcers reveal the intranuclear inclusion bodies or multinucleated giant cells, which are diagnostic (Fig. 15-3).[52] Viral culture and direct immunofluorescent staining of the vesicular fluid is also helpful.[58] Rectal biopsy may show crypt abscesses in up to 50% of patients.

Treatment

As acute attacks of HSV infection are usually self-limiting, traditional treatment was usually symptomatic including warm baths, local anesthetic ointments, and oral analgesics.[54] Attention to personal hygiene helps to prevent secondary infection of the ulcers.

Acyclovir is the only antiviral agent proven to be effective against HSV. Doses of 400 to 800 mg, five times per day for 7 days, have been found to reduce the duration of viral shedding, promote healing of the lesions,[59] and give more rapid resolution of rectal pain, discharge, and other symptoms of proctitis.[59–61] Although there is no evidence that this agent eradicates the virus,[49,51] the rate of relapse is reduced provided the drug is taken for life.[61–63] This is particularly relevant in AIDS patients, among whom recurrences are frequent. Oral doses of 200 to 400 mg, two to five times daily are suitable for prophylaxis.

Topical acyclovir is less effective than oral therapy but may be used up to 5 times daily either in conjunction with, or instead of oral treatment. Patients with severe infections may require intravenous acyclovir in doses of 5 mg/kg every 8 hours for 5 to 7 days. AIDS patients with HSV lesions resistant to acyclovir

Figure 15-2. Perianal herpes simplex virus infection in a butterfly distribution extending onto the coccyx. The vesicles have already coalesced and encrusted. (From Wexner,[204] with permission.)

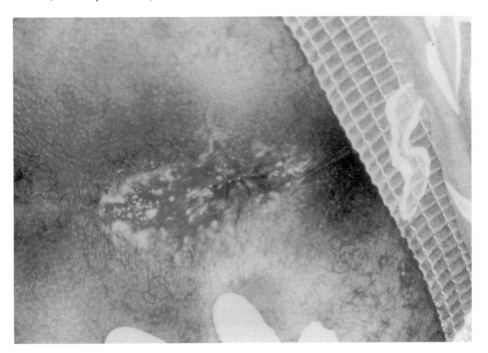

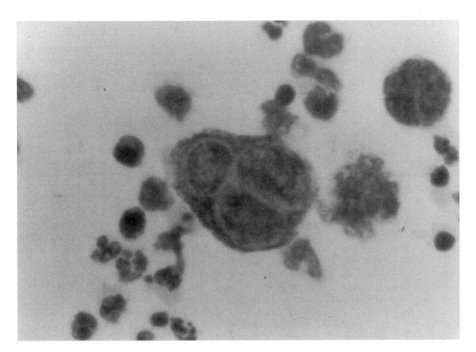

Figure 15-3. Microscopic identification of multinucleate giant cells from the cytologic scrapings of a perianal ulcer. (From Wexner,[204] with permission.)

may be treated with phosphonoformate (foscarnet) or vidarabine.[64–66]

CONDYLOMATA ACUMINATA

Condylomata acuminata is a perianal wart caused by the human papillomavirus (HPV) of which four types are usually sexually transmitted. Types 6 and 11 are usually benign, but types 16 and 18 are associated with the development of dysplasia and invasive carcinomas.[67,68] These warts should therefore be considered as potentially premalignant.

Incidence

Condylomata accuminata is the most frequent sexually transmitted disease seen by colorectal surgeons.[69] In the United States, the incidence increased fivefold between 1966 and 1981.[70] Warts may occur in women and heterosexual men, but again most commonly affected are homosexual or bisexual men, with up to 70% having the condition.[71] Indeed, between 50% and 75% of asymptomatic homosexual men may have anal condylomata.[9,72] Associated genital warts (vulval, vaginal, or cervical) are seen in 80% of affected women but in just 16% of affected men (penile).[73]

Transmission

Ninety percent of patients with anal condylomata admit to anal receptive intercourse.[73] The remainder is attributed to direct extension from the genital area.

Clinical Features

Pruritis ani, bleeding, discharge, persistent wetness, and pain are the usual symptoms.[74] External examination reveals single, pinkish-white warts that may coalesce and become a white macerated mass associated with a foul odor due to the warmth and moistness of the area (Fig. 15-4). Giant condylomata (Busche-Lowenstein's disease) are occasionally encountered

Figure 15-4. Extensive condylomata acuminata.

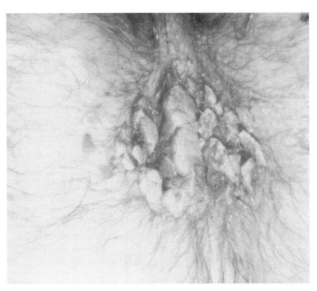

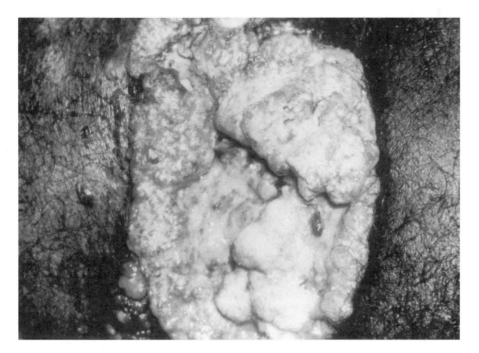

Figure 15-5. Buschke-Lowenstein's disease. (From Wexner,[69] with permission.)

(Fig. 15-5). These lesions enlarge relentlessly, forming a locally invasive but nonmetastasizing growth that may almost obliterate the anal canal. Histologically they appear benign but transformation into a squamous carcinoma has been reported, leading some to postulate that they may represent or contain a well-differentiated malignancy from its occurrence.[75]

Diagnosis

These lesions tend to be diagnosed by direct inspection and must therefore be distinguished from condylomata lata, molluscum contagiosum, and hypertrophied anal papillae. The broad lesions associated with secondary syphilis tend to be smoother, flatter, and moister, while the small lesions of molluscum are raised and centrally umbilicated. Hypertrophied papillae are less friable than are condylomata acuminata. Diagnosis can be aided by acetic acid wash, magnification, or colposcopy.

Anoscopy or proctosigmoidoscopy is imperative, as 84% of homosexual males have both perianal and intra-anal condylomata.[9] Furthermore, 10% of symptomatic patients have only intra-anal lesions.[9] Vaginal or penile examination should also be performed.

The diagnosis is confirmed on histology. A marked acanthosis of the epidermis with hyperplasia of the prickle cells is present. The cells of the upper prickle layer may become vacuolized (koilocytosis), and there is usually an underlying chronic inflammatory cell infiltrate.[76]

Treatment

Many types of therapy have been used in the treatment of condylomata, but none guarantee complete resolution of the condition.

Excision of all lesions, or at least representative and suspicious lesions, should be a part of all therapeutic approaches to confirm the diagnosis and exclude malignancy.[77] Excision can be performed under local, regional, or general anesthesia. Local infiltration of a 1:200,000 adrenaline solution reduces blood loss and serves to elevate and separate lesions, permitting accurate excision with minimal damage to the intervening skin

---

Some of the More Common Treatment Options for Condylomata Acuminata

Excision, (Destructive)

Surgical

Electrocautery

Cryotherapy

Laser

Medical

Podophyllin

Bichloroacetic acid

Immunotherapy

Autologous injection

Interferon
  Intramuscular
  Intralesional

Chemotherapy

5-fluorouracil

Bleomycin

Adapted from Wexner and Beck,[201] with permission.

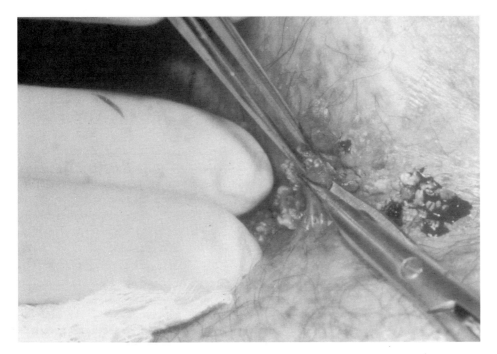

Figure 15-6. Excision of individual warts with fine scissors. Injection of 1:200,000 adrenaline helps to elevate the warts from normal skin.

(Fig. 15-6). Electrocautery applied to the base of the lesions helps to reduce postoperative hemorrhage. In most patients, a single operation is sufficient to remove all lesions. Postoperative bleeding is the most common complication (2 to 3%).

Podophyllin is cytotoxic to condylomata and very irritating to normal skin. As a result, careful application directly to the warts is necessary, and postapplication dusting with talcum powder is useful. A 25% solution applied in either liquid paraffin or tincture of benzoin is adequate, but the latter adheres more efficiently to the warts. Podophyllin cannot be used on intra-anal warts because of the risks of stenosis and fistula formation.[69] Single applications are seldom effective, and weekly or fortnightly treatments are recommended. As well as local complications, repeated use may be toxic to the gastrointestinal, hemopoeitic, hepatic, renal, respiratory, and central nervous systems. Furthermore, podophyllin treatment will produce dysplastic change within the condylomata that mimics carcinoma in situ. Repeated treatment with podophyllin has a lower initial success rate and a higher recurrence rate than surgical excision.[78]

Bichloroacetic acid can be used to destroy peri- and intraanal condylomata. Methods of application and complications are similar to those of podophyllin, but bichloroacetic acid is less irritating. Recurrence rates of 25 percent are reported.[79]

Electrocautery is an effective treatment and is widely used. Local, regional, or general anesthesia is required. The risks of deep burns and stenosis are reduced by careful attention to technique. A needle-tipped cautery should be used and held so that the current arcs onto the surface of the wart. Carbon dioxide lasers have been used to perform the same procedure but have not provided any clear advantage.[80] They are also more expensive and there is some concern about the transmission of viable virus particles that may be present in the resulting vapor.

Immunotherapy for the treatment of recurrent warts was introduced by Abcarian and colleagues.[73,81] Autologous vaccine is prepared from a sample of the patient's own condylomata and administered intramuscularly at weekly intervals over a 6-week period. Patients who are HIV-seropositive are not suitable candidates. No serious side effects have been reported, but minor local reactions may occur at the injection site in a few patients.[82] Success rates of 84 to 95% have been reported.[82–84]

Intramuscular[85,86] or intralesional[87] interferon-β has been proven to be of benefit in several controlled trials. Systemic administration of interferon is often accompanied by fever, headache, weakness, nausea, pain at the injection site, and a flulike syndrome.[86] Complete resolution has been reported in 51 to 82% of patients.

PARASITIC INFECTIONS

Parasitic infestations of the colon were previously uncommon in developed urban areas of the West. However, these conditions are now diagnosed with increasing regularity in the homosexual and bisexual male population.[88] These conditions include amebiasis, giardiasis, isosporiasis, and infections with *Enterobius vermicularis* and other helminths.[89–92] In fact, 25 to 70% of the homosexual population presenting with a diarrheal illness will have one or more protozoal organisms in their stool.[93,94]

Amebiasis

Entamoeba histolytica is the most common cause of parasitic colitis seen by surgeons in the United States and is endemic in certain parts of the world. The prevalence rate for infection among homosexual and bisexual men ranges from 20% to 32%.[95] Transmission in these groups occurs via oroanal intercourse with an infected partner. Some patients may be asymptomatic but others suffer abdominal pain, loose bloody stools, pyrexia, tenesmus, and malaise. Sigmoidoscopy may be normal but erythema, edema, friable mucosa, and typical hourglass ulcers may be seen. If the diagnosis is suspected but sigmoidoscopy is normal, colonoscopy should be performed, as the ulcers are most commonly seen in the cecum and terminal ileum. The diagnosis is confirmed by identifying cysts, which will be present in the stools of 9 out of 10 symptomatic patients.[7] The stool must be examined within 1 hour and antibiotics, mineral oil, or residual barium may give false-negative results.[7] Proctitis or dysentery is effectively treated by oral metronidazole, 750 mg three times daily for 10 days. In severe cases, oral diiodohydroxyquin, 650 mg three times daily, is given for 3 weeks following the metronidazole regimen.[74] Surgery is only indicated for complications such as toxic megacolon or perforation. These complications are thankfully rare, as surgery is associated with a 75% mortality.[96]

Giardiasis

Giardia lamblia is an intestinal flagellate that lives in the upper small intestine and biliary tract of infected individuals. The incidence of giardiasis is between 4% and 18% of the male homosexual population, where it is again transmitted through oroanal intercourse among infected partners.[92] These organisms do not infect the lower gastrointestinal tract but may still produce cramping, bloating, anorexia, weight loss, and a malabsorbtion syndrome with foul, loose stools. Almost all infected patients will have symptomatic enteritis.[92] Sigmoidoscopy is often normal but may demonstrate diffuse ulceration.[34] The diagnosis is confirmed by identification of the trophozites in a fresh stool specimen or in the scrapings from an ulcer base. Treatment with oral metronidazole, 750 mg, three times daily for 7 days, is usually sufficient to eradicate the organism.[74]

Cryptosporidiosis

In nonimmunocompromised patients, infection with *Cryptosporidium* produces a self-limiting colitis lasting up to 2 weeks. However, in the immunocompromised it may result in a life-threatening colitis,[97] and has been reported in 3% to 4% of those suffering from the acquired immune deficiency syndrome (AIDS).[98] The protozoans inhabit the microvilli and cause a profuse, often bloody, mucoid diarrhea resulting in electrolyte imbalance and severe dehydration.[99,100] Diagnosis is confirmed by identification of the oocytes in rectal biopsy specimens. Alternatively, the organisms may be seen on routine (Ziehl-Neelson) or modified acid-fast (Kinyoun) stain. Treatment is largely supportive, with rehydration and nutritional supplementation where necessary. Many antiparasitic agents, including metronidazole, thiabendazole, furazolidone, and spiramycin, have been tried but none have produced good results.[99]

Isosporiasis

The opportunistic protozoan *Isospora belli* has a much lower prevalence than does *Cryptosporidium*, occurring in less than 0.2% of patients with AIDS in the United States.[98] The clinical syndrome is similar to that caused by *Cryptosporidium* but the

diarrhea tends to be less profuse. The diagnosis is again confirmed by using a modified acid-fast stain of a fresh stool specimen, or by histologic examination of biopsy material. Seven days oral treatment with 160 mg trimethoprim/sulphamethoxazole 800 mg twice daily is usually sufficient to eradicate the disease.[101] However, as the rate of relapse is high, continued prophylaxis with these agents has been suggested.[98]

Shigella

Although *Shigella flexneri* was first reported as a common infection amongst homosexuals living in major urban centers of the United States,[102–104] the true incidence in this population remains unknown. Forty percent of asymptomatic homosexual men have at least one enteric pathogen, of which *Shigella* is the most common.[92] Furthermore, 30 to 50% of shigellosis in major American cities are within the homosexual population.[103–105] Sexual transmission is by direct or indirect fecooral contamination, and the organism is highly contagious.[34] Infection is characterized by a sudden onset of nausea, abdominal cramps, pyrexia, and bloody diarrhea.[106] Sigmoidoscopy reveals a diffuse hyperemia with friable mucosa and ulceration. The diagnosis is confirmed by stool culture. Rehydration, with intravenous fluids if required, is an important part of the treatment. Anticholinergic antidiarrheal agents should be avoided as they may exacerbate cramps, prolong bacterial shedding, and potentiate toxic megacolon.[107] The treatment of choice is either double-strength cotrimoxazole (trimethoprim 160 mg/sulphamethoxazole 800 mg) orally twice a day for 1 week, a single 1.5-g oral dose of tetracycline, or ampicillin, 500 mg orally four times a day for 1 week. Treatment should continue until cure is proven by repeated stool cultures.[34]

Campylobacter

Although the transmission of the campylobacter species by sexual means remains unproven, *Campylobacter jejuni*, *C. fetus*, and *C. intestinalis* are seen more frequently in homosexual men than in matched heterosexual controls.[34] Furthermore, *Campylobacter* has been cultured in 3% of asymptomatic homosexual men and in 6% of those with gastrointestinal symptoms.[92] Symptoms again include bloating, diarrhea, and a mucopurulent rectal discharge. Occasionally infection is associated with arthralgia, fever, and hepatosplenomegaly.[108,109] The nonspecific sigmoidoscopic findings are similar to those noted in *Shigella* infection and diagnosis is confirmed on stool culture. Most cases are self-limiting within 7 days,[108,109] but severe cases should be treated with erythromycin or tetracycline, 500 mg orally four times daily for 1 week.

ACQUIRED IMMUNODEFICIENCY SYNDROME

Incidence

In 1981, the Centers for Disease Control (CDC) in the United States reported an outbreak of *Pneumocystis carinii* pneumonia and Kaposi's sarcoma associated with an acquired immunodeficiency in young unmarried men.[110] By the end of 1981, 316 patients diagnosed with what became known as AIDS had been reported. As of March 1993, the CDC and the World Health

Organization had documented about 2.5 million cases of AIDS. There have been almost 300,000 AIDS cases in the United States and over 180,000 have died from the disease.[112]

The transmissible agent, a retrovirus, was identified first by Barré-Sinoussi and colleagues[113] and subsequently by Gallo and co-workers.[114] Initially designated as HTLV-III, it was renamed as the human immunodeficiency virus (HIV) in 1986. The CDC currently estimates that 1 in 250 persons in the United States has been infected with HIV.

In the United Kingdom, young homosexual males account for 87% of those with AIDS. In the United States, homosexual and bisexual men previously accounted for 75% of the reported cases of AIDS.[115] This percentage has decreased due to the increase amongst heterosexual patients and intravenous drug abusers.[112] Although affected men outnumber affected women nine to one, the overall proportion of women with the disease is slowly rising. The majority (71%) of AIDS cases in women are linked to intravenous drug abuse either directly or via a sexual partner.

Pathogenesis

After entering the body, HIV preferentially attacks T lymphocytes that carry the CD4 marker, eventually leading to their destruction. These lymphocytes are also known as helper T cells, and play a central role in cell-mediated immunity as well as a facilitative role in humoral immunity. Infection results not only in a decrease in their number but also in a decrease in their ability to recognize antigens. Macrophages also become less responsive, and B-cells produce fewer specific antibodies. These changes render the patient increasingly susceptible to infections and tumor development.

Transmission

HIV is transmitted via direct contact with infected body fluids of which blood, semen, and vaginal secretions have the highest concentration of the virus. Direct inoculation into the bloodstream via infected needles or blood products is the most efficient method of transmission. A single act of sexual intercourse with an infected partner carries a 1% probability of becoming infected. Different sexual acts carry different degrees of risk; anal receptive intercourse with ejaculation has the highest risk. The rectal mucosa is fragile and has an excellent blood supply. Small tears during intercourse may allow direct transmission of the virus into the blood stream. Unprotected vaginal sex is also a high-risk activity. Sexually transmitted diseases, such as syphilis, HPV, and chancroid, which result in open sores, will facilitate the transmission of the disease.

Natural History

Infection with HIV is usually accompanied by a short viral-like illness lasting 3 to 14 days. Some patients will then remain healthy for many years, as HIV has a long latency period, in common with other viruses of the lentivirus subgroup of retroviruses. Stress, poor nutrition, drug abuse, and other sexually transmitted diseases may act as cofactors to accelerate the onset of the disease. When symptoms from HIV infection eventually appear, they are similar to many other common viral illnesses.

Sexual Practices Associated with Increased Risk of Infection with HIV

Highest Risk Factors

Contact with infected sperm or blood

Receptive anal intercourse (especially with ejaculation)

Receptive vaginal intercourse (especially with ejaculation)

Fellatio involving contact with semen

Moderate/Significant Risk Factors

Insertive anal intercourse

Insertive vaginal intercourse

Brachloproctive eroticism

Use of enemas/rectal douches

Use of sexual devices

Oroanal contact

Fellatio without contact with semen

Lesser Risk Factors

Contact with urine

Mutual masturbation with ejaculation on partner

''Deep kissing''

Cunnilingus

Adapted from Glasel,[203] with permission.

However the resultant pyrexia, malaise, weight loss, night sweats, and lymphadenopathy do not resolve.

Diagnosis

HIV infection cannot be detected until antibodies to it have been produced by the body's immune system, a process known as seroconversion. Although this usually occurs within 2 to 6 weeks of initial exposure,[116,117] some early studies indicated that 5% of patients had not seroconverted by 6 months.[118,119] HIV antibody tests of greater sensitivity have demonstrated that such delayed seroconversion is unlikely.[120,121] Approximately 95% of patients will have an enzyme-lined immunosorbent assay (ELISA) against HIV antibody as the initial screening test. If a positive result is obtained, it is repeated and positivity confirmed by Western blotting. In combination these tests are 99% specific and sensitive.[122]

Prior to 1992 a diagnosis of AIDS was only made in those HIV-infected individuals who developed one or more indicator conditions specified by the CDC. This list initially contained only the most common clinical conditions associated with end-stage disease, such as *Pneumocystis carinii* pneumonia. However, as experience has grown, the catalogue of indicator conditions has expanded considerably. In 1993, the CDC also expanded the definition of AIDS to include those asymptomatic patients with a CD4 count above 200, indicating the importance of CD4 monitoring in the staging and management of the dis-

AIDS Indicator Conditions in the 1993 AIDS Surveillance Case Definition

Candidiasis of bronchi, trachea, or lung

Candidiasis, esophageal

Cervical cancer, invasive

Coccidiololdomycosis, disseminated of extrapulmonary

Cryptococcosis, extrapulmonary

Crytoposporidiosis, chronic intestinal (>1 month duration)

Cytomegalovirus disease (other than liver, spleen, or nodes)

Cytomegalovirus retinitis (with loss of vision)

Encephalopathy, HIV related

Herpes simplex, chronic ulcers (>1 month duration), or bronchitis, pneumonitis, or esophagitis

Histoplasmosis, disseminated or extrapulmonary

Isosporiasis, chronic, intestinal (>1 month duration)

Kaposi's sarcoma

Lymphoma, Burkitt's (or equivalent term)

Lymphoma, immunoblastic (or equivalent term)

Lymphoma, primary, of brain

Mycobacterium avium complex or M. kansasii, disseminated or extrapulmonary

Mycobacterium tuberculosis, any site (pulmonary or extrapulmonary)

Mycobacterium, other species or unidentified species, disseminated or extrapulmonary

Pneumocystis carinii pneumonia

Pneumonia, recurrent

Progressive multifocal leukoencephalopathy

Salmonella septicemia, recurrent

Toxoplasmosis of the brain

Wasting syndrome due to HIV

Adapted from Centers for Disease Control.[202]

ease. The new classification system is based on three clinical categories and the three CD4 cell ranges, resulting in a matrix of nine mutually exclusive categories (Table 15-4).

Prevalence of Colorectal Disease

High-risk homosexual males and AIDS patients regularly present to colorectal surgeons, as the lower gastrointestinal tract is the most frequently affected system in these patients.[58,123,124] In a study by Wexner et al.,[125] 34% of patients with AIDS had an anorectal condition during the course of their illness. Others have reported similar figures.[126–129] As a consequence, colorectal surgeons can be the first physicians to see patients, often before the diagnosis of AIDS is confirmed.[125] Homosexual men have the highest incidence of AIDS in Western countries. This cohort of patients is prone to develop opportunistic infections, viral infections, and tumors of the colorectum, not encountered in other patients.[130]

The reason for the increased risk of colorectal disease in homosexual and bisexual men with AIDS is unknown. The intestinal mucosa of these patients is known to contain decreased numbers of CD4 cells and increased numbers of suppressor T cells (CD8).[131] In addition there is some evidence that sperm alloantigens are the direct cause of this immune dysregulation.[132] Thus anoreceptive intercourse may not only predispose these patients to HIV infection but also to the colorectal manifestations of AIDS.

MYCOBACTERIUM AVIUM-INTRACELLULARE

Infection with the opportunistic organism *Mycobacterium avium-intracellulare* (MAI) has become more common with the onset of the AIDS epidemic. Furthermore, infected patients may remain in an asymptomatic carrier state, providing increased opportunity for transmission.

Clinical Features

Some patients may present with profuse watery diarrhea, dehydration, malabsorbtion, and severe abdominal pain. Other presentations include the presence of an abdominal mass due to infected nodes or psoas abscess,[124,133] obstruction,[134–136] perianal sepsis, or ulceration.[137] Purified protein derivative skin testing is positive in only 10 to 40% of cases, as these patients are predominately anergic.[106,133]

Radiographic evaluation of the small bowel and colon may easily be confused with Crohn's disease.[138] The diagnosis is often confirmed by colonoscopic ileal or colonic biopsy. Biopsy samples should be stained for acid-fast bacilli. The typical histologic features include macrophages filled with acid-fast mycobacteria[139] and blunted villi, shortened and widened by histiocyte infiltration. Granuloma formation is rare due to the absence of cell mediated immunity.[140]

Treatment

Medical treatment is usually disappointing as these organisms are often resistant to standard antituberculous therapy. Newer agents such as macrolide antibiotics, quinolones, and amikacin may eventually prove to be of benefit.[141,142]

CYTOMEGALOVIRUS

Cytomegalovirus (CMV) is endemic within the male homosexual population; 94% to 100% of healthy patients are seropositive.[143,144] Indeed, disseminated CMV has been noted at autopsy in 90% of AIDS victims.[97] CMV ileocolitis is the most common intestinal infection in AIDS patients, occurring in at least 10%.[145] Furthermore, CMV infection of the gastrointestinal tract is the initial manifestation that leads to the diagnosis of AIDS in 25% to 63% of patients.[146,147]

Clinical Features

Although CMV infection has been demonstrated in almost every organ, it does not always equate with symptoms. Proctocolitis however presents with diarrhea, fever, weight loss and

Table 15-4.   1993 Revised Classification System for HIV Infection for Adolescents and Adults[a]

CD4 + T-Cell Categories	(A) Asymptomatic Acute (Primary) HIV or Persistent Generalised Lymphadenopathy	(B) Symptomatic, Not A or C	(C) AIDS-Indicator Conditions
(1) >500	A1	B1	C1
(2) 200–499	A2	B2	C2
(3) <200	A3	B3	C3

[a] As of January 1, 1993 categories A3, B3, C1, C2, and C3 are reportable as AIDS.
Adapted from Centers for Disease Control.[202]

sometimes rectal bleeding.[148] The vasculitis caused by CMV infection may result in acute or chronic blood loss secondary to ulceration. Transmural infarction may cause perforation.

Diagnosis

Endoscopy reveals erythema, diffuse mucosal ulceration of varying degrees, and submucosal hemorrhage. The barium enema findings of diffuse or linear ulceration, granularity, skip lesions, and thumb-printing are nonspecific and can be confused with the appearances of Crohn's disease, ulcerative colitis, or ischemic colitis.[148,149] The diagnosis is confirmed histologically. Biopsies should be taken from multiple sites because of the multifocal nature of the ulceration.[150] Cecal biopsies have the highest diagnostic yield[146,147] and the overall sensitivity rate is 92%.[149] Histologic examination may reveal vasculitis, neutrophil infiltration, and large basophilic inclusion bodies that are pathognomonic of the disease. Granular cytoplasmic inclusions may also be seen (Fig. 15-7). Viral culture of the specimen may show the presence of CMV but is not specific for active infection.

Treatment

CMV proctocolitis often causes life-threatening hemorrhage or perforation requiring surgery. The results of surgery in this setting are poor. Wexner et al.[127] reported a 90% postoperative morbidity and a 30-day mortality rate of 71% in 7 patients who underwent emergent resection. Similar results have subsequently been reported by others.[151] As a metachronous perforation or bleed is not uncommon, and the risk of anastomotic dehiscence is high, subtotal colectomy with end ileostomy is the operation of choice.

Less severely ill patients, medically treated with 9-(1,3-dihydroxy-2-propoxynethyl) guanine (gancyclovir) or phosphonoformate (foscarnet) may have response rates as high as 85%, although cure is not possible.[145] Myeleosuppression, neutropenia, and thrombocytopenia may all result from treatment. Fur-

Figure 15-7.   Intranuclear inclusion bodies diagnostic of CMV infection. (From Wexner,[205] with permission.)

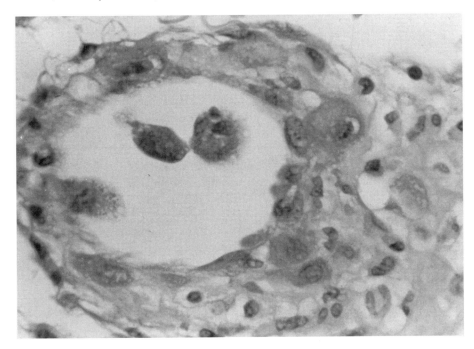

thermore, as these agents are only administered intravenously, usually via a permanent indwelling catheter, life-long maintenance treatment is required.[145] Careful counseling as to the benefits or otherwise of medication should be undertaken prior to commencement of therapy.

KAPOSI'S SARCOMA

Kaposi's sarcoma (KS) is the most common malignant tumor in patients with AIDS.[58] This endothelial tumor until recently was found almost exclusively in elderly Mediterranean males where it has a relatively benign course. In contrast to the 10 or 15 to 1 male to female ratio seen in this classic variant, AIDS-associated KS occurs with a male to female ratio of 50 to 1, most commonly in patients aged between 20 and 40 years.[152,153] Among homosexual and bisexual men with AIDS, 43% have KS,[154] which indeed is often the condition that leads to the diagnosis of the underlying syndrome.[147]

Clinical Features

This endothelial tumor may involve skin, mucosal surfaces, lymph nodes, or visceral organs.[155,156] Indeed, 25 to 75% of all AIDS patients have disseminated KS.[157-159] Gastrointestinal lesions may develop anywhere between mouth and anus but are more common in the upper alimentary tract than in the colon. They are usually asymptomatic but may present with bleeding, obstruction, perforation, or a protein-losing enteropathy.[160,161] Rectal KS may present with diarrhea, tenesmus, and bleeding[162] and patients often have other associated anorectal conditions.

At endoscopy, lesions are raised, round, sessile, red nodules ranging between 2 mm and 2 cm in diameter with the larger lesions having central umbilication (Fig. 15-8). The color is due to extravasated blood cells and hemosiderin deposits. In addition to this macular form, they may appear as submucosal ecchymoses or granulation tissue (Fig. 15-9). Due to the submucosal nature of the lesion, histopathologic confirmation of the diagnosis is often difficult.[140,158] Superficial biopsy is unhelpful,[159] and the use of an 8-mm biopsy forceps is recommended.[158,159] If a biopsy of sufficient depth is obtained, histology reveals spindle-shaped cells with central hemorrhage, extravasated red blood cells, and hemosiderin-laden macrophages.[158,163]

Radiographically, intestinal KS may be difficult to distinguish from Crohn's disease or adenocarcinoma because of the presence of plaques, nodules, strictures, and skip areas.

Treatment

Chemotherapy with single and multiple agents, radiation, and interferon have been disappointing.[164-167] However, with the exception of pulmonary KS, these lesions are rarely the immediate cause of death.[159,168,169] Gastrointestinal KS is a strong indication of a poor prognosis,[158] especially in the presence of a coexistent opportunistic infection. Patients with KS who do not have an opportunistic infection have an 80% 28-month survival whereas those with coexistent infection have a 20% 28-month survival.[170]

Surgical intervention is only indicated for complications. Resection should be limited to the diseased segment.

NON-HODGKIN'S LYMPHOMA

HIV patients have an increased incidence of malignant lymphomas. Although Hodgkin's lymphoma of the rectum has been noted in patients with AIDS, the majority of intestinal lym-

Figure 15-8. Nodular colorectal Kaposi's sarcoma. (From Wexner,[205] with permission.)

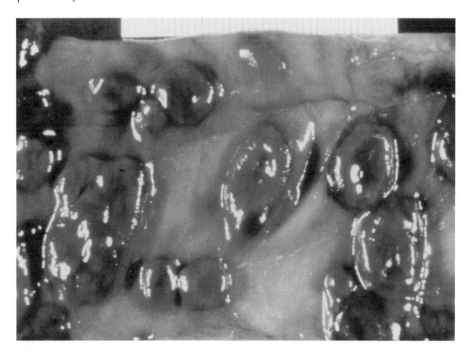

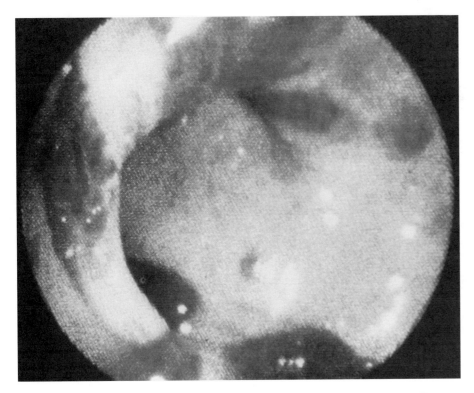

Figure 15-9. Colonic Kaposi's sarcoma presenting as submucosal ecchymoses. (From Wexner and Beck,[153] with permission.)

phomas in these patients are of the non-Hodgkin's variety.[171,172] Indeed, there is a considerable increase in the incidence of malignant non-Hodgkin's lymphoma in patients with AIDS,[173,174] of which the majority are high-grade B-cell lesions.[126,173] Impaired immunologic surveillance due to depression of the CD4 lymphocyte population is thought to play a causative role in their development,[175] and the Epstein-Barr virus has been implicated.[176] These tumors tend to be extranodular and aggressive in AIDS patients. In the gastrointestinal tract, the stomach is most frequently affected, with the rectum the next most common site.[172,173]

Clinical Features

Anorectal lymphomas often present with fever, tenesmus, and perirectal pain and thus are frequently misdiagnosed as perirectal abscesses.[177] Examination may reveal some erythema or induration in the perirectal area and patients are normally taken to the operating room for examination under anesthesia (Fig. 15-10). The presence of a mass mandates biopsy.

Gastrointestinal tract lymphomas may present as an abdominal mass, lower gastrointestinal hemorrhage, or obstruction.[136,151]

Treatment

These patients can be treated with combined chemotherapy,[173] often making surgery unnecessary.[126] One significant proviso, however, is that medical treatment may exacerbate the immunosuppression and advance the underlying disease state. Median survival is generally less than 12 months.[172,174] Surgical resection is aimed at removal of the tumor with adequate tumor-free margins. The decision to restore continuity should be made on an individual patient basis.

ANAL MALIGNANCIES

An increase in the incidence of cloagenic, squamous, and in situ carcinomas in homosexual and bisexual men, and especially in AIDS patients, has been noted by several authors.[77,178–181] Some authors have postulated that repeated anoreceptive intercourse is of itself a significant risk factor.[182,183] Others postulate that the transition from condylomata acuminatum to anal intraepithelial neoplasia (AIN) is analogous to that seen in the cervix in response to HPV infection.[184–187] This postulate is supported by the association between anal HPV infection and the presence of AIN[186] and squamous cell carcinoma.[188]

Clinical Features

In patients presenting with condylomata or other atypical mucosal lesions, biopsy is mandatory to confirm the diagnosis (Fig. 15-11). The most common site of atypia is the junction of the anal transitional zone and the rectal mucosa.[181] Diagnosis is confirmed histologically. Culture frequently reveals the presence of HPV 16 or 18,[188] but this is not required for confirmation of the diagnosis. The treatment of AIN remains controversial as the natural history of this condition is still unknown.[189] Furthermore, the use of cytology as a screening tool for the detection of AIN in high-risk populations has not been validated.[189]

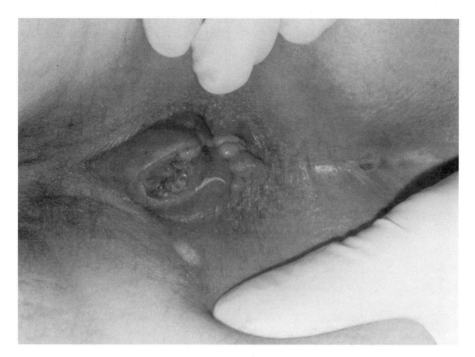

Figure 15-10. Perianal lymphoma often presents as a tender, indurated mass. (From Schmitt et al.,[194] with permission.)

Treatment

The currently excepted regime for the treatment of squamous cell carcinoma in the asymptomatic, HIV seropositive patient is one of combined chemotherapy and radiotherapy.[190] However, patients with advanced disease have already a poor prognosis and may not tolerate this treatment.

ANAL ULCERS

Many of the disease processes described so far may initially present as ulcers of the anorectum in patients with AIDS. Furthermore, many nonsexually transmitted conditions also occur, simple anal fissures being the commonest ulcerative process seen in these patients.[137] In addition to the conditions already

Figure 15-11. Florid condylomata acuminata with extensive carcinoma in situ lining large abscess cavity. (From Wexner et al.,[125] with permission.)

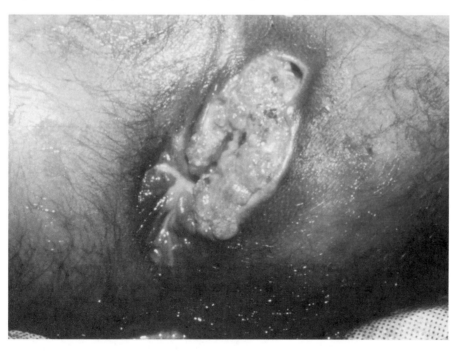

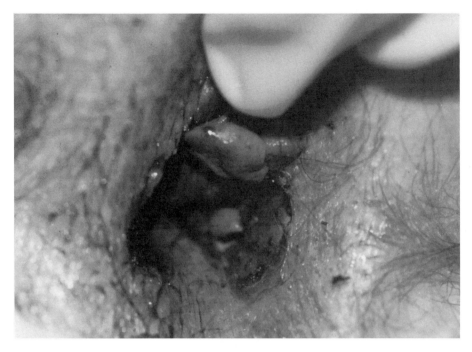

Figure 15-12. HIV-positive ulcer, posteriorly placed but wider and longer than a benign fissure.

Etiologies of Perianal Ulcers in HIV-Seropositive Patients

Benign

Fissure

Syphilis

Chancroid

Chlamydia

Lymphogranuloma venereum

Traumatic

Cytomegalovirus

Herpes simplex virus

Cryptococcus neoformans

Mycobacterium avium-intracellulare

Human immunodeficiency virus

Idiopathic

Malignant

Lymphoma

Kaposi's sarcoma

Squamous cell carcinoma

From Wexner,[204] with permission.

discussed, AIDS-specific ulcers also occur. No specific pathogen has been implicated in their etiology, but HIV particles and HPV 16 and 18 are often present.[137] These ulcers are longer and wider than benign fissures and are very erosive. They tend to be single, posteriorly placed, and occur more proximally in the anal canal (Fig. 15-12). Patients present with pain and pressure from retained pus and stool within the fissure. Operative debridement and intralesional depot steroid injection will relieve symptoms in the majority of patients.[137]

RISKS OF SURGERY IN AIDS PATIENTS

Risks of Anorectal Operations in AIDS Patients

Most anorectal operations in patients with HIV are relatively minor such as incision and drainage of small abscesses, transrectal biopsies, hemorrhoidectomy, sphincterotomy, and operations for fistula-in-ano. However, despite the relatively minor nature of these procedures, wound healing is a major problem.[125,191] Recently Consten and colleagues[192] have reported considerable improvement in symptoms in patients who had anal ulcers excised in combination with a mucosal advancement flap. Furthermore, because of the anal hypotonia often seen in homosexual patients,[193] sphincterotomy for fissure is often associated with the development of incontinence.[125,191] Preoperative manometry is useful in identifying those patients in whom sphincterotomy can be safely performed.[194]

The outcome of this operation in terms of morbidity, mortality, and recurrence is somewhat unpredictable. Some authors have stated that diminished numbers of CD4 cells do not reduce rates of wound healing[195] and should not be used as a reason to avoid surgery.[137] However, others have documented a correlation between reduced CD4 counts and decreased rates of wound healing and poorer prognosis.[196]

Risks of Intestinal Resections in AIDS Patients

Mortality and morbidity from intestinal resection in AIDS patients depends on the underlying pathology. The most common pathogen to cause complications requiring bowel resection is CMV. However, the results of emergent subtotal colectomy are poor, with up to a 71% 30-day mortality.[127] In general patients undergoing elective procedures have a better outcome than those who are operated on as an emergency. In general septic sequelae and death occur most frequently after anastomosis rather than diversion. The fashioning of a stoma is therefore recommended in all but the least severely immunocompromised patients.

Risks to Health Care Workers

The increased incidence of HIV infection means that surgeons and health care workers are not only exposed to patients suffering from the complications of AIDS, but also are called upon to treat those HIV-seropositive individuals who have not yet been diagnosed. However, the risk of transmission of HIV to health care workers is small. By February 1993, 32 health care workers in the United States were regarded by the CDC as having documented occupational transmission of HIV, 88% of whom had percutaneous exposure. Pooled data from 21 studies estimate that the risk associated with occupational exposure to HIV via percutaneous injury to be 0.2%. The CDC and several other organizations representing the interests of health care workers have recommended the adoption of what has become known as "universal precautions" for routine patient contact and additional protective measures for invasive procedures.[197-199] "Universal precautions" recommend the use of routine hand washing and the use of gowns, gloves, and masks when appropriate to prevent contamination of the skin or mucous membranes with bodily fluids, and the use of goggles to protect the eyes on occasions where splashing of bodily fluids is a potential hazard. These precautions also contain recommendations for the safe disposal of sharp objects and the correct cleansing of surfaces or equipment that have been in contact with bodily fluids.

Surgical procedures performed on known HIV-seropositive patients expose health care workers to increased risks. The use of waterproof gowns, goggles, and double gloving has been recommended.[200] Furthermore, to minimize the risk of inadvertent needle puncture, only the minimum number of experienced personnel required to safely complete the procedure should be present. Special filter masks should be worn to prevent inhalation of aerosolized particles that can be produced by the use of electrocautery or laser.

REFERENCES

1. Old Testament. Genesis 19:5
2. Wilcox RR (1981) The rectum as viewed by the venereologist. Br J Venereal Dis 57:1–6
3. Kinsey AC, Pomeroy WB, Martin LE (1948) pp. 650–651. In Sexual Behavior in the Human Male. WB Saunders, Philadelphia
4. Ostrow DG (1990) Homosexual behaviour and sexually transmitted diseases. pp. 61–69. In Holmes KK, Mårdh PA, Sparling PF, Wiesner PJ (eds): Sexually Transmitted Diseases. 2nd Ed. McGraw-Hill, New York
5. Kinsey AC, Pomeroy WB, Martin LE (1948) p. 610. In Sexual Behavior in the Human Male. WB Saunders, Philadelphia
6. Darrow WW, Barrett D, Jay K, Young A (1981) The gay report on sexually transmitted diseases. Am J Public Health 71:1004–1011
7. William DC (1980) The sexual transmission of parasitic infections in gay men. J Homosexuality 5:219–294
8. Filipe EV, Strauss SB, Beck EJ et al (1995) Sexual behaviour among London GUM clinic attenders: implications for HIV education. Int J STD AIDS 5:346–352
9. Sohn N, Robilotti JG (1977) The gay bowel syndrome: a review of colonic and rectal conditions in 200 male homosexuals. Am J Gastroenterol 67:478–483
10. Bolling DR (1977) Prevalence, goals and complications of heterosexual anal intercourse in a gynecological population. J Reprod Med 19:120–124
11. Kazal HL, Sohn N, Carrasco JI et al (1976) The gay bowel syndrome: clinicopathologic correlation in 260 cases. Ann Clin Lab Sci 6:184–192
12. Janda WM, Bonhoff M, Morgello JA, Lerner SA (1980) Prevalence and site-pathogen studies of *Neisseria meningitides* and *Neisseria gonohorrea* in homosexual men. JAMA 244:2060–2064
13. Baker RW, Peppercorn MA (1983) Gastrointestinal ailments of homosexual men. Medicine 61:390–405
14. British Cooperative Clinical Group (1973) Homosexuality and venereal disease in the United Kingdom. Br J Venereal Dis 49:329
15. Schmale JD, Martin JE, Domescik G (1969) Observations on the culture diagnosis of gonorrhoea in women. JAMA 210:312–314
16. Barlow D, Phillips I (1978) Gonorrhoea in women. Diagnostic, clinical and laboratory aspects. Lancet 1:761–764
17. Thin RN, Shaw EJ (1979) Diagnosis of gonorrhoea in women. Br J Venereal Dis 55:10–13
18. Klein EJ, Fisher LS, Chow AW, Guze ZB (1977) Anorectal gonococcal infections. Ann Int Med 86:340–346
19. Stansfield VA (1980) Diagnosis and management of anorectal gonorrhoea in women. Br J Venereal Dis 56:319–321
20. Judson FN (1983) Fear of AIDS and gonorrhoea rates in homosexual men. Lancet 2:159–160
21. Handsfield HH (1985) Decreasing incidence of gonorrhoea in homosexually active men—minimal effect on risk of AIDS. West J Med 143:469–470
22. Van den Hock JAR, van Galensens GJP, Continho RA (1990) Increase in unsafe homosexual behaviour. Lancet 2:179–180
23. Hunt AJ, Davies PM, Weatherburn P et al (1991) Changes in sexual behaviour in a large cohort of homosexual men in England and Wales 1988–1989. Br Med J 302:505–506
24. Kinghorn GR, Rashid S (1979) Prevalance of rectal and pha-

ryngeal infection in women with gonorrhoea in Sheffield. Br J Venereal Dis 55:408–410

25. Robbins RD, Sohn N, Weinstein MA (1983) Colorectal view of venereal disease. NY State J Med 47:323–327

26. Danielsson D, Johannisson G (1973) Culture diagnosis of gonorrhoea: a comparison of the yield with selective and non-selective gonococcal culture media inocculated in the clinic after transport of specimens. Acta Derm Venereol (Stockh) 53:75–80

27. Deherogada P (1977) Diagnosis of rectal gonorrhoea by blind anorectal swabs compared with direct vision swabs taken via proctoscope. Br J Venereal Dis 53:311–313

28. Daniel DC, Felman YM, Riccardi NB (1981) The utility of anoscopy in the rapid diagnosis of symptomatic anorectal gonorrhoea in men. Sex Transm Dis 8:16–17

29. Fluker JL, Deherogoda P, Platt DJ, Gerken A (1980) Rectal gonorrhoea in male homosexuals: presentation and therapy. Br J Venereal Dis 56:397–399

30. Centers for Disease Control (1987) Antibiotic-resistant strains of *Neisseria gonorrhoeae*: policy guidelines for detection, management and control. MMWR 36(suppl 5):1–18

31. Thin RN (1990) Early syphilis in the adult. pp. 221–230. In Holmes KK, Mårdh PA, Sparling PF, Wiesner PJ (eds): Sexually Transmitted Diseases. 2nd Ed. McGraw-Hill, New York

32. British Cooperative Clinical Group (1980) Homosexuality and venereal disease in the United Kingdom: a second study. Br J Venereal Dis 56:6–11

33. Catterall RD (1975) Sexually transmitted diseases of the anus and rectum. Clin Gastroenterol 4:659–669

34. Knapp JS, Zenilman JM, Thompson SE (1990) Gonorrhoea. pp. 512–522. In Morse SA, Moreland AA, Thompson SE (eds): Sexually Transmitted Diseases. JB Lippincott, Philadelphia

35. Goligher JC (1985) Sexually transmitted diseases. pp. 1033–1045. In Goligher JC (ed): Diseases of the Anus, Rectum and Colon, 5th Ed. Balliere-Tyndall, London

36. Hughes E, Cutherbertson AM, Killingback MK (1983) Venereal diseases of the anal canal and rectum. pp. 203–208. In Colorectal Surgery. Churchill Livingston, New York

37. Samenius B (1968) Primary syphillis of the anorectal region. Dis Colon Rectum 11:462–466

38. Akdamarr K, Martin RJ, Ichinase H (1977) Syphilitic proctitis. Dig Dis 22:701–704

39. Hart G (1986) Syphilis tests in diagnostic and therapeutic decision making. Ann Intern Med 104:368–376

40. Ronald AR, Albritton W (1990) Chancroid and *Haemophilus ducreyi*. pp. 263–271. In Holmes KK, Mårdh PA, Sparling PF, Wiesner PJ (eds): Sexually Transmitted Diseases. 2nd Ed. McGraw-Hill, New York

41. Holmes K (1981) The chlamydia epidemic. JAMA 245:1718–1723

42. Mc Millan A, Sommerville RG, McKee PMK (1981) Chlamydial infections in homosexual men: frequency of isolation of *Chlamydia trachomatis* from the urethra, anorectum and pharynx. Br J Venereal Dis 57:47–49

43. Quinn TC, Goodell SE, Mkrtichian EE et al (1981) *Chlamydia trachomatis* proctitis. N Engl J Med 305:195–200

44. Levine JS, Smith PD, Brugge WR (1980) Chronic proctitis

in male homosexuals due to lymphogranuloma venereum. Gastroenterology 79:563–565

45. Wang SP, Grayston JT, Alexander ER, Holmes KK (1975) A simplified microimmunofluorescent test with trachoma-lympho-granuloma venereum (*Chlamydia trachomatis*) antigen for use as a screening test for antibody. J Clin Microbiol 1:250–255

46. Handsfield HH (1982) Sexually transmitted disease. Hosp Pract 17:99–116

47. Perine PL, Osoba AO (1990) Lymphogranuloma venereum. pp. 195–204. In Holmes KK, Mårdh PA, Sparling PF, Wiesner PJ (eds): Sexually Transmitted Diseases. 2nd Ed. McGraw-Hill, New York

48. Goldmeier D (1979) Herpetic proctitis and sacral radiculomyelopathy in homosexual men. Br Med J 2:549

49. Corey L (1982) The diagnosis and treatment of genital herpes. JAMA 246:1041–1049

50. Goldmeier D (1980) Proctitis and herpes simplex virus in homosexual men. Br J Venereal Dis 56:111–114

51. Quinn TC, Corey L, Chaffee RG et al (1981) The etiology of anorectal infections in homosexual men. Am J Med 71:395–406

52. Goodell SE, Quinn TC, Mkrtichian E et al (1983) Herpes simplex virus proctitis in homosexual men: clinical, sigmoidoscopic and histopathological features. N Engl J Med 308:868–871

53. Nerurkar L, Goedert J, Wallen W et al (1983) Study of antiviral antibodies in sera of homosexual men. Fed Proc 42:6109

54. Jacobs E (1976) Anal infections caused by herpes simplex virus. Dis Colon Rectum 19:151–157

55. Wexner SD, Dailey TH (1986) Pruritis ani: diagnosis and management. Curr Concepts Skin Care 7:5–9

56. Samarasinghe PL, Oates JK, MacLennan IPB (1979) Herpetic proctitis and sacral radiculomyelopathy—a hazard for homosexual men. Br Med J 2:365–366

57. Baringer JR (1974) Recovery of herpes simplex virus from human sacral ganglions. N Engl J Med 291:828–830

58. Rotterdam H, Sommers SC (1985) Alimentary tract biopsy lesions in the acquired immune deficiency syndrome. Pathology 17:181–192

59. Rompalo AM, Mertz GJ, Davis LG et al (1988) Oral acyclovir for treatment of first-episode herpes simplex virus proctitis. JAMA 259:2879–2881

60. Whitely RJ, Levin M, Barton N et al (1984) Infections caused by herpes simplex virus in the immunocompromised host: natural history and topical acyclovir therapy. J Infect Dis 150:323–329

61. Mertz GJ, Jones CC, Mills J et al (1988) Long-term acyclovir suppression of frequently recurring genital herpes simplex virus infection. JAMA 1988:201–206

62. Douglas JM, Critchlow C, Benedetti et al (1984) A double-blind study of oral acyclovir for suppression of recurrences of genital herpes simplex virus infection. N Engl J Med 310:1551–1556

63. Straus SE, Takiff HE, Seidlin M et al (1984) Suppression of frequently recurring genital herpes. A placebo-controlled double-blind trial of oral acyclovir. N Engl J Med 310:1545–1550

64. Chatis PA, Miller CH, Schrager LE, Crumpacker CS (1989)

Successful treatment with foscarnet of an acyclovir-resistant mucocutaneous infection with herpes simplex virus in a patient with acquired immunodeficiency syndrome. N Engl J Med 320:297–300

65. Erlich KS, Mills J, Chatis P et al (1989) Acyclovir-resistant herpes simplex virus infections in patients with the acquired immunodeficiency syndrome. N Engl J Med 320:293–296

66. Wexner SD (1989) Treatment of AIDS patients with herpes simplex virus infections resistant to acyclovir. Colon Rectal Surg Outlook 2:1–2

67. Palmer JG, Shepherd NA, Jass JR et al (1987) Human papilloma virus type 16 DNA in anal squamous cell carcinoma. Lancet 2:42

68. Rudlinger R, Buchmann P (1989) HPV-16 positive Bowenoid papulosis and squamous cell carcinoma of the anus in an HIV-positive man. Dis Colon Rectum 32:1042–1045

69. Wexner SD (1990) Managing common anorectal sexually transmitted diseases. Infect Surg 9–48

70. Centers for Disease Control (1983) Condyloma acuminata: United States, 1966–1981: current trends. MMWR 32: 306–308

71. Car G, William DC (1977) Anal warts in a population of gay men in new York City. Sex Transm Dis 4:56–57

72. Schlappner OLA, Shaffer FA (1978) Anorectal condylomata acuminata: a missed part of the condylomata spectrum. Can Med Assoc J 118:172–173

73. Abcarian H, Sharon N (1977) The effectiveness of immunotherapy in the treatment of anal condyloma acuminatum. J Surg Res 22:231–236

74. Wexner SD (1990) Sexually transmitted diseases of the colon, rectum and anus. The challenge of the nineties. Dis Colon Rectum 33:1048–1062

75. Tessler AN, Applebaum SM (1982) The Busche-Loewenstein tumor. Urology 20:36–39

76. Connors RC, Ackerman AB (1976) Histologic pseudomalignancies of the skin. Arch Dermatol 112:1767–1780

77. Wexner SD, Milsom JW, Dailey TH (1987) The demographics of anal cancers are changing: identification of a high-risk population. Dis Colon Rectum 30:942–946

78. Jensen SL (1985) Comparison of podophyllin application with simple surgical excision in clearance and recurrence of perianal condyloma acuminatum. Lancet 2:1146–1148

79. Swerdlow DB, Salvati EP (1971) Condyloma acuminatum. Dis Colon Rectum 14:226–231

80. Billingham RP, Lewis FG (1982) Laser versus electrical cautery in the treatment of condylomata acuminata of the anus. Surg Gynecol Obstet 155:865–867

81. Abcarian H, Smith D, Sharon N (1976) The immunotherapy of anal condyloma acuminatum. Dis Colon Rectum 19: 237–244

82. Wiltz OH, Torregrosa M, Wiltz O (1995) Autogenous vaccine: the best therapy for perianal condyloma acuminata? Dis Colon Rectum 38:838–841

83. Abcarian H, Sharon N (1982) Long-term effectiveness of the immunotherapy of anal condyloma acuminatum. Dis Colon Rectum 25:648–651

84. Eftaiha MS, Amshel AL, Shonberg IL, Batshon B (1982) Giant and recurrent condyloma acuminata: appraisal of immunotherapy. Dis Colon Rectum 25:136–138

85. Schonfeld A, Schattner A, Crespi M et al (1984) Intramuscular human interferon β injections in treatmetn of condylomata acuminata. Lancet 1:1038–1042

86. Olmos L, Vilata J, Rodriguez Pichardo A et al (1994) Double-blind randomized clinical trial on the effect of interferon-beta in the treatment of condylomata acuminata. Int J STD AIDS 5:182–185

87. Reichman RC, Oakes D, Bonnez W et al (1988) Treatment of condyloma acuminatum with three different interferons administered intralesionally. A double-blind placebo-controlled trial. Ann Intern Med 108:675–679

88. Most H (1968) Manhattan: "A tropic isle?" Am J Trop Med Hyg 17:333–354

89. Dritz SK, Ainsworth TE, Back A (1977) Patterns of sexually transmitted enteric diseases in a city. Lancet 2:3–4

90. McMillan A (1978) Thread worms in homosexual males. Br Med J 1:367

91. Burnham WR, Reeve RS, Finch RG (1980) *Entamoeba histolytica* infection in male homosexuals. Gut 21:1097–1099

92. Quinn TC, Stamm WE, Goodell SE et al (1983) The polymicrobial origin of intestinal infections in homosexual men. N Engl J Med 309:576–582

93. William DC, Shookhoff HM, Felman YM, DeRamos SW (1978) High rates of enteric protozoal infections in selected homosexual men attending a venereal disease clinic. Sex Transm Dis 5:155–157

94. Phillips SC, Mildvan D, William DC et al (1981) Sexual transmission of enteric protozoa and helminths in a venereal-disease-clinic population. N Engl J Med 305:603–606

95. Pomerantz BM, Marr JS, Goldman WD (1980) Amebiasis in New York City 1958–1978: identification of the male homosexual high risk population. Bull NY Acad Med 56:232–244

96. Ellyson JH, Bezmalinovic Z, Parks SN, Lewis FR (1986) Necrotizing amebic colitis: a frequently fatal complication. Am J Surg 152:21–26

97. Quinn TC (1985) Gastrointestinal manifestations of AIDS. Pract Gastroenterol 9:23–34

98. Soave R (1988) Cryptosporidiosis and isosporiasis in patients with AIDS. Infect Dis Clin North Am 2:485–493

99. Soave R, Danner RL, Honig CL et al (1984) Cryptosporidiosis in homosexual men. Ann Intern Med 100:504–511

100. Currant WL, Reese NC, Ernst JV et al (1985) Human cryptosporidiosis in immunocompetent and immunodeficient persons. Studies of an outbreak and experimental transmission. N Eng J Med 308:1252–1257

101. DeHovitz JA, Pape JW, Boncy M, Johnston WD (1986) Clinical manifestations and therapy of *Isopora belli* infection in patients with the acquired immunodeficiency syndrome. N Engl J Med 315:87–90

102. Dritz SK, Back AF (1974) Shigella enteritis venereally transmitted. N Engl J Med 291:1194

103. Bader M, Pedersen AH, Williams R et al (1977) Venereal transmission of shigellosis in Seattle-King County. Sex Transm Dis 4:89–91

104. Allason-Jones E, Mindel A (1987) Sex and the bowel. Int J Colorectal Dis 2:32–37

105. William DC, Felman YM, Marr JS, Shookhoff HM (1977) Sexually transmitted enteric pathogensin male homosexual populations. NY State J Med 77:2050–2052

106. Chaisson RE (1988) Infections due to encapsulated bacteria,

salmonella, shigella and campylobacter. Infect Dis Clin North Am 2:475–484

107. DuPont HL, Hornick RB (1973) Adverse effect of lomotil therapy in shigellosis. JAMA 226:1525–1528

108. Guerrant RL, Lahita RG, Winn WC, Roberts RB (1978) Campylobacteriosis in man: pathogenic mechanisms and review of 91 blood-stream infections. Am J Med 65:584–592

109. Blaser MJ, LaForce FM, Wilson NA, Wang WL (1980) Reservoirs for human campylobacteriosis. J Infect Dis 141:665–669

110. Centers for Disease Control and Prevention (1981) Kaposi sarcoma and pneumocystis pneumonia among homosexual men. New York City and California. MMWR 30:305–308

111. Centers for Disease Control and Prevention (1981) Kaposi sarcoma and pneumocystis pneumonia among homosexual men. New York City and California. MMWR 30:305–308

112. Statistics from World Health Organization and Centers for Disease Control and Prevention (1993). AIDS; 7:1287–1291

113. Barré-Sinoussi F, Chermann J-C, Rey F et al (1983) Isolation of a T-lymphotrophic retrovirus from a patient at risk for acquired immune deficiency syndrome (AIDS). Science 220:868–870

114. Gallo RC, Salahuddin SZ, Popovic M (1984) Frequent detection and isolation of cytopathic retroviruses (HTLV-III) from patients with AIDS and at risk for AIDS. Science 224:500–502

115. Centers for Disease Control (1992) HIV/AIDS surveillance report. MMWR January:1–19

116. Bowen PA, Lobel SA, Caruana RJ et al (1988) Transmission of human immunodeficiency virus (HIV) by transplantation: clinical aspects and time course analysis of viral antigenemia and antibody production. Ann Intern Med 108:46–48

117. Courouce AM, Bouchardeau F, Jullien AM (1988) Blood transfusion and human immunodeficiency virus (HIV) antigen. Ann Intern Med 108:771–772

118. Ranki A, Valle SL, Krohn M et al (1987) Long latency precedes overt seroconversion in sexually transmitted human-immunodeficiency-virus infection. Lancet 2:589–593

119. Imagawa DT, Lee MH, Wolinsky SM et al (1989) Human immunodeficiency virus type 1 infection in homosexual men who remain seronegative for prolonged periods. N Engl J Med 320:1458–1462

120. Groopman JE, Caiazzo T, Thomas MA et al (1988) Lack of evidence of prolonged human immunodeficiency virus infection before antibody seroconversion. Blood 71:1752–1754

121. Zaaijer HL, Van Excel-Oehlers P, Kraaijeveld T et al (1992) Early detection of antibodies to HIV-1 by third generation assays. Lancet 340:770–772

122. Bylund DJ, Siegner WHM, Hooper DG (1992) Review of testing for human immunodeficiency virus. Clin Lab Med 12:305–333

123. Weber JN, Thom S, Barrison I, et al (1987) Cytomegalovirus colitis and oesophageal ulceration in the context of AIDS: Clinical manifestations and preliminary report of treatment with foscarnet (phosphonoformate). Gut 28:482–487

124. Waisman J, Rotterdam H, Niedt GN et al (1987) AIDS: an overview of the pathology. Pathol Res Pract 182:729–754

125. Wexner SD, Smithy WB, Milsom JW, Dailey TH (1986) The surgical management of anorectal diseases in AIDS and pre-AIDS patients. Dis Colon Rectum 29:719–723

126. Kaplan LD (1988) AIDS-associated lymphomas. Infect Dis Clin North Am 2:525–532

127. Wexner SD, Smithy WB, Trillo C et al (1988) Emergency colectomy for cytomegalovirus ileocolitis in patients with the acquired immune deficiency syndrome. Dis Colon Rectum 31:755–761

128. Beck DE, Jaso RG, Zajac RA (1990) Proctologic management of the HIV-positive patient. South Med J 83:900–903

129. Edwards P, Wodak A, Cooper DA et al (1990) The gastrointestinal manifestations of AIDS. Aust NZ J Med 20:141–148

130. Wolkomir AF, Barone JE, Hardy HW III, Cottone FJ (1990) Abdominal and anorectal surgery and the acquired immune deficiency syndrome in heterosexual intravenous drug users. Dis Colon Rectum 33:267–270

131. Rodgers VD, Kagnoff MF (1987) Gastrointestinal manifestations of the acquired immunodeficiency syndrome. West J Med 146:57–67

132. Mavligit GM, Talpaz M, Hsia FT et al (1984) Chronic immune stimulation by sperm alloantigens. JAMA 251:237–241

133. Rosengart TK, Coppa GF (1990) Abdominal mycobacterial infections in immunocompromised patients. Am J Surg 159:125–131

134. Haddad FS, Ghossain A, Sawaya E, Nelson AR (1987) Abdominal tuberculosis. Dis Colon Rectum 30:724–735

135. Burack JH, Mandel MS, Bizer LS et al (1989) Emergency abdominal operations in the patient with acquired immunodeficiency syndrome. Arch Surg 124:285–286

136. Deziel DJ, Hyser MJ, Doolas A et al (1990) Major abdominal operations in acquired immunodeficiency syndrome. Am Surg 65:445–450

137. Gottesman L (1995) Ulcerative disease of the anorectum in AIDS. Int J STD AIDS 6:4–6

138. Radin DR (1991) Intraabdominal *Mycobacterium tuberculosis* vs. *Mycobacterium avium intracellulare* infection in patients with AIDS: distinction based on CT findings. Am J Radiol 156:487–491

139. Cello JP (1988) Gastrointestinal manifestations of AIDS. Infect Dis Clin North Am 2:387–396

140. Cone LA, Woodard DR, Potts BE et al (1986) An update on the acquired immunodeficiency syndrome (AIDS): associated disorders of the alimentary tract. Dis Colon Rectum 29:60–64

141. Chiu J, Nussbaum J, Bozzette S et al (1990) Treatment of disseminated *Mycobacterium-avium* complex infection in AIDS with amikacin, ethambutol, rifampicin and ciprofloxacin. Ann Intern Med 113:358–361

142. Rathbun RC, Martin ES III, Eaton VE, Matthew EB (1991) Current and investigational therapies for AIDS-associated *Mycobacterium-avium* complex disease. Clin Pharm 10:280–291

143. Drew WL, Mintz L, Miner RC et al (1981) Prevalence of cytomegalovirus infection in homosexual men. J Infect Dis 143:188–192

144. Lange M, Klein EB, Kornfield H et al (1984) Cytomegalovirus isolation from healthy homosexual men. JAMA 252:1908–1910

145. Drew WL, Buhles W, Erlich KS (1988) Herpes virus infec-

tions (cytomegalovirus, herpes simplex virus, varicella-zoster virus). Infect Dis Clin North Am 2:495–509

146. Hinnant KL, Roterdam HZ, Bell ET, Tapper ML (1986) Cytomegalovirus infection of the alimentary tract: a clinicopathological correlation. Am J Gastroenterol 81:944–950

147. Dieterich DT, Rahmin M (1991) Cytomegalovirus colitis in AIDS: presentation in 44 patients and a review of the literature. J Acquir Immune Defic Synd 4 (suppl 1):S29–S35

148. Frager DH, Frager JD, Wolf EL et al (1986) Cytomegalovirus colitis in acquired immune deficiency syndrome: radiologic spectrum. Gastrointest Radiol 11:241–246

149. Culpepper-Morgan JA, Kotler DP, Scholes JV, Tierney AR (1987) Evaluation of diagnostic criteria for mucosal cytomegalic inclusion disease in the acquired immune deficiency syndrome. Am J Gastroenterol 82:1264–1270

150. Frank D, Raicht RF (1984) Intestinal perforation associated with cytomegalovirus infection in patients with acquired immune deficiency syndrome. Am J Gastroenterol 79:201–205

151. Wilson SE, Robinson G, Williams RA et al (1989) Acquired immune deficiency syndrome (AIDS): indications for abdominal sugery, pathology and outcome. Ann Surg 210:428–434

152. Reynolds WS, Windelmann RK, Soule EH (1965) Kaposi's sarcoma: clinicopathologic study with particular reference to its relationship to the reticuloendothelial system. Medicine 44:419–443

153. Wexner SD, Beck DE (1992) Acquired immunodeficiency syndrome. pp. 423–439. In Beck DE, Wexner SD (eds): Fundamentals of Anorectal Surgery. McGraw Hill, New York

154. Steis RG, Longo DL (1988) Clinical, biologic, and therapeutic aspects of malignancies associated with the acquired immunodeficiency syndrome: part 1. Ann Allergy 60:310–323

155. Hymes KB, Greene JB, Marcus A et al (1981) Kaposi's sarcoma in homosexual men—report of eight cases. Lancet 2:598–600

156. Friedman-Kien AE, Laubenstein LJ, Rubstein P et al (1982) Disseminated Kaposi's sarcoma in homosexual men. Ann Intern Med 86:693–700

157. Gottlieb MS, Groopman JE, Weinstein WM et al (1983) The acquired immunodeficiency syndrome. Ann Inter Med 99:208–220

158. Friedman SL, Wright TL, Altman DF (1985) Gastrointestinal Kaposi's sarcoma in patients with acquired immunodeficiency syndrome: endoscopic and autopsy findings. Gastroenterology 89:102–108

159. Mitsuyasu RT (1988) Kaposi's sarcoma in the acquired immunodeficiency syndrome. Infect Dis Clin North Am 2:511–523

160. Perrone V, Pergola M, Abate G et al (1981) Protein-losing enteropathy in a patient with generalized Kaposi's sarcoma. Cancer 47:588–591

161. Macho JR (1988) Gastrointestinal surgery in the AIDS patient. Gastroenterol Clin North Am 17:563–571

162. Lorenz HP, Wilson W, Leigh B, Schecter WP (1990) Kaposi's sarcoma of the rectum in patients with the acquired immunodeficiency syndrome. Am J Surg 160:681–683

163. Francis ND, Parkin JM, Weber J, Boylston AW (1986) Kaposi's sarcoma in acquired immune deficiency syndrome (AIDS). J Clin Pathol 39:469–474

164. Krown SE, Real FX, Cunningham-Rundles S et al (1983) Preliminary observations on the effect of recombinant leuko-

cyte A interferon in homosexual men with Kaposi's sarcoma. N Engl J Med 308:1071–1076

165. Volberding PA, Abrams DI, Conant M et al (1985) Vinblastine therapy for Kaposi's sarcoma in the acquired immunodeficiency syndrome. Ann Intern Med 103:335–338

166. Real FX, Oettgen HF, Krown SE (1986) Kaposi's sarcoma and the acquired immunodeficiency syndrome: treatment with high and low doses of recombinant leukocyte A interferon. J Clin Oncol 4:544–551

167. Gelmann EP, Longo D, Lane HC et al (1987) Combination chemotherapy of disseminated Kaposi's sarcoma in patients with the acquired immune deficiency syndrome. Am J Med 82:456–462

168. Meduri GU, Stover DE, Lee M et al (1985) Pulmonary Kaposi's sarcoma in the acquired immune deficiency syndrome. Clinical, radiographic, and pathologic manifestations. Am J Med 81:11–18

169. Kaplan LD, Wofsy CB, Volberding PA (1987) Treatment of patients with acquired immunodeficiency syndrome and associated manifestations. JAMA 257:1367–1374

170. Krigel RL, Friedman-Kien AE (1988) Kaposi's sarcoma in AIDS: diagnosis and treatment. pp. 245–261. In DeVita VT, Hellman S, Rosenberg SA (eds): AIDS: Etiology, Diagnosis, Treatment, and Prevention. 2nd Ed. JB Lippincott, Philadelphia

171. Coonley CJ, Strauss DJ, Filippa D (1984) Hodgkin's disease presenting with rectal symptoms. Cancer Invest 2:279–284

172. Joachim HL, Cooper ML, Hellman GC (1985) Lymphoma in men at high risk for acquired immune deficiency syndrome. Cancer 56:2831–2842

173. Ziegler JL, Beckstead JA, Volberding PA et al (1984) Non-Hodgkin's lymphoma in 90 homosexual men: relation to generalized lymphadenopathy and the acquired immunodeficiency syndrome. N Engl J Med 311:565–570

174. Lowenthal DA, Safai B, Koziner B (1987) Malignant neoplasia in AIDS. Infect Surg July:413–420

175. Groopman JE, Sullivan JL, Mulder C et al (1986) Pathogenesis of B-cell lymphoma in a patient with AIDS. Blood 67:612–615

176. Ziegler JL, Drew WL, Miner RC et al (1982) Outbreak of Burkitt's-like lymphoma in homosexual men. Lancet 2:631–633

177. Kaplan LD, Abrams DI, Feigal E et al (1989) AIDS-associated non-Hodgkin's lymphoma in San Francisco. JAMA 261:719–724

178. Cooper HS, Patchefsky AS, Marks G (1979) Cloacogenic carcinoma of the anorectum in homosexual men. An observation of four cases. Dis Colon Rectum 22:557–558

179. Croxson T, Chabon AB, Rorat E, Barash IM (1984) Intraepithelial carcinoma of the anus in homosexual men. Dis Colon Rectum 27:325–330

180. Daling JR, Weiss NS, Klopfenstein LL et al (1982) Correlates of homosexual behavior and the incidence of anal cancer. JAMA 247:1988–1990

181. Nash G, Allen W, Nash S (1986) Atypical lesions of the anal mucosa in homosexual men. JAMA 256:873–876

182. Peters RK, Mack TM (1983) Patterns of anal carcinoma by gender and marital status in Los Angeles County. Br J Cancer 48:629–636

183. Peters RK, Mack TM, Berstein L (1984) Parallels in the epi-

demiology of selected anogenital carcinomas. J Nat Cancer Inst 72:609–615

184. Syrjanen KJ (1986) Human papilloma virus (HPV) infections of the female genital tract and their associations with intraepithelial neoplasia and squamous cell carcinoma. Pathol Annu 21:53–89

185. Brescia RJ, Jenson B, Lancaster WD, Kkurman RJ (1986) The role of human papilloma viruses in the pathogenesis and histologic classification of precancerous lesions of the cervix. Hum Pathol 17:552–559

186. Scholefield JM, Sonnex C, Talbot IC et al (1989) Anal and cervical intraepithelial neoplasia: possible parallel. Lancet 1: 765–769

187. Melbye M, Sprogel P (1991) Aetiological parallel between anal cancer and cervical cancer. Lancet 338:657–659

188. Palmer JG, Scholefield JH, Coates PJ et al (1989) Anal cancer and human papillomaviruses. Dis Colon Rectum 32: 1016–1022

189. Surawitz CM, Critchlow C, Sayer J et al (1995) High grade anal dysplasia in visually normal mucosa in homosexual men: seven cases. Am J Gastroenterol 90:1776–1778

190. Scholefield JH, Northover JMA, Carr ND (1990) Male homosexuality, HIV infection and colorectal surgery. Br J Surg 77: 493–496

191. Carr ND, Mercey D, Slack WW (1989) Non-condylomatous perianal disease in homosexual men. Br J Surg 76:1064–1066

192. Consten ECJ, Slors FJM, Danner SA et al (1995) Local excision and mucosal advancement for anorectal ulceration in patients infected with human immunodeficiency virus. Br J Surg 82:891–894

193. Miles AJG, Allen-Mersh TG, Wastell C (1993) Effect of anoreceptive intercourse on anorectal function. J R Soc Med 86:144–147

194. Schmitt SL, Wexner SD, Nogueras JJ, Jagelman DG (1993) Is aggressive management of perianal ulcers in homosexual HIV-seropositive men justified? Dis Colon Rectum 36: 240–246

195. Safavi A, Gottesman L, Dailey TH (1991) Anorectal surgery in the HIV+ patient: update. Dis Colon Rectum 34:299–304

196. Consten ECJ, Slors FJM, Noten HJ (1995) Anorectal surgery in human immunodeficiency virus-infected patients: clinical outcome in relation to immune status. Dis Colon Rectum 38: 1169–1175

197. Fleming DO (1987) Hazard control of infectious agents. Occup Med 2:499–510

198. Lifson AR, Rutherford GW, Jaffe HW (1988) The natural history of human immunodeficiency virus infection. J Infect Dis 158:1360–1367

199. American Academy of Orthopaedic Surgeons (1989) Recommendations for the prevention of human immunodeficiency virus (HIV) transmission in the practice of orthopaedic surgery. Report of the AAOS task force on AIDS and Orthopaedic Surgery

200. Beck DE, Wexner SD (1990) AIDS and the colorectal surgeon. Part II: anorectal disease. Postgrad Adv Colorectal Surg 1–13

201. Wexner SD, Beck DE (1992) Sexually transmitted and infectious diseases. pp. 402–422. In Beck DE, Wexner SD (eds): Fundamentals of Anorectal Surgery. McGraw Hill, New York

202. Centers for Disease Control (1992) 1993 Revised classification system for HIV infection and expanded surveillance case definition for AIDS among adolescence and adults. MMWR 41(suppl 17):1–19

203. Glasel M (1988) High risk sexual practices in the transmission of AIDS. pp. 355–367, In DeVita VT, Hellman S, Rosenberg SA (eds): AIDS: Etiology, Diagnosis, Treatment, and Prevention. 2nd Ed. JB Lippincott, Philadelphia

204. Wexner SD (1989) AIDS: what the colorectal surgeon needs to know. Perspect Colon Rectal Surg 2:19–54

205. Wexner SD (1990) Cytomegalovirus ileocolitis and Kaposi's sarcoma in AIDS. pp. 217–222. In Fazio VW (ed): Current Therapy in Colon and Rectal Surgery. BC Decker, Toronto

16

MALIGNANT TUMORS

John Northover

Anal tumors are rare, accounting for no more than 1% of large bowel cancers. Due to their relative rarity the average general surgeon might see a new case only once every few years. For several reasons, however, they are presently a subject of interest beyond their numbers. First, modern combined modality therapy has taken the primary treatment of most epidermoid anal tumors away from surgeons, making them one of the first solid tumors for which surgery is no longer first-choice treatment. Second, much is now known about the etiology and natural history of epidermoid tumors, especially in relation to sexually transmitted viral exposure and to immunosuppression (particularly due to human immunodeficiency virus (HIV) infection). None of this can be said for the even rarer tumors—melanoma, Paget's disease, and adenocarcinoma.

Increasingly, surgeons are bystanders in the management of epidermoid tumors; nevertheless, there are several key tasks for the surgeon today, not least the treatment of recurrent tumors, so a thorough knowledge of the condition remains important. In melanoma, Paget's disease, and anal adenocarcinoma, surgeons continue to play a major part in patient care.

ANATOMY OF THE ANAL CANAL

The anal canal constitutes the final 4 cm of the alimentary tract. Traditionally the anal region is divided into the anal canal and the anal margin, although the definitions of these areas differ between disciplines. Anatomists see the canal as lying between the dentate line and the anal orifice, whereas surgically it is defined as lying between the pelvic floor and the anal verge. For pathologists, the canal has been defined as corresponding to the longitudinal extent of the internal anal sphincter.[1] Today this argument is less important as surgery plays a lesser role in treatment, but reports of surgical results from past decades are confused by this variation in definition.

Normal Histology

The upper canal above the dentate line is lined mainly by "colorectal" mucosa, indistinguishable from rectal mucosa; it is configured in 6 to 12 vertical folds or "columns," which terminate at the dentate line. At the line are a series of crypts, between the bases of the columns, into which drain about 10 anal glands, which fan out radially through the internal sphincter into the intersphincteric space. Below the dentate line the canal is lined by smooth nonkeratinizing squamous epithelium, devoid of sweat glands or other adnexae; this area may be referred to as the pecten (Fig. 16-1). Immediately above the dentate line—sometimes straddling it—and of variable extent is the transitional or junctional zone, lined by an epithelium of variable histology, but often very similar to urothelium (Figs. 16-2 and 16-3); it is here that many anal tumors may arise. The junctional zone, and to a lesser extent the pecten, harbor occasional melanocytes.

Anatomic Relations of the Anal Canal Epithelium

The anatomic relations of the epithelium are important when considering local spread of anal tumors. Immediately deep to the epithelium is a layer of connective tissue of variable density; below, and especially at, the dentate line, the lining epithelium is fairly tightly bound to the underlying internal anal sphincter, whereas above the line the attachment is looser, perhaps explaining the relative propensity for anal canal tumors to spread in the cephalad direction toward the rectum. Deep to the submucosa lies the internal anal sphincter, in its turn enveloped in the voluntary external sphincter. The deeper relations are described below.

Lateral Relations

The ischioanal fossae contain loose fat that is easily penetrated by invading tumor. Beyond this lies the side-wall, comprising the ischial tuberosities and the obturator internus muscles. At the upper extent of the ischiorectal fossae lies the muscular floor of the pelvis, fanning out from the upper extent of the external sphincter mechanism (puborectalis) to the bony sidewalls of the pelvis (Fig. 16-4).

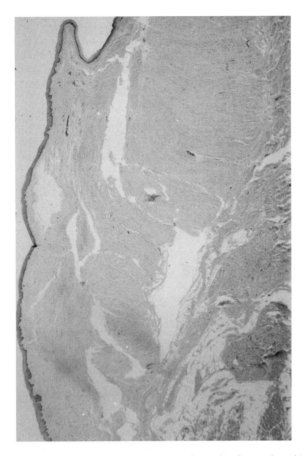

Figure 16-1. Histology, the pecten. The rather featureless skin of the pecten, devoid of adnexae, overlies the internal sphincter, and ends superiorly at a crypt at the dentate line.

Anterior Relations

In the male, the membranous urethra and penile bulb are closely applied to the anterior surface of the sphincters; in the female, the vagina and introitus are in close proximity.

Posterior Relations

The coccyx and distal sacrum, as well as the nerves issuing from them (perineal branch of S4 and the perforating cutaneous nerve to the lower buttock), lie immediately behind the posterior insertion of the external anal sphincter.

EPIDERMOID ANAL CANCERS

Pathology

Traditionally anal tumors have been divided into those arising from the anal canal and anal margin or verge. When surgery was the mainstay of treatment this division was important, as the type of surgery varied with the site of the lesion; today this division is less important.

Histology

Epidermoid anal tumors exhibit a range of histologic appearances. Lesions arising below the dentate line are typically squamous, whereas those arising above the dentate lining have been

assigned various names (transitional cell, basaloid, cloacogenic); all these lesions are generally regarded today as having a squamous cell origin.[2] To separate these tumors from those of glandular or melanocyte origin, they have become known collectively as *epidermoid carcinomas*. The squamous cell carcinoma is typically nonkeratinizing in the anal region, although keratin whorls may be seen, particularly in tumors arising at the anal verge (Fig. 16-5). Well-differentiated basaloid carcinomas comprise clumps of basophilic small cells, with a distinctive pattern of nuclear palisading at the periphery of the cell clumps. There may be central necrosis in these clumps, giving a Swiss cheese appearance (Fig. 16-6). Sometimes a resemblance to bladder tumor histology has led to use of the term *transitional cell carcinoma*. In less differentiated tumors these typical features are lost to a variable degree.

Patterns of Spread

Local spread of canal tumors is predominantly upward toward the lower rectum, such that it may appear that the lesion has arisen there. The tumor may invade deeply into and through the sphincters to involve contiguous structures, particularly the rectovaginal septum, vagina, or prostate.[3]

Lymphatic spread is predominantly to the mesorectal glands

Figure 16-2. Histology, the anal transition zone. Squamous epithelium covers the lip of a crypt, merging into the thinner transitional mucosa, which runs upwards for a variable distance in the proximal canal.

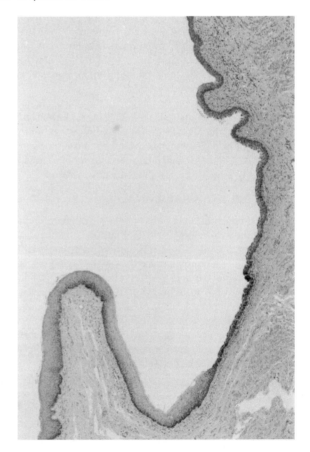

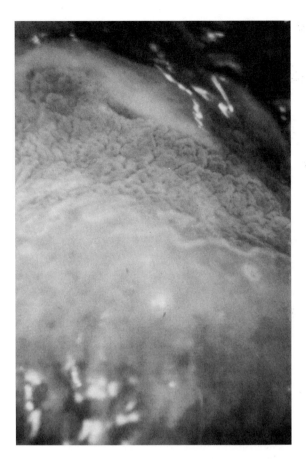

Figure 16-3. Endoscopic view, transitional zone. Seen through a proctoscope, using a ×10 colposcope, the transitional zone begins at a sharp demarcation, and has a deceptively villous appearance.

in canal tumors[4]; metastases were found in 40% of surgical specimens from St. Mark's Hospital,[1] and inguinal lymphadenopathy was found in 11% of St. Mark's cases, although only half of these were found on biopsy to be due to metastasis.[5]

Distant metastasis has been uncommon at the time of presentation in published series[5] but in the recent United Kingdom Coordinating Committee on Cancer Research (UKCCCR) therapy trial, 40% of those dying of anal cancer had distant spread at the time of death.[6] The principal sites of metastasis are the liver, lung, and bones.[7] Metastases have been described uncommonly in the kidney, adrenal gland, and brain.[3]

Premalignant Lesions

Several lesions are recognized as having the potential to undergo malignant change. The natural history of these lesions and their malignant potential is not clearly understood.

Anal Intraepithelial Neoplasia

The terms "Bowen's disease of the anus" and "leukoplakia" are best avoided, as they are confusing, convey no specific information, and are of uncertain malignant potential (Fig. 16-7).

The natural history of the various anogenital intraepithelial neoplasia is poorly understood. Cervical intraepithelial neoplasia and comparable lesions of the vulva, vagina, and anus, are graded I to III, depending on the proportion of the epithelial thickness affected; thus in grade III the whole thickness of the epithelium is dysplastic, an appearance sometimes referred to as carcinoma in situ (Fig. 16-8).

Anogenital human papillomavirus (HPV)-associated lesions may be identified using an operating microscope (colposcope) and the application of acetic acid to the epithelium.[8] Colposcopic examination may suggest the degree of dysplasia and permits targeted biopsy. Anal cytologic examination is sensitive but lacks specificity.[9] Histologic examination remains the diagnostic standard.[10]

High-grade anal intraepithelial lesions are characterized by hyperkeratosis, perhaps with epithelial pigmentation. Lesions may appear white, red, brown, or variegated. They may be flat or raised; ulceration is suggestive of invasive disease. Any suspicious area must be biopsied and examined histologically.

Multifocal anogenital intraepithelial neoplasia represents a challenging clinical problem.[11,12] Although the management of cervical lesions is well worked out, the natural history and significance of lesions at other sites makes the development of management strategies difficult at present.

Giant Condyloma (Bushke-Loewenstein Tumor)

Giant condyloma, a rare lesion, usually affects the penis or vulva but may sometimes grow at the anus.[1] Typically it has the shape of a cauliflower and may totally obscure the anus (Figs. 16-9 and 16-10). Fistulous tracks may develop with increasing local sepsis. They may invade locally but usually show no propensity for metastasis. Dysplastic change may occur, with progression to invasive malignancy in a few cases.

DEMOGRAPHY

Anal cancer is probably under-reported since some cases are misclassified as rectal tumors, and perianal tumors may be recorded as squamous carcinoma of the buttock skin. There is wide geographic variation although some data are misleading due to shortcomings in cancer registration. In the United Kingdom and the United States, the annual age-adjusted incidence is around 0.5 in 100,000.[13,14] A low incidence (0.2 cases in 100,000 of population) is reported in the Philippines, and the highest incidence (3.6 cases in 100,000) is reported in Geneva, Switzerland. In a recent study in Italy, anal cancers constituted 4% of large bowel cancers in females and 1.2% in males.[15]

The peak age for diagnosis is the late 50s, a decade earlier than colorectal cancer. In Los Angeles, Peters and Mack[16] showed an increasing incidence in men aged under 45 years, although no such change was demonstrated in older men or women at any age. Anal canal tumors are more common in women; at the margin they are more common in men.[17] This must be interpreted with caution since the anatomic distinction between anal canal and anal margin is often poorly defined.

In Denmark it appears that the absolute incidence is rising compared with 30 years ago; in women there has been a threefold increase, and in men the incidence has risen 1.5-fold[18]; similar increases have been reported from Sweden.[19] In North-

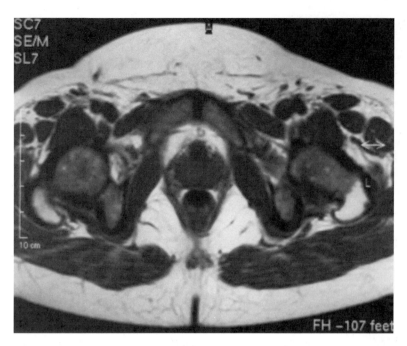

Figure 16-4. Anatomical relations of the anal canal in a male. This magnetic resonance scan shows the dark circular structure of the anal canal lying between the dense white areas of ischiorectal fat. The prostate and the contained urethra lie immediately in front of the canal, the two structures contained within the oblique V of the puborectalis.

east Brazil a high incidence of anal cancer is associated with a high incidence of cervical, vulval, and penile tumors. Within countries strong evidence exists of associated risk factors for anal and genital cancers in both men and women.[12,20–23] There seems little doubt that multifocal HPV infection underlies this phenomenon.[12]

The increasing incidence of HIV infection in the United States has been associated with conflicting reports of a corresponding rise in cases of anal and genital cancer and to more rapid progression of the natural history of the disease.[24] The balance of opinion strongly favors a direct association, although in Italy a careful study of tumors related to the acquired immu-

Figure 16-5. Histology, squamous cell carcinoma (SCC). This well differentiated tumor shows the keratin whorls invading the dermis; these are mainly seen in anal verge tumors.

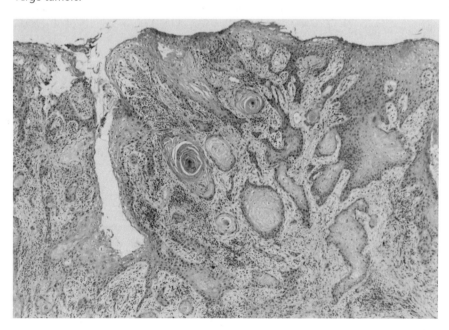

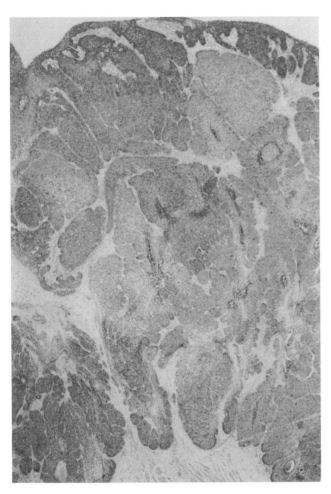

Figure 16-6. Histology, basaloid carcinoma. The discrete clumps of small cells, sometimes with central necrosis, are well demonstrated.

nodeficiency syndrome failed to confirm a rising risk of anal cancer.[25]

ETIOLOGY

For decades, anal cancer was said to be associated with poor hygiene and poverty, although the etiologic mechanisms underpinning these links were not known. Over the past 15 years, epidemiologic data have led to well-founded theories on the causation in at least a part of the case population.

Sexual Activity

In 1982, Austin[26] produced early data indicating that urban males in San Francisco were at excess risk for anal cancer compared with their suburban peers; no such difference was seen in women. It was suggested that the difference was related to the higher proportion of gay men living in the city, and that their sexual activity was giving effect to a risk factor. Around the same time, evidence was reported of excess risk in single males compared with their married peers (relative risk [RR], 6:1) and with women of any marital status.[16] A similar associa-

tion with marital status in males was shown in a British study.[27] Peters et al.[28] also found epidemiologic associations between cancers at several anogenital sites in California residents, suggesting common etiologic agents. Daling et al.[29] reported a great excess risk of anal cancer in men with a history of syphilis seropositivity; other cancer sites in men or any cancer site in women, including the anal region, showed no such association. They later published a case control study in which anal receptive intercourse (RR, 33) and genital wart infection (RR, 27) were found to be highly significant risk factors in men; in women, genital wart infection exhibited an association (RR, 22) and anal intercourse did not (RR, 2).[30] More recent data support an association with smoking, anogenital warts, and other anal lesions.[31]

Human Papillomaviruses

An epidemiologic association between a sexually transmissible agent and female genital cancer is well established. A venereal etiology for cervical cancer was first suggested 150 years ago, when it was noted that this tumor was rare in nuns. More recent data support this finding, but reliable information on individual sexual practices is difficult to assemble. Mathe[32] provided one of the earliest reports of the association of wart virus lesions in the mouth, larynx, esophagus, cervix, vulva, vagina, penis, and anus; he highlighted the occurrence of premalignant as well

Figure 16-7. Macroscopic view, "leukoplakia." Although this term is best avoided, it remains in common usage. The perianal skin, particularly posteriorly, is white; often the skin immediately around the white area appears erythematous, as seen here.

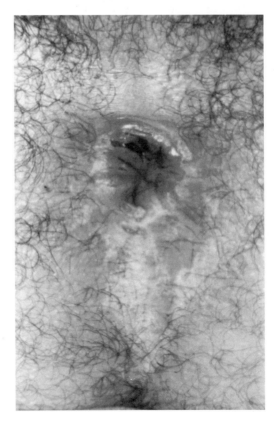

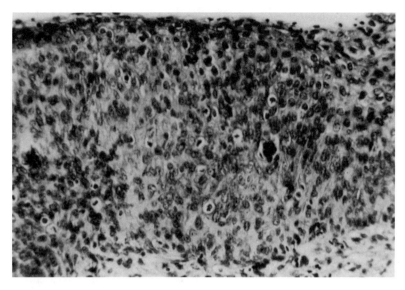

Figure 16-8. Histology, anal intra-epithelial neoplasia (AIN). In this lesion AIN grade III is seen, in which the whole thickness of the epithelium is occupied by dysplastic cells.

as cancerous lesions containing HPV 16 and 18 DNA, followed soon after by Gross and Gissmann.[33] Several groups had used nucleic acid hybridization techniques to demonstrate HPV type 16 DNA and, less commonly, types 18, 31, and 33 DNA, integrated into the genome in a high proportion of genital squamous cell carcinomas. Soon afterward DNA from the same HPV types was found in a significant proportion of anal squamous cell carcinomas.[34–38] The proportion of anal cancers containing HPV DNA has increased over the past several decades in parallel with an increasing prevalence of other HPV-associated disease.[39] These data indicate the high likelihood that sexually transmitted HPV predisposes to anal and other epidermal cancers. Case control studies have shown quite clearly that risks of developing anal cancer are increased in people who have suffered genital cancers previously (cervix, vagina, vulva, penis) or cancer at other squamous, sexually accessible sites (oral cavity and larynx) and vice versa.[20,40]

HPVs are DNA viruses. The more than 60 HPV types are associated with a wide variety of squamous epithelial lesions, ranging from the palmar and plantar warts caused by the relatively infectious HPV types 1 and 2, to the anogenital papillomaviruses, usually types 6 and 11, which are less infectious

Figure 16-9. Macroscopic view, giant condyloma. This lesion, about 10 cm in diameter, completely obscures the anus. Large veins can be seen on both buttocks, indicating the vascularity of the tumor, making its removal exciting.

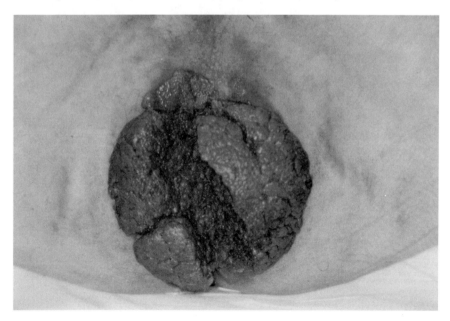

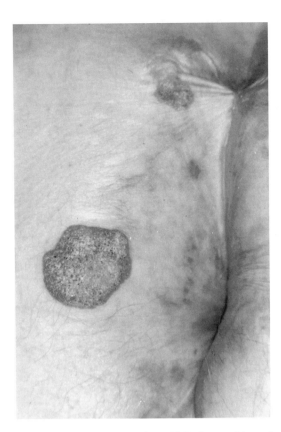

Figure 16-10. Macroscopic view, SCC after excision of giant condyloma. This picture was taken several years after excision and split skin grafting of the lesion seen in Figure 16-9. Discrete areas of malignancy have arisen lateral and anterolateral to the anus.

and are exclusively sexually transmissible. The epidemiology of anogenital papillomavirus infection is poorly understood, largely due to the social and moral taboos surrounding sexually transmitted diseases. HPV 16 carriage or previous infection may be quite common; whereas IgA antibodies to the E2 region of HPV 16 were present in 89% of anal cancer cases, they were found in the serum of as many as 24% of controls.[41] Overt lesions range from benign condylomata, through intraepithelial neoplasia, to invasive carcinoma.[42,43] The genital wart-associated types—6 and 11—may also be isolated from low-grade intraepithelial neoplasia. HPV types 16, 18, 31, and 33 are much less commonly associated with genital condylomata but are more often found in high-grade intraepithelial neoplasia and invasive carcinoma. The assertion that HPV infection, and hence anal cancer, only occur in those who practice anal intercourse is unlikely to be correct. Once one area of the anogenital epithelium is infected, spread throughout the anogenital tract occurs readily but probably remains occult in most individuals.[44]

Other Sexually Transmitted Diseases

Since carcinogenesis is a multistep process, papillomaviruses are likely to be only one of a number of factors in the pathogenesis of these tumors. Other potential co-carcinogens include other

sexually transmissible infective agents such as herpes simplex type II and chlamydia.

HIV Infection

The most important associated sexually transmitted disease is HIV infection. Howard and co-workers[45] described two cases of anal squamous cell carcinoma in young gay males infected with human T-cell leukemia virus III, suggesting that this condition had predisposed them to HPV infection. Soon anal cancer was seen as part of the spectrum of cancers occurring more frequently in the HIV-infected population.[38,46-48] Others have shown that anal dysplastic lesions are more common in HIV-infected individuals,[49] whereas others dispute the increased risk of anal cancer in HIV cases.[50]

Immunosuppression in Transplantation

If virally induced immunosuppression can predispose to anal cancer, it is perhaps not surprising that renal transplant recipients are at 100-fold increased risk of this tumor, as well as others in the anogenital region.[51] HPV has been implicated.[52]

Other Anorectal Diseases

An association has long been thought to exist between certain other anorectal conditions and epidermoid cancer.[1] A past history of hemorrhoids, fissure, or fistula were found to add to the risk of anal cancer in both heterosexual and homosexual men in California.[31] Evidence that anal Crohn's disease is a risk factor for epidermoid anal cancer is minimal.[53]

Smoking

Case control data suggest that smoking introduces an increased risk of anal cancer, just as has been shown for cervical cancer.[54] Moreover, women with a past history of anal cancer are at an excess risk of later development of lung cancer; this is taken as evidence for the effect of smoking in anal carcinogenesis.[55]

CLINICAL PRESENTATION

Symptoms

Seventy-five percent of cases are misdiagnosed as benign conditions initially, as the latter are so much more common.[56] The commonest symptoms are pain and bleeding, recorded in about 50% of cases;[5] a mass, pruritus, or discharge are reported by only around 25% of patients.[5] Advanced tumors may invade the sphincters (causing fecal incontinence) or the posterior vaginal wall, leading to vaginal discharge and, ultimately, fistulation.

Signs

At the anal margin, a malignant tumor usually has the appearance of a malignant ulcer (Fig. 16-11). Lesions within the canal are not visible initially (Fig. 16-12), although more extensive lesions may spread to the anal verge (Fig. 16-13), or extend via the ischiorectal fossa to the skin of the buttock.[57] Frequently, other benign perianal conditions such as condylomata or intra-

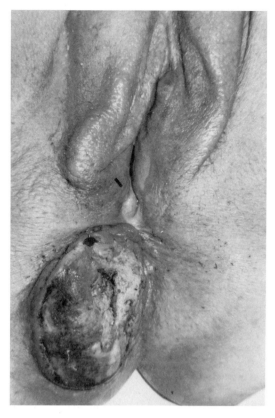

Figure 16-11. Macroscopic view, anal margin SCC. At the anal verge, SCC has the typical appearance of a malignant ulcer, as seen elsewhere on the body surface.

epithelial neoplasia are seen in association with anal cancer. Digital examination is often painful; if the tumor has extended into the sphincters, the characteristic induration may be felt around the anal canal on bidigital palpation. As anal cancer tends to spread upward, there may be involvement of the distal rectum, perhaps giving the impression that the lesion has arisen there. Involvement of the inferior mesenteric lymph nodes may be palpable easily, rather more so than in rectal cancer. Insertion of an endoscope may be impossible due to pain, but if an instrument can be passed, biopsy may be attempted.

In up to one-third of patients the inguinal lymph nodes are enlarged, although in only half of these will biopsy confirm metastatic spread—the rest are due to secondary infection[5]; therefore biopsy or fine needle aspiration is mandatory to confirm the presence of tumor if radical block dissection is contemplated. A routine search should be made for distant spread, although this is found in only a small minority at initial presentation.

INVESTIGATIONS

Ultrasound scanning can provide accurate information regarding sphincter involvement, although again insertion of the probe may be difficult or impossible due to pain[58] (Fig. 16-14). Computed tomography and magnetic resonance scanning may dem-

onstrate spread beyond the anal canal and allow a search for distant spread.[59]

Examination under anesthesia, preferably carried out jointly by the surgeon and radiotherapist, is usually required to allow biopsy and to afford optimum assessment of the degree of spread of a tumor prior to treatment planning.

Conventional serum tumor markers and some other measures of biologic activity have not been shown to help in estimating prognosis. There have been variable reports of the utility of DNA ploidy.[60,61] Goldman and colleagues[62] found that a raised preoperative titer of serum squamous cell carcinoma antigen (SCCAg) was associated with relapse after primary surgery; stage for stage, overall and tumor-specific survival were significantly related to preoperative SCCAg. Other workers have not found SCCAg useful as a preoperative prognostic factor, although a raised level correlated significantly when measured in postoperative follow-up.[63]

Staging

No staging system for anal cancer has been universally accepted, but that of Union International Contre le Cancer is the one most widely used for tumors of the anal canal, as follows[64]:

T1: <2 cm
T2: 2 ≤5 cm

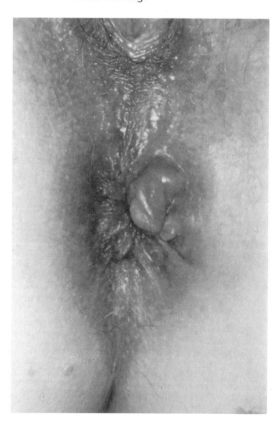

Figure 16-12. Macroscopic view, "invisible" anal canal tumor. In this case, the only external sign of the tumor within the anal canal is an oedematous skin tag.

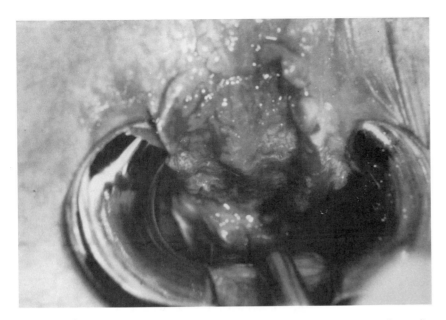

Figure 16-13. Macroscopic view, spreading anal canal tumor. An extensive malignant ulcer involves the anterior anal canal, extending downwards to the anal verge and upwards into the distal rectum.

T3: >5 cm
T4: invading adjacent organs (*not including sphincters*)
N0: no regional metastasis
N1: spread to perirectal nodes
N2: unilateral spread to internal iliac and/or inguinal nodes
N3: spread to perirectal and inguinal nodes and/or bilateral internal iliac and/or inguinal nodes

Figure 16-14. Ultrasound scan, anal canal tumor. With the patient in the supine position, a spreading anal canal tumor is seen in the right anterolateral quadrant, pushing the prostate forward.

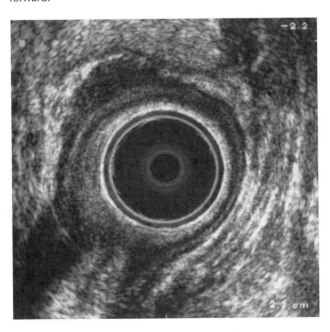

TREATMENT

Until relatively recently the treatment of anal cancer was carried out predominantly by surgeons; over the past 10 years it has become apparent that nonsurgical regimens—radiotherapy with or without chemotherapy—have key advantages over primary surgery in most cases. Before considering radiotherapy and chemotherapy, therefore, it is important to examine the background provided by several decades of surgical management.

Surgery as Primary Therapy

Several series from around the world were published during the 1980s, describing the results of surgery-based management during the preceding decades.[4,5,65–68] Lesions at the anal margin were treated mainly by local excision, and anal canal tumors were usually removed radically by abdominoperineal excision. Despite the commonly held view that anal cancer is predominantly a locoregional disease (and hence theoretically eradicable by surgery in most cases), the 5-year survival averaged around 55% in these series; the high rate of distant spread reported recently in patients in the UKCCCR trial may help to explain this.[69]

Anal Margin Tumors

The largest reported series was from St. Mark's Hospital, where 83 margin lesions were treated between 1948 and 1984.[5] Two-thirds of the patients were treated by local excision, of whom 65% survived for 5 years. All 11 cases managed by radical anorectal excision were treated with curative intent, but only 4 (36%) survived for 5 years. Overall, 5-year survival was 65% for T1 and T2 lesions; patients with T3 and T4 cancers fared significantly worse, with only 33% surviving for 5 years. The series reported from Copenhagen comprised 76 patients, 58 of whom were treated with curative intent, most by surgery.[67] Recurrence was locoregional in 23 of 24 cases of relapse. Of 32 patients treated by local excision only, 20 (63%) developed recurrent disease. In contrast to these results, the Memorial group in New York reported a corrected 88% 5-year survival following local excision, although many of their patients exhibited locoregional relapse, which often responded well to further local treatment.[65]

Anal Canal Cancer

Radical abdominoperineal excision of the rectum and anus was the preferred method of treatment for decades. Compared with margin cancer, anal canal cancer is more likely to be locally advanced at presentation[5] and to be associated with subsequent metastasis,[61] perhaps explaining the general preference for radical surgery. At the Mayo Clinic 188 cases were treated between 1950 and 1976.[4] Thirteen (7%) tumors were 2 cm or less and were treated by local excision with excellent results. Among 118 who underwent radical surgery, 4 died postoperatively, 46 developed recurrence, and 81(71%) survived for 5 years. Others had less favorable results, with 5-year survival ranging between 20 and 50+%

It was the realization that surgical results were so disappointing, while radiotherapists were able to boast of comparable survival figures and avoid a colostomy in most cases, that led surgeons to relinquish (slowly) their therapeutic monopoly and to pass patients on to their nonsurgical colleagues.

Current Role of the Surgeon

Today the surgeon still has several important roles in the modern care of anal cancer, some in primary management, others in the patient treated initially by nonsurgical means.

Initial Diagnosis

Most patients continue to present to surgeons, who are best suited to perform examination under anesthesia to confirm diagnosis and to stage the disease, with particular reference to any spread to contiguous organs and tissues. Ideally the radiotherapist should be present at such an examination; this is an opportunity to assess the tumor prior to planning treatment. If the tumor is found to involve the full thickness of the rectovaginal septum, the clinicians may agree that radiotherapeutic ablation of the tumor is most likely to result in a rectovaginal fistula, which may not be amenable to surgical repair after radiation treatment; in these circumstances primary radical surgery may be an appropriate choice. If they find that the sphincters are deeply invaded, it may nevertheless be reasonable to proceed on the nonsurgical path as continence is often perfectly adequate after tumor ablation in such cases. These decisions are best taken jointly at examination under anesthesia, followed by careful discussion and decision making with the patient.

Primary Management of Small Tumors at the Anal Margin

Small lesions at the anal margin are still best treated by local excision alone, thus avoiding protracted nonsurgical therapy. Some evidence shows that the risk of regional lymph node metastasis is not related to primary tumor size, which may explain the disappointing results sometimes reported after local excision; this conflicts with the Mayo view that tumor size is related to stage, accounting for their excellent results for local excision of small tumors.

Primary Therapy in Advanced Disease

Although Nigro's early experience of the dramatic effects of combined modality therapy (CMT) in advanced disease led to wider use of primary nonsurgical approaches, not all groups have been impressed by this approach in more advanced tumors; some felt that patients with advanced stage tumors should at least consider radical surgery as primary treatment, particularly as those developing recurrence after post-CMT salvage surgery could not then receive optimum radiotherapy.[70,71]

Surgery After Primary Nonsurgical Treatment

Treatment Complications or Relapse at the Primary Site

An important role for the surgeon comes after failure, either early or late, of primary nonsurgical treatment; in the recent UKCCCR trial, 50% of cases relapsed after complete remission using radiotherapy or combined modality therapy.[69] Four situations may confront the surgeon:

Residual tumor after CMT (around 10% of cases)
Complications of CMT
Incontinence or fistula after tumor resolution
Subsequent tumor recurrence

Histologic confirmation of tumor is mandatory to confirm the need for radical surgery. The appearance of the primary site can be misleading after combined modality therapy; in most patients complete remission is indicated by the tumor disappearing completely, although in some a lump may remain, occasionally indistinguishable from the primary tumor before therapy. Only generous biopsy will reveal whether the residual lump contains tumor or consists merely of inflammatory tissue.[72] Unfortunately the salvage rate for radical surgery in disease relapse after CMT may be poor—in a literature review in 1992, Zelnick and colleagues[70] found that 70% of reported cases had died within 3 years of salvage surgery; whether this was due to the biologic aggressiveness of this select group of cases, or whether these patients would have fared better if surgery had been used as primary treatment are open questions. Tanum[73] recently reported a more favorable outcome in a small Norwegian series—3-year survival in six of nine such patients. More comprehensive data will come from the UKCCCR trial.

A proportion of patients develop complications—radionecrosis, fistula, or incontinence—following radical radiation or combined therapy. Severe anal pain due to radionecrosis may necessitate either colostomy (in the hope that the lesion may heal after fecal diversion) or radical anorectal excision.

Occasionally a tumor is so locally extensive that the patient will be rendered incontinent as a consequence of primary tumor shrinkage, due to either breakdown of the rectovaginal septum

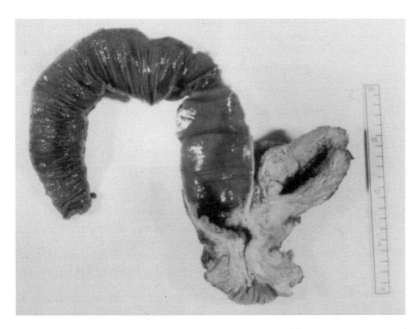

Figure 16-15. Pelvic exenteration specimen, removed for persistent tumor after combined modality therapy. An anterior wall canal tumor invading the prostate had not responded to CMT. Pelvic clearance led to a prospect of cure. Note the bladder hypertrophy due to chronic urinary obstruction.

or sphincter disruption by the tumor. Although rectovaginal fistula may be amenable to repair, sphincter dysfunction following radiotherapy is unlikely to improve with local surgery. Abdominoperineal excision may be required if these complications are not remedied by reparative surgery or if they are not considered worth the effort in individual cases.

Should clinical evidence of recurrent disease develop after initial resolution, biopsy is mandatory prior to surgical intervention. Although some regard surgical salvage in these circumstances as essentially palliative,[70,74] experience in the recent British trial and reports from other groups are less pessimistic.[69,73,75,76] Careful evaluation of the pattern and extent of recurrence should be undertaken to decide what form of treatment is indicated. The major decision relates to the possibility of attempting curative surgical ablation. Central pelvic recurrence without distant spread or sidewall involvement may be amenable to radical extirpation, perhaps requiring pelvic exenteration (Fig. 16-15). Apparently small volume, superficial, and isolated recurrence may be considered for local excision, although the risk of regional or distant spread must be considered before deciding on a local surgical approach.

Treatment of Inguinal Metastases

Inguinal lymphadenopathy is present in 10 to 25% of patients at initial presentation. Although this may be treated by radiotherapy, some argue for surgery; histologic confirmation is advisable before radical groin dissection, as up to 50% of cases of inguinal lymphadenopathy may be due to inflammation alone.[5]

Enlargement of groin nodes some time after primary therapy is most likely to be due to recurrent tumor[5]; radical groin dissection is indicated in this situation, with up to 50% 5-year survival.[4]

Operative Techniques

Local Procedures

Local procedures can be performed in either the lithotomy or the prone jackknife position.

Biopsy

Biopsy is required either for initial histologic assessment or for confirmation of tumor ablation following primary nonsurgical therapy. Careful thought must be given to the risk of radionecrosis at the site of biopsy in the post-treatment phase. Confirmatory biopsy is generally thought to be unnecessary if no clinical suspicion of residual disease exists.

A small sliver of tissue, no more than a few millimeters in diameter and depth, is taken from a representative site. In post-treatment assessment, if any suggestion of tumor deep to skin exists, it may be necessary to use a biopsy needle. If there is suspicion of residual or recurrent disease in the ischiorectal fossae or pelvis, this may be sampled either through the skin of the buttock or through the bowel wall, whichever is more appropriate.

Local Excision

Local excision should be reserved for the patient with a T1 tumor at the anal margin. Occasionally it may be applicable to an apparently localized and superficial perineal recurrence.[7]

To minimize bleeding and to provide an optimum view, the tumor is raised on a "bleb" of 1:200,000 adrenaline solution. An incision is made around the tumor 1 cm from its edge and is extended vertically through the subdermal tissues. The disc of tissue is removed by dissecting under the tumor in this plane; the specimen is then pinned out on a piece of cork so it can be placed in formalin in a well-oriented position for the pathologist.

The skin defect can be dealt with in several ways:

It can be left to heal by secondary intent (the usual approach)

If the wound cannot be closed completely, the skin edge can be advanced circumferentially and sutured to the fat

An advancement wedge from the buttock can be mobilized and advanced to the anal verge and lower canal. Flaps that include muscle can be used for more ambitious reconstructions if the sphincters have been compromised.[77]

Abdominoperineal Excision of the Anus and Rectum

Abdominoperineal excision does not differ in essence from that used for low rectal cancer. Several aspects deserve special mention.

Perineal Dissection

There must be adequate clearance of the lateral margins of the tumor, with the skin incision at least 2 cm lateral to the tumor. As it may have spread to a variable extent into the ischiorectal fat, it is important to be radical in the infralevator compartment, taking all the ischiorectal fat and detaching the levator muscles from the bony pelvic side walls.

Perineal Closure

In those patients operated on after radical radiotherapy (for initial treatment failure, radionecrosis, or later tumor recurrence), primary wound healing is less predictable than normal. If the wound edges are not sufficiently elastic to come together easily, or if the tissues are edematous or fibrotic, it is better to leave the wound open. If it fails subsequently to show signs of healing, it may be necessary to fashion a skin/muscle flap (a rectus abdominis flap preferably) as a secondary procedure to expedite healing.[78,79]

Radiotherapy Alone as Primary Treatment

Radiotherapists have long argued that they can treat anal tumors better than surgeons, offering similar survival prospects and with the advantage of stoma avoidance in most cases.[80] Like surgery, radiotherapy is a local treatment modality; like surgeons, radiotherapists have held on to the notion that this disease is predominantly a locoregional disease.[81] Surgeons were slow to hear the protestations of the radiotherapists. It was a surgeon, Norman Nigro,[82] reporting on the use of CMT in an attempt to make inoperable cases into candidates for surgical salvage, who began to turn the surgical community away from operation as first choice therapy. Before considering the role of CMT, however, it is necessary to look at the efficacy of radiotherapy alone.

Seventy years ago the mortality and morbidity of surgical treatment for anal carcinoma were sufficient to persuade some

surgeons to favor radiotherapy. By the 1930s, however, it was recognized that the low-voltage radiotherapy available frequently produced severe radionecrosis. Consequently there was a general move back to surgery, as it became safer—abdominoperineal excision for invading lesions and local excision for small growths became the standard treatment for the ensuing four decades, although radium implantation was being advocated for low-grade tumors in 1940.[83]

By the 1950s the development of the cobalt source generator and the more recent introduction of linear accelerators enabled radiotherapists to deliver more highly penetrating doses to more deeply placed structures with less superficial expenditure of energy. Radiation damage to surrounding tissues was consequently reduced, while effect on the tumor was enhanced. It became possible to treat both the primary tumor and its lymphatic drainage in the pelvis and groin in a single treatment volume.[81] Total radiation doses rose to 50 to 65 Gy, the limiting factors being toxic reactions in the perineal skin and mucosa of the distal bowel. Split course therapy, allowing recovery of the perineal skin, became widely used,[84] although some concern was voiced that the rest period might allow repopulation of the tumor volume by viable cancer tissue.[81] High-dose external beam radiotherapy alone was shown to offer survival rates of up to 75% at 3 years.[85–87]

Particularly in view of the perception of anal cancer as a localized disease, interstitial radiation went through a period of particular enthusiasm, although it is less used today. The main problem with this modality is the variation in dose around the implanted sources, so it found its main use in smaller distal tumors.[88] Papillon[89] tried to deal with dose inhomogeneity by fractionation, applying two treatments 2 months apart. He was able to achieve 5-year survival in two-thirds of patients treated in this way, with more than 90% achieving initial complete remission. Others reported less successful results, both in terms of cures and a significant level of radionecrosis.[90] A combination of interstitial and external beam therapy was held to exploit the advantages of additional therapy to the primary tumor while treating the regional lymphatic drainage adequately. Again, Papillon and his colleagues[85,89] produced the data on this approach, having followed initial external beam therapy by a boost of interstitial therapy to the primary site; they were able to produce high levels of complete remission and 5-year survivals while at the same time minimizing local treatment complications and hence retaining anal function in 90% of cases.

Combined Modality Therapy

It was an irony that radiotherapists were not the prime means by which surgeons were deflected away from surgery as first choice treatment for this tumor. As noted above, that distinction fell to a surgeon, Norman Nigro,[82] who sought through preoperative therapy to render three apparently inoperable tumors resectable. Using relatively low dose radiotherapy in combination with 5-fluorouracil (5-FU) and mitomycin C (a combination chosen empirically), he was surprised to obtain complete remissions in all three cases. In the two who accepted subsequent abdominoperineal excision, the surgical specimens were tumor free; the third patient declined surgery and remained disease free. Thus began the era of what came to be known as CMT (radiation and chemotherapy combined) with surgery available as salvage treatment if needed. The classical Nigro regimen consisted of 30 Gy of external beam irradiation over a period of 3 weeks. A bolus of mitomycin C was given on day 1, and 5-FU was delivered in a synchronous, continuous 4-day infusion during the first week of radiotherapy. After completion of radiotherapy, a further infusion of 5-FU was administered, with the intention of proceeding to abdominoperineal excision 6 weeks later.

Nigro's[91] experience over the ensuing 10 years bore out his early enthusiasm. As he became more confident, he no longer pressed his patients to undergo radical surgery routinely, initially confining himself to excising the site of the primary tumor after CMT. Later he dropped even this relatively minor surgical step if the primary site looked and felt normal after treatment, although it took time for many of his American surgical colleagues to accept this degree of reduced intervention.

A variety of similar techniques have since been described, aiming either to increase radiosensitivity (and hence improve the prospects for local control) or to act outside the pelvis at distant sites of potential spread. Most regimens have used synchronous therapy, and others have sought to use higher doses of each modality sequentially.[92] With wider experience, it became clear that higher doses of radiotherapy (45 to 60 Gy) should be applied, usually split into two courses to minimize morbidity. Chemotherapy comprised intravenous infusion of 5-FU at the beginning and end of the first radiotherapy course, and a single bolus of mitomycin C given on the first day of treatment. Others have used alternative chemotherapeutic agents. Modifications of chemotherapy dosage and prophylactic antibiotic therapy were necessary in elderly or frail patients and in those with extensive ulcerated tumors.

All the reported series described encouraging results, but it remained a matter for debate whether similar levels of local tumor control and survival could be achieved without chemotherapy, perhaps thereby avoiding some morbidity.[93] Cummings et al.[94] retrospectively compared patients treated by radiotherapy over a 20-year period with another group treated more recently with combined therapy. Local control had been maintained 6 months after treatment in 60% of radiation patients compared with 94% of those who had received CMT. Later his group made a noncontrol comparison of several regimens; they found that local control and 5-year survival were broadly comparable after radiation with or without 5-FU (around 58 and 66%, respectively), but if mitomycin C was added, superior results were achieved for both these parameters (86 and 77%).[95,96] Other data, again from noncontrol series, and therefore open to the same biases that may have affected Cummings' series, showed no advantage (survival, local control, toxicity) through the addition of the 5-FU/mitomycin C regimen to radiation.[97]

In the late 1980s a randomized trial designed to answer this question was launched by the UKCCCR; it was set up to assess relative efficacy in local control of the tumor and hence avoidance of colostomy.[6] The regimens compared in this study represented what was seen to be optimum therapy at the time of trial design. Radiotherapy dosage was identical in the two arms, employing 45 Gy through opposed anterior and posterior fields over 4 to 5 weeks. The recommended target volume included the inguinal lymph nodes; the superior field margin was the midpelvic line. The whole perineum was included, and the peri-

anal region was boulused. Six weeks after therapy, response was assessed; if a 50% or greater response had been achieved, a boost course of radiotherapy was delivered as either 15 Gy to the perineum with electrons or photons, or by iridium 192 implant to 25 Gy. Chemotherapy comprised 5-FU and mitomycin C. 5-FU was administered by continuous infusion either as 1,000 mg/m^2 on days 1 to 4 or 750 mg/m^2 on days 1 to 5 at the consistent choice of individual oncologists. A second course of 5-FU was given during the final week of the radiotherapy course. Mitomycin C was administered at a dose of 12 mg/m^2 by intravenous bolus on day 1 only. For patients with significant intercurrent illness and those aged over 80, a reduced dose regimen was recommended for both drugs. Antibiotic prophylaxis was used in all CMT patients and for any receiving radiotherapy alone with frank sepsis in their tumor.

This trial recruited 585 patients and showed a significant improvement in local control in the CMT arm: 36% had developed local treatment failure 3 to 5 years after CMT compared with 59% in the radiotherapy arm (relative risk, 0.54, 95% = CI 0.42–0.69, $P < 0.0001$)[69]; most cases of local failure were treated by salvage surgery. There was no difference in overall 3-year survival (CMT, 65%; radiotherapy, 58%), whereas the cancer-related mortality was significantly less after CMT (28% versus 39%, $P = 0.02$). Forty percent of those dying due to anal cancer showed evidence of distant spread. There was no statistically significant difference in morbidity between the two regimens, although several deaths were attributable to chemotherapy; early experience of septicemic deaths led to recommendations for dose reductions in the elderly and frail, and to the introduction of prophylactic antibiotics. No deaths could be attributed to 5-FU cardiotoxicity. Mitomycin C is probably an important component of the regimen; an RTOG/Eastern Cooperative Oncology Group intergroup trial recently demonstrated that the drug combination led to significantly fewer local failures and better disease-free survival than 5-FU alone.[98] The local control and survival rates in the UKCCCR trial are somewhat inferior to those reported from smaller nonrandomized series, but they reflect the results achievable at multiple centers across a large population. At present, therefore, the combined modality regimen used in the UKCCCR trial should be seen as the standard regimen in the management of epidermoid anal cancer.

Future Prospects

The management of anal epidermoid carcinoma has changed dramatically over the past decade, although the survival rate has probably not altered substantially as a result of the move away from surgery as first choice therapy. A key question for the future must be whether survival can be improved. Two groups have reported promising, although nonrandomized, results using cisplatinum instead of mitomycin C in CMT.[99,100] In esophageal carcinoma, a regimen including radiotherapy, 5-FU, cisplatinum, and mitomycin C has proved to be only moderately toxic.[101] The UKCCCR plans to test this regimen in comparison with standard CMT. In addition, the high level of distant disease at death in the previous UKCCCR trial has highlighted this aspect of the disease; further courses of chemotherapy following complete remission are to be compared with no "adjuvant" therapy in an attempt to alter this outcome.

A further area of combined modality management that warrants attention is the problem of treatment-induced morbidity and the functional deficit that may follow radical radiotherapy to the pelvis.

It is heartening that evidence shows clearly that the mutilation of surgery in years past can be avoided in many cases of this rare disease. An important task that must not be overlooked is to inform all those managing this condition of these benefits so that surgery is avoided more uniformly. Moreover, if we are to tackle the higher prevalence of the disease in some parts of the world, particularly South America, increased efforts are required to minimize transmission of oncogenic HPV types in the hope that this may prevent some cases.

RARER ANAL TUMORS

Perianal Paget's Disease

Perianal Paget's disease is exceedingly rare. St. Mark's Hospital reported only eight cases seen over a 60-year period.[102] Only 100 cases had been recorded in the world literature until 1990, although at least 25 more cases were reported since then, often associated with investigation of the cellular origin of this odd lesion. First described by Sir James Paget[103] in 1874 as a breast lesion, similar findings in the perianal area were reported 20 years later.[104]

Clinical Features

The commonest symptom is pruritus, usually associated with bleeding and a lump at the anal verge. Some will complain of soiling or a change in bowel habit. On examination there may be a raised lesion or well-demarcated rash that may be erythematous, oozing, or scaling (Fig. 16-16). The mean age is around the seventh decade with no apparent gender difference. In most cases—perhaps 50 to 80%—there is an underlying adenocarcinoma, usually of the rectum, although the lesion may rarely be in a distant organ.[105]

Histopathology

The characteristic feature is the finding in the perianal squamous epithelium of large rounded cells with abundant, pale cytoplasm and a large nucleus often situated peripherally (Fig. 16-17). Although these cells resemble signet ring cells, they usually contain less mucus and have a different histochemical staining pattern[102]; it is important to distinguish true Paget's disease from pagetoid spread of signet ring cells from a nearby adenocarcinoma. Paget's cells are probably of apocrine origin; when unassociated with adenocarcinoma elsewhere, perianal Paget's disease is usually a low-grade neoplastic lesion. If the staining pattern differs from the usual, in particular if apocrine markers are absent, it is more likely that the lesion is associated with an underlying adenocarcinoma.[102,106] Clinically occult Paget's disease may be found on histologic examination following rectal excision for carcinoma.[107,108] Conversely, Paget's disease with no apparent associated malignancy may be followed several years later by the development of an adenocarcinoma.[102,109,110]

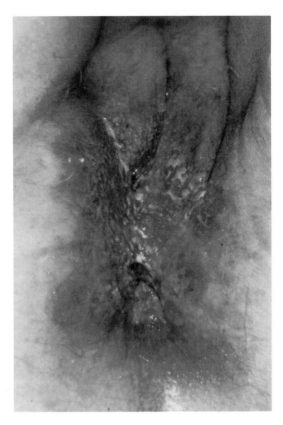

Figure 16-16. Macroscopic view, perianal Paget's disease. This shows a typical appearance in perianal Paget's disease, with variegated darkly reddened skin and distortion of the anus.

Management

The diagnosis is made by biopsy under general anesthesia; as the true extent of the lesion may not be apparent macroscopically, several biopsies are necessary around the apparent periphery of the lesion.[111]

A staging system for this disease has been described as a basis for deciding on appropriate treatment.[111] Broadly, treatment depends on whether there is an associated adenocarcinoma; thus a careful search for such a lesion is required initially. If the lesion appears isolated, wide local excision, with or without skin graft, is sufficient.[102,109,112] A margin of at least 1 cm of normal skin is taken, the deep margin of excision extending down to the underlying sphincter muscle; excision should reach up to the dentate line, or higher if the lesion extends to this level. In some cases, local spread within the anus may be sufficient to require abdominoperineal excision, even in the absence of an associated adenocarcinoma.[111]

If rectal cancer is present, abdominoperineal excision is indicated, whatever the level of the lesion within the rectum; particular care is needed in the perineal dissection to ensure wide excision of the perianal lesion. In patients with widespread or recurrent disease there have been reports of success using chemotherapy and radiotherapy.[113,114] Photodynamic therapy has been used in similar circumstances.[115]

Long-term follow-up is required in this condition, as local

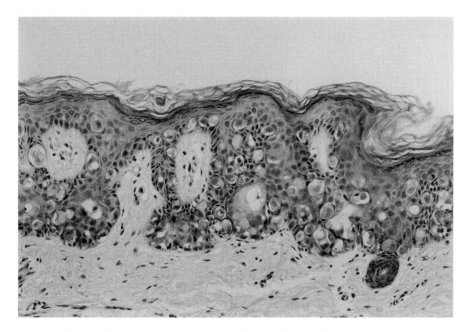

Figure 16-17. Histology, perianal Paget's disease. Classical "Paget's cells" are seen singly and in clumps within the perianal skin.

recurrence may occur many years later, also with the risk of later metastatic spread.[102,109,116]

Prognosis

In stage I disease long-term disease-free survival is usual. In those with associated adenocarcinoma without evidence of metastasis at the time of primary surgery, 5-year survival rates of around 50% can be expected.[109]

Melanoma

Incidence

Melanoma is very rare, accounting for just 1% of malignant tumors of the anal canal. Around 600 cases have been recorded in the medical literature since the first case report in 1854.[117] Sweden and Israel each yielded less than 50 cases in 15 and 20 years, respectively.[118,119] There are only a few series with more than a handful of cases from which to draw general conclusions regarding the behaviour of this tumor and upon which guidelines for management can be based.[120–122]

Some series have demonstrated a predominance in females.[118,122,123] Mean age for this condition is in the late 50s.[120] The condition affects European Jews more frequently than other groups in Israel.[119] Registry data from the United States show the condition to be more common north of latitude 40°N.[123]

Clinical Features

The lesion may mimic a thrombosed external pile due to its color (Fig. 16-18), although amelanotic tumors also occur, constituting 25% of cases in one series.[122] The commonest symptom at presentation is bleeding.[118] It has a very poor prognosis—most patients die rapidly from distant spread. In a series

Figure 16-18. Macroscopic view, melanoma. Looking much like a thrombosed external pile, this tumor has breached the skin within the anal canal, but is spreading subcutaneously posteriorly.

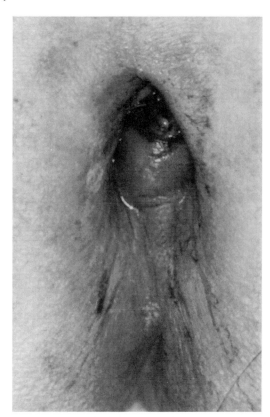

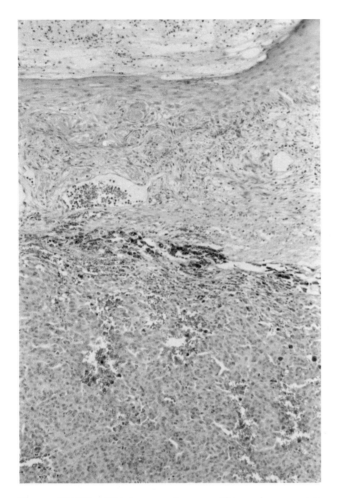

Figure 16-19. Histology, melanoma. This melanoma, predominantly amelanotic, is spreading widely deep to the dermis.

of 21 cases reported from St. Mark's Hospital, there were no long-term survivors, while Wanebo et al.[124] recorded a 5-year survival rate of just 8%.[121]

Pathology

Melanocytes are found in the squamous zone and to a lesser extent in the transitional zone of the anal canal[125]; presumably, therefore, malignant melanoma arises in these areas, although the tumor is often sufficiently advanced at presentation to make ascertainment of its anatomic origin difficult.[126] Histologically, melanoma at this site resembles the lesion in other primary sites (Fig. 16-19). The main cell types are polygonal and spindle cells.[1] The presence of tumor giant cells may assist in differential diagnosis. At least one-third of cases have involved lymph nodes at presentation,[127] whereas a similar proportion have manifest distant spread at that time.[118]

Management

Some variation in the approach to this exceedingly aggressive disease is possible. At St. Mark's Hospital, the condition was so uniformly poor in outlook that radical surgery was aban-

doned in favor of palliative local excision more than 30 years ago.[121] Others have reported that radical surgery offers no survival advantage.[128,129] At the M.D. Anderson Hospital, local recurrence was less frequent after radical surgery, but this did not translate into any survival advantage.[130] In the Roswell Park and Memorial Sloan-Kettering series, survival was superior in those subjected to radical rather than local surgery.[120,131] The Swedish experience was dismal, but the authors pointed out that tumor sizes were smaller in those treated by local excision, so the unfavorable outcome from abdominoperineal excision might be due at least in part to selection bias.[118] Goldman and his colleagues[118] concluded that radical surgery should be considered in the absence of evidence of distant metastasis, and others recommend local excision only.[121,130]

In this author's limited experience, local symptoms may be sufficiently distressing during the inexorable advance of the disease that colostomy or palliative abdominoperineal excision may become necessary in some cases.

Figure 16-20. Histology, adenocarcinoma arising in a fistula-in-ano. The mouth of this fistula, lined by squamous epithelium, contains a plug of mucopus. On its left wall and spreading downwards and to the right, and containing mucous lakes, are areas of darker staining adenocarcinoma cells.

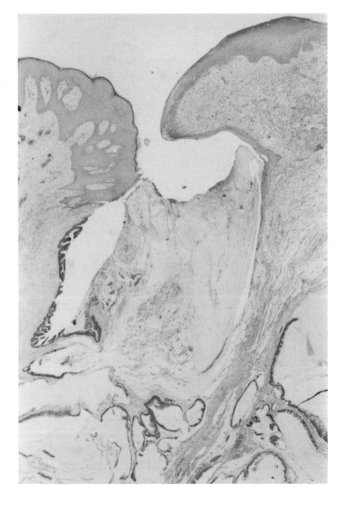

Prognosis

The outcome in this disease is far worse than in any other tumor type in the anorectal region. Median survival is around 12 to 18 months.[118,130] Several series report no long-term survivors,[121,122,128] whereas in others up to 25% of favorable cases survived for 5 years.[120,131] The one ray of hope comes from Weinstock's[123] population-based registry review, which suggests that the prognosis may have improved over the past 15 years.

Adenocarcinoma

Adenocarcinoma, a rare tumor, may be difficult to ascribe with confidence to the anal canal—almost certainly most adenocarcinomas growing down the anal canal and perhaps out through the orifice have arisen in the distal rectum. There are, however, two particular lesions that certainly arise in the anal canal.

Anal Gland Carcinoma

Anal gland carcinoma, which is excessively rare, is usually a flat, submucosal tumor that spreads circumferentially to cause stenosis. Histologically it closely resembles anal gland mucosa.

Mucinous Adenocarcinoma Arising in a Chronic Fistula-in-ano

Mucinous adenocarcinoma arising in a chronic fistula-in-ano presents in a patient with longstanding perianal sepsis. The pattern of the fistulous disease may have become complex and may be associated with an increasing mucous discharge. These tumors are usually well differentiated and are associated with mucous pools in the surrounding tissues (Fig. 16-20); it is important to make the distinction from chronic fistula that has become lined with benign colorectal mucosa.[1]

Anal adenocarcinoma is treated in the same way as low rectal cancer, with radical surgery as the mainstay. The prognosis is poor despite radical treatment.[132]

REFERENCES

1. Morson B, Dawson I (1990) Morson and Dawson's Gastrointestinal Pathology. Blackwell, Oxford
2. Williams G, Talbot I (1994) Anal carcinoma—a histological review. Histopathology 25:507–516
3. Klotz R Jr, Pamukcoglu T, Souilliard D (1967) Transitional cloacogenic carcinoma of the anal canal. Clinicopathologic study of three hundred seventy-three cases. Cancer 20:1727–1745
4. Boman B, Moertel C, O'Connell M et al (1984) Carcinoma of the anal canal. A clinical and pathologic study of 188 cases. Cancer 54:114–125
5. Pinna Pintor M, Northover JMA, Nicholls RJ (1989) Squamous cell carcinoma of the anus at one hospital from 1948 to 1984. Br J Surg 76:806–810
6. UKCCCR Anal Cancer Working Party (1989) Protocol—prospective randomised trial of combined modality therapy v. radiation alone in the management of anal cancer. United Kingdom Coordination Committee on Cancer Research.
7. Greenall M, Magill G, Quan S, DeCosse J (1986) Recurrent epidermoid cancer of the anus. Cancer 57:1437–1441
8. Scholefield J, Sonnex C, Talbot I et al (1989) Anal and cervical intraepithelial neoplasia: possible parallel. Lancet 2:765–769
9. de Ruiter A, Carter P, Katz D et al (1994) A comparison of cytology and histology to detect anal intraepithelial neoplasia. Genitourin Med 70:22–25
10. Scholefield JH, Palmer JG, Shepherd NA et al (1990) Clinical and pathological correlates of HPV type 16 DNA in anal cancer. Int J Colorectal Dis 5:219–222
11. Koutsky LA, Wolner HP (1989) Genital papillomavirus infections: current knowledge and future prospects. Obstet Gynecol Clin North Am 16:541–564
12. Scholefield J, Hickson W, Smith J (1992) Anal intraepithelial neoplasia: part of a multifocal disease process. Lancet 340:1271–1273
13. Office-of-Population-Censuses-and-Surveys (1988) Cancer Statistics Registrations. HMSO, London
14. Young J, Percey C, Asire A (1981) Surveillance, Epidemiology, and End Results, 1973–77. National Institutes of Health, Public Health Service, Bethesda, MD
15. Levi F, La Vecchia C, Randimbisson L et al (1991) Patterns of large bowel cancer by subsite, age, sex and marital status. Tumori 77:246–251
16. Peters R, Mack T (1983) Patterns of anal carcinoma by gender and marital status in Los Angeles County. Br J Cancer 48:629–636
17. Jarrett W (1988) Cancer and AIDS; the contribution of comparative medicine. Vet Rec 123:34–36
18. Oriel J (1989) Human papillomaviruses and anal cancer. Genitourin Med 65:213–215
19. Goldman S, Glimelius B, Nilsson B, Pahlman L (1989) Incidence of anal epidermoid carcinoma in Sweden 1970–1984. Acta Chir Scand 155:191–197
20. Melbye M, Sprogel P (1991) Aetiological parallel between anal cancer and cervical cancer. Lancet 338:657–659
21. Daling J, Sherman K (1992) Relationship between human papillomavirus infection and tumours of anogenital sites other than the cervix. IARC Sci Publ 119:223–241
22. Rabkin C, Biggar R, Melbye M, Curtis R (1992) Second primary cancers following anai and cervical carcinoma: evidence of shared etiologic factors. Am J Epidemiol 136:54–58
23. Ogunbiyi O, Scholefield J, Robertson G et al (1994) Anal human papillomavirus infection and squamous neoplasia in patients with invasive vulvar cancer. Obstet Gynaecol 83:212–216
24. Milburn P, Brandsma J, Goldsman C et al (1988) disseminated warts and evolving squamous cell carcinoma in a patient with acquired immunodeficiency syndrome. J Am Acad Dermatol 19:401–405
25. Monfardini S, Vaccher E, Lazzarin A et al (1990) Characterization of AIDS-associated tumors in Italy: report of 435 cases of an IVDA-based series. Cancer Detect Prev 14:391–393

26. Austin D (1982) Etiologic clues from descriptive epidemiology; squamous carcinoma of the anus. Natl Cancer Inst Monogr 62:89–90

27. Scholefield JH, Thornton JH, Cuzick J, Northover JM (1990) Anal cancer and marital status. Br J Cancer 62:286–288

28. Peters R, Mack T, Bernstein L (1984) Parallels in the epidemiology of selected anogenital carcinomas. J Natil Cancer Institute 72:609–615

29. Daling J, Weiss N, Klopfenstein L (1982) Correlates of homosexual behaviour and the incidence of anal cancer. JAMA 247:1988–1990

30. Daling J, Weiss N, Hislop P (1987) Sexual practices, sexually transmitted diseases and the incidence of anal cancer. N Engl J Med 317:973–977

31. Holly EA, Whittemore AS, Aston DA et al (1989) Anal cancer incidence: genital warts, anal fissure or fistula, hemorrhoids, and smoking. J Natl Cancer Inst 81:1726–1731

32. Mathe G (1985) La prévention des cancers génito-anaux et bucco-laryngo-oesophagiens à virus transmis sexuellement. Biomed Pharmacother 39:253–262

33. Gross G, Gissmann L (1986) Urogenitale und anale Papillomavirusinfektionen. Hautarzt 37:587–596

34. Rudlinger R (1988) Warzen im ausseren anogenitalbereich, unter spezieller berucksichtigung von HIV-positiven patienten. Anogenitale warzen. Schweiz Rundschau Med Prax 77: 1202–1207

35. Palmer J, Scholefield J, Coates P et al (1989) Anal cancer and human papillomaviruses. Dis Colon Rectum 32:1016–1022

36. Beckmann A, Daling J, Sherman K et al (1989) Human papillomavirus infection and anal cancer. Int J Cancer 43: 1042–1049

37. Gal A, Saul S, Stoler M (1989) In situ hybridization analysis of human papillomavirus in anal squamous cell carcinoma. Mod Pathol 2:439–443

38. Palefsky JM, Holly EA, Gonzales J (1991) Detection of human papillomavirus DNA in anal intraepithelial neoplasia and anal cancer. Cancer Res 51:1014–1019

39. Scholefield JH, McIntyre P, Palmer JG et al (1990a) DNA hybridisation of routinely processed tissue for detecting HPV DNA in anal squamous cell carcinomas over 40 years. J Clin Pathol 43:133–136

40. Melbye M, Palefsky J, Gonzales J et al (1990) Immune status as a determinant of human papillomavirus detection and its association with anal epithelial abnormalities. Int J Cancer 46:203–206

41. Heino P, Goldman S, Lagerstedt U, Dillner J (1993) Molecular and serological studies of human papillomavirus among patients with anal epidermoid carcinoma. Int J Cancer 53: 377–381

42. Taxy J, Gupta P, Gupta J, Shah K (1989) Anal cancer. Microscopic condyloma and tissue demonstration of human papillomavirus capsid antigen and viral DNA. Arch Pathol Lab Med 113:1127–1131

43. De Schryver A, Meheus A (1990) Epidemiology of sexually transmitted diseases: the global picture. Bull WHO 68: 639–654

44. Syrjanen K, Syrjanen S, von Krogh G (1988) Anal condylomas in homosexual/bisexual and heterosexual males II. Histopathological and virological assessment. p. 127. In: VIIth International Papillomavirus Workshop.

45. Howard L, Paterson-Brown S, Weber J et al (1986) Squamous carcinoma of the anus in young homosexual men with T helper depletion. Genitourin Med 62:393–395

46. Safai B, Lynfield R, Lowenthal D, Koziner B (1987) Cancers associated with HIV infection. Anticancer Res 7:1055–1067

47. Lorenz H, Wilson W, Leigh B (1991) Squamous cell carcinoma of the anus and HIV infection. Dis Colon Rectum 34: 336–338

48. Melbye M, Cote T, Kessler L et al (1994) High incidence of anal cancer among AIDS patients. The AIDS/Cancer Working Group. Lancet 343:636–639

49. Carter P, de Ruiter A, Whatrup C et al (1995) Human immunodeficiency virus infection and genital warts as risk factors for anal intraepithelial neoplasia in homosexual men. Br J Surg 82:473–474.

50. Rabkin C, Yellin F (1994) Cancer incidence in a population with a high prevalence of infection with human immunodeficiency virus type 1. J Natl Cancer Inst 86:1711–1716

51. Penn I (1986) Cancers of the anogenital region in renal transplant patients. Analysis of 65 cases. Cancer 58:611–616

52. Manias D, Ostrow R, McGlennen R et al (1989) Characterization of integrated human papilloma virus type 11 DNA in primary and metastatic tumors from a renal transplant recipient. Cancer Res 49:2514–2519

53. Gilbert J, Mann C, Scholefield J, Domizio P (1991) The aetiology and surgery of carcinoma of the anus, rectum and sigmoid colon in Crohn's disease. Negative correlation with human papilloma virus type 16 (HPV 16). Eur J Surg Oncol 17:507–513

54. Daling J, Sherman K, Hislop T et al (1992) Cigarette smoking and the risk of anogenital cancer. Am J Epidemiol 135: 180–189

55. Frisch M, Melbye M (1995) Risk of lung cancer in pre- and postmenopausal women with ano-genital malignancies. Int J Cancer 62:508–511

56. Edwards A, Morus L, Foster M, Griffith G (1991) Anal cancer: the case for earlier diagnosis. J R Soc Med 84:395–397

57. Nelson R, Prasad M, Abcarian H (1985) Anal carcinoma presenting as a perirectal abscess or fistula. Arch Surg 120: 632–635

58. Goldman S, Norming U, Svensson C, Glimelius B (1991) transanorectal ultrasonography in the staging of anal epidermoid carcinoma. Int J Color Dis 6:152–157

59. Scherrer A, Reboul F, Martin D et al (1990) CT of malignant anal canal tumors. Radiographics 10:433–453

60. Scott N, Beart R Jr, Weiland L et al (1989) Carcinoma of the anal canal and flow cytometric DNA analysis. Br J Cancer 60:56–58

61. Shepherd N, Scholefield J, Love S et al (1990) Prognostic factors in anal squamous cell carcinoma: a multivariate analysis of clinical, pathological and flow cytometric parameters in 235 cases. 16:545–555

62. Goldman S, Svensson C, Bronnergard M et al (1993) Prognostic significance of serum concentration of squamous cell carcinoma antigen in anal epidermoid carcinoma. Int J Color Dis 8:98–102

63. Fontana X, Lagrange J, Francois E et al (1991) Evaluation of the 'squamous cell carcinoma antigen' as a marker of epidermoid cancer of the anal canal. Ann Gastroenterol Hepatol Paris 27:293–296

64. Speissl B, Beahrs O, Hermanek P et al (eds) (1989) TNM Atlas. Illustrated Guide to the TNM/pTNM Classification of Malignant Tumours. Springer-Verlag, Berlin

65. Greenall M, Quan S, Stearns M (1985) Epidermoid cancer of the anal margin. Pathologic features, treatment and clinical results. Am J Surg 149:95–101

66. Pyper P, Parks T (1985) The results of surgery for epidermoid carcinoma of the anus. Br J Surg 72:712–714

67. Jensen S, Hagen K, Harling H (1988) Long term prognosis after radical treatment for squamous call carcinoma of the anal canal and anal margin. Dis Colon Rectum 31:273–278

68. Brown D, Oglesby A, Scott D, Dayton M (1988) Squamous cell carcinoma of the anus: a twenty-five year retrospective. Am Surg 54:337–342

69. UKCCCR Anal-Cancer Trial Working Party (1996) Epidermoid anal cancer: results from the UKCCCR randomised trial of radiotherapy alone versus radiotherapy, 5-fluorouracil and mitomycin-C. Lancet 348:1049–1054

70. Zelnick R, Haas P, Ajlouni M et al (1992) Results of abdominoperineal resections for failure after combination chemotherapy and radiation therapy for anal canal cancers. Dis Colon Rectum 35:574–578

71. O'Brien P, Williams M, Jenrette J, Pitre B (1993) Combined modality therapy in the treatment of epidermoid carcinoma of the anus at the Medical University of South Carolina. J South Carolina Med Assoc 89:333–336

72. Northover J (1988) Place de la chirurgie dans le cancer épidermoide de l'anus. Lyon Chir 87:82–84

73. Tanum G (1993) Treatment of relapsing anal carcinoma. Acta Oncol 32:33–35

74. Herrera L, Luna P, Garcia C (1995) Surgical therapy of recurrent epidermoid carcinoma of the anal canal. In: Cancer of the Colon, Rectum and Anus. McGraw-Hill, New York, pp. 1043–1050

75. Longo W, Vernava A, Wade T et al (1994) Recurrent squamous cell carcinoma of the anal canal. Predictors of initial treatment failure and results of salvage therapy. Ann Surg 220:40–49

76. Ellenhorn J, Enker W, Quan S (1994) Salvage abdominoperineal resection following combined chemotherapy and radiotherapy for epidermoid carcinoma of the anus. Ann Surg Oncol 1:105–110

77. Hoffman MS, LaPolla JP, Roberts WS et al (1990) Use of local flaps for primary anal reconstruction following perianal resection for neoplasia. Gynecol Oncol 36:348–352

78. Zoetmulder F, Baris G (1995) Wide resection and reconstruction preserving fecal continence in recurrent anal cancer: report of three cases. Dis Colon Rectum 38:80–84

79. Waterhouse N, Northover J (1993) Reconstructive surgery of the groin and perineum. pp. 10–22. Modern Coloproctology: Surgical Grand Rounds from St Mark's Hospital. Edward Arnold, London

80. Papillon J, Mayer M, Montbarbon J et al (1983) A new approach to the management of epidermoid carcinoma of the anal canal. Cancer 51:1830–1837

81. Cummings B (1995) Anal cancer: radiation, with and without chemotherapy pp. 1025–1042. In: Cancer of the Colon, Rectum and Anus. McGraw-Hill, New York

82. Nigro N, Vaitkevicius V, Considine JB (1974) Combined therapy for cancer of the anal canal: a preliminary report. Dis Colon Rectum 17:354–356

83. Gabriel W (1940) Squamous cell carcinoma of the anus and anal canal: an analysis of 55 cases. Proc R Soc Med 34:139–160

84. Eschwege F, Lasser P, Chavy A (1985) Squamous cell carcinoma of the anal canal: treatment by external beam irradiation. Radiother Oncol 3:145–150

85. Papillon J, Montbarbon J (1987) Epidermoid carcinoma of the anal canal: a series of 276 cases. Dis Colon Rectum 30:324–333

86. Doggett S, Green J, Cantril S (1988) Effect of radiation therapy alone for limited squamous cell carcinoma of the anal canal. Int J Radiat Oncol Biol Phys 15:1069–1072

87. Schlienger M, Krzirsch C, Pene F (1989) Epidermoid carcinoma of the anal canal: treatment results and prognostic variables in a series of 242 cases. Int J Radiat Oncol Biol Phys 17:1141–1151

88. Cummings B (1982) The place of radiation therapy in the treatment of carcinoma of the anal canal. Cancer Treat Rev 9:125–147

89. Papillon J (1982) Rectal and Anal Cancer. Springer-Verlag, Berlin

90. James R, Pointon R, Martin S (1985) Local radiotherapy in management of squamous carcinoma of the anus. Br J Surg 72:282–285

91. Nigro N (1984) An evaluation of combined therapy for squamous cell cancer of the anal canal. Dis Colon Rectum 27:763–766

92. Steel G (1988) The search for therapeutic gain in the combination of radiotherapy and chemotherapy. Radiother Oncol 11:31–35

93. Tannock IF (1989) Combined modality treatment with radiotherapy and chemotherapy. Radiother Oncol 16:83–101

94. Cummings B, Keane T, Thomas G, et al (1984) Results and toxicity of the treatment of anal canal carcinoma by radiation therapy or radiation therapy and chemotherapy. Cancer 54:2062–2068

95. Cummings B, Keane T, O'Sullivan B, et al (1991) Epidermoid anal cancer: treatment with radiation alone or by radiation with 5-fluorouracil with and without mitomycin C. Int J Radiat Oncol Biol Phys 21:1115–1125

96. Cummings B, Keane T, O'Sullivan B, et al (1993) Mitomycin in anal canal carcinoma. Oncology, suppl. 1, 50:63–69

97. Allal A, Kurtz J, Pipard G et al (1993) Chemotherapy versus radiotherapy alone for anal cancer: a retrospective comparison. Int J Radiat Oncol Biol Phys 27:59–66

98. RTOG (1994) Is mitomycin C necessary in the chemoradiation regimen for anal canal carcinoma? Interim results of a phase III randomized intergroup study. ASTRO Proc

99. Gerard J, Romestaing P, Mahe M, Salerno N (1991) Cancer of the anal canal. The role of the combination of 5FU and cisplatinum. Lyon Chir 87:74–76

100. Rich T, Ajani J, Morrison W et al (1993) Chemoradiation of anal cancer: radiation plus continuous infusion of 5-fluorouracil with or without cisplatin. Radiother Oncol 27:209–215

101. Stewart F, Harkins B, Han S, Daniel T (1989) Cisplatin, 5-FU, mitomycin C and concurrent radiation therapy with and without esophagectomy for esophageal carcinoma. Cancer 64:622–628

102. Armitage N, Jass J, Richman P et al (1989) Paget's disease of the anus: a clinicopathological study. Br J Surg 76:60–63

103. Paget J (1874) On disease of the mammary areola preceding cancer of the mammary gland. St Bartholomew Hosp Res Lond 10:87–89

104. Darier J Couillard P (1983) On a case of Paget's disease of the perineo-anal scrotal region. Soc Franc Dermatol Syph 4: 25–31

105. Neumann R (1986) Extramammary Paget's disease associated with stomach cancer. Hautarzt 37:586–570

106. Merot Y, Mazoujian G, Pinkus G (1985) "Extramammary Paget's disease of the perianal and perineal regions. Evidence of apocrine derivation. Arch Dermatol 121:750–752

107. Lertprasertsuke N, Tsutsumi Y (1991) Latent perianal Paget's disease associated with mucin-producing rectal adenocarcinoma. Acta Pathol Jpn 41:386–393

108. Sasaki M, Terada T, Nakanuma Y et al (1990) Anorectal mucinous adenocarcinoma associated with latent perianal Paget's disease. Am J Gastroenterol 85:199–202

109. Jensen S, Sjolin K, Shokouh-Amiri M et al (1988) Paget's disease of the anal margin. Br J Surg 75:1089–1092

110. Goldman S, Ihre T, Lagerstedt U, Svennson C (1992) Perianal Paget's disease: report of five case. Int J Color Dis 7:167–169

111. Shutze W, Gleysteen J (1990) Perianal Paget's disease. Classification and review of management: report of two cases. Dis Colon Rectum 33:502–507

112. Beck D, Fazio V (1987) Perianal Paget's disease. Dis Colon Rectum 30:263–266

113. Secco G, Lapertosa G, Sertoli M et al (1984) Perianal Paget's disease; case report of an elderly patient treated with polychemotherapy and radiotherapy. Tumori 70:381–383

114. Thirlby R, Hammer C, Galagan K et al (1990) Perianal Paget's disease: successful treatment with combined chemoradiotherapy. Report of a case. Dis Colon Rectum 33:150–152

115. Petrelli N, Cebollero J, Rodriguez-Bigas M, Mang T (1992) Photodynamic therapy in the management of neoplasms of the perianal skin. Arch Surg 127:1436–1438

116. Beck D, Fazio V (1989) Premalignant lesions of the anal margin. South Med J 82:470–474

117. Quan S (1995) Anorectal melanoma. pp. 1069–1071. In: Cancer of the Colon, Rectum and Anus. McGraw-Hill New York

118. Goldman S, Glimelius B, Pahlman L (1990) Anorectal malignant melanoma in Sweden. Report of 49 cases. Dis Colon Rectum 33:874–877

119. Siegal B, Cohen D, Jacob E (1983) Surgical treatment of anorectal melanomas. Am J Surg 146:336–338

120. Brady M, Kavolius J, Quan S (1995) Anorectal melanoma. A 64 year experience at Memorial Sloan-Kettering Cancer Center. Dis Colon Rectum 38:146–151

121. Ward M, Romano G, Nicholls RJ (1986) The surgical treatment of anorectal malignant melanoma. Br J Surg 73:68–69

122. Antoniuk P, Tjandra J, Webb B et al (1993) Anorectal malignant melanoma has a poor prognosis. Int J Color Dis 8:81–86

123. Weinstock M (1993) Epidemiology and prognosis of anorectal melanoma. Gastroenterology 104:174–178

124. Wanebo H, Woodruff J, Farr G, Quan S (1981) Anorectal melanoma. Cancer 47:1891–1900

125. Clemmensen O, Fenger C (1991) Melanocytes in the anal canal epithelium. Histopathology 18:237–241

126. Fenger C, Neilsen V (1986) Precancerous changes in the anal canal epithelium in resection specimens. Acta Pathol Microbiol Immunol Scand A 94:63–69

127. Garcia-Olmo D, Pellicer-Franco E, Morales-Cuenca G et al (1990) Cancer of the anus: incidence and behaviour of melanoma in our series. Rev Esp Enferm Dig 77:269–273

128. Slingluff C, Seigler H (1992) Anorectal melanoma: clinical characteristics and the role of abdominoperineal resection. Ann Plast Surg 28:85–88

129. Wong J, Cagle L, Storm F, Morton D (1987) Natural history of surgically treated mucosal melanoma. Am J Surg 154: 54–57

130. Ross M, Pezzi T, Meurer D et al: (1990) Patterns of failure in anorectal melanoma. A guide to surgical therapy. Arch Surg 125:313–316

131. Konstadoulakis M, Ricaniadis N, Walsh D, Karakousis C (1995) Malignant melanoma of the anorectal region. J Surg Oncol 58:118–120

132. Basik M, Rodriguez-Bigas M, Penetrante R, Petrelli N (1995) Prognosis and recurrence patterns of anal adenocarcinoma. Am J Surg 169:233–237

17

PERIANAL DERMATOLOGY

Richard M. Devine

Not infrequently, patients referred to the proctologist for "hemorrhoids" turn out to have a perianal dermatologic disorder. These dermatologic problems are the result of a variety of infectious, neoplastic, or inflammatory disorders that may be localized to the perianal area or may be a manifestation of a systemic disease. When confronted with a perianal skin change, the proctologist should be able to evaluate the problem appropriately so the correct diagnosis is made and appropriate treatment initiated.

Neoplastic changes, perianal Crohn's disease, idiopathic pruritus, and sexually transmitted diseases including herpes simplex and problems seen in patients positive for the human immunodeficiency virus are covered elsewhere in the text. This chapter focuses on those skin problems that are not unique to the perineum but may involve that area.

HIDRADENITIS SUPPURATIVA

Hidradenitis suppurativa is characterized by chronic recurrent suppurative infections in the apocrine gland-bearing skin areas, primarily in the axillae, groin, and anogenital regions.

The human skin contains two types of sweat glands, the eccrine glands and the apocrine glands. The eccrine glands and the apocrine glands are both simple tubular structures. The eccrine glands are located throughout the body and open directly on the skin. The apocrine glands lie deep beneath the skin surface, are located primarily in the axillae, groin, and perineal regions, and open into hair follicles. The eccrine glands' function is to control body temperature. The apocrine glands probably represent vestigial organs in humans, but in other mammals they have mating and protective functions.

In 1955, Shelley and Cahn[1] described the experimental production of hidradenitis by manual epilation of an area in the axillae of 12 men and then application of a belladonna adhesive tape. The belladonna created anhidrosis of the apocrine glands. Three of the 12 subjects developed deep tender nodules that on histologic examination demonstrated plugging of the apocrine sweat duct, dilatation of the duct, and severe inflammatory changes confined to a single apocrine gland. The adjacent hair

follicles and deeper eccrine glands appeared normal. If the process was left to continue, the gland would rupture and the infection would spread to other glands. Shelley and Cahn's[1] work formed the basis for the theory that obstruction of the apocrine duct is the initiating event in the development of hidradenitis.

In recent years, however, this view on the pathogenesis of hidradenitis has been questioned. Evidence against this theory is the fact that histologic examination of areas involved with hidradenitis (inframammary, inguinal, upper thigh, and buttock areas) fails to show any apocrine glands, and examination of axillary tissue shows that the predominant lesions are epithelial lined cysts of follicular origin, often with absence of inflammation in the adjacent apocrine gland.[2] The location of hidradenitis corresponds to the location of the apocrine glands, but it also corresponds to the distribution of terminal hair follicles dependent on low concentrations of androgens. Thus, it may be occlusion and infection of these hair follicles that is the primary event in hidradenitis, with secondary infection of the surrounding apocrine glands.

Clinical Manifestations

The clinical manifestations of hidradenitis suppurativa do not appear until after puberty, and the disease occurs in both men and women. The earliest form of the disease is a localized, firm, tender swelling that does not point. As the disease progresses the indurated area increases in size, becomes erythematous and painful, and will eventually drain spontaneously. The hallmark of hidradenitis is chronic relapse with recurrent swelling and drainage in the affected areas. With recurrent infection chronic sinus tracts are formed, fibrosis increases, and the apocrine glands are destroyed. At this point, the disease will have the typical appearance of multiple pitted scars, which lead to dermal sinus tracts. Histologically, the affected areas demonstrate acute and chronic inflammatory changes in the dermis and subdermal layers with prominent fibrosis. Cystic structures lined by stratified squamous epithelium and epithelial lined sinus

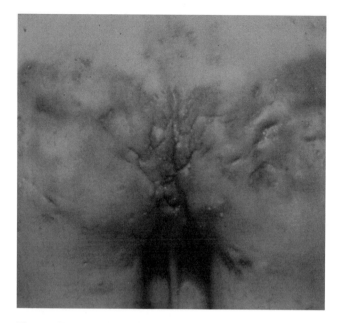

Figure 17-1. Hidradenitis suppurativa.

tracts may also be observed. In the perineum, the most common organisms isolated are staphylococcus and streptococcus species. Highet et al.[3] studied the bacteriology of 32 patients with perineal suppurative hidradenitis and found *Streptococcus milleri* in 21 of 32 patients. Other common organisms are *Staphylococcus aureus*, anaerobic streptococci, *Proteus*, and *Bacteroides* species. Bendahan et al.,[4] in Tel Aviv, found evidence of *Chlamydia trachomatis* infection by direct immunofluorescent studies in six of seven consecutive patients treated for hidradenitis, although this organism could not be identified in purulent skin discharge. In 10 controls with cryptogenic perianal abscesses, only 2 had serologic evidence of chlamydial infection.[4]

The diagnosis is usually not difficult. The recurrent nature of the disease with its characteristic scarring, sinus tract formation, and location is unique to hidradenitis (Figs. 17-1 and 17-2; see also Plate 17-1, 17-2). Other perineal fistulous dis-

Figure 17-2. Hidradenitis suppurativa.

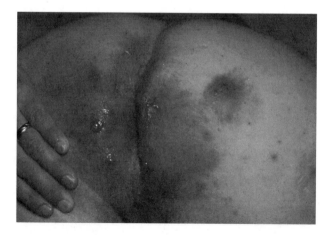

eases such as Crohn's disease, infected sebaceous cysts, perirectal abscess, pilonidal sinus, actinomycosis, tuberculosis, and lymphogranuloma inguinale should be in the differential diagnosis. If sinus tracts extend to the dentate line, the diagnosis of hidradenitis should be suspect. Hidradenitis and Crohn's disease can be present in the same patient. In 61 patients with a diagnosis of hidradenitis suppurativa seen at the Cleveland Clinic over an 8-year period, 38% also had a diagnosis of Crohn's disease.[5]

Treatment

Only in very early lesions without sinus tract formation or scarring is medical treatment alone beneficial. Almost all cases seen by the colon and rectal surgeon will involve at least some areas of subcutaneous purulence with draining sinus tracts that require surgical treatment. In these cases, antibiotics should be used as an adjunct to surgery. Recommended antibiotics include minocycline, ciprofloxacin, cephalosporin or clindamycin. Ideally, the choice of antibiotic should be directed by cultures of purulent drainage.

Two main surgical techniques are used to treat perianal hidradenitis: wide local excision or extensive "deroofing" of sinus tracts.

Thornton and Abcarian and the Lahey Clinic group are proponents of wide local excision. Thornton and Abcarian[6] reported the results of treatment in 107 patients with perianal or perineal hidradenitis suppurativa. All but 4 of the patients were black. In all patients, the involved area was excised down to normal fat or fascia, and the wounds were left open to heal by secondary intention. The open wound was treated with Sitz baths four times a day and gauze dressings. Twenty-two percent of the patients had large wounds (more than 5 cm in any dimension), yet a diverting colostomy was used in only one case, and skin grafting was not used in any patient. The average hospital stay was 7.2 days, with no mortality, and only four patients developed a recurrence within the 5-year period of the study.

The Lahey Clinic reported a retrospective analysis of 43 patients (90% male), all of whom were white.[7] Thirty-one of the patients were treated by wide local excision. Only two patients were diverted with a colostomy and only two had split-thickness skin grafting. Both of the skin grafts failed. They felt that wide local excision was more successful in preventing recurrence than incision and drainage or local unroofing, but the number of patients treated with local unroofing was small.

Williams et al.[8] report on two cases of neglected perianal hidradenitis that had progressed to involve the whole buttock area bilaterally. These patients were both treated with wide local excision and split-thickness grafting. One patient also had fecal diversion with a colostomy. Both skin grafts healed without difficulty. These two cases represent one end of the spectrum of perianal hidradenitis. Most cases are not this extensive and do not require skin grafting, even though it may be necessary in very extensive cases.

Culp[9] and Brown et al.[10] advocate a less radical surgical approach of "deroofing" all sinus tracts rather than excising them. Patients are examined under a general anesthetic. All tracts are very carefully delineated with a malleable probe, to explore their extent and communications. The skin overlying these tracts is excised, but the base of the tract, which is epithelialized, is left in place. Any areas of granulation tissue are removed with a curette. To prevent recurrence, it is important to probe all areas that may represent sinus tracts very carefully. Firm, indurated areas should be unroofed even if a tract into them cannot be found because these areas will almost always contain an infected cavity. Culp[9] reported follow-up of 1 to 7 years in 30 patients with minimal recurrence. The advantage of this technique is faster healing.

Squamous cell carcinoma is a rare complication of hidradenitis suppurativa. In a review of 16 cases, all the squamous cell cancers arose in the perianal or buttock area.[8] The time interval between the initial diagnosis of hidradenitis and the diagnosis of cancer was an average of 16 years. Wide local excision was the more frequent surgical approach, although some patients had an abdominal perineal excision. Nine patients developed recurrent disease, and 7 of these died of cancer.

PERIANAL TUBERCULOSIS

Tubercular involvement of the anus is a rare manifestation of gastrointestinal tuberculosis. There is no typical appearance of anal tuberculosis. It can present as a verrucous growth extending into the anal canal, as a perianal ulceration, or as multiple perianal fistulas. Because the gastrointestinal tract is often involved, it is difficult to distinguish this entity from Crohn's disease.[11]

When evaluating perianal ulcers or fistulous disease, tests to rule out tuberculosis should be performed when dealing with patients at increased risk of infection, such as immigrants from undeveloped nations or immunocompromised patients. An abnormal chest radiograph or positive tuberculosis skin test should also raise the index of suspicion. To rule out tuberculosis, a chest radiograph, tuberculin skin test, and sputum test for acid-fast bacteria should be done. Drainage from the perianal abscess should be stained for acid-fast material and cultured. Any anal lesions should be biopsied for histopathology, acid-fast staining, and cultures. Treatment is standard antituberculosis chemotherapy.

PSORIASIS

It is not uncommon for psoriasis to involve the intergluteal cleft and perianal regions. Farber and Nall[12] found that 44% of patients with psoriasis reported perianal involvement. Occasionally psoriasis will present as an isolated lesion in the perianal area or the gluteal cleft, which is considered a form of inverse or flexural psoriasis, a type that predominantly affects skin folds and flexures. It is thought that irritation secondary to fecal contamination and maceration in the perianal area gives rise to the psoriatic plaque.

Perianal psoriasis usually presents as a well-demarcated erythematous patch (Fig. 17-3; see also Plate 17-3). Perianal involvement can result in fissuring, which can be painful. In the patient with a known diagnosis of psoriasis or one who has characteristic lesions on other areas of the body (elbows, knees), the diagnosis is straightforward; when other lesions are not present, the diagnosis can be difficult. To confirm the diagnosis a punch biopsy of the involved skin can be done. Histologic findings include epidermal microabscesses, persistence of the nuclei

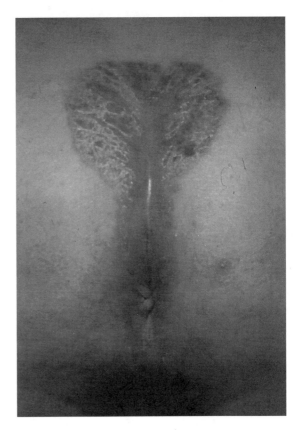

Figure 17-3. Psoriasis.

of the keratinocytes into the superficial stratum corneum layer of the skin, elongation of the dermal papilla, and diffuse hyperplasia and thickening of the epidermal spinosum layer with elongation of the rete ridges.

The simplest form of treatment for perianal psoriasis is the topical use of medium-strength corticosteroids.

TINEA CRURIS

Tinea cruris is a superficial fungal infection of the skin that most often occurs in the inguinal region of men, but the perianal region can also be involved. The usual pattern is a gradually progressing, sharply bordered, raised, reddened patch (Fig. 17-4; see also Plate 17-4). The most common organisms isolated in the United States today are *Trichophyton mentagrophytes* and *Trichophyton rubrum*.

The diagnosis can be made by seeing hyphae on a potassium hydroxide (KOH) preparation. A small scraping is taken of the scaling area and this is placed on a glass slide. A drop of 10 to 20% KOH is placed on the scale followed by a coverslip. The slide is gently heated and then examined under the microscope. The diagnosis can also be confirmed by culturing the affected area for fungal organisms.

Treatment consists of topical powder or creams containing an imidazole. Most commonly used are miconazole, clotrimazole, and ketoconazole. The fungal organisms thrive in an environment that is warm and moist, so the wearing of loose fitting clothing that provides for better air circulation may prevent recurrence.

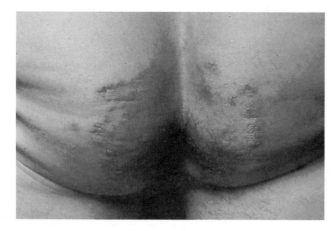

Figure 17-4. Tinea cruris.

Other diseases to consider in the differential diagnosis include psoriasis, candida, and erythrasma.

CANDIDIASIS

Candidiasis is an acute or chronic infection of the skin with the yeastlike fungus of the *Candida* genus. *Candida albicans* is the most common. Candidal infections can involve many different areas of the body, including the nails, mouth, mucocutaneous surfaces, and skin. The cutaneous folds, including the intergluteal cleft, are highly susceptible to infection with *C. albicans*.

Interiginous infection with *C. albicans* presents as a very red edematous lesion with a creamy exudate (Fig. 17-5; see also Plate 17-5). The main rash may be surrounded by satellite pustules. Symptoms are burning and itching.

Diagnosis can be established by a KOH preparation and culture of the exudate. Treatment includes daily washing with a gentle soap and twice daily application of a topical agent containing an antifungal agent such as clotrimazole, ketoconazole, miconazole, or nystatin.

PINWORMS

Infection with the intestinal roundworm *Enterobius vermicularis* is very common and has caused perianal pruritus for over 10,000 years.[13] It is a thread-like white worm 3 to 12 mm in

Figure 17-5. Candidiasis.

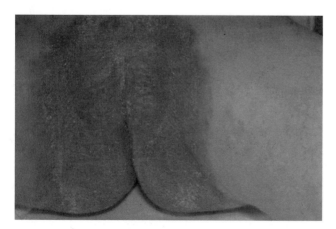

length. Infection occurs when the eggs of the worm are ingested. Following ingestion the adult worms of both sexes develop in the distal small bowel and proximal colon. The adult female lays thousands of eggs before it migrates out the anus. The eggs can remain viable for up to 20 days in cool moist conditions and can be found in house dust and bed linens.[14]

The peak incidence of infection occurs in children between the ages of 5 and 14. The main symptom is intense perianal and perineal pruritus. This occurs most often at night and is related to the migration of the female worm through the anal canal.

The diagnosis is established using a kit containing sticky cellulose tape. The tape is applied to the perianal skin in the morning before bathing and is then returned to the lab where it is examined for the presence of eggs. Occasionally the diagnosis is made when the adult female worm is observed as it protrudes through the anal canal.

Treatment consists of a single doses of mebendazole, 100 mg, or a single dose of pyrantel pamoate 11 mg/kg up to a maximum of 1 g.

LICHEN SCLEROSUS ET ATROPHICUS

Lichen sclerosus et atrophicus is a benign skin lesion that can affect any area of the body but is most commonly seen on the vulvar and penile skin. It is less common in men, and it usually does not involve the perianal skin in males.[15] In women, however, approximately 40 to 45% of those with vulvar lichen sclerosus et atrophicus will have perianal involvement as well.[16] The age of onset is fairly equally distributed between the third and eighth decades, but it can be seen at any age.

The gross appearance is characterized by pale macules or papules that eventually coalesce to form wrinkled plaques (Fig. 17-6; See also Plate 17-6). With time, thinning of the skin becomes more marked, with some degree of hypopigmentation. Telangiectasias may be prominent. The most common symptoms are burning and itching; stenosis of the introitus may occasionally result. Squamous cell carcinoma of the vulva or perineum has been found in about 5% of affected women.[16]

The most prominent histologic features are edema of the upper dermis with homogenization of the collagen. The epidermis is atrophic, and the rete ridges become flattened. There is hyperkeratosis, with the thick layer of keratin often thicker than the epidermis.

Asymptomatic patients do not need treatment. The most common treatment for symptomatic patients is topical corticosteroid cream. Two percent testosterone propionate topically has also been used with good results, although the benefits may not be seen for 3 to 4 months.[17]

Because of the small but definite risk of associated cancer, the patient should be seen annually or semiannually. Any unusual appearing areas or nonhealing ulcers should be biopsied to rule out cancer.

CONTACT DERMATITIS

Perianal contact dermatitis is probably the most common cause of perianal skin irritation. Contact dermatitis can be due to an allergic reaction to the presence of an allergen or it can be caused by prolonged exposure to an irritating substance.

A diaper rash is an example of a dermatitis due to prolonged

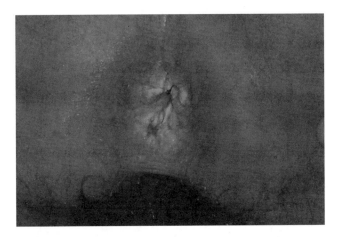

Figure 17-7. Lichen planus.

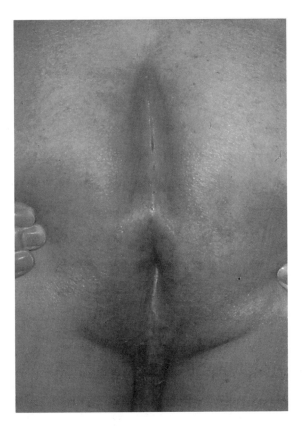

Figure 17-6. Lichen sclerosus et atrophicus.

exposure to an irritant. In adults, prolonged exposure of the perianal skin to fecal material can cause an irritant reaction. Anal pathology such as fissures, hemorrhoids, and enlarged papillae can cause anal discharge and soiling that will predispose to irritant contact dermatitis as well as to infection with *Candida* or other fungi.

Allergic contact dermatitis can be caused by a variety of substances. Soaps, toilet paper, feminine sprays, topical anesthetics, and proprietary creams and ointments all contain substances that may cause an allergic reaction in some patients.[18]

Evaluation of the patient should include a careful history to see what possible substances the patient may be using that may be a source of an allergic reaction. A careful examination of the anal area is done to rule out underlying anal pathology that may be the source of the irritation. Cultures and KOH smears can be done to rule out infection with fungi.

If there is underlying anal pathology, surgical treatment will often resolve the problem.[19] If an allergic reaction is suspected, simply eliminating the suspected offending substance may result in improvement. In more difficult cases or to confirm the diagnosis of contact allergy, the patient could be referred to a dermatologist for patch testing. Improved anal hygiene will help patients with irritant dermatitis. It is essential to cleanse the perianal area of fecal material after a bowel movement. Mild soap in water is best, but if this is impractical, the use of Tucks perianal pads or Balneol ointment is recommended.

LICHEN PLANUS

Lichen planus is a relatively common skin disorder that can affect any area of the body. The most common sites of involvement are the flexures of the wrists or the skin above the ankles. In 40% of patients, skin lesions and mucous membrane involvement, particularly of the oral cavity, occur together.

The characteristic skin lesions of lichen planus are reddish blue papules with a fine scale (Fig. 17-7; see also Plate 17-7). In chronic cases, the papules can coalesce to form hypertrophic plaques. The degree of pruritus varies but can be intense in some patients.

The most characteristic histologic finding is a layer of lymphohistiocytic infiltrate adjacent to the epidermis. The epidermis shows hyperkeratosis, and the rete ridges are elongated.

Lichen planus should be suspected by the proctologist when perianal lesions are seen in conjunction with other skin and oral lesions. The diagnosis is made by skin biopsy, which should be done to rule out the presence of squamous cell cancer. Differential diagnosis includes perianal psoriasis, squamous cell cancer, and lichen sclerosis et atrophicus.

REFERENCES

1. Shelley WB, Cahn MM (1995) The pathogenesis of hidradenitis suppurativa in man. Arch Dermatol 72:562–565
2. Yu CCW, Book MG (1990) Hidradenitis suppurativa: a disease of follicular epithelium, rather than apocrine glands. Br J Dermatol 122:763–769
3. Highet AS, Warren RE, Weekes AJ (1988) Bacteriology and antibiotic treatment of perineal suppurative hidradenitis. Arch Dermatol 124:1047–1051
4. Bendahan J, Paran H, Kolman S et al (1992) The possible role of Chlamydia trachomatis in perineal suppurative hidradenitis. Eur J Surg 158:213–215
5. Church JM, Fazio VW, Lavery IC et al (1993) The differential diagnosis and comorbidity of hidradenitis suppurativa and perianal Crohn's disease. Colon Dis 8:117–119
6. Thornton JP, Abcarin H (1978) Surgical treatment of perianal and perineal hidradenitis suppurative. Dis Colon Rectum 21:573–577
7. Wiltz O, Schuetz DJ, Murray JJ (1990) Perianal hidradenitis

suppurativa, the Lahey Clinic experience. Dis Colon Rectum 33:731–174

8. Williams SY, Busby RC, Demuth RJ, Nelson H (1991) Perineal hidradenitis suppurativa: presentation of two unusual complications and a review. Ann Plast Surg 26:456–463

9. Culp CE (1983) Chronic hidradenitis suppurativa of the anal canal, a surgical skin disease. Dis Colon Rectum 26:669–676

10. Brown SCW, Kazzazi N, Lord PH (1986) Surgical treatment of perineal hidradenitis suppurativa with special reference to recognition of the perianal form. Br J Surg 73:978–980

11. Harland RW, Varkey B (1992) Anal tuberculosis: report of two cases and literature review. Am J Gastroenterol 87:1488–1491

12. Farber EM, Nall L (1992) Perianal and intergluteal psoriasis. Cutis 50:336–338

13. Fry GF, Moore JG (1969) Enterobius vermicularis: 10,000-year-old human infection. Science 166:1620

14. Matsen JM, Turner JA (1969) Reinfection in enterobiasis (pinworm infection). simultaneous treatment of family members. Am J Dis Child 118:576–581

15. Myrick Thomas RH, Ridley CM, McGivvon DH, Black MM (1988) Lichen sclerosus et atrophicus and autoimmunity—a study of 350 women. Br J Dermatol 118:41–46

16. Hart WR, Norris HJ, Helwig HB (1975) Relation of lichen sclerosus et atrophicus of the vulva to development of carcinoma. Obstet Gynecol 45:369–377

17. Tremaine RDL, Miller RAW (1989) Lichen sclerosus et atrophicus. Int J Dermatol 28:10–16

18. DeGrout AC, Baar TJM, Terpstra H, Weyland JW (1991) Contact allergy to moist toilet paper. Contact Dermatitis 24:135–136

19. Pirone E, Infantino A, Masin A et al (1992) Can proctologic procedures resolve perianal pruritus and mycosis? A prospective study of 23 cases. Int J Color Dis 7:18–20

18

EPIDEMIOLOGY AND ETIOLOGY

Lisa Boardman
William E. Karnes, Jr.

Adenocarcinoma of the colorectum is the third most frequent malignant neoplasm worldwide, with approximately 570,000 new cases a year. As a cause of cancer-related death, colorectal carcinoma ranks second behind lung cancer in developed Western societies and ranks eighth in underdeveloped countries.[1] In Western Europe and the United States, colorectal cancer ranks third behind lung and breast cancer in women and third behind lung and prostate cancer in men. Each year in the United States, approximately 150,000 new cases of colon carcinoma are diagnosed, and approximately 57,000 individuals die of the disease.[2] Those who are cured benefit from early diagnosis and curative surgical resection. Those who are diagnosed too late for curative resection face little chance of cure by available treatments.

A modest recent decline in colorectal cancer mortality in the United States has been attributed to earlier diagnosis, clearance of polyps found on screening examinations, and improvements in adjuvant chemotherapy.[3] Still, nearly 40 to 45% of new patients die of their disease.[2] More effective approaches to the prevention, early detection, and treatment of colon carcinoma are clearly needed. Accomplishment of these goals will require a deeper understanding of the environmental and endogenous factors that influence risk and of the biologic and genetic processes responsible for colorectal carcinogenesis. This chapter reviews current epidemiologic, biologic, and genetic data as it relates to the etiology of colorectal carcinoma. Where appropriate, the implications of these data for current screening and diagnostic and treatment strategies are discussed.

EPIDEMIOLOGY AND ENVIRONMENTAL ETIOLOGY

Sporadic colorectal carcinoma is a disease of Western society (Fig. 18-1). The variable geographic incidence of colorectal carcinoma is most impressive for left-sided lesions. Left-sided carcinomas predominate in countries with a high incidence of colon carcinoma, and right-sided lesions predominate in coun-

tries with a low incidence.[4] Rectal carcinomas seem to follow a similar geographic pattern as left-sided colon carcinomas. However, in contrast to left-sided colon carcinomas, whose incidence has increased and then plateaued in the United States, rectal carcinomas have shown a declining incidence.[5,6] Overall, colorectal cancer affects men and women approximately equally, although the relative incidences of colon versus rectal cancers are 2:1 in males and 3:1 in females. The relative contributions of specific oncogenes and tumor suppressor gene abnormalities in adenomatous polyps and carcinomas also differ between proximal and distal colon carcinomas, suggesting different etiologies.[7] Most epidemiological studies have not considered these differences between right-versus left-sided colorectal carcinomas.

The geographic prevalences of colorectal carcinoma are strikingly similar to those of breast carcinoma, suggesting common risk factors[8] (Fig. 18-2A). In contrast, the geographic prevalences of gastric and colorectal carcinoma are negatively correlated (Fig. 18-2B). For all three cancers, immigrants gradually acquire (over 2 to 3 decades) the risk of the country to which they move.[9–11] Within a geographic region, populations tied together by strong ethnic, religious, or cultural traditions and who maintain isolated and distinct lifestyles exhibit risks that often differ significantly from those of the surrounding population.[11–13] Coincident with industrialization and the adoption of modern Western lifestyles in the late 19th century, the prevalence of colorectal cancer increased dramatically in Western society.[14] Japan is experiencing a similar trend in colorectal and breast cancer prevalence as its population adopts Western life-style changes.[15]

Compared with populations at low risk for colorectal carcinoma, Westerners have smaller, less frequent bowel movements; have higher percent body fat; are more sedentary; have fewer children; eat more fat, red meat, and refined carbohydrates; and eat less fiber-containing vegetables and fruit. Since

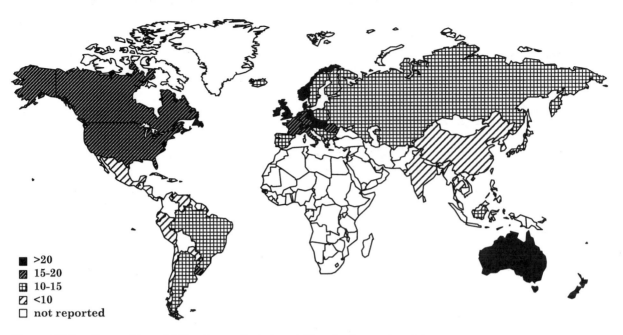

Figure 18-1. Geographic variability of age-adjusted mortality rates from colorectal carcinoma per 100,000 population in 50 countries. (Data from Boring et al.[2])

these characteristics so tightly co-segregate between at-risk populations, it is not surprising that international correlative studies have shown each of these factors to be associated with increased risk of colorectal carcinoma. Even carefully performed analytical case controlled and cohort studies have had a difficult time in separating independent effects.

Burkitt[16] hypothesized that the extremely low incidence of colon cancer in residents of rural Bantu, Africa, was related to their high-fiber and low-fat diets. Indeed, along with the increase in colorectal carcinoma incidence in the United States during the past 70 to 80 years has been an increase in fat and meat intake and reduction in dietary fiber.[17] The recent increase in the incidence of colorectal carcinoma in Japan (130% increase since 1985) has been accompanied by similar changes in diet, particularly fat, which has increased from 10 to 25% of energy over the same period.[18] As a result of these observations, diet has become a major focus of epidemiologic studies seeking to understand the geographic variability of colorectal cancer prevalence. The cancer-initiating and promoting effects of dietary components is under current investigation in animal, human, and in vitro studies.[19]

Fat

In Western societies 40% or more of daily caloric intake is in the form of fat, whereas fat represents only 10 to 25% of caloric intake in underdeveloped countries.[20,21] A dose-related cancer-promoting effect is seen as dietary fat increases from 10 to 40% of caloric intake in animal studies.[22] Based on food disappearance data of the Food and Agriculture Organization, a strong correlation is seen between the geographic incidence of colorectal carcinoma and mean fat or cholesterol intake per capita[23,24] (Fig. 18-3). International and national subgroup correlative studies agree with these observations,[25,26] as do most case

control studies.[29–34] However, several cohort studies failed to show a positive correlation between meat or fat intake and colorectal cancer. In fact, two cohort studies found an inverse relationship (see reviews of these studies and references in Refs. 27 and 28.) Different fats may pose variable risks, with some forms even being protective.[35–37] Most studies made no attempt to dissect forms of fat in their analysis.

Animal and human studies have attempted to elucidate if and how high-fat diets contribute to colon carcinogenesis. High dietary fats cause increased mucosal proliferation and increased intraluminal bile acids in animals.[34,38] Certain fats and bile acids are cytotoxic, genotoxic, capable of stimulating colonocyte proliferation, and can alter metabolism of carcinogens and promote carcinogen-induced tumors in animals.[36,39–44] In humans, adenoma size and degree of dysplasia are associated with increased fecal and serum concentrations of bile acids known to act as tumor promoters in animals.[45–49] The lithocholic acid/deoxycholic acid ratio in stool has been associated with colorectal cancer risk,[50] and the cholodeoxycholic acid/cholic acid ratio in duodenal bile has been shown to correlate with colorectal cancer and adenoma size.[51,52] By contrast, omega-3 fatty acids from fish oil reduce colonic mucosal proliferative indices and polyp formation in humans[38] and reduce the incidence of colon cancer induced by azoxymethane in rats.[37]

Fiber

Epidemiologic investigations of the role of fiber in colorectal carcinoma risk are complicated by its multiple forms and difficulties in quantitation of intake. Nonanalytical correlative studies have shown a significant relationship between increased fiber intake and reduced colon cancer risk.[53,54] Case control studies that utilize standardized measures of fiber intake have shown significant negative associations between dietary fiber

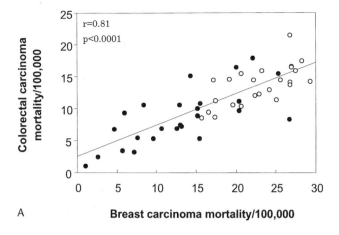

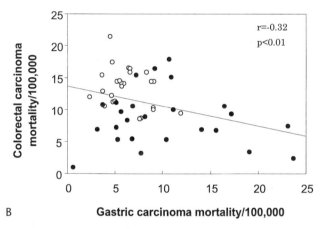

Figure 18-2. (**A**) Correlation between age-adjusted mortality rates in 100,000 population from 50 countries for colorectal and breast carcinoma (r = 0.81, *P* < 0.0001). Western and non-Western countries are represented by open and closed circles, respectively. (**B**) Correlation between age-adjusted mortality rates in 100,000 population from 50 countries for colorectal and gastric carcinoma (r = 0.32, *P* < 0.01). Western and non-Western countries are represented by open and closed circles, respectively. (Data from Boring et al.[2])

intake, particularly from vegetable sources, and the rate of colorectal carcinoma.[55,56] Two cohort studies showed protective effects of fruit intake but no specific effect of other dietary fiber.[57] Meta-analysis of selected studies has verified a significant correlation between fiber and incidence of colorectal cancer.[54]

Fiber is broadly defined as plant cellular material resistant to digestion and includes polysaccharides (cellulose, hemicellulose, gums, and pectin) and the nonpolysaccharide lignin. Some are entirely digested by colonic bacteria (pectin), whereas others remain unaltered in the colon (lignin). Dietary fiber increases stool bulk and reduces fecal transit time. Fiber dilutes carcinogens, binds and alters the metabolism of bile acids known to promote carcinogen-induced colon cancer in animals,[58] and causes alterations in fecal pH, bacterial flora, short-chain fatty acids, and colonocyte proliferative indices.[59] Each type of fiber causes its own physiologic effects. Finally, many high-fiber vegetables are rich in antioxidants and anticancer micronutri-

ents that may directly counteract endogenous carcinogens. Thus, the apparent protective role of fiber may, in part, reflect nonfiber co-constituents.

Calcium

Like fiber, calcium has an apparent protective effect against colon carcinogenesis. A prospective 19-year longitudinal study of 1,954 men in the United States found an inverse relationship between dietary calcium intake and colorectal carcinoma.[60] Additional case control studies have shown similar results.[30,61] By contrast, a prospective study of Japanese men in Hawaii[62] and a case control study in Italy showed no significant association.[63]

Calcium has multiple effects that may contribute to its apparent protective effects against colon carcinogenesis. Calcium binds known animal model promoters of colon carcinoma (bile acids and fatty acids),[44,64–67] inhibits colon epithelial cell proliferation, reduces the cytotoxic potential of fecal water, and protects animals from developing colon tumors following exposure to carcinogens.[68] Extracellular calcium plays a critical role in proliferation and differentiation in cell and tissue culture.[69–72] In rats, supplementary calcium and vitamin D reduces proliferative indices of the colonic mucosa and causes a trend toward reduced number of colon tumors in carcinogen-treated animals.[73] The relative hyperproliferation of colonic crypt cells seen in patients with adenomas or colon cancer is significantly reduced by intake of 2,500 mg/day of calcium orally.[74]

Miscellaneous Dietary and Endogenous Factors

A number of other dietary factors have been examined including total energy intake, beer, vitamins, other micronutrients, food additives, and method of food preparation. Total caloric intake has been shown to be related to colorectal carcinoma risk.[31,56] Excessive beer drinking has been associated with a relative risk of 1.7 for rectal but not colon cancer in a cohort[75] and a case control study.[76] Of six cohort and case control studies examining the effects of coffee, two showed relative risk above unity, and four suggested a protective effect.[77,78] Historic parallels

Figure 18-3. Correlation between estimates of cholesterol consumption and colorectal carcinoma mortality rates in 100,000 population from 20 industrialized countries (r = 0.86, *P* < 0.001). (Data from Liu et al.[23])

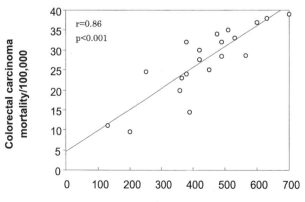

between the use of nitrate as a food preservative and the appearance of colorectal carcinoma have been observed.[15] In a Swedish case control study, heavily browned fried meat was shown to be a more important determinant of risk than meat intake alone.[79] Such foods may increase the colonic load of carcinogenic pyrolysis products and heterocyclic amines.[79,80] Finally, acetylator status and P450 genotypes in a given individual may influence proper metabolism of dietary carcinogens and affect risk of colon cancer.[81]

Future Studies

Although existing epidemiologic and experimental studies support recommendations to reduce dietary fat and increase dietary fiber, the component risk and protective elements of the diet are not clearly defined. Continuing human and animal studies are needed that focus on the effects of individual and combined dietary components. Key to these studies will be the identification and validation of intermediate markers of premalignant change. Among these are proliferative indices, aberrant crypts, adenomas, and genetic and cellular markers. By examining earlier events in colon carcinogenesis, studies may uncover promising new information over a shorter time frame than is possible if colorectal cancer is the end point.

COLON CARCINOGENESIS

Morphologic and Histopathologic Sequence

Normal Mucosa-Polyp Sequence

The morphologic sequence of events leading to colon cancer is thought to begin with abnormal proliferation of colonocytes in anatomic patches followed by dysplastic microadenomas and adenomas, increasing dysplasia, carcinoma, and metastasis. Normal colonic mucosa is rapidly and continuously renewed. Homeostasis is maintained by a balance between cell division and cell loss. Normally, the proliferating population of cells is confined to the lower third of the crypts.[82] New cells are thought to arise from stem cells located deep in the crypts. Resulting daughter cells migrate up the crypts, rapidly differentiate, and lose replicative function (Fig. 18-4).

In animal models, exposure to carcinogens causes proliferative activity to extend to the luminal surface. Affected cells fail to differentiate and appear not to undergo apoptosis appropriately. This leads to focal outgrowths of dysplastic mucosa (adenomas) characterized by infolding of crypts and/or formation of polypoid structures with tubular, tubulovillous, or villous histologic features. Prior to development of macroscopic polyps, some crypts show distinctive changes that can be visualized microscopically after staining with methylene blue.[83] Compared with normal crypts, these aberrant crypt foci (ACF) are larger and have a thicker mucosal lining and enlarged pericryptal zones[84] (Fig. 18-4).

In humans, adenomas and colorectal carcinomas are reported to arise from patches of mucosa that exhibit abnormal cell proliferation and maturation, referred to as field defects.[85] Similarly, aberrant crypts are particularly common in patients with adenomas and colorectal carcinoma.[86] Although it has not been

proved, field defects may represent patches of mucosa containing high densities of ACFs.

Like adenomas, ACFs in humans often have K-*ras* and adenomatous polyposis coli (APC) mutations but rarely have p53 mutations, suggesting that they represent the earliest precursors of colorectal carcinoma in humans.[87–90] As such, they may be ideal markers for the evaluation of new preventive strategies including dietary interventions and drug therapies designed to reduce adenoma formation and cancer. Most ACFs, however, do not exhibit dysplasia and may represent pre-hyperplastic polyps as opposed to pre-adenomas.[91] Current work is focusing on defining the natural history of ACFs and their subclassifications. Finally, while ACFs are relatively easy to identify and quantitate in ex vivo colon specimens, no convenient method exists for measuring ACF densities in situ, and they are rarely found on random biopsies. In the future, they may be identifiable using special magnifying colonoscopes in conjunction with special staining of the mucosa.

Adenoma-Carcinoma Sequence

Sixty to 70% of polyps are adenomas. The rest are hyperplastic, lipomas, hamartomas, or inflammatory polyps that are not considered to present significant risk for subsequent colorectal cancer.[92] The widely accepted belief that most sporadic colon cancers arise from adenomas is based on several lines of evidence: (1) adenoma remnants are occasionally found in resected cancers[93]; (2) colorectal cancer is inevitable in familial adenomatous polyposis (FAP), which is characterized by hundreds to thousands of adenomas[94]; (3) acquired genetic abnormalities common to adenomas are carried over into cancers[95]; and (4) clearance of adenomas reduces risk of subsequent colorectal cancer.[96–98] This latter evidence is a particularly relevant outcome of the National Polyp Study.[96,99]

The multicenter National Polyp Study followed a cohort of 1,418 patients for an average of 5.9 years. The incidence of colorectal cancer in patients undergoing repeated colonoscopic polypectomy was significantly lower than expected based on three reference groups (Fig. 18-5). The first reference group included 226 patients ascertained retrospectively at the Mayo Clinic for an average of 9 years who declined surgical polypectomy after barium enema detected polyps beyond the reach of a proctoscope.[100] The second reference group came from a St. Mark's Hospital retrospective analysis of 1,618 patients followed for 14 years after excision of rectal adenomas.[101] The third reference group included average-risk people registered in the Surveillance, Epidemiology, and End Result (SEER) program of the National Cancer Institute that evaluates incidence rates of colorectal cancer.[102] Compared with these three reference groups, the percent reduction in the incidence of colorectal cancer in those undergoing periodic clearance of adenomas was 90, 88, and 76%, respectively.

In the United States and Western Europe, the incidence of both adenomas and colorectal carcinomas increases with age. By age 40, 10 to 20% of individuals have at least one colorectal adenoma.[103] Fifty percent of these will have two or more adenomas. These data suggest that within a population there is a subgroup of "polyp formers." At present, "polyp formers" can only be recognized by structural studies of the colon such as colonoscopy or combined flexible sigmoidoscopy and barium

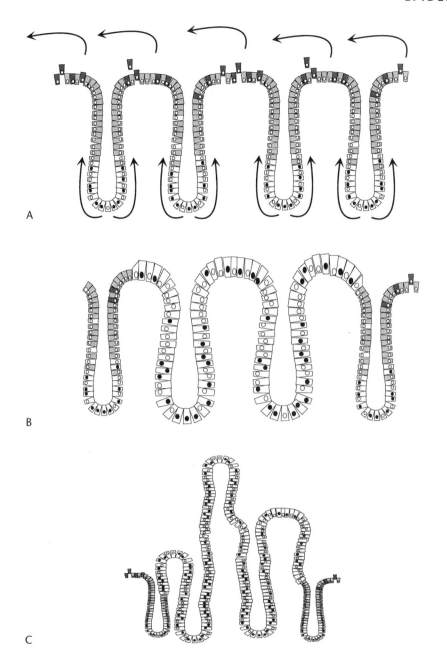

Figure 18-4. Proposed histopathologic changes leading from normal mucosa to dysplastic microadenoma. In normal mucosa (**A**) dividing cells (black nuclei) are restricted to the lower third of the crypt. Daughter cells migrate up the crypts, lose replicative function (white nuclei), and differentiate (gray cells). As cells reach the surface, they undergo senescence and shedding into the lumen (dark gray cells). A balance between cell renewal and cell loss maintains normal mucosal structure. In aberrant crypts (**B**) cells (presumably of clonal origin) maintain replicative function throughout the crypts and fail to differentiate or undergo apoptosis appropriately. The imbalance between cell renewal and cell loss leads to an outgrowth of dysplastic cells (microadenoma) (**C**) and eventually a visible adenoma.

enema. In the future, novel stool markers and other noninvasive diagnostic procedures such as "virtual colonoscopy" utilizing computed tomography with three-dimensional reconstruction of the colon will permit identification of high-risk "polyp formers" who will most benefit from colonoscopic surveillence and polyp clearance.[104]

The cumulative lifetime risk of colorectal cancer is 6%.[105] The huge discrepancy between the prevalence of adenomas and colorectal carcinomas indicates that most adenomas do not progress to cancer within one's lifetime. However, certain features of adenomas predict subsequent risk of colorectal cancer including polyp size greater than 1 cm, muliplicity, villous or

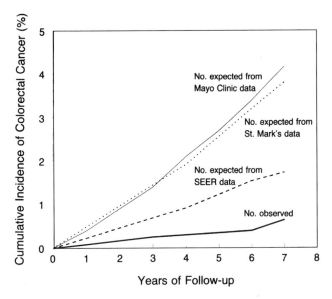

Figure 18-5. The observed cumulative incidence of of colorectal cancer in the National Polyp Study cohort compared with three reference groups described in the text. (From Winawer,[166] with permission.)

tubulovillous histology, and increasing levels of dysplasia.[101] For adenomas destined to become malignant, the interval between adenoma and carcinoma appears to be approximately 5 years.[96] After clearance of polyps by colonoscopic polypectomy, 30% of individuals can be expected to redevelop polyps on subsequent examinations.

Together these data support a surveillence strategy of yearly colonoscopies and polypectomies for patients with recurring large or multiple adenomas, tubulovillous or villous histologies, or moderate to severe dysplasia. For individuals with single, small tubular adenomas with low-grade dysplasia, follow-up colonoscopies can be delayed 3 to 5 years depending on their prior polyp history. When clearance of polyps is maintained between surveillance colonoscopies, intervals can be lengthened. As patients reach advanced ages, the risk/benefit ratio of this strategy increases and should be altered accordingly, particularly when longevity is threatened by other chronic diseases.

Dysplasia-Carcinoma Sequence

Not all colon cancers arise from adenomas. In chronic ulcerative colitis (CUC), Crohn's disease, flat adenomatous disease, and perhaps some cases of hereditary nonpolyposis colorectal cancer (HNPCC) colorectal cancer, develops when dysplasia arises in nonpolypoid mucosa. Since adenomas are dysplastic by definition, the term dysplasia-cancer sequence may be a more inclusive description than adenoma-carcinoma sequence.[106]

Ulcerative Colitis

Patients with ulcerative colitis, and to a lesser extent Crohn's disease, have an increased risk of colon cancer.[107] The cumulative risk of developing colorectal cancer in patients with ulcera-

tive colitis and pancolitis is 5 to 10% at 20 years and 12 to 20% at 30 years.[108] Colorectal cancer risk is inversely related to age of onset of ulcerative colitis and decreases by 50% for each of the following age-of-onset categories: younger than 15, 15 to 29, and each decade between 30 and 60 years.[109] The genetic etiologies of colorectal cancer in ulcerative colitis may be distinct from that of sporadic colorectal cancer. Several studies suggest a lower incidence of K-*ras* and APC mutations in ulcerative colitis-associated colon cancers, and relatively early appearance of *p53* mutations compared with sporadic colorectal neoplasms.[110–112] However, a recent study suggests that K-*ras* and APC mutations are common and appear early in the dysplasia-cancer sequence.[113] Approximately 20% of dysplastic lesions and colorectal cancers in ulcerative colitis show microsatellite instability, suggesting a role for defective mismatch repair mechanisms.[114,115]

Flat Adenoma

Flat adenomas, originally described in 1984 by Muto et al.,[93] are associated with an increased risk of malignant transformation compared with normal mucosa. These flat, often translucent, lesions can be difficult to detect endoscopically. The degree of dysplasia and risk of malignancy increases in lesions greater than 6 mm in diameter and in those with a central depression.[106,116] Histologic features may be tubular, tubulovillous, or villous. Flat adenomas frequently occur synchronously and metchronously with exophytic sporadic adenomas.

A Genetic Sequence

Colorectal cancer results from the accumulation of somatic mutations affecting several cancer-related genes. An estimated 5 to 15% of colorectal cancers develop in the setting of an inherited germline mutation of a cancer-related gene. Even in these cases, in which every cell in the body contains a mutant cancer-related gene, somatic mutations of additional cancer-related genes must occur before a cancer is formed. We have learned much about the genes that are important in colon carcinogenesis and we are beginning to learn more about the processes responsible for the accumulation of somatic mutations required for colorectal carcinogenesis.

DNA is at greatest risk of mutation during DNA synthesis when a new strand of DNA is synthesized from an unwound parental DNA template. At this vulnerable time, DNA may be damaged by strand breaks, chemical alterations, or base pair mismatching, among others. Although mutations are inevitable over time, intrinsic mechanisms that recognize and repair DNA damage are sufficient to prevent a significant rate of new mutations in progeny cells under normal circumstances. These mechanisms may be stressed beyond their capacity in the presence of environmental mutagens, particularly under conditions of excessive cellular proliferation (DNA synthesis). The rate of new mutations and their propagation into a clonal population can also increase through failure of mechanisms that recognize and repair damaged DNA or that delete DNA-damaged cells from the population. Each of these processes is involved in colon carcinogenesis whether occurring in the setting of an inherited predisposition or sporadically.

Clues From Inherited Colorectal Cancer Syndromes

Inherited cancer predisposition syndromes (covered in greater detail in Chapter 21) involve the heterozygous loss or dysfunctional mutation of a tumor suppressor gene in the germline. A sporadic mutation of the second allele leads to complete loss of the tumor suppressor's function and sets the stage for cancer development (Knudson's two-hit hypothesis).[117] Knudson's[117] two-hit hypothesis appears to play a role in two inherited conditions that predispose to colorectal carcinoma, HNPCC and FAP.

In HNPCC, the germline mutation affects one allele of a family of genes encoding mismatch repair enzymes that help ensure DNA replication fidelity (hMSH2, hMLH1, and hPMS1).[118,119] HNPCC accounts for at least 5% of new colorectal cancer cases each year.[71] Most colon cancers in this condition show somatic loss or mutation of the second HNPCC allele. The somatic "second hit" renders mismatch repair mechanisms dysfunctional leading to accelerated passage through a sequence of additional cancer-related gene mutations.

FAP is caused by a germline mutation of the APC gene. As many as 20% of cases represent spontaneous new mutations and have no family history of polyposis.[120] FAP is characterized by hundreds to thousands of adenomas by the third decade of life and the inevitable development of colorectal cancer if prophylactic colectomy is not performed.[94] Each of the thousands of polyps shows somatic mutations to the second normal APC allele.

In both FAP and HNPCC the "first hit" already affects every cell in the body. In sporadic colon carcinoma, the inital "hit" must occur first by chance and the "second hit" must affect one of the clonal progeny possessing the "first hit." Thus, the chance over time of patients with FAP and HNPCC developing colorectal carcinoma is exceedingly high compared with those without germline mutations.

Genetics of Sporadic Colorectal Tumorogenesis

Probably many mutational pathways lead toward colorectal carcinoma. It is also likely that the sequential order of mutations can be variable. In cells destined to become sporadic colorectal cancers, we presume that normal mechanisms for ensuring DNA fidelity are intact prior to the initating step. The initiating events must therefore occur through environmental influences that either directly cause mutations (mutagens) or cause increased susceptibility to mutations (increased proliferation). The earliest genetic abnormalities seen in sporadic adenomatous polyps affect APC (63%) and/or K-ras (30 to 50% of medium to large polyps)[121,122] (Fig. 18-6). Although the function of the APC gene product is unknown, its loss of function is associated with the characteristic features of adenomatous polyps: retention of replicative function and failure of terminal differentiation. K-ras encodes a protein (p21ras) that helps transmit proliferative signals from growth factor receptors to the nucleus.[123] Mutations affecting any one of three codons of K-ras (12, 13, and 61) lead to a constitutively and dominantly active p21ras product that generates proliferative signals independent of normal regulatory mechanisms.[123] Thus, a cell with an activating K-ras mutation or loss of APC function, or both, acquires a growth advantage compared with its neighbors, leading to clonal enlargement of adenomatous polyps. The increased pro-

portion of cells undergoing DNA synthesis in polyps compared with normal mucosa renders them more vulnerable to a second mutational hit. As the number of mutant APC and K-ras-bearing clones increases, the chance of additional "hits" toward cancer increases further.

Eventually a member of the clonal population of cells in an adenomatous polyp may sustain additional hits to genes such as DCC or p53. The DCC locus on chromosome 18q is lost in 70 to 85% of late-stage adenomas and colorectal carcinomas.[124] Normal DCC suppresses malignant phenotypes, but its mechanism of action is unknown. Loss of the p53 locus on 17p is rare in adenomas but is found in approximately 75% of colorectal carcinomas.[125] Normal p53 becomes activated by DNA damage and functions to induce programmed cell death (apoptosis) or to arrest the cell cycle at the G1/S interface prior to DNA synthesis.[126] Normal p53 thus provides a cell an opportunity to commit suicide or to repair its DNA prior to propagating mutations to its progeny. A cell with a single mutant p53 allele loses some of this ability through "dominant negative" effects and becomes an efficient conduit for propagation of additional mutations to cancer-related genes.[127] This is enhanced further by loss of the second p53 allele. Eventually, a complement of mutations to several cancer-related genes will occur, leading to the autonomous and invasive phenotype of frank malignancy.

The progression from normal colonocyte to frank malignancy outlined above illustrates several important concepts: (1) mutations are an ongoing and inevitable process that is accelerated by increased proliferation, exogenous mutagens, and dysfunction of processes that recognize and repair DNA or induce apoptosis in response to irreparable DNA damage; (2) chance dictates whether a given cell that has suffered a "first hit" will sustain a critical complement of second, third, fourth, and so forth "hits" required for carcinogenesis; (3) this chance is multiplied by the number of cells containing critical "first hits" and further increases if "first hits" affect mechanisms of DNA damage recognition, repair, or "weeding out" of DNA-damaged cells. Risk of cancer development is therefore highest for germline mutations in which every cell in the colon has a "first hit" and in large clonal adenomas composed of millions of identical clones containing critical "first hits."

BIOLOGY OF COLON CANCER CELLS

Autonomy and Immortality

Cancer cells in culture show evidence of aberrant regulation of growth and apoptosis when compared with normal cells. Normal cells require a complex mixture of exogenously supplied soluble as well as surface-bound growth/attachment/survival factors to enable proliferation and survival in culture. By contrast, most cancer cells show complete or partial independence of exogenously supplied soluble or fixed substrate signals.[128] They can be passaged indefinitely and are less responsive to apoptosis-inducing signals.[129] The characteristic features of cancer cells (autonomy, anchorage independence, and immortality) can occur when cancer cells produce their own growth and survival factors (autocrine/paracrine), or when they acquire aberrant signals downstream of receptor-ligand interactions that (1) stimulate cell growth constitutively (activated oncogenes); (2) fail to suppress proliferative signals; and/or (3) fail to stimu-

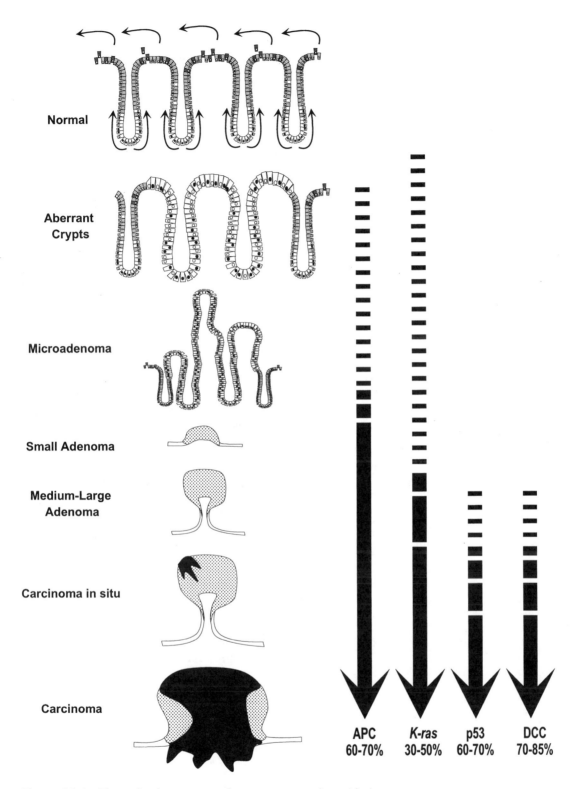

Normal

Aberrant
Crypts

Microadenoma

Small Adenoma

Medium-Large
Adenoma

Carcinoma in situ

Carcinoma

APC
60-70%

K-ras
30-50%

p53
60-70%

DCC
70-85%

Figure 18-6. The molecular sequence of events corresponding with the histopathologic changes leading to colorectal carcinoma includes the appearance of *APC* and K-*ras* mutations in aberrant crypts. The frequency of *APC* mutations increases as the sequence reaches the small adenoma phase. K-*ras* mutations become most frequent in the late adenoma phase. Finally, as colorectal carcinomas arise, the frequency of *p53* and *DCC* mutations increases. Arrows represent the increasing frequencies of mutations in each gene. The percentages of advanced colorectal carcinomas that harbor mutations in each gene are shown at the bottom of each arrow.

late apoptotic signaling. The latter two mechanisms involve failure of tumor suppressor and apoptosis-promoting signals.[130]

Autonomous proliferation reflects aberrant proliferative signals important for tumor growth in vivo.[128] In colon cancer, as well as many other cancers, autonomous growth results from either ligand-dependent (autocrine/paracrine) or ligand-independent mechanisms.[131] Several growth factors and their receptors have been implicated in the regulation of colon carcinoma and adenoma growth.[132] For example, essentially all colon cancer and adenoma cell lines and tumors co-express epidermal growth factor receptor (EGFR) and its ligand, transforming growth factor-α (TGF-α).[133–137] In many cases, autonomous growth and tumorogenicity of these cells are sensitive to disruption of this autocrine loop by blocking antibodies or antisense constructs that prevent expression of EGFR or TGF-α.[131,138–141] However, a proportion of colon cancer cell lines proliferate independently of this autocrine loop.[131,140]

Ligand-independent autonomous proliferation requires activation of proliferative signals downstream of ligand interactions with cell surface receptors. Activation could theoretically occur at any point along proliferative signal transduction pathways, from the receptor to the nucleus. Many of the genes whose products participate in proliferative signaling were originally discovered as oncogenes (mutant or aberrantly expressed genes defined by their ability to induce a transformed phenotype when expressed in normal cells).[141a] Oncogenes and tumor suppressor genes known to be important in colon carcinogenesis likely play key roles in this phenomenon.[129]

Role of Colorectal Cancer-Related Genes in the Biology of Colorectal Cancer Cells

K-ras

Activating mutations of K-ras appear to be an early event in colon carcinogenesis. Thirty to 50% of medium to large adenomas and colon carcinomas have activating mutations of K-ras.[122] Interestingly, ACF appear to exhibit activating K-ras mutations more frequently than do small adenomas.[87,89,90,125,142] The protein product of K-ras, p21ras, is a GTP-binding protein with endogenous GTPase activity. Point mutations affecting codons 12, 13, or 61 impart a constitutively active GTP-bound state that causes transformation as well as ligand-independent proliferation when introduced into normal cells.[123] By contrast, normal p21ras activity is tightly controlled by several proteins that regulate shuttling between its active GTP and inactive GDP bound state. Many of these regulators bind to and are substrates of receptors with intrinsic tyrosine kinase activity (RTKs), including EGFR, by virtue of their src homology domains (SH2 domains). p21ras, therefore, directs proliferative and transforming signals from activated RTKs, whereas its oncogenic form is capable of generating these signals independently of receptor activation.[123] As described above, this effect could lead to clonal and focal outgrowths of continuously replicating cells (aberrant crypts, microadenomas, and adenomas).

APC

The earliest genetic abnormality in adenomas arising in FAP is loss of both APC alleles. APC mutations are also seen in 60 to 70% of early sporadic polyps.[121] Loss of APC function must,

therefore, be a prerequisite for adenoma formation in FAP. The function of APC has not been determined. Since adenomas are characterized by unrestricted cell division and failure of proper differentiation, normal APC must play a critical role in directing progeny of stem cells along a path of terminal differentiation and loss of replicative function. When APC function is lost, normal mucosal renewal mechanisms are lost, leading to the clonal expansion of replicative cells.

p53

p53 is the most frequently altered gene in human cancers,[143] occurring in approximately 60% of carcinomas.[144] p53 plays a critical role in halting cell cycle progression at G0/G1 or inducing apoptosis in response to DNA damage. DNA damage induces wild-type p53, which, in turn, activates transcription of inhibitors of the cell cycle-dependent kinase complex, including WAF-1[126,145] and GADD45.[146] WAF-1 inhibits cell cycle-dependent kinases,[147] whereas GADD45 and WAF-1 both bind to and likely inhibit the replication function of proliferating cell nuclear antigen.[88,148] p53 also suppresses expression of bcl-2, a gene whose product is important for preventing apoptosis.[149] Cells with loss of p53 function fail to induce WAF-1, GADD45, G1/S cell cycle arrest, or apoptosis in response to DNA damage.[126] The lost opportunity to repair or destroy damaged genes prior to replication results in genomic instability.[150–152] In this way, loss of p53 function may contribute to neoplastic transformation. The tumor suppressor activity of p53 has thus been equated to its function as a "guardian of the genome."[153]

Approximately one-third of mutations affecting p53 in cancers occur without loss of heterozygosity, suggesting either "dominant negative" or "gain of function" activity of the mutant allele.[127] The "dominant negative" hypothesis is supported by observations that wild-type p53 protein forms heteroligomers with mutant p53 proteins leading to loss of wild-type transactivation function.[154,155] The "gain of function" hypothesis is supported by observations that some mutant forms of p53 exhibit oncogenic characteristics when introduced into cells that lack p53.[156–158] Such mutants can act alone or in conjunction with oncogenes to induce tumorogenicity, increase plating efficiency, or allow for autonomous proliferation.[157,159] The multiple functions of p53 in growth regulation and protection against propogation of DNA-damaged cells suggest its critical role as gate-keeper in carcinogenesis.

DCC and MCC

The DCC locus on chromosome 18q is lost in 70 to 85% of late-stage adenomas and colorectal carcinomas.[124] DCC is an extremely large gene that encodes an enormous transmembrane protein with some similarities to the neural adhesion molecule family of proteins, suggesting a role in cell-cell contact and communication.[124,160] Introduction of 18q into colon cancer cells with loss of DCC results in reversion of their tumorgenic phenotype.[161] Further studies are required to elucidate the role of DCC loss in colon cancer and its mechanism of action.

The mutated colorectal cancer (MCC) gene is located close to the APC gene and encodes a protein with some structural similarities to APC.[162,163] Its function, however, is unknown.

Somatic mutations of *MCC* are found in only 10 to 15% of colorectal carcinomas.[162]

Mismatch Repair Genes

Approximately 13 to 17% of sporadic colorectal cancers exhibit microsatellite instability, which may or may not be related to defective mismatch repair mechanisms involving genes implicated in HNPCC (*hMSH2, hMLH1*, and *hPMS1*).[164] Colon cancer cell lines that exhibit microsatellite instability often show mutations of type II TGF-β receptor. These cell lines fail to show normal inhibition of growth in response to TGF-β.[165] Thus, defective function of mismatch repair genes may contribute to colon carcinogenesis by allowing for mutations to key growth modulatory genes.

THE FUTURE

During the past decade, an explosion of new information has advanced our knowledge concerning the natural history, genetics, biology, and environmental factors associated with colon carcinogenesis. The long-term outcome of this expanding body of knowledge will be the prevention and effective treatment of colon cancer. Before this can happen, answers to questions on several fronts are needed: (1) what are the component carcinogenic and protective constituents of diet and the environment; (2) through what mechanisms do dietary factors and putative chemopreventative agents (e.g., nonsteroidal anti-inflammatory drugs) influence colon carcinogenesis; (3) through what mechanisms do mutations of colorectal cancer-associated genes contribute to colon carcinogenesis; (4) what intermediate markers are best predictive of colorectal cancer risk; and (5) what screening tests are most cost effective for identifying populations at risk?

As these questions are elucidated, populations at risk will be identified for which preventive strategies can be implemented. Eventually, gene therapy may be the standard for cancer prevention in individuals with inherited colorectal cancer syndromes. However, pharmacologic interventions are likely to be the mainstay for prevention and treatment of colorectal cancer for years to come. As the aberrant cell-signaling pathways responsible for abnormal growth (as well as failure of differentiation and apoptosis) are elucidated, targeted therapies will be developed that correct underlying defects or prevent them from occurring.

REFERENCES

1. Granoth A et al (1988) Time trends in mortality from cancer. WHO/CAN 88.5
2. Boring CC, Squires TS, Tong T (1993) Cancer statistics. CA 43:7–26
3. Chu KC, Kramer BS, Smart CR (1991) Analysis of the role of cancer prevention and control measures in reducing cancer mortality. J Natl Cancer Inst 83:1636–1643
4. Weisburger JH (1991) Causes, relevant mechanisms, and prevention of large bowel cancer. Semin Oncol 18:316–336
5. Greenwald P (1992) Colon cancer overview. Cancer 70:1206–1215
6. Devesa SS, Chow WH (1993) Variation in colorectal cancer incidence in the United States by subsite of origin. Cancer 71:3819–3826
7. Delattre O, Olschwang S, Law DJ et al (1989) Multiple genetic alterations in distal and proximal colorectal cancer. Lancet 2:353–356
8. Howell MA (1976) The association between colorectal cancer and breast cancer. J Chron Dis 29:243–261
9. Henderson BE (1990) Summary report of the sixth symposium on cancer registries and epidemiology in the Pacific basin. J Natl Cancer Inst 82:1186–1190
10. McMichael AJ, McCall MG, Hartshorne JM, Woodings TL (1980) Patterns of gastrointestinal cancer in European migrants to Australia: the role of dietary change. Int J Cancer 25:431–437
11. Thomas DB, Karagas MR (1987) Cancer in first and second generation Americans. Cancer Res 47:5771–5776
12. Snowdon DA (1988) Animal product consumption and mortality because of all causes combined, coronary heart disease, stroke, diabetes, and cancer in Seventh-Day Adventists. Am J Clin Nutr 48:739–748
13. Slattery ML, West DW, Robison LM et al (1990) Tobacco, alcohol, coffee, and caffeine as risk factors for colon cancer in a low risk population. Epidemiology 1:141–145
14. Lauer K (1991) The history of nitrite in human nutrition: a contribution from German cookery books. J Clin Epidemiol 44:261–264
15. Weisburger JH, Wynder EL (1987) Etiology of colorectal cancer with emphasis on mechanisms of action and prevention. pp. 197–220. In: Important Advances in Oncology. Lippincott-Raven, Philadelphia
16. Burkitt DP (1971) Epidemiology of cancer of the colon and rectum. Cancer 28:3–13
17. Anonymous (1982) Diet, Nutrition and Cancer. National Academy Press, Washington, DC
18. Willett W (1989) The search for the cause of breast and colon cancer. Nature 338:389–394
19. Potter JD (1992) Reconciling the epidemiology, physiology, and molecular biology of colon cancer. JAMA 268:1573–1577
20. Anonymous (1985) Nutrition and Your Health: Dietary Guidelines for Americans. US Department of Agriculture/US Department of Health and Human Services
21. Anonymous (1983) Household Food Consumption and Expenditure. Annual Report of the Food Survey Committee
22. Reddy BS (1992) Dietary fat and colon cancer: animal model studies. Lipids 27:807–813
23. Liu K, Stamler J, Moss D (1979) Dietary cholesterol, fat, and fiber, and colon-cancer mortality: an analysis of international data. Lancet 2:782
24. Carroll KK, Khor HT (1975) Dietary fat in relation to tumorigenesis. Prog Biochem Pharmacol 10:308–353
25. Rose DP, Boyer AP, Wynder EL (1986) International comparison of mortality rates of cancer of the breast, ovary, prostate and colon and per capita food consumption. Cancer 58:2363–2371

26. Armstrong B, Doll R (1977) Environmental factors and cancer incidence and mortality in different countries with special reference to dietary practices. Int J Cancer 15:617–631

27. Kolonel L (1987) Fat and colon cancer: how firm is the epidemiologic evidence? Am J Clin Nutr 45:336–341

28. Vogel VG, McPherson RS (1989) Dietary epidemiology of colon cancer. Hematol Oncol Clin North Am 3:35–63

29. Willett WC, Stampfer MJ, Colditz GA (1990) Relation of meat, fat, and fiber intake to the risk of colon cancer in a prospective study among women. N Engl J Med 323:1664–1672

30. Peters RK, Pike MC, Garabrant D, Mack TM (1992) Diet and colon cancer in Los Angeles County, California. Cancer Causes Control 3:457–473

31. Kono S, Imanishi K, Shinchi K, Yanai F (1993) Relationship of diet to small and large adenomas of the sigmoid colon. Jpn J Cancer Res 84:13–19

32. Neugut AI, Garbowski GC, Lee WC et al (1993) Dietary risk factors for the incidence and recurrence of colorectal adenomatous polyps. Ann Intern Med 118:91–95

33. Steinmetz KA, Potter JD (1993) Food-group consumption and colon cancer in the Adelaide Case-Control Study. II. Meat, poultry, seafood, dairy foods and eggs. Int J Cancer 53:720–727

34. Iscovich JM, L'Abbe KA, Castelleto R et al (1992) Colon cancer in Argentina. I: Risk from intake of dietary items. Int J Cancer 51:851–857

35. Kromhout D (1990) The importance of N-6 and N-3 fatty acids in carcinogenesis. Med Oncol Tumor Pharmacother 7:173–176

36. Reddy BS, Burill C, Rigotly J (1991) Effects of diets high in omega-3 and omega-6 fatty acids on initiation and post initiation stages of colon carcinogenesis. Cancer Res 51:487–491

37. Enig NG et al (1978) Dietary fat and cancer trends: a critique. Fed Proc 37:2215–2220

38. Anti M, Marra G, Armelo D et al (1992) Effect of omega-fatty acids on rectal mucosal cell proliferation in subjects at risk for colon cancer. Gastroenterology 103:883–891

39. Kandell RL, Bernstein C (1991) Bile salt/acid induction of DNA damage in bacterial and mammalian cells: implications for colon cancer. Nutr Cancer 16:227–238

40. McMichael AJ, Potter JD (1985) Host factors in carcinogenesis: certain bile-acid metabolic profiles that selectively increase the risk of proximal colon cancer. J Natl Cancer Inst 75:185–191

41. Tempero M (1986) Bile acids, ornithine decarboxylase, and cell proliferation in colon cancer: a review. Dig Dis 4:49–56

42. Rafter JJ, Eng VW, Furrer R et al (1986) Effect of dietary calcium and pH on the mucosal damage produced by deoxycholic acid on the rat colon. Gut 27:1320–1329

43. Wargovich M, Eng VW, Newmark HL et al (1983) Calcium ameliorates the toxic effect of deoxycholic acid on colonic epithelium. Carcinogenesis 4:125–127

44. Broitman S et al (1977) Polyunsaturated fat, cholesterol and large bowel tumorigenesis. Cancer 40:2455

45. Hill MJ (1985) Biochemical approaches to the intervention of large bowel cancer. Prog Clin Biol Res 186:263–276

46. Bayerdorffer E, Mannes GA, Richter WO et al (1993) Increased serum deoxycholic acid levels in men with colorectal adenomas. Gastroenterology 104:145–151

47. Hill MJ (1986) Microbes and Human Carcinogenesis. Edward Arnold, London

48. Hill MJ, Melville DM, Lennard Jones JE (1987) Faecal bile acids, dysplasia, and carcinoma in ulcerative colitis. Lancet 2:185–186

49. Hill MJ (1989) Colorectal bacteria in colorectal carcinogenesis. pp. 160–176. In: Colorectal Cancer, Springer-Verlag, Heidelberg

50. Owen RW, Dodo M, Thompson MH et al (1992) The faecal ratio of lithocholic to deoxycholic acid may be an important aetiological factor in colorectal cancer. Eur J Cancer Clin Oncol 19:1307

51. Moorehead RJ, Campbell GR, Donaldson JD et al (1987) Relationship between duodenal bile acids and colorectal cancer. Gut 28:1454–1459

52. Mullan FJ, Wilson HK, Majury CW et al (1990) Bile acids and the increased risk of colorectal tumours after truncal vagotomy. Br J Surg 77:1085–1090

53. Trock B, Unza E, Greenwald P (1990) Dietary fiber, vegetables, and colon cancer: critical review and meta-analysis of epidemiologic evidence. J Natl Cancer Inst 82:650–661

54. Trock BJ, Lanza E, Greenwald P (1990) High fiber diet and colon cancer: a critical review. Prog Clin Biol Res 346:145–157

55. Boland CR, Kolars JC (1992) Fiber and colon cancer: the weight of the evidence. Gastroenterology 103:1964–1967

56. Iscovich JM, L'Abbe KA, Castelleto R et al (1992) Colon cancer in Argentina. II: Risk from fibre, fat and nutrients. Int J Cancer 51:858–861

57. Ausman LM (1993) Fiber and colon cancer: does the current evidence justify a preventive policy? Nutr Rev 51:57–63

58. Korpela JT, Korpela R, Adlercreutz H (1992) Fecal bile acid metabolic pattern after administration of different types of bread. Gastroenterology 103:1246–1253

59. Klurfeld DM (1992) Dietary fiber-mediated mechanisms in carcinogenesis. Cancer Res, suppl. 52: 2055s–2059s

60. Garland C, Barrett-Conner E, Rossof AH (1985) Dietary vitamin D and calcium and risk of colorectal cancer: a 19-year prospective study in men. Lancet 1:307–309

61. Sorenson AW, Slattery ML, Ford MH (1988) Calcium and colon cancer: a review. Nutr Cancer 11:135–145

62. Heilbrun LK, Hankin JH, Nomura AMY, Stemmermann GN (1986) Colon cancer and dietary fat, phosphorus, and calcium in Hawaiian-Japanese men. Am J Clin Nutr 43:306–309

63. Negri E, La Vecchia C, D'Avanzo B, Franceschi S (1990) Calcium, dairy products, and colorectal cancer. Nutr Cancer 13:255–262

64. Welberg JW, Kleibeuker JH, Van der Meer R (1991) Calcium and the prevention of colon cancer. Scand J Gastroenterol [Suppl] 188P52-9.52–59

65. Wargovich MJ, Lynch PM, Levin B (1991) Modulating effects of calcium in animal models of colon carcinogenesis and short-term studies in subjects at increased risk for colon cancer. Am J Clin Nutr 54:202S–205S

66. Newmark HL, Wargovich MJ, Bruce WR (1984) Colon cancer and dietary fat, phosphate and calcium: a hypothesis. J Natl Cancer Inst 72:1323–1325

67. Newmark HL, Lipkin M (1992) Calcium, vitamin D, and colon cancer. Cancer Res 52:2067s–2070s

68. Lapre JA, De Vries HT, Koeman JH, Van der Meer R (1993) The antiproliferative effect of dietary calcium on colonic epithelium is mediated by luminal surfactants and dependent on the type of dietary fat. Cancer Res 53:784–789

69. Yuspa SH, Kilkenny AE, Steiner PM, Roop DR (1989) Expression of murine epidermal differentiation markers is tightly regulated by restricted extracellular calcium concentrations in vitro. J Cell Biol 109:1207–1217

70. Babcock MS, Marino MR, Gunning WT III, Stoner GD (1983) Clonal growth and serial propagation of rat esophageal epithelial cells. In Vitro 19:403–415

71. Whitfield JF, Boynton AL, MacManus JP et al (1979) The regulation of cell proliferation by calcium and cyclic AMP. Mol Cell Biochem 27:155–179

72. Buset M, Lipkin M, Winawer S (1986) Inhibition of human colonic epithelial cell proliferation in vivo and in vitro by calcium. Cancer Res 46:5426–5430

73. Beaty MM, Lee EY, Glauert HP (1993) Influence of dietary calcium and vitamin D on colon epithelial cell proliferation and 1,2-dimethylhydrazine-induced colon carcinogenesis in rats fed high fat diets. J Nutr 123:144–152

74. Barsoum GH, Hendrickse C, Winslet MC et al (1992) Reduction of mucosal crypt cell proliferation in patients with colorectal adenomatous polyps by dietary calcium supplementation. Br J Surg 79:581–583

75. Carstensen JM, Bygren LO, Hatschek T (1990) Cancer incidence among Swedish brewery workers. Int J Cancer 45:393–396

76. Riboli E, Cornee J, Macquart Moulin G et al (1991) Cancer and polyps of the colorectum and lifetime consumption of beer and other alcoholic beverages. Am J Epidemiol 134:157–166

77. La Vecchia C (1990) Epidemiological evidence on coffee and digestive tract cancers: a review. Dig Dis 8:281–286

78. Rosenberg L (1990) Coffee and tea consumption in relation to the risk of large bowel cancer: a review of epidemiologic studies. Cancer Lett 52:163–171

79. Gerhardsson de Verdier M, Hagman U, Peters RK (1991) Meat, cooking methods and colorectal cancer: a case-referent study in Stockholm. Int J Cancer 49:520–525

80. Bruce WR (1987) Recent hypotheses for the origin of colon cancer. Cancer Res 47:4237–4242

81. Smith CA, Moss JE, Gough AC et al (1992) Molecular genetic analysis of the cytochrome P450 debrisoquine hydroxylase locus and association with cancer susceptibility. Environ Health Perspect 98:107–112

82. Lipkin M (1985) Growth and development of gastrointestinal cells. Annu Rev Physiol 47:175–197

83. Bird RP (1987) Observation and quantification of aberrant crypts in the murine colon treated with a colon carcinogen: preliminary findings. Cancer Lett 37:147–151

84. McLellan EA, Bird RP (1988) Specificity study to evaluate induction of aberrant crypts in murine colons. Cancer Res 48:6183–6186

85. Winawer SJ, Zauber AG, Stewart ET, O'Brien MJ (1991) The natural history of colorectal cancer: opportunities for intervention. Cancer 67:1143–1149

86. Pretlow TP, O'Riordan MA, Pretlow TG, Stellato TA (1992) Aberrant crypts in human colonic mucosa: putative preneoplastic lesions. J Cell Biochem,-suppl. 16G:55–62

87. Jen J, Powell SM, Papadopoulos N et al (1994) Molecular determinants of dysplasia in colorectal lesions. Cancer Res 54:5523–5526

88. Smith ML, Chen IT, Zhan QM et al (1994) Interaction of the p53-regulated protein GADD45 with proliferating cell nuclear antigen. Science 266:1376–1380

89. Roncucci L, Stamp D, Medline A et al (1995) Identification and quantification of aberrant crypt foci and microadenomas in the human colon. Frequent and characteristic K-ras activation in aberrant crypt foci of colon. Is there preference among K-ras mutants for malignant progression? Hum Pathol 75:1527–1533

90. Yamashita N, Minamoto T, Ochiai A et al (1995) Frequent and characteristic K-ras activation and absence of p53 protein accumulation in aberrant crypt foci of the colon. Gastroenterology 108:434–440

91. Laumann R, Jucker M, Tesch H (1992) Point mutations in the conserved regions of the p53 tumour suppressor gene do not account for the transforming process in the Jurkat acute lymphoblastic leukemia T-cells. Leukemia 6:227–228

92. Muto T, Bussey HJ, Morson BC (1975) The evolution of cancer of the colon and rectum. Cancer 36:2251–2270

93. Muto T, Kamiya J, Sawada T et al (1984) Small "flat elevation" of the large bowel with special reference to clinicopathological features. Stomach Intest 19:1359–1366

94. Burt RW, Bishop DT, Lynch HT (1990) Risk and surveillance of individuals with heritable factors for colorectal cancer. Bull WHO 68:655–665

95. Fearon ET, Vogelstein B (1990) A genetic model for colorectal tumorigenesis. Cell 61:759–767

96. Winawer SJ, Zauber AG, Diaz B (1987) The National Polyp Study: temporal sequence of evolving colorectal cancer from the normal colon. Gastrointest Endosc 33:A167

97. Gilbertson VA (1974) Proctosigmoidoscopy and polypectomy in reducing the incidence of rectal cancer. Cancer 34:936

98. Murakanni R, Tsukuma H, Kanamori S et al (1990) Natural history of colorectal polyps and the effect of polypectomy on occurrence of subsequent cancer. Int J Cancer 46:159–164

99. Winawer SJ, Zauber AG, O'Brien MJ et al (1992) The national polyp study: design, methods, and characteristic of patients with newly diagnosed polyps. Cancer 70:1236–1245

100. Stryker SJ, Wolff BG, Culp CE (1987) Natural history of untreated colonic polyps. Gastroenterology 93:1009–1013

101. Atkin WS, Morson BC, Cuzick J (1992) Long-term risk of colorectal cancer after excision of rectosigmoid adenomas. N Engl J Med 326:658–662

102. Gloeckler-Reis LA, Hankey BF, Edwards BK (1990) Cancer Statistics Review, 1973–1987. Dept of Health and Human Services, Bethesda, MD

103. Eddy TM (1990) Screening for colorectal cancer. Ann Intern Med 113:377

104. Hara AK, Johnson CD, Reed JE et al (1996) Detection of colorectal polyps by computed tomographic colography: feasibility of a novel technique. Gastroenterology 110:

105. Anonymous (1983) American Cancer Society: Cancer Facts and Figures. American Cancer Society, New York

106. Watanabe T, Sawada T, Kubota Y et al (1993) Malignant potential in flat elevations. Dis Colon Rectum 36:548–553

107. Gillen CD, Walmsley RS, Prior P (1994) Ulcerative colitis and Crohn's disease: a comparison of the colorectal cancer risk in extensive colitis. Gut 35:1590–1592

108. Levin B (1992) Inflammatory bowel disease and colon cancer. Cancer 70:1313–1316

109. Ekbom A, Helmick C, Zach M, Adami HO (1990) Ulcerative colitis and colorectal cancer. N Engl J Med 323:1228–1233

110. Tarmin L, Yin J, Harpaz N et al (1995) Adenomatous polyposis coli gene mutations in ulcerative colitis-associated dysplasias and cancers versus sporadic colon neoplasms. Cancer Res 55:2035–2038

111. Burmer GC, Levine DS, Kulander BG (1990) c-Ki-ras mutations in chronic ulcerative colitis and sporadic colon carcinoma. Gastroenterology 99:416–420

112. Burmer GC, Crispin DA, Kolli VR et al (1991) Frequent loss of a p53 allele in carcinomas and their precursors in ulcerative colitis. Cancer Commun 3:167–172

113. Redston MS, Papadopoulos N, Caldas C (1995) Common occurrence of APC and K-ras gene mutations in the spectrum of colitis-associated neoplasias. Gastroenterology 108: 383–392

114. Kern SE, Redston M, Seymour AB et al (1994) Molecular genetic profiles of colitis-associated neoplasms. Gastroenterology 107:420–428

115. Suzuki H, Harpaz N, Tarmin L et al (1994) Microsatellite instability in ulcerative colitis-associated colorectal dysplasias and cancers. Cancer Res 54:4841–4844

116. Jaramillo E, Watanbe M, Slezak P, Rubio C (1995) Flat neoplastic lesions of the colon and rectum detected by high-resolution video endoscopy and chromoscopy. Gastrointest Endoscopy 42:114–122

117. Knudson AGJ (1971) Mutation and cancer: statistical study of retinoblastoma. Proc Natl Acad Sci USA 68:820–823

118. Leach FS, Nicolaides NC, Papadopoulos N et al (1993) Mutations of a mutS homolog in hereditary nonpolyposis colorectal cancer. Cell 75:1215–1225

119. Fishel R, Lescoe MK, Rao MRS et al (1993) The human mutator gene homolog msh2 and its association with hereditary nonpolyposis colon cancer. Cell 75:1027–1038

120. Powell SM, Petersen GM, Krush AJ et al (1990) Molecular diagnosis of familial adenomatous polyposis. New Engl J Med 33:52–55

121. Powell SM, Zilz N, Beazer-Barclay Y et al (1992) APC mutations occur early during colorectal tumorogenesis. Nature 359:235–237

122. Elder JT, Tavakkol A, Klein SB (1990) Protooncogene expression in normal and psoriatic skin. J Invest Dermatol 94:19–25

123. Bos JL (1989) ras oncogenes in human cancer: a review. Cancer Res 49:4682–4689

124. Hedrick L, Cho KR, Fearon ER (1994) The DCC gene product in cellular differentiation and colorectal tumorigenesis. Genes Dev 8:1174–1183

125. Vogelstein B, Fearon ET, Hamilton SR et al (1988) Genetic alterations during colorectal-tumor development. N Engl J Med 319:525

126. el-Deiry WS, Tokino T, Velculescu VE et al (1993) WAF1, a potential mediator of p53 tumor suppression. Cell 75: 817–825

127. Caron de Fromentel C, Soussi T (1992) TP53 tumor suppressor gene: a model for investigating human mutagenesis. Genes Chromosomes Cancer 4:1–15

128. Rozengurt E (1992) Growth factors and cell proliferation. Curr Opin Cell Biol 4:161–165

129. Hoffman B, Liebermann DA (1994) Molecular controls of apoptosis: differentiation/growth arrest primary response genes, proto-oncogenes, and tumor suppressor genes as positive and negative modulators. Oncogene 9:1807–1812

130. Bishop JM (1991) Molecular themes in oncogenesis. Cell 64: 235–248

131. Karnes WE Jr, Walsh JH, Wu SV et al (1992) Autonomous proliferation of colon carcinoma cells that co-express transforming growth factor-alpha and its receptor: variable effects of receptor-blocking antibody. Gastroenterology 102: 474–485

132. Karnes WE Jr (1994) Growth factors and gastrointestinal malignancies. pp. 825–850. In Gut Peptides—Biochemistry and Physiology. Lippincott-Raven, Philadelphia

133. Coffey RJ, Goustin AS, Soderquist AM et al (1987) Transforming growth factor alpha and beta expression in human colon cancer lines: implications for an autocrine model. Cancer Res 47:4590–4594

134. Anzano MA, Rieman D, Prichett W et al (1989) Growth factor production by human colon carcinoma cell lines. Cancer Res 49:2898–2904

135. Hanauske AR, Buchok J, Scheithauer W, Von Hoff DD (1987) Human colon cancer cell lines secrete alpha TGF-like activity. Br J Cancer 55:57–59

136. Watkins LF, Brattain MG, Levine AE (1988) Modulation of a high molecular weight form of transforming growth factor-alpha in human colon carcinoma cell lines. Cancer Lett 40: 59–70

137. Liu C, Woo A, Tsao MS (1990) Expression of transforming growth factor-alpha in primary human colon and lung carcinomas. Br J Cancer 62:425–429

138. Ito M, Yoshida K, Kyo E et al (1990) Expression of several growth factors and their receptor genes in human colon carcinomas. Virchows Arch [B] 59:173–178

139. Rodeck U, Williams N, Murthy U, Herlyn M (1990) Monoclonal antibody 425 inhibits growth stimulation of carcinoma cells by exogenous EGF and tumor-derived EGF/TGF-alpha. J Cell Biochem 44:69–79

140. Watkins LF, Levine AE (1991) Differential role of transforming growth factor-alpha in two human colon-carcinoma cell lines. Int J Cancer 47:455–460

141. Sizeland AM, Burgess AW (1991) The proliferative and morphologic responses of a colon carcinoma cell line (LIM 1215) require the production of two autocrine factors. Mol Cell Biol 11:4005–4014

141a. Cantley LC, Auger KR, Carpenter C et al (1991) Oncogenes and signal transduction. Cell 64:281–302

142. Smith AJ, Stern HS, Penner M et al (1994) Somatic APC and K-ras codon 12 mutations in aberrant crypt foci from human colons. Cancer Res 54:5527–5530

143. Levine AJ (1993) The tumor suppressor genes. Annu Rev Biochem 62:623–651

144. Vogelstein B (1990) Cancer. A deadly inheritance. Nature 348:681–682

145. Nelson WG, Kastan MB (1994) DNA strand breaks—the DNA template alterations that trigger p53-dependent DNA damage response pathways. Mol Cell Biol 14:1815–1823

146. Kastan MB, Zhan Q, el Deiry WS et al (1992) A mammalian cell cycle checkpoint pathway utilizing p53 and GADD45 is defective in ataxia-telangiectasia. Cell 71:587–597

147. Dulic V, Kaufmann WK, Wilson SJ et al (1994) p53-dependent inhibition of cyclin-dependent kinase activities in human fibroblasts during radiation-induced G1 arrest. Cell 76:1013–1023

148. Chen JJ, Jackson PK, Kirschner MW, Dutta A (1995) Separate domains of p21 involved in the inhibition of CDK kinase and PCNA. Nature 374:386–388

149. Miyashita T, Harigai M, Hanada M, Reed JC (1994) Identification of a p53-dependent negative response element in the bcl-2 gene. Cancer Res 54:3131–3135

150. Hartwell L (1992) Defects in a cell cycle checkpoint may be responsible for the genomic instability of cancer cells. Cell 71:543–546

151. Yin Y, Tainsky MA, Bischoff FZ (1992) Wild-type p53 restores cell cycle control and inhibits gene amplification in cells with mutant p53 alleles. Cell 70:937–948

152. Livingstone LR, White A, Sprouse J (1992) Altered cell cycle arrest and gene amplification potential accompany loss of wild-type p53. Cell 70:923–935

153. Lane DP (1992) Cancer. p53, guardian of the genome. Nature 358:15–16

154. Milner J, Medcalf EA (1991) Cotranslation of activated mutant p53 with wild type drives the wild-type p53 protein into the mutant conformation. Cell 65:765–774

155. Milner J, Medcalf EA, Cook AC (1991) Tumor suppressor p53: analysis of wild-type and mutant p53 complexes. Mol Cell Biol 11:12–19

156. Ponchel F, Puisieux A, Tabone E et al (1994) Hepatocarcinoma-specific mutant p53-249ser induces mitotic activity but has no effect on transforming growth factor beta-1-mediated apoptosis. Cancer Res 54:2064–2068

157. Dittmer D, Pati S, Zambetti G et al (1993) Gain of function mutations in p53. Nature Genet 4:42–46

158. Shaulsky G, Goldfinger N, Ben-Ze'ev A, Rotter V (1990) Nuclear accumulation of p53 protein is mediated by several nuclear localization signals and plays a role in tumorigenesis. Mol Cell Biol 10:6565–6577

159. Peacock JW, Benchimol S (1994) Mutation of the endogenous p53 gene in cell transformed by hpv-16 E7 and EJ c-ras confers a growth advantage involving an autocrine mechanism. EMBO J 13:1084–1092

160. Cho KR, Oliner JD, Simons JW et al (1994) The DCC gene—structural analysis and mutations in colorectal carcinomas. Genomics 19:525–531

161. Tanaka D, Oshimura M, Kikuchi R et al (1991) Suppression of tumorogenicity in human colon carcinoma cells by introduction of normal chromosome 5 or 18. Nature 349:340

162. Kinzler KW, Nilbert MC, Su LK et al (1991) Identification of FAP locus genes from chromosome 5q21. Science 253:661–665

163. Kinzler KW, Nilbert MC, Vogelstein B et al (1991) Identification of a gene located at chromosome 5q21 that is mutated in colorectal cancers. Science 251:1366–1370

164. Lothe RA, Peltomaki P, Meling GI et al (1993) Genomic instability in colorectal cancer—relationship to clinicopathological variables and family history. Cancer Res 53:5849–5852

165. Markowitz S, Wang J, Myeroff L et al (1995) Inactivation of the type II TGF-beta receptor in colon cancer cells with microsatellite instability. Science 268:1336–1338

166. Winawer SJ, Zauber AG, Ho MN et al (1993) Prevention of 1colorectal cancer by colonoscopic polypectomy. N Engl J Med 329:1977–1981

19

PATHOLOGY

Neil A. Shepherd

Colorectal carcinoma has the second highest cancer mortality after lung cancer in the United Kingdom and United States. Of all human cancers, it is probably best understood in terms of etiopathogenesis, predisposing factors, pathologic antecedents, molecular genetics, and mode of spread. Our understanding of colorectal carcinogenesis has been particularly aided by the availability of tissues for pathologic and molecular study, as primary excisional surgery has remained the treatment of choice over many years and because of the existence of an excellent human model for the adenoma-carcinoma sequence, namely, familial adenomatous polyposis (FAP). Unfortunately, the management (especially pathologic diagnosis and surgical treatment) and prognosis of the disease has changed little despite advances in surgical technique and adjuvant therapy. Thus, while colorectal cancer is relatively predictable in its spread, further understanding of its molecular basis is required before major advances in its management and prognosis will occur.

Adenocarcinomas and their benign predecessors, the adenomatous polyps, are by far the most important neoplastic entities in the large intestine. Other benign tumors are rarely clinically significant. Adenocarcinoma accounts for more than 90% of all primary malignancies of the large bowel. Other malignant tumors (e.g., other forms of carcinoma including those with neuroendocrine differentiation, the sarcomas, malignant lymphoma, malignant melanoma, and secondary tumors) tend to present in a similar manner to adenocarcinoma and are usually treated by primary excisional surgery; however, because of their relative rarity, such tumors have relatively poorly defined management strategies.

ADENOMAS

The adenoma is a benign neoplasm of colorectal epithelium. Although most adenomas are polyps, it should be emphasized that the term polyp is purely descriptive, referring to a lesion or mass projecting from an epithelial surface, and does not necessarily imply a neoplastic lesion. The diagnosis of a polyp is made by histopathologic examination. By definition adenomas are dysplastic and premalignant. It is now well established that the adenoma-carcinoma sequence (see below) is the most important pathway for the genesis of colorectal cancer. Adenomas are much commoner in an elderly population: prevalence rates vary from 2 to 70% depending on whether such an analysis is colonoscopic or an autopsy study and on the age of the patient group.[1]

Adenomas themselves are seldom of clinical significance. Only the much larger lesions will cause hemorrhage and anemia or electrolyte disturbances as a result of excessive mucus secretion. Their importance lies in their premalignant potential. Such potential is relative; small adenomas can be assumed to be in an early stage of neoplastic development on both morphologic and molecular biologic evidence; studies of FAP patients, adenoma follow-up, and autopsy investigations have shown that only a small portion of adenomas will become malignant.

Macroscopic Features

Smaller adenomas are usually sessile and appear slightly redder than the adjacent mucosa. As they increase in size, they become more polypoid and pedunculated, and surface nodularity becomes obvious. Larger adenomas may still be pedunculated but may contain villous areas; in these the adenoma has a velvety, papillary surface. Much larger villous tumors tend to carpet the mucosa diffusely and may be more sessile (Fig. 19-1; see also Plate 19-1). A wide spectrum of appearances is seen in the resected colons of polyposis patients because of the varying period of development of the polyps.

Microscopic Features

The three morphologic subtypes (tubular, villous, and tubulovillous) are distinguished by microscopic appearance. Tubular adenomas consist of tightly packed tubules with variable amounts of lamina propria, the latter often considerably reduced compared with normal mucosa. The tubules may show branching,

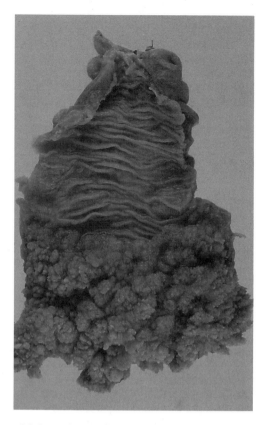

Figure 19-1. A large villous adenoma of the rectum treated by anterior resection. It shows the typical carpeting velvety appearance.

budding, and dilatation, the latter particularly when a pedunculated polyp has been subject to mechanical forces. On the other hand, villous adenomas show an exophytic morphology in which the dysplastic epithelium is thrown into folds rather than villi (the term "villous" is strictly be a misnomer) lined by dysplastic epithelium and containing a central core of lamina propria.

Adenomas are by definition dysplastic. Dysplasia has been defined as "an unequivocal neoplastic alteration of the colorectal epithelium."[2] Thus all adenomas show a disordered epithelial cell growth pattern with a failure of maturation and differentiation extending from the basal zone of the crypt to the surface of the lesion. Most small tubular adenomas show mild dysplasia (Fig. 19-2A; See also Plate 19-2A), with the entire tubule being lined by epithelium that is morphologically similar to that seen in the normal basal proliferative zone.[3] The nuclei are enlarged, oval, and hyperchromatic, but their orientation remains toward the basement membrane (Fig. 19-2A; See also Plate 19-2A). In moderate dysplasia the nuclear features are only a little more advanced, but polarity is less well preserved, with characteristic stratification (Fig. 19-2B; see also plate 19-2B). In severe dysplasia, polarity is lost altogether, and cytologic changes are much more pronounced, the nuclei being enlarged and spheroidal with an open chromatin pattern and prominent nucleoli (Fig. 19-2C). In severe dysplasia, distinct architectural abnormalities are seen, with complex branching of dysplastic tubules and cribriform change. In other organs, such advanced cytologic and architectural abnormality would

warrant a diagnosis of carcinoma in situ or even intramucosal carcinoma. In many countries such a diagnosis is used (as in the TNM classification; pathologic stage pTis), but such a tumor does not appear to have any metastatic potential, one factor here being the relative paucity of intramucosal lymphatics in the colorectum.[4] It is preferable that terms such as carcinoma in situ and intramucosal carcinoma not be applied to large intestinal pathology, as they may precipitate unnecessary radical surgery.[5]

Cancer Risk, Malignancy in Adenomatous Polyps, and Epithelial Misplacement

The frequency of severe dysplasia increases with size of polyp and amount of villosity within individual adenomas. Size, amount of villosity, and grade of dysplasia are the three most important morphologic risk factors for malignancy both within an individual polyp and for the development of malignancy elsewhere in the colon.[6] Occasionally, in larger polyps, both pedunculated and sessile, small foci of invasive adenocarcinoma are seen.

The presence of invasive adenocarcinoma within an endoscopically removed polyp is the subject of some controversy with regard to subsequent management. The literature indicates that endoscopic removal is adequate treatment for cancer arising in a polyp if the adenocarcinoma is not poorly differentiated, does not show involvement of vascular spaces, and is well clear of the line of excision as indicated by an eosinophilic coagulative necrosis zone due to diathermy.[7,8] More recent data would suggest that such conservatism in management is appropriate even if vascular involvement exists, as submucosal venous involvement does not appear to be a significant factor in the genesis of metastatic disease.[9] Nevertheless, I am well aware of several cases in which such criteria have been fulfilled, yet resection was carried out and metastatic disease demonstrated in local lymph nodes. It is recommended that each case be judged on its own merits, particularly if the patient is relatively young and fit, in which case subsequent limited resection may well be justified.

Epithelial misplacement or pseudoinvasion is a close mimic of invasive adenocarcinoma in pedunculated adenomas (especially of the sigmoid colon), which are more likely to undergo torsion, ischemia, and architectural distortion.[10] In this situation the dysplastic epithelium may become displaced within the submucosa and may closely mimic invasive malignancy. Useful pathologic discriminators for a diagnosis of epithelial displacement include the retention of lamina propria around dysplastic glands, a lack of morphologic features of malignancy in the epithelium, and signs to indicate mucosal ischemia and hemorrhage, especially hemosiderin deposition.

Flat/Depressed Adenomas

Current interest exists in the so-called flat or depressed adenoma.[11] Such adenomas are unusual, accounting for less than 2% of the total, and are difficult to identify endoscopically. They are often only diagnosed at the time of intestinal resection. The interest relates to the apparent higher grade of dysplasia given their small size and possible differing genetic evolution, the latter suggested by a relative absence of K-*ras* mutations

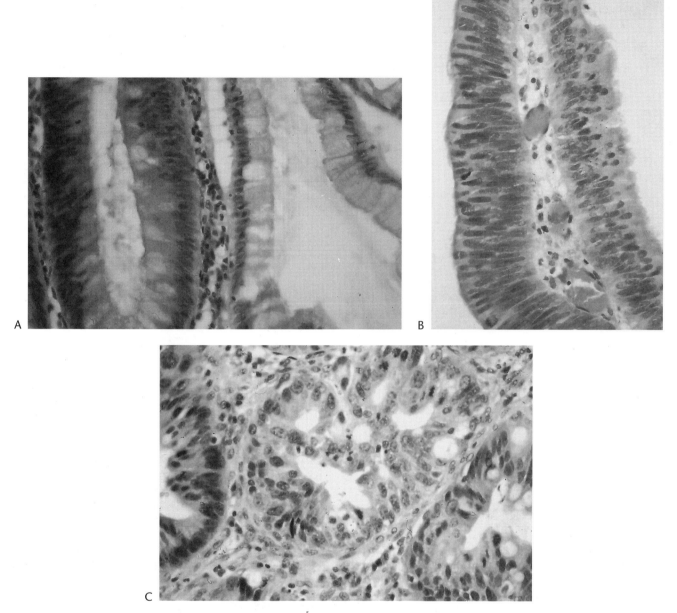

Figure 19-2. Dysplasia in adenomatous polyps. (**A**) Mild dysplasia in a tubular adenoma (left) contrasts with normal mucosa (right). Nuclei are enlarged, oval, and hyperchromatic, but their orientation is toward the basement membrane. (**B**) Moderate dysplasia in a villous adenoma with typical nuclear stratification. (**C**) Severe dysplasia with enlarged pale-staining nuclei and loss of polarity and architectural abnormality (H&E, × 200.)

compared with their more standard counterparts.[12] Furthermore, they appear to develop by an unusual horizontal mode with partial involvement of adjacent crypts.[13]

THE ADENOMA-CARCINOMA SEQUENCE

Most adenocarcinomas of the colon and rectum are generally considered to arise in pre-existing adenomas. Notable exceptions include carcinoma arising in inflammatory bowel disease,

in which "dysplasia" is a recognizable premalignant lesion (see Ch. 18), and de novo lesions.[2] Occasional examples of the latter have been described, but it is difficult if not impossible to document such lesions definitely, as carcinomas very often destroy the associated adenoma from which they arose.[14]

Adenomas have been shown to be clonal and, allied to certain morphologic features, particularly universal dysplasia, can be accepted as representing a neoplasm. Molecular biologic changes that have been demonstrated in colorectal carcinogene-

Evidence For and Against the Adenoma-Carcinoma Sequence

For

Epidemiologic evidence

1. Similar distribution of adenomas and carcinomas in the colon and rectum
2. Adenomas increase in frequency within carcinoma-bearing colons
3. Similar frequencies of adenomas and carcinomas in regions with high and low rates of colorectal neoplasia
4. Removing adenomas reduces the risk of carcinoma
5. Some untreated adenomas eventually become malignant
6. Severe dysplasia more common in adenomas of patients with synchronous and metachronous carcinoma

Pathologic evidence

1. Untreated polyposis patients eventually develop carcinomas in one of their adenomas
2. Many carcinomas show adjacent adenomatous tissue
3. Very few small carcinomas described without adjacent adenomatous component
4. Evidence of direct transformation from adenoma to carcinoma
5. Similar histochemical and immunohistochemical properties of adenomas and carcinomas

Experimental evidence

1. Mutagenic chemicals induce both adenomas and carcinomas in experimental animals
2. In vitro adenoma cells can eventually develop phenotypic features of malignant cells

Molecular evidence

1. Adenomas show intermediate properties between normal and carcinomatous cells, particularly in terms of DNA content
2. Adenomas share molecular genetic mutations of carcinoma
3. Increasing genetic mutations correlate with increasing grade of adenoma and finally carcinoma

Against

1. Carcinomas may arise in flat nonadenomatous mucosa and in inflammatory bowel disease
2. No adenomatous areas in some small nonulcerated carcinomas
3. Failure to disclose carcinoma in the great majority of adenomas
4. Differing epidemiology of adenomas and carcinomas in a small minority of studies

sis are not strictly within the compass of this chapter (see Ch. 18) but data from such genetic studies have further strengthened the evidence for the adenoma-carcinoma sequence.[15] Thus adenomas represent several stages (of increasing size and dysplasia) in the neoplastic progression toward colorectal cancer, in which increasing genetic mutations have occurred.[16,17] For instance, mutations of the *APC* gene (the mutated gene in familial adenomatous polyposis) occur relatively early, whereas *p53* mutations underpin the progression of large severely dysplastic adenomas toward frank malignancy.[18]

Pathologically, examples of the sequence are seen regularly: mild dysplastic adenomas harbor foci of more severe dysplasia, and areas of adenocarcinoma arise in large tubulovillous adenomas. The evidence for the adenoma-carcinoma sequence has been reviewed elsewhere[19] but morphologic studies (particularly in polyposis) and more recent molecular biologic evidence have strengthened the belief that this is the most important pathway for the genesis of colorectal cancer. The accompanying box summarizes the evidence for and against the adenoma-carcinoma sequence.

ADENOCARCINOMA

Pathology

Biopsy Diagnosis of Colorectal Cancer

Biopsy diagnosis is essentially a confirmatory exercise, the clinician being already suspicious of malignancy in most cases. A notable exception is stricture formation, in which the endoscopic features of malignancy may not be obvious. As resection is the almost inevitable consequence of a diagnosis of malignancy, diligence on the part of the pathologist is important. The controversies about the legitimacy of a diagnosis of adenocarcinoma in situ and intramucosal carcinoma have already been mentioned (see above). The diagnosis of malignancy requires evidence of invasion across the muscularis mucosae into the submucosa by neoplastic glands or cells, or both. This is usually associated with a stromal or desmoplastic reaction. Normally the cytologic features of malignant epithelium are different from those of adenomas and thus the stromal and cytologic features readily enable the pathologist to differentiate normally sited or misplaced adenomatous epithelium from invasive malignancy. Pathologic mimics of adenocarcinoma on biopsy are well recognized and include epithelial misplacement and colitis cystica profunda, the mucosal prolapse (solitary ulcer) syndrome, and endometriosis.

Of secondary importance in biopsy pathology is the typing and grading of colorectal cancer. Almost 90% of malignancies will be of the standard adenocarcinomatous type. About 10% will be of the mucinous type, which is more common in the right colon. Nevertheless, it should be emphasized that morphologic diversity and heterogeneity are common in colorectal cancer; the superficial parts of a mucinous carcinoma, seen on biopsy, will often show features more akin to those of standard adenocarcinoma. Equally, grading on biopsy is beset by similar problems with heterogeneity. Whereas both typing and grading may be a guide to tumor spread and behavior, neither can be considered definitive on biopsy material.

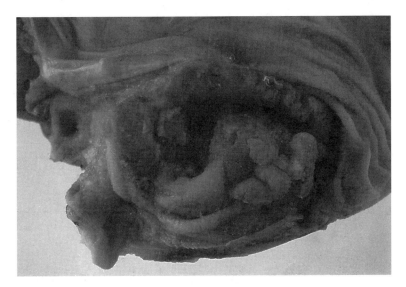

Figure 19-3. A carcinoma of the cecum resected by right hemicolectomy. The tumor shows characteristic rolled everted edges and central ulceration.

Of more importance for the patient's immediate management is confirmation that the tumor does not represent a rare form of neoplasm in which primary excisional surgery may not be indicated. For instance, anal carcinomas may present as low rectal tumors because of anatomic considerations and yet the primary treatment of anal squamous cell carcinoma is radiotherapy or chemotherapy (or both) rather than surgery. Equally, secondary tumors, leukemia, and lymphoma may simulate primary carcinoma endoscopically and, once again, primary surgery may not be appropriate.

Macroscopic Features and Pathologic Assessment of Resection Specimens

About 40% of all cancers of the large intestine arise in the rectum and approximately 35% in the sigmoid colon. Of the remainder of the colon, the cecum and ascending colon are favored sites. The macroscopic features are not particularly influenced by the site of the tumor, although stricturing cancers are more common in the colon than in the rectum. Most carcinomas are large ulcerating lesions with rolled and everted edges (Fig. 19-3; see also Plate 19-3). Circumferential involvement is common and is likely to lead to large bowel obstruction. Protuberant tumors tend to be smaller and well differentiated. Nevertheless, size and appearance are relatively poor correlates with tumor behavior and prognosis. Large tumors may be slow growing and indolent, whereas small buttonlike carcinomas can show early involvement of extramural blood vessels and metastatic disease.

The cut surface of the cancer characteristically shows firm, pale homogeneous tumor tissue often with zones of necrosis. Mucoid change correlates with mucinous histology and occurs in about 10% of tumors, with a predilection for the right colon. Long segment strictures due to carcinoma are caused by diffusely infiltrative poorly differentiated carcinomas.

The pathologic assessment of a colorectal specimen is greatly facilitated by receipt of the specimen fresh, appropriate orienta-

tion of the open specimen on a cork board, and adequate fixation.[20] This particularly aids in assessment of resection margins in rectal cancer and the dissection of lymph nodes. Pathologic assessment concentrates on those parameters of importance to prognostication. The accompanying box lists the aims of dissection and tissue sampling for microscopy. The importance of meticulous technique at the time of specimen dissection cannot be overemphasized: it is more important for the pathologist to

---

The Aims of Dissection and Tissue Sampling for Microscopy

1. Description
   Specimen length
   Distance of tumor from closer margin
   Tumor size: axial length versus maximum circumference
   Relation to deep margin and peritoneum
   Associated lesions—polyps, inflammation, and so forth
   Unassociated lesions—diverticula, and so forth
2. Identification of mesorectal margin (if present) with gelatin/India ink
3. Dissection of mesentery in lymphatic drainage field of tumor and removal of all lymph nodes by traditional methods of dissection or fat clearance
4. Sagittal 2-mm slices through entire tumor
5. Two blocks (minimum) taken from where tumor is closest to the mesorectal margin and/or the peritoneal surface
6. Block of tumor and proximal/distal margin only if tumor is within 2 cm of the margin
7. Minimum of six tumor blocks to assuage the problems of heterogeneity

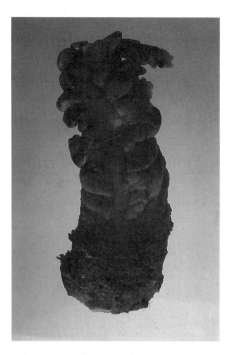

Figure 19-4. An anterior resection specimen fixed and the mesorectal margin then painted with a colored gelatin mixture. This enables the deep (radial, circumferential, mesorectal) margin to be accurately identified histologically.

spend time at the dissecting table rather than at the microscope when assessing a colorectal cancer. All lymph nodes should be removed, as increasing the lymph node harvest undoubtedly increases the number of lymph node-positive cases.[21] It remains controversial whether this is best achieved by routine dissection or by fat clearance methods.[20,22,23] Both methods have advantages and detractions, and no clear evidence shows that fat clearance methods result in significant differences in patient management or prognosis.

In rectal cancer, assessment of depth of spread within the mesorectum[24] and analysis of the proximity of the tumor to the mesorectal (deep, radial, circumferential) margin[25–27] is of supreme importance. The mesorectal margin should be identified by painting it with colored gelatin (Fig. 19-4; see also Plate 19-4). In upper rectal cancer and colonic cancer, the closeness of the tumor to the peritoneal surface is also an important feature to identify those patients likely to develop pelvic and intraperitoneal recurrence and for prognostic purposes.[28,29] Pathologists should not waste valuable resources assessing proximal and distal margins of a colorectal cancer resection specimen except when the tumor is within 2 cm of that margin but should instead concentrate on the much more important deep or mesorectal margin.[30]

Microscopic Features

Most colorectal cancers are adenocarcinomas in which tubular morphology is clearly identified. Grading is determined chiefly by such tubular differentiation.[31] About 60% of all standard carcinomas are of a moderate grade in which tubular morphology is readily identified but tubules are irregular or poorly

formed. Twenty percent of carcinomas are well differentiated in that tubules are regular and well formed, and a further 20% are poorly differentiated, with little or no tubule formation. Grading is applied to the area of the tumor with the most poorly differentiated features. In general, grade correlates very well with spread and stage of tumor, although whether grade has any independent prognostic significance in the face of the more powerful staging parameters is controversial.[32,33]

Some carcinomas, particularly from the right colon, show large lakes of mucin in which tumorous epithelium floats: these tumors are designated mucinous type. Controversies exist concerning the definition of mucinous carcinoma, although most would now accept a mucin content in excess of 50% of the total volume of that tumor as a reasonable definition.[34–36] The distinction is of some importance because mucinous tumors have been shown to have a worse prognosis, and their presence in younger patients, particularly in the right colon, may indicate the hereditary nonpolyposis colorectal cancer syndrome (see Ch. 21).[37,38] A smaller proportion will show intracellular mucin secretion producing the characteristic signet ring cell morphology. Such tumors tend to occur in younger individuals, may not show an associated adenomatous component, and may arise as a result of genetic pathways different from those of other commoner adenocarcinomas of the colorectum.[39] They are associated with extensive local spread, long segment stricturing, and a particularly gloomy prognosis.

Spread and Prognostic Factors

Malignant tumors can spread in several different ways, and each mode of spread has an influence on prognosis. A combination of modes of spread may be used to stage a tumor to provide useful information for prognosis and also for further management of the individual patient. The prognostic utility of pathologic parameters in colorectal cancer has become somewhat confused because many different parameters have been shown to have some independent prognostic influence in the myriad investigations that have been performed.[40,41] Only local spread, lymphatic spread, mesorectal margin involvement, and peritoneal involvement have consistently provided useful predictive values, and currently the only pathologic parameter that is a major determinant of adjuvant therapy is stage, usually defined by the Dukes staging classification. Nevertheless, recent advances in our understanding of the spread of carcinoma and its influence on local recurrence, distant recurrence, and patient outcome have major implications for the future of adjuvant therapy.

Local Spread

The prognostic power of the extent of local spread, through the bowel wall and beyond, is undisputed.[24,42,43] In general, tumors have a relatively good prognosis if they are retained within the wall of the bowel. This is demarcated by the outer border of the muscularis propria. The extent of mesorectal spread is also of important predictive value.[24,44] Histologically demonstrated involvement of the mesorectal margin is of strong independent prognostic significance and is a powerful predictor of subsequent local recurrence, particularly in those patient groups in which complete mesorectal resection has not been practiced.[25–27] Local recurrence itself is a poor prognostic feature, the great majority of patients dying rapidly after presentation with local recurrence.[45] Heald[46] has championed the practice of complete mesorectal excision and has shown that this is associated with a low rate of local recurrence in rectal cancer, indicating the importance of extent of spread and involvement of mesorectal margins in the development of local recurrence.[47] Few studies of the extent of local spread in colonic cancer have been performed, but it appears that involvement of the peritoneal surface (see below) is a more important assessment.[28,48] Local spread beyond the rectum and colon will inevitably lead to involvement of contiguous organs, particularly the bladder and uterus in rectal and sigmoid cancer and the small intestine in colonic cancer. Extensive spread to other luminal viscera may result in fistula formation.

Lymphatic Spread

Local lymph node involvement has been shown to be the most important independent prognostic indicator in both rectal[43] and colonic[38] cancer. Such nodal involvement is the basis of all prognostic classifications in colorectal cancer, indicating the need for meticulous dissection of all lymph nodes in a specimen. The number of involved nodes,[31,49] the position of the involved nodes,[50] and the status of the high tie node[28,42] are all of major prognostic influence. Some have advocated the use of cytokeratin immunohistochemistry to detect nodal micrometastases and thus assign more cases to a higher stage.[51]

Venous Spread

Cases that show spread in thick-walled extramural veins have a significantly worse prognosis[52,53] (Fig. 19-5; see also Plate 19-5). Surprisingly, submucosal venous involvement does not seem to be associated with a worse prognosis,[53] and even extramural spread has little independent prognostic significance in curative cases.[29,43] Variations in the assessment of this parameter may help to explain some of these ambiguities; it is currently recommended that this parameter always be recorded.[21]

Peritoneal Spread

Even though at least half of the surface area of the colon and up to 25% (in women) of that of the rectum (16% in men) is invested in peritoneum, the prognostic influence of local peritoneal involvement has been neglected. This assessment is included in the Australian Clinico-Pathological System (ACPS) of staging, but its influence is lessened because of the progressive nature of this system (i.e., the significance of local spread is lost if lymph nodes are involved).[54] Serosal involvement also features in the pTNM system.[21,55] In our hands, local peritoneal involvement is very common in colonic cancer (55% of all cases) and is the most powerful independent prognostic parameter in colonic cancer.[48] It is also of some prognostic value in rectal cancer and is a consistent predictor of cases that subsequently recur in the peritoneal cavity.[29,48] We believe that it also accounts for a small proportion of local recurrences in the pelvis in cases of upper rectal and sigmoid cancer. Support for the powerful prognostic influence of this parameter is provided by the ACPS studies.[28]

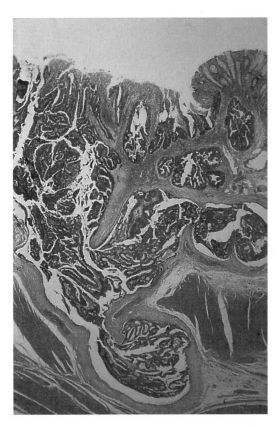

Figure 19-5. A well-differentiated adenocarcinoma of the colon showing spread into a thick-walled intramural vein. This feature is associated with both local recurrence and a poor prognosis. (H&E × 10.)

Implantation Metastasis

Colorectal cancer cells are regularly shed into the lumen of the bowel; these can be demonstrated both proximal and distal to the tumor and are seemingly still viable.[56] Thus it is of no great surprise that these cells can implant on a "raw" surface and form a tumor mass. Such a phenomenon accounts for a small proportion of local recurrences, particularly if the bowel lumen has not been satisfactorily washed out at the time of surgery.[48] Furthermore, occasional examples of this phenomenon are seen particularly in the region of the anal canal and at colostomy sites after previous colorectal cancer resection.

Other Morphologic Prognostic Factors

Although the prognostic value of the quality of the advancing margin (circumscribed versus diffuse infiltration) and lymphocytic infiltrate at the advancing margin (marked versus sparse) had been previously demonstrated, it was Jass et al.[43] who popularized these variables in colorectal cancer assessment. About 75% of rectal cancers show a well- or moderately well-circumscribed advancing margin, whereas between 10 and 20% show a well-defined lamina of lymphocytes at the advancing margin (Fig. 19-6; see also Plate 19-6). Both these features are prognostically favorable and form part of the Jass prognostic classification for rectal cancer. The value of lymphocytic infiltrate as a

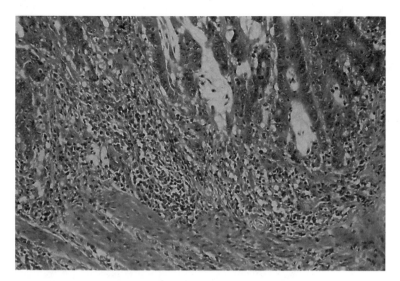

Figure 19-6. The advancing margin of a moderately differentiated adenocarcinoma of the colon. The margin is well circumscribed and is associated with a marked lymphocytic infiltrate. Both features are favorable prognostic parameters in colorectal cancer. (H&E × 50.)

prognostic marker has been questioned because of poor interobserver agreement[57,58] and the absence of independent prognostic significance in colonic[38] and colorectal cancer.[59] Graham and Appelman[60] drew attention to the identification of lymphoid aggregates, in a Crohn's-like pattern at the junction of the muscularis propria and the subserosa, close to colorectal cancer. This feature may have more prognostic importance than the lymphocytic reaction at the advancing margin, being of significant independent prognostic importance in one study.[59]

Other parameters that have been accorded prognostic value by some but are thought to be of dubious value in routine use are the presence of synchronous adenomas in a colorectal cancer,[61] intratumoral fibrosis,[62] intratumoral necrosis, and perineural spread.[63] Extramural tumor nodules, not obviously in lymph nodes, are associated with a poor prognosis, but this parameter has not been subjected to rigorous study.[59]

Molecular Parameters and Other Laboratory Techniques

Many investigators have attempted to relate diverse biologic features of colorectal cancer cells with prognosis,[32,33] especially using molecular biologic techniques[32,33]; the literature is full of studies demonstrating correlations of tumor behavior with such genetic and other abnormalities. For instance, in the late 1980s, ploidy as defined by flow cytometry was especially popular as a prognostic tool (in the literature at least), but few units, if any, are using flow cytometry routinely now. Many studies have purported to demonstrate the usefulness of molecular prognostic factors. The current situation is well illustrated by *p53* overexpression/mutation. A literature review would suggest that in *p53* analysis we have an excellent diagnostic and prognostic marker for colorectal neoplasia, yet closer examination shows that many authors disagree and that routine use cannot be recommended. This is not to deny the enormous importance of molecular biology for future diagnosis, management, and

possible prevention of colorectal neoplasia. At present, pathologists must rely on routine specimen analysis for accurate prognostic assessment.[41]

STAGING

Dr. Cuthbert Dukes[64] is credited with the most simple, workable, and useful prognostic classification of colorectal cancer. His ABC system combines spread through the bowel wall with local lymph node involvement and provides such useful clinical information that it, or modifications of it, is still the single most important determinant of the decision to administer adjuvant therapy after surgery. Indeed, throughout the world, it is the system most commonly used by pathologists.[65] Dr. Dukes modified his ABC system to provide further information about lymph node involvement by including an assessment of the highest lymph node status.[42] Many others have modified the Dukes system, and these schemes have been applied to both rectal and colonic cancer (Table 19-1).

The Dukes classification has been abused by wholesale misunderstandings, largely propagated by the development of classifications using similar terminology.[33] Dukes has been credited with stages (such as D) that he did not present. Although the Dukes classification is simple to use and reproducible, it nevertheless falls short of the quintessential classification. Only about 16% of rectal cancer patients have Dukes A carcinomas and a confident prediction of cure; this total falls to about 5% in colonic cancer. Less than 10% of patients have C2 tumors, for which a cancer-related death is to be expected. The B stage includes tumors with variable local extent having correspondingly variable cancer-specific end points. Nevertheless, there is no doubt that the advantages of simplicity and applicability outweigh such shortcomings, and the many modifications of the Dukes system (Table 19-1) have little added value. All are more complicated and thus more difficult to commit to memory; none has achieved anything like universal acceptance.

Table 19-1. Pathological Staging Systems of Colorectal Cancer

Author	Site of Tumors	Terminology
Dukes, 1932	Rectum	ABC
Kirklin et al, 1949	Sigmoid and rectum	Mod ABC
Astler and Coller, 1954	Colon and rectum	Mod ABC
Dukes and Bussey, 1958	Rectum	Mod ABC
ACPS, 1976	Colon and rectum	Mod ABC
GITSG, 1984	Colon and rectum	Mod ABC
Jass et al, 1987	Rectum	Weighted scores
UICC/pTNM 1995 (revised)	Colon and rectum	TNM

Abbreviations: Mod, modified; GITSG, Gastrointestinal Tumour Study Group (1975); ACPS, Australian Clinico-Pathological Staging[54,96]; UICC, Union International Contre le Cancer; pTNM, UICC pathologic cancer staging system.[32]

The Kirklin-Dockerty[66] and Astler and Coller[67] modifications deviate from the Dukes classification by dividing up local penetration of the bowel wall and introducing intramucosal carcinoma. The Astler-Coller system does, however, introduce one subgroup with useful prognostic value[68,69]: this is the C1 stage in their classification, which represents tumors with lymph node involvement but without direct spread in continuity through the bowel wall. This tumor has a cumulative prognosis equivalent to that of Dukes B carcinomas.[69]

The Gastrointestinal Tumor Study Group classification[49] is more complicated than the aforementioned systems and is relatively insensitive at predicting death from cancer.[70] It is the first system to introduce the number of involved lymph nodes as a prognostic parameter; subsequent studies have demonstrated the strong predictive value of dividing lymph node involvement into two groups (one to four and more than four).[43,70]

The ACPS employs the original Dukes classification but adds additional information, including whether tumor has been left behind at the time of operation or whether metastases are present (stage D).[54] The ACPS system also incorporates important assessments such as serosal invasion (stage B2) and apical node involvement (stage C2, as in the Dukes-Bussey system).[71] The system has been subject to prospective analysis over many years, is relatively simple, and has demonstrated advantages over other systems.[28,72] It suffers, like all systems before it, from of its sequential nature, unfortunately. The system is seldom used in the Northern Hemisphere; this is a pity because it has many advantages over other, more complicated staging systems.

Jass and his colleagues[43] based their prognostic classification of rectal cancer on the work of Dukes but used multivariate analysis to select variables of independent prognostic value. Lymph node involvement and spread through the bowel wall are incorporated, but in addition the quality of the invasive border and the lymphocytic infiltrate at this margin are included as strong independent prognostic indicators. Thus the system is not strictly a staging classification because it combines staging parameters with these ''biologic'' factors. The Jass classification has its supporters and detractors.[73–75] Assessment of the lymphocytic infiltrate at advancing margins has been associated with weak interobserver consistency,[57,58] although others have demonstrated acceptable levels of observer agreement.[38,74,76] The system is apparently not as useful in the colon as in the rectum.[38] More recently it has been suggested that the system has a doubtful advantage over other staging classifications.[58,59] The jury is still out over the Jass classification, but it would be fair to state that its usefulness in clinical practice is not as great as initial expectations led us to believe.

The TNM classification of the Union International Contre le Cancer is energetically promoted in United States and Germany and is becoming more popular in the United Kingdom.[21,55] Some have asserted that it is too complex for routine usage, but it would be folly to ignore a system that has such strong backing from many powerful cancer bodies. Its major advantages are its dual structure using the same principles in clinical and pathologic classification, its international uniformity, and the fact that similar systems can be used for most organs.[55] However, there can be no doubt that, compared with the Dukes system and even some of its modifications, it is complex and difficult to commit to memory, especially as it is being continually modified.[77,78]

As with many other organ systems, pathologists are left with several staging systems and even more prognostic parameters that apparently should be assessed and recorded. If uniformity of pathologic assessment is to be achieved internationally, then it is imperative that a uniform staging system be adopted that is simple and useful. One could also argue that separate systems should be introduced for colon and rectum, as local spread beyond the bowel wall (toward the mesorectal margin in rectal cancer and the peritoneal surface in colonic cancer) have very different implications.[33] An inspection of Table 19-1 will demonstrate the disregard for these differences in that most of the staging systems blithely combine rectum and colon in their analyses. What is required is an internationally acceptable system upon which to judge the efficacy of subsequent management strategies that allows prediction of local recurrence and prognosis using the smallest number of independent prognostic parameters and is not tied to Dukes-type systems, which, by their progressive nature, cannot be all-encompassing.[33,41]

OTHER PRIMARY CARCINOMAS OF THE LARGE INTESTINE

More than 99% of carcinomas of the colon and rectum are adenocarcinomas; 10% are of the mucinous subtype. Primary adenosquamous carcinomas, pure squamous cell carcinomas, small cell undifferentiated (oat cell) carcinomas, and so-called undifferentiated carcinomas are all described in the colon and rectum but are very rare. It seems that they all have a worse prognosis than the standard adenocarcinoma.

NEUROENDOCRINE TUMORS

Pure neuroendocrine tumors (carcinoids) are relatively uncommon in the large intestine, but neuroendocrine differentiation is not an unusual feature of primary adenocarcinoma of the colorectum. Carcinomas with such neuroendocrine differentiation have a significantly worse prognosis than those without.[79,80] Pure carcinoids are most commonly located in the cecum or rectum. The cecum is a midgut derivative, and carci-

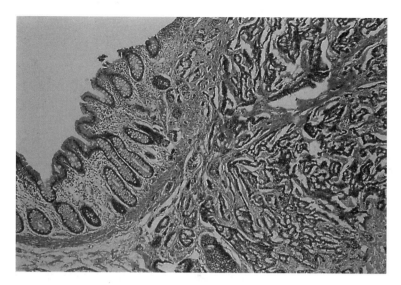

Figure 19-7. A typical benign rectal carcinoid tumor. The lesion is primarily submucosal, although there is involvement of the overlying mucosa and the tumor shows the characteristic palisading, ribboning pattern of hindgut carcinoids. (H&E × 25.)

noid tumors arising here disclose pathologic and behavioral features comparable to those that arise in the small intestine.[81] Such tumors are usually large, with significant metastatic potential. Like ileal carcinoids, although less commonly, cecal endocrine tumors may secrete vasoactive hormones such as 5-hydroxytryptamine and are a rare cause of the carcinoid syndrome, when metastases to the liver have occurred. Histologically, cecal carcinoids show the classic pattern seen in appendiceal and ileal carcinoid tumors, although a tubular morphology may occur.

The rectum is the most common site of endocrine tumors of the large intestine. Most of these lesions are small, submucosal nodules, less than 1 cm in diameter, and are often distinctly yellow on endoscopic examination[82] (Fig. 19-7; see also plate 19-7). They are almost always asymptomatic and are usually discovered as an incidental finding during investigation for other anorectal conditions. Rectal carcinoids in patients with ulcerative colitis are well recognized, and they appear to occur as a complication of endocrine cell hyperplasia, a common pathologic sequela to colitis.[83] Small submucosal rectal carcinoids are adequately treated by local excision, and local recurrence is most unusual.[84] Histologically, rectal carcinoids show the characteristic palisading, ribboning pattern of hindgut carcinoids (Fig. 19-7). Occasionally malignant hindgut carcinoids occur, and these show the same ribboning pattern, although solid, almost anaplastic foci are a typical feature of these aggressive rapidly metastasizing tumors. Further pathologic features that aid in the diagnosis of malignant carcinoids of the more distal colon and rectum are the size of the tumor (greater than 2 cm in diameter), ulceration, spread in the muscularis propria, extensive necrosis, and an infiltrating growth pattern.[82]

BENIGN CONNECTIVE TISSUE TUMORS AND THE SARCOMAS

Smooth muscle tumors are the most common connective tissue tumors of the gastrointestinal tract, although they occur more in the upper gut than in the large bowel. There is some debate about the histogenesis of many of these tumors in that evidence of smooth muscle derivation is not always forthcoming, and some may represent neural tumors[85]: the terminology of gastrointestinal stromal tumors of the gut is preferred by some. The rectum is the most common site for smooth muscle/stromal tumors within the large bowel. Most originate from the muscularis propria, but occasionally they arise from the muscularis mucosae and present as small mobile submucosal nodules. Usually they present as a polypoid intraluminal tumor, an intramural tumor, or a subserosal tumor. Ulceration of the mucosa is commonly seen with larger tumors and is not necessarily indicative of malignancy. On sectioning, smooth muscle/stromal tumors are firm and show the whorled pattern typical of such fibroid tissue. Discriminators of malignancy include size, ulceration, necrosis, and, most importantly, cytologic guides such as mitotic activity, proliferation index, and aneuploidy.[86] Tumors with mitotic counts in excess of 10/50 high power fields (hpf) should be regarded as leiomyosarcomas/malignant stromal tumors and are prone to substantial metastatic potential. Nevertheless, these tumors are unpredictable, with a variable survival rate after apparently curative surgery. Late metastatic disease, often after 10 years, is a characteristic feature of leiomyosarcoma.

Benign fatty tumors (lipomas) of the large intestine are submucosal tumors and are more common in the right colon than the distal colon and rectum (Fig. 19-8; see also Plate 19.8). Sometimes they are multiple. Small lipomas are not unusual in endoscopic practice, but are almost always asymptomatic. Larger tumors may cause hemorrhage and are also liable to intussusception, causing acute or subacute intestinal obstruction[87] (Fig. 19-8). On angiography, colonic lipomas can mimic the appearances of angioectasia. Liposarcoma is usually found as a retroperitoneal/pelvic soft tissue tumor and secondarily involves the large bowel. Lipohyperplasia of the ileocecal valve is not strictly a neoplasm, but it may mimic one, especially on barium enema. Histologically, there is an excess of adipose

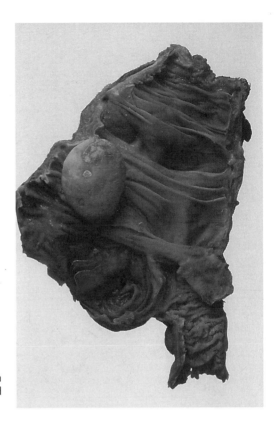

Figure 19-8. A pedunculated lipoma, 7 cm in diameter, of the ascending colon treated by right hemicolectomy. There is ulceration of the surface and there had been early intussusception.

tissue in the submucosa without the lobulation indicative of a lipoma.

Classical neural tumors, namely, neurilemmoma and neurofibroma, are decidedly unusual in the colon and rectum, although in some hands the more common gastrointestinal stromal tumors display evidence of neural differentiation in an appreciable percentage of cases.[85] Solitary diffuse neurofibroma may arise in the mucosa of the colon. Plexiform neurofibromas originate in the submucosa or in the myenteric plexus, most developing in patients with von Recklinghausen's disease. Intestinal ganglioneuromatosis may cause polypoid and stricturing lesions of the intestine, although these are much more common in the small bowel.[88]

Blood vessel tumors include both benign and malignant varieties. Cavernous hemangioma may be considered as a congenital anomaly or hamartoma and usually presents in childhood or early adulthood. It occurs most often in the rectum and sigmoid colon and presents with rectal hemorrhage. Although all blood vessels in the involved segment show dilatation, those in the submucosa are the most markedly affected. Isolated case reports exist of primary intestinal hemangiosarcoma, but colorectal involvement by Kaposi's sarcoma is not uncommon in the context of the acquired immunodeficiency syndrome (AIDS).[89] The sarcoma presents as a bluish submucosal nodule, particularly in the lower rectum, may be large enough to produce a polypoid mass, and is often multiple.

MALIGNANT LYMPHOMA AND LEUKEMIA

Lymphoma occurring in the large bowel is usually the result of secondary spread from nodal disease, and primary lymphoma of the colon and rectum represents only 0.5% of primary malig-

nant neoplasms. As would be expected from the distribution of lymphoid tissue within the large intestine, the commonest sites of lymphoma are the cecum and rectum.[90,91] Primary Hodgkin's disease is vanishingly rare, and the great majority of primary lymphomas are non-Hodgkin's lymphomas of B-cell phenotype. Primary colorectal malignant lymphoma may present as a localized lesion, as multicentric lymphoma, or as malignant lymphomatous polyposis. Localized primary B-cell lymphoma of the large intestine is a recognized complication of chronic ulcerative colitis.[92] Histologically, these tumors show features typical of tumors of mucosa-associated lymphoid tissue; a characteristic feature of these polymorphic lymphomas is the presence of tumor cells infiltrating and destroying the crypt epithelium. This feature is known as the lymphoepithelial lesion. There are occasional reports of large intestinal lymphoma complicating Crohn's disease.[92]

Grade and stage of primary B-cell lymphomas are both important in management and prognosis.[93] High-grade lymphomas are infiltrative tumors that involve long segments of the bowel and may be multicentric. They rapidly efface the muscularis propria, leading to fissuring ulceration and perforation. Low-grade tumors are less infiltrative and may remain localized for long periods. Excisional surgery is probably the management of choice for these low-grade tumors, whereas this may be inappropriate for high-grade lesions unless clinical staging is favorable. High-grade B-cell lymphoma of lymphoblastic and diffuse large cell types arising in the anorectal region are well described in AIDS patients.[94] Malignant lymphomatous polyposis has characteristic macroscopic features (Fig. 19-9; see also Plate 19-9). It comprises about 25% of all primary colorectal lymphomas and histologically shows the features of

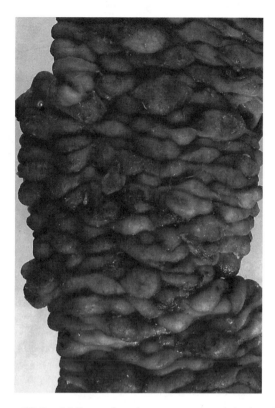

Figure 19-9. Malignant lymphomatous polyposis in the colon. The mucosal surface is festooned with numerous, often pedunculated, polyps of variable size. The polyps are usually much larger and more coalescent than those seen in other polyposis syndromes. Predominant involvement of the ileocecal region is characteristic of this condition.

a mantle zone/centrocytic lymphoma (and thus is of the low-grade B-cell type).[93,95] Because of its multifocality, surgery is usually inappropriate and the prognosis dismal.

Burkitt's lymphoma occurs in the terminal ileum in children and may secondarily involve the cecum. Secondary nodal lymphoma affecting the large intestine often presents with multiple lesions, and often long segments of the bowel are affected with deep infiltration of the bowel wall. Finally, deposits of leuke-

mia, especially acute myelogenous leukemia, may be found in the bowel; very occasionally such masses are the presenting feature of the disease.

MALIGNANT MELANOMA, SECONDARY MALIGNANCY, AND OTHER RARE NEOPLASMS

Malignant melanoma accounts for 10 to 15% of primary malignant tumors of the anus but is very rare as an unequivocally primary tumor of the rectum. Anorectal melanomas are usually of the nodular type. The clinical presentation is that of a large protuberant or ulcerating mass that often extends into the lower rectum, as most anorectal melanomas are centered above the dentate line. Extensive local spread into perianal and perirectal tissues and involvement of hemorrhoidal lymph nodes is usual. In common with melanomas of mucous membranes elsewhere, two major histologic subtypes are seen: epithelioid and spindle cell melanoma. Many of these tumors lack melanin pigment, and the diagnosis is often unsuspected clinically. The prognosis of anorectal melanoma is appalling, and most patients die within a year of presentation.

Metastatic disease to the colon and rectum is commonly demonstrated at autopsy but is only rarely of any clinical significance. Diffuse-type gastric carcinoma and direct spread from carcinomas of the prostate, cervix, and bladder are most often seen in the rectum. Metastatic lobular carcinoma of the breast and metastatic malignant melanoma have a particular affinity for the intestines, the latter presenting as submucosal polypoid masses that cause subacute obstruction, sometimes by intussusception.

Tumors arising in the connective tissues between the sacrum and the anus and rectum may occasionally manifest as anorectal tumors. Retrorectal cystic hamartoma (anal gland cyst hamartoma; tailgut cyst) presents in this way and may be confused both macroscopically and histologically with benign cystic teratoma of the sacrococcygeal region. Inclusion epidermal and dermoid cysts also occur in the presacral space. The sacrococcygeal region is the commonest site of chordoma and myxopapillary ependymoma. More rarely neurilemmoma, hemangiopericytoma, papillary ependymoma, and benign and malignant tumors of bone and cartilage may involve this area and encroach on the anorectum.

REFERENCES

1. Morson BC, Dawson IMP, Day DW (1990) Benign epithelial tumours and polyps. pp. 563–596. In: Morson & Dawson's Gastrointestinal Pathology. 3rd Ed. Blackwell Scientific Publications, Oxford
2. Riddell RH, Goldman H, Ransohoff D et al (1983) Dysplasia in inflammatory bowel disease. Standardised classification with provisional clinical application. Hum Pathol 14:931–966
3. Fenoglio CM, Kaye GI, Lane N (1973) Distribution of human colonic lymphatics in normal, hyperplastic and adenomatous tissue. Gastroenterology 64:51–66
4. Konishi F, Morson BC (1982) Pathology of colorectal adenomas: a colonoscopic survey. J Clin Pathol 35:830–841
5. Morson BC, Dawson IMP, Day DW (1990) Benign epithelial tumours and polyps. p. 567. In: Morson & Dawson's Gastrointestinal Pathology. 3rd Ed. Blackwell Scientific Publications, Oxford
6. O'Brien MJ, Winawer SJ, Zauber AG et al (1990) The National Polyp Study. Patient and polyp characteristics associated with high grade dysplasia in colorectal adenomas. Gastroenterology 98:371–379
7. Morson BC, Whiteway JE, Jones EA (1984) Histopathology and prognosis of malignant colorectal polyps treated by endoscopic polypectomy. Gut 25:437–444
8. Muller S, Chesner IM, Egan MJ (1989) Significance of venous and lymphatic invasion in malignant polyps of the colon and rectum. Gut 30:1385–1391

9. Geraghty JM, Williams CB, Talbot IC (1991) Malignant colo-rectal polyps: venous invasion and successful treatment by en-doscopic polypectomy. Gut 32:774–778

10. Muto T, Bussey HJR, Morson BC (1973) Pseudocarcinoma-tous invasion in adenomatous polyps of the colon and rectum. J Clin Pathol 26:25–31

11. Muto T, Kamiya J, Sawada T et al (1985) Small ''flat ade-noma'' of the large bowel with special reference to its clinico-pathological features. Dis Colon Rectum 28:847–851

12. Fujimori T, Satonaka K, Yamamura IY et al (1994) Non-in-volvement of ras mutations in flat colorectal adenomas and carcinomas. Int J Cancer 57:51–55

13. Kubota O, Kino I (1995) Depressed adenomas of the colon in familial adenomatous polyposis. Histology, immunohisto-chemical detection of proliferating cell nuclear antigen (PCNA) and analysis of background mucosa. Am J Surg Pathol 19:318–327

14. Desigan G, Wang M, Alberti-Flor J (1985) *De novo* carcinoma of the rectum: a case report. Am J Gastroenterol 80:553–556

15. Fearon ER (1994) Molecular genetic studies of the adenoma-carcinoma sequence. Adv Intern Med 39:123–147

16. Fearon ER, Vogelstein B (1990) A genetic model for colorectal tumorigenesis. Cell 61:759–767

17. Hamilton SR (1992) The adenoma: adenocarcinoma sequence in the large bowel: variations on a theme. J Cell Biochem (suppl) 16:41–46

18. Scott N, Quirke P (1993) Molecular biology of colorectal neo-plasia. Gut 34:289–292

19. Fenoglio-Preiser CM, Pascal RR (1989) The adenoma-carci-noma sequence. pp. 754–756. In Whitehead R (ed): Gastroin-testinal and Oesophageal Pathology. Churchill Livingstone, Edinburgh

20. Sheffield JP, Talbot IC (1992) Gross examination of the large intestine. J Clin Pathol 45:751–755

21. Hermanek P, Henson DE, Hutter RVP, Sobin LH (eds) (1993) UICC TNM Supplement. A Commentary on Uniform Use. Springer-Verlag, Berlin

22. Jass JR, Miller K, Northover JMA (1986) Fat clearance method versus manual dissection of lymph nodes in specimens of rectal cancer. Int J Color Dis 1:155–156

23. Cawthorn SJ, Gibbs NM, Marks CG (1986) Clearance tech-nique for the detection of lymph nodes in colorectal cancer. Br J Surg 73:58–60

24. Cawthorn SJ, Parums DV, Gibbs NM et al (1991) Extent of mesorectal spread and involvement of lateral resection margin as prognostic factors after surgery for rectal cancer. Lancet 335:1055–1059

25. Quirke P, Dixon MF, Durdey P, Williams NS (1986) Local recurrence of rectal adenocarcinoma due to inadequate surgical resection. Histopathological study of lateral tumour spread and surgical excision. Lancet 2:996–999

26. Ng IO, Luk IS, Yuen ST et al (1993) Surgical lateral clearance in resected rectal carcinomas. A multivariate analysis of clini-copathologic features. Cancer 71:1972–1976

27. Adam IJ, Mohamdee MO, Martin IG et al (1994) Role of circumferential margin involvement in the local recurrence of rectal cancer. Lancet 344:707–710

28. Newland RC, Dent OF, Lyttle MN (1994) Pathologic determi-nants of survival associated with colorectal cancer with lymph node metastases. A multivariate analysis of 579 patients. Can-cer 73:2076–2082

29. Shepherd NA, Baxter KJ, Love SB (1995) Influence of local peritoneal involvement on local recurrence and prognosis in rectal cancer. J Clin Pathol 48:849–855

30. Cross SS, Bull AD, Smith JHF (1989) Is there any justification for the routine examination of bowel resection margins in colo-rectal adenocarcinoma? J Clin Pathol 42:1040–1042

31. Jass JR, Atkin WS, Cuzick J (1986) The grading of rectal cancer: historical perspectives and a multivariate analysis of 447 cases. Histopathology 10:437–459

32. Hermanek P, Sobin LH (1995) Colorectal carcinoma. pp. 64–79. In: Prognostic Factors in Cancer. Springer-Verlag, Berlin

33. Shepherd NA (1995) Pathological prognostic factors in colo-rectal cancer. pp. 115–141. In Kirkham N, Lemoine NR (eds): Progress in Pathology. Churchill Livingstone, Edinburgh

34. Pihl E, Nairn RC, Hughes ESR et al (1980) Mucinous colo-rectal carcinoma: immunopathology and prognosis. Pathology 12:439–447

35. Umpleby HC, Ranson DL, Williamson RCN (1985) Peculiari-ties of mucinous colorectal carcinoma. Br J Surg 72:715–718

36. Green JB, Timmcke AE, Mitchell WT (1993) Mucinous carci-noma — just another colon cancer? Dis Colon Rectum 36: 49–54

37. Sasaki O, Atkin WS, Jass JR (1987) Mucinous carcinoma of the rectum. Histopathology 11:259–272

38. Shepherd NA, Saraga EP, Love SB, Jass JR (1989) Prognostic factors in colonic cancer. Histopathology 14:613–620

39. Morson BC, Dawson IMP, Day DW (1990) Malignant epithe-lial tumours. pp. 609–610. In: Morson & Dawson's Gastroin-testinal Pathology. 3rd Ed. Blackwell Scientific Publications. Oxford

40. Deans GT, Parks TG, Rowlands BJ, Spence RA (1992) Prog-nostic factors in colorectal cancer. Br J Surg 79:608–613

41. Jass JR (1995) Prognostic factors in rectal cancer. Eur J Cancer 31:862–863

42. Dukes CE, Bussey HJR (1958) The spread of rectal cancer and its effect on prognosis. Br J Cancer 12:1016–1023

43. Jass JR, Love SB, Northover JMA (1987) A new prognostic classification of rectal cancer. Lancet 1:1303–1306

44. Scott N, Jackson P, Al-Jaberi T et al (1995) Total mesorectal excision and local recurrence: a study of tumour spread in the mesorectum distal to rectal cancer. Br J Surg 82:1031–1033

45. Abulafi AM, Williams NS (1994) Local recurrence of colo-rectal cancer: the problem, mechanisms, management and ad-juvant therapy. Br J Surg 81:7–19

46. Heald RJ, Ryall RDH (1986) Recurrence and survival after total mesorectal excision for rectal cancer. Lancet 1: 1479–1482

47. Macfarlane JK, Ryall RDH, Heald RJ (1993) Mesorectal exci-sion for rectal cancer. Lancet 341:457–460

48. Shepherd NA, Baxter KJ, Love SB (1997) The prognostic in-fluence of local peritoneal involvement in colonic cancer: a prospective evaluation. Gastroenterology (in press)

49. Gastrointestinal Tumor Study Group (1984) Adjuvant therapy of colon cancer — results of a prospectively randomized trial. N Engl J Med 310:737–743

50. Shida H, Ban K, Matsumoto M (1992) Prognostic significance of location of lymph node metastases in colorectal cancer. Dis Colon Rectum 35:1046–1050

51. Greenson JK, Isenhart CE, Rice R (1994) Identification of occult micrometastases in pericolic lymph nodes of Dukes B

colorectal cancer patients using monoclonal antibodies against cytokeratin and CC49. Correlation with long term survival. Cancer 73:563–569

52. Grinnell RS (1950) The spread of carcinoma of the colon and rectum. Cancer 3:640–653

53. Talbot IC, Ritchie S, Leighton MH (1980) The clinical significance of invasion of veins by rectal cancer. Br J Surg 67:439–442

54. Newland RC, Chapuis PH, Pheils MT, MacPherson JG (1981) The relationship of survival to staging and grading of colorectal carcinoma. A prospective study of 503 cases. Cancer 47:1424–1429

55. Hermanek P, Sobin LH (eds) (1992) UICC TNM Classification of Malignant Tumours. 4th Ed. 2nd Rev. Springer-Verlag, Berlin

56. Umpleby HC, Williamson RCN (1984) Viability of exfoliated colorectal carcinoma cells. Br J Surg 71:659–663

57. Dundas SAC, Laing RW, O'Cathain A (1988) Feasibility of new prognostic classification for rectal cancer. J Clin Pathol 41:1273–1276

58. Deans GT, Heatley M, Anderson N et al (1994) Jass' classification revisited. J Am Coll Surg 179:11–17

59. Harrison JC, Dean PJ, El-Zeky F, van der Zwaag R (1994) From Dukes through Jass: pathological prognostic indicators in rectal cancer. Hum Pathol 25:498–505

60. Graham DM, Appelman HD (1990) Crohn's-like lymphoid reaction and colorectal cancer: a potential histologic prognosticator. Mod Pathol 3:332–335

61. Kronborg O, Hage E, Fenger C, Deichgraeber E (1986) Do synchronous adenomas influence prognosis after radical surgery for colorectal cancer? A prospective study. Int J Color Dis 1:99–103

62. Halvorsen TB, Seim E (1989) Association between invasiveness, inflammatory reaction, desmoplasia and survival in colorectal cancer. J Clin Pathol 42:162–166

63. Shirouzu K, Isomoto H, Kakegawa T (1993) Prognostic evaluation of perineural invasion in rectal cancer. Am J Surg 165:233–237

64. Dukes CE (1932) The classification of cancer of the rectum. J Pathol Bacteriol 35:323–332

65. Fenoglio-Preiser CM, Pascal RR (1989) Other tumours of the large intestine. pp. 747–768. In Whitehead R (ed): Gastrointestinal and Oesophageal Pathology. Churchill Livingstone, Edinburgh

66. Kirklin MD, Dockerty MB, Waugh JM (1949) The role of the peritoneal reflection in the prognosis of carcinoma of the rectum and sigmoid colon. Surg Gynecol Obstet 88:326–331

67. Astler VB, Coller FA (1954) The prognostic significance of direct extension of carcinoma of the colon and rectum. Ann Surg 139:846–851

68. Wolmark N, Fisher B, Wieand HS (1986) The prognostic value of the modifications of the Dukes C class of colorectal cancer. An analysis of the NSABP clinical trials. Ann Surg 203:5–22

69. Jass JR, Love SB (1989) Prognostic value of direct spread in Dukes' C cases of rectal cancer. Dis Colon Rectum 32:477–480

70. Nathanson SD, Schultz L, Tilley B, Kambouris A (1986) Carcinomas of the colon and rectum. A comparison of staging classifications. Am J Surg 52:428–433

71. Newland RC, Chapuis PH, Smyth EJ (1987) The prognostic value of substaging colorectal carcinoma. A prospective study of 1117 cases with standardised pathology. Cancer 60:852–857

72. Chapuis PH, Fisher R, Dent OF et al (1985) The relationship between different staging methods and survival in colorectal carcinoma. Dis Colon Rectum 28:158–161

73. Fisher ER, Robinsky B, Sass R, Fisher B (1989) Relative prognostic value of the Dukes and the Jass systems in rectal cancer. Dis Colon Rectum 32:944–949

74. Secco GB, Fardelli R, Campora E et al (1990) Prognostic value of the Jass histopathologic system in left colon and rectal cancer: a multivariate analysis. Digestion 47:71–80

75. Kubota Y, Petras RE, Easley KA (1992) Ki-67 determined growth fraction versus standard staging and grading parameters in colorectal carcinoma. Cancer 70:2602–2609

76. Di Giorgio A, Botti C, Tocchi A et al (1992) The influence of tumour lymphocytic infiltration on long term survival of surgically treated colorectal cancer patients. Int Surg 77:256–260

77. Kyriakos M (1985) The President's cancer, the Dukes classification and confusion. Arch Pathol Lab Med 109:1063–1065

78. Kyriakos M (1986) The President's cancer, the Dukes classification and confusion, reply. Arch Pathol Lab Med 110:365–366

79. Hamada Y, Oishi A, Shoji T (1992) Endocrine cells and prognosis in patients with colorectal carcinoma. Cancer 69:2641–2646

80. de Bruine AP, Wiggers T, Beek C et al (1993) Endocrine cells in colorectal adenocarcinomas: incidence, hormone profile and prognostic relevance. Int J Cancer 54:765–71

81. Spread C, Berkel H, Jewell J (1994) Colon carcinoid tumours: a population-based study. Dis Colon Rectum 37:482–491

82. Burke M, Shepherd NA, Mann CV (1987) Rectal and anal carcinoid tumours. Br J Surg 74:358–361

83. Gledhill A, Hall PA, Cruse JP, Pollock DJ (1986) Enteroendocrine cell hyperplasia, carcinoid tumours and adenocarcinoma in longstanding ulcerative colitis. Histopathology 10:501–508

84. Loftus JP, van Heerden JE (1995) Surgical management of gastrointestinal carcinoid tumours. Adv Surg 28:317–326

85. Newman PL, Wadden C, Fletcher CD (1991) Gastrointestinal stromal tumours: correlation of immunophenotype with clinicopathological features. J Pathol 164:107–117

86. Yu CC, Fletcher CD, Newman PL (1992) A comparison of proliferating cell nuclear antigen (PCNA) immunostaining, nucleolar organizer region (AgNOR) staining and histological grading in gastrointestinal stromal tumours. J Pathol 166:147–152

87. Siddiqui MN, Garnham JR (1993) Submucosal lipoma of the colon with intussusception. Postgrad Med J 69:497

88. Carney JA, Go VLW, Sizemore GW, Hayles AB (1976) Alimentary tract ganglioneuromatosis. N Engl J Med 295:1287

89. Friedman SL, Wright TL, Altman DF (1985) Gastrointestinal Kaposi's sarcoma in patients with AIDS. Gastroenterology 89:102–108

90. Richards MA (1986) Lymphoma of the colon and rectum. Postgrad Med J 62:615–620

91. Zighelboim J, Larson MV (1994) Primary colonic lymphoma: clinical presentation, histopathologic features and outcome with combination chemotherapy. J Clin Gastroenterol 18:291–297

92. Shepherd NA, Hall PA, Williams GT et al (1989) Primary

malignant lymphoma of the large intestine complicating chronic inflammatory bowel disease. Histopathology 15: 325–337

93. Shepherd NA, Hall PA, Coates PJ, Levison DA (1988) Primary malignant lymphoma of the colon and rectum. A histopathological and immunohistochemical study of 45 cases with clinicopathological correlations. Histopathology 12:235–252

94. Reynolds P, Saunders LP, Layefsky ME, Lemp GF (1993) The spectrum of AIDS-associated malignancies in San Francisco 1980–7. Am J Epidemiol 137:19–30

95. Isaacson PG, Maclennan KA, Subbuswamy SG (1984) Multiple lymphomatous polyposis of the gastrointestinal tract. Histopathology 8:641–656

96. Davis NC, Newland RC (1983) Terminology and classification of colorectal adenocarcinoma: the Australian clinico-pathological staging system. Aust NZ J Surg 53:211–222

20

CANCER PREVENTION

SCREENING

Paul J. Finan

Colorectal cancer remains an important cause of morbidity and mortality throughout the developed world. National statistics continue to show not only the high incidence of this disease, with over 25,000 and 155,000 new cases annually in the United Kingdom and the United States, respectively,[1,2] but also a continuing high mortality. Five-year survival figures vary from 20%[3] to 36%.[4] Technical advances and improvements in perioperative care may be expected to reduce the 30-day mortality rate to some extent but it remains clear that the reason for this high mortality is the advanced stage of the disease at presentation. Over 20% of cases have documented overt or occult metastases[5,6] and the recent interest in adjuvant chemotherapy attests to the commonly held belief that microscopic spread of the disease at the time of surgery is common and hence the adoption of multimodality therapy for this disease.

It is not surprising, therefore, that over the past 25 years there have been renewed efforts to diagnose colorectal cancer at an earlier stage in the hope of improving overall survival. The magnitude of this problem itself would warrant these efforts but a combination of a better understanding of the disease, successful interventions, often nonsurgical, and improved surgical and medical therapies has led to colorectal cancer joining other common cancers as a disease that is suitable for screening.[7]

Screening may be defined as "the presumptive identification of unrecognized disease or defect by the application of tests, examinations, or other procedures that can be applied rapidly." Screening tests distinguish apparently well people who probably have the disease from those who probably do not.[3] There are many factors that contribute to an effective screening program and these are outlined in the accompanying box.[9]

It can be seen that colorectal cancer as a disease fulfills many of these requirements but several will only be known following the completion of well-conducted controlled trials, many of which are outlined later in this chapter.

From the statistics previously mentioned, it is clear that colorectal cancer is an important cause of morbidity and mortality. Within the general population, however, there is a variation of risk that will, of necessity, alter individual lifetime risk and hence the appropriateness of screening. Increased risk may be due to both inherited and noninherited factors, many of which are included in the accompanying box. Bond[10] has drawn a distinction between screening and surveillance and such a distinction is important to state at this stage. Screening is the application of a simple and inexpensive test to people in the general population at average risk for developing colorectal cancer, whereas surveillance identifies subjects who are at an increased risk by virtue of factors mentioned in the box and because of this increased risk they are offered direct evaluation of the whole colon on a regular basis. Surveillance of high-risk groups is discussed at the end of this chapter but most of the discussion is confined to screening of the average risk population.

Perhaps the most relevant statistic in colorectal cancer as applied to screening is that this is a disease of the elderly. In a recent study of colorectal cancer over a 2-year period in the Yorkshire region, Hall et al.[11] noted only 2% were under the age of 45 years and figures from the Office of Population Censuses and Surveys (OPCS)[4] 1987 show only 9% to be under the age of 55. This preponderance of disease within the older age groups to some extent governs the timing of screening. Efforts to detect the disease in the population below 55 years when there are no other risk factors such as family history, are clearly not going to be successful.

There has been a general acceptance over the past 10 to 20 years of the natural progression from normal epithelium to precancerous polyps and ultimately on to malignant tumors.[12,13] This hypothesis has been mirrored by a similar progression of changes at a molecular level.[14] Pathologic studies have noted the almost inevitable occurrence of colorectal cancer in untreated cases of familial adenomatous polyposis, evidence of residual adenomatous tissue within malignant tumors, and perhaps most important, the report on progression of untreated benign polyps to malignant tumors.[15] Although controlled trials of adenoma removal are not considered ethical, there remains good evidence that colonoscopic polypectomy will protect

Guidelines for an Effective Screening Program

1. The disease under investigation should be an important cause of morbidity and mortality.
2. The natural history of the disease should be understood.
3. Treatment of early stage disease should produce an improvement in survival.
4. The screening tests should have an acceptable sensitivity and specificity.
5. The proposed tests should be acceptable to the general population.
6. Facilities to make the diagnosis (where the screening test is not itself diagnostic) and treat the early stage/premalignant stage of the disease should be available.
7. There should be strong evidence that the screening tests can result in reduced morbidity and mortality in the targeted population.
8. The benefits of screening must outweigh any disadvantages.
9. The individual benefits should be achieved at a reasonable cost.
10. If implemented, the program must be audited to ensure that the expected benefit is observed in practice.

(From Wilson and Jungner,[9] with permission.)

Risk Factors for Colorectal Neoplasia

No Inherited Predisposition

Age
Colorectal adenomas
Colorectal carcinoma
Inflammatory bowel disease
Previous cholecystectomy
Previous surgery for peptic ulcer disease
Previous ureterocolonic diversion

Inherited Predisposition

Adenomatous polyposis coli (APC)
HNPCC or Lynch syndromes (I & II)
Turcot's syndrome
Muir-Torre syndrome
Juvenile polyposis
Peutz-Jeghers syndrome
Gorlin syndrome
Cowden's disease

against the subsequent development of colorectal cancer both in the experience of individuals[16] and in multicenter studies, for example, the National Polyp Study.[17] Interestingly, these studies offer two general approaches to screening strategies for colorectal cancer including the identification of early, treatable colorectal cancer and, secondly, the identification of premalignant lesions that if removed, interrupt the progression of these polyps to malignant tumors.

The results of treatment of colorectal cancer are, to a large extent, governed by the stage of disease at presentation.[18] These are excellent when the tumor remains within the bowel wall. There are, however, statistical biases in any assessment of long-term survival and any apparent success in treating early detected disease should be subjected to controlled clinical trial. *Lead time bias* is the time between recognition of the disease by screening and when the disease would have been detected clinically. Clearly for slowly progressive diseases this may be considerable. Thus it is entirely possible that the only result of a screening program is to detect the disease earlier without altering overall mortality. *Length time bias* reflects the fact that slowly growing tumors are more likely to be detected within a screening program. Both these biases demonstrate the need for properly controlled trials to show the effect on mortality by the disease.

Finally, tests for screening have to be inexpensive, acceptable with a high compliance, and able to be repeated. They must have both a high sensitivity and specificity. Sensitivity is defined as the proportion of affected persons that are correctly identified by the test in question and specificity as the proportion of nonaffected individuals who are not identified by the test. While they both should be high, they are often inversely correlated. A fall in sensitivity will miss disease within the population, giving false reassurance. A fall in specificity will lead to unnecessary investigation of people with financial and psychological cost.

SCREENING TECHNIQUES

Three screening techniques have been used with varying degrees of success. These include symptom questionnaires, endoscopic studies, and testing of feces for the presence of occult blood.

Symptom Questionnaires

Direct questioning for symptoms of bowel cancer (e.g., bleeding, diarrhea, altered bowel habit, and abdominal pain), were investigated within the Nottingham Screening Project. One thousand five hundred thirty-three individuals were offered both symptom questionnaire and fecal occult blood testing and 34.3% returned both. The questionnaire was considered positive in 24.4% of cases but subsequent investigation for malignant disease revealed no cancers and only one adenomatous polyp. There were 12 positive occult blood tests within the group, of whom 4 had symptoms and 8 did not. Investigation of these patients revealed 4 with polyps and 2 with cancer. Interestingly, those individuals with cancers and 3 with adenomas had no symptoms. It was concluded that not only were bowel symptoms common within the community but they were a poor predictor of neoplastic disease.[19]

A similar study was completed to determine the prevalence

of large bowel symptoms in the adult population over the age of 40. Bleeding within the previous 6 months was reported by 12.4% of persons questioned and although no cancers were detected several adenomas were. The authors concluded that a self-completed questionnaire enhanced fecal occult blood testing.[20] In these two studies compliance (37% to 50%) was poor. It seems therefore that the questionnaire approach to symptoms is of little value as a screening tool for colorectal cancer.

Endoscopic Techniques

The left-sided predominance of colorectal tumors with 40% lying within reach of the rigid sigmoidoscope has led to the recommendation that examination by rigid and flexible sigmoidoscopy is of value in screening. To date, however, there are no randomized control studies to support this approach. Hertz et al.[21] reported a study of the use of rigid sigmoidoscopy at the Strang Cancer Prevention Clinic in New York. Eighty-one percent of tumors detected were of Dukes' B stage or less and the overall survival was 88% at 15 years.

A similar study reported the value of rigid sigmoidoscopy in over 21,000 subjects who had an initial rigid sigmoidoscopy with follow-up amounting to nearly 100,000 patient years.[22,23] At the first evaluation 27 malignancies were identified. Subsequently only 13 were detected of which 12 were of Dukes' stage A, representing an 85% reduction in the expected incidence of rectal cancers in this population over the same time period.

Two case-control studies are frequently quoted as offering further evidence of the value of periodic endoscopic examination of the rectum. One suggested a 77% reduction in the risk of developing rectal and distal sigmoid carcinomas following sigmoidoscopy. However, the authors also observed a reduction in the expected incidence of more proximal lesions, which is difficult to explain given the limited endoscopic examination.[24] A further careful case control study from the Kaiser Permanente Medical Care program recorded similar findings.[25] Two hundred sixty patients dying of rectal carcinoma were compared with 868 controls. It was noted that screening sigmoidoscopy had been performed in 8.8% of the patients dying of rectal carcinoma as compared with 24.2% in the control group. They calculated that following rigid sigmoidoscopy there was a 59% reduction in the risk of death from distal colorectal malignant disease. This "protective" effect was found even if the rigid examination had been performed several years previously. Finally, a study from St. Mark's Hospital has examined the incidence of rectal cancer in over 1,500 patients undergoing rigid sigmoidoscopy over a 30-year period and having been found to have polyps. No further follow-up had been conducted and they found that rectal tumors were uncommon following complete removal of rectal adenoma and those that did arise were following incomplete removal. The size of rectal polyp reflected the apparent risk to the remaining colonic epithelium beyond the reach of the rigid sigmoidoscope.[26] The 60-cm flexible sigmoidoscope could be an acceptable instrument for screening for distal colorectal malignancy. No controlled trials have been performed; however, the pooled results of 14 studies involving 11,000 distal colorectal examinations showed that of 30 cancers detected 24 were still localized at diagnosis.[27] Proposals for controlled trials of flexible sigmoidoscopy to screen for colorectal cancer in the average-risk general population are being

considered both in the UK[28] and the United States under the auspices of the National Cancer Institute. Issues that will determine the success of such an approach include compliance for a procedure that is invasive, the appropriate frequency of testing, and the cost, including that of full colonoscopy in a proportion of cases depending on the flexible sigmoidoscopic findings. Currently, full colonoscopy should probably be reserved for screening in high-risk individuals, for example, those with a strong family history and those who have previously had large adenomas removed. No controlled trials of its use in screening of average-risk individuals exist. Perhaps some idea of the problems of using what would be a highly specific and sensitive test are noted in a recent study from Indiana, where 5,000 physicians, dentists, and spouses were invited to undergo screening colonoscopy. Only 305 responded (6%) and although polyps were found in 25% of cases, only 13 of 104 adenomas were over 1 cm in size. Two Dukes' stage A cancers were found.[29]

Fecal Occult Blood Testing

Fecal occult blood testing has probably received more attention than any other method of colorectal cancer screening with several well-controlled prospective randomized trials within the general population.

The basis for the test is that the normal physiologic blood loss (up to 2 ml/day) is increased in the presence of colorectal neoplasms. This increase may be detected using a variety of methods although most of the large trials have been based on the Guaiac-impregnated paper method (e.g., Hemoccult). The Guaiac turns blue when oxidized and will do so when exposed to the pseudoperoxidase activity of hemoglobin. It is not specific for human hemoglobin and large amounts of ingested red meat may lead to false-positive results as may foods that contain naturally occurring peroxidase (e.g., broccoli, cauliflower). Similarly, false-negative results may be caused by the ingestion of vitamin C.[30] The optimal dietary conditions have been explored by Macrae.[31] In an early study of the use of Guaiac-impregnated test paper, 11 of 12 (silent) colon cancers were found to be positive in at least one of three fecal occult blood tests.[32] Many studies have concentrated on the test conditions required to maximize the sensitivity and specificity. Within a fecal occult blood testing program, testing for 3 days or 6 days was compared.[33] Compliance fell in those who where offered 6-day testing (from 57.8% to 53.9%) and although the positivity rate increased significantly (1.69% versus 1.29%) there was no significant increase in the yield of neoplasms and there was an inevitable increase in the number of colonoscopies.

There is often a delay between applying feces to the Hemoccult and testing in the laboratory, if, for example, the test kit is posted. This may result in dessication and rehydration of the slides with a drop of water has been recommended. An Italian study noted a significant increase in the positivity of the test from 3.1% to 5% with no obvious fall in specificity or positive predictive value.[34] Others have also found an increased sensitivity by rehydration but accompanied by a fall in specificity and, therefore, an increase in the overall cost of the screening program.[35] Although Hemoccult has been the most intensively tested method worldwide, other Guaiac-based tests have been compared with sensitivities ranging from 65% to 90%. In general, as the sensitivity increases, the specificity falls.[36] Other approaches that have not been fully evaluated in screening programs include immunologic tests that are highly specific for human hemoglobin and assays that are designed to detect porphyrins (a breakdown product of heme).[37-39]

Testing of feces for cellular abnormalities such as fecal mutant DNA or protein products[40,41] may develop in the future but, at present, occult blood tests remain the basis of the many uncontrolled and, more recently, well-constructed controlled trials of population screening.

Some evidence of the effectiveness of fecal occult blood screening in reducing mortality has come from a case control study from the Kaiser Permanente Medical Care Programme.[42] A group of 486 persons developing fatal colorectal cancer over 50 years of age was compared with 727 age- and sex-matched controls. There was the suggestion of a 20% to 30% reduction in mortality in patients exposed to fecal occult blood testing. The odds ratio was lowest during the first year after the most recent occult blood test and the authors suggested annual or biennial screening might lower population risk from colorectal cancer.

The results of several randomized trials of population screening are available. Not all are the same in design, some being self-selecting, others population-based, and some use different methodologies (e.g., rehydration) and others combine occult blood testing with other screening strategies (e.g., rigid sigmoidoscopy). Despite this variability, some comparisons of sensitivity and specificity can be made, as can estimates of neoplastic yield, and each trial deserves further comment.

Memorial-Sloan Kettering Study

The Memorial-Sloan Kettering study[42a] examined fecal occult blood testing within the context of a preventative medical program. Those attending a clinic were already being offered a comprehensive medical examination and sigmoidoscopy. Over 20,000 subjects were enrolled. They were randomized to have clinical examination and sigmoidoscopy versus the same plus fecal occult blood testing. The stated end points included compliance for fecal occult blood testing, the number of cancers detected and mortality rate, and the compliance for further investigation when the occult blood test was positive. The subjects were entered into two studies: those that were already undergoing health screening (AS) and those presenting for initial study (IS). Compliance initially was good, being between 70% (AS) and 80% (IS). However, this fell on subsequent rescreens to 56% (AS) and 20% (IS). Positive rates for Hemoccult were 1.4% (AS) and 2.6% (IS). The predictive value for neoplasia and cancer in the initial study trial was 36% (AS) and 17% (IS) and there was a difference in the incidence of Dukes' A and B cases, being 69% in the study group compared with 35% in the control group. Owing to the poor compliance on rescreening, no such stage shift was noted at repeated examinations. Although there was a highly significant difference in long-term survival between the study and control groups of the (IS) trial (70% versus 48%), the difference in reduction of colorectal cancer mortality just failed to reach statistical significance.

The authors concluded that methods to improve compliance should be investigated, that positivity for fecal occult blood testing was strongly age-dependent, being rare below the age of 50 years, that subsequent investigation should be by colonoscopy, and that there was a marked stage shift of detected tumors at initial screen. Although lead time and length time bias could

not be excluded, the observed reduction in mortality was probably a consequence of adding fecal occult blood testing to sigmoidoscopy.

Minnesota Study

The Minnesota Study,[35,43] like the Memorial-Sloan Kettering Study, was not a true population study but a comparison of annual and biennial Hemoccult screening compared with a control group within a volunteer-based screening program. The study commenced in 1975 and enrolled over 45,000 subjects. Initial compliance was approximately 80%. Rehydration of slides was introduced during this study, resulting in the increase in positivity from 2.4% to 9.8%, an increase in sensitivity from 80.8% to 92.2% and a decrease in specificity from 97.7% to 90.4%. Although there was a high proportion of Dukes' A and B cases (approximately 65%) this was no different from the proportion of similar tumors in the control group.

This study has reported on mortality from colorectal cancer. With 13 years of follow-up there was a significant (33%) reduction in mortality in the annually screened versus control group. A much smaller reduction was noted in the biennially screened group. There have, however, been criticisms of some aspects of this study. In particular, the high colonoscopy rate among the screened group, largely owing to the high positivity rate associated with rehydration, resulted in 38% of the annually screened subjects having a colonoscopy. This should be taken into consideration when noting mortality rates from other studies.

Goteborg Study

The Goteborg Study[44,45] offered Hemoccult testing to subjects between 60 and 64 years of age. There were 27,700 subjects of whom half were offered 3-day fecal occult blood testing and then rescreens 2 years later. Compliance was 66% at initial screen and 58% at rescreening. Like the Minnesota study, the test group had rehydration of the slides with an increase in positivity from 1.9% to 5.8%. All slides in the rescreening study were rehydrated. Sixty-one carcinomas were found in the test group and only 20 in the control group. Of the 61, 16 were detected at first screen, 19 at second screen, and there were 16 interval cancers. There was only a slight shift to more favorable tumors in the screened group (Dukes' A and B, 46% versus 40%), and at follow-up this difference was lost and, indeed, there were slightly more Dukes' A and B tumors in the control group.[45] This fact, together with the false-negative rate for the carcinomas of 44% at first screen, would indicate that a reduction in mortality is unlikely to be seen from this study.

Burgundy Study

The Burgundy Study[46,47] is a large study of 94,000 subjects between the ages of 45 and 74 years. This was not a true randomized controlled trial but screening was done by geographic areas. Initial compliance for the 47,150 who were offered the test was 52% although the rate varied from 80% to 30% depending on how the test was presented to the subjects. The overall positive rate was 2.1% and of the 23 tumors detected in the screened group, 18 were Dukes' stage A or B. No mortality data from this study are available.

Danish Study

The Danish Study[48,49] is a true population-based controlled trial of screening using Hemoccult. Sixty thousand subjects between 45 and 74 years of age were recruited and initial compliance was 67%. Like other studies, the positive rate was only 1.1% but this was using unrehydrated slides. There were 37 cancers detected in the screened group of which 51% were Dukes' stage A. Only 2% of the control group have similar early lesions. A reduction in mortality from colorectal cancer of 18% did not achieve statistical significance and longer term follow-up from this study is awaited.[49a]

Nottingham Study

The Nottingham Study[50,50a] is the largest of the occult blood studies and is a true population-based study. Over 150,000 subjects were included, of whom half were offered fecal occult blood screening. The initial compliance was 53.4% and the positivity rate was 2.1%. Eleven percent of the positive results led to a diagnosis of cancer of which 46% were Dukes' stage A. Rescreening at 2-year intervals has revealed a further 132 cancers, 37% of which were Dukes' stage A. Of the 893 cancers detected within the study group, roughly one-quarter were screen detected, one-quarter were interval cancers presenting between screens, and one-half were in noncompliers. Overall, within the control group, 856 cancers have been noted. At a median follow-up of 7.8 years, 360 persons have died from colorectal cancer in the study group compared with 420 in the control group, representing a 15% reduction in mortality from colorectal cancer (Hardcastle JD, personal communication). Interestingly, this figure is of a similar order to that obtained from the Danish study.

There are many excellent reviews of screening for colorectal cancer using occult blood testing.[51-55] Until recently there has been only indirect evidence of likely benefit. However, as trials report the reduction in mortality from colorectal cancer in screened groups it will become increasingly important to consider the introduction of occult blood testing on a national basis.[49a,50a,55a]

Surveillance of High-Risk Individuals

There are several groups in which there is an increased lifetime risk of the development of colorectal cancer (see Box). As previously stated, efforts to detect neoplastic change in these groups should more strictly be termed ''surveillance'' rather than ''screening.'' Owing to the increased risk it is unethical

to perform controlled trials and cancer prevention protocols, have concentrated on trying to obtain guidelines as to the frequency of examination which is usually by colonoscopy.

Family History of Colorectal Cancer

Several studies have shown an increase in the lifetime risk of developing colorectal cancer when an affected first-degree relative has also had the disease.[56-59] Furthermore, it is becoming increasingly evident that there is an increased risk, depending on the strength of family history.[60] Surveillance of family members has been carried out using flexible sigmoidoscopy[61] and colonoscopy[62,63] and although no firm conclusions have been reached, it may be that endoscopy can be tailored to the perceived risk to result in effective surveillance.[64]

A controlled prospective study of colonoscopic screening for neoplasms included 181 asymptomatic first-degree relatives of colorectal cancer patients and 83 asymptomatic controls.[65] Adenomatous polyps were detected in 14.4% of the former and 8.4% of the latter. If there was more than one first-degree relative the number of adenomas increased to 23.8%. No cancers were found in this study and many of the adenomas were small and probably of little significance.[65]

Colonoscopic surveillance is, however, mandatory in those few well-characterized nonpolyposis families where there is dominant inheritance, for example, hereditary nonpolyposis colorectal cancer. These families are considerably rarer than was first thought and probably represent only 0.5% to 2% of all cases of colorectal cancer. When they are identified colonoscopic surveillance is recommended and guidelines have recently been suggested.[66] A critical review of the literature on screening for relatives of patients with colorectal cancer has recently been published.[67]

Inflammatory bowel disease confers an increased risk of colorectal neoplasia, particularly when total and long-standing.[68] Again, although surveillance by colonoscopy is widely used there is little information from well-conducted control series regarding the frequency of such examinations. In one recent study, very few cases of malignancy were detected directly as a result of colonoscopy.[69]

In conclusion, the high prevalence of colorectal cancer within the general population demands that efforts are made to reduce the incidence by secondary prevention through removal of premalignant lesions. There may soon be substantial evidence from the trials available to recommend screening of the general population by fecal occult blood testing. Surveillance of high-risk groups is clearly needed and research here should concentrate on studies that offer guidelines as to the best modality of screening and its frequency.

REFERENCES

1. Office of Population Censuses and Surveys (1993) Cancer Statistics: Registrations. England Wales 1988. Series MB1 19 HMSO
2. American Cancer Society (1990) Cancer Facts & Figures. American Cancer Society, New York
3. Slaney G (1971) Results of treatment of carcinoma of the colon and rectum. Mod Trends Surg 3:69
4. Office of Population Censuses and Surveys (1988) OPCS Monitor, MB1 88/1, HMSO, London
5. Gill PG, Morris PJ (1978) The survival of patients with colorectal cancer treated in the regional hospital. Br J Surg 65:17–20
6. Finlay IG, McArdle CS (1986) Occult hepatic metastases in colorectal carcinoma. Br J Surg 73:732–735
7. Winawer SJ (1995) Surveillance overview. pp. 26–271. In Cohen AM, Winawer SJ, Friedman MA, Gunderson LL, (eds): Cancer of the Colon Rectum and Anus. McGraw Hill, New York

8. United States Commission on Chronic Ulcers (1997) Chronic Ulcers in the United States. p. 267 Vol. 1. Harvard University Press, Cambridge

9. Wilson JMG, Jungner G (1968) Principles and Practice of Screening for Disease. WHO, Geneva (Public Health Papers No. 34)

10. Bond JH (1995) Screening and early detection. pp. 149–157. In Wanebo HJ (ed): Colorectal Cancer, Mosby, St. Louis

11. Hall NR, Finan PJ, Ward B et al (1994) Genetic susceptibility to colorectal cancer in patients under 45 years of age. Br J Surg 81:1485–1489

12. Morson BC (1974) Evolution of cancer of the colon and rectum. Cancer 34:845–849

13. Muto T, Bussey HJR, Morson B (1975) The evolution of cancer of the colon and rectum. Cancer 36:2251–2270

14. Vogelstein B, Fearon ER, Hamilton SR et al (1988) Genetic alterations during colorectal tumour development. N Engl J Med 319:525–532

15. Stryker SJ, Wolff BG, Culp CE et al (1987) Natural history of untreated colonic polyps. Gastroenterology 93:1009–1013

16. Meager AP, Stuart M (1994) Does colonoscopic polypectomy reduce the incidence of colorectal carcinoma? Aust NZ J Surg 64:400–404

17. Winawer SJ, Zauber AG, Ho MN et al (1993) Prevention of colorectal cancer by colonoscopic polypectomy. N Engl J Med 329:1977–1981

18. Dukes CE (1932) The classification of cancer of the rectum. J Pathol Bacteriol 35:323–332

19. Farrands PA, Hardcastle JD (1984) Colorectal screening by a self-completion questionnaire. Gut 25:445–447

20. Silman AJ, Mitchell P, Nicholls RJ et al (1983) Self-reported dark red bleeding as a marker comparable with occult blood testing and screening for large bowel nooplasms. Br J Surg 70:721–724

21. Hertz RE, Deddish MR, Day E (1960) Value of period examination in detecting cancer of the rectum and colon. Postgrad Med 27:290

22. Gilbertson VA (1974) Proctosigmoidoscopy and polypectomy in reducing the incidence of rectal cancer. Cancer 34:936–939

23. Gilbertson VA, Nelms JM (1978) The prevention of invasive cancer of the rectum. Cancer 41:1137

24. Newcomb PA, Norfleet RG, Surawicz TS et al (1992) Screening sigmoidoscopy and colorectal cancer mortality. J Natl Cancer Inst 84:1572–1575

25. Selby JV, Friedman GD, Quesenbury CP, Weiss NS (1992) A case control study of screening sigmoidoscopy and mortality from colorectal cancer. N Engl J Med 326:653–657

26. Atkin WS, Morson BC, Cuzick J (1992) Long-term risk of colorectal cancer after excision of rectosigmoid adenomas. N Engl J Med 326:658–662

27. Selby JA (1995) Clinical trials of screening sigmoidoscopy. pp. 291–301. In Cohen AM, Winawer SJ, Freedman MA, Gunderson LL (eds): Cancer of the Colon Rectum and Anus. McGraw-Hill, New York

28. Atkin WS, Cuzick J, Northover JM, Whynes DK (1993) Prevention of colorectal cancer by once only sigmoidoscopy. Lancet 341:736–740

29. Rex DX, Lehman GA, Hawes RH (1991) Screening colonoscopy in asymptomatic average risk persons with negative faecal occult blood tests. Gastroenterology 100:64–67

30. Joffe RM, Kasten B, Yeung DS et al (1975) False-negative stool occult blood tests caused by ingestion of ascorbic acid (Vit C). Ann Intern Med 83:824–826

31. Macrae FA, St John BJB, Caligiore P et al (1992) Optimal dietary conditions for haemoccult blood testing. Gastroenterology 82:899–903

32. Greegor DH (1971) Occult blood testing for the detection of asymptomatic colon cancer. Cancer 28:131–134

33. Thomas WM, Pye G, Hardcastle JD, Mangham CM (1990) Faecal occult blood screening for colorectal neoplasia: a randomised trial of three days or six days of tests. Br J Surg 77:277–279

34. Castiglione G, Biagini M, Barchielli A et al (1993) Effects of rehydration on Guaiac-based faecal occult blood testing in colorectal cancer screening. Br J Cancer 67:1142–1144

35. Mandel JS, Bond JH, Bradley M et al (1989) Sensitivity, specificity and positive predictivity of the haemoccult test in screening for colorectal cancers. University of Minnesota's Colon Cancer Control Study. Gastroenterology 972:597–600

36. Aldercreutz H, Partenen P, Virkola P et al (1984) Five Guaiac-based tests for occult blood in faeces compared in vitro and in vivo. Scand J Clin Lab Invest 44:519–528

37. St John DJB, Yeung GP, McHutchinson JG (1992) Comparison of the specificity and sensitivy of haemoccult and haemoquant in screening for colorectal neoplasia. Ann Int Med 117:376–382

38. Pye G, Jackson J, Thomas WM, Hardcastle JD (1990) Comparison of colo-screen self-test and haemoccult faecal occult blood tests in the detection of colorectal cancer in symptomatic patients. Br J Surg 70:630–631

39. Thomas WM, Hardcastle JD, Pye G (1992) Chemical and immunological testing for faecal occult blood: a comparison of two tests in symptomatic patients. Br J Cancer 65:618–620

40. Sidransky D, Tokino T, Hamilton SR et al (1992) Identification of ras oncogene mutations in the stool of patients with curable colorectal cancer. Science 256:102–105

41. Smith-Ravin J, England J, Talbot IC, Bodmer W (1995) Detection of C-Ki-ras mutations in faecal specimens from sporadic colorectal cancer patients. Gut 36:81–86

42. Selby JV, Friedman GD, Quesenbury CP, Weiss NS (1993) Effects of faecal occult blood testing on mortality from colorectal cancer. A case control study. Ann Intern Med 118:1–6

42a. Winawer SJ, Flehinger BJ, Schottenfeld D, Miller DG (1993) Screening for colorectal cancer with faecal occult blood testing and sigmoidoscopy. J Natl Cancer Inst 85:1311–1318

43. Mandel JS, Bond JH, Church TR (1993) Reducing mortality from colorectal cancer by screening for faecal occult blood. N Engl J Med 328:1365–1371

44. Kewenter J, Bjork S, Haglind E et al (1988) Screening and rescreening for colorectal cancer: a control trial of faecal occult blood testing in 27,700 subjects. Cancer 62:645–651

45. Kewenter J, Brevinge H, Engaras B et al (1994) Follow-up after screening for colorectal neoplasms with faecal occult blood testing in a control trial. Dis Colon Rectum 37:115–119

46. Faivre J (1989) Preliminary results of a mass screening programme for colorectal cancer in France. pp. 94–101 In Hardcastle JD (ed): Screening for Colorectal Cancer. Normed Verlag, Englewood NJ

47. Faivre J, Arveux P, Milan C et al (1991) Participation in mass screening for colorectal cancer: results of screening and rescreening from the Burgundy Study. Eur J Cancer Prev 1:49

48. Kronborg O, Fenger C, Sondergaard O et al (1987) Initial mass screening for colorectal cancer with faecal occult blood test. Scand J Gastroenterol 22:677–686

49. Kronborg O, Fenger C, Worm J et al (1992) Causes of death during the first five years of a randomised trial of mass screening for colorectal cancer with faecal occult blood test. Scand J Gastroenterol 27:47–52

49a.Kronborg O, Fenger C, Olsen J et al (1996) Randomised study of screening for colorectal cancer with fecal-occult-blood test. Lancet 348:1467–1471

50. Hardcastle JD, Thomas WM, Chamberlain J (1989) Randomised control trial of faecal occult blood screening for colorectal cancer: the results of the first 107, 349 subjects. Lancet 1:1160–1164

50a.Hardcastle JD, Chamberlain JO, Robinson MHE et al (1996) Randomized controlled trial of fecal-occult-blood screening for colorectal cancer. Lancet 348:1472–1477

51. Simon JB (1985) Occult blood screening for colorectal carcinoma: a critical review. Gastroenterology 88:820–837

52. Simon JB (1987) The pros and cons of faecal occult blood testing for colorectal neoplasms. Cancer Metastasis Rev 6:397–411

53. Hardcastle JD, Pye G (1989) Screening for colorectal cancer: a critical review. World J Surg 13:38–44

54. Alquist DA (1992) Occult blood screening: Obstacles to effectiveness. Cancer 70:1259–1265

55. Winawer SJ, Bond JH (1995) Faecal occult blood tests: screening trials. pp. 279–290. In Cohen AM, Winawer SJ, Friedman MA, Gunderson LL (eds): Cancer of the Colon Rectum and Anus. McGraw Hill, New York

55a.Liebeman D, Sleisenger MH (1996) Is it time to recommend screening for colorectal cancer? Lancet 348:1463–1464

56. Maire P, Morichau-Beauchant M, Drucker J et al (1984) Familiar prevalence of colorectal cancer: a 3-year case-control study. Gastroenterol Clin Biol 8:22–27

57. Ponz de Leon M. Antonioli A, Ascari A et al (1987) Incidence and familial occurrence of colorectal cancer and polyps in a health-care district of Northern Italy. Cancer 60:2848–2859

58. Bonelli I, Martines H, Conio M (1988) Family history of colorectal cancer as a risk factor for benign and malignant tumours of the large bowel. A case-control study. Int J Cancer 41:513–517

59. Stephenson BM, Finan PJ, Gascoyne J et al (1991) Frequency of familial colorectal cancer. Br J Surg 78:1162–1166

60. Lovett E (1976) Family studies in cancer of the colon and rectum. Br J Surg 63:13–18

61. Rozen P, Fireman Z, Terdiman R et al (1981) Selective screening for colorectal tumours in the Tel-Aviv area: relevance of epidemiology and family history. Cancer 47:827–831

62. Baker JW, Gathright JB, Timke AE et al (1990) Colonoscopic screening of asymptomatic patients with a family history of colon cancer. Dis Col Rectum 33:926–930

63. Luchtefeld MA, Syverson D, Solfelt M et al (1991) Is colonoscopic screening appropriate in asymptomatic patients with family history of colon cancer? Dis Colon Rectum 34:763–768

64. Stephenson BM, Murday VA, Finan PJ et al (1993) Feasibility of family-based screening for colorectal neoplasia: experience in one general surgical practice. Gut 34:96–100

65. Guillem JG, Forde KA, Treat MR et al (1992) Colonoscopic screening for neoplasms in asymptomatic first-degree relatives of colon cancer patients. A controlled prospective study. Dis Colon and Rectum 35:523–529

66. Winawer SJ, St John DJ, Bond JH et al (1995) Prevention of colorectal cancer: guidelines based on new data. Bull WHO 73(1):7–10

67. Brewer DA, Fung CL-S, Chapuis PH, Bokey EL (1994) Should relatives of patients with colorectal cancer be screened? A critical review of the literature. Dis Colon Rectum 37:1328–1337

68. Lennard-Jones JE, Melville DM, Morson BC et al (1990) Precancer and cancer in extensive ulcerative colitis: findings among 401 patients over 22 years. Gut 31:800

69. Axon ATR (1994) Cancer surveillance in ulcerative colitis—a time for reappraisal. Gut 35:587–589

FOLLOW-UP AFTER SURGERY FOR COLORECTAL NEOPLASIA

Ole Kronborg

ADENOMA

Patients with colorectal adenomas have a two- to sixfold increased risk of developing carcinoma according to case-control studies.[1-3] This risk remains increased when all visible adenomas have been removed although to a lesser degree.[2] It is possible to reduce mortality from colorectal cancer by repeated colonoscopy and polypectomy, but the optimal intervals between endoscopies are not known and the examinations themselves carry a small risk of complications that may be lethal. The incidence of colorectal cancer may also be reduced by removing adenomas,[4-6] but to what degree is not fully known and there may be a large proportion of adenoma patients who will not benefit from surveillance.

The Adenoma-Carcinoma Sequence

Adenomas are accepted as precursors of most cases of colorectal cancer but only a small proportion actually becomes invasive. The substantial classic evidence for the evolution from adenoma to carcinoma[7] is presented in the accompanying box. The final proof is lacking. In animal studies it has been demonstrated that an adenoma cell line may be transformed by exposure to a carcinogen and produce carcinoma when injected in athymic nude mice.[8] The Mayo Clinic study of untreated polyps[9] suggested a risk of invasive cancer of 24% within 20 years of radiologic detection of a polyp of at least 1 cm in diameter.

However, even a biopsy from a polyp left in situ, showing adenoma, does not exclude the presence of carcinoma in another part of the polyp, and what was thought to be cancer following removal of a previous adenoma may have been an invasive cancer from the beginning. The evidence for the adenoma-carcinoma sequence, nevertheless, is overwhelming.

This is less convincing for the de novo carcinoma theory, suggesting that colorectal cancer may develop without a preceding adenoma. Small flat adenomas may easily be overlooked, making it difficult to estimate relationships between size of adenoma and cancer risk within the adenoma. It is generally claimed that the risk is higher in large adenomas, but endoscopists may have been less aware of small adenomas.

Japanese workers have looked for the small flat adenomas with magnifying colonoscopes and found that they may be severely dysplastic,[10–12] and even contain carcinoma. It is likely, however, that the frequency of the latter has been overstated in Japan, where severe dysplasia within the mucosa is considered to be carcinoma in contrast to others who would regard this as severe dysplasia in a benign adenoma. A hereditary flat multiple adenoma syndrome has been described,[13] but patients with sporadic flat adenomas probably are more frequent.

Unfortunately, it is still not possible to predict which adenoma will become invasive and 20 to 30 adenomas have to be removed to prevent one carcinoma.[14,15] Genetic models for the adenoma-carcinoma sequence have been produced,[16,17] but so far it has not been possible to select persons at high risk of sporadic carcinoma using genetic probes. Mutations of the *ras*

oncogene are more frequent in large than in small adenomas. DNA content in adenomas, as measured by flow cytometry, is related to dysplasia, but the predictive value for colorectal cancer is unknown.[18]

The incidence of aneuploidy also seems to increase with severity of dysplasia in flat adenomas.[19] Expression of cancer-associated antigens in adenomas has not been fully evaluated,[20] but like different enzymes they support the adenoma-carcinoma sequence. Most small adenomas probably grow slowly or not at all.[21] A Norwegian study[22] suggested that at least 2 years were necessary for an adenoma to reach a diameter of 5 mm from an initial size of 2 mm. The National Polyp Study (NPS) in the United States[5] reported the average age in patients with adenomas to be 60 years and 67 years for those with colorectal cancer, suggesting a slow rate of progression of the adenoma-carcinoma sequence and stressing the need to identify persons with the highest risk to avoid too many unnecessary endoscopies.

Clinical Consequences

Prospective studies have been in progress for more than a decade to investigate the consequences of interrupting the adenoma-carcinoma sequence by removing all visible polyps from the colon and rectum.[23,24] Colonoscopy is preferred as the means of identification, but when incomplete it should be supplemented by double-contrast barium enema (DCBE). Colonoscopy should be complete in at least 95% of the examinations and has the highest diagnostic sensitivity for adenomas.[25] To obtain a clean colon, repeated examinations may be required before long-term surveillance is considered. Inadequate bowel preparation, piecemeal removal of adenomas, and possible missed multiple adenomas, all make it necessary to repeat the endoscopy.[26] Multiple adenomas at repeated colonoscopy, located over a large length of colon, indicate the necessity for subtotal colectomy, unless severe complicating diseases are present making frequent colonoscopy the best method of management.

Piecemeal removal of a single large sessile adenoma makes it necessary to re-examine no more than that area of the large bowel. This policy has been followed rigorously in one prospective program,[23] whereas the National Polyp Study[24] included a 1-year colonoscopy in one-half of the patients, the other half having their first surveillance at 3 years. The piecemeal technique makes it difficult for the pathologist to determine whether the adenoma has been removed completely and the presence of carcinoma may be undetected.[27,28] Another reason for repeating the colonoscopy is if the endoscopist has found the initial examination difficult. In this circumstance, it is preferable to repeat the examination.

The National Polyp Study is a multicenter trial and was initiated in 1980 to follow up patients who had adenomas of less than 3 cm in diameter removed.[24] After an initial complete colonoscopy with polypectomy, the patients were randomized to surveillance colonoscopy and barium enema at 1 and 3 years (699 patients) and at 3 years (719 patients). The proportions of patients with significant neoplasia including a new adenoma above more than 1 cm in diameter, severe dysplasia, or carcinoma were the same (3.3%) within the first 3 years. A multivariate analysis revealed the only independent significant risk factor to be the number of initial adenomas. The study suggested a reduced incidence of cancer compared with that of a normal population.[5]

The Funen Adenoma Study was initiated in 1978 and is an ongoing one-center study. It includes patients under 78 years of age with adenoma(s), regardless of size and method of removal, who had been subjected to complete colonoscopy with a resulting clean colon.[30] A total of 1,675 patients were included and 1,080 were randomized to different surveillance intervals. Patients with pedunculated and small sessile adenomas were re-examined at two (332 patients) or four yearly (341 patients) intervals, respectively. Another group of 542 patients with similar adenomas were followed with colorectal examinations every 3 years. Proportions of patients with new adenomas above 1 cm in diameter, severe dysplasia, villous morphology, or carcinoma were 5.2% and 8.6%, respectively, at 4 years and 8.6% and 17.4% at 8 years, but none of the differences was statistically significant (Fig. 20-1). The presence of more than two adenomas at the initial examination was the only factor associated with a higher risk of new significant neoplasia, confirming the experience of the NPS[29] and previous studies.[32,33] Three patients developed cancer within 2,404 person-years among the 673 patients, a similar proportion to that in a Danish normal population (RR = 0.9).

Patients with sessile adenomas greater than 5 mm in diameter have been randomized to varying surveillance intervals of 6, 12, and 24 months in the Funen Adenoma Study. The unpublished data of 230 patients suggest a higher risk of new significant neoplasia than in those with pedunculated and small sessile adenomas (Fig. 20-1). The intervals may, however, be prolonged to 2 years without a significant increase in risk of advanced pathology. Besides actual invasion, advanced pathology includes severe dysplasia, which is subject to interobserver variation.[14,34] Including all types of adenomas in the Funen Adenoma Study up to 1992, 10 patients developed invasion among 1,056 patients followed. This was similar to that expected in a sex- and age-matched normal population. In these patients the staged distribution was, however, more favorable and only one patient has died of cancer. This is significantly less than the number of expected deaths (6.7 deaths).[6]

Most adenomas detected on surveillance examinations are small (less than 1 cm), tubular, and only mildly dysplastic, but they are fairly equally distributed in the colon and rectum.[35] One-half are situated above the reach of the 60-cm flexible sigmoidoscope, making full colonoscopy necessary to secure a clean colon in all patients.[36] There is a tendency toward clustering with new adenomas appearing more often than expected by chance in the area of the original adenoma.[37] Residual stalks after previous polypectomy may be mistaken for a new adenoma, but this diagnostic problem is of minor importance.[38]

Within 10 years the risk of a new adenoma occurring is approximately 50%.[27,32] Patients at high risk of new adenoma formation may have the highest risk of cancer.[39,40] Short intervals between surveillance colonoscopies to obtain a clean colon may reduce the risk, but again the optimal timing is not known. Another reason for using colonoscopic surveillance is to identify the presence of flat adenomas, which otherwise may be overseen with the result that severe dysplasia may be missed.[11,12] Figures from St. Mark's Hospital[41] have suggested, however, that patients with small tubular adenomas in the rectum and rectosigmoid area removed during rigid proctoscopy have a very small risk of developing colonic cancer later. Thus only 4 of 776 patients with a follow-up ranging from 2 to 23 years did so in spite of no colonoscopic surveillance program. In this study, however, patients with colorectal cancer occurring within the first 2 years were excluded as well as the group of

Figure 20-1. Cumulated hazard of significant neoplasia during surveillance of patients with previous adenomas. Grey line, initial large sessile or villous adenomas, black line, initial pedunculated and small sessile tubular and tubulovillous adenomas.

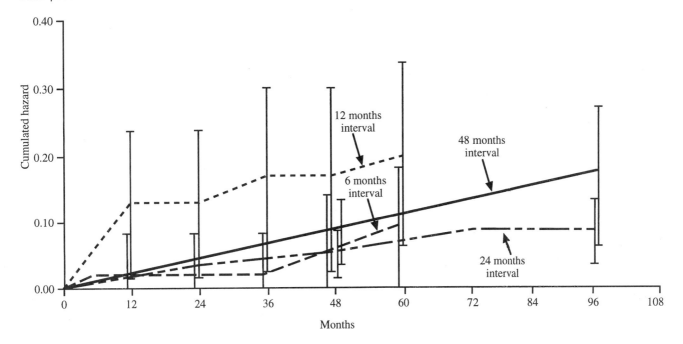

patients having full colonoscopy. The study was similar to another retrospective trial from the Mayo Clinic,[42] which demonstrated no increased risk of cancer in 751 patients followed for 10,000 person-years after removal of polyps of less than 1 cm in diameter without histologic confirmation of adenoma. A similar finding among 133 patients with a single tubular adenoma less than 1 cm in diameter was reported in the Kaiser Permanente Study.[43]

There is some evidence that the risk of new adenoma formation may decrease after 4 years of surveillance,[44,45] but these figures are based on results from the precolonoscopic era. By contrast, evidence from more recent publications does not suggest a decrease with time.[29,31,35]

Surveillance methods other than colonoscopy have been tried, but without much success. The DCBE studied by the NPS had a very low sensitivity. Fecal occult blood tests such as Hemoccult II have a sensitivity for adenomas over 1 cm in diameter of only 25%, but in no more than 5% to 10% of smaller adenomas,[23,46] which do not bleed and are usually detected by chance. More sensitive tests, including the immunochemical Heme-Select test, will detect no more than 45% of adenomas larger than 1 cm.[47] A new possible marker of colorectal neoplasia, Calprotectin, the cytosol protein in granulocytes, has been detected in increased concentrations in feces from 32 of 40 patients with adenomas.[48] In the future, it may be possible to screen fecal samples for a number of mutations with the hope of obtaining a higher sensitivity for adenoma detection.

Acceptability and compliance for colonoscopy are high.[49] This is not surprising as the patients are told that they have a possible precursor of cancer. Unfortunately, colonoscopy is not without complications but they should be minimal by avoiding colonoscopy in patients with severe disabling diseases and by adequate training of endoscopists. If the complication rate is unacceptably high, this may compromise any possible reduction in mortality from cancer. In one surveillance program of 1,818 colonoscopies, one patient died owing to a sigmoid perforation,[49] a mortality figure similar to that reported in other large series.[50,51] The total number of severe complications demanding surgery in an adenoma surveillance program in the author's teaching center is given in Table 20-1. Before the colonoscopic era, colotomy with polypectomy carried a much higher risk of

complications,[52] but then only patients with adenomas of at least 1 cm in diameter were subjected to this treatment.

Compliance may decrease with increasing length of intervals between planned colonoscopies. More than 3 years is probably too long and even 3 years as recommended by many authors requires intensive reminding before the examination.[26] A colonoscopic follow-up allows assessment of factors other than the state of the colon. Dietary supplements including calcium, fiber, vitamins, and the taking of nonsteroidal anti-inflammatory drugs are being currently evaluated by randomized study.[53,54] The number of patients followed would have to be enormous to allow useful conclusions. Smoking probably increases the risk of new adenoma formation,[55,56] whereas coffee may reduce it.[55] The possible influence of alcohol is uncertain.

There is little information on the growth rate of polyps and factors that might affect it. Measurement of polyps deliberately left behind has not been carried out after the polyps become more than 1 cm in diameter.[22] Measurement of epithelial proliferation by $_3$H-thymidin incorporation and autoradiography might give useful information on the effect of some factors, for example diet, on growth.[57,58]

Adenoma surveillance by endoscopy at intervals of a few years may seem realistic at present, but the situation will change dramatically if screening with flexible sigmoidoscopy in persons above 50 years of age becomes routine. This could generate a surveillance population, which may amount to 10% to 20% of the normal population.[59,60] Most endoscopy units would not be able to meet such a demand,[61] having other diagnostic and therapeutic obligations and it is therefore mandatory to obtain a more targeted selection of high-risk groups for colorectal cancer. One possibility would be to exclude from surveillance programs persons with a single small tubular adenoma without severe dysplasia,[62] but a randomized study is necessary before such a policy can be justified. It seems reasonable to discontinue surveillance after a certain age. Individuals who have a clean colon at 75 years have a very low risk of dying from colorectal cancer later.[63]

Practical Guidelines

In patients with adenoma, steps should be taken to obtain a clean colon either by full colonoscopy or limited flexible sigmoidoscopy and DCBE. Thus another colonoscopy should be carried out within 3 months in patients with multiple adenomas or where the endoscopist does not feel confident that a clean colon had been obtained initially. Where an adenoma has been removed piecemeal another endoscopy is necessary within 3 months to determine whether there is any residual adenoma or carcinoma. In this circumstance only the area of the polypectomy needs to be re-examined.

Having secured an initially clean colon, long-term surveillance should include colonoscopy every 3 years where originally a pedunculated or small sessile tubular or tubulovillous adenoma had been removed. A surveillance interval of 2 years should be applied to patients who have initially undergone removal of a villous or large sessile adenoma above 5 mm in diameter.

The approach using flexible sigmoidoscopy combined with barium enema is less accurate than total colonoscopy. It may,

Table 20-1. Complications From Colonoscopy in the Adenoma Surveillance Program at Odense University Hospital, 1978–1994

	Number	%
Diagnostic colonoscopy	4,311	
Colonic perforation	9	0.21
Suture alone	6	
Suture + colostomy	3	
Death	1	0.02
Therapeutic colonoscopy	1,901	
Colonic perforation	5	0.26
Suture alone	4	
Suture + colostomy	1	
Death	1	0.05
Bleeding needing colotomy	1	0.05

however, be necessary when full colonoscopy is not possible owing to technical difficulty or patient preference.

A surveillance program should not be continued in patients older than 75 years provided they have a clean colon or a severe disabling disease is present.

CARCINOMA

The possible benefit of detecting asymptomatic recurrence after "curative" surgery is probably small.[64] Nevertheless this strategy may lead to more recurrences being resectable,[65,67] and in a few cases long-term survival may result.[68] Prospective evidence to support this approach is scarce, however. Only two major trials have been initiated to study the possible benefits of different methods of surveillance.[69,70] Recurrence develops in approximately one-half of all patients. In most of these cases this appears within the first 2 years.

The risk of a metachronous lesion developing is at least 5% over a 10-year period after a previous resection of a sporadic cancer. Endoscopy with removal of any adenoma should theoretically reduce the risk, and the detection and removal of an asymptomatic early carcinoma may also increase long-term survival.

Symptoms seldom appear before the recurrence or metachronous tumor becomes advanced. Even asymptomatic recurrence may not be curable and a surveillance policy including colonoscopy, liver biopsy, and second look surgery is not without risk.

Methods of Surveillance

Recurrence in the pelvis after anterior resection may be detected by digital exploration. Although in males a mass in the perineum may be difficult to palpate, in women recurrence can often be detected by vaginal examination after abdominoperineal excision. The general abdominal examination has a low sensitivity. When liver metastases or an abdominal mass are palpable it is usually too late for salvage surgery to be possible. A minority of recurrences detected by clinical examination may, however, be removable surgically.

Endoscopy may detect intraluminal recurrence. Occasionally this may be truly anastomotic but more commonly it is the result of penetration of the mucosa by extraluminal recurrence invading the lumen. Colonoscopy is the method of choice to detect metachronous tumors and to treat them if small.

Patients having an incomplete colonoscopy before surgery should have the examination repeated shortly after to avoid any overlooked synchronous neoplasm. A long-term surveillance by colonoscopy at 3- to 5-year intervals is generally accepted practice although its value in reducing mortality has not been proved. Most metachronous carcinomas can be treated by curative surgery,[65,71,72] and polypectomy of adenomas may reduce the subsequent incidence of carcinoma.[73] It has been suggested that a metachronous carcinoma being detected at surveillance probably has a better prognosis than large bowel cancer presenting with symptoms.[74]

Colonoscopy is usually easy to perform after colorectal surgery,[46] but some patients are difficult to colonoscope or refuse the examination. In this circumstance the combination of DCBE with flexible sigmoidoscopy is a valuable second option. The sensitivity of barium enema is less than that of colonoscopy

and a radiologic diagnosis of a polyp makes a colonoscopy necessary.

Simple laboratory tests including hemoglobin, albumin, and erythrocyte sedimentation estimations rate may be useful. Their value in detecting early recurrence has not been assessed but is likely to be poor.[64] Fecal occult blood tests are of little value, because most early local recurrences are extraluminal. This test may detect metachronous cancers and large adenomas. Any positive test should be followed by colonoscopy.[64]

Measurement of serum enzymes including alkaline phosphatase, glumatic oxaloacetic and pyruvic transaminases, alanin-amino transferase, lactate dehydrogenase, and gamma transpeptidase and gamma glutamyl transpeptidase is widely used. Their sensitivity for detection of small and limited liver metastases is, however, very low. The same is true for serum bilirubin. Levels of α-fetoprotein have not been useful in detecting resectable recurrence. Other potential markers are IgA- and IgM-associated secretory compound and prostaglandin E_2, the latter for liver as well as lung metastases.[75] These again are of limited value.

The literature on carcinoembryonic antigen (CEA) is extensive but no prospective study has demonstrated its value in reducing mortality. Most reviews suggest it is of little use,[76–78] but not all.[66,79,80] Increased levels are found in no more than 25% of patients with early colorectal cancer and 20% do not express CEA. It is doubtful whether CEA levels are related to DNA ploidy,[81] which again is an unreliable indicator of tumor aggressiveness.[82] CEA has some prognostic value and no reduction of an elevated preoperative CEA within the first 6 weeks after surgery suggests the presence of persisting tumor. Sequential measurements at monthly intervals have been recommended to evaluate doubling time, which together with slope analysis may differentiate to some degree between local recurrence and distant metastases.[83,84] Patients with recurrence detected by a rise in CEA may have local recurrence alone in no more than 20% to 30% of the cases.[67] Second look surgery should be contemplated before CEA rises above 10 ng/ml provided further tests do not show inoperability.[85] The rise may occur 4 to 6 months before clinical symptoms develop in more than 25% to 50% of the patients,[69,76,84,86,87] thus estimations at longer intervals, for example, 2 to 3 months, may reduce this figure.

A CEA-directed surveillance program may be expensive[88] and only one major randomized study has been performed to evaluate the possible influence on mortality; the final results have not yet been published. A meta-analysis of retrospective data has suggested a 9% better 5-year survival when an intensive surveillance includes CEA measurements, compared with no surveillance at all.[68] CEA is, however, a poor predictor for resectability of liver metastases.[89]

Other serum markers including CA 19-9, CA 50, CA 195, and TPA have less predictive value than CEA. The combined use of different markers may increase sensitivity but at the expense of a fall in specificity.[64] Acute-phase reactant proteins have been shown to increase the predictive value of CEA.[90] Diagnostic accuracy also may be increased by radioimmunodetection of the recurrence by monoclonal anti-CEA antibodies.[91]

Ultrasonography, computed tomography (CT), and magnetic resonance imaging (MRI) will detect liver metastases above 2 cm in diameter with a high degree of accuracy.[92] Ultrasound is the least expensive test but interobserver variation is large.

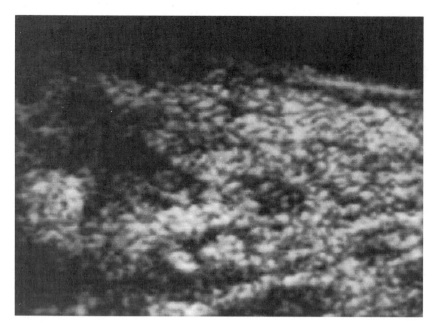

Figure 20-2. Local recurrence as detected by a linear ultrasound probe. Normal figuration of the layers of the rectal wall is in the upper right quadrant.

It may be more specific in the presence of benign cystic lesions and is probably the most frequently used examination. CT is more accurate than ultrasound in detecting local recurrence and lymph node metastases but an early postoperative CT is necessary for comparison with late examinations.[93] The imaging techniques, including immunoscintigraphy,[94] should probably not be used as initial screening examinations for recurrence but so far none of them has been evaluated in large randomized trials. A comparison of CT of the liver and chest radiographs at 5 years with annual examinations showed no differences in mortality.[95]

The value of endoluminal ultrasound, whether performed blindly in the rectum or guided by the colonoscope in follow-up is still uncertain. Local recurrence is difficult to differentiate from fibrosis (Fig. 20-2), and the technique of ultrasonographic-guided biopsy is not optimal in the colon.[64]

CT and conventional tomography are both more accurate in detecting lung metastases than chest radiographs.[72] Bone scintigraphy should not be used for surveillance, because bone metastases are uncommon, and when they occur the disease is incurable. The same is true for brain metastases.

Second-look surgery has been abandoned as a screening method for abdominal recurrence and should be performed only when other examinations suggest resectable disease. Intraoperative ultrasound is highly sensitive for liver metastases (Fig. 20-3). Radioimmuno-guided second look procedures may reduce the number of superfluous resections in patients with recurrence in more than one area.[96] However, interim results from the one large randomized CEA trial suggest no survival advantage by patients undergoing CEA-prompted second look surgery,[97] confirming the results from a large retrospective study.[88]

Selection of Patients

At the present time, the benefit of a planned surveillance program is uncertain and an attempt should be made to select pa-tients with the highest probability of it being advantageous. Elderly patients above 75 years with other disabling disease should not be followed, even when they have had curative treatment. The risk of recurrence may be high but they are unlikely to survive major surgery for recurrence, and metachronous carcinoma is very rare within the first 5 years.

Below 75 years, surveillance is probably not necessary for patients with an early lesion (Dukes' A), owing to the very good prognosis. However, they should have colonoscopy every

Figure 20-3. Liver metastasis (1 cm in diameter) as shown by intraoperative ultrasound examination.

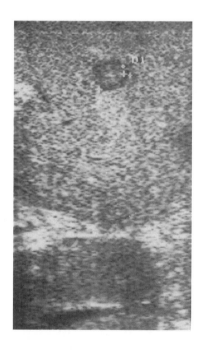

3 to 5 years to detect a metachronous neoplasm. An exception might be patients who have had a curative local removal of a small rectal carcinoma. Follow-up by digital rectal examination and proctoscopy during the first 5 years at intervals initially of 3 to 6 months should be performed.[98]

Patients with a synchronous neoplasm, whether a carcinoma or adenoma, carry a high risk of developing a metachronous neoplasm and should be followed by colonoscopy every 2 years,[99] having obtained an initially clean colon. Multiple neoplasms that cannot be treated by colonoscopic snare removal should have a subtotal colectomy, and endoscopic surveillance can then be limited to sigmoidoscopy. The same policy is followed in patients with the hereditary nonpolyposis colorectal cancer (HNPCC) syndrome.[100]

Patients without intercurrent disabling disease, having had curative surgery for Dukes' stage B and C lesions, should be selected for a surveillance program. Using the most sensitive markers for early recurrence, survival after curative surgery will theoretically be maximized. This group of patients is large and heterogeneous in that it can be subdivided in smaller clinicopathologic groups with very different prognoses. A number of histopathologic criteria may be used to assess risk and recently genotyping has become possible.[101] The subdivisions may influence the choice of initial adjuvant therapy and the intensity of any surveillance program.

In summary the aim of surveillance of patients after curative surgery is to detect early recurrence or metachronous neoplasia. There is some evidence that this strategy is beneficial in terms of survival. Programs for detection of symptomatic recurrent carcinoma have, however, shown very little benefit.

REFERENCES

1. Kune GA, Kune S, Watson LF (1987) History of colorectal polypectomy and risk of subsequent colorectal cancer. Br J Surg 74:1064–1065

2. Murakami R, Tsukuma H, Kanamori S et al (1990) Natural history of colorectal polyps and the effect of polypectomy on occurrence of subsequent cancer. Int J Cancer 46:159–164

3. Simons BD, Morrison AS, Lev R, Verhoek-Oftedahl W (1992) Relationship of polyps to cancer of the large intestine. J Natl Cancer Inst 84:962–966

4. Gilbertsen VA, Nelms JM (1978) The prevention of invasive cancer of the rectum. Cancer 41:1137–1139

5. Winawer SJ, Zauber AG, Ho MN et al (1993) Prevention of colorectal cancer by colonoscopic polypectomy. N Engl J Med 329:1977–1981

6. Joergensen OD, Kronborg O, Fenger C (1993) The Funen Adenoma Follow-up Study. Incidence and death from colorectal carcinoma in an adenoma surveillance program. Scand J Gastroenterol 28:869–874

7. Hill MJ, Morson BC, Bussey HJR (1978) Etiology of adenoma-carcinoma sequence in large bowel. Lancet 1:245–247

8. Manning AM, Williams AC, Game SM, Paraskeva C (1991) Differential sensitivity of human colonic adenoma and carcinoma cells to transforming growth factor β (TGF-β): conversion of an adenoma cell line to a tumorigenic phenotype is accompanied by a reduced response to the inhibitory effects of TGF-β. Oncogene 6:1471–1476

9. Stryker SJ, Wolff BG, Culp CE et al (1987) Natural history of untreated colonic polyps. Gastroenterology 93:1009–1013

10. Takemoto T, Sakari N (1987) High-magnification endoscopy. pp. 220–230. In Sivak MV (ed): Gastroenterologic Endoscopy. 1st Ed. WB Saunders, Philadelphia,

11. Adachi M, Muto T, Okinaga K, Morioka Y (1991) Clinicopathologic features of the flat adenoma. Dis Colon Rectum 34:981–986

12. Wolber R, Owen D (1991) Flat adenomas of the colon. Hum Pathol 22:70–74

13. Lynch HT, Smyrk TC, Watson P et al (1992) Hereditary flat adenoma syndrome: a variant of familial adenomatous polyposis? Dis Colon Rectum 35:411–421

14. Jass JR (1989) Do all colorectal carcinomas arise in preexisting adenomas? World J Surg 13:45–51

15. Eide T (1991) Natural history of adenomas. World J Surg 15:3–6

16. Mulder JW, Offerhaus GJA, Feyter EP et al (1992) The relationship of quantitative nuclear morphology to molecular genetic alterations in the adenoma-carcinoma sequence of the large bowel. Am J Pathol 141:797–804

17. Cho KR, Vogelstein B (1992) Genetic alterations in the adenoma-carcinoma sequence. Cancer 70:1727–1731

18. Goh HS, Jass JR (1986) DNA content and the adenoma-carcinoma sequence in the colorectum. J Clin Pathol 39:387–392

19. Muto T, Masaki T, Suzuki K (1991) DNA ploidy pattern of flat adenomas of the large bowel. Dis Colon Rectum 34:696–698

20. Salem RR, Wolf BC, Sears HF et al (1993) Expression of colorectal carcinoma-associated antigens in colonic polyps. J Surg Research 55:249–255

21. Knoernschild HE (1963) Growth rate and malignant potential of colonic polyps: early results. Surgical Forum 14:137–138

22. Hofstad B, Vatn M, Larsen S, Osnes M (1994) Growth of colorectal polyps: recovery and evaluation of unresected polyps of less than 10 mm, 1 year after detection. Scand J Gastroenterol 29:640–645

23. Kronborg O, Hage E, Deichgraeber E (1981) The clean colon. A prospective, partly randomized study of the effectiveness of repeated examinations of the colon after polypectomy and radical surgery for cancer. Scand J Gastroenterol 16:879–884

24. Winawer SJ, Zauber AG, O'Brien MJ et al (1992) The national polyp study. Design, methods, and characteristics of patients with newly diagnosed polyps. Cancer 70:1236–1245

25. Williams CB, Macrae FA, Bartram CI (1982) A prospective study of diagnostic methods in adenoma follow-up. Endoscopy 14:74–78

26. Winawer SJ, O'Brien MJ, Way JD et al (1990) Risk and surveillance of individuals with colorectal polyps. Bull WHO 68:789–795

27. Kronborg O (1989) The Funen adenoma follow-up study. pp. 38–43. In Hardcastle JD (ed): Proceedings of an International Meeting Organised by The United Kingdom Co-ordinating Committee on Cancer Research: screening for Colorectal Cancer. Normed Verlag, Hamburg

28. Walsh RM, Ackroyd FW, Shellito PC (1992) Endoscopic

resection of large sessile colorectal polyps. Gastrointest Endosc 38:303–309

29. Winawer SJ, Zauber AG, O'Brien MJ et al (1993) Randomized comparison of surveillance intervals after colonoscopic removal of newly diagnosed adenomatous polyps. N Engl J Med 328:901–906

30. Joergensen O, Kronborg O, Fenger C (1993) The Funen Adenoma Follow-up Study. Characteristics of patients and initial adenomas in relation to severe dysplasia. Scand J Gastroenterol 28:239–243

31. Joergensen OD, Kronborg O, Fenger C (1995) The Funen Adenoma Follow-up Study. A randomized surveillance study of patients with pedunculated and small sessile tubular and tubulovillous adenomas. Scand J Gastroenterol 30

32. Kirsner JB, Rider JA, Moeller HC et al (1960) Polyps of the colon and rectum. Statistical analysis of a long term follow-up study. Gastroenterology 39:178–182

33. Minopoulus GJ, McIntyre RLE, Lee ECG, Kettlewell MGW (1983) Colonoscopic polypectomy in a regional teaching hospital. Br J Surg 70:51–53

34. Brown LJR, Smeeton NC, Dixon MF (1985) Assessment of dysplasia in colorectal adenomas: an observer variation and morphometric study. J Clin Pathol 38:174–179

35. Kronborg O (1991) Follow-up surveillance in patients with adenomas. J Gastroenterol Hepatol 6:552–553

36. Woolfson IK, Eckholdt GJ, Wetzel CR et al (1990) Usefulness of performing colonoscopy one year after endoscopic polypectomy. Dis Colon Rectum 33:389–393

37. Cappell MS, Forde KA (1989) Spatial clustering of multiple hyperplastic, adenomatous, and malignant colonic polyps in individual patients. Dis Colon Rectum 32:641–652

38. Kelly JK, MacCannell KL, Price LM, Hershfield NB (1987) Residual stalks of pedunculated adenomas. J Clin Gastroenterol 9:227–231

39. Christiansen J, Kirkegaard P, Ibsen J (1979) Prognosis after treatment of villous adenomas of the colon and rectum. Ann Surg 189:404–408

40. Lofti AM, Spencer RJ, Ilstrup DM, Melton LJ (1986) Colorectal polyps and the risk of subsequent carcinoma. Mayo Clin Proc 61:337–343

41. Atkin W, Morson BC, Cuzick J (1992) Long-term risk of colorectal cancer after excision of rectosigmoid adenomas. N Engl J Med 326:658–662

42. Spencer RJ, Melton LJ, Ready RL, Ilstrup DM (1984) Treatment of small colorectal polyps: a population-based study of the risk of subsequent carcinoma. Mayo Clin Proc 59:305–310

43. Grossman S, Milos ML, Tekawa IS, Jewell NP (1989) Colonoscopic screening of persons with suspected risk factors for colon cancer: II. past history of colorectal neoplasms. Gastroenterology 96:299–306

44. Hudson AT, Muldoon JP (1965) Is long-term follow up of rectal polyps justifiable? Dis Colon Rectum 8:369–371

45. Henry LG, Condon RE, Schulte WJ et al (1975) Risk of recurrence of colon polyps. Ann Surg 182:511–515

46. Jahn H, Joergensen OD, Kronborg O, Fenger C (1992) Can Hemoccult-II replace colonoscopy in surveillance after radical surgery for colorectal cancer and after polypectomy? Dis Colon Rectum 35:253–256

47. Robinson MHE, Kronborg O, Williams CB et al (1995) A study of faecal occult blood testing and colonoscopy in the surveillance of subjects at high risk of colorectal neoplasia. Br J Surg 82:318–320

48. Røseth AG, Kristinsson J, Fagerhol MK et al (1993) Faecal Calprotectin: a novel test for the diagnosis of colorectal cancer? Scand J Gastroenterol 28:1073–1076

49. Kronborg O, Fenger C (1987) Prognostic evaluation of planned follow-up in patients with colorectal adenomas. Int J Colorect Dis 2:203–207

50. Macrae FA, Tan KG, Williams CB (1983) Towards safer colonoscopy; a report on the complications of 5000 diagnostic or therapeutic colonoscopies. Gut 24:376–383

51. Jentschura D, Raute M, Winter J et al (1994) Complications in endoscopy of the lower gastrointestinal tract. Therapy and prognosis. Surg Endosc 8:672–676

52. Kleinfeld G, Gump FE (1960) Complications of colotomy and polypectomy. Surg Gyn Obstet 111:726–728

53. Armitage NCM (1991) Intervention studies in adenoma patients. World J Surg 15:29–34

54. Faivre J, Boutron M-C, Doyon F et al (1993) The ECP calcium fibre polyp prevention study preliminary report. Eur J Cancer Prev 2:99–106

55. Olsen J, Kronborg O (1993) Coffee, tobacco and alcohol as risk factors for cancer and adenoma of the large intestine. Int J Epidemiol 22:398–402

56. Jacobson JS, Neugut AI, Murray T et al (1994) Cigarette smoking and other behavioral risk factors for recurrence of colorectal adenomatous polyps (New York City, NY, USA). Cancer Causes Control 5:215–220

57. Paganelli GM, Biasco G, Santucci R et al (1991) Rectal cell proliferation and colorectal cancer risk level in patients with nonfamilial adenomatous polyps of the large bowel. Cancer 68:2451–2454

58. Anti M, Marra G, Armelao F et al (1993) Rectal epithelial cell proliferation patterns as predictors of adenomatous colorectal polyp recurrence. Gut 34:525–530

59. Hoff G (1987) Colorectal polyps. Clinical implications: screening and cancer prevention. Scand J Gastroenterol 22:769–775

60. Kronborg O, Joergensen OD, Fenger C (1994) Advantages and drawbacks of adding flexible 60 cm sigmoidoscopy to Hemoccult-II in screening for colorectal neoplasia. 3rd UEGW Oslo, publication no. 181:p.A41 (Abstract)

61. Ransohoff DF, Lang CA, Kuo HS (1991) Colonoscopic surveillance after polypectomy: considerations of cost effectiveness. Ann Intern Med 114:177–182

62. Bond JH (1993) Polyp guidelines: diagnosis, treatment, and surveillance for patients with nonfamilial colorectal polyps. Ann Intern Med 119:836–843

63. Williams CB, Bedenne L (1990) Management of colorectal polyps: is all the effort worthwhile? J Gastroenterol Hepatol 1:144–165

64. Kronborg O (1994) Optimal follow-up in colorectal cancer patients: what tests and how often? Sem Surg Oncol 10:217–224

65. Ovaska JT, Järvinen HJ, Mecklin JP (1989) The value of a follow-up programme after radical surgery for colorectal carcinoma. Scand J Gastroenterol 24:416–422

66. Minton J, Chivinsky AH (1989) CEA directed second-look

surgery for colon and rectal cancer. Ann Chir Gynaecol 78: 32–37

67. Quentmeier A, Schlag P, Smok M, Herfarth Ch (1990) Re-operation for recurrent colorectal cancer: the importance of early diagnosis for resectability and survival. Eur Surg Oncol 16:319–325

68. Bruinvels DJ, Stiggelbout AM, Kievit J et al (1994) Follow up of patients with colorectal cancer. A meta-analysis. Ann Surg 219:174–182

69. Northover JMA (1985) Carcinoembryonic antigen and recurrent colorectal cancer. Br J Surg, (suppl). 72:44–46

70. Kronborg O, Fenger C, Deichgraeber E, Hansen L (1988) Follow-up after radical surgery for colorectal cancer; design of a randomized study. Scand J Gastroenterol, suppl. 149: 159–162

71. Kronborg O, Fenger C, Deichgraeber E (1991) Colonoscopy after radical surgery for colorectal cancer. A ten-year prospective investigation of 309 patients. Ugeskr Laeger 153: 503–506

72. Kelly CJ, Daly JM (1992) Colorectal cancer. Principles of postoperative follow-up. Cancer 70:1397–1408

73. Cali RL, Pitsch RM, Thorson AG et al (1993) Cumulative incidence of metachronous colorectal cancer. Dis Col Rectum 36:388–393

74. Kronborg O, Hage E, Deichgraeber E (1983) The remaining colon after radical surgery for colorectal cancer. The first three years of a prospective study. Dis Colon Rectum 26: 172–176

75. Narisawa T, Kusaka H, Yamazaki Y et al (1990) Relationship between blood plasma prostaglandin E_2 and liver and lung metastases in colorectal cancer. Dis Colon Rectum 33: 840–845

76. Carlsson U, Stewenius J, Ekelund G et al (1983) Is CEA analysis of value in screening for recurrences after surgery for colorectal carcinoma? Dis Colon Rectum 26:369–373

77. Ballantyne GH, Modlin IM (1988) Postoperative follow-up for colorectal cancer. Who are we kidding? J Clin Gastroenterol 10:359–364

78. Kievit J, Velde CJH van de (1990) Utility and cost of carcinoembryonic antigen monitoring in colon cancer follow-up evaluation. A Markov analysis. Cancer 65:2580–2587

79. Sugarbaker PH (1990) Surgical decision making for large bowel cancer metastatic to the liver. Radiology 174:621–626

80. Himal HS (1991) Anastomotic recurrence of carcinoma of the colon and rectum. The value of endoscopy and serum CEA levels. Am Surg 57:334–337

81. Kouri M, Pyrhönen S, Mecklin JP et al (1991) Serum carcinoembryonic antigen and DNA ploidy in colorectal carcinoma. Scand J Gastroenterol 26:812–818

82. Offerhaus GJA, Feyter EP de, Cornelisse CJ et al (1992) The relationship of DNA aneuploidy to molecular genetic alterations in colorectal carcinoma. Gastroenterology 102: 1612–1619

83. Boey J, Cheung HC, Lai CK, Wong J (1984) A prospective evaluation of serum carcinoembryonic antigen (CEA) levels in the management of colorectal carcinoma. World J Surg 8: 279–286

84. Staab HJ, Anderer FA, Stumpf E et al (1985) Eight-four potential second-look operations based on sequential carcinoembryonic antigen determinations and clinical investigations in patients with recurrent gastrointestinal cancer. Am J Surg 149:198–204

85. Minton JP, Hoehn JL, Gerber DM et al (1985) Results of a 400-patient carcinoembryonic antigen second-look colorectal cancer study. Cancer 55:1284–1290

86. Finlay JG, McArdle CS (1983) Role of carcinoembryonic antigen in detection of asymptomatic disseminated disease in colorectal carcinoma. BMJ 286:1242–1244

87. Rocklin MS, Slomski CA, Watne AL (1990) Postoperative surveillance of patients with carcinoma of the colon and rectum. Am Surg 56:22–27

88. Moertel CG, Fleming TR, MacDonald JS et al (1993) An evaluation of the carcinoembryonic antigen (CEA) test for monitoring patients with resected colon cancer. JAMA 270: 943–947

89. Steele G, Bleday R, Mayer RJ et al (1991) A prospective evaluation of hepatic resection for colorectal carcinoma metastases to the liver: Gastrointestinal Tumor Study Group Protocol 6584. J Clin Oncol 9:1105–1112

90. Walker C, Gray BN (1983) Acute-phase reactant proteins and carcinoembryonic antigen in cancer of the colon and rectum. Cancer 52:150–154

91. Begent RHJ, Keep P, Searle F et al (1986) Radioimmunolocalization and selection for surgery in recurrent colorectal cancer. Br J Surg 73:64–67

92. Charnsangavej C (1993) New imaging modalities for follow-up of colorectal carcinoma. Cancer 71:4236–4240

93. Wanebo HJ, Llaneras M, Martin T, Kaiser D (1989) Prospective monitoring trial for carcinoma of colon and rectum after surgical resection. Surg Gynecol Obstet 169:479–487

94. Doerr RJ, Herrera L, Abdel-Nabi H (1993) In-111 Cyt-103 monoclonal antibody imaging in patients with suspected recurrent colorectal cancer. Cancer 71:4241–4247

95. McCall JL, Black RB, Rich CA et al (1994) The value of serum carcinoembryonic antigen in predicting recurrent disease following curative resection of colorectal cancer. Dis Colon Rectum 37:875–881

96. Martin EW, Carey LC (1991) Second-look surgery for colorectal cancer. The second time around. Ann Surg 214: 321–327

97. Northover J, Houghton J, Lennon T (1994) CEA to detect recurrence of colon cancer. JAMA 272:31

98. Sugarbaker PH (1986) Symposium. The management of recurrent colorectal cancer. Int J Colorect Dis 1:133–151

99. Bussey HR, Wallace MH, Morson BC (1967) Metachronous carcinoma of the large intestine and intestinal polyps. Proc R Soc Med 60:208–211

100. Mecklin J-P, Järvinen H (1993) Treatment and follow-up strategies in hereditary nonpolyposis colorectal carcinoma. Dis Colon Rectum 36:927–929

101. Finkelstein SD, Sayegh R, Christensen S, Swalsky PA (1993) Genotypic classification of colorectal adenocarcinoma. Cancer 71:3827–3838

21

POLYPS AND POLYPOSIS SYNDROMES

BENIGN NEOPLASMS

R. John Nicholls

A polyp is defined as an abnormal elevation from an epithelial surface. It is therefore a morphologic entity that says nothing of the pathologic nature of the lesion. This can only be obtained by histopathologic examination and a classification of large bowel polyps is given in chapter 19. Polyps may be single or multiple. Each pathologic category can be associated with a polyposis syndrome in which the total count of polyps in the large bowel exceeds 100. Usually the number is considerably more than this.

There are numerous types of colorectal polyps including adenoma, hamartoma, metaplastic, and rarer examples such as lymphoma. Lipoma is a fairly common benign neoplasm and is not a mucosal lesion. Inflammatory polyps are seen in patients with inflammatory bowel disease or bilharzia. Patients with pneumatosis intestinalis may sometimes be misdiagnosed as having intestinal polyps.

The most important distinction in polyp type lies between neoplastic and non-neoplastic (see accompanying box). Although the rare hamartomatous polyps have some malignant potential the true neoplastic benign polyp, the adenoma, is by far the most important in this respect.

Metaplastic polyps are common and are not in themselves thought to be premalignant. However, pathologists do on occasion find remnants of metaplastic polyps in colorectal cancer, suggesting the possibility that they may be associated with neoplasia.[1] In the rare condition of giant metaplastic polyposis, there may be many quite large metaplastic polyps of up to 2 cm in diameter.[2] A mistaken diagnosis of familial adenomatous polyposis may be made unless preoperative histology is obtained.

There are two sorts of hamartomatous intestinal polyps. These include those that lack smooth muscle as seen in juvenile polyps and juvenile polyposis, and those that have smooth muscle as seen in the Peutz-Jeghers syndrome. Juvenile polyps may also occur in adults. They usually present with colicky abdominal pain, bleeding, intussusception, or sometimes even the passage per anum of the polyp itself (which, lacking smooth mus-

cle, does not seem to have a firm attachment to the intestinal wall). Until very recently juvenile polyps were not thought to be serious so far as the long-term risk of malignancy is concerned, but opinion has now changed and a very definite risk of intestinal malignancy has been demonstrated.[3]

The Peutz-Jeghers syndrome is an autosomal-dominant condition characterized by mucocutaneous pigmentation and intestinal hamartomas. The pigmentation may be seen not only around and inside the mouth and anus, but also on the palms of the hands and on the soles of the feet. Polyps may occur in the stomach, duodenum, and small as well as large bowel. Many patients present at a young age with intussusception and by early adult life may have undergone a number of laparotomies.

A number of authors have found an excessive rate of gastrointestinal malignancy in the Peutz-Jeghers syndrome. Some of this may have been caused by overdiagnosis of malignancy in Peutz-Jeghers polyps. This can arise when epithelial displacement beneath the muscularis mucosae, which is quite commonly seen in the Peutz-Jeghers syndrome, is reported as malignant invasion.[4] Despite this, there is a very definite risk of death from malignancy in the Peutz-Jeghers syndrome. About half of the recorded cancers are found outside the gastrointestinal tract and arise in sites such as the breast, ovary, cervix, and testis.[5,6]

ADENOMA

The malignant potential depends on the morphology, size, and histologic degree of differentiation. The treatment is linked to these three factors. Almost all adenomas of the colon can be removed by endoscopic smear polypectomy. This is because they are usually pedunculated and therefore amenable to this technique. Surgical treatment of adenomas may become necessary when the base of the polyp is too wide for snaring, increasing the risk of incomplete removal or perforation of the bowel wall. Suspicion of malignancy may also indicate surgery. Multiple adenomas not controlled by snare polypectomy can be treated by colectomy. The different approaches of surgical treatment are described.

Classification of Polyps

Non-neoplastic

Metaplastic (hyperplastic)

Inflammatory

Hamartomatous
  Peutz-Jeghers
  Juvenile

Neoplastic

Adenoma

Adenocarcinoma

Surgical management of large bowel adenomas can be applied to two generally different situations: first, where an adenoma is too proximal for endoanal access, and, second, where it is accessible via an endoanal approach. The former concerns lesions in the rectosigmoid region and colon; the latter involves most adenomas in the rectum.

Sessile adenomas tend to occur most commonly in the rectum and are usually accessible to endoanal techniques of removal. Where they occur beyond the range of endoanal removal, formal surgical resection is required. In all cases, an assessment of the possibility of malignant invasion having taken place must be made.

Incidence

Adenoma is common in patients over the age of 55 years, having been reported in one third of such individuals.[7] The incidence is difficult to establish and figures available largely come from autopsy studies. These have shown considerable variation. Clarke et al.[8] have reported remarkable differences in Scotland, Japan, and Scandinavia. There was a range from 10 (Finland) to nearly 40 (Aberdeen) per 100,000, with Norway, Japan, and Brazil lying between these extremes. There is an increase in the prevalence of adenomas according to age and this correlates closely with the incidence of carcinoma.[7] There are however, epidemiologic inconsistencies in the relationship between adenoma and carcinoma. For example, adenomas are seen more frequently in males.[7-11] Although the sex ratio for carcinoma is closer to equality, there is also an interesting disparity between the anatomic location of adenomas and cancer. Adenomas are mostly found in the sigmoid colon and less so in the rectum than the incidence of rectal carcinoma might indicate.[8] The reason for this is unknown. It may be that rectal adenomas when they occur are more likely to undergo malignant change or that some rectal carcinomas are not preceded by adenomas that can be recognized as such by morphologic appearance. This highlights the important distinction between the "polyp-carcinoma" sequence and "adenoma-carcinoma" sequence. The data supporting the concept of "de novo" carcinoma can be resolved if it is appreciated that carcinoma, being an epithelial lesion, must originate from an area of mucosal dysplasia whether this is manifested by a morphologically evident lesion or not.

Risk of Malignancy

Adenomas may be tubular, tubulovillous, or villous. The risk of malignant change depends on the amount of villousness in the polyp, the number, and the size. Large (greater than 2 cm) villous adenomas have a high chance of being malignant, whereas small tubular adenomas, particularly when they are single, impart a very low lifetime risk of malignancy.

There is evidence that most adenomas do not become malignant. Patients with a rectal adenoma are not necessarily at high risk of developing carcinoma more proximally.[11] In patients with small tubular adenomas of less than 10 mm in diameter removed by sigmoidoscopy, the risk of malignancy was not increased. It was increased, however, by a factor of four in those with a large sessile adenoma. In the cohort of patients studied, 90% of colonic carcinomas that ultimately developed were in this group. Studies such as these have introduced the concept of the "high" and "low" risk adenoma. This has major implications for follow-up (see Ch. 20). The evidence available to date indicates that small non-poorly differentiated adenomas that are sporadic do not require long-term surveillance.[13-15]

Most clinicians, however, would recommend that finding an adenoma in a patient means that a colonoscopy will be necessary in order not only to treat that polyp but also to exclude any others. Following colonoscopic polypectomy it has become accepted practice to repeat the colonoscopy after a short interval until the colon is found to be clean of polyps, and then annually for subsequent follow-up. There is no general agreement on the optimal regime for follow-up and the evidence that such a strategy protects against cancer and reduces mortality is not strong at the present time. A program of either three or five yearly colonoscopies according to the perceived risk is advocated by some: three yearly when the polyps have been large or have had a villous component, or have been very numerous, and five yearly when they have been small, single, and tubular.[16]

The finding of more than 100 adenomas in the large bowel indicates a diagnosis of familial adenomatous polyposis. This autosomal-dominant condition is associated with a gene deletion on chromosome 5.[17] Cancer appears to be virtually inevitable at some stage in the patient's life. Gardner[18] observed osteomas and cysts in such patients, and later described a number of other abnormalities, including adenomas, in the upper gastrointestinal tract. Many patients have congenital hypertrophy of the retinal pigment epithelium.[19,20] If the search is keen enough, most patients with familial adenomatous polyposis will be found to have some or all of these extraintestinal stigmata. This means that there is little value in separating familial adenomatous polyposis from Gardner's syndrome and it is probably wise now to cease using the latter term.

Patients either present as sporadic cases or are the offspring of a known family with the disease. Clearly it is always important to screen relatives, although rectal examination in children can wait until they are 12 or 13 years old.

Treatment

Colon

The majority of benign polyps in the colon can be removed by endoscopic snare polypectomy; however, in about 5% of cases, this is not feasible, usually because the base is too wide for snaring. Although some endoscopists would adopt a piecemeal removal technique, others would fear incomplete removal and also perforation. As a rough guide, a base of 25 mm or more should be an indication for formal surgical removal. Sessile villous adenomas are the best example of this type of morphology. In the colon, they tend to be in the cecum. Although the surgical clearance need not be radical owing to the presumption that the lesion is benign, it is prudent to take this wider, because malignant invasion cannot be excluded prior to histopathologic examination of the surgical specimen.

The second circumstance in which surgery is preferred to endoscopic removal is where there is a suspicion before treatment of malignant invasion whatever the size of the lesion. Features suggesting the possibility can be assessed to some extent during colonoscopy and on examination of biopsy material. Ulceration, size itself, and histologic grade showing poor differentiation are important risk factors. In addition, the barium enema can be helpful. Drawing-in of the profile of the bowel wall at the base of the polyp as seen by distortion of the barium mucosal shadow at this point strongly suggests invasion.

When the suspicion of malignancy is high, it is safer in an adequately fit patient to carry out a surgical resection. In this circumstance, a radical operation should be performed with as full a lymphovascular clearance as is anatomically possible.

The Malignant Adenoma

Surgery may also be necessary after endoscopic snare removal of an adenoma subsequently found by the pathologist to show invasion through the muscularis mucosa. Here one is dealing with an established cancer and two questions must then be considered; the completeness of removal and the perceived risk of regional lymphadenopathy.

Morson et al.[21] reviewed the outcome after snare polypectomy of a malignant polyp, classifying histologic local clearance into three categories. These included excision complete, excision doubtfully complete, and excision incomplete. In a series of 60 patients with malignant adenoma, 14 underwent a subsequent major surgical resection on the basis of the histologic findings, but in only 2 of these was any residual tumor found. One subsequently developed metastatic disease but the remainder were tumor-free at 5 years. In the 46 patients who did not undergo further treatment, there was no known case of a recurrent cancer. Six patients died; in 5 of these there was no evidence of recurrence, death being due to nonmalignant disease, and in the sixth case the cause of death was unknown. Overall, there was 1 known cancer death in 60 of these patients followed for 5 years, giving a cancer-specific death rate of 1.7%. In another study, malignant invasion was reported in 3.5% in a series of 676 adenomas removed by snare polypectomy. Of these, 7 underwent surgical resection and in only 2 was lymph node involvement found.[22]

Although there is a very low incidence of regional spread in this particular selected group of carcinomas, Morson and colleagues concluded from their study that cases in which excision was doubtfully complete may, in fact, be complete owing to tissue destruction by diathermy at the margin of excision during polypectomy. In addition to those with complete excision, they considered tumors confined to the intestinal wall not showing histologic evidence of vascular invasion nor anaplasia

also to be suitable for snare polypectomy alone without surgical resection.

Further support for this policy came from a report by Christie,[23] who reviewed 106 cases of malignant adenoma. Sixty-two underwent polypectomy alone, only 1 of whom developed recurrence and died. Of the 44 who underwent colectomy, 26 had had a preceding polypectomy. None of the surgical patients died of malignancy. In the subgroup of 48 patients with sessile tumors, 18 had a surgical resection ab initio. Of these, there was one case with lymph node involvement. Fifteen patients had endoscopic snare excision only and a further 15 had snare excision followed by surgery. Of these, 5 had persisting local disease, but only 1 had lymph node metastases.

The same author reviewed the literature on treatment of malignant adenomas, which included 11 studies on the subject. There were 244 patients who underwent surgery, of whom more than one-half had been preceded by an endoscopic polypectomy. Among these, there was residual tumor present in 27 cases, of whom 18 had nodal involvement. Eleven subsequently died of metastatic disease. In addition, there were 259 patients who underwent polypectomy only based on Morson's criteria. Subsequently 3 died, but it was pointed out that in these cases the criteria were not strictly observed.

More recent reports of the outcome of management of malignant adenomas treated by polypectomy help to refine the indication for continued observation or immediate surgical resection. Cooper et al.[24] followed 140 patients who had had removal of an adenoma with malignant invasion. Histopathologic criteria of lymphatic or venous invasion and an inadequate margin of clearance of the tumor were regarded as indications of an adverse outcome. Cancer-specific failure was related to the findings as follows: histology unfavorable 14 of 71 (19.7%), uncertain 2 of 23(8.6%), and favorable 0 of 46(0%). In the 104 patients who underwent surgical resection, 13 had lymphadenopathy. Histologic lymphatic invasion was shown to relate significantly to adverse outcome. Furthermore a resection margin of less than 1 mm also could be related to treatment failure. In the few cases (5) with venous invasion an adverse outcome occurred in 3, suggesting that this finding should also be regarded as an indication for surgical resection. Volk et al.[25] reported similar results. In a series of 47 patients with a malignant adenoma, there were 16 with favorable histology. This was defined as a histologic grade not poorly differentiated and a resection margin of 2 mm or more. None of these cases developed treatment failure at a follow-up of 30 months. In contrast, 10 of the 30 patients with unfavorable histology experienced failure of the policy of local excision. Of these 21(70%) had had a surgical resection. In 6 residual carcinoma was demonstrated on histologic examination all of who were disease-free after resection at a follow-up interval of 29 to 97 months. One further patient having a resection died of metastatic disease. These results show the importance of setting histologic criteria for continued observation and for taking surgical action when they are not fulfilled. A further useful indication of residual disease after polypectomy that the pathologist can give to the clinician is a statement of the depth of invasion. Nivatvongs et al.[26] showed that invasion into the submucosa beyond the level of the base of the adenoma is associated with a higher incidence (27%) of regional lymphadenopathy.

Hackelsberger et al.[27] have had a similar experience in 86 patients with malignant adenoma, defined as pT1 on pathologic examination. Thirty-four were regarded to have features conferring high risk and all went on to have a surgical resection. Residual tumor was found in 5, including lymphadenopathy in 2. None of the 42 patients having pathologic features denoting low risk had further trouble at a reasonable follow-up interval.

Malignant invasion was reported in 3.4% of a series of 676 adenomas removed by snare polypectomy. Of these, 7 underwent a subsequent surgical resection and in only 2 was an involved lymph node found.[21] In a series of 60 patients with malignant adenoma, 14 underwent a subsequent major surgical resection on the basis of histologic findings, but in only two of these was any residual tumor found. One of these subsequently developed metastatic disease but the remainder were tumor-free at 5 years. In the 46 patients who did not undergo further treatment, there was no known case of a recurrent cancer. Overall, the cancer-specific death rate was 2%.[21]

The morphology of the adenoma is also an important indicator of the possibility of malignant invasion and regional lymphadenopathy. This is discussed more fully in Chapter 39 but Muto et al.[28] have shown that a flat adenoma greater than 10 mm in diameter is more likely to contain malignant invasion than a polypoid exophytic lesion.

The evidence to date indicates that the policy of snare polypectomy for adenomas subsequently shown to have malignant invasion on histopathologic examination is justified under certain circumstances. These include an adequate margin of resection (more than 2 mm at least), absence of poor differentiation, and absence of lymphatic or venous invasion. These criteria are almost identical to those that pertain to surgical local excision as discussed in Chapter 39.

In cases with multiple adenomas insufficiently numerous to be deemed familial adenomatous polyposis, surgery may be necessary owing to the failure of endoscopic snare polypectomy to control adenoma development. It is not possible to be dogmatic on the indication for surgery in these uncommon cases. Factors including the presence of a synchronous carcinoma, the extent of any villous change, and previous endoscopic removal that may have failed owing to technical difficulty may well influence the decision to operate. The operation is likely to involve either a colectomy with ileorectal anastomosis if the rectum is relatively spared, or a restorative proctocolectomy with ileal reservoir if there is fairly extensive colonic and rectal involvement, the latter of which cannot be managed by local means.

Rectum

Sessile tumors of villous type are most common in the rectum. They vary in size from small (a few millimeters) to complete involvement of the entire rectal mucosa. Unless small enough for snare polypectomy, surgical removal should be undertaken. The choice of procedure will depend on the size, particularly the longitudinal extent and the distance from the anal verge.

Growths that are accessible to endoanal removal include almost all in the lower and some in the middle third of the rectum. The technique of submucosal excision is satisfactory for most of these lesions. Large circumferential villous adenomas extending too proximal for safe endoanal access will require abdominal removal, usually by anterior resection. Intestinal continuity by coloanal anastomosis after anal mucosectomy may be necessary if the distal border of the tumor extends into the upper anal canal. For smaller lesions too proximal for conventional endoanal removal transanal endoscopic microsurgery (TEM) may be the most appropriate treatment to avoid an abdominal operation.

Assessment of Malignant Invasion

It is essential to determine as far as possible whether malignant invasion has occurred. Malignancy is defined histopathologically by the presence of invasion of dysplastic tissue from the mucosa into the submucosa, the anatomic boundary separating these layers being the muscularis mucosae.

Clinical examination by digital and sigmoidoscopic means will determine the size and morphology of the tumor, whether sessile or pedunculated. An adenoma with a diameter of 10 mm at its base has only about a 1% chance of containing a focus of invasion whereas when this increases to more than 25 mm, the risk of invasive cancer rises to around 20% or more.[29,30] Although it is true that villous morphology as determined histologically is associated with a much higher risk than a tubular adenoma, in practice a preoperative biopsy from a rectal adenoma is not advisable because it is unlikely to be taken from an area of invasion. The correct strategy should be to carry out a complete excision of the lesion, which can then be examined by the pathologist in its entirety. A villous morphology is more likely if the growth is sessile, extensive, frondlike, and associated with excessive mucus production.

The principal sign of malignancy on digital examination is hardness. The growth should be carefully palpated with the aim of detecting an area of induration. This is a sensitive method for detecting malignancy in the pristine case but induration can be due to fibrosis where the tumor has previously been treated by diathermy fulguration or surgery.

In the last 10 years, rectal endoluminal ultrasound has been developed to a point where invasion can be detected with a sensitivity of more than 90% of clinically evident carcinoma.[31,32] Here its main value is to distinguish a carcinoma that is confined to the rectal wall from one that has penetrated the muscularis propria. In the case of villous adenoma, ultrasound is less accurate in identifying the presence of a focus of invasion into the submucosa. Clinical examination remains the mainstay of assessment.

Adenoma With Invasion. In cases of adenoma with evident malignant invasion, the choice of operation will depend on the level of the lesion from the anal verge and is discussed in detail in Chapter 39 in the section on local excision. If anterior resection is feasible, then this is the procedure of choice. Where the lesion is in the lower rectum, the choice lies between a total anorectal extirpation or local excision. This choice will depend on the extent of the malignant invasion both in terms of depth and surface area. It will also be influenced by any evidence of regional lymphadenopathy. At the present time, digital palpation, although only about 50% sensitive,[33] is as useful as any other method of assessment. Ultrasound and computed tomography can detect enlarged nodes but cannot determine their content any more accurately than digital examination. Where malignant invasion is evident, a biopsy of the hard area should be undertaken to assess the histologic grade. If poorly differentiated, a major resection is preferred to a local excision.

Adenoma Without Invasion. Benign adenomas in the rectum, unless very extensive, can be removed by local excision. In all patients, full examination of the large bowel is mandatory. Polypoid adenomas should be removed by colonoscopic snare polypectomy along with any synchronous polyps in the colon. In the uncommon circumstance of malignant invasion of the stalk being reported by the pathologist, or if excision of the polyp was incomplete, then a surgical resection of the area of rectal wall at the base of the polyp should be carried out. The resulting specimen must be submitted for histologic examination. Further action should be determined according to the criteria for local excision.

Submucous Excision

Endoanal Approach

An adenoma 25 mm or more in diameter not suitable for snare polypectomy should be removed by local submucous excision when it is in range of an endoanal approach. It is suitable for most growths up to 10 cm from the anal verge. In some cases, lesions more proximal can be treated where the rectum is mobile and the configuration of the buttocks allows access. The upper level of accessibility is somewhat variable depending on the mobility of the rectum. Sometimes it is possible to produce sufficient intussusception of the rectum by traction to enable adenomas as proximal as the rectosigmoid junction to be removed. Thus, the feasibility depends considerably on the build of the patient. In a doubtful case it is reasonable after discussion with the patient to attempt endoanal removal. If this proves not to be possible, then an abdominal operation can be carried out immediately. Circumferential extent is not a contraindication to submucosal excision. It is possible using the submucosal excision technique to remove large villous adenomas, including those that are circumferential, provided there is adequate longitudinal access.

The pathology of a noninvasive adenoma permits complete removal by dissection in the submucosal plane. The technique described by Parks[34] uses the principle of injection of saline into the submucosal plane to separate the mucosa bearing the lesion from the underlying circular layer of the muscularis propria.

Operative Technique

Endoanal surgery requires certain conditions to minimize the difficulty of working in a confined space. The principles are common to all surgery and, because of their simplicity, are of the most basic importance. First, the position of the patient should be such as to allow the surgeon to be comfortable sitting upright without having to bend or strain. The lithotomy position with about 30° of Trendelenberg tilt is the most suitable, but the key is to ensure elevation of the operating table to bring the anus level with the surgeon's eyes when sitting comfortably. The second condition is lighting. Background illumination should be replaced by a high-intensity headlight. The third is the availability of suitable instruments. They should all be long to avoid the hands obscuring the field. The scissors should be sharp-tipped. This will enable great precision in dissection without the tips slipping back from the tissues. Suction is not necessary and can traumatize the mucosa, impairing vision. Keeping the field free of blood by applying swabs held on dissecting forceps is preferable. Exposure using an anal retractor that will open up the lower rectum can be achieved with various models. Parks' design gives good access to the lower rectum, particularly when the third blade is added. The Eisenhammer speculum has the advantage of having rigid, nonflexible blades that diverge giving good exposure as the instrument is opened. A Mayo table placed between the surgeon and the patient is essential. The towel covering it should be folded up and clipped to the perineal skin.

The retractor is inserted and the lower rectum exposed. This is achieved by placing stay sutures into the mucosa about 10 mm away from the edge of the tumor encompassing its entire circumference (Fig 21-1). The submucosal plane is then infiltrated by an injection of saline containing adrenaiine in a dilution of 1:300,000. The mucosa is elevated from the muscularis propria and the adrenaline reduces bleeding owing to its vasoconstrictor effect. Excision then starts at the lower border of the tumor using sharp scissor dissection (Fig. 21-2). An incision is made parallel to the lower edge of the tumor into normal mucosa to give a 10-mm margin of clearance. The edematous submucosal space is then entered and this plane is developed, identifying the fibers of the circular muscle of the rectum. As the tumor is gradually freed, the mucosal excision is continued laterally around each side until the upper margin is reached. Appropriate traction on the stay sutures facilitates exposure and submucosal vessels are coagulated with diathermy (Fig. 21-3). Dissection with the diathermy cautery can be almost bloodless.

With a circumferential lesion, the same principle is adopted to remove a cylinder of mucosa. In cases where the tumor extends more than about 8 cm proximal to the anus, difficulties of exposure can be encountered. It may be possible to prolapse the upper rectum downward by traction on the stay sutures. In some cases, for example, in thin elderly females, lesions as high as the rectosigmoid junction may come down to the anal level to allow safe submucosal removal. In others, particularly in males with muscular buttocks, it may be impossible to gain access. Further dissection can be dangerous and in this circumstance an abdominal approach should be undertaken.

Occasionally during the dissection the submucosal plane is found to be obliterated at a certain point. This suggests the possibility of a focal area of malignant invasion. The operator should then circumvent the dilemma by taking the dissection through the full thickness of the rectal wall at this point. The resulting defect in the rectal wall is then repaired. Even in cases in which the rectal wall is not breached, the mucosal defect left after excision is closed to ensure hemostasis.

The excised specimen must be oriented for the pathologist. A convenient method for doing so is to pin it out onto a cork board, recreating as far as possible its gross morphology. The cork is then placed upside down in a container of formalin (10%) and the specimen is allowed to fix for 24 hours (Fig. 21-4).

Postoperatively, the patient is given a mild laxative and can be discharged from the hospital when the bowels are open. Complications include hemorrhage, which can be reactionary or secondary, and urinary retention. If the pathologist finds malignant invasion, further action is dependent on certain factors.

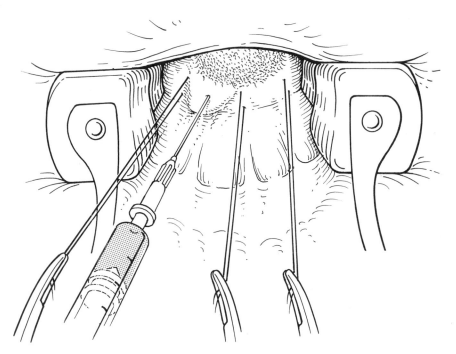

Figure 21-1. Exposure of lower rectum. Infiltration of the submucosa with saline and adreniline (1:300,000) solution after placement of stay sutures.

These include the completeness of excision at the point of invasion and the histologic grade. Incomplete excision or a poorly differentiated grade are indications for major surgery forthwith (Ch. 39).

Posterior Approaches

It is also possible to carry out the procedure via a posterior rectotomy as described originally by Kraske[35] and subsequently modified by division of the sphincters by D'Allaines[36] and more

recently by Mason.[37] The original operation described by Kraske involved removal of the coccyx and part of the sacrum. Subsequent developments have avoided this step by division of the puborectalis and external sphincter,[36,37] or removal of the coccyx with avoidance of sphincter division through a transverse excision.[38]

All give good exposure to the lower rectum but less so to the middle and upper rectum. They all involve opening the rectum to remove the adenoma. This has the disadvantage of risking local implantation of carcinoma should a focus of malig-

Figure 21-2. Submucosal excision of adenoma.

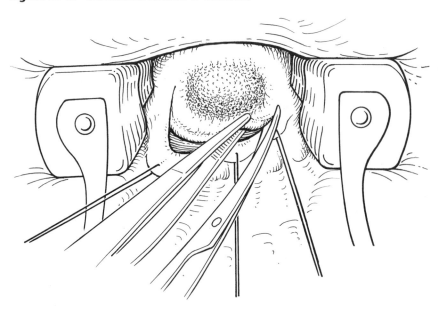

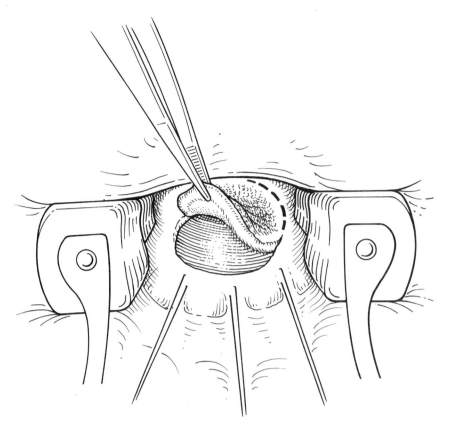

Figure 21-3. Completion of excision. Note fibers of circular muscle of rectum in base of wound.

nant invasion be present in the adenoma. It is known that perforation of the rectum or colon during surgery for carcinoma significantly increases the rate of local recurrence.[39] A deliberate surgical perforation as occurs with all posterior techniques must increase this risk.

It is difficult to judge the present place of the posterior approach. Adenomas of the lower rectum can almost all be removed endoanally and those more proximal by a major restorative resection. Perhaps the posterior approach should be reserved for the occasional adenoma inaccessible to endoanal removal in a patient unfit to tolerate major surgery.

Posterior techniques involve division of the levator to expose Waldeyer's fascia and the mesorectum anteriorly. The lower rectum is mobilized by lateral dissection and opened. The ade-

Figure 21-4. Excised specimen pinned onto cork board for fixation before histopathologic examination.

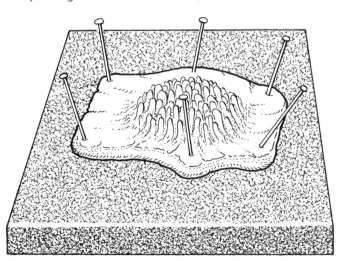

noma is then removed by submucosal excision as already described and presented to the pathologist in a similar manner. The rectotomy is closed and the rest of the wound is closed in layers. With the transsphincteric operation, the divided edges of the levator ani, puborectalis, and external sphincter are repaired individually.

Transanal Endoscopic Microsurgery

Buess has developed a technique that enables surgery on the rectum to be carried out via a closed endoanal approach.[40] Special instruments are required and these are manipulated by the operator through a closed endoscopic system. The equipment includes an operating rectoscope with a 40-mm outside diameter with a gas insufflation facility and stereoscopic optical system. The instruments, including scissors, forceps, needle holder, and diathermy probes, are inserted through dedicated ports and manipulated externally. With this technique, it is possible to carry out submucosal or full-thickness excision with suture closure of the defect. Buess et al.[40] reported the results of 75 patients, 68 with an adenoma and 7 with a carcinoma, with lesions from 4 to 22 cm from the anal verge. Complications occurred in 3 (4%) patients and included perforation (1), bleeding (1), and wound dehiscence (1). There was no mortality. For a further discussion of this technique see Chapter 39.

Follow-Up

Patients should be followed postoperatively to detect recurrence or the development of metachronous adenomas or carcinoma. This should probably be done annually and includes a colonoscopy with particular attention to the site of previous removal and the presence of any new adenoma. In a series of 24 patients treated by submucosal excision, the recurrence rate of adenoma in the vicinity of the surgical scar at 2 years was 15%.[41] It was somewhat less in a larger series of 30 patients in whom a focus of malignant invasion was present in 5 (17%) cases, where excision was extended to full-thickness removal of the rectal wall at the site of focal malignant invasion. At a mean follow-up of 3 years from treatment, 3 (10%) recurrent adenomas had occurred. Each case was amenable to subsequent local excision.[42] In a much larger series of 174 patients with a villous tumor of the colon or rectum treated over a 5-year period, Christiansen et al,[43] reported a 30% recurrence rate at 5 years. Recurrences in the vicinity of the original lesion can usually be treated by another submucous removal. If small, diathermy or laser destruction[44] should be attempted.

Anterior Resection

For adenomas too proximal for endoanal removal and too large for safe TEM, anterior resection is indicated. This operation avoids the difficulties of inadequate visualization due to bleeding that may occur when access from below is difficult. It also has the merit of achieving a satisfactory local and regional clearance where malignant invasion proves subsequently to be present.

In cases with an adenoma so extensive as to involve most of the rectum, major resection should also be attempted. Where a large adenoma extends down to or beyond the anorectal junction, a combination of anterior resection and endoanal stripping for the most distal mucosa can be used. The anal sphincter mechanism is preserved and intestinal continuity restored by a coloanal anastomosis. This reconstruction can be made after forming a colonic reservoir or simply by using a straight limb of descending colon.

Technique

Technical aspects of standard anterior resection are well described. The principles adopted for an adenoma are no different from carcinoma. The abdomen is opened and the rectum mobilized to the level of the pelvic floor. Judging the level of the lower border of the tumor to ensure complete removal may be difficult, because the lesion is often too soft to be palpable through the rectal wall from the outside. It may be necessary, therefore, to pass a sigmoidoscope before division of the gut to be sure there is adequate distal clearance. Before division of the rectum, the surgeon dissects the most distal portion of the adenoma via an endoanal approach to a point above the level of abdominal mobilization. The technique used is identical to that described for submucosal excision. Having achieved distal mobilization, the rectum is divided at the level of the anorectal junction and the specimen is removed. The splenic flexure is mobilized and the left colon brought down within the anal canal. An endoanal anastomosis is then made between colon and the anal epithelium using interrupted sutures, taking the full thickness of the former and an ample bite of the latter. The operation is covered with a diverting loop stoma, which is closed some 8 weeks later provided anastomotic healing is satisfactory.

Complications include anastomotic breakdown which occurs in 5% to 30% of cases, but only in a minority (5%) is it not possible to close the stoma.[45] Function is satisfactory in the majority with an average frequency of defecation of around 3 times per 24 hours but with a range of 1 to 8. Some improvement in this can be achieved by adding a colonic reservoir to the reconstruction.[46] This reduces the likelihood of high stool frequency with a range extending up to about 4 times per 24 hours.[47-49] Long-term results in terms of local recurrence have not been reported after this procedure.

REFERENCES

1. Ansher AF, Lewis JH, Fleischer DE et al (1989) Hyperplastic colonic polyps as a marker for adenomatous colonic polyps. Am J Gastroenterol 84:113
2. Williams GT, Arthur JF, Bussey HJR, Morson BC (1980) Metaplastic polyps and polyposis of the colorectum. Histopathology 4:155–170
3. Jass JR, Williams CB, Morson BC, Bussey HJR (1987) Juvenile polyposis—a precancerous condition. Gut 28:A1367
4. Shepherd NA, Bussey HJR, Jass JR (1987) Epithelial misplacement in Peutz-Jeghers polyps: a diagnostic pitfall. Am J Surg Pathol 11:743–749
5. Giardiello FM, Welsh SB, Hamilton SR et al (1987) Increased

risk of cancer in Peutz-Jeghers syndrome. *N Engl J Med* 316: 1511–1514

6. Spigelman AD, Murday J, Phillips RKS (1989) Cancer and the Peutz-Jeghers syndrome. *Gut* 30:1588–1590

7. Eide TJ (1991) Natural history of adenomas. World J Surg 15: 3–6

8. Clark JC, Collan Y, Eide TJ et al (1985) Prevalence of polyps in autopsy scans from areas with varying incidence of large bowel cancer. Int J Cancer 36:179

9. Sato E, Ouchi A, Sasano N, Ishidate T (1976) Polyps and diverticulosis of large bowel in autopsy population of Akita prefecture compared with Miyagi. Cancer 37:1316

10. Rickert RR, Auerbach O, Garfunkel L et al (1979) Adenomatous lesions of the large bowel. An autopsy survey. Cancer 43: 1847

11. Williams AR, Balasooriya BAW, Day DW (1982) Polyps and cancer of the large bowel; a necropsy study in Liverpool. Gut 23:835

12. Atkin WS, Morson BC, Cuzick J (1992) Long term risk of colorectal cancer after excision of recto sigmoid adenomas. N Engl J Med 326:658–662

13. Grossman S, Milos ML, Tikawa IS, Jewell NP (1989) Colonoscopic screening of persons with suspected risk factors of colon cancer II. Past history of colorectal neoplasms. Gastroenterology 96:299–306

14. Gatterschi B, Costantini M, Bruzzi P et al (1991) Univariate and multivariate analyses of the relationship between adenocarcinoma and solitary and multiple adenomas in colorectal adenoma patients. Int J Cancer 49:509–512

15. Zarchy TM, Ersholt D (1994) Do characteristics of adenomas on flexible sigmoidoscopy predict advances in baseline colonoscopy? Gastroenterology 106:1501–1504

16. Williams CB (1985) Polyp follow-up: how, who for and how often? Br J Surg 72:525–526

17. Bailey CJ, Bodmer WK, Bussey HJR et al (1987) Localization of the gene for familial adenomatous polyposis on chromosome 5. Nature 328:614–616

18. Gardner EJ (1951) A genetic and clinical study of intestinal polyposis predisposing factor for carcinoma of the colon and rectum. Am J Human Genet 3:167

19. Berk T, Cohen Z, McLeod RS, Parker JA (1988) Congenital hypertrophy of the retinal pigment epithelium as a marker for familial adenomatous polyposis. Dis Colon Rectum 51: 253–257

20. Blair NP, Temple CL Hypertrophy of the retinal pigment epithelium associated with Gardner's syndrome. Am J

21. Morson BC, Whiteway JE, Jones FA et al (1984) Histopathology and prognosis of malignant colorectal polyps treated by endoscopic polypectomy. Gut 25:437

22. Nivatvongs S, Goldberg SM (1978) Management of patients who have polyps containing invasive carcinoma removed via colonoscopy. Dis Colon Rectum 21:8

23. Christie JP (1988) Polypectomy or colectomy? Management of 106 consecutively encountered colorectal polyps. Am Surg 54:93

24. Cooper HS, Deppish LM, Gourley WK et al (1995) Endoscopically removed malignant colorectal polyps clinicopathological correlations. Gastroenterology 108:1657–1665

25. Volk EE, Goldblum JR, Petras RE et al (1995) Management and outcome of patients with invasive carcinoma arising in colorectal polyps. Gastroenterology 109:1801–1807

26. Nivatvongs S, Rojanasakul A, Reimann HM et al (1989) The

27. Hackelsberger A, Fruhmorgen P, Weiler H et al (1995) Endoscopic polypectomy and management of colorectal adenomas with invasive carcinoma. Endoscopy 27:153–158

28. Muto T, Kamiya J, Sawada T et al (1985) Small flat adenoma of the large bowel with special reference to its clinicopatholgoical features. Dis Colon Rectum 28:847–851

29. Gillespie PE, Chambers TJ, Chan KW, Williams CB (1979) Colonic adenomas—a colonoscopic survey. Gut 20:240

30. Muto T, Bussey HJR, Morson BC (1975) The evolution of cancer of the colon and rectum. Cancer 36:2251

31. Hildebrand T, Feifel G, Schwarz HP, Scherr O (1986) Endorectal ultrasound: instrumentation and clinical aspects. Int J Colorectal Dis 1:203

32. Beynon J, Foy DMA, Roe AM et al (1986) Endoluminal ultrasound in the assessment of local invasion in rectal cancer. Br J Surg 73:474

33. Nicholls RJ, Mason AY, Morson BC et al (1982) The clinical staging of rectal cancer. Br J Surg 69:404

34. Parks AG, (1966) Benign tumours of the rectum. pp. 541–548. In Roe C, Smith R, Morgan CN (eds): Clinical Surgery. Vol. 10, Abdomen, Rectum and Anus. London, Butterworths

35. Kraske P (1885) Zur Extirpation hochsitzender Mast darmkrebse. Verh Gas Chir 14:464, 1885

36. D'Allaines F (1956) Die chirurgische Behandlung des Rektum Karzinomas. Leipzig, Barth

37. Mason AY (1975) Malignant tumours of the rectum: local excision. Clin Gastroenterol 4:582, 1975

38. Localio SA, Gouge TH, Ransom JHC (1978) Abdomino-sacral resection for carcinoma of the midrectum; 10 years experience. Ann Surg 188:745

39. Phillips RKS, Hittinger R, Blesovsky L et al (1984) Local recurrence following "curative" surgery for large bowel cancer. The overall picture. Br J Surg 71:12

40. Buess G, Kipfmuller K, Narnhus M (1987) Endoscopic microscopy of rectal tumours. Endoscopy, 19, suppl. 1:38

41. Thomson JPS (1977) Treatment of sessile villous and tubular adenomas of the rectum. Experience of St. Mark's Hospital 1963–1972. Dis Colon Rectum 20:467

42. Parks AG, Stuart AE (1973) The management of villous tumours of the large bowel. Br J Surg 60:688

43. Christiansen J, Kirkegaard P, Ibsen J (1979) Prognosis after treatment of villous adenomas of the colon and rectum. Ann Surg 189:404

44. Krasner N (1989) Laser therapy in the management of benign and malignant tumours in the colon and rectum. Int J Colorectal Dis 4:2

45. Parks AG, Percy JP (1982) Resection and sutured colo-anal anastomosis for rectal cancer. Br J Surg 69:301

46. Lazorthes F, Farges P, Chiotasso P et al (1986) Resection of the rectum with construction of a colonic reservoir and coloanal anastomosis for carcinoma of the rectum. Br J Surg 73:136

47. Parc R, Tiret E, Frileaux P et al (1986) Resection and coloanal anastomosis with colonic reservoir for rectal carcinoma. Br J Surg 73:139

48. Nicholls RJ, Lubowski DZ, Donaldson D (1988) Comparison of colonic reservoir and straight colo-anal reconstruction after rectal excision. Br J Surg 75:318

49. Seow Choen F, Goh HS (1995) Prospective randomised trial comparing J colonic pouch-anal anastomoses and straight coloanal reconstruction. Br J Surg 82:608–610

HEREDITARY GASTROINTESTINAL POLYPOSIS SYNDROMES

Theresa Berk

Zane Cohen

Classification of gastrointestinal polyposis syndromes, both familial and nonfamilial, is determined by histology, which, in turn, is a prerequisite for appropriate patient management. The descriptive term "polyp" has been used generically for benign and malignant tumors although not all polyps are tumors. Polyp syndromes may be misclassified clinically because of their rarity or microscopically due to the lack of histologic confirmation.

Although the adenoma-carcinoma sequence[1] has been well described for the neoplastic syndrome, familial adenomatous polyposis (FAP), seemingly innocuous non-neoplastic polyp syndromes may carry an associated cancer risk. Goodman et al.[2] proposed an evolutionary pathogenetic link. It begins with a genetic and/or environmental promoter in the gastrointestinal tract, resulting in localized mucosal hyperplasia and eventual small hyperplastic polyps. Inflammation and cystic dilatation lead to hamartomas and further epithelial atypia. Adenomatous characteristics may appear within the hamartomas. Depending on the severity of epithelial dysplasia, the metamorphosis to adenoma and frank carcinoma complete the chain. The overlap of histologic boundaries is evident and it may be that the clinical distinctions will not be as significant as any molecular similarities. Unfortunately, the lack of known genetic defects responsible for rare hamartomatous syndromes has prevented prognostic management strategies from being developed.

Following a description of gastrointestinal polyp syndromes, the FAP model will demonstrate a paradigm for genetic technology in current diagnosis. The impact of genetic registers in guiding policy issues for predictive testing in FAP will be outlined. Studies quoted in this chapter are for the most part registry-based to indicate the value of long-term consistent ascertainment. Management issues in FAP will address surgical options and the debate of prophylaxis versus clinical indications, therapeutic treatment for extracolonic manifestations, and long-term cancer risk.

GASTROINTESTINAL POLYP SYNDROMES

Inflammatory Polyposis

Until the introduction of the microscope and the development of histopathology in the 1860s, there was no distinction between pseudopolyps caused by inflammation and those with no obvious trauma. Inflammatory polyposis is the most common sequelae of ulcerative colitis but also occurs in Crohn's disease, diverticulitis, and parasitic conditions.

Lymphoid polyps, generally 1 to 2 mm in diameter, are enlarged lymphoid follicles and may develop in response to mucosal or submucosal inflammation, often in the ileum and lower rectum of adolescents and young adults.[3] Radiologically, lymphoid polyps resemble adenomas in FAP, leading occasionally to inappropriate colectomy when not biopsied.[4] This scenario is of particular concern when it occurs in first-degree relatives from families with a documented history of FAP.

Metaplastic Polyposis

First described in 1980, these 1 to 5-mm hyperplastic lesions are characterized by a pale serrated appearance and no dysplasia.[5] Clinically, metaplastic polyposis has been confused with FAP due to the large numbers of polyps, averaging from 50 to 100, visualized on radiographs. Reports of both synchronous adenomas and adenocarcinoma in metaplastic polyps larger than 1-cm have suggested that size may be indicative of a separate syndrome, serrated adenomatous polyposis, with a spectrum of morphologic change.[6]

Hamartomatous Syndromes

The following disorders all include polyps, recognized as hamartomas, composed of normal intestinal epithelium that is present in abnormal amount and configuration.

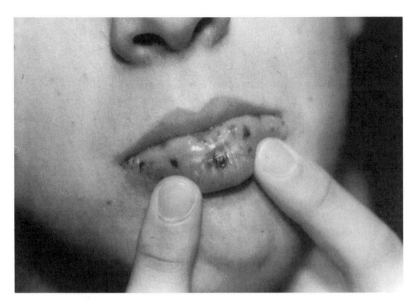

Figure 21-5. Lip pigmentation in a patient with Peutz-Jeghers syndrome.

Peutz-Jeghers Syndrome

First described by Hutchinson in 1896[7] but clarified by Peutz in 1921[8] and by Jeghers et al. in 1949,[9] Peutz-Jeghers syndrome (PJS) is a combination of skin pigmentation and hamartomatous gastrointestinal polyps. The brown/black melanin lesions are congenital, mostly perioral (Fig. 21-5), buccal, and on the dorsal aspects of the fingers and toes. The danger of basing a diagnosis on these lesions is their tendency to fade with age. In our center, two siblings from the Far East, both in their 30s, were misdiagnosed with an inflammatory parasitic disease because of the absence of the telltale freckling. Clinical history revealed that both patients were born with strongly pigmented features on the lips. Although harmless, excessive freckling can cause psychosocial problems for afflicted adolescents, many of whom are now successfully treated by laser.

From 50 to 100 polyps may develop after puberty. Because they occur predominantly in the small intestine and range in size from 1 to 5 cm, the most common presenting symptom is small bowel intussusception with abdominal cramping and bleeding leading to obstruction and severe anemia. Occasionally, obstruction may occur in the colon.[10] In many patients with PJS, occult bleeding may be significant and require transfusion. Between chronic obstructive episodes, patients remain otherwise asymptomatic. Current approaches by some registries include clearing gastroduodenal and colonic polyps larger than 0.5 mm by endoscopy and by intraoperative endoscopy for polyps larger than 15 mm.[11]

The cancer risk in PJS has been widely debated.[12–14] The unusual histologic presentation of normal epithelium overlapping muscle may create a misinterpretation of cancer. However, two recent registry series did find evidence of long-term intestinal and extraintestinal cancer, which obviously has implications for patient management. The first review from Johns Hopkins Hospital of 31 patients in 13 PJS families recorded 15 of 31 (48%) of patients with cancer, identified an average of 25 years after their PJS diagnosis.[15] Of interest is that 11 of 15 (73%) of patients, age range 38 to 60 years, had cancers of the

pancreas, breast, or ovary—areas without synchronous hamartomas. Comparing those 15 cancers with age- and sex-matched general population cancer incidence rates in the United States, an 18-fold increase was recorded. The second review from St. Mark's Hospital identified 16 of 72 (22%) of patients with cancer and a mortality rate of 94% in 15 of 16 patients.[11] The average age of death was 38 years. The relative risk of dying of cancer was 48% by age 57. Interestingly, in the first series, 4 of 15 cancers were gastrointestinal but no cancer was found within hamartomas. One family was reported with both hamartomas and adenomas. In the second series, 9 of 16 patients were diagnosed with gastrointestinal cancer and 4 of 16 had cancer within hamartomas. Again, the hypothesis of a genetic predisposition or cyclical evolution is raised.

Screening of PJS patients for intestinal and extraintestinal malignancy may be most effective when confined to those cancers with the highest incidence and easiest intervention. Biennial colonoscopy, gastroduodenoscopy, and small bowel enema for gastrointestinal cancers have been advocated by registries involved in long-term follow-up and epidemiologic studies on PJS patients. For affected women at risk for gynecologic malignancies, annual cervical biopsy with biennial pelvic ultrasound and mammography may be suggested. For prepubertal boys with PJS, testicular ultrasound has been carried out.[11] Alternatively, screening may be initiated for other family members with PJS only when an extraintestinal cancer is diagnosed.

PJS is an autosomal-dominant disorder that occurs in both patients with and without a family history. Management of affected families may be easier in the future with the localization of the Peutz-Jeghers syndrome gene.[16a] One-time colonoscopy and gastroscopy is presently recommended for the unaffected parents and siblings of a patient with PJS.

Juvenile Polyposis

Solitary juvenile polyps, once known as mucus retention polyps from their cystic appearance, are common in children, particularly in the rectum. The rarer florid form, juvenile polyposis

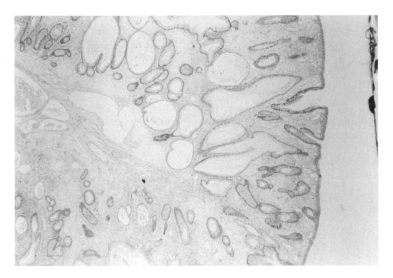

Figure 21-6. Juvenile polyp—microscopic appearance.

(JP), has historically been mistaken for FAP from 1882 when the polyps of two siblings were described by Cripps.[16] Histologically, these 5- to 50-mm hamartomas lack smooth muscle, with only one epithelial cell layer that is easily inflamed and results in rectal bleeding[17] (Fig. 21-6). Questions about how to define JP, described more fully by McColl et al. in 1964,[18] have been complicated by the finding of adenomas within, and contiguous to, juvenile polyps as well as adenocarcinoma. Associated congenital anomalies include heart defects, hydrocephalus, malrotation of the gut, cleft palate, and polydactyly. JP is often diagnosed in adolescence or early adulthood. Clinicians may find it difficult to distinguish JP from solitary juvenile polyps in children but the tendency is for true cases to present with more polyps at an earlier age. The general criteria include five juvenile gastrointestinal polyps but that limit may drop to three in someone with a confirmed family history of JP. From 50 to 200 juvenile polyps may develop, mostly in the colon and stomach, hence the initial confusion with FAP. However, polyps in JP are traditionally less clustered and the colonic mucosa between polyps more histologically normal than in FAP.[19]

Concerns about cancer risk in JP occurred despite its initial classification as a non-neoplastic syndrome.[20,21] Until associated adenocarcinoma was found, patients were not monitored closely for epithelial dysplasia which, according to Jass,[19] occurs in approximately 47% of JP patients. One registry case referred as an FAP patient died of rectal cancer. In this case, juvenile polyps with contiguous adenomas and adenocarcinoma were confirmed on histologic review. In the interim, one of two affected children was born with a ventricular septal defect and has since developed juvenile polyps.[4] A St. Mark's Hospital Registry review recorded 18 of 87 (21%) patients, age range 15 to 59 years, with JP and colorectal cancer, the majority of whom had already undergone colectomy.[19] The Helsinki Registry reported 5 of 18 (28%) similarly affected patients, age range 37 to 49 years. In this series, gastric cancer was also observed.[22]

The association with juvenile gastric polyps and epithelial dysplasia reinforces the need for both colonoscopy and upper gastrointestinal tract screening. Follow-up intervals are determined by polyp number, grade, and size. In the absence of a family history, one-time colonoscopy is suggested for at-risk parents and siblings of affected patients.

Is prophylactic colectomy and ileorectal anastomosis indicated for JP? Based on the St. Mark's Hospital series, patients who were cancer-free when registered had a cumulative cancer risk of 68% by age 60.[19] More effective and easier management of the rectal remnant, better cancer prevention, and increased patient compliance with sigmoidoscopy rather than colonoscopy are potential surgical benefits. However, in the absence of clinical indications, at present there is not enough long-term cancer data available to recommend prophylactic colectomy in this patient population.

JP is believed to be an autosomal-dominant disorder. According to Jarvinen,[22] the incidence of isolated cases of JP ranges from 43% to 75%, leading to speculation that more new mutations may exist than are now known for FAP.[22] Recent linkage analysis studies have excluded tumor-suppressor genes APC (adenomatous polyposis coli) and MCC (mutated in colorectal cancer).[23,24] Jass[19] has observed an inflammatory process and overgrowth of the epithelium that is most vulnerable early in life and less so with advancing age. A genetic defect controlling both foundation-supporting tissues and epithelium may account for the variable congenital defects as well as variable polyp expression in JP.[19] A recent report of a mixed polyposis syndrome with atypical juvenile polyps, adenomas, and adenocarcinoma describes how the anomaly was mapped to a new locus, unrelated to the APC gene.[25] It is anticipated that these anomalous families will provide molecular clues to their etiology.

Cronkhite-Canada Syndrome

Cronkhite-Canada syndrome, first described in 1955, refers to 1- to 2-mm hamartomatous polyps of the gastrointestinal tract, specifically the stomach and colon, along with ectodermal changes, namely, hair loss, nail atrophy, and skin pigmentation.[26] Of note, adenomas and colorectal carcinoma have been observed.[27] The most common symptoms are intussusception and gastrointestinal bleeding. Mortality is proportional to the degree of the most common complication, diarrhea, which may result in malabsorption and protein-losing enteropathy. Treatment is generally therapeutic with nutritional and electrolyte support, antibiotics, or steroids. Speculation about its etiology includes an infectious process, immunity impairment, or nutritional deficiency disorder. Cronkhite-Canada syndrome has been suggested as a variant of JP, despite its adult onset and lack of hereditary pattern.

Ruvalcaba-Myhre-Smith Syndrome

Reported in 1980, Ruvalcaba-Myhre-Smith syndrome refers to hamartomas of the colon and ileum, pigmentation of the penis, and macrocephaly. In some cases, developmental delay, lipid storage disorder, and prominent corneal nerves have been recorded.[28] Typical presenting symptoms include bleeding and abdominal pain due to ulceration or obstruction, often in childhood. There is no strong evidence of gastric/small bowel polyps or gastrointestinal cancer. Histologically, the hamartomas appear to be juvenile polyps and this syndrome may be another variant of JP.[29,30]

Cowden's Disease

Cowden's disease, also known as multiple hamartoma syndrome when reported in 1963, is characterized by multiple 1- to 4-mm connective tissue polyps of the skin and gastrointestinal tract, notably the rectosigmoid region.[31] Developmental anomalies may occur. Most commonly, papillomas of the face and oral areas as well as keratoses of the extremities are seen. Other skin lesions include pigment changes, lipomas, hemangiomas, and neuromas. The colorectal cancer risk is not known but adenomas and colonic adenocarcinoma have been reported. Histologically, an admixture of lymphoid, inflammatory, and juvenile polyps has been recorded. Screening with colonoscopy, gastroscopy, and small bowel enema is contingent on number, size, and grade of polyp involvement. Breast and thyroid adenomas or cancers have raised concerns with regard to breast and thyroid screening.[32] However, despite its autosomal-dominant mode of inheritance, neither the incidence nor the etiology of Cowden's disease is known.

Neoplastic Syndromes

Familial Adenomatous Polyposis

Although FAP accounts for less than 1% of all colorectal cancers, it has provided knowledge about carcinogenesis in the general population and about colon cancer in particular. The first report of FAP by Sklifosovski in 1881[33] was followed by discovery of its genetic origin,[34] association with cancer,[35] and autosomal-dominant mode of inheritance.[36]

Histologically, FAP is characterized by multiple adenomas, averaging less than 5 mm in diameter, the oft-cited number of 100 varying according to the age of the patient. Because puberty is the general age of onset, an adolescent with less than 10 adenomas and a confirmed family history of FAP must be considered as affected. There is no histologic difference between adenomas in FAP and those in the general population, but clinically, both number and transition are distinct. Controversy about apparent rectal sparing in FAP has sparked the search for and identification of microadenomas in grossly normal rectal mu-

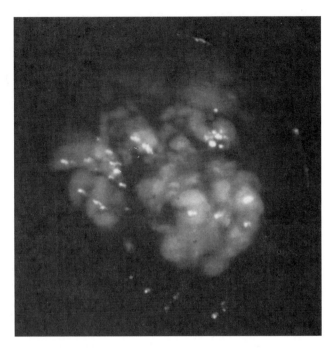

Figure 21-7. Colonoscopic appearance of adenomas in familial adenomatous polyposis.

cosa. This emphasizes the potential role of random biopsy on either flexible or rigid sigmoidoscopy[37] (Figs. 21-7 to 21-9).

Prompted by a mortality rate of greater than 90% in early cases of FAP, pathologic research began on the natural history of the adenoma.[38] Morson and Bussey[39] identified a progressive sequence of epithelial dysplasia with adenomatous tissue at the margins of intestinal cancers, establishing the adenoma as a cancer precursor. Based on their St. Mark's Hospital series of 617 cases, the average diagnosed patient with FAP already had cancer by age 39 years.[38] Their findings would have implications for the management of solitary colorectal cancer in the future. The difference is highlighted in the approximate 25-year earlier age span between the diagnosis of bowel cancer in FAP patients and in the general population. Recent studies have shown that screening of at-risk first-degree relatives establishes a diagnosis by age 16 years[40] and treatment by age 20 years.[41]

In 1951, Gardner described a triad of skin, soft tissue, and bony lesions, all benign, in FAP patients, prompting a subset of the disease to be called Gardner's syndrome.[42] Investigators continued to search beyond the colon for associated lesions such as pigmented retinal lesions, which were a useful predictor for FAP prior to molecular testing.[43] As colorectal cancer mortality declined in at-risk screened patients, additional lesions, many of them malignant, were being diagnosed in affected families. The growing list nullified a standardized definition of Gardner's syndrome. There was no observable pattern within a family for what became known as extracolonic manifestations (ECM) and the eponym created confusion about appropriate management as well as greater anxiety for the ''different'' affected relative. Over the years, clinicians have realized that there is no distinction between the pathology of the colorectal adenomas in affected patients. Acknowledgment of familial polyposis as a systemic disorder was prompted by the formation of an international body in 1985, the Leeds Castle Polyposis

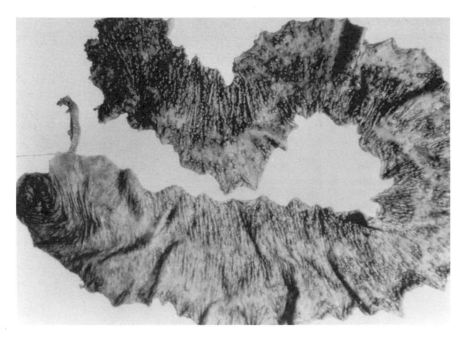

Figure 21-8. Gross appearance of surgical specimen in familial adenomatous polyposis.

Group (LCPG), to promote education and research on FAP.[44] The eponymic debate was resolved in 1991 when the genetic defect was found to be identical for all affected patients.[45] Indeed, there is neither clinical nor molecular significance to the term Gardner's syndrome.

Attenuated Adenomatous Polyposis

Our registry has observed a subset of patients whose phenotype did not quite fit with classic FAP, in that there was a later age of onset of both adenomas and cancer, from age 40 upward; adenomas were fewer in number, often sessile, and 1 to 2 mm in diameter, with apparent rectal sparing. Other observations included fundic gland polyps, occasional duodenal adenomas, and the consistent absence of pigmented retinal lesions.[46,47]

In 1992, this variant was linked to the APC gene and it became clear that the spectrum of the FAP phenotype was enlarging.[48] The inherited predisposition for what became known as attenuated adenomatous polyposis may be overlooked in asymptomatic family members with few adenomas and low expressivity of the gene defect. Consequently, it may be as-

Figure 21-9. Detailed view of surgical specimen in familial adenomatous polyposis.

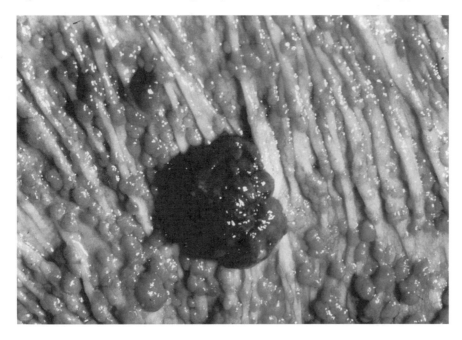

sumed that symptomatic presenting patients are isolated cases. It has been further speculated that a second modifier gene, either linked or not linked to the APC gene, may account for the heterogeneity in numbers of adenomas. A modifier gene might alter the function of the normal APC gene to suppress adenoma formation. This theory might also apply to those in the general population who develop solitary adenomas in later life that evolve to colorectal cancer.[49]

THE IMPACT OF GENETIC REGISTERS

The concept of treating the family as a patient through generational study with the goal of cancer prevention was formalized with the first FAP Registry in 1925. It was planned by pathologist Cuthbert Dukes as a research protocol to describe the histology of colorectal adenomas and was developed by Dick Bussey,[38] setting the standard for successive FAP family study centers. The benefit of focusing on preventive rather than acute care by screening first-degree relatives would not be evident for some years to come. A dramatic reduction of colorectal mortality, generally from 62% in probands to 8% in the call-up children and siblings, has become a registry pattern.[50] This can be contrasted with a 35% incidence of bowel cancer in a center currently treating FAP patients without a registry.[51] Bulow et al.[52] recently reported a 10-year cumulative survival of 94% in call-up cases compared to 41% in probands. Among the advantages of a centralized family study center are the avoidance of record duplication, the option to connect family branches or trace new at-risk family members, and improved survival with local follow-up by monitoring the natural history of FAP.

The registry approach varies by geography, such that stable populations in Denmark, the Netherlands, and Japan have developed national registers with greater than 90% data accession.[53–55] Other parts of Europe, the Far East, Australia, the United States, and Canada have more heterogeneous populations and develop regional centers.[56,57] The need for local registers has been emphasized for reliable epidemiologic data regarding the incidence of FAP, approximately 1 in 10,000.[58,59] The proportion of isolated cases of FAP ranges from 22% to 46% in registry-based studies.[60,61] Penetrance has been calculated as close to 100% by age 40, according to Bisgaard et al.[60] who recently reviewed 156 at-risk children born from 1920 to 1949 who had undergone regular sigmoidoscopy. Eighty-two of 156 children were affected by age 40 and 74 of 156 children over age 40 were clear on clinical follow-up. Reproductive fitness was estimated at 0.87 by comparing these children with those of unaffected age- and sex-matched parents.

The Leeds Castle Polyposis Group now comprises 52 registers in 20 countries. The opportunity to improve standards of care for FAP patients through cooperative study has often been registry-based, resulting in studies on the incidence of upper gastrointestinal tract cancer,[62] the risk of rectal cancer postcolectomy,[63] the Concerted Action Polyposis Prevention chemoprevention study of resistant starch and aspirin for proven APC gene carriers,[64] and, finally, landmark molecular research.[65] A protocol for newly established FAP registries is now available.[66,67]

FAP is one of the few genetic syndromes for which service testing is available and the multidisciplinary approach of a reg-

ister (surgeon, gastroenterologist, pathologist, counselor/social worker, and researchers) can ensure that families receive education and support. Registries can assume an advocacy role to establish health policy for predictive testing, based on their unique liaison between patients and the community.

FAMILIAL ADENOMATOUS POLYPOSIS

Clinical Screening

Early detailed registry pedigrees provided generational proof that the majority of children and siblings are diagnosed from age 15 years to age 25 years.[68] Consequently, screening guidelines were established from age 10 years to age 14 years.[50,69] In our registry, and others, introducing children to the FAP clinic prior to examination is important. FAP clinics are arranged so that both affected family members and at-risk adolescents and siblings can be together, each receiving individual care with generalized support. Flexible sigmoidoscopy remains the screening standard because it is minimally invasive, allows for biopsy, and is generally acceptable to the adolescent. The use of barium enema is discouraged because of the propensity to overlook early-stage 1- to 2-mm adenomas. Colonoscopy is reserved for a positive diagnosis of FAP. One of the major drawbacks to screening has been the lack of compliance by patients subjected to excessive screening. The danger of delaying flexible sigmoidoscopy to early adulthood is twofold: refusal by the typically asymptomatic and body-conscious 20-year-old for a perceived invasive technique; and the risk of bowel cancer in exceptional patients with carpeting of polyps in their colon or rectum.

Follow-up is recommended every 2 years until age 35 and every 3 to 5 years thereafter for at-risk first-degree relatives who have not undergone predictive testing or who are uninformative subsequent to DNA analysis.

Molecular Screening

The discovery of the APC gene on chromosome 5q21–22 marked a turning point in the management of FAP and in the understanding of the earliest molecular stage of colon tumorigenesis in the general population.[70] APC mutations in this extremely large gene with 8,538 nucleotides and 15 exons may result in benign colorectal tumors in approximately 30% of the Western population.[71–73] In the past 5 years, more than 700 genetic mutations have been recognized in the APC gene, the focus being on mutations producing a truncated version of the gene product that inactivates the gene.[74,75] These germline mutations tend to cluster in discrete regions in the first half of the gene and are associated with severity of colorectal adenomas,[76] congenital retinal lesions,[77] and later age of onset.[49]

Genetic heterogeneity has been reported in three unrelated families with a purported although atypical clinical diagnosis of FAP but no APC gene mutation.[78,79] Studies by Paul et al.[80] and Giardiello et al.[81] have demonstrated the heterogeneous clinical nature of extracolonic manifestations, even in families with identical APC mutations. This has led to speculation that environmental factors or interactions between the APC gene and other modifier genes may account for such genotype-phenotype differences. For example, Hamilton[82] has found no correlation between the actual number of colorectal cancers, which is low, and of adenomas, which is high, in FAP. Thus, the adenoma-carcinoma sequence occurs in a comparative minority of polyps, perhaps influenced by a modifier gene, recently identified by Dietrich et al.[83] in a mouse model, called the Multiple Intestinal Neoplasia (MIN) mouse. The discovery of morphologically similar adenomas to those of FAP patients may expedite gene mapping of potential modifiers.[84]

Direct Mutation Analysis and Linkage Analysis

Molecular testing for FAP is currently offered by direct mutation analysis and by indirect linkage analysis. Powell et al.[85] introduced the in vitro synthesized protein (IVSP) assay, which looks directly at the truncated protein product of the APC gene. This technique may account for up to 82% of genetic mutations and requires a single affected individual, thereby making it effective for isolated cases.[85] Because APC mutations may be spread out across the entire coding region in some FAP patients, a combination approach using the IVSP assay and chemical cleavage analysis may be used to target the underlying mutation once a truncating mutation is found.[86]

Linkage analysis requires at least two affected family members, using molecular markers that are closely linked and flanking the APC gene to determine the inheritance pattern. The closer the genetic distance between the markers, the higher the risk. Genetic risk estimates from greater than 95% to 99% probability can be offered in families where such markers are informative. Linkage analysis is possible with archival tissue specimens, an option previously denied families with deceased affected members and only at-risk surviving children.[87] This is a more labor-intensive process and has been found effective in 88% of informative families.[88] The presence or absence of congenital retinal lesions, along with linkage analysis results, may provide some families with a more accurate risk assessment.[61,89]

Screening Guidelines

The clinical protocol for an at-risk individual with a positive APC mutation in our registry and others is biennial flexible sigmoidoscopy until adenomas are diagnosed, followed by colonoscopy until adenoma progression warrants colectomy.[89,90] Patients in whom an APC mutation cannot be identified but who have several affected and available relatives may be informative for molecular linkage. Patients with greater than 95% risk will be monitored with annual flexible sigmoidoscopy. Patients with less than 5% risk will have a baseline flexible sigmoidoscopy at age 10 years and follow-up every 3 to 5 years. Those at intermediate risk, that is, from 5% to 95%, will follow the clinical regimen described earlier. Concerns about sampling errors in centers where commercial laboratories do predictive testing have caused some clinicians to continue clinical screening, irrespective of negative molecular findings, or to select targeted intervals at age 18, 25, and 35 years.[91] In our registry, and others where quality control is maintained with an on-site laboratory, children and siblings who do not carry the APC gene mutation, confirmed on consecutive samples, are not clinically screened for FAP.[88] Patients are counseled about the approximate 5% population risk for colorectal cancer from the age of 50 years.

We initiated a cost-effectiveness study comparing at-risk family members undergoing traditional screening and predictive testing. Direct health care resources for both strategies were measured. Flexible sigmoidoscopy for an at-risk family member, every 2 years from age 10 to age 35 and every 3 years from age 35 to age 50, would cost $8,031 (1995 Canadian dollars). Genetic analysis would amount to $5,161. Annual flexible sigmoidoscopy for APC-gene positive patients would raise that cost to $7,483. Indirect costs such as traveling, time off work, or accommodation were not included in this analysis, which focused on direct procedural related costs. A recent National Cancer Institute Workshop on genetic screening advocated pre- and posttest genetic counseling for at-risk family members so that such issues can be addressed without bias. Quality of life concerns will factor heavily in future risk-benefit analyses of predictive testing in FAP and related hereditary cancer syndromes. In particular, the testing of minors and in vitro testing has been discussed for adult-onset cancer-related disease.[92] In cases where there is no proven medical benefit to the prepubertal child, predictive testing is timed to coincide with the onset of flexible sigmoidoscopy.

Colorectum

Surgery

Timing for Colectomy

With the advent of molecular diagnosis for FAP, the question of prophylactic colectomy is being raised, not in the traditional clinical context, but for positive gene carriers who may not yet have developed adenomas.[93] However, surgical intervention in the absence of clinical indicators, such as more than 10 to 20 grossly visible adenomas, moderate or severe dysplasia, or polyps larger than 5 to 10 mm in diameter, is not currently advocated by our registry or other large centers.[94] FAP is a chronic systemic disorder and patient compliance with long-term surveillance is often contingent on the surgical experience of other affected family members. Consequently, once patients are clinically diagnosed, it is important to tailor the timing of surgery to the individual.[95] In a recent review of newly diagnosed offspring in our registry, 29 of 46 patients (46%) underwent colectomy by age 20, median age 15. It has been our experience that deferring clinically indicated surgery beyond age 20 may result in refusal by the young adult, who is often asymptomatic and removed from parental influence. Unlike inflammatory bowel disease, FAP is a covert disease and it is more commonly the isolated cases that present with symptoms such as rectal bleeding/anemia, diarrhea, or crampy abdominal pain. The isolated cases tend to be diagnosed at a later age, often with moderate to severe dysplasia or even adenocarcinoma.

Colectomy and Ileorectal Anastomosis

Colectomy and ileorectal anastomosis (IRA) is our preferred operative procedure, provided that there is relative rectal sparing of polyps, a rectal cancer does not exist, and that the patient understands the need for future follow-up. Although colectomy and IRA has been standard primary management for FAP in most centers for the past 70 years, controversy about the rectal remnant has grown in recent years. Thomson[44] reviewed the LCPG experience of nine international registries and found 55.8% of 960 patients underwent colectomy and IRA with a morbidity rate of 7.8% and an operative mortality of 1.1%. This contrasts with 9.8% who had restorative proctocolectomy (RPC) with a morbidity rate of 34% and no intraoperative deaths.

One of the major potential risks following colectomy and IRA is the subsequent development of rectal cancer. Contributing risk factors have included a greater than 12 cm length of remaining rectum, length of time (more than 10 years postcolectomy), age greater than 40 years, or preoperative carpeting of polyps in the rectum.[96,97] Debinski et al.[98] reviewed 258 of 317 (81%) of patients after IRA (age range 12 to 64 years) and reported a 2.3-fold risk for rectal cancer and for synchronous cancers in patients with more than 1,000 adenomas. This risk correlated with increased age.

A recent LCPG study found the cumulative incidence of rectal cancer after IRA to be 13.1% at 26 years.[63] In one cohort of 50 patients from 11 registries, the median age at rectal cancer diagnosis was 46 years and the median interval from IRA was 11 years. The median distance from the anal verge to the cancer was 15.0 cm. The frequency of sigmoidoscopy (range less than 6 months to greater than 2 years) was not significant for staging or survival. In a second cohort of 35 patients from the Scandinavian Registry, the relative risk for rectal cancer was 5.2% by age 50 years and 14.1% by age 60 years, emphasizing increased age as a risk factor. The combined mortality risk for primary rectal cancer was 1% at 10 years and 2% at 15 years.

Other registry findings reported a 7% to 24% cumulative risk of rectal cancer by age 50 years and a 29% risk by age 60 years.[96,99,100] In our center, 3 of 104 (3%) of colectomy and IRA patients, age range 56 to 63 years, developed rectal cancer at a mean interval of 26 years. One of the three patients had a Dukes' stage C cancer of the sigmoid colon at the time of colectomy. Following proctectomy in these three patients, there has been no mortality. To decrease the relatively small cancer risk, RPC can be used as an alternate primary procedure or staged following colectomy and IRA.[99] At the present time, we offer colectomy and IRA as a preferred operation to patients who have relative sparing of the rectum with no evidence of dysplasia, as this procedure has a consistently better functional outcome and lower morbidity than RPC.

Restorative Proctocolectomy

General indications for RPC are more than 20 adenomas in the distal 10 cm of rectum and noncompliance with ongoing rectal surveillance. Mesenteric desmoid tumor at the time of surgery may make RPC technically impossible. Purported benefits include restoration of gastrointestinal continuity and sphincter control and, most important, elimination of all at-risk or diseased colorectal mucosa.[101] Total mucosectomy with a hand-sewn ileoanal anastomosis and a loop ileostomy is our preferred option if RPC is undertaken.

Reports of adenocarcinoma after RPC have raised questions about preserving 1 cm of anal canal mucosa to achieve a potentially improved functional result.[102] When using RPC for FAP patients, total mucosectomy is the preferred management. However, Fazio et al.[103] perform a stapled anastomosis while leaving intact only the anal transition zone. They reserve the hand-sewn anastomosis for patients with severe dysplasia and cancer of the middle or upper rectum or colon. Any residual rectal mucosa in FAP patients following RPC requires careful follow-up.[104] Further, ileal mucosa in the neorectum is susceptible to polyp formation, as indicated by Nugent et al.,[105] who identified ileal adenomas from 1 to 7 years postoperatively in 5 of 38 (13%) RPC patients. Thus, the reservoir should be screened for the development of adenomas at serial intervals.

The functional RPC results on 62 FAP patients from the Cleveland Clinic Registry were reviewed from 1983 to 1993, 16 of 62 patients having had previous IRA.[103] Diverting ileostomies were performed in 50 of 60 (80%) patients. Among the more common complications were seepage and increased bowel movements requiring medication while only 5 of 62 (8%) patients were diagnosed with pouchitis. Quality of life was rated as good or excellent by 38 of 40 (95%) of these patients. In another series, the incidence of pouchitis was only 10% in 39 FAP patients and 33% in the same number of ulcerative colitis patients.[106] It is well known that the incidence of pouchitis following RPC is substantially lower in FAP patients than in ulcerative colitis patients.

The use of a one-stage pouch or two-stage procedure with protective loop ileostomy, again, is controversial. Beart and Welling[97] reviewed 48 of 55 FAP patients with ileostomy and 7 of 55 patients without ileostomy from 1981 to 1986, none of whom developed sepsis after RPC. However, small bowel obstruction occurred in 8 of 55 patients and surgery was required in 3 of 8 patients.

In our center, comparison of 104 patients with IRA and 40 patients with RPC, mean age 34, demonstrated more complications related to bowel function in the RPC group. There were no significant differences in quality of life data, although 71 of 104 (68%) IRA patients rated their physical well-being as excellent, compared to 18 of 40 (45%) of RPC patients. Emotional health was rated as 72% for IRA and 55% for RPC (Table 21-1).

Anorectal function in adolescents and young adults has been measured by Perrault et al.,[107] who followed seven FAP patients, median age 16 years, with the two-stage RPC. No complications were reported. Ziv et al.[108] examined the results of 17 adolescents with IRA and 7 adolescents with RPC, age range 10 to 19 years, with a follow-up from 4 to 95 months. Aside

Table 21-1. Comparison of Functional Results for Restorative Proctocolectomy (RPC) and Ileorectal Anastomosis (IRA) Patients in the Steve Atanas Stavro Familial Gastrointestinal Cancer Registry

	RPC N = 40 (%)	IRA N = 104 (%)
Leakage	6 (15)	3 (3)
SBO	12 (30)	16 (15)
Bowel movements	13 (33)	18 (17)
Continence		
Day	22 (55)	87 (84)
Night	14 (35)	87 (84)

Abbreviation: SBO, small bowel obstruction.

from increased operating time and hospital stay for RPC (12 versus 7 days), no significant differences in functional or qualitative results were noted. The surgical indications did not differ for adults or adolescents but consideration should be given to the delay in return to school with a longer recovery time, particularly if a two-stage procedure is contemplated. Intensive pre- and postoperative education is suggested to address body image concerns following any abdominal operative procedure, more so when a temporary or permanent stoma is required.

The Role of Proctocolectomy and Continent Ileostomy

Prior to the use of the continent ileostomy or RPC, total proctocolectomy and Brooke ileostomy was, and still is, considered a curative procedure when colectomy and IRA are not feasible. However, the continent ileostomy is usually not the preferred procedure for adolescents or young adults who are desmoid- or cancer-free. Indications for total proctocolectomy include the presence of cancer in the lower one-third of the rectum or the finding of desmoid tumor at the time of surgery. Construction of a nipple valve for a continent ileostomy is technically obviated by a desmoid tumor. Preoperatively, these patients should be counseled for a permanent ileostomy in the event that a continent ileostomy cannot be completed. Because the surgical decision is made intraoperatively, without the benefit of prior knowledge by the patient, adaptation and recovery may otherwise be protracted. Involvement by the enterostomal therapist is essential.

Following construction of a permanent conventional ileostomy or a continent ileostomy, continued surveillance is important. Reports of inflammatory stomal polyps are more common than those of stomal adenomas and can be fulgurized as indicated. However, isolated reports of adenocarcinoma in the stoma highlight the need for ileoscopy and early biopsy of all stomal lesions in symptomatic patients.[109–111] The risk appears to increase with time, in some cases, up to 25 years postoperatively.[112] If severe dysplasia is found on stomal biopsy, further resective surgery is indicated.

The continent ileostomy may be used more commonly today for patients who are experiencing mechanical or psychosocial difficulties with a Brooke ileostomy. Revision rates continue to range from 10% to 30%, mainly due to valve slippage or enterocutaneous fistulae.[97]

Postoperative Management

Surveillance Postcolectomy

All patients with colectomy and IRA require life-long sigmoidoscopy of the rectal remnant. The exact surveillance interval depends on the number of polyps in the rectum. Generally, we recommend surveillance every 6 months to 1 year. For dense adenomas, fulgurization and follow-up every 3 months is performed. Given the rectal cancer risk from age 50, decreasing the interval to 4 months and using a rigid sigmoidoscope for more clarity has been suggested in some centers whereas others may opt for RPC at this time.[41] Annual endoscopy for potential pouch and ileostomy adenomas is recommended for patients with restorative proctocolectomy, Brooke ileostomy, or continent ileostomy.

Regression of Adenomas

Polyp regression, first reported by Hubbard,[114] may occur as early as 5 months postcolectomy. Nicholls et al.[115] measured mucosal proliferation before and after IRA. Cell proliferation rates decreased as early as 6 weeks postcolectomy and IRA in 16 patients, examined up to 2 years postoperatively. The opportunity for chemoprevention during this period may prevent adenoma recurrence. Clinicians must be vigilant in surveying patients with initial spontaneous regression of rectal adenomas due to long-term risk. Adenomas may recur either spontaneously or after discontinuing chemoprevention.

The Role of Sulindac in the Rectum

As a prostaglandin inhibitor, sulindac is metabolized in the colon by bacterial fecal flora to its active component sulfide. It is maintained at a concentrated plasma level in the colon but not the small intestine.[116] Interval rectal cancer while on closely monitored sulindac has recently been reported.[117,118] It should be emphasized that despite its potential to cause polyp regression in targeted groups, sulindac should not replace surgery when indicated.

In three randomized placebo-controlled registry studies, using oral dosages of sulindac up to 400 mg daily, patients pre- or postcolectomy were monitored from 6 to 9 months.[119–121] Nugent et al.[119] noted a significant drop in cell proliferation and a corresponding decrease in rectal adenomas for 5 of 7 postcolectomy patients, as opposed to those on placebo who were unchanged or worse. Labayle et al.[120] reported rectal adenoma regression in 9 of 10 postcolectomy patients after 4 months, irrespective of initial number or size of adenomas. However, recurrence was observed less than 4 months after discontinuing sulindac.

Giardiello et al.[121] demonstrated that both the number and size of rectal adenomas were significantly reduced in eight patients with intact colons at 9 months following administration of the drug. However, cell proliferation was not affected and a follow-up study revealed that the colonic epithelium reacted to sulindac because of cell loss from programmed cell death or apoptosis.[122] This finding has been confirmed in our center and may provide valuable insight for the manipulation of the colonic epithelium at an early cellular level. To potentially minimize side effects of oral sulindac, the use of rectal sulindac therapy was reported by Winde et al.[123] Dosage was tapered from 300 mg at 6 weeks to the targeted dose of 50 mg daily as the number of polyps declined over 33 months of therapy. Complete polyp regression was achieved in 9 of 15 postcolectomy patients at 6 weeks and in 12 of 15 patients at 24 weeks with no polyp recurrence.

FAP-Associated Disease

Given the chronic nature of FAP, extracolonic screening must be prioritized for those lesions with the highest morbidity and mortality or for their prognostic significance. Patient compliance with peripheral screening may be limited by the perceived severity of associated lesions. Consequently, the focus remains on tempering both the number and type of examinations for ECM. FAP registry studies have identified desmoid tumors

Table 21-2. Mortality Findings for Extracolonic Death in FAP

Author	Desmoid Tumor (%)	Duodenal Cancer (%)
Arvanitis et al.[124]	11/36 (31)	8/36 (22.2)
Belchetz et al.[125]	12/140 (9)	7/140 (5)
Bertario et al.[126]	8/137 (6)	
Herrera-Ornelas et al.[127]	3/16 (19)	
Iwama et al.[128]	8/71 (11)	11/23 (48)
Nugent et al.[129]	5/53 (9.4)	11/53 (21)

(from 6% to 31%) and periampullary cancers (from 5% to 22%) to be the most common extracolonic causes of mortality[124–129] (Table 21-2). This section focuses on current approaches to management of these lesions. It is followed by a description of specific extracolonic sites where precursor lesions may allow for early diagnosis of FAP.

Gastrointestinal Disease

Stomach

Hyperplastic gastric polyps, from 1 to 5 mm, may be present in the fundus of up to 60% of patients.[130] The often diffuse appearance of fundic gland polyps (Fig 21-10) has caused patients to be inappropriately referred for gastrectomy, despite their generally benign histology (Fig. 21-11). Patients in our registry are gastroscoped from age 25 years and, if normal or if only fundic gland polyps are identified on biopsy, 5-year follow-up is recommended.

Although infrequent, gastric adenomas can occur in the antrum. There have been only five cases of antral gastric adenomas identified in our center. Iwama et al.[128] described polyps from 12 of 27 (44%) patients who died from gastric cancer, emphasiz-

Figure 21-10. Endoscopic appearance of fundic gland polyps.

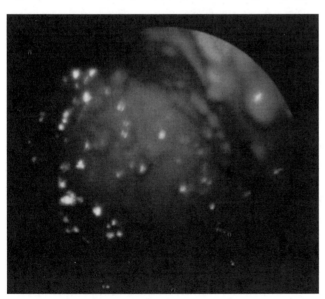

ing the increased incidence of gastric neoplasia in the Far East. However, Western registries, including our own, report only anecdotal cases.[131,132] The comparable incidence of fundic gland polyps in the east and the west suggests a shared genetic etiology whereas the rise in gastric cancer suggests environmental modifiers.[130]

The search for genetic markers was stimulated by the finding of somatic APC mutations in gastric adenomas.[133] In our registry, one 67-year-old patient developed hypoproteinemia while being monitored for hyperplastic fundic gland polyps. A giant 11 × 8 × 3.5 cm hyperplastic tumor with severe dysplasia but no adenocarcinoma was identified.[134] Interestingly, a K-*ras* mutation was identified in the dysplastic regions of this tumor, suggesting a progressive molecular chain of events that may lead to the development of adenocarcinoma.

Jejunum

Routine screening is not recommended for jejunal adenomas, occasionally noted on small bowel enteroclysis, due to the low risk of adenocarcinoma. Five of 1,255 (.4%) cases of jejunal cancer, including two primaries in our center, were documented in the recent LCPG study of 10 registries.[62,131] The use of push-type endoscopy with a longer fiberscope may detect lesions in the proximal jejunum.[135] It has been speculated that some metastatic adenocarcinoma cases without a clear primary may reflect missed jejunal neoplasia in the proximal jejunum.[136]

Duodenal Neoplasms

The LCPG reported 29 cases of duodenal cancer and 10 cases of ampullary cancer in 57 of 1,255 (5%) FAP patients.[62] Adenomatous tissue found within, or contiguous to, these cancers reinforces the theory of an adenoma-carcinoma sequence in the duodenum[137] (Fig. 21-12). The incidence of duodenal cancer in the general population was determined to be only 1 in 880,000 by Offerhaus et al.,[131] using available surveillance, epidemiology, and end results (SEER) data from 1969 to 1987. The absolute risk for duodenal and periampullary cancer in FAP was calculated as 1 in 1,697 person-years, which is also extremely low. This incidence is borne out by 16 of 790 (2%) patients with ampullary cancer in our center and 1 of 310 (.3%) patients in the Scandinavian study.[52] In the St. Mark's Hospital series, two confirmed and four suspected cases of duodenal cancer were noted in 106 follow-up patients, a mean of 46 months (range 6 to 79 months) after initial screening.[136]

Risk Factors

The carcinogenic effect of bile, particularly in the ampulla and upper duodenum where bile is highly saturated, has been implicated in duodenal tumorigenesis.[138] Nugent et al.[139] reported epithelial dysplasia in 8 of 20 cholecystectomy specimens in FAP cases, implicating the proximity of the gallbladder mucosa exposed to this bile.

A family history of duodenal neoplasia is a risk factor that may be overlooked when initiating screening protocols. In our center, there was statistical correlation between the age of the patient and family history of periampullary adenomas in 132 endoscoped patients and 12 related autopsy cases from 74 FAP

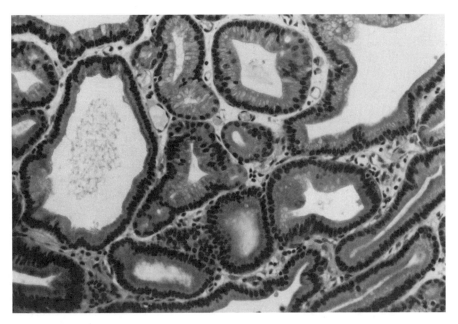

Figure 21-11. Fundic gland polyp—microscopic appearance. Regenerative epithelial cells with abundant cytoplasm.

families.[140] No genotype-phenotype correlation was confirmed. Risk assessment by familial segregation may allow for more cost-effective long-term surveillance of the upper gastrointestinal tract.

Staging

To classify patients by morphology and histology, some centers have adopted a staging system based on that of Spigelman.[138] Bulow et al.[141] found that the more advanced the dysplasia,

Figure 21-12. Endoscopic appearance of duodenal adenomas.

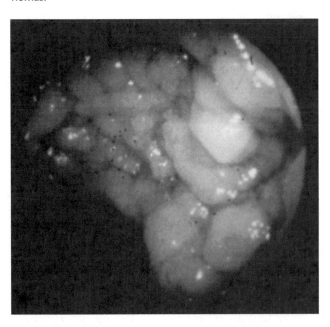

size, type, and number of duodenal adenomas, the longer the interval from FAP diagnosis. In a recent update on the St. Mark's Hospital series, Debinski et al.[136] reported that 130 of 200 (65%) patients had mild duodenal disease compared to 70 of 200 (35%) who were classified as more severe. In our center, side-viewing endoscopy is initiated from age 25 years, at which time patients are classified with no/minimal, moderate, or severe gastroduodenal disease and recalled accordingly (Table 21-3). Because the growth of duodenal adenomas is slower than in the colorectum, screening intervals are arbitrary at present and await further understanding of their natural history.

Surveillance

Unlike colorectal adenomas, the development of generally smaller than 5 mm tubular adenomas in the duodenum appears to be incremental with age greater than 40 years. Two registry series compared retrospective and prospective results for duodenal polyposis, noting disease progression on forward- and side-viewing endoscopy.[130,142] In the St. Mark's Hospital series, 21 of 52 (40%) patients, mean age 43 years at first endoscopy, showed a change in follow-up ranging from 2 to 4 years.[142] In the Cleveland Clinic series, 163 of 247 (66%) patients, mean

Table 21-3. Endoscopy Screening Guidelines in the Steve Atanas Stavro Familial Gastrointestinal Cancer Registry

Adenoma Category	Repeat Interval
1. 0	5 years
2. <1–2 mm	3 years
3. 2–10 mm	6 months to 1 year
4. >10 mm	Surgical resection

age 34 years, had duodenal adenomas prior to 1986, while an increase to 88% was recorded from 1986 to 1990.[130] A lower incidence of duodenal adenomas in 199 of 310 (64%) patients, mean age 37 years, may reflect the use of a forward-viewing scope in a five-center Scandinavian trial.[52] Grossly normal duodenal tissue is frequently identified as adenoma on histology, reinforcing the need for random sampling.[52,130,132,143]

Management

The results of surgical treatment have been mixed and follow-up too short to validate the long-term duodenal cancer risk. The rate of recurrence was high after snare polypectomy or duodenotomy with polypectomy in three major registries.[130,144] Pancreas-sparing duodenectomy was successfully performed in five patients with large villous adenomas and no pancreatic involvement or cancer.[145] In our center, endoscopic resection or surgery has been reserved for otherwise intractable duodenal neoplasia, characterized by size larger than 1 cm, villous architecture, and severe dysplasia. Four patients with severe duodenal dysplasia underwent surgical ampullectomy or pancreaticoduodenectomy and three-fourths of patients had polyp recurrence as early as 6 months postoperatively. Despite frequent monitoring, one additional patient with acute coronary disease developed Dukes' stage C adenocarcinoma and died after local duodenal resection.

The use of photodynamic therapy may be appropriate in patients who are not surgical candidates and can benefit from debulking of large duodenal adenomas, thereby reducing the potential for dysplasia.[146] Both laser and fulgurization of lesions may have a role but the danger of stricturing and pancreatitis must balance an aggressive medical approach.

The Role of Sulindac in the Duodenum

In the one randomized trial, reported by Nugent et al.[119] to assess the impact of sulindac on duodenal polyps, initial results did not indicate any significant regression. Debinski et al.[147] suggested that the inclusion of polyps greater than or equal to 3 mm may have biased their results. On review, polyps less than or equal to 2 mm regressed in 9 of 11 patients and in 4 of 12 placebo patients. Two of 11 patients had increased polyps on sulindac compared to 5 of 12 placebo patients. Large, or moderately, or severely dysplastic adenomas may be the result of cumulative somatic mutations. Both early APC and later K-ras mutations have been demonstrated in 7 of 19 periampullary adenomas smaller than 1 cm and larger than 1 cm in our center.[148,149] Nugent[150] has suggested that sulindac may be most effective in polyps smaller than 5 mm with only early APC mutations. In our registry, eight patients with greater than 10-mm adenomas were started on 150 mg of sulindac, twice daily, with a mean follow-up of 7 months. No polyp regression was noted. While on therapy, one patient developed an invasive periampullary cancer and two patients had increased polyp growth requiring surgery. The role of nosteroidal anti-inflammatory agents such as sulindac or sulindac analogs may be more effective when confined to small adenomas in the duodenum. Clearly, chemoprevention may be more effective in the long-term management of duodenal disease but at present more randomized controlled trials are needed.

Desmoid Tumor

In our center, 85 of 950 (9%) patients (52 female, 33 male) have been diagnosed with desmoid tumor (49 mesenteric, 18 abdominal wall, 15 combined, 3 extraintestinal). Nineteen of 85 (22.3%) patients have died, reflecting the increased mortality risk from desmoid tumors in FAP. Gurbuz et al.[151] performed a person-year analysis, using 83 of 825 patients with desmoid tumor and found the incidence of desmoid tumor in FAP to be 852 times that of the general population. Non-FAP desmoid tumor may occur postpartum in the abdominal wall. FAP desmoid tumors, ranging from 1 to 30 cm in diameter, are generally abdominal (Fig. 21-13), although extraintestinal sites such as the thigh, scapula, breast, and buttock may be affected. Mesenteric tumors account for an extremely high morbidity with invasion or compression of vital tissue in the intestine or urinary tract. In our series of 40 patients with mesenteric desmoid tumor, small bowel obstruction (11) and hydronephrosis (9) were the most common complications.[152]

Computed tomography (CT) scans not only monitor desmoid tumor growth but also identify features associated with a poor prognosis, particularly for mesenteric masses (list of features follows): size larger than 10 cm; several mesenteric tumors; small bowel displacement; and bilateral ureteric obstruction.[153] Spontaneous abdominal desmoid tumors, either prior to or at the time of colectomy, have been reported in 17% to 33% of series with less than 100 patients.[151,154–157] Isolated cases of desmoid tumor should be screened for FAP.

Risk Factors

Risk factors for desmoid tumor associated with FAP include prior surgery, young age at colectomy, family history of desmoid tumor, and childbearing. The role of surgery in promoting desmoid tumor, generally from 1 to 3 years after colectomy, has been mentioned from 69% to 83% of the time in registry series with desmoid tumors.[156–158] The danger of mesenteric desmoid tumor postcolectomy and IRA may be a factor in deciding on this type of surgery. It is possible that the development of a desmoid tumor or desmoplastic reaction following colectomy and IRA may be a technical barrier to subsequent RPC or Kock pouch. Penna et al.[157] reported 5 of 12 patients with desmoid tumor who died, including 3 patients with rectal cancer and 1 patient with duodenal cancer who were treated by laparotomy alone. Desmoplastic reaction may be frequently observed during colectomy (Fig. 21-14). It appears as a diffuse plaque like growth that, again, may prevent the creation of a pelvic pouch due to mesenteric shortening. It may also prevent a surgeon from performing a Kock pouch or creating a nipple valve due to the thickened mesentery.

Farmer et al.[154] have suggested that the younger the patient at colectomy (less than 25 years), the more aggressive the desmoid disease and the greater the mortality compared to the more indolent course in those older than 25 years. Jarvinen[155] reported the mean age at colectomy for patients with desmoid tumor to be 26.1 years whereas those without desmoid tumor had a mean age of 38 years. Gurbuz et al.[151] noted a trend for a shorter interval between colectomy and diagnosis of desmoid tumor in 10 of 14 patients younger than 30 years. In our center, 12 of 19 deaths were due to mesenteric desmoid tumor (Fig.

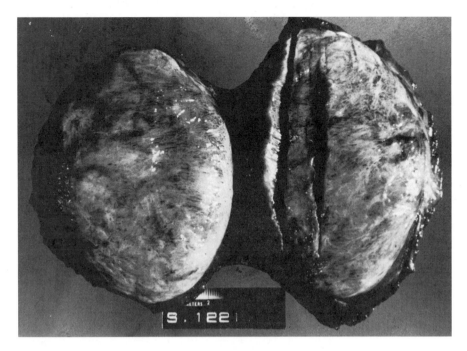

Figure 21-13. Abdominal wall desmoid tumor.

21-15). Eight of 12 patients were younger than 30 years, range 15 to 28 years, at desmoid tumor diagnosis and there was a mean of 3.1 years between colectomy and desmoid tumor. Among the remaining four patients, range 33 to 39 years at desmoid tumor diagnosis, the lag time was similar at 3 years. However, survival in the younger than 30-year-old patients was shorter with 29 years as the mean age of death compared to 45 years in the older than 30-year-old patients. Excluded from this group were seven desmoid tumor patients who died an average of 11 years after desmoid tumor diagnosis from cancer of the rectum (3), duodenum (2), brain (1), and thyroid (1).

An intrafamilial correlation for desmoid tumor was observed by Gurbuz et al.[151] in 15 families with 49 of 83 (59%) patients with desmoid tumor. The relative risk for desmoid tumor in a first-degree relative was 2.5 times that of an affected patient without a family history of desmoid tumor. Reports of desmoid tumor families with two or more affected members have raised questions about the number required for such a definition.[67,155]

Figure 21-14. Desmoplastic reaction in the mesentery.

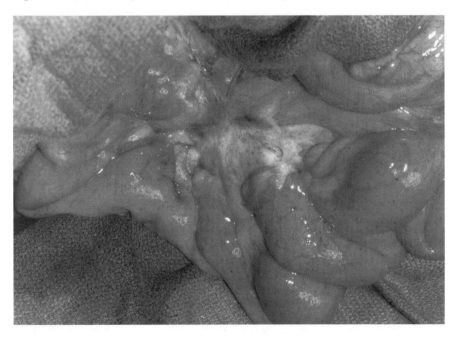

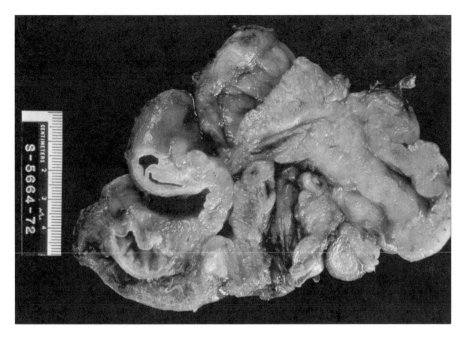

Figure 21-15. Mesenteric desmoid tumor.

Church[67] has proposed that families be limited to those with available data on more than three affected members and more than 30% with desmoid tumors. In the Cleveland Clinic Registry, 8 of 278 (3%) families meet these criteria. In our center, 5 of 239 (2%) families have at least three relatives with desmoid tumor while overall, 38 of 85 patients from 15 families are affected. In these high-risk families, timing colectomy 5 to 10 years later for newly diagnosed adolescents without large or extensive adenomas may be one option to delay the potential sequelae of desmoid tumors.[128,155]

The direct association between pregnancy and desmoid tumor development or progression, although clear in the non-FAP population, remains controversial and has not been proven in registry series.[151,154–156] In our center, although 43 of 52 women had conceived prior to desmoid diagnosis, only two women experienced significant desmoid tumor growth postpartum.

Surgery

A distinction is necessary between surgery for abdominal wall and mesenteric desmoid tumor. Abdominal wall desmoid tumors are generally encapsulated (Fig. 21-9) and are more readily excised than the more dense mesenteric mass with an undefined margin (Fig. 21-11). Specifically, excision may be recommended for smaller than 10-cm diameter abdominal wall desmoid tumors with at least a 2-cm clearance margin.[67,109,159] If required, a mesh repair will allow for closure of the abdominal wall defect. In our series, 17 of 18 patients with abdominal wall desmoids have survived from 1 to 35 years after laparotomy, despite high recurrence rates.

Surgery for mesenteric desmoid tumor is dangerous because it may compromise the major arteries, induce recurrence, and increase morbidity and mortality.[158] A total of 20 operative procedures, including small bowel transplantation, were performed on our 12 mortality cases of mesenteric desmoid tumor.

Postoperative complications range from short bowel syndrome to enteric fistula or intra-abdominal abscess.[156] Surgery may be indicated for small bowel obstruction in order to bypass segments of bowel. One should be very hesitant about trying to completely excise desmoid tumors due to the extremely high morbidity and/or mortality. In fact, in almost all cases of symptomatic mesenteric desmoid tumor, one should attempt medical therapy before considering a surgical approach.

Medical Treatment

There is no standardized therapeutic or chemopreventive protocol for these heterogeneous tumors, which vary by severity and individual response. Several registries have adopted the combination of tamoxifen (Nolvadex) and sulindac (Clinoril), with dosages varying from 10 to 40 mg tamoxifen and 150 to 200 mg sulindac, twice daily.[67,156,160] In our center, responses to the anti-estrogen, tamoxifen, or its analog, toremifene, reported by Brooks et al.[161] have been variable. Only one of three patients on toremifene has achieved no increase in their desmoid tumors over 3 years whereas the remaining patients experienced significant progression. An adverse effect was noted in one patient who developed retinopathy.

Due to our lack of success with conventional agents, we initiated a chemotherapy program for patients with severe disease. Five acutely symptomatic patients were placed on a regimen of doxorubicin and dacarbazine, described by Lynch et al.[162] Due to toxicity, the doxorubicin was replaced by carboplatin after reaching prescribed dosage and treatment was maintained from 10 to 23 months.[163] Treatment intervals were tapered to decrease cumulative marrow damage and treatment was not discontinued until patients were stable over a 6-month period. The goal of stabilization or tumor regression was achieved in four patients, each of whom had mesenteric desmoids larger than 10 cm in diameter. In one patient with ureteric obstruction, a 12-cm × 10-cm mass was reduced to a 5.9-cm cystic collection that was drained and follow-up CT scan confirmed complete resolution. This regimen was carried out on an outpatient basis and patients were monitored with 3-monthly CT scans. Due to the potential severity and sequelae of associated side effects, administration of the drug and follow-up by an oncologist is a requisite. Complications encountered included thrombocytopenia, febrile neutropenia, axillary thrombosis, and mucositis. However, all complications were managed conservatively and no deaths have occurred in this difficult patient group. Although the risk of recurrence remains, cytotoxic chemotherapy offers another option to patients with intractable desmoid tumors.

Although somatic and germline mutations of the APC gene were confirmed in FAP desmoid tumors, no genotype-phenotype correlation has been identified.[151,164,165] As yet unnamed modifier genes may be responsible for a defect in regulating connective tissue formation, which manifests as desmoid tumor.

Associated Benign Extracolonic Manifestations

Retinal Lesions

In isolated cases, at-risk children with deceased affected relatives, or families uninformative for direct mutation and indirect linkage analysis, the diagnosis of retinal lesions may be clinically significant. The ocular trait appears in up to 65% of affected families.[166,167] Characteristically, multiple bilateral pigmented ovals are surrounded by a pale halo and appear to be the sole congenital lesions in FAP[168] (Fig. 21-16). Histologically, these are hypertrophied cells without malignant potential.[168,169] Retinal lesions, often around the retinal periphery, may be missed without detailed fundoscopy by an ophthalmolo-

gist and should not be confused with unilateral isolated pigmented dots in the general population. Correlation between the degree of retinal pigmentation and the APC gene mutation site by Olschwang et al.[77] may explain why some families are positive (after exon 9) for retinal lesions whereas others are negative (before exon 9). In our center and others, combining the ophthalmologic and molecular findings may refine risk assessment for at-risk first-degree relatives.[4,88] However, children who are negative on fundoscopy from an otherwise positive for retinal lesions FAP family cannot be assumed to be risk free. In our center, two such cases, both adolescents, proved to be the exceptions and were confirmed as FAP after two negative sigmoidoscopies, underlining the need for pretest counseling of affected parent and child.

Cutaneous and Subcutaneous Lesions

Epidermoid cysts on the scalp, face, or extremities of an at-risk child is indicative of FAP and screening should be initiated to confirm the diagnosis.[38,40] Affected parents with a similar history of cysts in childhood are often cognizant of their significance and will ask for biopsy and flexible sigmoidoscopy. Although generally innocuous, cyst removal may be indicated for cosmesis.

Osteomas of the jaw or skull bones may precede the onset of colorectal adenomas. Abnormal dentition may include cysts, supernumerary teeth, excessive decay, or early loss of up to a full set of teeth.[40] Orthopantomography or skull series have not been proven as useful screening tools due to the variability of these lesions.[170] However, local referrals by knowledgeable oral surgeons may result in early diagnosis of FAP. In our center, one isolated case with mandibular osteomas at age 17 years was asymptomatic when she underwent bowel screening and

Figure 21-16. Hypertrophic pigmented and depigmented retinal lesions in familial adenomatous polyposis.

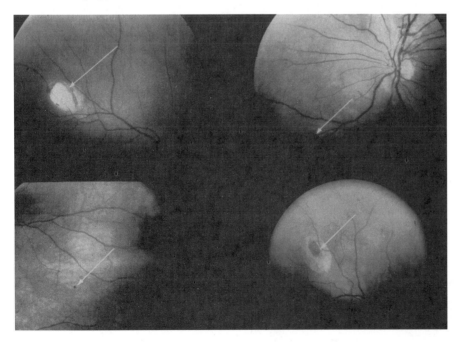

was confirmed with FAP. Recurrent mandibular osteomas may warrant excision and can be problematic for the patient. Both cysts and osteomas may be stigmatizing for patients as the overt reminder of their otherwise invisible disorder.

Associated Malignant Extracolonic Manifestations

From a prognostic perspective, the recognition of liver, thyroid, or brain neoplasms may alert the clinician to screen at-risk children or siblings with these lesions for FAP.

Hepatoblastoma

The risk of hepatoblastoma in FAP was evaluated by Giardiello et al.[171] and found to be 1 of 305 person-years, based on seven cases, all less than 5 years of age. Among 5 of 7 deaths in this series, each child had an affected parent but died before puberty and the potential onset of FAP. The two surviving patients went on to develop FAP. A recent review noted that 11 of 25 such patients survived childhood hepatoblastoma, 7 of whom were later diagnosed with FAP.[172] Hepatoblastoma has been reported in more than one affected family member, prompting researchers to seek its unknown molecular basis.[173,174]

Thyroid Cancer

Young women less than 35 years are at greatest risk to develop papillary thyroid carcinoma and generally undergo successful thyroidectomy, according to a recent review of 20 cases by Plail et al.[175] There is no correlation between the timing of diagnosis of thyroid disease and FAP, although in our center 8 of 9 women had FAP prior to their thyroid cancer. Bulow et al.[176] report a 10-year survival rate of 91% to 94%. The relative risk of thyroid cancer has been calculated as 100- to 160-fold over that of the general population in two European series[175,176] with an absolute lifetime risk of 2% in an American series.[177] No specific germline mutations have yet been identified.[178]

Brain Tumor

The association between FAP and brain tumor was clarified in a recent molecular study by Hamilton et al.,[179] demonstrating medulloblastoma in 11 of 14 patients from 10 FAP families.

The relative risk of brain tumor was 92 times that of the general population. Familial clustering of brain tumors was observed in 4 of 10 families but no correlation was found between onset of brain tumor and FAP or between genotype and phenotype. Regular flexible sigmoidoscopy is strongly recommended in patients with medulloblastoma from FAP families. In our registry, one referred patient was diagnosed with medulloblastoma at age 22 years while second-degree relatives had FAP. The neoplasm was perceived as an isolated event because her 42-year-old parent did not have FAP at the time. APC mutation was later confirmed and a clinical diagnosis followed in mother and daughter within 3 years.

The study by Hamilton et al.[179] answered part of the controversy surrounding patients presenting with variations of the FAP phenotype and brain tumor, that is, an autosomal-recessive inheritance pattern or the pleiotropic manifestation of a germline APC mutation.[180–182] Molecular genetics was used to define the disorder of central nervous system tumor and colorectal adenomas, referred to as Turcot's syndrome.[183] Autopsy material from the original case was reviewed and contained a mutant DNA mismatch-repair gene found in hereditary nonpolyposis colorectal cancer (HNPCC). The danger of labeling families by clinical findings alone is evidenced by two siblings in our center, diagnosed with Turcot's syndrome and then FAP on the basis of medulloblastoma in one case (age 6), rectal cancer and café-au-lait spots in the second case (age 11), and colorectal adenomas in both. The development of lymphoma at age 17 years in the sibling with brain tumor did not fit with the described phenotype. Evidence by Hamilton et al.[179] of a germline mutation in a DNA-mismatch repair gene confirmed the HNPCC diagnosis and enabled clinicians to adjust the follow-up protocol accordingly.

SUMMARY

A review of hereditary gastrointestinal polyp syndromes has focused on familial adenomatous polyposis because of the accrued long-term data available. A registry perspective was used to highlight a multidisciplinary approach to cancer prevention and to recommend both medical and surgical management strategies. Molecular technology will alter the conventional approach to screening and treatment for all polyposis syndromes by individualized risk assessment.

REFERENCES

1. Morson B (1974) The polyp-cancer sequence in the large bowel. Proc R Soc Med 67:451–457
2. Goodman ZD, Yardley JH, Milligan FD (1979) Pathogenesis of colonic polyps in multiple juvenile polyposis—report of a case associated with gastric polyps and carcinoma of the rectum. Cancer 43:1906–1913
3. Shepherd NA, Bussey HJR (1990) Polyposis syndromes—an update. Curr Topics Pathol 81:323–351
4. Berk T, Cohen Z, McLeod RS, Cullen JB (1987) Surgery based on misdiagnosis of adenomatous polyposis—the Canadian polyposis registry experience. Dis Colon Rectum 30:588–590
5. Williams GT, Arthur JF, Bussey HJR, Morson BC (1980) Metaplastic polyps and polyposis of the colorectum. Histopathology 4:155–170
6. Torlakovic E, Snover DC (1996) Serrated adenomatous polyposis in humans. Gastroenterology 110:748–755
7. Hutchinson J (1896) Pigmentation of lips and mouth. Arch Surg 7:290–291
8. Peutz JLA (1921) Very remarkable case of familial polyposis of mucous membrane of intestinal tract and nasopharynx accompanied by peculiar pigmentation of skin and mucous membrane. Nederlandsch Maandschr Geneerk 10:134–146
9. Jeghers H, McKusick VA, Katz KH (1949) Generalized intestinal polyposis and melanin spots of the oral mucosa, lips and digits. N Engl J Med 241:993–1005

10. McAllister AJ, Richards KF (1977) Peutz-Jeghers syndrome—experience with twenty patients in five generations. Am J Surg 134:717–720

11. Spigelman AD, Phillips RKS (1994) Peutz-Jeghers syndrome. pp. 188–202. In Phillips RKS, Spigelman AD, Thomson JPS (eds): Familial Adenomatous Polyposis and Other Polyposis Syndromes. Edward Arnold, London

12. Utsunomiya J, Gocho H, Miyanaga T (1974) Peutz-Jeghers syndrome: its natural course and management. Johns Hopkins Med J 136:71–82

13. Linos DA, Dozois RR, Dahlin DC, Bartholomew LG (1981) Does Peutz-Jeghers syndrome predispose to gastrointestinal malignancy? A later look. Arch Surg 116:1182–1184

14. Hizawa K, Iida M, Matsumoto T et al (1993) Cancer in Peutz-Jeghers syndrome. Cancer 72: 2777–2781

15. Giardiello FM, Welsh SB, Hamilton SR et al (1987) Increased risk of cancer in the Peutz-Jeghers syndrome. New Engl J Med 316:1511–1514

16. Cripps WH (1882) Two cases of disseminated polypus of the rectum. Trans Pathol Soc London 33:165–168

16a.Hemminki A, Tomlinson I, Markie D et al (1997) Localization of a susceptibility locus for Peutz-Jeghers syndrome to 1qp using comparative genomic hybridization and targeted linkage analysis. Nat Genet 15:87–90

17. Desai DC, Neale KF, Talbot IC et al (1995) Juvenile polyposis. Br J Surg 82:14–17

18. McColl I, Bussey HJR, Veale AMO, Morson BC (1964) Juvenile polyposis coli. Proc R Soc Med 57:896–897

19. Jass JR (1994) Juvenile polyposis. pp. 203–214. In Phillips RKS, Spigelman AD, Thomson JPS (eds): Familial Adenomatous Polyposis and Other Polyposis Syndromes. Edward Arnold, London

20. Giardiello FM, Offerhaus JGA (1995) Phenotype and cancer risk of various polyposis syndromes. Eur J Cancer 31A: 1085–1087

21. Subramony C, Scott-Conner EH, Skelton D, Hall TJ (1990) Familial juvenile polyposis—study of a kindred: evolution of polyps and relationship to gastrointestinal carcinoma. Am J Clin Pathol 102:91–97

22. Jarvinen HJ (1993) Juvenile gastrointestinal polyposis. Probl Gen Surg 10:749–757

23. Petersen GM, Brown J, Bu X et al (1990) Genetic linkage study of juvenile polyposis: preliminary analysis. pp. 431–432. In Utsunomiya J, Lynch HT (eds): Hereditary Colorectal Cancer (Proceedings of the Fourth International Symposium on Colorectal Cancer). Springer-Verlag, Tokyo

24. Leggett BA, Thomas LR, Knight N et al (1993) Exclusion of APC and MCC as the gene defect in one family with familial juvenile polyposis. Gastroenterology 105: 1313–1316

25. Thomas HJW, Whitelaw SC, Cottrell SE et al (1996) Genetic mapping of the hereditary mixed polyposis syndrome to chromosome 6q. Am J Hum Genet 58:770–776

26. Cronkhite LW Jr, Canada WJ (1955) Generalized polyposis—an unusual syndrome of polyposis, pigmentation, alopecia, and onychotrophia. N Engl J Med 252:1011–1015

27. Rappaport LB, Sperling HV, Stavrides A (1986) Colon cancer in the Cronkhite-Canada syndrome. J Clin Gastroenterol 8: 199

28. Ruvalcaba RH, Myhre S, Smith DW (1980) Sotos syndrome with intestinal polyposis and pigmentary changes of the genitalia. Clin Genet 18:413–416

29. Finan MC, Ray MK (1989) Gastrointestinal polyposis syndromes. Dermatol Clin 7:419–434

30. Flaherty MJ, Haggitt RC (1993) Peutz-Jeghers, Ruvalcaba-Myhre-Smith, and Devon Family syndromes. Probl Gen Surg 10:724–730

31. Lloyd KM, Dennis M (1963) Cowden's disease: a possible new symptom complex with multiple system involvement. Ann Intern Med 58:136–142

32. Salem OS, Steck WD (1983) Cowden's disease (multiple hamartoma and neoplasia syndrome). J Am Acad Dermatol 8: 686–696

33. Sklifosovski NV (1881) Polyadenoma tractus intestinalis. Vrach 2:55–57

34. Bickersteth RA (1890) Case from Mr. Smith's ward—multiple polypi of the rectum occurring in a mother and child. St. Bartholomew's Hosp Rep 26:299–300

35. Smith T (1887) Three cases of multiple polypi of the lower bowel occurring in one family. St. Bartholomew's Hosp Rep 23:225–229

36. Cockayne EA (1927) Heredity in relation to cancer. Cancer Rev 2:337–347

37. Bradburn DM, Gunn A, Hastings A et al (1991) Histological detection of microadenomas in the diagnosis of familial adenomatous polyposis. Br J Surg 78:1394–1395

38. Bussey HJR (1975) Familial Polyposis Coli. The Johns Hopkins University Press, Baltimore and London

39. Morson BC, Bussey HJR (1970) Predisposing causes of intestinal cancer. In: Current Problems in Surgery. Year Book Medical Publishing, Chicago

40. Bulow S (1987) Familial polyposis coli—a clinical and epidemiological study (thesis). Danish Med Bull 34:1–15

41. Nugent KP, Northover J (1994) Total colectomy and ileorectal anastomosis. pp. 79–91. In Phillips RKS, Spigelman AD, Thomson JPS (eds): Familial Adenomatous Polyposis and Other Polyposis Syndromes. Edward Arnold, London

42. Gardner EJ (1951) A genetic and clinical study of intestinal polyposis, a predisposing factor for carcinoma of the colon and rectum. Am J Hum Genet 3:167–176

43. Blair NP, Trempe CL (1980) Hypertrophy of the retinal pigment epithelium associated with Gardner's Syndrome. Am J Ophthalmol 90:661–667

44. Thomson JPS (1988) Leeds castle polyposis group meeting. Dis Colon Rectum 31:613–616

45. Nishisho I, Nakamura Y, Miyoshi Y et al (1991) Mutations of chromosome 5q21 genes in FAP and colorectal cancer patients. Science 253:665–669

46. Lynch HT, Smyrk T, Lanspa SJ et al (1993) Upper gastrointestinal manifestations in families with hereditary flat adenoma syndrome. Cancer 71:2709–2714

47. Lynch HT, Smyrk T, McGinn T et al (1995) Attenuated familial adenomatous polyposis (AFAP)—a phenotypically and genotypically distinctive variant of FAP. Cancer 76: 2424–2433

48. Spirio L, Otterud B, Stauffer D et al (1992) Linkage of a variant or attenuated form of adenomatous polyposis coli to the adenomatous polyposis coli (APC) locus. Am J Hum Genet 51: 92–100

49. Spirio L, Olschwang S, Groden J et al (1993) Alleles of the

APC gene: an attenuated form of familial polyposis. Cell 75: 951–957

50. Berk T, Stern H (1993) Screening, management and surveillance for families with familial adenomatous polyposis. Gastrointest Endosc Clin North Am 3:725–736

51. Goldberg PA, Madden MV, du Toit E et al (1995) The outcome of familial adenomatous polyposis in the absence of a polyposis registry. South Afr Med J 85:272–276

52. Bulow S, Bulow C, Nielsen TF et al (1995) Centralized registration, prophylactic examination, and treatment. Results in improved prognosis in familial adenomatous polyposis. Scand J Gastroenterol 30:989–993

53. Bulow S (1990) Surveillance of Danish families with adenomatous polyposis: results of the Danish polyposis register. pp. 45–50. In: Hereditary Colorectal Cancer (Proceedings of the Fourth International Symposium on Colorectal Cancer). Springer-Verlag, Tokyo

54. Griffioen G, Vasen HFA, den Hartog Hager FCA (1990) Value of registration in the identification and surveillance of familial adenomatous polyposis in the Netherlands. pp. 57–62. In Utsonomiya J, Lynch HT (eds): Hereditary Colorectal Cancer (Proceedings of the Fourth International Symposium on Colorectal Cancer). Springer-Verlag, Tokyo

55. Iwama T, Mishima Y, Utsunomiya J (1990) Current status of the registration of familial adenomatous polyposis at the polyposis center in Japan. pp. 63–69. In Utsunomiya J, Lynch HT (eds): Hereditary Colorectal Cancer (Proceedings of the Fourth International Symposium on Colorectal Cancer). Springer-Verlag, Tokyo

56. De Pietri S, Sassatelli R, Roncucci L et al (1995) Clinical and biologic features of adenomatosis coli in northern Italy. Scand J Gastroenterol 30:771–779

57. Morton DG, Macdonald F, Haydon J et al (1993) Screening practice for familial adenomatous polyposis: the potential for regional registries. Br J Surg 80:255–258

58. Bulow S, Holm NV, Hauge M (1986) The incidence and prevalence of familial polyposis coli in Denmark. Scand J Soc Med 14:67–74

59. Jarvinen HJ (1992) Epidemiology of familial adenomatous polyposis in Finland: impact of family screening on the colorectal cancer rate and survival. Gut 33:357–360

60. Bisgaard ML, Fenger K, Bulow S et al (1994) Familial adenomatous polyposis (FAP): frequency, penetrance, and mutation rate. Hum Mutat 3:121–125

61. Maher ER, Barton DE, Slatter R et al (1993) Evaluation of molecular genetic diagnosis in the management of familial adenomatous polyposis coli: a population based study. J Med Genet 30:675–678

62. Jagelman DG, DeCosse JJ, Bussey HJR, and The Leeds Castle Polyposis Group (1988) Upper gastrointestinal cancer in familial adenomatous polyposis. Lancet 21:1149–1151

63. De Cosse JJ, Bulow S, Neale K et al (1992) Rectal cancer risk in patients treated for familial adenomatous polyposis. Br J Surg 79:1372–1375

64. Burn J, Chapman PD, Mathers J et al (1995) The protocol for a European double-blind trial of aspirin and resistant starch in familial adenomatous polyposis: the CAPP study. Eur J Cancer 31A:1385–1386

65. Herrera L, Kakati S, Gibas L et al (1986) Brief clinical report: Gardner syndrome in a man with an interstitial deletion of 5q. Am J Med Genet 25:473–476

66. Bulow S, Burn J, Neale K et al (1993) The establishment of a polyposis register. Int J Colorectal Dis 8:34–38

67. Church JM, McGannon E (1995) A polyposis registry: how to set one up and make it work. Semin Colon Rectal Surg 6: 48–54

68. Bussey HJR (1990) Historical developments in familial adenomatous polyposis. pp. 1–7. In Phillips RKS, Spigelman AD, Thomson JPS (eds): Familial Adenomatous Polyposis. Alan R. Liss, London

69. Neale K, Ritchie S, Thomson JPS (1990) Screening of offspring of patients with familial adenomatous polyposis: the St. Mark's hospital polyposis register experience. pp. 61–66. In: Herrera L (ed): Familial Adenomatous Polyposis. Alan R. Liss, New York

70. Bodmer WF, Bailey CJ, Bodmer J et al (1987) Localization of the gene for familial adenomatous polyposis on chromosome 5. Nature 328 (August):614–616

71. Groden J, Thliveris A, Samowitz W et al (1991) Identification and characterization of the familial adenomatous polyposis coli gene. Cell 66:589–600

72. Kinzler KW, Nilbert MC, Su L-K et al (1991) Identification of FAP locus genes from chromosome 5q21. Science 253: 661–665

73. Su L-K, Vogelstein B, Kinzler KW (1993) Association of the APC tumor suppressor protein with catenins. Science 262: 1734–1737

74. Beroud C, Soussi T (1996) APC gene: database of germline and somatic mutations in human tumors and cell line. Nucleic Acids Res 24:121–124

75. Xia L, St. Denis KA, Bapat B (1995) Evidence for a novel exon in the coding region of the adenomatous polyposis coli (APC) gene. Genomics 28:589–591

76. Nagase H, Miyoshi Y, Horii A et al (1992) Correlation between the location of germ-line mutations in the APC gene and the number of colorectal polyps in familial adenomatous polyposis patients. Cancer Res 52:4055–4057

77. Olschwang S, Tiret A, Laurent-Pulg P et al (1993) Restriction of ocular fundus lesions to a specific subgroup of APC mutations in adenomatous polyposis coli patients. Cell 75: 959–968

78. Tops CMJ, van der Klift HM, van der Luijt RB et al (1993) Nonallelic heterogeneity of familial adenomatous polyposis. Am J Med Genet 47:563–567

79. Stella A, Resta N, Gentile M et al (1993) Exclusion of the APC gene as the cause of a variant form of familial adenomatous polyposis (FAP). Am J Hum Genet 53:1031–1037

80. Paul P, Letteboer T, Gelbert L et al (1993) Identical APC exon 15 mutations result in a variable phenotype in familial adenomatous polyposis. Hum Mol Genet 2:925–931

81. Giardiello FM, Krush AJ, Petersen GM et al (1994) Phenotypic variability of familial adenomatous polyposis in 11 unrelated families with identical APC gene mutation. Gastroenterology 106:1542–1547

82. Hamilton SR (1992) The adenoma-adenocarcinoma sequence in the large bowel: variations on a theme. J Cell Biochem, suppl. 16G:41–46

83. Dietrich WF, Lander ES, Smith JS et al (1993) Genetic identi-

fication of Mom-1, a major modifier locus affecting Min-induced intestinal neoplasia in the mouse. Cell 75:631–639

84. Moser AR, Pitot HC, Dove WF (1990) A dominant mutation that predisposes to multiple intestinal neoplasia in the mouse. Science 247:322–324

85. Powell SM, Petersen GM, Krush AJ et al (1993) Molecular diagnosis of familial adenomatous polyposis. N Engl J Med 329:1982–1987

86. Prosser J, Condie A, Wright M et al (1994) APC mutation analysis by chemical cleavage of mismatch and a protein truncation assay in familial adenomatous polyposis. Br J Cancer 70:841–846

87. Bapat B, Mitri A, Greenberg CR (1993) Improved predictive carrier testing for familial adenomatous polyposis using DNA from a single archival specimen and polymorphic markers with multiple alleles. Hum Pathol 24:1376–1379

88. Caspari R, Friedl W, Boker T et al (1993) Predictive diagnosis in familial adenomatous polyposis: evaluation of molecular genetic and ophthalmologic methods. Z Gastroenterol 31:646–652

89. Bapat BV, Parker JA, Berk T et al (1994) Combined use of molecular and biomarkers for presymptomatic carrier risk assessment in familial adenomatous polyposis: implications for screening guidelines. Dis Colon Rectum 37:165–171

90. Petersen GM (1995) Genetic counseling and predictive genetic testing in familial adenomatous polyposis. Semin Colon Rectal Surg 6:55–60

91. Petersen GM, Francomano C, Kinzler K, Nakamura Y (1993) Presymptomatic direct detection of adenomatous polyposis coli (APC) gene mutations in familial adenomatous polyposis. Hum Genet 91:307–311

92. Wertz DC, Fanos JH, Reilly PR (1994) Genetic testing for children and adolescents—who decides?. JAMA 272:875–881

93. De Cosse JJ (1995) Surgical prophylaxis of familial colon cancer: prevention of death from familial colorectal cancer. J Natl Cancer Inst Monographs 17:31–32

94. Petersen GM, Boyd PA (1995) Gene tests and counselling for colorectal cancer risk: lessons from familial polyposis. J Nat Cancer Inst Monographs 17:67–71

95. Jarvinen HJ (1990) Timing of prophylactic surgery for patients with familial adenomatous polyposis. pp. 209–214. In Herrera L (ed): Familial Adenomatous Polyposis. Alan R. Liss, New York

96. Iwama T, Mishima Y (1994) Factors affecting the risk of rectal cancer following rectum-preserving surgery in patients with familial adenomatous polyposis. Dis Colon Rectum 37:1024–1026

97. Beart RW Jr, Welling DR (1990) Surgical alternatives in the treatment of familial adenomatous polyposis. pp. 199–208. In Herrera L (ed): Familial Adenomatous Polyposis. Alan R. Liss, New York

98. Debinski HS, Love S, Spigelman AD, Phillips RKS (1996) Colorectal polyp counts and cancer risk in familial adenomatous polyposis. Gastroenterology 110:1028–1030

99. Nugent KP, Phillips RKS (1992) Rectal cancer risk in older patients with familial adenomatous polyposis and an ileorectal anastomosis: a cause for concern. Br J Surg 79:1204–1206

100. Sarre RG, Jagelman DG, Beck GJ et al (1987) Colectomy with ileorectal anastomosis for familial adenomatous polyposis: the risk of rectal cancer. Surgery 101:20–26

101. Berk T, Bulow S, Cohen Z et al (1991) Surgical aspects of familial adenomatous polyposis. pp. 52–67. In Nicholls RJ, Mortensen NJ McC, Northover JMA: Topics in Colorectal Disease. Springer-Verlag, Berlin

102. Hoehner JC, Metcalf AM (1994) Development of invasive adenocarcinoma following colectomy with ileoanal anastomosis for familial polyposis coli—report of a case. Dis Colon Rectum 37:824–828

103. Fazio VW, Church J, Cohen Z, Hawley P (1995) Symposium: familial polyposis. Contemp Surg 47:46–58

104. Wolfstein IH, Bat L, Neumann G (1982) Regeneration of rectal mucosa and recurrent polyposis coli after total colectomy and ileoanal anastomosis. Arch Surg 117:1241–1242

105. Nugent KP, Spigelman AD, Nicholls RJ et al (1993) Pouch adenomas in patients with familial adenomatous polyposis. Br J Surg 80:1620

106. Tjandra JJ, Fazio VW, Church JM et al (1993) Similar functional results after restorative proctocolectomy in patients with familial adenomatous polyposis and mucosal ulcerative colitis. Am J Surg 165:322–325

107. Perrault J, Telander RL, Zinsmeister AR, Kaufman B (1988) The endorectal pull-through procedure in children and young adults: a follow-up study. J Pediatr Gastroenterol Nutr 7:89–94

108. Ziv Y, Church JM, Oakley JR et al (1995) Surgery for the teenager with familial adenomatous polyposis: ileo-rectal anastomosis or restorative proctocolectomy? Int J Colorectal Dis 10:6–9

109. Jagelman DG (1990) Evaluation of the gastrointestinal tract in patients with familial adenomatous polyposis pp. 97–100. In: Familial Adenomatous Polyposis. Alan R. Liss, New York

110. Gilson TP, Sollenberger LL (1992) Adenocarcinoma of an ileostomy in a patient with familial adenomatous polyposis—report of a case. Dis Colon Rectum 35:261–265

111. Johnson JA, Talton DS, Poole GV (1993) Adenocarcinoma of a Brooke ileostomy for adenomatous polyposis coli. Am J Gastroenterol 88:1122–1124

112. Suarez V, Alexander-Williams J, O'Connor HJ (1988) Carcinoma developing in ileostomies after 25 or more years. Gastroenterology 95:205–208

113. Mullen P, Behrens C, Chalmera T et al (1995) Barnett continent intestinal reservoir. Multicenter experience with an alternative to the Brooke ileostomy. Dis Colon Rectum 38:573–582

114. Hubbard TB (1957) Familial polyposis of the colon: the fate of the retained rectum after colectomy in children. Am Surg 23:577–586

115. Nicholls RJ, Springall RG, Gallagher P (1988) Regression of rectal adenomas after colectomy and ileorectal anastomosis for familial adenomatous polyposis. Br Med J 296:1707–1708

116. Giardiello FM (1994) Sulindac and polyp regression. Cancer Metast Rev 13:279–283

117. Niv Y, Fraser GM (1994) Adenocarcinoma in the rectal segment in familial polyposis coli is not prevented by sulindac therapy. Gastroenterology 107:854–857

118. Lynch HT, Thorson AG, Smyrk T (1995) Rectal cancer after prolonged sulindac chemoprevention. Cancer 75:936–938

119. Nugent KP, Farmer KCR, Spigelman AD et al (1993) Randomized controlled trial of the effect of sulindac on duodenal and rectal polyposis and cell proliferation in patients with familial adenomatous polyposis. Br J Surg 80:1618–1619

120. Labayle D, Fischer D, Vielh P et al (1991) Sulindac causes regression of rectal polyps in familial adenomatous polyposis. Gastroenterology 101:635–639

121. Giardiello FM, Hamilton SR, Krush AJ et al (1993) Treatment of colonic and rectal adenomas with sulindac in familial adenomatous polyposis. N Engl J Med 328:1313–1316

122. Pasricha PJ, Bedi A, O'Connor K et al (1995) The effects of sulindac on colorectal proliferation and apoptosis in familial adenomatous polyposis. Gastroenterology 109:994–998

123. Winde G, Schmid KW, Schlegel W et al (1995) Complete reversion and prevention of rectal adenomas in colectomized patients with familial adenomatous polyposis by rectal low-dose sulindac maintenance treatment. Dis Colon Rectum 38:813–830

124. Arvanitis ML, Jagelman DG, Fazio VW et al (1990) Mortality in patients with familial adenomatous polyposis. Dis Colon Rectum 33:639–642

125. Belchetz LA, Berk T, Bapat BV et al (1996) Changing causes of mortality in patients with familial adenomatous polyposis. Dis Colon Rectum (in press)

126. Bertario L, Presciuttini S, Sala P et al (1994) Causes of death and postsurgical survival in familial adenomatous polyposis: results from the Italian registry. Sem Surg Oncol 10:225–234

127. Herrera-Ornelas L, Elsiah S, Petrelli N, Mittelman A (1987) Causes of death in patients with familial polyposis coli (FPC). Semin Surg Oncol 3:109–117

128. Iwama T, Mishima Y, Utsunomiya J (1993) The impact of familial adenomatous polyposis on the tumorigenesis and mortality at the several organs. Ann Surg 217:101–108

129. Nugent KP, Spigelman AD, Phillips RKS (1993) Life expectancy after colectomy and ileorectal anastomosis for familial adenomatous polyposis. Dis Colon Rectum 36:1059–1062

130. Church JM, McGannon E, Hull-Boiner S et al (1992) Gastroduodenal polyps in patients with familial adenomatous polyposis. Dis Colon Rectum 35:1170–1173

131. Offerhaus GJA, Giardiello FM, Krush AJ et al (1992) The risk of upper gastrointestinal cancer in familial adenomatous polyposis. Gastroenterology 102:1980–1982

132. Goedde TA, Rodriguez-Bigas L, Herrera L, Petrelli NJ (1992) Gastroduodenal polyps in familial adenomatous polyposis. Surg Oncol 1:357–361

133. Nakatsuru S, Yanagisawa A, Furukawa et al (1993) Somatic mutations of the APC gene in precancerous lesion of the stomach. Hum Mol Genet 2:1463–1465

134. Odze RD, Quinn PS, Terrault NA et al (1993) Advanced gastroduodenal polyposis with RAS mutations in a patient with familial adenomatous polyposis. Human Pathol 24:442–448

135. Bertoni G, Sassatelli R, Tansini P et al (1993) Jejunal polyps in familial adenomatous polyposis assessed by push-type endoscopy. J Clin Gastroenterol 17:343–348

136. Debinski HS, Spigelman AD, Hatfield A et al (1995) Upper intestinal surveillance in familial adenomatous polyposis. Eur J Cancer 31A:1149–1153

137. Spigelman AD, Talbot IC, Penna C et al (1994) Evidence for adenoma-carcinoma sequence in the duodenum of patients with familial adenomatous polyposis. J Clin Pathol 37:709–710

138. Spigelman AD, Williams CB, Talbot IC et al (1989) Lancet 2:783–785

139. Nugent KP, Spigelman AD, Talbot IC, Phillips RKS (1994) Gallbladder dysplasia in patients with familial adenomatous polyposis. Br J Surg 81:291–292

140. Sanabria JR, Croxford R, Berk TC et al (1996) Familial segregation in the occurrence and severity of periampullary neoplasms in familial adenomatous polyposis. Am J Surg 171:136–141

141. Bulow S, Alm T, Fausa O et al (1995) Duodenal adenomatosis in familial adenomatous polyposis. Int J Colorectal Dis 10:43–46

142. Nugent KP, Spigelman AD, Williams CB et al (1993) Follow-up in familial adenomatous polyposis. Lancet 341:1225

143. Domizio P, Talbot IC, Spigelman AD et al (1990) Upper gastrointestinal pathology in familial adenomatous polyposis: results from a prospective study of 102 patients. J Clin Pathol 43:738–743

144. Penna C, Phillips RKS, Tiret E, Spigelman AD (1993) Surgical polypectomy of duodenal adenomas in familial adenomatous polyposis: experience of two European centres. Br J Surg 80:1027–1029

145. Chung RS, Church JM, vanStolk R (1995) Pancreas-sparing duodenectomy: indications, surgical technique and results. Surgery 117:254–259

146. Mlkvy P, Messmann H, Debinski H et al (1995) Photodynamic therapy for polyps in familial adenomatous polyposis—a pilot study. Eur J Cancer 31A:1160–1165

147. Debinski HS, Trojan J, Nugent KP et al (1995) Effect of sulindac on small polyps in familial adenomatous polyposis. Lancet 345:855–856

148. Gallinger S, Vivona AA, Odze RD et al (1995) Somatic APC and K-ras codon 12 mutations in periampullary adenomas and carcinomas from familial adenomatous polyposis patients. Oncogene 10:1875–1878

149. Bapat B, Odze R, Mitri A et al (1993) Identification of somatic APC gene mutations in periampullary adenomas in a patient with familial adenomatous polyposis (FAP). Hum Mol Genet 2:1957–1959

150. Nugent KP (1995) Colorectal cancer: surgical prophylaxis and chemoprevention. Ann R Coll Surg Engl 77:372–376

151. Gurbuz AK, Giardiello FM, Petersen GM et al (1994) Desmoid tumours in familial adenomatous polyposis. Gut 35:377–381

152. Berk T, Cohen Z, McLeod RS, Stern HS (1992) Management of mesenteric desmoid tumours in familial adenomatous polyposis. Can J Surg 35:393–395

153. Brooks AP, Reznek RH, Nugent K et al (1994) CT appearances of desmoid tumours in familial adenomatous polyposis: further observations. Clin Radiol 49:601–607

154. Farmer KCR, Hawley PR, Phillips RKS (1994) Desmoid disease. pp. 128–142. In Phillips RKS, Spigelman AD, Thomson JPS (eds): Familial Adenomatous Polyposis and Other Polyposis Syndromes. Edward Arnold, London

155. Jarvinen HJ (1987) Desmoid disease as a part of familial adenomatous polyposis coli. Acta Chir Scand 153:379–383

156. Lofti AM, Dozois RR, Gordon H et al (1989) Mesenteric fibromatosis complicating familial adenomatous polyposis:

predisposing factors and results of treatment. Int J Colorectal Dis 4:30–36

157. Penna C, Tiret E, Parc R et al (1993) Operation and abdominal desmoid tumors in familial adenomatous polyposis. Surg Gynecol Obstet 177:263–268

158. Rodriguez-Bigas MA, Mahoney MC, Karakousis CP, Petrelli NJ (1994) Desmoid tumors in patients with familial adenomatous polyposis. Cancer 74:1270–1274

159. Fazio VW, Ziv Y, Church JM et al (1995) Ileal pouch-anal anastomoses complications and function in 1005 patients. Ann Surg 222:120–127

160. Tsukada K, Church JM, Jagelman DG et al (1992) Noncytotoxic drug therapy for intra-abdominal desmoid tumor in patients with familial adenomatous polyposis. Dis Colon Rectum 35:29–33

161. Brooks MD, Ebbs SR, Colletta AA, Baum M (1992) Desmoid tumours treated with triphenylethylenes. Eur J Cancer 28A: 1014–1018

162. Lynch HT, Fitzgibbons R Jr, Chong S et al (1994) Use of doxorubicin and dacarbazine for the management of unresectable intra-abdominal desmoid tumours in Gardner's syndrome. Dis Colon Rectum 37:260–267

163. Hamilton L, Blackstein M, Berk T et al (1996) Chemotherapy for desmoid tumours in association with familial adenomatous polyposis—a report of three cases. Can Med Assoc J (in press)

164. Miyaki M, Konishi M, Kikuchi-Yanoshita R et al (1993) Coexistence of somatic and germ-line mutations of APC gene in desmoid tumors from patients with familial adenomatous polyposis. Cancer Res 53:5079–5082

165. Sen-Gupta S, Van der Luijt RB, Bowles LV et al (1993) Somatic mutation of APC gene in desmoid tumour in familial adenomatous polyposis. Lancet 342:552–553

166. Heyen F, Jagelman DG, Romania A et al (1990) Predictive value of congenital hypertrophy of the retinal pigment epithelium as a clinical marker for familial adenomatous polyposis. Dis Colon Rectum 33:1003–1008

167. Hodgson SV, Bishop DT, Jay B (1994) Genetic heterogeneity of congenital hypertrophy of the retinal pigment epithelium (CHRPE) in families with familial adenomatous polyposis. J Med Genet 31:55–58

168. Traboulsi EI, Krush AJ, Gardner EJ et al (1987) Prevalence and importance of pigmented ocular fundus lesions in Gardner's syndrome. N Engl J Med 316:661–667

169. Parker JA, Kalnins VI, Deck JHN et al (1990) Histopathological features of congenital fundus lesions in familial adenomatous polyposis. Can J Ophthalmol 25:159–163

170. Woods RJ, Sarre RG, Ctercteko GC et al (1989) Occult radiologic changes in the skull and jaw in familial adenomatous polyposis coli. Dis Colon Rectum 32:304–306

171. Giardiello FM, Offerhaus JA, Krush AJ et al (1991) Risk of hepatoblastoma in familial adenomatous polyposis. J Pediatr 119:766–768

172. Garber JE, Li FP, Kingston KE et al (1988) Hepatoblastoma and familial adenomatous polyposis. J Natl Cancer Inst 80: 1626–1628

173. Bernstein IT, Bulow S, Mauritzen K (1992) Hepatoblastoma in two cousins in a family with adenomatous polyposis. Dis Colon Rectum 35:373–374

174. Ding S-F, Michail NE, Habib NA (1994) Genetic changes in hepatoblastoma. J Hepatol 20:672–675

175. Plail RO, Bussey HJR, Glazer G, Thomson JPS (1987) Adenomatous polyposis: an association with carcinoma of the thyroid. Br J Surg 74:377–380

176. Bulow S, Holm NV, Mellemgaard A (1988) Papillary thyroid carcinoma in Danish patients with familial adenomatous polyposis. Int J Colorectal Dis 3:29–31

177. Giardiello FM, Offerhaus GJA, Lee DH et al (1993) Increased risk of thyroid and pancreatic carcinoma in familial adenomatous polyposis. Gut 34:1394–1396

178. Colletta G, Sciacchitano S, Palmirotta R et al (1994) Analysis of adenomatous polyposis coli gene in thyroid tumours. Br J Cancer 70:1085–1088

179. Hamilton SR, Liu B, Parsons RE et al (1995) The molecular basis of Turcot's Syndrome. N Engl J Med 332:839–847

180. Lasser DM, DeViro DC, Garvin J, Wilhelmsen KC (1994) Turcot's syndrome: evidence for linkage to the adenomatous polyposis coli (APC) locus. Neurology 44:1083–1086

181. Itoh H, Hirata K, Ohsato K (1993) Turcot's syndrome and familial adenomatous polyposis associated with brain tumor: review of related literature. Int J Colorectal Dis 8:87–94

182. Tops CMJ, Vasen HFA, van Berge Henegouwen G et al (1992) Genetic evidence that Turcot syndrome is not allelic to familial adenomatous polyposis. Am J Med Genet 43: 888–893

183. Turcot J, Després JP, St. Pierre F (1959) Malignant tumors of the central nervous system associated with familial polyposis of the colon: report of two cases. Dis Colon Rectum 2: 465–468

22

SURGERY FOR COLONIC CARCINOMA

Peter W. Marcello
David J. Schoetz, Jr.

Carcinoma of the colon is a substantial cause of suffering and death around the world. In the United States alone, colorectal carcinoma accounts for an annual estimated 138,200 new cases, 73.4% of these being carcinoma of the colon. Of these 100,000 cases, 47.5% of patients will ultimately die of their disease. Colorectal carcinoma accounts for 10% of cancers in men and is the third most common cause of cancer deaths in men after lung and prostate carcinomas. In women, colorectal carcinoma is responsible for 12% of cancer cases and is third in producing deaths in women after breast and lung carcinoma.[1] Globally, many countries have higher age-adjusted death rates than the United States, including Canada, the United Kingdom, Western Europe, Australia, and New Zealand.

Although some unusual forms of carcinoma of the colon exist, for the majority of individuals, the cancer is an adenocarcinoma with one of its variants. As has been discussed by other authors in this text, the pathophysiology of carcinoma of the colon is a combination of genetic factors that predispose to the development of carcinoma when initiated by environmental influences. Because of the relatively long duration of time involved in the progression of a benign polyp to an invasive malignancy, an opportunity is available for screening programs to be developed that intervene during the precancerous phase. Identification of individuals at risk for the development of colorectal carcinoma and assignment of relative risk categories will permit application of screening and surveillance programs that should decrease the incidence of carcinoma of the colon and also identify the tumor at an earlier stage so that survival after definitive treatment improves.

Carcinoma of the colon can affect any part of the colon. The distribution of carcinoma of the colon in a series from the Lahey Clinic is seen in Figure 22-1, reflecting a series of 344 consecutive patients seen from 1972 to 1976.[2] For purposes of this chapter, carcinoma of the colon will refer to the anatomic colon and the rectosigmoid. Carcinoma of the rectum, which repre-

sents a different challenge because of the narrow confines of the pelvis, is discussed in Chapter 23.

CLINICAL PRESENTATIONS

Despite the advent of aggressive screening programs, most patients with carcinoma of the colon have symptoms on presentation that prompt investigations that ultimately reveal the diagnosis. In a series of 11,655 cases of carcinoma of the colon,[3] abdominal pain was the most common symptom, occurring in 46.8% of patients. Rectal bleeding was present in 29.6%; unexplained anemia occurred in 17.8%. Change in bowel habits is a frequent complaint, with constipation in 20.3% and diarrhea in 16.2%. Obstruction resulting from progressive luminal narrowing is a late symptom, as is the presence of an abdominal mass.

Rectal bleeding as a symptom always requires thorough investigation. Although overt rectal bleeding is most often from an anorectal source, such as internal hemorrhoids, bright red bleeding may also be from a left-sided colorectal neoplasm. In a series of 145 consecutive patients presenting to a family practitioner with complaints of rectal bleeding,[4] thorough colonic and anorectal investigation discovered a carcinoma in 10%. Consequently, all patients with bright red rectal bleeding must have a complete history and anorectal examination, with appropriate colonic investigations as indicated.

Occult gastrointestinal bleeding may be found as the source for iron deficiency anemia. If a patient has microcytic anemia on presentation that proves to be caused by iron deficiency, complete endoscopic evaluation of the gastrointestinal tract should be undertaken with the expectation that a primary colonic lesion is the most likely source. One series[5] documented 11% of patients with iron deficiency to have primary colorectal carcinoma.

Clinical presentation is determined in part by the site of the tumor in the colon. Since the 1920s, a substantial shift has been

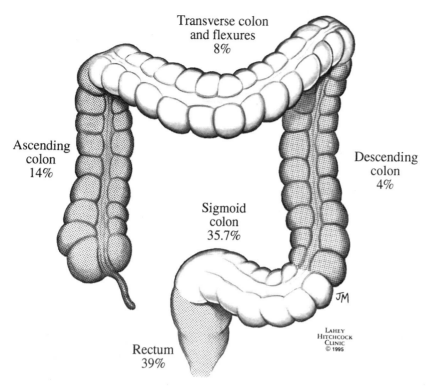

Transverse colon
and flexures
8%

Ascending
colon
14%

Descending
colon
4%

Sigmoid
colon
35.7%

Rectum
39%

LAHEY
HITCHCOCK
CLINIC
© 1995

Figure 22-1. Distribution of colorectal carcinomas among 344 patients treated at the Lahey Clinic from 1972 to 1976. (By permission of Lahey Hitchcock Clinic.)

noted in the distribution of carcinoma from the rectum and sigmoid toward the right colon.[6] In addition to the obvious implications for the most effective screening programs, the changing anatomic distributions have an impact on the symptoms mandating colonic investigation. Because right-sided carcinomas do not often cause obstructive symptoms and bleed slowly, they are likely to be discovered at a later stage; similarly, distal colon carcinomas are likely to cause symptoms and thus be found at an earlier stage. These speculations were confirmed by the Large Bowel Cancer Project in the United Kingdom,[7] in which carcinomas of the right colon were more likely to be poorly differentiated and at a more advanced stage than carcinomas of the left colon. Despite this, the survival rate after surgical removal of right colon carcinoma was better than that after removal of left-sided tumors.

Although it might be surmised that a delay in treatment would adversely affect survival, review of the available literature indicates that individuals who do not seek prompt attention for symptoms fare as well as those who are immediately evaluated.[8] The reasons for this observation are not clear and certainly cannot be the basis for physician-generated delay in evaluating patients with symptoms suggestive of the possibility of colon carcinoma.

The mean age of patients with colon carcinoma is usually in the 60s. Debate has centered around the prognostic significance of colon carcinoma in young persons. Although it is generally accepted that the incidence of colorectal carcinoma is rising in younger individuals, colon carcinoma in individuals without genetic or disease-related risk factors is unusual before 45 years of age. In a series of 85 patients aged 40 years or younger

treated for colorectal carcinoma, the stage-adjusted survival was the same after surgical resection compared with older age groups.[9] However, the percentage of poorly differentiated tumors is higher, and more advanced tumors are found in younger patients,[10] perhaps accounting for the overall poorer survival of the young cohort.

Patients older than 70 years have the same cancer-specific survival as their younger counterparts.[8] Advances in perioperative management of medical conditions, combined with the overall improvement in the health of older persons, have resulted in better operative survival and equivalent cancer cures in the aging population. Tumors in older patients have a tendency to be right sided and more locally advanced. The operative mortality rate is higher in patients older than 75 years because of the presence of underlying cardiovascular disease.[11]

Obstruction of the colon by carcinoma implies a more advanced tumor and has usually been identified as a poor prognostic variable. In a series of 156 patients with obstruction, hospital mortality was twice that of the nonobstructed group and ability to perform a potentially curative resection was only 58%.[12] The overall 5-year survival rate was only 18% compared with 40% in the uncomplicated cancer resection group. Other authors[13,14] have subsequently confirmed these observations, with higher postoperative morbidity and mortality rates and fewer survivals. Nevertheless, despite the poorer prognosis, the stage-adjusted survival rate is near enough to that of patients with nonobstructing carcinomas that multistaged or aggressive single-stage resections should be performed whenever technically feasible.

Perforation is the most lethal complication of colon carcinoma. Colonic perforation may occur at the site of the tumor or may occur proximal to an obstructing lesion. It is the perforated tumor that is associated with the higher morbidity and mortality of colonic perforation, with a significantly reduced cancer survival. In a series from the Medical College of Virginia,[12] the operative mortality rate associated with perforated carcinoma was 30%, and the crude 5-year survival rate was only 7%.

EVALUATION

History

When confronted with a patient with symptoms suggestive of the possibility of underlying carcinoma of the colon, the first step is to perform a complete history and physical examination. Associated symptoms that may help to support the diagnosis should be sought. A previous history of colorectal carcinoma makes the likelihood of a second carcinoma higher than in the general population.[15] Furthermore, a previous history of an adenomatous polyp is associated with a higher incidence of colorectal carcinoma; in one representative series,[16] the incidence of colorectal carcinoma in patients with previous neoplastic polyps was sixfold greater than in patients without polyps.

After a specific disease-oriented history, the presence of serious medical illnesses that may alter preoperative preparation and perioperative management should be sought. Patients in the usual age group for colon carcinoma are likely to have such illnesses as hypertension, atherosclerotic disease, pulmonary diseases, and diabetes. A previous history of deep venous thrombosis of the lower extremities with or without an associated pulmonary embolism mandates preoperative investigation and prophylaxis during operation. Bleeding episodes in the past should prompt a more detailed history and appropriate laboratory investigations to exclude the presence of an underlying coagulopathy. Any significant medical illnesses should be noted.

Surgical procedures in the past, particularly intestinal operations, are of potential importance in planning operative strategy because they may alter the planned intervention. Gynecologic procedures, especially if performed through the abdomen, must be documented. Ovarian metastases and primary ovarian disease may be anticipated in a percentage of women with carcinoma of the colon.

A detailed list of all medications currently being taken and knowledge regarding recent ingestion of aspirin and nonsteroidal anti-inflammatory agents, which may alter platelet function, should be recorded. Allergies to medications, particularly antibiotics, and physical agents, such as iodine and tape, must be known before operation to prepare the patient properly for surgical intervention.

Social history should include the patient's occupation and questions about lifestyle; this portion of the history is an excellent time to establish rapport with the patient because many life experiences are shared and may form the basis for a conversation not directly related to the potentially difficult medical problem being evaluated and its psychologic connotations. Smoking history and alcohol usage should be documented because they are potentially important in both diagnosis and management.

Physical Examination

Physical examination should include a general impression of the overall physical and emotional health of the individual. Patients with advanced malignancies that have resulted in significant weight loss may exhibit this feature on general inspection. Anxiety is readily apparent during social interactions. Routine vital signs are recorded, including pulse, blood pressure, respiratory rate, and temperature. Jaundice should be excluded by inspection of the sclera. Pallor is readily apparent in the conjunctiva. Both supraclavicular fossas should be palpated carefully because lymphatic metastases may be present in these areas with advanced disease. Abdominal examination should seek the presence of hepatomegaly and an abdominal mass; if found, the character of the liver or mass should be described in detail, and appropriate alterations in the preoperative evaluation should be made. A palpable abdominal mass may be movable or fixed to either the abdominal wall or surrounding viscera. In women, a thorough pelvic examination should be performed. Rectal examination is essential; random testing for occult blood in the stool should be part of the examination only when the diagnosis of carcinoma is not known because carcinomas may bleed irregularly. Although subsequent investigations will evaluate the entire colon and rectum, a digital rectal examination can exclude the presence of a synchronous distal rectal tumor; also, the presence of a shelf of tumor in the cul-de-sac anterior to the rectum indicates the presence of advanced intra-abdominal carcinomatosis in the presence of a primary carcinoma of the colon.

Diagnostic Tests

When the physical examination has been completed, the next step is to perform a series of diagnostic maneuvers to establish the diagnosis. When lower gastrointestinal tract endoscopy can be performed easily in the office, either rigid sigmoidoscopy or flexible sigmoidoscopy combined with anoscopy for more accurate examination of the anal canal can be performed at the time of the initial consultation using disposable enemas as mechanical preparation. If not, this evaluation should be scheduled early in the evaluation by a skilled endoscopist in an appropriate setting. Advantages of rigid sigmoidoscopy include ease of performance and relatively low cost. Flexible sigmoidoscopy, on the other hand, permits examination of three times greater length of the distal large bowel with a concomitant significant increase in the diagnostic yield.[17] This test is particularly important because the distribution of carcinoma of the colon shifts more proximally. Regardless of which type of lower endoscopy is chosen, it is imperative to evaluate the anal canal thoroughly by anoscopy. Bright red rectal bleeding is most often from hemorrhoids. Furthermore, neoplasms of the anal canal and distal rectum can easily escape detection with instruments designed to evaluate the more proximal bowel.

Laboratory investigations should be tailored to the individual but should include a hematocrit and hemoglobin; microcytic anemia is frequent with right-sided carcinoma of the colon. Liver function tests are routinely obtained but are not often helpful; elevations of the bilirubin, serum glutamic oxaloacetic transaminase, and alkaline phosphatase levels may dictate additional preoperative testing. Routine coagulation testing is unnecessary; a detailed history will provide indication for any specific hematologic tests. Baseline renal function should be evaluated, and a blood glucose test in the fasting state is a reasonable screening test for diabetes mellitus. Most anesthesiologists will insist on some other testing, depending on age and comorbid conditions. Electrocardiography and radiography of the chest are necessary for persons more than 40 years of age. Isolated pulmonary metastases from carcinoma of the colon are unusual, and the possibility probably does not justify routine radiography of the chest as much as the potential screening value for unanticipated problems in the chest and as a baseline for possible postoperative pulmonary problems. In this age of cost containment, it is advisable to examine critically the value of all tests previously obtained routinely.[18]

Complete examination of the colon should be performed whenever possible. Synchronous lesions are present in about 3.5% of patients.[19] The most appropriate method of accomplishing complete colonic evaluation is the subject of considerable debate, especially with the desire to curtail costs. Early after the introduction of the colonoscope in 1969, comparisons of the new instrument with the standard single-column barium enema study indicated that the tests were interchangeable for the detection of carcinoma.[20] Because the air-contrast barium enema study is associated with a greater accuracy for the detection of small polyps, radiologists maintained that the double-contrast study was at least equivalent to colonoscopy at a lower cost.[21] As experience with the colonoscope increased, the impression was that the two tests were complementary; the flexures and the right colon were not as well visualized by colonoscopy as by air-contrast barium enema. Currently, it is generally accepted that the colonoscope is the preferred method of clearing the colon of synchronous lesions before a planned colon resection for carcinoma. Single-column barium study missed carcinomas in 22% of a series of 176 patients, whereas the air-contrast barium enema study missed carcinomas in 27% of the same series.[22] Furthermore, the incidence of missed synchronous benign polyps with both radiographic studies was high compared with total colonoscopy.

When the diagnosis of carcinoma of the colon has not been established but the colonic symptoms are being evaluated with the suspicion of an underlying colonic malignancy, total colonoscopy is most likely to provide the diagnosis in the presence of a primary colonic problem.[23] Were it not for the greater cost of total colonoscopy, undoubtedly, for most patients over the age of 40 years with colonic symptoms, total colonoscopy would be the preferred initial investigation. At present, all patients with a known diagnosis of carcinoma of the colon should undergo total colonoscopy.

At times the tumor does not permit passage of a colonoscope proximally because of luminal compromise. In this circumstance, the proximal colon may be examined by the radiologist with barium studies combined with fluoroscopy. Because intraoperative palpation of the colon is notoriously inaccurate for the detection of tumors, a preoperative barium enema study would be helpful. Care must be taken not to force barium through a high-grade stenosis of the colon because subsequent dehydration of the barium may precipitate a complete colonic obstruction. If it is impossible to perform any evaluation of the colon before operation, plans should be made for detailed intraoperative palpation and colonoscopy within 3 to 6 months after complete resection of the index carcinoma.

In addition to the laboratory investigations mentioned earlier, preoperative blood studies should include carcinoembryonic antigen (CEA). When it was initially described, it was hoped that this circulating glycoprotein would be specific for colorectal carcinoma; subsequently, it has become known that the test is nonspecific for this lesion or any other condition. However, elevation of the level over 5 ng/ml is often seen in advanced disease.[29] Furthermore, a greatly elevated level is often indicative of distant metastatic disease and may alter the preoperative investigations and the intraoperative conduct. If the CEA level is elevated preoperatively, a repeat test should be obtained 2 to 4 weeks after curative resection to act as a baseline for subsequent follow-up studies.

Radiography Testing

Considerable controversy exists regarding the extent of preoperative radiographic testing. Chest radiographs are obtained primarily to search for cardiac and pulmonary disorders that may affect the conduct of anesthesia and postoperative management rather than for colon cancer–related purposes; pulmonary metastases are unusual. Abnormalities discovered on chest radiography may indicate additional testing.

Computed tomography (CT) of the chest is reserved for specific indications and cannot be justified routinely. Abdominal CT is more frequently performed; the proposed justification for this study is the high incidence of abnormalities detected in patients with carcinoma of the colon. In a series of 158 patients with carcinoma of the colon or rectum,[25] 35% were found to have serious abnormalities that altered the preoperative or intraoperative management. The converse argument is that less expensive tests are available to screen for occult metastases based on history, physical examination, and laboratory testing.

Ultrasonography of the liver is reasonably accurate for lesions more than 2 cm in size, which is the lower limit of sensitivity of CT scanning, with less cost. Unquestionably, patients with occult hepatic metastases comprise a higher percentage of total patients undergoing supposed curative resections for colorectal carcinoma than was once thought.[26] Whether the addition of routine preoperative CT will alter overall survival has not been proven, and the addition of routine intraoperative ultrasonography for more thorough exploration of solid organs has yet to be reported as a necessary part of operative strategy for all colorectal resections for carcinoma. Intraoperative ultrasonography may be of benefit in patients with full-thickness tumors (T3 or T4), whereas occult hepatic metastases are identified in 10% to 12% of cases.[27]

In an attempt to improve preoperative staging, radiolabeled monoclonal antibodies to various antigenic portions of the tumor have been developed and are under study both for preoperative evaluation of primary carcinomas of the colon and for diagnosis and treatment of recurrent colon carcinomas.[28] Most of the available data has been generated from a hand-held gamma camera system and radioactive iodine-labeled antibodies to CEA. Proponents of the routine application of this system suggest that the use of this system in resections of both primary and recurrent carcinoma of the colon leads to the discovery of occult tumor deposits that, if removed, should increase tumor survival.[29] As tumor specificity of these antibodies improves, permitting greater accuracy in detecting metastases preoperatively, it is probable that this technology will be part of the routine preoperative and intraoperative management of patients with carcinoma of the colon. Of even greater benefit would be a reliable preoperative whole-body imaging system based on monoclonal antibodies that would direct the surgeon intraoperatively.

With the increasing use of intrarectal ultrasonography in the preoperative assessment of depth of invasion in rectal tumors, permitting a more stage-specific treatment plan, it is not surprising that similar technology is being developed for application with flexible delivery systems, such as endoscopes. Preoperative staging of the degree of wall invasion of primary colonic malignancies indicates an accuracy of 70% to 80% in accurately predicting the local tumor stage, with insufficient resolution for accurate prediction of nodal involvement in most instances.[30]

OPERATIVE PREPARATION

After the preoperative investigations have been completed, appropriate plans must be made for the operation itself. Patients undergoing elective resection can undergo outpatient mechanical bowel preparation, consuming clear liquids only for the day before the operation, and then purging the colon with either 4 L of polyethylene glycol solution over 4 hours or by consuming two doses of oral Fleet Phospho-Soda (C.B. Fleet Co., Inc., Lynchburg, VA). After the completion of the mechanical preparation, two doses of oral antibiotics are administered at 7 PM and 11 PM the evening before operation. This amended dosage schedule is required because the effect of the antibiotics will be lessened if they are taken during the mechanical cleansing. Because many antibiotic regimens are acceptable, the choice should be based on the need to treat both aerobic and anaerobic bacteria. Neomycin (1 g) and metronidazole (2 g) is an inexpensive and well-tolerated combination that is effective. Nothing by mouth should be taken after midnight.

In patients with serious obstruction, the oral cathartic route may not be tolerated and may actually precipitate an acute obstructive episode. When the obstruction is partial, the preparation can be administered more slowly in the hope of achieving mechanical cleansing. Complete obstruction and signs of perforation are contraindications to the performance of preoperative mechanical preparation.

Despite pressures to decrease the total hospital stay, resulting in a higher percentage of patients undergoing their preparation on an outpatient basis, some circumstances should suggest the need for inpatient preparation. Elderly persons and those with significant underlying medical illnesses that may be aggravated by bowel preparation should be admitted the day before operation so that close nursing supervision can ensure adherence to the regimen. Mechanical cleansing is the single most important factor that decreases the incidence of septic complications and should be a high priority.

Because mechanical preparation tends to dehydrate those who undergo it, a period of hydration should be instituted before the induction of general anesthesia. In patients who undergo outpatient preparation, a higher intraoperative and postoperative fluid requirement must be anticipated.[31] It is increasingly possible to provide outpatient hydration by either home health services or by having the patient come to the hospital several hours before the scheduled operation to undergo a period of intravenous fluid replacement.

Intravenous antibiotics should be administered prophylactically within 1 hour of the skin incision. As with oral antibiotic combinations, a number of drugs are acceptable. With prophylactic antibiotics, the number of doses should be kept to a minimum, and a heightened awareness of cost should be kept in mind in making choices. Allergies will, in part, dictate the possible options as will the presence of a condition, such as valvular heart disease or intravascular prostheses, that may require a specific or expanded spectrum of coverage.[32]

Thromboembolism is a potentially serious complication of abdominal surgery. Use of either pneumatic compression stockings or subcutaneous heparin should be instituted before the induction of anesthesia and continued until the patient is fully ambulatory in the postoperative period. Neither of these regimens is foolproof in the prevention of deep venous thrombosis or pulmonary embolism. Early aggressive ambulation is a key part of postoperative management that further diminishes the complications of venous stasis.

Type of skin preparation and instrumentation are a matter of personal and institutional preference. After induction of anesthesia, an indwelling catheter should be placed into the urinary bladder to permit displacement of the bladder from the operative field and more immediate monitoring of urine output. Placement of an orogastric tube to decompress the stomach is also performed; this tube can be removed before return of consciousness, and insertion in the postoperative period because of ileus or obstruction is unusual. Incisions that afford access to the entire peritoneal cavity should be chosen; most often, this is a vertical midline. Before the resection is started, a thorough exploration of the abdomen is carried out, with particular reference to the liver, the cul-de-sac, the peritoneal surfaces and omentum, and the para-aortic area. When the presence of disease outside the bounds of the proposed operation is excluded, attention is directed to the colonic resection itself.

OPERATIVE RESECTION

Surgical intervention remains the mainstay of therapy for carcinoma of the colon. Resection of the involved segment of colon should be performed whenever possible. The surgeon should characterize clearly whether the resection has been considered *curative*, in which all of the obvious disease has been resected along with involved lymph nodes and any contiguous structures, or *palliative*, in which residual local, regional, or distant disease is present at the termination of the operative procedure. The importance of this distinction cannot be overestimated because the potential need for additional therapies postoperatively will be determined in part by the nature of the resection. Palliative resections are of value in preventing obstruction and continued blood loss; these symptoms may detract substantially from the quality of life, even though the disease is not cured by removal of the involved bowel.

Principles of curative resection of carcinoma of the colon include removal of the tumor with a minimum proximal and distal margin of 5 cm in case of intramural tumor spread. In fact, it is nearly always possible to excise considerably more of the colon than the minimum because of the length and potential mobility of the intra-abdominal colon. Extent of resection is determined by the need to remove the lymphovascular pedicle supplying the involved segment of colon because the potential presence of nodal metastases requires high ligation of the arterial and venous supply.[33] Modern anatomic principles have generally been accepted and are outlined in Figures 22-2 to 22-4.

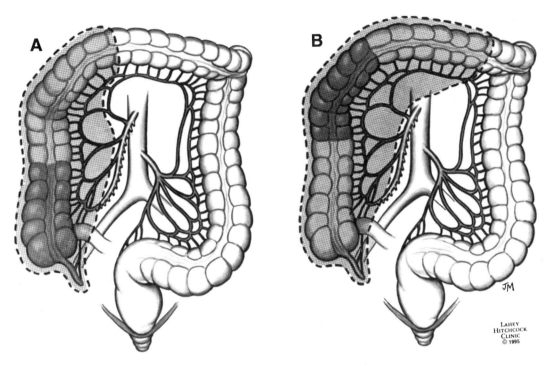

Figure 22-2. Recommended surgical resection for carcinomas of the right colon and hepatic flexure. (By permission of Lahey Hitchcock Clinic.)

Figure 22-3. Recommended surgical resection for carcinomas of the transverse colon and splenic flexure. (By permission of Lahey Hitchcock Clinic.)

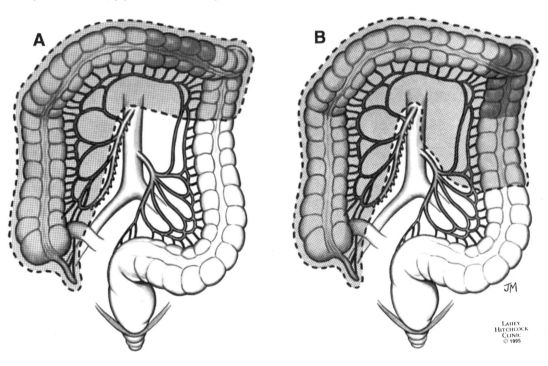

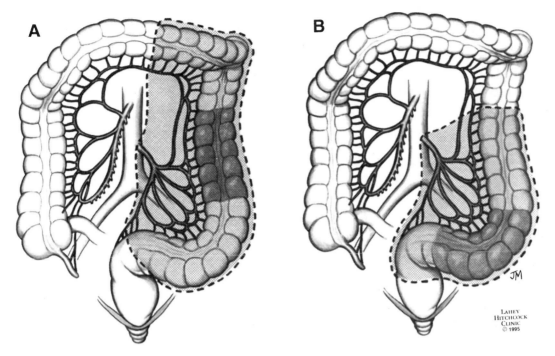

Figure 22-4. Recommended surgical resection for carcinomas of the left and sigmoid colon. (By permission of Lahey Hitchcock Clinic.)

Tumors of the cecum and ascending colon are treated by right hemicolectomy, with ligation of the ileocolic, right colic, and the right branch of the middle colic arteries and veins (Fig. 22-2). Tumors of the distal ascending colon and hepatic flexure are treated by extended right hemicolectomy, which requires ligation of the middle colic vessels at their origin (Fig. 22-2). Carcinomas of the transverse colon and splenic flexure should best be treated with subtotal colectomy, with anastomosis of the ileum to the descending colon while dividing the left colic artery at its origin (Fig. 22-3). Carcinomas of the descending and sigmoid colon are treated by left hemicolectomy, with ligation of the left branch of the middle colic and division of the inferior mesenteric artery (Fig. 22-4).

Re-establishment of gastrointestinal tract continuity is by anastomosis with any technique that maintains the principle of a tension-free and well-vascularized anastomosis. This may be accomplished by sutures or staples or biofragmentable anastomotic rings. Suture techniques may be single or double layered, absorbable or permanent material and interrupted or continuous stitches. Clinically significant anastomotic leakage is present in less than 3% of intra-abdominal colonic or ileocolonic anastomoses in the elective situation regardless of the technique as long as the above-mentioned principles are followed.[34]

CONTROVERSIES IN RESECTIONAL TECHNIQUE

"No-Touch" Technique

The basis of the "no-touch" technique is isolation and ligation of the lymphovascular pedicle before mobilization of the tumor-bearing segment of colon. The premise of the technique is that manipulation of the carcinoma during resection may result in tumor embolization into the draining veins. Studies from the 1950s demonstrated tumor emboli in the portal venous system after standard colon resection. Fisher and Turnbull[35] retrieved viable tumor cells in the mesenteric venous blood in 8 of 25 resected specimens of colorectal carcinoma.

The no-touch technique was popularized by Turnbull and associates[36] as a means of reducing the likelihood of tumor dissemination. In 1967, Turnbull compared his results using the no-touch technique in 664 patients with the results in 232 patients treated by five colleagues at the Cleveland Clinic using conventional techniques. Crude 5-year survival rates for all stages were 51% for the no-touch technique and 35% for conventional techniques. The difference in survival rates was greatest for patients with Dukes' stage C carcinomas (58% vs. 28%). Turnbull believed the survival advantage was related directly to the operative technique and advocated the routine use of the no-touch technique.

This report was criticized on several issues: The study was a retrospective trial with historical controls, there was no survival advantage for patients with Dukes' stage A and B disease, carcinomas with contiguous organ involvement were grouped with metastatic lesions and listed as stage D, and far fewer annual operations were performed by the five surgeons in the conventional group.

A reappraisal of the no-touch technique using a multi-institutional prospectively randomized trial was reported by Wiggers et al. in 1988.[37] Of their patients, 117 were in the no-touch group and 119 were in the control group, all with resectable tumors. None of the patients received postoperative chemotherapy. Perioperative morbidity was similar in both groups, and no difference in local recurrence was identified. Overall 5-year survival rates were 59.8% for the no-touch group and 56.3% for the control group. Although not statistically significant, a trend toward a less extensive and a delayed presentation of distant metastases was apparent in the no-touch group. This was noted particularly when tumors demonstrated angioinvasive growth. Liver metastases developed less frequently in the no-touch group when angioinvasion (2.5% vs. 7%) or when lymph node metastases (4.3% vs. 8.4%) was present in the resected specimen. Although these data suggested a possible benefit to the no-touch technique, no significant differences in survival were identified. Further prospective evaluation of the no-touch technique will not likely occur, especially with the routine application of chemotherapy for patients with node-positive colonic carcinoma. The no-touch technique is not widely practiced and is best left to the discretion of the operating surgeon.

Extended Lymphadenectomy

The extent of colon resection and lymphadenectomy for curative resection of colonic carcinoma is based on the anatomic boundaries that encompass the tumor-bearing segment of involved bowel. An understanding of the vascular and lymphatic anatomy of the colon is essential for establishing an effective operative strategy. Extended mesenteric resection offers the theoretical advantage of enhanced clearance of lymph nodes with metastatic deposits, which improves the chances of cure. Previously, lymph node metastases were thought to progress in a stepwise fashion along the lymphatic chain, from epicolic to paracolic nodes, and on to intermediate and principal nodes. It is now known that metastases may "skip" a nodal chain and present more proximally. Advocates of radial mesenteric resection believe more extensive resection is necessary to remove all potential tumor-bearing nodes. Enker et al.[38] reported improved survival in patients undergoing extended colonic mesenteric resection, although other authors[39] have shown no advantage.

The true value of complete mesenteric resection lies in more accurate tumor staging. Because of inadequacies in perioperative lymph node assessment, one cannot reliably predict at the time of surgery whether lymph node involvement has occurred. Because nodal status bears heavily on both patient prognosis and recommendations for adjuvant chemotherapy, extended lymph node resection would more accurately stage nodal involvement. The downstaging of patients with isolated proximal nodes would improve survival of patients with both stage II and stage III carcinomas. For solid tumors, the evolving concept of regional lymph nodes as "indicators" rather than "governors" of survival has been touted by Cady.[40] In cases of breast, prostate, bladder, and cervical carcinoma, lymph node status bears important prognostic and therapeutic information and less on actual extended survival. With further development of adjuvant therapy for colorectal carcinoma, a similar philosophy toward lymph node status may evolve.

High Ligation of the Inferior Mesenteric Artery

As with tumors of the more proximal colon, the extent of resection for carcinomas of the rectosigmoid follows the principles of blood supply and lymphatic drainage. The boundaries of the proximal margin of resection have been a topic of considerable debate. The main controversy revolves around the level of vas-

cular ligation of the inferior mesenteric artery. Whether the inferior mesenteric artery should be ligated at its origin ("high" ligation) or beyond the branch of the left colic artery ("low" ligation; Fig. 22-5) has been argued since the turn of the century. In 1908, Miles[41] described the abdominoperineal resection that required ligation of the inferior mesenteric artery to the level of the left colic artery. In the same year, Moynihan[42] reported resection of the distal sigmoid and rectum with ligation of the inferior mesenteric artery at the aorta without untoward effects on the vascularity of the proximal bowel. In a study of 179 patients by Grinnell,[43] metastatic lymph nodes were identified between the level of the left colic artery and the point of ligation of the inferior mesenteric artery at the aorta in 19 patients (10.7%). In a follow-up study of these 19 patients, 16 died with residual cancer and 1 patient was alive with recurrent disease. One patient was lost to follow-up review and the other died of an accident soon after the operation. Grinnell concluded that high ligation did not confer a survival advantage if the most proximal lymph nodes were involved. Numerous other studies have evaluated the role of "high" ligation and are summarized in Table 22-1. No study has shown a significantly improved survival rate with high ligation of the inferior mesenteric artery, except for the improved survival advantage of 13.8% for sigmoid carcinomas in the study by Rosi et al.[44] It is our current practice not to perform high ligation of the inferior mesenteric artery routinely in the resection of rectosigmoid carcinomas.

Laparoscopic Surgery for Colonic Carcinoma

With the advances in both laparoscopic technology and operative technique, enthusiasm for the use of laparoscopic-assisted resections for malignant lesions of the colon and rectum has been increasing. Early reports revealed that laparoscopically assisted colon resections could be performed safely, with complication rates similar to open procedures.[45,46] Most reports noted earlier return of gastrointestinal tract function, a reduction in postoperative pain and narcotic requirement, a shorter length of stay, and earlier resumption of normal activities compared with open procedures.[47,48] Whether laparoscopic procedures can adhere to the same oncologic principles as open colorectal resections remains to be seen. Results after laparoscopic resections for malignancy are still early.

Table 22-1. Comparison of High Versus Low Ligation of Inferior Mesenteric Artery for Colorectal Carcinoma

Source	No. of Patients	Mortality (%)	Survival Advantage (%)
Rosi et al.[44] (1962)	137	2.2	6.8 (13.8)[a]
Grinnell[43] (1965)	179	6.2	5.7
Pezim & Nicholls[115] (1984)	1,370	2.2	None
Surtrees et al.[116] (1990)	250[b]	NA	None
Corder et al.[117] (1992)	143	0	None

Abbreviation: NA, not applicable.
[a] Sigmoid lesions only.
[b] Stage III tumors only.

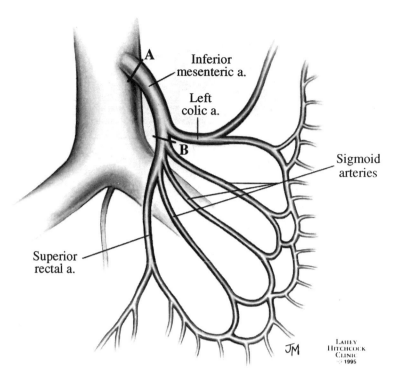

Figure 22-5. Point of division of the inferior mesenteric artery during resection of rectosigmoid carcinomas. (**A**) "High" ligation of the inferior mesenteric artery involves division of the inferior mesenteric artery at its origin from the aorta. (**B**) "Low" ligation of the inferior mesenteric artery preserves the left colic artery. High ligation of the inferior mesenteric artery does not appear to offer a survival advantage over division of the inferior mesenteric artery beyond the origin of the left colic artery. (By permission of Lahey Hitchcock Clinic.)

Of grave concern are the increasing numbers of reports of recurrence of disease at the site of insertion of the trocar after resection for carcinoma of the colon.[49–51] More than 33 cases of port site recurrences have been documented in the literature.[51] The majority appear to occur early in a surgeon's laparoscopic experience, usually within the first 20 procedures. Recurrences at the site of insertion of the trocar may occur in port sites other than that used to remove the specimen, suggesting aerosolization of tumor cells with creation or release of the pneumoperitoneum. It must be remembered that recurrence occasionally occurs at the wound site after open procedures. In a recent review[52] of 1,711 conventional colorectal resections, recurrence of disease at the wound site was documented in 11 cases (0.6%). The true incidence of recurrent disease at the wound site after laparoscopic colonic resections for malignancy is unknown but will need to be evaluated critically in future reports.

POSTOPERATIVE CARE AND COMPLICATIONS

The postoperative management of patients after colonic resection is the same for both benign and malignant disease. The role of perioperative antibiotics, prophylaxis against thromboembolism, and use of urinary catheters has been discussed previously. Currently, patient-controlled analgesia with or without intramuscular ketorolac tromethamine (Toradol, Syntex Labo-

ratories, Palo Alto, CA) is the preferred method of control of postoperative pain at our institution. We encourage ambulation of all patients within the first 24 hours after operation. The routine use of a nasogastric tube after elective colonic resection should be discouraged; the historic dogma of mandatory nasogastric decompression until resolution of ileus is outdated. In a recent survey,[53] only 30% of members of the American Society of Colon and Rectal Surgeons still routinely use nasogastric tubes. Current prospective evaluations of postoperative nasogastric tube decompression have failed to show a benefit in either resolution of ileus or prevention of postoperative emesis.[54,55] Additionally, extended follow-up studies of these patients have failed to demonstrate an increased incidence of incisional hernia related to postoperative bowel distension.[56]

The progression of postoperative diet has also recently been challenged. Previously, oral intake was withheld after elective gastrointestinal tract surgery until bowel function had resumed, usually within 3 to 5 days of the procedure. With the advent of laparoscopic procedures, postoperative diet has been advanced more quickly without untoward effect. This has resulted in prospective evaluation of postoperative feeding after open colonic resection. Several trials of early postoperative feeding, with resumption of clear liquid diet on the first postoperative day followed by regular diet as tolerated, have shown that it is safe and can be tolerated by the majority of patients.[57,58] This has not, however, always translated into a shorter length of hospitalization. In the study from Cleveland Clinic Florida,[58] 161 patients undergoing colorectal procedures were equally randomized to "early" feeding and "traditional" feeding groups. In comparison between early and traditionally fed groups, postoperative emesis occurred in 21% and 14%, nasogastric tube reinsertion in 11% and 10%, and length of hospitalization 6.2 and 6.8 days, respectively. Although the early fed group tolerated regular diet on an average 2.4 days before the traditionally fed group, this did not significantly decrease the length of stay. At present, we selectively advance diet beyond conventional teaching after uncomplicated procedures, depending on the length and extent of the operation and the surgeon's preference.

The mortality rate after resection of colorectal carcinoma ranges from 1% to 6% and is dependent on whether the operation is elective or emergent, the patient's age, and comorbidity.[2,3,59–61] The experience of the operating surgeon has also been correlated with patient mortality rates. Of interest is the recent report[61] comparing the operative mortality rate experience of board certified colorectal surgeons and other institutional general surgeons who performed 2,805 colorectal operations for both benign and malignant disease from 1989 to 1994. The overall mortality rate in 1,565 cases carried out by colorectal surgeons was 1.4% in contrast to 7.3% mortality rate among other surgeons in 1,240 cases. Mortality rate among colorectal surgeons was also comparatively lower as patient severity of illness increased. Further auditing of outcome databases will need to be reviewed before any widespread conclusions can be drawn.

The incidence of postoperative complications after colorectal resection ranges from 30% to 40%. Respiratory and cardiac complications, along with wound infections, are most frequent. Clinically significant anastomotic leakage occurs in 1% to 3% of procedures and is higher for emergency procedures and rectal resections.

COMPLICATED CARCINOMAS

Synchronous Carcinomas or Polyps

The identification of one or more benign adenomatous polyps in association with a carcinoma of the colon or rectum is well known. Synchronous polyps are found in 30% to 40% of patients with colorectal carcinoma.[62,63] The incidence of synchronous polyps in one study[63] was higher for right-sided carcinomas (47%) compared with left-sided lesions (22%). Ideally, these benign lesions should be identified and excised during preoperative colonoscopy because they are often undetectable at the time of surgery. Larger polyps that cannot be removed safely endoscopically, may be resected with the primary carcinoma if nearby or by either a separate colotomy and polypectomy or resection if distant from the index lesion. If colotomy is planned, the exact location of the adenoma should be identified clearly by either fluoroscopic examination during colonoscopy or air-contrast barium enema. Alternatively, the bowel adjacent to the polyp may be tattooed in four quadrants with india ink at the time of colonoscopy. Determination of the location of the colonic polyp by the level of insertion of the colonoscope is notoriously inaccurate and should not be relied on unless the polyp is adjacent to a well-defined colonoscopic landmark.

Approximately 2% to 5% of patients who have colorectal

carcinoma on presentation will have a synchronous carcinoma.[19,62,64] These synchronous lesions tend to be early staged carcinomas, underscoring the importance of their detection at the time of initial diagnosis. In the study from St. Mark's,[64] 75% of synchronous carcinomas were classified as Dukes' stage A and were moderately to well-differentiated tumors in 90%. Surgical resection requires adherence to the same oncologic principles for each carcinoma. For two colonic primaries, subtotal colectomy will often be required. For separate colonic and rectal carcinomas, resection must be individualized, depending on tumor location, need for adjuvant therapy, and patient comorbidity and sphincter function.

Contiguous Organ Involvement

Before the 1940s, extension of colorectal tumors into adjacent structures was deemed incurable. Turnbull et al.[36] described these lesions as metastatic and classified them as Dukes' stage D. In 1946, Sugarbaker[65] reported the results of 132 surgical resections for colorectal carcinoma of which one-third required en bloc resection. The 1-year to 5-year survival rate in this group was 56%, and on that basis he recommended radical resection if contiguous organ involvement was present. The validity of multivisceral resections with curative intent for locally advanced colorectal carcinoma has been demonstrated repeatedly over the past half century.[66–75]

Contiguous organ involvement occurs in 5.5% to 16.7% of patients with colorectal carcinoma.[73] Carcinoma of the colon most often involves the abdominal wall, small intestine, and bladder, whereas tumors of the rectosigmoid invade the uterus and ovary, posterior vaginal wall, and bladder. At operation it is nearly impossible to differentiate between extension into adjacent solid organs or adhesion to contiguous structures from paraneoplastic inflammation. Therefore, when direct extension is suspected, the surrounding tissues should be removed en bloc if technically feasible. In about 48% to 84% of contiguous organ resections, malignant invasion is microscopically confirmed. Survival is greatly impacted if tumor planes are violated intraoperatively. Gall et al.[69] reported long-term survival in only 17% of patients without en bloc resection compared with 49% of patients with contiguous resection. Likewise, the outcome of patients with contiguous organ involvement is similar to that of patients with transmural penetration of tumor without local invasion if the margins of surgical resection are clear. Two recent studies[74,75] of en bloc resection have confirmed these findings, with acceptable morbidity and mortality. When the carcinoma is deemed unresectable by the operating surgeon, a palliative procedure should be performed. In the presence of diffuse carcinomatosis, a limited sleeve resection of the primary tumor is appropriate to prevent continued intestinal blood loss and impending obstruction of the involved colonic segment. For unresectable tumors with extensive local invasion, enteroenterostomy may prevent eventual obstruction. If an internal bypass procedure is performed, it should be at least 20 cm both proximally and distally from the tumor. One should try to avoid construction of a stoma if a suitable internal bypass is feasible.

Obstructing and Perforated Carcinomas

The incidence of colonic obstruction in patients with colorectal carcinoma varies from 8% to 21% and is the most common cause of adult large bowel obstruction. If a medical emergency, the diagnosis may not be known preoperatively. Patients may have varying degrees of obstruction on presentation, usually involving the left side of the colon or rectum. The severity of illness depends mainly on the competency of the ileocecal valve. If the valve remains competent, preventing decompression into the small bowel, perforation can occur.[76]

Perforation associated with colorectal carcinoma may arise from the primary lesion itself or less commonly from the more proximal bowel. As with obstructing carcinomas, patients with these carcinomas often are seen emergently. The tumor may perforate locally (resulting in abscess formation), freely into the peritoneal cavity, or into adjacent structures. Prognosis is generally worse in this group compared with patients undergoing elective resections. Perioperative mortality ranges from 30% to 40% and has not improved even in recent series.[77–80]

In a review of 2,004 patients with colorectal carcinoma, Welch and Donaldson[78] found 118 cases (5.9%) with perforation. Tumors were freely perforated in 42%, localized by abscess formation in 42%, and had fistulized into adjacent structures in 16%. Resection was performed in 94 patients; however, in only 52 patients was resection believed to be curative. The overall 5-year survival rate was dismal (15%) and was better for patients who underwent resection with curative intent (36%).

Perforation may also occur inadvertently during curative resection of colorectal carcinoma, which carries grave consequences on both patient survival and recurrence. In a review of 174 resections with intraoperative spillage, surgical injury to bowel occurred at the level of the tumor in 67 cases and remote to the carcinoma in 107 cases.[81] As anticipated, local recurrence was considerably higher and 5-year survival poorer if the tumor was perforated (65% and 13%, respectively) compared with visceral injury away from the lesion (36% and 41%, respectively).

Obstructive carcinomas also tend to be of more advanced stage and carry a significantly higher perioperative morbidity and mortality in comparison to nonobstructive lesions.[12,14,82,83] Various operative procedures are described for the management of patients with obstructing colonic carcinoma. Historically, a three-stage procedure, including proximal colostomy, resection of primary tumor, and colostomy closure, was performed. This procedure results in significant morbidity, prolonged hospitalization, poor survival, and failure to restore intestinal continuity in up to 40% of patients.[84] Subtotal colectomy with primary anastomosis has been advocated by some, but it will drastically reduce the water-absorbing surface of the colon, leaving some elderly patients incontinent because of a higher daily stool volume.[76] Another option is to resect the obstructing primary, with construction of an end colostomy and either Hartmann pouch or mucus fistula. A second procedure will be required for closure of the colostomy.

Primary resection with immediate on-table lavage is well described for obstructing colonic carcinoma.[85–87] The unprepared colon may be cleansed by use of an antegrade irrigation system. In a review of 73 consecutive cases of colonic obstruction, on-table lavage with primary anastomosis was achieved in 60 cases (82%), with a perioperative mortality of 7% and anastomotic leakage in 4 cases (7%).

Primary resection and anastomosis may also be protected by use of the Coloshield (Deknatel Inc., Fall River, MA), an intracolonic bypass tube, which temporarily covers the area of anastomosis. This was initially reported by Ravo and coworkers[88] for the management of perforated diverticulitis and has since been used in cases of obstructing rectosigmoid carcinomas.

Whether patients with obstructing carcinoma of the colon should be treated by resection or emergency colostomy followed by resection has been the study of considerable debate over the past two decades. Many studies are retrospective in design and offer conflicting viewpoints.[13,14,25,82–84] Recently, a randomized prospective trial of emergency colostomy versus staged resection was completed.[89] Fifty-eight patients were treated by diverting colostomy and 63 by resection and end colostomy. The perioperative mortality rate was similar in both groups (12.7% with resection and 13.7% with diversion). With the exception of a reduced incidence of postoperative wound infection in patients who underwent resection, morbidity was not significantly different. As might be anticipated, patients undergoing diversion had a significantly lower requirement for transfusion and shorter length of hospital stay. Patients in the diverted group were also more likely to have restoration of intestinal continuity (91%) compared with patients with initial resection (72%). This likely relates to the reluctance of the surgeon to perform anastomotic surgery after the carcinoma has been cured in patients who also have severe concurrent illness. Overall recurrence and survival rates were similar in both groups. Whether a one-, two-, or three-stage procedure is performed in patients with obstructing carcinoma remains the discretion of the operating surgeon. Finally, stenting of an obstructing left colon lesion is now possible, permitting decompression and mechanical preparation of the colon, and conversion from an emergent to elective single-stage resection of the carcinoma.[90] The use of self-expanding metal stents is well described for relief of obstruction of the esophagus and biliary tree. Similarly, these stents may be placed endoscopically across short distal colonic strictures and obstructing carcinomas. Although the treatment of colonic perforations has yet to be described with this technique, the routine application of these stents requires further investigation.

Noncontiguous Disease

Liver Metastases

Carcinomas of the colon and rectum will metastasize to the liver in about 35% of patients, with roughly one half (10% to 20%) identified at the time of primary resection. The liver also is identified as one of the involved sites in 75% to 80% of patients with recurrent colorectal carcinoma. To date, hepatic resection of metastatic lesions offers the best chance of cure. Local and systemic chemotherapy for liver metastases has failed to improve long-term survival.[91]

Only one multi-institutional prospective trial[92] has documented the efficacy of hepatic resection of colorectal metastases. In this trial performed by the Gastrointestinal Tumor Study Group (GITSG 6584), 150 patients with hepatic metastases underwent exploration. The 30-day surgical mortality rate was 2.7%, and complications were noted in 13%. Curative resection (clear margins of resection) was carried out in 46%, noncurative resection in 12%, and the lesions were deemed unresectable in 42%. Median survival was 37 months in the curative group, 21 months in the noncurative group, and 16 months in the unresectable group. Noncurative resection provided no benefit to asymptomatic patients. Factors affecting survival after hepatic resection of colorectal metastases include primary tumor grade and stage, the interval between resection of the primary tumor and discovery of hepatic metastasis, number of metastases, preoperative CEA values, and margins of surgical resection.[91-94]

Resection of synchronous liver metastases may safely be combined with colonic resection without appreciable additional morbidity.[95,96] If extended hepatectomy or bilobar resection of hepatic metastases is warranted, the primary tumor should be excised first, followed by later elective hepatic resection.

A recent alternative to resection of liver metastases is cryosurgery. Liver lesions are subjected to two freeze-thaw cycles of liquid nitrogen delivered by insulated probes. The area subjected to the freeze-thaw process is monitored continuously by intraoperative ultrasonography. Long-term efficacy of cryoablation has been documented for selective patients with colorectal metastases.[97]

Ovarian Metastasis

Ovarian metastasis has been identified in 2% to 10% of women with colorectal carcinoma.[73,98] Avenues of potential spread include peritoneal seeding, hematogenous and lymphatic spread, or direct extension. Tumor implants are often identified deep in the ovarian stroma, with an intact and normal-appearing capsule. Controversy persists over the role of prophylactic oophorectomy at the time of colorectal resection. To date, no randomized prospective trial has been conducted to determine the benefit of prophylactic resection. It seems reasonable at present to recommend the removal of any abnormal-appearing ovary regardless of the patient's age. Also, prophylactic bilateral salpingo-oophorectomy should be considered in postmenopausal women to excise occult metastases and prevent the subsequent development of ovarian carcinoma.

Lung Metastasis

Pulmonary metastasis will develop from a colorectal primary in about 10% of patients.[91] In the majority of patients (90%), the disease will have spread to other organs. A solitary nodule in a patient with a history of colorectal carcinoma has an equal chance of representing a lung primary or metastatic colon lesion. As with isolated hepatic metastases, the only hope of cure is by resection. After identification of a solitary lesion on follow-up radiography of the chest, CT of the chest is warranted. Previous chest films should be reviewed for comparison. Abdominal CT and colonoscopy to exclude an extrapulmonary recurrent lesion should be performed before resection of the lung lesion.

The collective results of pulmonary resection in 335 patients from 12 series was reviewed by Brister et al.[99] The overall survival rate was 70% at 2 years and 30% at 5 years, with no long-term survivors among patients who did not undergo resection. Although few in number, patients with isolated pulmonary metastasis should undergo resection if technically feasible.

PROGNOSTIC INDICATORS

A variety of clinical and pathologic factors have been shown to affect patient survival significantly. Of all the variables analyzed, pathologic stage, including depth of tumor penetration through the bowel wall and presence and number of lymph node metastases, remains the most reliable predictor of both tumor recurrence and patient survival.[100-102] Other independent pathologic factors include degree of cellular differentiation and blood vessel, lymphatic, and perineural invasion. More recent studies have examined specific cytologic and genetic characteristics of colorectal carcinomas for further stratification of patients with intermediate risk in whom outcome is less certain. DNA content, proliferative index, chromosomal deletions, presence of tumor suppressor genes, and production of cellular enzymes may carry prognostic significance.[103-105] Clinical factors associated with patient survival and recurrence include patient age, gender, race, and presence of obstruction or perforation. Tumor location within the colon has not repeatedly demonstrated independent prognostic significance.

Transfusion and Survival

Numerous retrospective studies have identified perioperative transfusion of blood products as a negative prognostic indicator of both patient survival and tumor recurrence.[106-108] Whether this is a primary affect of the transfusion on immune function or a secondary indicator of extensive primary disease remains uncertain. Because the development of a neoplasm is somewhat dependent on the host's immunity, factors that alter immunity could facilitate tumor growth or recurrence. It has been shown clearly in both experimental models and clinical studies that immune function is depressed after homologous blood transfusion. Immunosuppression after transfusion primarily relates to an alteration in blood lymphocyte function. The immunologic changes associated with blood transfusion include inhibition of the lymphocyte's response to antigens, increased suppressor activity, decreased natural killer cytotoxicity, and decreased number of helper T cells.

For every negative report on blood transfusion and surgery for colorectal carcinoma another shows no significant influence on survival or recurrence. The major flaws with these reports are their small sample size and retrospective study design. However, a meta-analysis of some 20 papers representing more than 5,300 patients supported the hypothesis of blood transfusion as a poor prognostic variable independent of other factors.[108]

Two reports have prospectively evaluated the role of autologous transfusions and lymphocyte-depleted transfusions in surgery for colorectal carcinoma. Transfusion of these blood products should not theoretically result in the same level of host immunosuppression. In a randomized trial of 475 patients with colorectal carcinoma from the Netherlands,[109] patients received either allogenic transfusions (236 patients) or autologous transfusions (239 patients) as needed. In 423 patients undergoing curative resection, patient and tumor characteristics were similar in both groups. At 4 years, the recurrence rate was 66% for the allogenic-transfusion group and 63% for the autologous-transfusion group. The recurrence rate was higher among patients who required any transfusion, regardless of the type, in comparison to patients who did not require transfusion. The authors concluded that the poorer prognosis associated with transfusion may relate more to the circumstances necessitating their use rather than their immunosuppressive actions.

The use of leukocyte-depleted transfusions was prospectively evaluated in a randomized trial.[110] In theory, transfusions devoid of leukocytes should result in fewer immunologic alterations and therefore better cancer prognosis. Among 697 randomized patients undergoing curative resections, the use of leukocyte-depleted transfusions did not improve either patient survival or tumor recurrence. Cancer recurrence rates were not influenced by the need for blood transfusion of either type. However, the 3-year survival was significantly lower for patient's requiring any transfusion (69%) compared with patients not receiving transfusion (81%).

At present, the literature remains divided on the prognostic importance of perioperative blood transfusion after curative resection of colorectal carcinoma. A final answer awaits further laboratory and clinical research.

LOCAL RECURRENCE

After curative resection of colonic carcinoma, locally recurrent disease will develop in 5% to 19% of patients, usually within 2 years of the original resection.[111-114] Patients may have obstructive symptoms, intestinal bleeding, weight loss, a newly noted mass, or they may remain asymptomatic. If the tumor is identified at endoscopy, the luminal appearance often represents only the "tip of the iceberg" because these tumors often have considerable local invasion when discovered. Recurrent disease may develop because of luminal tumor implantation at the suture line at the time of original resection, inadequate margins of the initial resection, or recurrence in the bed of the original resection, or the lesion may represent the development of metachronous carcinoma adjacent to the suture line.

At least half of patients who have a local recurrent lesion will have concurrent distant disease, obviating the possibility of cure. Surgical options include resection if technically feasible or bypass if locally advanced and symptomatic. If identified at surveillance endoscopy without evidence of distant disease, repeated resection offers the only chance of cure. Factors associated with local recurrence include stage and differentiation of the primary tumor, presence of obstruction or perforation at the initial resection, and margins of resection.

REFERENCES

1. Wingo PA, Tong T, Bolden S (1995) Cancer statistics, 1995. CA Cancer J Clin 45:8–30
2. deLeon ML, Schoetz DJ Jr, Coller JA, Veidenheimer MC (1987) Colorectal cancer: Lahey Clinic experience, 1972–1976: an analysis of prognostic indicators. Dis Colon Rectum 30:237–242
3. Evans JT, Vana J, Aronoff BL et al (1978) Management and survival of carcinoma of the colon: results of a national survey by the American College of Surgeons. Ann Surg 188:716–720
4. Goulston KJ, Cook I, Dent OF (1986) How important is rectal bleeding in the diagnosis of bowel cancer and polyps? Lancet 2:261–265
5. Rockey DC, Cello JP (1993) Evaluation of the gastrointestinal tract in patients with iron-deficiency anemia. N Engl J Med 329:1691–1695
6. Cady B, Persson AV, Monson DO, Maunz DL (1974) Changing patterns of colorectal carcinoma. Cancer 33:422–426
7. Aldridge MC, Phillips RKS, Hittinger R et al (1986) Influence of tumour site on presentation, management and subsequent outcome in large bowel cancer. Br J Surg 73:663–670
8. Sugarbaker PH (1981) Carcinoma of the colon—prognosis and operative choice. Curr Prob Surg 18:762–764
9. Umpleby HC, Williamson RCN (1984) Carcinoma of the large bowel in the first four decades. Br J Surg 71:272–277
10. Behbehani A, Sakwa M, Ehrlichman R et al (1985) Colorectal carcinoma in patients under age 40. Ann Surg 202:610–614
11. Payne JE, Chapuis PH, Pheils MT (1986) Surgery for large bowel cancer in people aged 75 years and older. Dis Colon Rectum 29:733–737
12. Kelley WE Jr, Brown PW, Lawrence W Jr, Terz JJ (1981) Penetrating, obstructing, and perforating carcinomas of the colon and rectum. Arch Surg 116:381–384
13. Phillips RKS, Hittinger R, Fry JS, Fielding LP (1985) Malignant large bowel obstruction. Br J Surg 72:296–302
14. Serpell JW, McDermott FT, Katrivessis H, Hughes ESR (1989) Obstructing carcinomas of the colon. Br J Surg 76:965–969
15. Evers BM, Mullins RJ, Matthews TH et al (1988) Multiple adenocarcinomas of the colon and rectum: an analysis of incidences and current trends. Dis Colon Rectum 31:518–522
16. Kune GA, Kune S, Watson LF (1987) History of colorectal polypectomy and risk of subsequent colorectal cancer. Br J Surg 74:1064–1065
17. Marks G, Boggs HW, Castro AF et al (1979) Sigmoidoscopic examinations with rigid and flexible fiberoptic sigmoidoscopes in the surgeon's office; a comparative prospective study of effectiveness in 1,012 cases. Dis Colon Rectum 22:162–168
18. Marcello PW, Roberts PL (1996) "Routine" preoperative studies: which studies in which patients? Surg Clin North Am 76:11–23
19. Heald RJ, Bussey HJR (1975) Clinical experiences at St. Mark's Hospital with multiple synchronous cancers of the colon and rectum. Dis Colon Rectum 18:6–10
20. Loose HWC, Williams CB (1974) Barium enema versus colonoscopy. Proc R Soc Med 67:1033–1037
21. Thoeni RF, Menuck L (1977) Comparison of barium enema and colonoscopy in the detection of small colonic polyps. Radiology 124:631–635
22. Thorson AG, Christensen MA, Davis SJ (1986) The role of colonoscopy in the assessment of patients with colorectal cancer. Dis Colon Rectum 29:306–311
23. Neugut AI, Garbowski GC, Waye JD et al (1993) Diagnostic yield of colorectal neoplasia with colonoscopy for abdominal pain, change in bowel habits, and rectal bleeding. Am J Gastroenterol 88:1179–1183
24. Moertel CG, O'Fallon JR, Go VLW et al (1986) The preoperative carcinoembryonic antigen test in the diagnosis, staging, and prognosis of colorectal cancer. Cancer 58:603–610

25. Kerner BA, Oliver GC, Eisenstat TE et al (1993) Is preoperative computerized tomography useful in assessing patients with colorectal carcinoma? Dis Colon Rectum 36:1050–1053

26. Finlay IG, McArdle CS (1986) Occult hepatic metastases in colorectal carcinoma. Br J Surg 73:732–735

27. Stone MD, Kane R, Bothe A Jr (1994) Intraoperative ultrasound imaging of the liver at the time of colorectal cancer resection. Arch Surg 129:431–436

28. Arnold MW, Schneebaum S, Berens A et al (1992) Radioimmunoguided surgery challenges traditional decision making in patients with primary colorectal cancer. Surgery 112:624–630

29. Arnold MW, Schneebaum S, Berens A et al (1992) Intraoperative detection of colorectal cancer with radioimmunoguided surgery and CC49, a second-generation monoclonal antibody. Ann Surg 216:627–632

30. Boyce GA, Sivak MV Jr (1991) New approaches to the diagnosis of malignant and premalignant lesions: colonoscopic endosonography and laser-induced fluorescence spectroscopy. Semin Colon Rectal Surg 2:17–21

31. Lee EC, Roberts PL, Taranto R et al (1996) Inpatient vs. outpatient bowel preparation for elective colorectal surgery. Dis Colon Rectum 39:369–373

32. American Society of Colon and Rectal Surgeons, the Standards Task Force (1992) Practice parameters for antibiotic prophylaxis—supporting documentation. Dis Colon Rectum 35:278–285

33. Stearns MW Jr, Schottenfeld D (1971) Techniques for the surgical management of colon cancer. Cancer 28:165–169

34. Didolkar MS, Reed WP, Elias EG et al (1986) A prospective randomized study of sutured versus stapled bowel anastomoses in patients with cancer. Cancer 57:456–460

35. Fisher ER, Turnbull RB Jr (1955) The cytologic demonstration and significance of tumor cells in the mesenteric venous blood in patients with colorectal carcinoma. Surg Gynecol Obstet 100:102–108

36. Turnbull RB Jr, Kyle K, Watson FR, Spratt J (1967) Cancer of the colon: the influence of the no-touch isolation technic on survival rates. Ann Surg 166:420–427

37. Wiggers T, Jeekel J, Arends JW et al (1988) No-touch isolation technique in colon cancer: a controlled prospective trial. Br J Surg 75:409–415

38. Enker WE, Laffer UT, Block GE (1979) Enhanced survival of patients with colon and rectal cancer is based upon wide anatomic resection. Ann Surg 190:350–360

39. Sugarbaker PH, Corlew S (1982) Influence of surgical techniques on survival in patients with colorectal cancer: a review. Dis Colon Rectum 25:545–557

40. Cady B (1984) Lymph node metastases: indicators, but not governors of survival. Arch Surg 119:1067–1072

41. Miles WE (1908) A method of performing abdominoperineal excision for carcinoma of the rectum and of the terminal portion of the pelvic colon. Lancet 2:1812–1813

42. Moynihan BGA (1908) The surgical treatment of cancer of the sigmoid flexure and rectum with especial reference to the principles to be observed. Surg Gynecol Obstet 6:463–466

43. Grinnell RS (1965) Results of ligation of inferior mesenteric artery at the aorta in resections of carcinoma of the descending and sigmoid colon and rectum. Surg Gynecol Obstet 120:1031–1036

44. Rosi PA, Cahill WJ, Carey J (1962) A ten year study of hemicolectomy in the treatment of carcinoma of the left half of the colon. Surg Gynecol Obstet 114:15–24

45. Phillips EH, Franklin M, Carroll BJ et al (1992) Laparoscopic colectomy. Ann Surg 216:703–707

46. Hoffman GC, Baker JW, Fitchett CW, Vansant JH (1994) Laparoscopic-assisted colectomy: initial experience. Ann Surg 219:732–743

47. Falk PM, Beart RW Jr, Wexner SD et al (1993) Laparoscopic colectomy: a critical appraisal. Dis Colon Rectum 36:28–34

48. Ortega AE, Beart RW Jr, Steele GD Jr et al (1995) Laparoscopic bowel surgery registry: preliminary results. Dis Colon Rectum 38:681–686

49. Berends FJ, Kazemier G, Bonjer HJ, Lange JF (1994) Subcutaneous metastases after laparoscopic colectomy, letter. Lancet 344:58

50. Cirocco WC, Schwartzman A, Golub RW (1994) Abdominal wall recurrence after laparoscopic colectomy for colon cancer. Surgery 116:842–846

51. Wexner SD, Cohen SM (1995) Port site metastases after laparoscopic colorectal surgery for cure of malignancy. Br J Surg 82:295–298

52. Reilly WT, Nelson H, Schroeder G et al (1996) Wound recurrence following conventional treatment of colorectal cancer. Dis Colon Rectum 39:200–207

53. Golub RW, Cirocco WC, Golub R (1994) Current trends in gastric decompression: a survey of the American Society of Colon and Rectal Surgeons, abstracted. Dis Colon Rectum 37:P48

54. Wolff BG, Pemberton JH, van Heerden JA et al (1989) Elective colon and rectal surgery without nasogastric decompression: a prospective, randomized trial. Ann Surg 209:670–675

55. Savassi-Rocha PR, Conceicao SA, Ferreira JT et al (1992) Evaluation of the routine use of nasogastric tube in digestive operation by a prospective controlled study. Surg Gynecol Obstet 174:317–320

56. Otchy DP, Wolff BG, vanHeerden JA et al (1995) Does the avoidance of nasogastric decompression following elective abdominal colorectal surgery affect the incidence of incisional hernia? Results of a prospective, randomized trial. Dis Colon Rectum 38:604–608

57. Bufo AJ, Feldman S, Daniels GA, Lieberman RC (1994) Early postoperative feeding. Dis Colon Rectum 37:1260–1265

58. Reissman P, Teoh TA, Cohen SM et al (1995) Is early oral feeding safe after elective colorectal surgery? A prospective randomized trial. Ann Surg 222:73–77

59. Bokey EL, Chapuis PH, Fung C, Hughes WJ et al (1995) Postoperative morbidity and mortality following resection of the colon and rectum for cancer. Dis Colon Rectum 38:480–487

60. The Consultant Surgeons and Pathologists of the Lothian and Borders Health Board (1995) Lothian and Borders large bowel cancer project: immediate outcome after surgery. Br J Surg 82:888–890

61. Rosen L, Stasik JJ Jr, Reed JF (1996) Variations in colon and rectal surgical mortality: comparison of specialties with a state-legislated database. Dis Colon Rectum 39:129–135

62. Chu DZ, Giacco G, Martin RG, Guinee VF (1986) The signif-

icance of synchronous carcinoma and polyps in the colon and rectum. Cancer 57:445–450

63. Slater G, Fleshner P, Aufses AH Jr (1988) Colorectal cancer location and synchronous adenomas. Am J Gastroenterol 83: 832–836

64. Finan PJ, Ritchie JK, Hawley PR (1987) Synchronous and 'early' metachronous carcinomas of the colon and rectum. Br J Surg 74:945–947

65. Sugarbaker ED (1946) Coincident removal of additional structures in resections for carcinoma of the colon and rectum. Ann Surg 123:1036–1046

66. Jensen HE, Balslev I, Nielsen J (1970) Extensive surgery in the treatment of carcinoma of the colon. Acta Chir Scand 136:431–434

67. Polk HC Jr (1972) Extended resection for selected adenocarcinomas of the large bowel. Ann Surg 175:892–899

68. McGlone TP, Bernie WA, Elliot DW (1982) Survival following extended operations for extracolonic invasion by colon cancer. Arch Surg 117:595–599

69. Gall FP, Tonak J, Altendorf A (1987) Multivisceral resections in colorectal cancer. Dis Colon Rectum 30:337–341

70. Landmann DD, Fazio VW, Lavery IC et al (1989) En bloc resection for contiguous upper abdominal invasion by adeno-carcinoma of the colon. Dis Colon Rectum 32:669–672

71. Eisenberg SB, Kraybill WG, Lopez MJ (1990) Long-term results of surgical resection of locally advanced colorectal carcinoma. Surgery 108:779–786

72. Kroneman H, Castelein A, Jeekel J (1991) En bloc resection of colon carcinoma adherent to other organs: an efficacious treatment? Dis Colon Rectum 34:780–783

73. Staniunas RJ, Schoetz DJ Jr (1993) Extended resection for carcinoma of the colon and rectum. Surg Clin North Am 73: 117–129

74. Izbicki JR, Hosch SB, Knoefel WT et al (1995) Extended resections are beneficial for patients with locally advanced colorectal cancer. Dis Colon Rectum 38:1251–1256

75. Poeze M, Houbiers JGA, van de Velde CJH et al (1995) Radical resection of locally advanced colorectal cancer. Br J Surg 82:1386–1390

76. Padmanabhan A, Fielding LP (1991) Surgery of locally advanced colon cancer. Semin Colon Rectal Surg 2:43–47

77. Glenn F, McSherry CK (1971) Obstruction and perforation in colo-rectal cancer. Ann Surg 173:983–992

78. Welch JP, Donaldson GA (1974) Perforative carcinoma of colon and rectum. Ann Surg 180:734–740

79. Peloquin AB (1975) Factors influencing survival with complete obstruction and perforation of colorectal cancers. Dis Colon Rectum 18:11–21

80. Runkel NS, Schlag P, Schwarz V, Herfarth C (1991) Outcome after emergency surgery for cancer of the large intestine. Br J Surg 78:183–188

81. Slanetz CA Jr (1984) The effect of inadvertent intraoperative perforation on survival and recurrence in colorectal cancer. Dis Colon Rectum 27:792–797

82. Vigder L, Tzur N, Huber M et al (1985) Management of obstructive carcinoma of the left colon: comparative study of staged and primary resection. Arch Surg 120:825–828

83. Scott NA, Jeacock J, Kingston RD (1995) Risk factors in patients presenting as an emergency with colorectal cancer. Br J Surg 82:321–323

84. Deans GT, Krukowski ZH, Irwin ST (1994) Malignant obstruction of the left colon. Br J Surg 81:1270–1276

85. Murray JJ, Schoetz DJ Jr, Coller JA et al, (1991) Intraoperative colonic lavage and primary anastomosis in nonelective colon resection. Dis Colon Rectum 34:527–531

86. Tan SG, Nambiar R, Rauff A et al (1991) Primary resection and anastomosis in obstructed descending colon due to cancer. Arch Surg 126:748–751

87. Stewart J, Diament RH, Brennan TG (1993) Management of obstructing lesions of the left colon by resection, on-table lavage, and primary anastomosis. Surgery 114:502–505

88. Ravo B, Mishrick A, Addei K et al (1987) The treatment of perforated diverticulitis by one-stage intracolonic bypass procedure. Surgery 102:771–776

89. Kronborg O (1995) Acute obstruction from tumour in the left colon without spread: a randomized trial of emergency colostomy versus resection. Int J Colorectal Dis 10:1–5

90. Tejero E, Mainar A, Fernandez L et al (1995) New procedure for relief of malignant obstruction of the left colon. Br J Surg 82:34–35

91. Asbun HJ, Hughes KS (1993) Management of recurrent and metastatic colorectal carcinoma. Surg Clin North Am 73: 145–166

92. Steele G Jr, Bleday R, Mayer RJ et al (1991) A prospective evaluation of hepatic resection for colorectal carcinoma metastases to the liver: Gastrointestinal Study Group Protocol 6584. J Clin Oncol 9:1105–1112

93. Cady B, Stone MD, McDermott WV Jr et al (1992) Technical and biological factors in disease-free survival after hepatic resection for colorectal cancer metastases. Arch Surg 127: 561–569

94. Scheele J, Stang R, Altendorf-Hofmann A, Paul M (1995) Resection of colorectal liver metastases. World J Surg 19: 59–71

95. Jatzko G, Wette V, Müller M et al (1991) Simultaneous resection of colorectal carcinoma and synchronous liver metastases in a district hospital. Int J Colorectal Dis 6:111–114

96. Vogt P, Raab R, Ringe B, Pichlmayr R (1991) Resection of synchronous liver metastases from colorectal cancer. World J Surg 15:62–67

97. Ravikumar TS, Kane R, Cady B et al (1991) A 5-year study of cryosurgery in the treatment of liver tumors. Arch Surg 126:1520–1524

98. MacKeigan JM, Ferguson JA (1979) Prophylactic oophorectomy and colorectal cancer in premenopausal patients. Dis Colon Rectum 22:401–405

99. Brister SJ, de Varennes B, Gordon PH et al (1988) Contemporary operative management of pulmonary metastases of colorectal origin. Dis Colon Rectum 31:786–792

100. Phillips RKS, Hittinger R, Blesovsky L et al (1984) Large bowel cancer: surgical pathology and its relationship to survival. Br J Surg 71:604–610

101. Steinberg SM, Barwick KW, Stablein DM (1986) Importance of tumor pathology and morphology in patients with surgically resected colon cancer: findings from the Gastrointestinal Tumor Study Group. Cancer 58:1340–1345

102. Steinberg SM, Barkin JS, Kaplan RS, Stablein DM (1986) Prognostic indicators of colon tumors: the Gastrointestinal Tumor Study Group experience. Cancer 57:1866–1870

103. Witzig TE, Loprinzi CL, Gonchoroff NJ et al (1991) DNA

ploidy and cell kinetic measurements as predictors of recurrence and survival in stages B2 and colorectal adenocarcinoma. Cancer 68:879–888

104. Jen J, Kim H, Piantadosi S et al (1994) Allelic loss of chromosome 18q and prognosis in colorectal cancer. N Engl J Med 331:213–221

105. Jessup JM, Lavin PT, Andrews CW et al (1995) Sucrase-isomaltase is an independent prognostic marker for colorectal carcinoma. Dis Colon Rectum 38:1257–1264

106. Arnoux R, Corman J, Péloquin A et al (1988) Adverse effect of blood transfusions on patient survival after resection of rectal cancer. Can J Surg 31:121–125

107. Beynon J, Davies PW, Billings PJ et al (1989) Perioperative blood transfusion increases the risk of recurrence in colorectal cancer. Dis Colon Rectum 32:975–979

108. Chung M, Steinmetz OK, Gordon PH (1993) Perioperative blood transfusion and outcome after resection for colorectal carcinoma. Br J Surg 80:427–432

109. Busch ORC, Hop WCJ, Hoynck van Papendrecht MAW et al (1993) Blood transfusions and prognosis in colorectal cancer. N Engl J Med 328:1372–1376

110. Houbiers JGA, van de Watering LMG, Hermans J et al (1994) Randomised controlled trial comparing transfusion of leuco-cyte-depleted or buffy-coat-depleted blood in surgery for colorectal cancer. Lancet 344:573–578

111. Phillips RKS, Hittinger R, Blesovsky L et al, (1984) Local recurrence following 'curative' surgery for large bowel cancer: I. The overall picture. Br J Surg 71:12–16

112. Willett CG, Tepper JE, Cohen AM et al (1984) Failure patterns following curative resection of colonic carcinoma. Ann Surg 200:685–690

113. Umpleby HC, Williamson RCN (1987) Anastomotic recurrence in large bowel cancer. Br J Surg 74:873–878

114. Galandiuk S, Wieand HS, Moertel CG et al (1992) Patterns of recurrence after curative resection of carcinoma of the colon and rectum. Surg Gynecol Obstet 174:27–32

115. Pezim ME, Nicholls RJ (1984) Survival after high or low ligation of the inferior mesenteric artery during curative surgery for rectal cancer. Ann Surg 200:729–733

116. Surtees P, Ritchie JK, Phillips RKS (1990) High versus low ligation of the inferior mesenteric artery in rectal cancer. Br J Surg 77:618–621

117. Corder AP, Karanjia ND, Williams JD, Heald RJ (1992) Flush aortic tie versus selective preservation of the ascending left colic artery in low anterior resection for rectal carcinoma. Br J Surg 79:680–682

23

SURGERY FOR RECTAL CARCINOMA

R. John Nicholls

To understand the management of rectal carcinoma, it is fundamental for the clinician to be conversant with the pathology. Treatment decisions must be made based on the perceived pathologic extent of the disease. Preoperative staging is the key to management. In making this assessment, the clinician has available the results of the clinical examination, imaging, and histopathologic features such as grading. The aim is to predict as accurately as possible the extent of the disease in the individual patient as would be seen by the pathologist in carrying out a full examination.

By far the most important factor that determines outcome is dissemination. If present, then treatment is palliative in almost all cases. Where there is no evidence of dissemination on preoperative assessment, treatment decisions depend on the pathologic factors that might relate to future local treatment failure. In this circumstance there are several options, including various operations, radiotherapy, and chemotherapy.

The pathologic features of primary adenocarcinoma discussed in Chapter 19 can be summarized as being related to two aspects: the likelihood of regional or general dissemination already having occurred and the likelihood of locoregional recurrence developing after treatment. These considerations apply to any rectal carcinoma, from the most extensive lesion to one that is small and mobile.

The absence of dissemination poses various questions. For the locally extensive lesion, is preoperative radiotherapy indicated? Is the tumor at a level sufficiently proximal to the anorectal junction to be able to be removed by a sphincter-conserving operation? Does an apparent locally nonextensive tumor permit a local rather than a major form of removal? These questions can be answered only by pathologic knowledge. The clinician's task is to make such judgments as accurately as possible preoperatively.

Although present management is the result of these basic considerations, at a secondary, albeit important, level are the issues of complications and quality of life. The overriding consideration must, however, remain locoregional control of the tumor.

HISTORY

In the 19th century rectal carcinoma was excised by surgeons without any objective regard to pathology including dissemination or local extent. From the mid-19th century attempts to remove rectal carcinoma were reported along with others that aimed only to palliate through defunctioning. John of Arderne was familiar with the disease but had no means of treating it. The first perineal removal of a rectal cancer is attributed to Jean Faget[1] who carried out the procedure in 1739 on a patient who had developed perforation with abscess formation. Jacques Lisfranc[2] performed his first removal in 1826. This was a limited and doubtless horrific procedure that left the patient, if he survived, with a perineal wound discharging feces uncontrollably. Nine cases were published in 1833 by Pinault and were generally considered to be palliative. With the introduction of anesthesia and antisepsis Verneuil[3] revived the operation, which he performed from the 1870s onward.[4] There was a high mortality from these procedures and little is known of the long-term outcome. The perineal approach was the only available technique before general advances in surgery made abdominal removal feasible.

The description of the posterior approach to the rectum by Kraske[5] opened up new possibilities and this method retained its popularity well into the 20th century owing to the lower morbidity compared with the subsequently described abdominal procedures. Kraske described two cases of rectal carcinoma removed posteriorly. In one an intersphincteric removal of the rectum was carried out with permanent colostomy. In the other an anastomosis between the proximal and distal rectum was made after removal of the segment bearing the tumor. Within a short period, this latter case had encouraged surgeons to develop techniques for anastomosis. These include the Durchzug technique of Hochenegg,[6-8] who was in Vienna with Kraske before the latter left for the Chair of Surgery in Fribourg, and the eversion technique described by Maunsell[9] and Weir.[10]

The next major innovation was the introduction by Miles of the abdominoperineal excision of the rectum.[11] He based this on the pathologic appreciation of lymph node spread aiming at the concept of radical surgery inspired by Halstead. His anatomicopathologic distribution of regional lymphadenopathy was not in line with the modern view in that involvement distal to the level of the tumor was regarded by Miles as being an important route of spread. The operation itself had a high mortality, approaching 50%, but it ultimately became established owing to its oncologic merit as surgical management improved. Nevertheless for the next 20 to 30 years posterior resection was still favored by many surgeons as a safe option.

In the latter years of the second decade of the 20th century, anterior as opposed to posterior resection began to be undertaken and this gained popularity.[12-15] Initially the operation was applied to growths in the rectosigmoid, not the rectum, which were still generally treated by abdominoperineal resection even into the 1950s and 1960s in some units.

Anterior resection was encouraged by two important developments. The first was by Westhues[16,17] and Dukes,[18] who studied the extent of infiltration of rectal carcinoma distal to the lower border of the tumor. It was found to be limited, giving justification not only to anterior resection for proximal rectal growths but also to its greater application for tumors more distal. The second was a remarkable analysis of cancer-specific outcome, morbidity, and mortality following posterior resection compared with abdominoperineal resection of the rectum. In this Kirschner[19] showed the former to be more effective in cancer cure but more hazardous in immediate survival. He went on to speculate correctly that as surgery and anesthesia became safer, so the more radical approach would become the preferred method. This classic paper quite possibly may not have had the worldwide dissemination that it deserved at the time.

The subsequent history of rectal cancer surgery up to the 1940s included the appreciation that resectability was an essential requirement for long-term survival and the further development of total rectal excision including the synchronous combined approach[19,20] and the extension of anterior resection of growths in the upper and middle rectum. Eighty years ago local excision for selected tumors had been advocated[21] with indications very similar to those that would be accepted today.

The combination of pathology and surgery in creating strategies for cancer treatment was a vital step that occurred in the 1920s. Virchow had changed the face of medicine with his book *Cellular Pathologie*.[22] By the end of the 19th century much was known concerning histopathologic factors relating to prognosis.[23] Surgery was the therapeutic response to this knowledge by attempting to overreach the locoregional spread identified by the histopathologist. The pathologic classification of Dukes[18] gave a degree of objectivity that influenced the extent of surgical resection. This first example of tumor staging could be applied to most tumors for which surgery had a therapeutic role.

Between the 1920s and the late 1970s, numerous techniques of colorectal and coloanal anastomosis were described. The pull-through procedure of Hochenegg was further modified in the 1920s by D'Allaines,[24] Babcock,[13] Bacon,[14] Black,[25] Turnbull and Cuthbertson,[26] Cutait and Figlioni,[27] and Cutait et al.,[28] who described methods of low anastomosis drawing the colon down through the anal canal. These operations resulted in varying degrees of acceptable function but as far as can be seen, they were equally satisfactory regarding cancer-specific survival. In

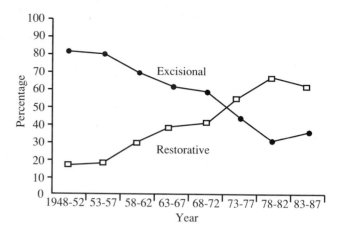

Figure 23-1. The changing relationship between total rectal excision and sphincter conservation. St. Mark's Hospital 1948 to 1987.

the early 1960s endoanal anastomosis was described[29] and also direct anastomosis using a posterior approach without[30] or with[31] division of the anal sphincters. Coloanal anastomosis was thus realized. The subsequent development of stapling made low anastomosis more attractive to surgeons in general with the result that there has been a considerable reduction in the number of total rectal excisions performed in favor of restorative procedures (Fig. 23-1).

SURVIVAL

The surgery of rectal cancer has three aims, which include adequate locoregional clearance of the tumor, minimal complications, and acceptable bowel function. Improvements in surgical technique and the awareness of the importance of adequate margins of excision to reduce the chance of local treatment failure have demonstrated a surgeon-related determinant on cancer-

Figure 23-2. The relationship between long-term survival and Dukes' pathologic stage including dissemination (D).

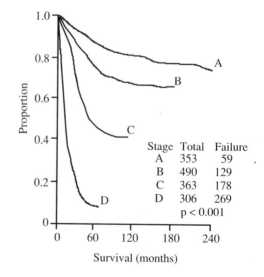

Stage	Total	Failure
A	353	59
B	490	129
C	363	178
D	306	269
		$p < 0.001$

specific outcome. Although surgery and radiotherapy can both influence the rate of local treatment failure, the pathology of the tumor itself is the most important factor for cancer-specific outcome both of survival (Fig. 23-2) and local recurrence. These factors have been described in detail in Chapter 19

Pathologic Factors

Dissemination

The overriding pathologic variable influencing survival is dissemination. Because they are locoregional treatment modalities, surgery and radiotherapy have no influence on metastatic disease. At presentation 10% to 30% patients with large bowel cancer will already have metastases; the range in the reported series is a function of the proportion of cases with obstruction or perforation, which are generally associated with a more advanced tumor.[32-34] In the group of patients with rectal cancer operated on for cure, over 40% will ultimately die with metastases.[35] The study of Finlay and McArdle[36] used the findings of computed tomography (CT) with 15-mm cuts to demonstrate a group of patients with hepatic metastases not detectable by routine CT. There were 71 patients in the study of whom 17 (24%) were shown to have occult hepatic metastases. Of these, 16 (93%) died within 5 years compared with 5 (9.5%) of the 54 without. Unfortunately such intensive scanning is not practicable for routine use but other forms of imaging, for example magnetic resonance imaging (MRI) or radionuclide scintigraphy, have not so far improved on CT. The preoperative estimation of distant stage is neither sufficiently specific nor sensitive to reflect accurately the clinicopathologic situation.

A more refined identification of dissemination would considerably improve the strategy of management by facilitating selection of patients for chemotherapy. It would also increase the power of clinical trials. Under certain circumstances the presence of defined disseminated disease may influence the choice of surgery or even whether it should be used at all.

Locoregional Spread

Dukes and Bussey[37] in their classic study were the first to attempt to identify the pathologic importance of local spread on prognosis. In an analysis of 2,447 patients having surgical removal of the primary disease, these authors identified a subgroup of 523 operation survivors without lymphatic metastases and with a growth penetrating the bowel wall. Corrected 5-year survival rates for growths with extramural spread to a slight or a moderate or extensive degree were 89.7% and 57.0%. They concluded that local spread had an important influence on survival. Gilchrist and David[38] had previously demonstrated a relationship between level of tumor and survival. In a series of 137 patients 5-year survival after surgery for intraperitoneal growths was 75% and for extraperitoneal growths 65.2%.

General Statement on Survival

Survival is related to pathologic and surgical variables. The most important of the former is stage, including dissemination as the major determinant. Local stage is related to resectability although there appears to be a significant surgical component to this factor. In a prospective study of outcome after clinico-

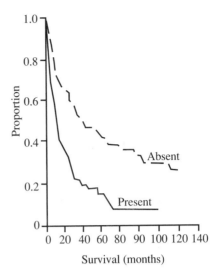

Figure 23-3. The influence of histologic grade on survival. (From Chapuis et al.,[42] with permission.)

pathologic staging of 503 patients followed over a period of 7.5 years, unresected or inadequately resected tumor along with positive lymph node status were found to be the most important influences on survival.[39] There is no evidence that extended lymphadenectomy improves survival, but adequate local clearance by surgery with adjuvant radiotherapy in selected cases may (see below).

There have been many attempts to assess the relative importance of locoregional pathologic factors that might influence survival. Techniques of multivariate analysis have been applied to surgical series from which pathologic staging and grading data are available. The accuracy of outcome depends not only on the accuracy of the pathology but also on the clinical data, a point emphasized by Fielding[40,41] reporting on the conclusions of an American Society of Colon and Rectal Surgeons Committee that examined staging. Chapuis et al.[42] in a multivariate analysis of 709 patients showed clinicopathologic stage to be the most important variable, but other factors including local spread, lymph node metastases, histologic grade, (Fig. 23-3), and venous invasion (Fig. 23-4) also were independently related to survival. This study did not consider the end point of local recurrence.

Surgical Factors

Operability

Resection of the primary tumor is the most important surgical factor that determines survival.

Patient Unfit for Surgery

The tumor may be inoperable if the patient is thought to be unfit for surgery. In an aging population this is an important consideration. There are many reports of elective surgery for large bowel cancer showing an increase in surgical mortality and morbidity with age. Fielding et al.[43] have shown a remarkable rise in mortality after the seventh decade from 3% (39 of 1,363) of patients under 70 years to 12% (141 of 1,147) over

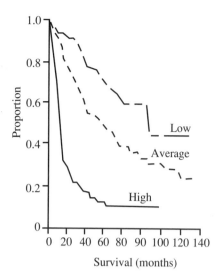

Figure 23-4. The influence of venous invasion on survival. (From Chapuis et al.,[42] with permission.)

70 years. Many older people have significant intercurrent disease that increases the risk of surgery. Stomas in the frail and aged are often not accepted[44] and poor eyesight and arthritis can make management difficult.

Possible alternatives to surgery in controlling local symptoms include radiotherapy, transanal resection,[45] electrocoagulation, and laser destruction.[46,47] The first two can be useful in palliation where life expectancy is short, for example where there is dissemination. Electrocoagulation is practiced little today but was strongly advocated in the past.[48] There are few data on its effectiveness, however. Laser treatment for large bowel cancer to palliate symptoms has been disappointing. Several sessions over weeks to months may be necessary and symptoms often persist.[47,49]

Surgery is the most effective means of relieving symptoms, and even in patients with disseminated disease there is subjective evidence of improvement and general well-being after removal of the primary tumor.

The decision on operability must be made on clinical grounds taking numerous factors into account. These include the fitness and age of the patient, the presence of dissemination, and the severity of the symptoms. Few patients today are too unfit for general anesthesia or are unlikely to tolerate abdominal surgery. In high-risk cases, for example, patients with severe cardiovascular disease especially in the aged, it may be safer to limit the extent of surgery to minimize the possibility of serious complications. For example, Hartmann's operation may be preferable to a low anterior resection, which has a potential anastomotic failure rate of about 15%. With regard to symptoms, the presence of intestinal obstruction will override other considerations with relief being obligatory. There are therefore no absolute guidelines on general operability. Judgments must depend on the circumstances of the individual case in the light of the surgeon's experience.

Tumour Unresected

Slaney[50] in a classic study reviewed the outcome of treatment of large bowel cancer in a series of 12,494 cases operated on between 1950 and 1961 recorded by the Birmingham Regional Cancer Registry. This represented as many as 98% of all cases occurring in the region with a total population of around 5 million. Survival at 5 years was only 20.5% and there was little change throughout the period. Only about 50% of patients had a radical or curative operation and about one-fifth were so advanced that no resection was possible at all. This contrasts with resectability rates for rectal cancer of over 90% reported from specialist centers.[35,51] A relationship between survival and the proportion of patients having a curative operation can be demonstrated with unresectability being a major factor responsible for noncurative surgery[52] (Fig. 23-5).

Although advanced local spread at presentation is likely to be the most important factor responsible for nonresectability, there is also a surgeon-related factor. This is difficult to quantify but an attempt to do so was made by Peloquin.[53] In a retrospective study of cancer-specific outcome following surgery for large bowel cancer at one hospital over a 24-year period, there was evidence that eight "aggressive" surgeons achieved a higher resectability rate (91.6%) than did eight "conservative" surgeons (72%). These proportions were significantly correlated with respective survival rates of 152 of 323 (47%) and 87 of 248 (35%).

More recently McArdle and Hole[54] drew similar conclusions from a retrospective review of the treatment of large bowel cancer by surgery from 1974 to 1979 at one hospital. Besides demonstrating considerable differences in morbidity and cancer specific end points among the 16 surgeons active during the period, the proportion of patients undergoing curative surgery ranged from 40% to 76%. There has been a rise in resectability over the first half of the century. Grinnell[55] determined the resectability rate during the years 1916 to 1920 and 1946 to 1950 and reported this to have risen from 50% to 92%. Others[56] reported similar data. At St. Mark's Hospital the resection rate rose from 46.5% in 1928 to 1932 to 93.2% from 1953 to 1972.[35] It is now uncommon for a tumor to be so locally extensive as to be unresectable; resectability should be over 90%.[35,51]

Figure 23-5. Relationship of the proportion of radical operations and survival among all patients seen with large bowel cancer and various symptoms. (From Nicholls,[52] with permission.)

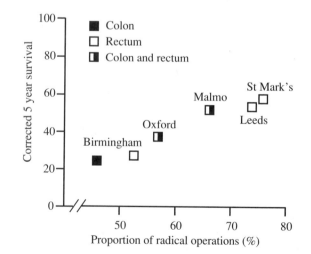

Regional Clearance

Both regional lymphadenopathy[57,58] and extramural venous invasion[59] worsen the prognosis. Theoretically the anatomic extent of removal of the lymphovascular pedicle should influence outcome. Lymphatic spread may take place along the inferior mesenteric axis or to the internal iliac nodes via the "middle" rectal pedicle.[60–62] It is, however, difficult to determine from the literature whether surgical attempts to remove these results in improved survival.

Level of Ligation of the Lymphovascular Pedicle

In the 1950s it was suggested that the level of ligation in the inferior mesenteric arterial pedicle could influence long-term survival. It was speculated that in a few cases, ligation at the level of its origin (high tie) might convert what would have been a Dukes' C2 tumor were the lesion to have been made at a lower level (low tie) into a Dukes' C1 case. If this were so then the prognosis would be enhanced by high tie. There have been no prospective randomized studies to answer this question. Some information is available from retrospective reviews. In one of these, patients undergoing curative anterior resection were divided into two groups according to the level of ligation, (high or low). When stratifying for Dukes' stage no difference was found.[63] A subsequent study using the same database again showed no advantage for Dukes' C cases treated by curative anterior resection whether the inferior mesenteric artery was ligated above or below the branch of the left colic artery.[64] The difficulty with such studies is not only their retrospective nature but also the very real problem of knowing exactly what was done at the time of surgery. Furthermore, other factors, such as dissemination or local extent as well as surgical technique, may override any possible influence that an extra centimeter or two of mesentery may have.

"No Touch" Technique

Turnbull et al.[65] advocated the so-called "no touch" technique. This consisted of immediate division of the lymphovascular pedicle before beginning mobilization of the tumor. The 5-year survival rate in the 896 patients so treated was greater than in a group of over 2,000 patients not having this manipulation. In a large multicenter, randomized, controlled clinical trial there was, however, no difference; 117 patients underwent early ligation and 119 a conventional dissection. Five-year survival rates in the two groups were 40.1% and 43.7% respectively.[66] There is therefore no objective evidence to support the value of early ligation with the "no touch" technique.

Pelvic Lymphadenopathy

Following the demonstration by Sauer and Bacon[60] of internal iliac node involvement in some cases with lower middle third rectal carcinoma, Deddish and Stearns[67] adopted a surgical policy of pelvic lymphadenectomy in patients undergoing total rectal excision at Memorial Hospital, New York. Of 122 patients, 11 had evidence of lymphatic metastases on examination of the resected specimen. This incidence of 12% was similar to that recorded by Sauer and Bacon. Only two of these patients

had extended survival, however, and in the light of the morbidity encountered it was felt that lymphadenectomy was of little value. The same database has more recently been reviewed.[68] This retrospective study showed no difference in pelvic local recurrence rates among 192 patients having a lymphadenectomy (29%) and 220 not having had this procedure (29%).

Despite these negative data, pelvic lymphadenectomy has been strongly advocated by Japanese surgeons. The technique adopted included removal of the mesenteric and extramesenteric lymphatic drainage through a formal dissection from just below the third part of the duodenum, taking all nodal tissue from the aorta and vena cava and continuing this into the internal iliac system, obturator fossa, and the lateral vesicle tissues. This subject has recently been reviewed by Scholefield and Northover.[69] In a study of 231 patients having pelvic lymphadenectomy,[70] positive nodes were found in 42 (18.1%). In the 114 patients with Dukes' C tumors, the incidence was 36% (42 of 114). Disease-free survival at 5 years in all patients was 69.4%. In the 42 with involved lateral nodes it was 49%. Twenty-seven patients developed local recurrence including 25 of 114 with Dukes' C and only 2 of 84 with Dukes' B tumors. The price paid for such extended surgery was a high incidence of urinary and sexual complications owing to autonomic nerve damage. Hojo et al.[71] reported urinary difficulties in just under 40% of 437 patients. Impotence occurred in 76% of males under the age of 60. Attempts to preserve the integrity of pelvic autonomic nerves may reduce this incidence but it still represents a significant drawback to the technique.[62]

Not all reports from Japan have shown a survival benefit for lateral pelvic lymph node dissection. In the report of Moreira et al.[72] a retrospective comparison was made of 95 patients having a lateral pelvic node dissection and 83 who did not. Of the former, 10 (11%) were found to have involved lateral pelvic nodes and all had a Dukes' C tumor. Respective 5-year survival rates in the lymphadenectomy and nonlymphadenectomy groups were 76% and 72% and local recurrence rates were 9% and 16%. There was no statistical difference between these proportions.

There have been no randomized clinical trials to test the value of extended lymphadenectomy, which therefore remains sub judice. Even if surgeons are prepared to perform this maneuver the identification of lymphadenopathy in nonresected cases is too inaccurate to allow histopathologic comparability between the lymphadenectomized and nonlymphadenectomized groups.

LOCAL RECURRENCE

Local recurrence is the cancer-specific end point most applicable to surgery. It is influenced by pathologic and surgical factors and can be reduced by radiotherapy. The autopsy study from Malmo has shown that local recurrence at death is almost always associated with dissemination.[73]

Incidence

The incidence of local recurrence in surgical series varies considerably from less than 5% to over 30%.[74–76] Thus, rates of below 10%, provided they are carefully annotated, are well below the average. Most multicenter trials in which local recurrence has been recorded report rates of around 20%. In the classic study from Malmo[73] a cohort of 960 patients representing 94% of all patients developing large bowel cancer in the region were treated in the Department of Surgery between 1958 and 1967. Of these 7.7% were inoperable and 66.7% were operated on for cure. The highly developed social system in Sweden allowed almost complete tracking of the patients and the autopsy rate of 83.1% permitted the most accurate analysis of the distribution of the disease at death available in the literature. Of the 960 patients, 635 had died. Of these 528 (83.1%) had had an autopsy. These included 267 patients treated for cure. Sixty of these were tumor free, having died from other than cancer causes. Of the 207 remaining patients, 110 had local recurrence and 195 had dissemination. In only eight cases of local recurrence was there no evidence of dissemination. Thus 93% of local recurrences were found to coexist with dissemination. Although the distribution of tumor at death may not be a reflection of the situation during life, the observation that local recurrence rarely occurs in isolation is in line with the results of adjuvant radiotherapy trials and of salvage surgery for recurrence in which distant failure has been the main cause of death. The message from this high-quality analysis is that local recurrence at death, at least, only rarely occurs without simultaneous dissemination.

Variability

The wide range of incidence of local recurrence may be due to three factors: accuracy and duration of follow-up, differences in the distinction between locally palliative and curative clearance, and surgical technique.

It is only in the last 10 years that local recurrence has been specifically looked for. The early randomized trials of preoperative radiotherapy carried out at Memorial Hospital,[77] and by the Veterans Administration Adjuvant Surgical Group[78] were unable to report on local recurrence because at that time only survival was the chosen end point. Imaging techniques including CT and more recently MRI have helped to identify local recurrence, and endoluminal ultrasound has been used to identify anastomotic recurrence after anterior resection. While emphasizing the importance of technique, Heald[79] has helped to make surgeons aware of the importance of local recurrence; several adjuvant trials of radiotherapy had, however, already recognized the necessity to record this as an end point.[80–84] Furthermore, Phillips et al.[74] in an important paper revealed the factors leading to local recurrence based on data obtained from the Large Bowel Cancer Project. This involved 94 surgeons in 23 hospitals in the United Kingdom and gave a picture of treatment, complications, and local recurrence following surgery. Although not truly epidemiologic, this and the Malmo study have been influential in focusing surgeons on outcomes after treatment for large bowel cancer.

The incidence of reported local recurrence depends on the denominator used.[85] It is higher in patients with disseminated disease and in palliative cases in general. The judgment that a ''curative'' resection has been performed may involve some degree of subjectivity on the part of the surgeon. Thus where one surgeon has a high threshold in deciding whether local clearance has been complete, local recurrence will be less than that of another whose threshold is lower. The distinction between the locally palliative and locally curative case is crucial in

enabling comparison between surgical series. Local recurrence rates are almost always given in series of patients having a curative operation. The Concord Hospital clinicopathologic staging system[42] recognizes the importance of the assessment of local disease at operation. In practice most cases considered by the surgeon to have had an incomplete local clearance are confirmed by the pathologist's examination. When the latter states, however, that the surgical margins are complete, the prognosis is still poor indicating that a surgical assessment of incomplete clearance should be taken to mean that the case is locally palliative.[86]

McCall et al.[76] have reviewed the world literature on local recurrence from 1982 to 1992. They selected publications reporting a minimum of 50 patients having surgery for rectal cancer treated for cure and without having had adjuvant therapy. There were 51 articles reporting a total of 10,465 patients. The data were analyzed with stratification for Dukes' stage and type of procedure, whether total rectal excision or anterior resection. Patients having total mesorectal excision and extended pelvic lymphadenopathy were also analyzed when this information was available.

Local recurrence rates ranged from 3% to 50% with a median of 18.5% (Table 23-1). On pooling data from all the publications the median rate was 18.8%. Of the 6,188 patients for whom information on type of operation was available, local recurrence after anterior resection (3,577 patients) was 16.2% and after total rectal excision (2,601 patients) 19.3%. A total of 1,033 patients had total mesorectal excision with a local recurrence rate of 7.1%. There was no difference in the spectrum of pathologic stage in this group when compared with the rest of the

Table 23-1. Local Recurrence Rates Reported in the Literature

1st Author	Year	No. of Patients	Local Recurrence Rate (%)
Adloff[223]	1984	113	32
Balslev[82]	1986	247	18
Carlsson[224]	1987		
Series I		100	24
Series II		231	38
Cawthorn[225]	1990	122	7
Gerard[84]	1988	175	28
GTSG[141]	1985 (controls)	58	24
Hojo[71]	1989		
Extended		192	14
Standard		245	19
Karanjia[226]	1990	152	3
Lasson[227]	1984	102	16
Localio[212]	1983	360	13
McDermott[114]	1985	934	20
Pahlman[228]	1984	197	38
Phillips[74,75]	1984	848	15
Pollett[89]	1983	334	7
Stockholm[80]	1987	274	20
Williams[106]	1984	148	17
Zirngibl[229]	1990	1,153	23

(Modified from McCall et al.,[76] with permission.)

series, but the follow-up was somewhat shorter although not significantly so.

Although such an analysis suffers from the major defect of data control, the large number of patients gives a general picture of the present reported state regarding local recurrence. It confirms the variance of this cancer-specific end point and hints at the possible benefit of total mesorectal excision.

Locoregional Pathologic Spread

Morson et al.[87] were the first to show that the pathologic variables of local spread and height of lesion were related to local recurrence being found to be greatest in patients with tumors in the lower rectum having extensive extrarectal spread. This is likely due to the proximity of the tumor being closer to the pelvic wall laterally, the sacrum posteriorly, and the urogenital system anteriorly, whereas a tumor in the upper rectum is further away from any of these structures. Morson et al.[87] also speculated that local recurrence might often occur as a result of unresected involved lymph nodes on the side wall of the pelvis. This question has already been discussed and is compatible with the occurrence of lateral pelvic lymphadenopathy in 10% to over 30% of cases and its relationship to local recurrence.

Direct local spread in continuity with the tumor occurs not only laterally but also distally within the rectal wall. In most cases this is limited to less than 10 mm and historically the appreciation of this fact[16,57] gave the rationale for the development of anterior resection. Only occasionally is distal intramural spread greater than 10 mm and these are usually cases with a poorly differentiated tumor. There is evidence that a distal margin of less than 10 mm after anterior resection may be associated with local recurrence,[75,83] and in such cases no patient will survive for any useful length of time.[89]

Local spread not in continuity with the tumor has been described by Heald.[90] Careful sectioning of the mesorectum has shown the presence of tumor nests that may lie well below the level of the distal border of the primary growth (Fig. 23-6). This finding has been considered a common reason for local recurrence and has led to the emphasis of the importance of total mesorectum excision.[79] There is, however, little direct histopathologic information to allow an assessment of the prevalence of this form of spread.

Histologic Grade

The histologic grade of the tumor has an important influence on both survival and local recurrence. Grading on preoperative biopsy is, however, liable to observer error. In a study that compared the grade assessed by a panel of pathologists examining the same set of slides, Blenkinsopp et al.[91] reported useful concordance only for poorly differentiated tumors. There was considerable variation in the diagnosis of well-differentiated growths. Preoperative grading in 42 patients found to have a poorly differentiated tumor on examination of the excised specimen was accurate in only 17%, giving a false-negative rate of about 58%.[92] Despite these difficulties in interpretation, histologic grade as recorded in practice can be shown to relate to local recurrence. In a group of 848 patients with rectal cancer of whom 370 had an anterior resection and 478 a total rectal excision, local recurrence rates were 18% and 12%, respec-

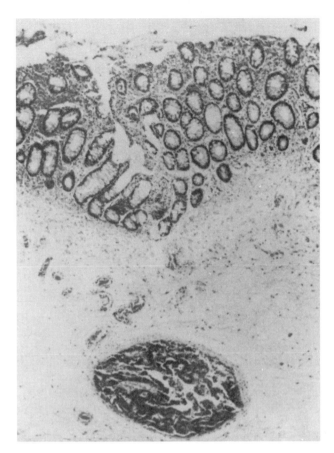

Figure 23-6. Isolated nest of adenocarcinoma distant from the primary tumor lying distally within the mesorectum. (From Heald et al.,[40] with permission.)

tively. Histologic grade was positively correlated with local recurrence. Dukes' A and C tumors after anterior resection led to local recurrence in 10.3% and 19.2% of cases, respectively. The equivalent rates after total rectal excision were 13.6% and 34.5%.[74,75] Poorly differentiated tumors are more likely to exhibit distal intramural spread[93–95] (see below). Regional lymphadenopathy and dissemination are also positively correlated.

Surgical Factors Influencing Local Recurrence

The variability of local recurrence rates reported by different surgeons even within the same institution[53,54] suggests the importance of technique. This can be divided into two components including locoregional clearance and the avoidance of implantation. Curative surgery aims to remove all cancer from the patient. It will always include the primary tumor with a suitable surrounding region of normal tissue and in most cases removal of the lymphovascular pedicle also.

Clearance Margins

The extent of the local clearance must be determined by the pathologic features of the primary tumor. Direct local spread occurs circumferentially and distally and discontinuous spread may involve the mesorectum. Quirke et al.[96] demonstrated the importance of achieving clear lateral margins. In a series of 51 patients who survived anterior resection, tumor was found at the lateral margin in 13 of whom 11 developed clinical local recurrence within 2 years. This was compared with only one case in the 38 patients who did not have lateral involvement.

Although the concept of wide local removal can be traced back to Halstead and authors at various times have emphasized its importance,[97] the message from the study of Quirke et al. is twofold. First, locally extensive tumors in which achieving a clear circumferential margin may be difficult should be identified preoperatively and radiotherapy considered. Second, during the dissection, the surgeon should be constantly aware of the importance of achieving circumferential clearance. In most cases this is realized by dissection in the anatomic plane just outside the fascia propria. However, where the tumor extends locally into the perirectal fat or has involved neighboring organs, a deliberate wide dissection must be taken to achieve adequate local removal.

In the early 1950s Quer et al.[93] and Grinnell[94] published evidence showing that intramural spread of tumor distal to the lower border of the tumor was absent or very limited in most cases. When more than 1 to 2 cm, the tumor was likely to be poorly differentiated. The classic study by Goligher et al.,[98] which was one of the first formal investigations of local recurrence, reported this complication in 16 of 151 operative survivors of anterior resection. These cases were added to by nine others referred, giving a total of 25 available for study. In 15 of these, local recurrence was unexpected in being neither a new primary nor the result of obvious residual disease. Here the authors concluded that the evidence indicated that recurrence had been due to implantation. In the same article they also reported the results of careful pathologic study in 1,500 consecutive patients having rectal excision. They found "metastatic" involvement below the level of the growth in only 98 (6.5%) specimens. In 68 of these a margin of clearance of 1 inch (2.54 cm) would have removed them. More extensive distal spread occurred only in the remaining 30 or 3% of the total. The authors reported direct intramural spread to a greater distance distally in a few cases and it was for this reason that the 2 inch or "5 cm rule" evolved. Applied strictly, this meant that anterior resection was acceptable for growths lying 5 cm above the anorectal junction. Given the length of the anal canal of 3 to 4 cm, this would have limited restorative procedure to tumors at more than 8 or 9 cm from the anal verge, therefore excluding all growths in the lower and some in the midrectum.

Surgical developments of anastomotic technique including coloanal procedures and particularly stapled anastomosis have forced surgeons and pathologists to revise their thinking on the "5 cm rule." Retrospective studies[89,99] showed no difference in survival according to the distal margin of clearance. Williams et al.[100] in a clinicopathologic study examined 50 abdominoperineal rectal excision specimens and found no distal intramural spread in 38 (76%) of patients. Only five patients had spread of more than 1 cm all of whom had a poorly differentiated Dukes' C tumor and all died of metastases within 3 years. A comparison of patients having had an anterior resection showed no difference in survival or local recurrence in the 48 with a margin less than 5 cm and the 31 in whom the margin was greater. In a similar study there was no difference in survival according to lengths of distal margin of more than 5, 2 to 5,

and less than 2 cm. Furthermore, no patient with intramural spread greater than 10 mm survived long term.[89]

There are, however, limits to the safety margin beyond which local recurrence is more likely. With the introduction of stapling, reports of high local recurrence rates of over 30% within 1 to 2 years appeared.[101] Phillips et al.[75] demonstrated a notable incidence of local recurrence after anterior resection where the margin was less than 10 mm compared with total rectal excision for growths at a similar level. Hermanek[102] supported the view that local recurrence is related to the length of the distal margin of clearance and that when less than 20 mm the risk increases markedly.

It would be reasonable at the present time to regard 25 mm as an acceptable length of distal bowel, which combines adequate intramural cancer clearance in almost all cases with the maximum opportunity for sphincter preservation.

The Mesorectum

Discontinuous spread into the mesorectum to form circumscribed nests of tumor was shown to occur by Heald et al.[90] They described six cases in which histopathologic examination of the mesorectum showed foci of adenocarcinoma often well distal to the lower border of the tumor (Fig. 23-6). The presence of this potential source of local recurrence has led to the doctrine that total mesorectal excision should accompany anterior resection as a routine in the belief that local recurrence will be minimized or prevented. Histopathologic detection of such small areas is difficult and requires close section of the mesorectum and painstaking study of the sections by the histopathologist. The incidence and localization of these nests has therefore been somewhat uncertain.

Some light has recently been shed on this. In a detailed prospective histopathologic study of 14 curative anterior resection specimens in which mesorectal excision had been performed and a further six total excisions, adenocarcinoma was found in the mesorectum distal to the lower border of the tumor in five (25%) cases. Of these only one patient was alive and disease free at 5 years. Two patients had died of metastases and two had developed local recurrence. This contrasted with only two failures in the 15 who did not have evidence of distal mesorectal spread. Although the site of treatment failure in these was not given, the data suggest on small numbers that mesenteric involvement confers a worse risk.[103]

Total mesorectal excision has been advocated as a routine component of anterior resection because with this approach local recurrence rates of less than 5% have been reported.[104] This maneuver cannot, however, eradicate local recurrence because this occurs after total rectal excision in which all mesorectum is removed (Table 23-2). Furthermore, it will not deal with metastatic nodes on the lateral pelvic wall, which are known to occur in 10% to 30% of cases (see above).

A randomized prospective clinical trial should theoretically answer the question whether total mesorectal excision leads to lower local recurrence compared with conventional anterior resection but the methodologic problems are considerable. Such a trial would have to be multicentric to achieve adequate accrual over a significant short period of time. It is very difficult to standardize a precise surgical technique to be used by different surgeons. Surgeons may themselves already be convinced of

Table 23-2. Local Recurrence After Anterior Resection and Total Rectal Excision

Authors	Operation	No. of Patients	Local Recurrence (%)
Stearns & Binkley[230]	TRE	131	53
Gilbertson[231]	TRE	89	36
Morson et al.[87]	TRE	1,115	12
Pilipshen et al.[232]	TRE	330	30
Lasson et al.[227]	TRE	62	16
Williams & Johnston[106]	TRE	83	8
	AR	71	11
Luke et al.[233]	TRE	80	22
	AR	44	23
Phillips et al.[74,75]	TRE	478	12
	AR	370	18

Abbreviations: TRE, total rectal excision; AR, anterior resection.

the desirability of total mesorectal excision and may not be prepared to accept the protocol of randomization. Pathologic factors are also difficult to standardize. A trial has nevertheless been initiated (Pahlman, personal communication) but results will not be available for some time.

Recurrence in the pelvis occurs after total rectal excision in which all the mesorectum is excised.[67,87,105–107] A certain incidence of involved nodes in the lateral pelvic wall has been demonstrated in all studies analyzing this question.[69] Anterior resection does not include removal of this source of recurrence. In the light of this information total mesorectal excision cannot be the final answer to eliminating local recurrence. It is reasonable, however, to conclude that it will optimize the results of anterior resection by minimizing local recurrence although it will not abolish it. This technique would seem to be indicated for growths in the middle and lower rectum. If so, this will necessitate an anastomosis between the colon and the lowest part of the rectum or the upper anal canal.

Removal of the rectum requiring a low anastomosis may be the explanation for the finding by Akyol et al.[108] of a higher local recurrence rate after a hand-sutured compared with a stapled anastomosis. In a prospective randomized trial of 294 patients surviving curative anterior resection, 142 underwent a manual and 152 a stapled anastomosis. Respective local recurrence rates were 31 of 142 and 18 of 152. Furthermore, the relative cancer-specific mortality was also significantly different, the risk being 50% less in the stapled compared with the hand-sutured group.

Implantation

Access to the peritoneum or the anastomosis by cancer cells may arise during perforation of the tumor by virtue of its own growth or by contamination at the time of surgery. Perforation was found by Phillips et al.[74] to be associated with a significantly high level of local recurrence. Local recurrence occurred

in 269 (13%) of 2,076 patients in whom the tumor was not perforated intraoperatively compared with 40 (28%) of 144 patients in whom it was. Perforation confers palliative status on the operation. Some cases of local recurrence are due to implantation at the anastomosis of viable tumor cells. This was the main theme of Goligher et al.[98] who considered about one-half of ''unexpected'' recurrences to be due to this cause.

Umpleby and Williamson[109] have reviewed this subject and quote an incidence of suture line recurrence of 5% to 15% of patients.[110–114] Such recurrences may be due to invasion of extramural tumor into the anastomotic area or to implantation of viable tumor cells at the time of surgery. Alternatively malignant transformation of proliferating mucosa at the anastomotic site might occur.

Rosenberg et al.[115] studied the viability of shed intraluminal cancer cells. They used various means of assessment of viability including exclusion of trypan blue, tritiated thymidine uptake, and positive tissue culture and were unable to demonstrate viability. They concluded that exfoliated cells were unlikely to be a major cause of anastomotic recurrence. Umpleby et al.[116] subsequently demonstrated that such cells were viable both in intraluminal washings and at resection margins. These authors were able to induce viable tumors on inoculation of intraluminal preparations in 6 of 17 T-cell-depleted mice. Clinically, implantation can occur in wounds or raw surfaces well away from the original tumor. Reports of recurrence at colostomy sites,[117] hemorrhoidectomy wounds,[118] and more recently port site recurrence after laparoscopic surgery for carcinoma[119] clearly show that implantation can occur.

There is some evidence that irrigation of the rectal stump and the proximal divided colon with a cancericidal solution before constructing the anastomosis can result in a low anastomotic recurrence rate.[120,121] A 10% incidence for suture line recurrence when irrigation was not used was reduced to zero in 101 subsequent patients who were irrigated[121] and a similar reduction from 13% to 3% occurred following the introduction of mercuric perchloride solution irrigation at St. Mark's Hospital.[120] There is some evidence from animal studies that suture line recurrence may be promoted by the presence of metal staples.[122] This may be a mechanical effect with viable cells being forced into the tissues by the staples or there may be some local biological effect produced by the staples. Umpleby and Williamson[123] studied the effectiveness of different irrigants in causing death of exfoliated cancer cells. Mercuric perchloride, chlorhexadine-cetrimide, and povidone-iodine were all effective and more reliable than sterile water.

Irrigation of the rectal stump should be an essential step during anterior resection. In cases where the anastomosis will be constructed using the double staple technique, irrigation should precede the application of the distal transverse staple line. Because exfoliated cancer cells can be viable, it is a fair presumption that perforation results in local contamination with implantation and subsequent growth. The conclusion must be that perforation or any other form of contamination during surgery significantly worsens the prognosis and in some units its occurrence is regarded to confer palliative status to such cases. Table 23-3 gives a summary of various factors involved in local recurrence from data from the Large Bowel Cancer Project.[75]

Table 23-3. Risk Factors for Local Recurrence Large Bowel Cancer

	No.	Local Recurrence (%)
Dukes		
A	263	10 (3.8)
B	1,198	154 (12.9)
C	749	143 (18.0)
Histologic grade		
Well	578	66 (11.4)
Moderate	1,330	181 (13.6)
Poor	265	55 (20.8)
Obstruction		
Absent	1,940	249 (12.8)
Present	280	60 (21.4)
Perforation		
Absent	2,076	269 (13.0)
Present	144	40 (27.8)
Tumor mobility		
Mobile	1,574	171 (10.9)
Not mobile	646	138 (21.4)

(From Phillips et al.,[74] with permission.)

CHOICE OF TREATMENT

The treatment of rectal cancer requires a combined approach. Surgery is the mainstay but adjuvant radiotherapy has now been shown to reduce local recurrence in selected cases. The effect of chemotherapy in reducing long-term mortality is uncertain but recent trials indicate that it may now have a place in routine practice in selected cases.

The most important factor determining the choice of operation is the level of the tumor. Growths in the upper rectum with the lower border lying at 12 cm or more from the anal verge should be treated by anterior resection. If the tumor is locally extensive radiotherapy should be given. For tumors in the middle and lower rectum there are several options requiring decisions preoperatively. These include whether radiotherapy should be added and whether total rectal excision or a restorative procedure should be advised. Restorative surgery can be divided into anterior resection and local excision.

Preoperative Staging

The choice of treatment will depend on the presence or absence of dissemination and the anticipated possibility of local recurrence. The aim of preoperative staging is to determine the pathologic extent of the tumor before treatment as accurately as possible. At the locoregional level, this should be to anticipate the pathologic stage that the pathologist will discover on examining the excised specimen. The available means of doing so include digital palpation of the tumor and imaging by pelvic and endoluminal ultrasonography, CT, and MRI. Radioimmunoscintigraphy is not yet sufficiently reliable to be part of current practice. Recommendations on the protocol of recording of information in cases of rectal cancer have been made by the United Kingdom Coordinating Committee on Cancer Research (UKCCCR).[124]

Dissemination

The identification of metastatic disease before treatment may influence the choice of operation or the selection of radiotherapy under certain circumstances. Patients with a solitary metastasis have a 20% to 50% prospect of 5-year survival following hepatic resection.[125,126] These cases are rare, however, amounting to around 5% of all patients with metastatic disease, and there is no imperative to identify them preoperatively as the presence of a solitary metastasis is unlikely to influence the choice of treatment.

It may do so, however, where there are multiple bilobar metastases. Such patients have a median survival of no more than 18 months and in many cases of less than 12 months.[127] A low anterior resection in such cases may not be the best form of palliation. Complications including anastomotic breakdown are three times more likely in the palliative than in the curative case.[128] Thus serious morbidity is likely. Anastomotic breakdown in the early postoperative period may require further operation with establishment of a stoma that will require subsequent closure provided the patient's general condition permits. Having recovered from major surgery patients having a low colorectal or coloanal anastomosis may well suffer from poor bowel function for several months. These possibilities might mean that a patient with a life expectancy of only a few months could spend much of this time afflicted by morbidity with extended hospitalization and poor function.

Patients with a middle or lower third carcinoma with extensive metastatic disease may therefore be treated more satisfactorily by Hartmann's operation. Local excision may occasionally be justifiable in those rare cases where the local features of the primary tumor are suitable to this approach. Alternatively other forms of local treatment (e.g., radiotherapy) may be used in this palliative situation. It can control local symptoms of pain and bleeding for periods of several weeks to months.[129]

In most patients with disseminated rectal cancer, the choice of treatment is made on the basis of the locoregional state. The knowledge of dissemination before treatment will affect the decisions in only a small proportion of patients and thus the routine use of preoperative imaging to look for metastatic disease is a matter for debate.

Locoregional Extent

Locoregional staging requires careful and experienced digital examination of the tumor. Such an assessment is, however, limited and can usefully be amplified by imaging techniques using endoluminal ultrasound or CT or MRI. MRI has been reported to have a high sensitivity in detecting penetration of the rectal wall but intraluminal ultrasound is as accurate and much less expensive.[130–132] Combining these methods, it is possible to identify two main clinicopathologic groups, including the locally extensive tumor and the locally not extensive tumor, which are potentially suitable for local treatment. Preoperative determination of lymph node status is inaccurate. Imaging including CT and ultrasonography[132] can detect enlarged nodes as can digital examination[133] in about 50% of patients. In a comparative study of ultrasound versus MRI, the former proved to be more accurate.[132] Sensitivity and specificity may, however, be poor for tumor involvement although the picture may change with the use of endoluminal MRI.[134] It is noteworthy that about 30% of metastatic nodes are 5 mm or less in diameter.[135] There is no means at present of assessing the mesorectum preoperatively for the presence of tumor nests. Thus locoregional staging is essentially an exercise in the assessment of level and local extent.

Digital examination is capable of identifying two broad groups of tumor. These include locally extensive and locally not extensive. The clinical staging system developed by Mason[136] is unable in practice to identify all the four stages he described, but it can differentiate with an accuracy of about 80% tumors with a low chance of subsequent local recurrence from those with a high chance (i.e., locally not extensive and locally extensive). In a prospective study of 54 patients with palpable rectal cancer staged clinically, 22 were judged to be locally not extensive. Only two had died of cancer in 5 years and none had developed local recurrence. Of the 32 patients staged as having a locally advanced tumor, 6 (19%) developed local recurrence.[137] There was also a correlation between the number of quadrants within the rectum occupied by the tumor and the categories of locally not extensive and locally extensive.

Tumors can thus be usefully designated as clinical stage I and clinical stage II, respectively. These stages do not correspond with any of the conventional pathologic staging systems but they can predict local recurrence more reliably than any present pathologic staging system. The reason for this is that the pathologic stage of pT3 (equivalent to Dukes' B or Astler Coller B2) is extremely heterogeneous. It includes tumors that have just penetrated the rectal wall with very low local recurrence rates and those that have extended well out into the extramural tissue with high local recurrence rates. The heterogeneity of stage T3 renders the pathologic (pT) and ultrasonic (uT) equivalents as being of very limited value in determining the risk of subsequent local recurrence. Reference to Figure 23-7 shows how the subdivision of clinical stages I and II cuts across conventional pathologic and ultrasound staging systems and by so doing increases the sensitivity for treatment selection.

Clinical stage I includes stages T1, T2, and the less extensive T3. In this group, 5-year survival is high and local recurrence low. Clinical stage II includes the more extensive stage T3 and stage T4. For these, 5-year survival is low and local recurrence high (Fig. 23-7). This clinical staging system supported by imaging gives the best opportunity for selecting, on the one hand, patients with a high prospect of local recurrence and for whom preoperative radiotherapy is indicated, and on the other those early carcinomas potentially suitable for local treatment.

Radiotherapy

Although radiotherapy is discussed more fully in Chapter 24, it is nevertheless important to consider its role in the manage-

Figure 23-7. Local staging of rectal carcinoma. Comparison of clinical, histopathologic, and ultrasound stage.

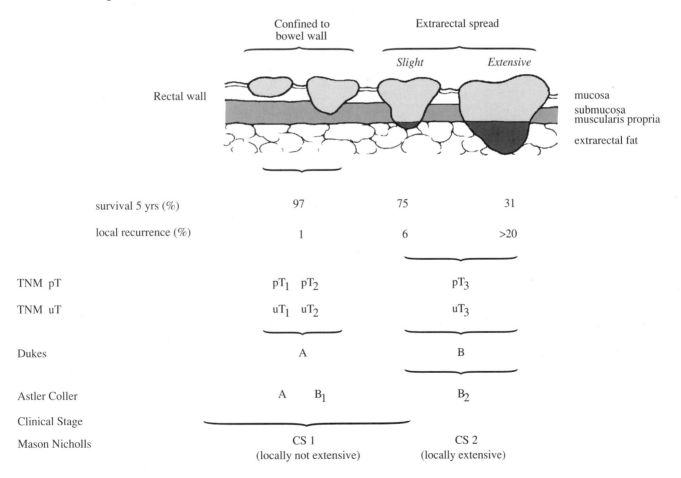

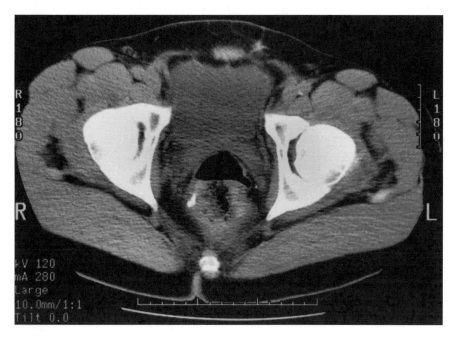

Figure 23-8. CT scan showing locally advanced tumor. Extrarectal spread well shown. Indication for preoperative radiotherapy.

ment of rectal carcinoma when faced with the choice of treatment.

Adjuvant Radiotherapy

There are now several trials that demonstrate that preoperative radiotherapy reduces local recurrence when followed by surgery. The randomized controlled trial carried out at Memorial Hospital[77] was the first of a sequence of studies examining the role of adjuvant radiotherapy. In this study no difference in survival or in the incidence of nodal metastases was found but local recurrence was not examined as an end point. The Veterans' Administration Hospitals Trial[78] was reported to show an improved 5-year survival rate in the irradiated group (40%) compared with the nonirradiated (28%) but again local recurrence rates were not reported. This was also true of the subsequent Veterans' Administration Surgical Adjuvant Group Study in which a higher dose (3,150 cGy) was used with no comment on local recurrence.[138] Other trials of the 1970s and 1980s[139,140] also did not examine local recurrence as an end point.

There are now, however, several trials that show that preoperative radiotherapy reduces local recurrence.[81,83,84] The published results indicate that preoperative radiotherapy is more effective than postoperative. With postoperative radiotherapy, cancer-specific results have been disappointing and morbidity has been higher.[82,191] Postoperative radiotherapy can damage the colonic segment brought down to an anastomosis and is more likely to cause small bowel enteropathy. These considerations should be taken into account when planning treatment.

The available evidence indicates that local recurrence is reduced by preoperative radiotherapy. Perhaps its effect is by sterilization of tumor metastases and lateral pelvic wall nodes, plus achieving a similar effect to that proposed by advocates of lateral pelvic lymphadenectomy while at the same time avoiding the local morbidity caused by surgery.

Locally Advanced Tumor

There is now much information to indicate that radiotherapy is beneficial in converting a case deemed by the surgeon to be inoperable at presentation into one that becomes operable. Such growths are identified on clinical examination as being fixed and CT scan is essential to define the local extent (Fig. 23-8).

In a series of 72 tumors considered to be inoperable, it was possible to resect 28 after high-dose radiotherapy. Unfortunately only 3 (10%) of these patients survived for 5 years and of the 28, 19 exhibited subsequent local recurrence.[142] It is noteworthy that 6 (14%) of the 44 unresectable patients survived 5 years. In contrast the same approach did appear to improve survival. James and Schofield[143] reported 42 patients with an inoperable carcinoma at presentation. Of these, 18 became operable and the median survival in this group was 25 months compared with 7 months in the unresected patients. Others[144,145] have reported a similar experience in rendering an initially inoperable tumor operable.

SURGERY

Choice of Operation

Total Rectal Excision or Sphincter-Preserving Procedure

With improvements in anastomotic technique and greater understanding of pathologic spread of the tumor, anterior resection has become increasingly applied to cancers in the middle rectum and in some cases in the lower rectum. It is now the operation of choice in the majority of cases. The factors that govern this decision include level of the tumor, local extent, and the presence or absence of disseminated disease. The last of these has already been discussed. All are pathologic factors and they take precedence over clinical considerations including general fitness of the patient, age and build, and the patient's wishes. The surgeon must be guided by interpretation of the pathology of the tumor and must bear in mind the fact that local recurrence with few exceptions is incurable. Thus the patient's wishes should be secondary to these overriding considerations.

Given the inaccuracy of preoperative assessment of regional lymphadenopathy, the choice between anterior resection and total rectal excision depends largely on the distal margin of clearance and the degree of local penetration. Clearly sphincter function must be adequate for a restorative procedure. Based on these criteria, anterior resection is now offered to most patients with cancer of the middle and in some cases lower third of the rectum. For those in the upper third, anterior resection should be advised in almost every case.

Standard anterior resection does not remove the entire mesorectum. Although complete mesorectal clearance does not abol-ish local recurrence, it appears likely to optimize the capability of anterior resection to achieve local tumor clearance.

There is evidence, however, that a distal margin of clearance of 10 mm or less may be associated with a greater incidence of local recurrence than if the patient had had a total rectal excision.[75] If the margin is 25 mm or more, then there appears to be no compromise of survival or local clearance. This means that most tumors of 6 cm or more from the anal verge or 2 or 3 cm above the anorectal junction are suitable for restorative resection (Fig. 23-9). Comparing tumors of similar stage, survival after anterior resection and total rectal excision is not significantly different.[106,107,146] Given the potential of total mesorectal excision to minimize local recurrence, there is a strong argument that any tumor of the middle or lower third of the rectum should be treated by a total rectal excision. This will therefore require a coloanal anastomosis as the routine form of restoration of intestinal continuity. The addition of a colonic

Figure 23-9. Distal surgical margin for anterior resection for rectal carcinoma.

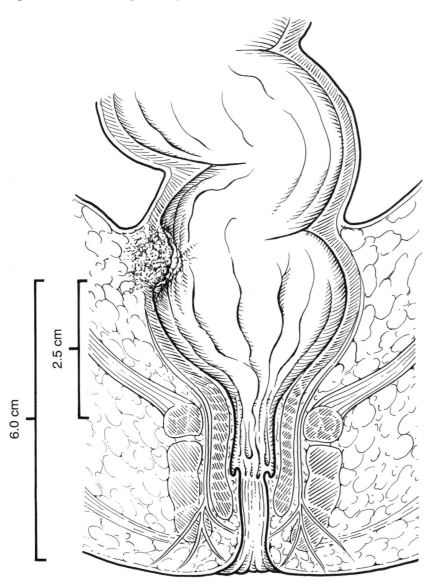

pouch (see below) to this reconstruction will optimize function. Accordingly, the traditional view of low anterior resection should now be modified to comprise total rectal excision with coloanal colonic pouch reconstruction as the standard major restorative operation for tumors of the mid- and lower rectum.[147]

The Early Rectal Tumor

A few patients are amenable to local excision but they comprise only about 5% of the total and must be selected very carefully. Despite the capacity of transanal endoscopic microsurgery to remove tumors in the middle and upper rectum, local excision should essentially remain an option for low growths in patients who otherwise would require a total excision of the anorectum. This approach is based on the premise that a tumor confined to the rectal wall has a low likelihood of simultaneous lymph node metastasis. Morson et al.[148] showed that a carcinoma confined to the rectal wall has a less than 10% chance of coexisting lymph node metastases. The original criteria of Morson et al.[148] should be revised, however, in the light of a multivariate analysis of a large group of radical operation specimens.[88] Nodal involvement as the end point was found in 263 (22%) well-, 1,196 (41.5%) moderately, and 252 (77%) poorly differentiated tumors. Lymphatic invasion was highly likely (78.3%) to be associated with nodal metastases compared with only 23.5% when it was not. When confined to the submucosa, lymph node metastases were present in only 4.9% of cases but this incidence gradually rose even within the T2 group such that invasion of the inner and outer muscularis propria conferred different risks (Fig. 23-10). As a result of these findings Hermanek has recommended local excision only in the low-risk group of PT1 and some PT2 lesions. In case selection endorectal ultrasonography is an essential adjuvant to digital examination. The respective accuracies in assessing penetration of the rectal wall are approx-

Table 23-4.   Criteria for Local Excision

Preoperative
  Digital examination
    Tumor ≤3 cm, mobile not ulcerated
  Ultrasound: uT1, ?uT2
  Histologic grade: well differentiated
Postoperative
  Histopathologic examination
    Local extent: pT1 (low risk pT2)[a]
    Histologic grade: well differentiated
    Excision complete
    No lymphatic or venous invasion
Subsequent clinical decision
  Major resection or surveillance depending on postoperative histopathologic examination

---

[a] Data from Hermanek and Gall,[158] Morson et al.,[148] and Hermanek.[88]

imately 95%[130] and 80%.[133] Tumors suitable for local excision must be accessible, small, and confined to the rectal wall. They should not show an anaplastic histology.[88,148] Although modern technology affords access to the upper rectum, for example, transanal endoscopic microsurgery,[149,150] and increases the scope for local excision, the rules of case selection based on the local pathology must still apply.

Many of the criteria defined by Morson et al.[148] and amplified by Hermanek[88] had already been detailed by Lockhart Mummery in 1914, who stated that a tumor suitable for local excision should be ''quite small and localized to the bowel in cases where a more extensive operation is for some reason or other impossible.''[21] The only more recent additions to these requirements are histologic grade and the morphology of the tumor (Table 23-4).

The relationship between morphology and treatment failure has not been considered until recently. Nicholls[151] has reported evidence to indicate that treatment failure after local excision is related to morphology. Between 1948 and 1985, 161 patients underwent local excision for rectal cancer at one hospital. Of these 78 had a polypoid exophytic growth, 46 malignant invasion within a sessile villous adenoma, 16 a raised flat adenocarcinoma, and 21 an ulcerating carcinoma. Cancer-specific survival was clearly related to the morphology. Of the 78 exophytic tumors, 75 patients (96%) were alive at 5 years and 3 had died, all of cancer. Of the 46 sessile adenomas with malignant invasion, 39 patients (88%) were alive at 5 years. Four had died and three were lost to follow-up. Two of the deaths were among the four T3 tumors in this group. Six (37%) of the 16 patients with raised flat adenocarcinoma had died of cancer. These included two T1, one T2, and three T3 stage tumors. Five-year survival in the 21 patients with an ulcerating carcinoma was low. Only six (30%) of these patients were alive and 14 had died. One patient was lost to follow-up. Of the 14 patients, 7 died of cancer. Thus the cancer-specific death rate in this group was 33%. These data show the importance of morphology, which is a feature easily detected by simple digital examination. They also show that ulcerated or flat adenocarcinomas should not be treated by local excision. Histopathologic examination of the excised specimen is an integral part of the policy of local excision. If any of the criteria in Table 23-4 are not fulfilled,

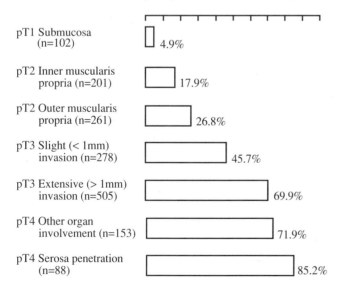

Figure 23-10.   Frequency of regional lymph node metastases in rectal carcinoma related to the depth of invasion from the study of curative operative specimens. (Data from Erlangen Tumour Centre and University Surgical Clinic 1969–1990.[88])

pT1 Submucosa (n=102)   4.9%
pT2 Inner muscularis propria (n=201)   17.9%
pT2 Outer muscularis propria (n=261)   26.8%
pT3 Slight (< 1mm) invasion (n=278)   45.7%
pT3 Extensive (> 1mm) invasion (n=505)   69.9%
pT4 Other organ involvement (n=153)   71.9%
pT4 Serosa penetration (n=88)   85.2%

then a major resection of the rectum should be advised. This will usually be total excision.

Outcome of Local Excision

Biggers and Beart[152] reported a large series from the Mayo Clinic of 234 patients treated for local excision of whom 93 had a T1 and 141 a T2 tumor. Local failure occurred in 19% of these. A similar overall rate (23%) was reported by Killingback.[153] In a careful analysis, he reviewed 63 cases of local excision out of a total of 493 patients with rectal cancer treated personally between 1969 and 1984. Of these, 25 with malignant polyps diagnosed subsequently on pathologic examination of the resected specimen were excluded. In the remaining patients available for follow-up treated intentionally by local excision for a known carcinoma, nine developed local recurrence and seven (18%) died. Of the nine only five were suitable for a subsequent salvage operation of whom three died. Thus the policy of Morson seemed to be of questionable value in his experience. In contrast, Whiteway et al.[154] in a review of 27 patients with an ulcerating carcinoma, reported a cancer-specific mortality of zero when the policy of subsequent major surgery following pathologic examination of the local excision specimen had been fulfilled. There was one operative death and in the remaining 26 patients, two refused further surgery despite being advised to undergo it; both died of cancer. In the remaining 24 patients, 5 underwent subsequent major surgery, 2 of whom died of cancer. None of the 19 patients with satisfactory pathology had further surgery and all were tumor free at 5 years. Thus cancer failure occurred in 2 (8%) of the 24 patients in whom the policy was fulfilled.

The report from St. Mark's Hospital of Lock et al.[155] of 110 patients treated between 1948 and 1973 by local excision indicated that local recurrence was low with only six late failures. The pictures was somewhat different when the expanded series extending from 1948 to 1984 was subsequently analyzed.[156] Of 167 patients, reliable follow-up data over 5 years were available in 152. The authors made little comment on morphology but showed that histologic grade was a major factor in determining prognosis. Local failure occurred in only 1 (2%) of 56 well-differentiated tumors. In contrast, of the 81 patients with a moderately differentiated tumor, death occurred in 12 (19%) of the 64 who did not undergo further surgery. There were too few poorly differentiated tumors (15) to draw useful conclusions although surprisingly six of the nine who had no further surgery survived long term. There was an indication from this analysis that the indications for local excision had been extended beyond the original criteria.

These results and those of others[157] emphasize the importance of case selection, indicating that local excision should be applied to well-differentiated tumors and those of T1 stage (early carcinoma of Hermanek and Gall[158]) unless the clinician is forced by the patient's wish or frailty to contemplate otherwise.

Using such limited criteria, Hermanek and Gall[158] in a series of 249 early carcinomas (comprising 9.3% of all patients treated for rectal carcinoma between 1969 and 1983 in the unit) reported 5-year survival rates of 95% in the 53 patients having local excision and 100% in the 130 patients having a major resection for tumors of the same pT stage.

Buess et al.[159] have reported a series of 74 patients with rectal cancer treated by transanal microscopic endosurgery. Of these, 47 were of T1, 21 T2, and 6 T3 local stage. At a mean follow-

Figure 23-11. The Lloyd-Davies/Trendelenburg position.

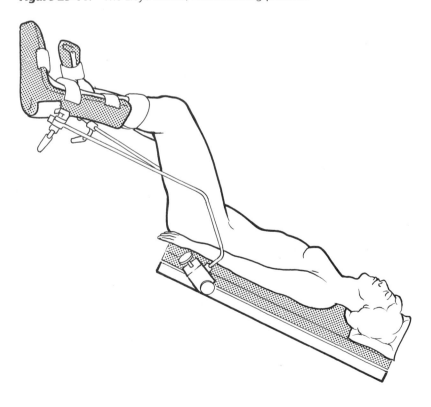

up of 14 months, 4 were reported to have recurred. It is clear that full and accurate long-term follow-up is essential to enable a proper assessment of this technique, particularly in view of the distribution of T stage in the series. More important will be the cancer-specific results obtained by other units and the long-term outcome. In 433 patients with cancer treated in 44 centers,[160] the complication rate appeared to be related to the experience of the surgeon with an overall rate of under 5% and a mortality of less than 1%. Complications of this technique may, however, be severe. In a series of 251 patients, there were five perforations and four rectovaginal fistulae as well as two cardiorespiratory deaths.[161]

The reviews of Graham et al.[162] and Banerjee et al.[163] offer an extensive bibliography on the subject of local treatment.

TECHNIQUE

Preoperative Preparation and Anesthesia

Routine preoperative assessment of cardiorespiratory status, correction of anemia, and bowel preparation in all cases except those with obstruction should be carried out. The use of an oral laxative agent produces a satisfactory colon in around 80% of cases. Counseling of patients likely to need a stoma is essential and the position of the stoma should be marked on the skin.

Antibiotic cover should be given during induction of anesthesia. A simple intravenous injection of an agent effective against anaerobes (metronidazole, tinidazole) combined with an antibiotic against gram-positive organisms (aminoglycoside or cephalosporin) is sufficient to achieve optimal prophylaxis against wound infection. General anesthesia with muscle relaxation and ventilation should be used unless the patient is judged too unfit. In this circumstance, regional anesthesia with general sedation will be necessary.

The Operation

Laparotomy

With the patient in the Trendelenburg position modified by Lloyd Davies, simultaneous access to the abdomen and perineum is achieved (Fig. 23-11). Some surgeons prefer to turn

Figure 23-12. Identification of the right presacral nerve. The fascia propria of the rectum invests the mesorectum.

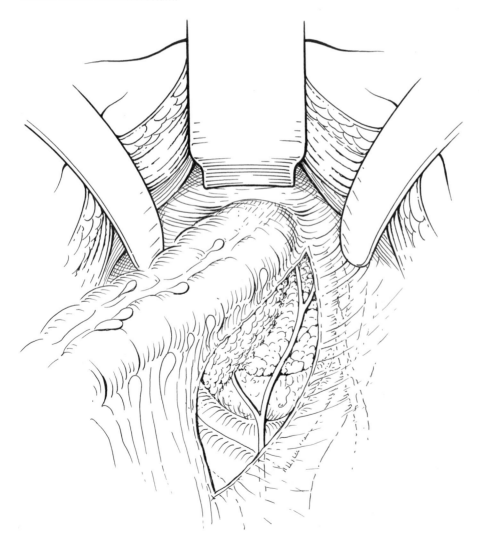

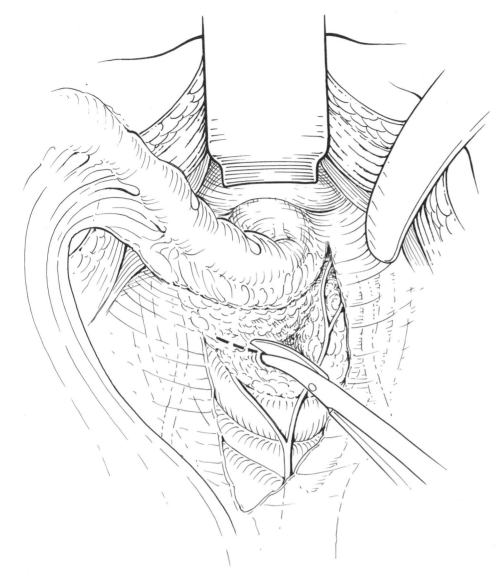

Figure 23-13. The presacral dissection continued. Division of the fascia of Waldeyer.

the patient into the left lateral or jackknife position after an initial abdominal phase. With the abdominosacral approach used by Localio et al.,[30] the patient is placed obliquely to enable simultaneous approaches.

A midline incision is satisfactory for most purposes. It is easy to make, does not encroach on any future stoma site, and gives good access to the abdominal contents. It is often possible to perform the operation through a small incision. If this proves to be impossible, a midline incision is easy to extend. With modern suture materials and closure techniques, the incidence of dehiscence or late herniation is acceptable compared with other incisions. Transverse incisions are favored by some surgeons. They are well tolerated and heal well.

On opening the abdomen a full assessment of the contents with particular reference to dissemination, especially to the peritoneum or liver, to synchronous lesions, and the primary tumor itself should be made.

Anterior Resection

There is no dogmatic order in which the steps of the operation should be performed. It is, however, usually convenient to begin with the rectal phase of the dissection.

The Rectal Dissection

The sigmoid colon is mobilized by division of the lateral peritoneum. As the dissection proceeds, posteriorly the gonadal vessels and the ureter will in turn be seen. Continuing toward the midline, the left iliac vein and left presacral nerve will be identified. Dissection is then made on the right of the sigmoid with division of the peritoneum laterally from the level of the origin of the inferior mesenteric artery down to the level of the recto-vaginal or rectovesical reflexion. The right ureter can usually be seen through the peritoneum and is easily avoided. Development of the plane created on the right results in entry into the presacral space. This lies posterior to the fascia propia of the rectum and anterior to the presacral fascia and the right presacral nerve (Fig. 23-12). Once entered the dissection is continued toward the left to complete the exposure of the presacral space on both sides.

At this stage the dissection is continued proximally toward the inferior mesenteric artery and vein. Both vessels are divided, the artery at its origin from the aorta and the vein at a suitable point toward its entry into the splenic vein.

The pelvic dissection is then resumed with the development of the presacral space by scissor dissection. In doing so, the presacral nerves should be pushed laterally where they hug the rectum. The presacral dissection should maintain the fascia propia of the rectum intact as it is continued distally. Toward the lower sacral level, the fascia of Waldeyer will be encountered and should be divided (Fig. 23-13). This will enable the mobilization from the lower rectum and pelvic floor muscles down to the level of the anorectal junction and therefore to the distal limit of the mesorectum.

Attention is then turned to the anterior dissection. The peritoneum is divided on the left side to the level of its anterior reflexion and a transverse incision is made joining the distal extension of each lateral division. In the male, this should be made anterior to the peritoneal reflexion immediately over the seminal vesicles (Fig. 23-14). Gentle displacement posteriorly

by blunt dissection will separate the vesicles, vasa differentia, and the prostate anateriorly from the fascia of Denonvilliers posteriorly. In contrast with the rectal dissection for benign disease, Denonvilliers fascia should not be divided. The dissection is therefore continued as far as is necessary to achieve adequate distal clearance (Fig. 23-15).

In the female the transverse division of peritoneum should also be made anterior to the reflexion of the peritoneum in the Pouch of Douglas. The plane between the vagina and rectum is, however, more difficult to find than its equivalent in the male. It lies between the postvaginal venous plexus and the fascia of Denonvilliers and becomes apparent when the posterior vaginal wall is displaced anteriorly by blunt dissection (Fig. 23-16).

During the dissection the location of the tumor is constantly assessed by palpation. Where invasion is felt to extend beyond the anatomic plane, it must be circumvented by a more extensive dissection at that point. The distal margin of the tumor will be felt through the rectal wall and the dissection should be taken at least 25 mm further (Fig. 23-16). When level with the lower border of the tumor, the surgeon must avoid any tendency to dissect obliquely into the mesorectum; the anatomic plane between rectum and pelvic floor should be maintained well beyond. In low anterior resection, the bowel should be divided at the anorectal junction to ensure removal of the entire mesorectum.

Figure 23-14. Anterior dissection in the male. Incision of the peritoneum overlying the base of the bladder and seminal vesicles. This is the safest approach to the fascia of Denonvilliers.

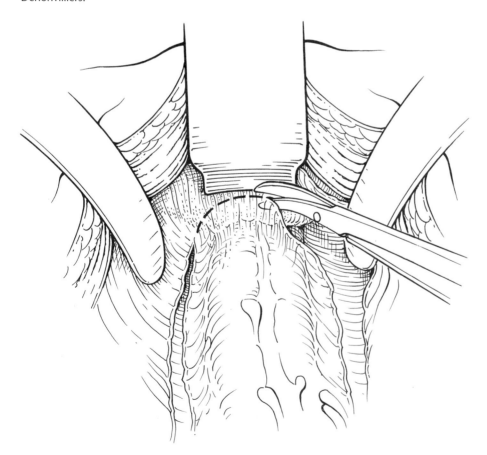

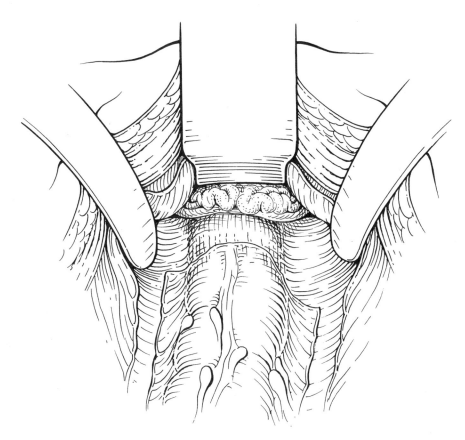

Figure 23-15. Exposure of fascia of Denonvilliers.

Figure 23-16. Anterior dissection in the female showing the posterior vaginal wall with venous plexus and fascia of Denonvilliers.

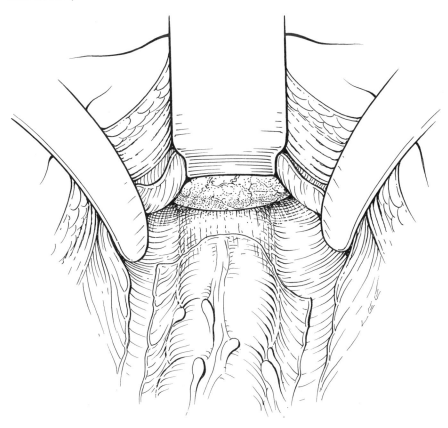

Having mobilized to an adequate level of distal clearance, a transverse crushing clamp is applied to the rectum. The distal stump is then irrigated with a suitable cancericidal solution.

Mobilization of the Colon

Adequate mobility of the left colon is essential for low anterior resection. Tension on the anastomosis is one of the main reasons for breakdown. In most cases it will be necessary to mobilize the splenic flexure. This can be difficult where the flexure is closely applied to the spleen or where there are adhesions between the greater omentum and the splenic capsule. The key to this dissection is the development of the plane between the greater omentum and colon (Fig. 23-17). Care must be taken to avoid traction on the omentum during this stage for fear of causing injury to the spleen. In difficult cases a careful dissection alternating between the lateral aspect of the left colon and the omentocolic plane in the distal transverse colon will gradually liberate the flexure.

Limitation of mobility is caused by the mesocolic vessels. In most cases it will be necessary to divide all those derived from the inferior mesenteric artery. Thus not only the inferior mesenteric itself but also the upper left colic artery and vein should be taken (Fig. 23-18). Division will leave the left colon perfused entirely by the middle colic artery via the marginal artery. The colon is divided at a level that will give an adequate length to descend to the level of the anastomosis while avoiding any area of diverticular disease.

Removal of the Specimen

Following division of the bowel proximally, the mode of distal division will depend on the intended anastomotic technique. In all cases, however, irrigation of the anorectal stump with a cancerocidal solution is obligatory.

Where the double-staple technique[164] is to be used, a transverse stapling instrument is applied to the rectal wall just distal to the clamp. In a narrow pelvis this can be difficult and the manufacturers supply various modifications that can make this step easier. If the 60-mm (Ethicon Ltd.) or 55-mm (US Surgical) staplers are too wide for the pelvis, models with a 30-mm head are available. Care must be taken, however, to ensure that the entire width of bowel is included within the instrument before

Figure 23-17. Mobilization of the splenic flexure. Dissection of the plane between greater omentum and colon to gain exposure to colosplenic fascia.

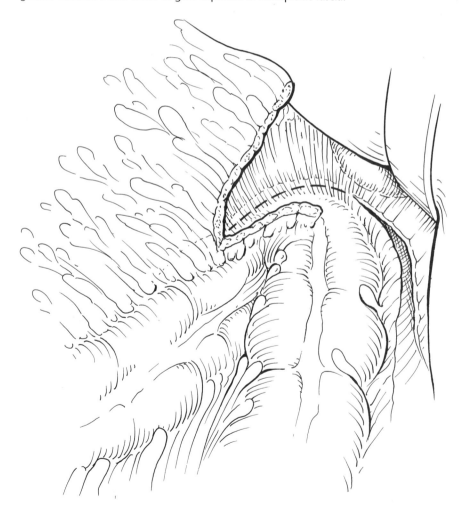

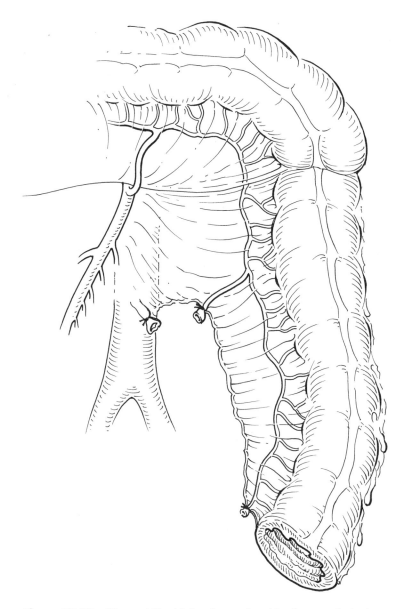

Figure 23-18. The mobilized left colon perfused by the marginal artery.

firing and those staplers that have a pin engagement mechanism are more satisfactory in this regard. Staplers with mobility in two planes (Roticulator, Auto-sutures) can be useful but are more expensive.

Whatever type of anastomosis is to be used, the bowel is divided immediately below the crushing clamp. This can be done with a long-handled scalpel or electrocautery. Removal of the specimen is an important moment during anterior resection because it is essential to ensure that the clamp does not slip, causing contamination. Before division, packs should be placed in the pelvis around the bowel and the division should be carried out without there being any tension between the clamp and the rectal wall. The surgeon should support with one hand the clamp and rectum together while the division is taking place (Fig. 23-19). The liberated specimen should then be carefully removed from the pelvis into a receptacle again without traction on the clamp.

Anastomosis

The choice between a hand-sutured or stapled anastomosis depends on the preference of the surgeon. Clinical trials of various techniques have not shown any to be significantly superior. Stapling is easier than a hand suture in cases of very low anastomosis. The double-staple technique has the advantage of simplicity but there is the risk of leakage from the ends of the transverse suture lying lateral to the anastomosis.

General principles for anastomotic technique include vascularity, lack of tension, and avoidance of contamination. Vascularity of the distal rectum is almost never in doubt. The colonic end, which is usually perfused only by the marginal artery, must be carefully assessed for viability. A healthy color with pink arterial bleeding from the submucosa indicates adequate perfusion. Any degree of tension should be avoided. Further mobilization of the left colon with division of any restraining vessel

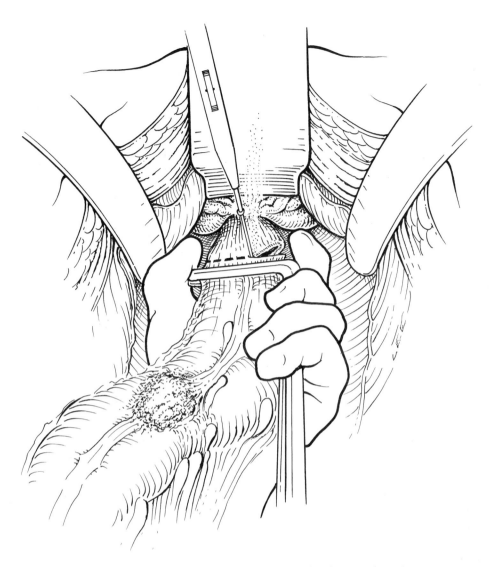

Figure 23-19.   Division of the rectum below the clamp. The clamp and specimen are supported by the surgeon's hand.

while ensuring adequate perfusion may be necessary if there is any doubt.

Hand-Sutured Anastomosis.   Given the evidence that no particular technique is superior, a double- or single-layer suture, interrupted or continuous, using absorbable or nonabsorbable material may all be used. The choice is usually determined by the surgeon's preference. The only variable that has been shown to be associated with anastomotic failure is the individual surgeon.[165]

Technical aspects of importance include the creation of an inverting anastomosis, taking ample amounts of bowel wall with each suture and placing them a correct distance apart (approximately 4 mm). If access to the distal rectum is difficult, the anastomosis is easier using an interrupted single-layer technique. The sutures of the posterior layer are inserted into the colon above and the rectum below before tying. When the row is complete, the colon is then pushed distally along the sutures to the level of the anastomosis and the sutures are tied (Fig.

23-20). The anterior layer is then completed using interrupted sutures preferably placed extramucosally (Lembert) to ensure inversion.

If access to the rectal stump is easy, the anastomosis can be made approximating the colon to the rectum with the first suture and continuing along the posterior wall tying and cutting sutures in turn. The first suture should always be placed in the mesenteric border of the colon and therefore on the right side of the rectum.

Stapled Anastomosis.   Circular stapling instruments were introduced in the late 1970s. The first machines had been developed in the Soviet Union and early trials in the West[166–168] produced encouraging results with a low rate of anastomotic failure. However, the Russian instrument was difficult to use, requiring the insertion of each staple into the head of the instrument by the theater staff before sterilization. Instruments with improved engineering and disposable heads rapidly became available. Using these it is possible to perform an anastomosis at

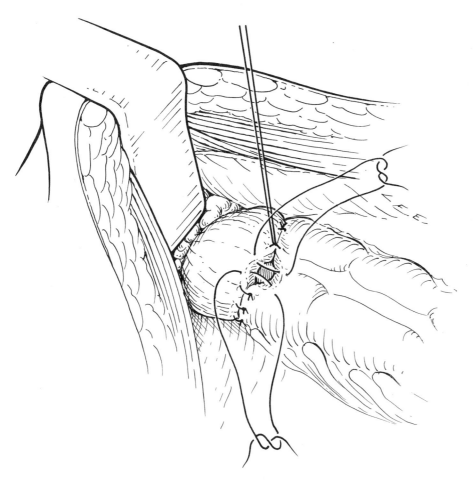

Figure 23-20. Hand-sutured anastomosis using a single-layer extramucosal interrupted technique.

the level of the lowest part of the rectum or anal canal. Circular staplers are available with different head sizes. In general the largest available should be selected. In deciding on size, the diameter of the colon can be assessed using sizers of different diameters provided by the manufacturers.

Single-Staple Technique. The single-staple technique was the first method to be described. Following removal of the specimen, a pursestring suture is placed in the distal rectum (Fig. 23-21) and the proximal colon. The instrument is then inserted per anum and the anvil opened from the head by operating the wing nut screw mechanism on the handle of the instrument. This displacement then permits the distal pursestring to be tied over the rectal stump. The head is then maneuvered over the colon and the proximal pursestring tied. The wing nut is then turned to close the instrument approximating the head and the anvil. When the markings on the instrument indicate that approximation has occurred, the instrument is fired. The head and anvil are then separated by a short distance on unscrewing the wing nut and the instrument is removed per anum by gentle traction combined with rotational and angular movement. Modern instruments are equipped with an adjustable depth of staple mechanism.

Points of technical importance include the use of suture, the distance and depth of placement of the pursestring bites, ensur-

ing the pursestring suture is tied right up to the shaft of the instrument, avoidance of damage to the internal sphincter on inserting the instrument, approximation of head and anvil without incorporating other tissues such as mesenteric fat or the posterior vaginal wall, and gentle extraction. A proline 0 gauge suture is the most satisfactory. It slides easily through the tissues and is sufficiently strong to minimize the possibility of fracture during tying. The pursestring suture should be placed through the entire thickness of the bowel wall about 4 mm apart and 4 mm along its longitudinal length. If the anorectal stump is too short, the pursestring can be inserted per anum although this somewhat defeats the purpose of abdominal stapled anastomosis.

Tying the distal pursestring suture on the rectum can be a difficult maneuver. There is the risk of breaking the suture or jamming. On gentle tightening the bowel should be gathererd to the shaft. A gap posteriorly may occur if the instrument is angled too anteriorly. This can be felt with the tip of the index finger (Fig. 23-22).

In patients with a rigid anal canal, insertion may be difficult. Under this circumstance, a gentle two-finger dilatation may be justified. Before closure of the instrument, the surgeon should clear any excessive mesenteric fat from the shoulder of the head and anvil and protect the anastomosis with a hand placed around it to prevent other tissue from becoming incorporated. Removal

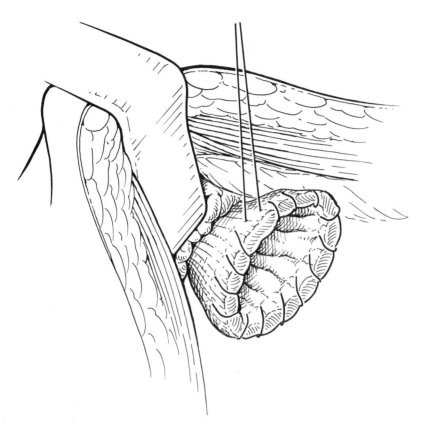

Figure 23-21. Single-staple technique. Insertion of pursestring suture using 0 proline material closed at 4 mm intervals laterally and at 4 mm from the edge of the bowel.

can be difficult. The knife may not cut cleanly and an initial rotation through 90° and then 180° to 360° of the instrument will release any remaining intact tissue. The safest method of removal is manually in which the surgeon takes the instrument with the left hand while gently holding the anastomosis per abdomen with the right (Fig. 23-23).

The head of the removed instrument is then dismantled and the rings of rectum and colon (doughnuts) are inspected. Each must be complete and should include muscularis propria as well as mucosa. The doughnuts should be labeled proximal (colonic) and distal (rectal) and sent in separate pots for histologic examination.

Double-Staple Technique. The double-staple technique[164] simplified stapling[169] by avoiding the distal pursestring and was made possible by modification of the circular stapling instrument in two ways. First, the head was made detachable from the anvil and second the shaft within the anvil was supplied with a sharp trocar.

Having applied the transverse stapler to the rectal stump and removed the specimen after irrigation, the head is detached from the instrument, which is then inserted through the anus into the rectal stump. The detached head is then placed in the colon and secured by a pursestring suture. The trocar on the head is then advanced by screwing the wing nut until it penetrates the rectal stump. The trocar is then removed and the male fitting on the head is engaged into the female fitting on the distal shaft. The instrument is then closed and the subsequent procedure is similar to that of a single-staple technique.

Points of particular importance include the correct application of the transverse staples, the avoidance of tearing of the rectal stump when advancing the trocar, and penetration of the rectal stump by the trocar close to the transverse suture.

Transverse stapling instruments with an adjustable depth of staple are preferable because an excessive tension on the staples may be a cause of breakdown. The headless instrument is often difficult to insert into the anus owing to the wide shoulder of the anvil. Careful angulation with a rotary motion will often be necessary to achieve this without damaging the anal canal. During this maneuver, the abdominal surgeon should protect the rectal stump with a hand to oppose any sudden upward movements of the anvil as it overcomes the resistance of the anal canal to enter the rectal stump. As the trocar begins to penetrate the rectal stump on operating the wing nut, it is helpful to supply countertraction per abdomen on each side of the point of penetration using a curved artery forceps slightly opened (Fig. 23-24). Penetration of the trocar close to the transverse stapled line minimizes the possibility of ischemia of any part of the distal stump.

Air Test. The integrity of the anstomosis should be determined by the injection of air per anum with the anastomosis under liquid such as normal saline or povidone iodine instilled in the pelvis per abdomen. The appearance of bubbles indicates a defect. The air test, although initially recommended for stapled anastomosis, is just as readily applicable to the hand-sutured variety. Any defect can be repaired immediately with a suture.[169]

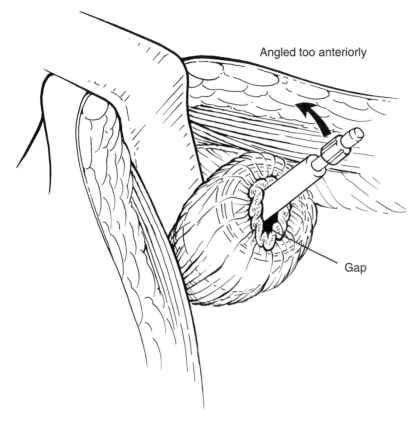

Figure 23-22. Single-stapled anastomosis. Posterior gap on tightening the pursestring suture when the stapler is angled too anteriorly.

Figure 23-23. A safe method of removal of the stapler using a bimanual technique.

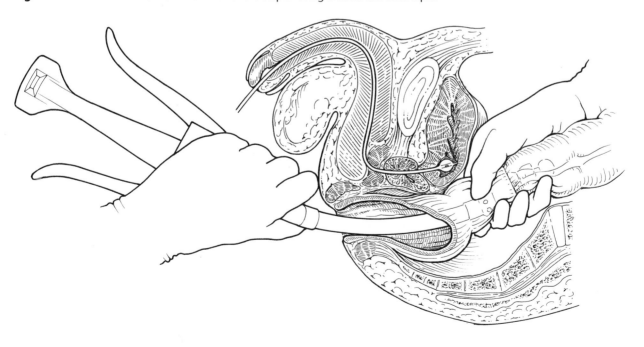

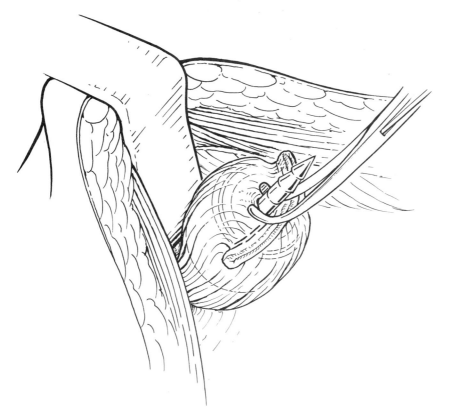

Figure 23-24. Double-staple technique. Penetration of the rectal stump by the trocar using countertraction applied by curved artery forceps on the stapled rectal stump.

Endoanal Anastomosis. Hand-sutured endoanal coloanal anastomosis was described by Parks.[29] It enables restoration of intestinal continuity as far distally as is possible. Although stapling can also do so, the ability to perform a hand-sutured anastomosis should be an essential part of the colon and rectal surgeon's capability. Not all cases are suitable for stapling and occasional technical difficulties can occur. To be able to salvage a failed or impossible stapled anastomosis by hand suturing is indispensible. The colon must be mobilized adequately to descend to the anus. This is usually easy and involves the careful division of vessels as described above. Adequate mobility almost always requires ligation of all vessels to the left colon leaving perfusion by the marginal artery via the middle colic artery.

The anastomosis is carried out by the surgeon seated between the patient's legs. The table should be raised bringing the anus level with the head of the operator with about 30° of Trendelenburg tilt. Although not essential, a headlight is extremely useful allowing easy vision into the upper anal canal and lower rectum (Fig. 23-25).

Various retractors are satisfactory for exposing the anal canal including the Eisenhammer, Gelpi, or Lone Star models. The Eisenhammer retractor is strong giving excellent exposure and can be removed and reinserted with ease. In so doing, the anal dilatation time can be minimized. Long instruments allow the field to be visualized without being obscured by the hands and the use of swabs is preferable to suction.

Coloanal anastomosis is only necessary where division of

the anorectum leaves the stump short enough. This is usually at the level of the anorectal junction. In most cases, it is not difficult to insert sutures at this level. In these a simple anastomosis directly between the colon and the divided edge of the anal stump should be carried out. In some cases, for example in males with muscular buttocks and a funnel type of perineum, the anorectal junction may be too inaccessible to achieve a safe suture.

Under this circumstance, the anastomsis can be facilitated by a mucosectomy of the anal stump to the dentate line. Advancement of the anastomosis by the 2 or so cm achieved by this maneuver can make an enormous difference to the ease of execution. The mucosectomy is performed by sharp scissor dissection after elevation of the mucosa from the underlying internal sphincter facilitated by the submucosal injection of a solution of adrenaline (1 in 300,000) in saline.

The anastomosis itself starts with the placement of two sutures into the mesenteric and antimesenteric border of the colon from the abdomen. A suture with a strong small needle is recommended. A 25-mm taper cut needle mounted on a 2-0 polyglactin suture is very satisfactory (Ethicon Ltd.). Each suture is then passed down through the pelvis to be drawn through the anus by the perineal operator (Fig. 23-26). Using the anal retractor for exposure, the antimesenteric suture is then placed into the anal canal at the upper level of the divided mucosa in the 3 o'clock position. It is then tied and the mesenteric suture is placed at 9 o'clock in the anal canal and also tied (Fig. 23-27). By this maneuver the colon is approximated to the anal canal.

Anterior and posterior sutures are then placed fixing the anastomosis in the four cardinal positions. The diagonal sectors are then closed with two or three sutures in each (Fig. 23-28). This technique is identical to that used for manual ileoanal anastomosis.

Coloanal Colonic Pouch. Bowel frequency following a straight coloanal procedure is unpredictable.[170] Recent experience[171] has shown that this is particularly true for females. Function may be improved by construction of a reservoir from the terminal part of the colon.[172–175] This is made as a J-construction from the terminal 12 cm of colon. The single passage of a long linear stapler will create a two-limbed reservoir of about 6 cm per limb as advised by Lazorthes. The end of the colon is closed with a conventional transverse stapler (Fig. 23-29). The resulting coloanal anastomosis (Fig. 23-30) will be side to end in type and can be made either by stapling or by hand suture. The functional advantages afforded by this modification have encouraged its increasing use.

Other Techniques of Low Anastomosis. Kraske[5] described two patients with rectal cancer removed via a posterior parasacral approach. In one of these he carried out a direct colorectal anastomosis. Modifications of this approach combined with an abdominal dissection have been described (see above).

The technique developed by Localio et al.[30] includes an abdominal dissection with the patient placed in an oblique lateral

Figure 23-25. Coloanal anastomosis. General setup.

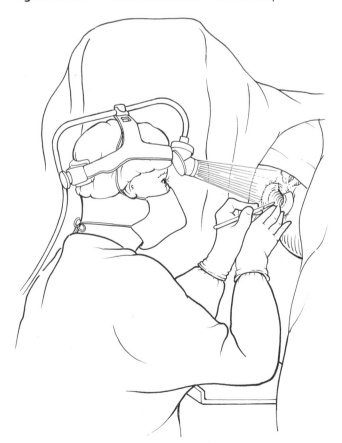

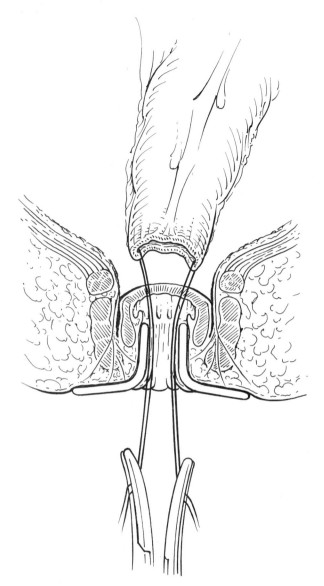

Figure 23-26. Coloanal anastomosis. Delivery of colon to the anal level.

position to allow simultaneous exposure of the sacrum. Following mobilization of the rectum, the lower part of the sacrum and coccyx is removed to gain access to the pelvis. The bowel is then divided below the level of the tumor and the specimen removed. A direct anastomosis between colon and the distal anorectal stump is made directly through the posterior approach. The wound is then closed. The Mason technique[31] is similar but posterior access is enhanced by division of the sphincters, which are then repaired in layers after the anastomosis is completed.

With the introduction of stapling and the availability of hand-sutured endoanal anastomosis, these techniques are now not greatly used.

On-Table Lavage. In cases with a considerable amount of fecal loading in the colon, on-table lavage should be carried out. This largely applies to patients with obstruction in the emer-

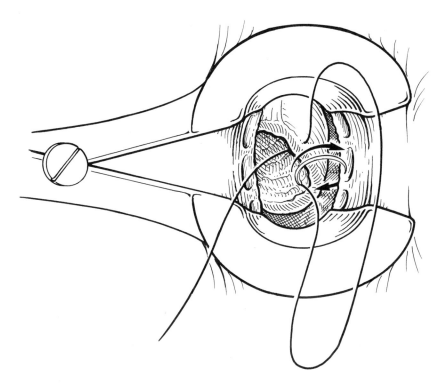

Figure 23-27.   Coloanal anastomosis. Insertion of the 3 o'clock suture.

Figure 23-28.   The completed coloanal anastomosis.

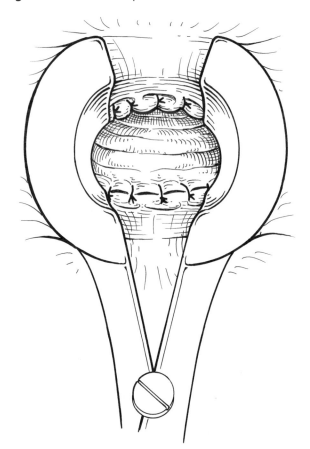

gency setting. However, not infrequently during an elective operation, preparation may be poor owing to a subclinically obstructing tumor or to failure of the bowel preparation.

The procedure involves the insertion of a retaining catheter (a Foley catheter is the most suitable) into the proximal colon and corrugated wide-bore tubing into the distal end of the colon after division of the bowel in preparation for removal of the specimen (Fig. 23-31). Some operative descriptions recommend placement of the proximal catheter into the terminal ileum, but it is safer to carry out an appendicectomy and insert the catheter through its base. If the surgeon intends to leave the catheter in situ during the postoperative period, then it is essential to use this second route. Under these circumstances, the cecum should be sutured around the catheter to the parietal peritoneum to seal off the area. Anesthetic tubing is the most satisfactory for intubation of the distal colon; its corrugations allow the tube to be well secured by a stout tie. The tubing is draped over the side of the patient into a sealed plastic bag. The Foley catheter is connected to an intravenous infusion-giving set and the colon is then irrigated with normal saline until the effluent is clear.

The tube is removed from the distal colon and the bowel cut back to viable tissue for the anastomosis. The Foley catheter is either immediately removed with closure of the cecum or left in situ for 7 to 10 days postoperatively.

The technique has been associated with a low mortality and leak rate when used in obstructive cases.[176–178] In a collected group of 122 patients of whom 20 had intestinal obstruction, a clinical anastomotic leakage rate of 4.8% was reported.[178]

Total Rectal Excision

The technique of rectal mobilizaton for total rectal excision differs importantly from anterior resection. The stoma and perineal wound create special difficulties.

Stoma Siting

The patient has to live with the stoma for the rest of his or her life. Correct siting preoperatively is essential. The stoma site should be placed away from bony prominences, skin creases, and scars (including the umbilicus) and brought out through the rectus abdominus muscle. This function is best carried out by the stoma therapist, and having marked the site preoperatively, it is helpful to apply a colostomy appliance to allow the patient to assess whether the location is satisfactory. In obese patients a higher siting may be necessary to allow the stoma to be visible when the patient is upright. The stoma should lie below the belt line but if placed too low, the appliance may be disturbed by movements during hip flexion.

The Operation

The anus should be closed with a suture before starting (Fig. 23-32). This is best done with a long curved hand needle. Inserted through the perianal skin in the midline anteriorly, the

Figure 23-29. Colonic reservoir construction.

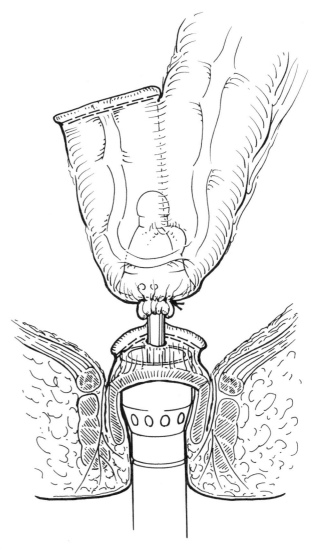

Figure 23-30. Coloanal stapled anastomosis.

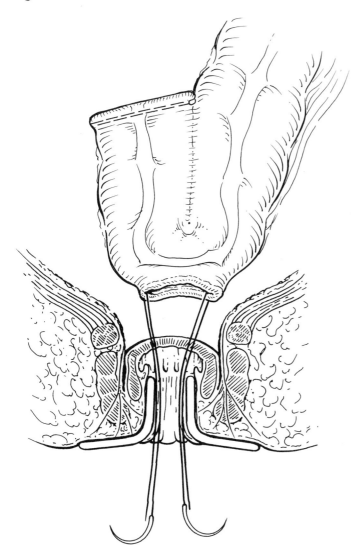

tip of the needle is advanced around the anus to emerge through an exit point in the midline posteriorly. The needle is withdrawn from the tissues and then reinserted through the same point and passed around the left side of the anus to exit through the anterior point where the suture was originally inserted. It is then tied taking care to ensure that the closure is watertight. Correct closure of the anus is essential to prevent contamination of the operative field.

There are good reasons for making the stoma trephine before opening the abdomen. The fascial planes of the anterior abdominal wall are undisturbed and the surgeon is likely to take more care in its creation at the beginning than at the end of the operation. A disc of skin centered around the marked point measuring 25 mm in diameter is made. The subcutaneous fat is retracted and Scarpa's fascia is divided. A cruciate incision is made in the anterior rectus sheath to a diameter of one-and-a-half fingers. The rectus abdominus muscles are parted longitudinally without division and the posterior rectal sheath and peritoneum are then divided. Care is taken to avoid damage to the inferior epigastric vessels (Fig. 23-33).

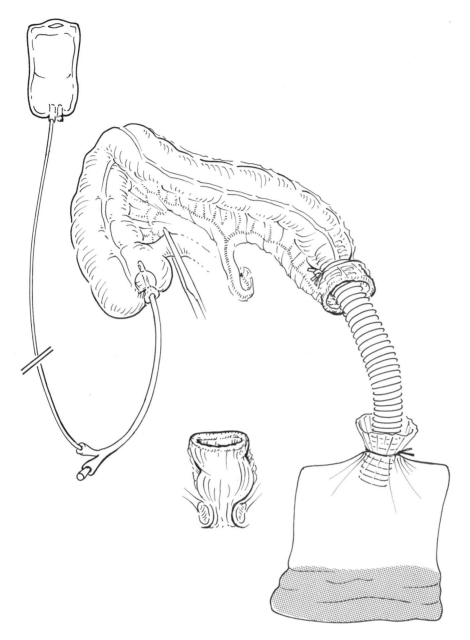

Figure 23-31. On-table lavage.

The abdomen is then opened. Division of the colon can be carried out before or after rectal mobilization. It is not necessary to mobilize the entire left colon as for low anterior resection. The point of division of the sigmoid colon to ensure a suitable colostomy without tension lies level with the symphysis pubis on gently drawing the sigmoid colon downward.

Closure of the lateral peritoneal space is carried out by most surgeons. It is easy to do using a pursestring suture between the lateral peritoneum and the peritoneal edge of the left colon. Closure of the space gives some support to the stoma itself.

The clamped end of the divided colon is delivered through the trephine. The mucocutaneous suture to create the stoma is made after the abdomen is closed. A length of about 10 mm of colon projecting proud from the skin should be the goal. A mucocutaneous suture using a subcuticular (intradermal) technique avoids the punctate cutaneous scars created by a full-thickness skin suture.

Rectal Mobilization

The technique of rectal mobilization is identical to that for anterior resection except down to the level of the midpelvis where Waldeyer's fascia is encountered. At this point the abdominal dissection should stop because the aim of total rectal excision is to remove a cylinder of tissue including the rectum and entire

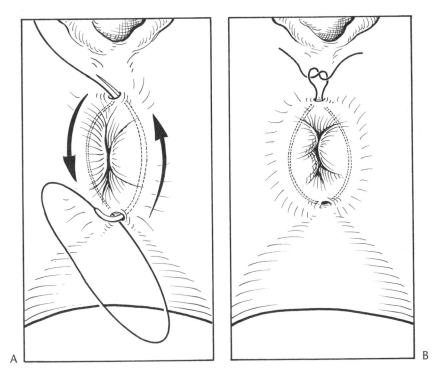

Figure 23-32. (**A & B**) Total rectal excision. Method of insertion of anal stitch.

Figure 23-33. (**A–D**) Total rectal excision. Creation of the abdominal stoma.

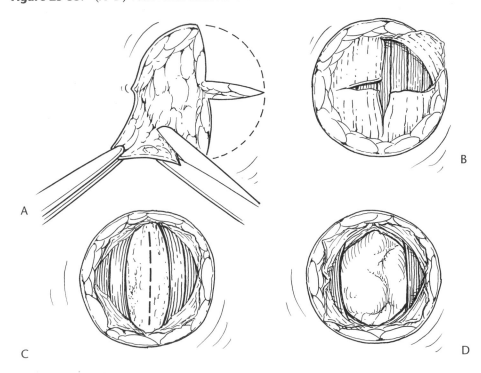

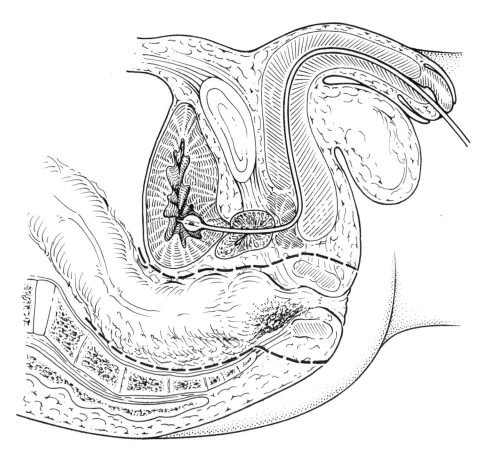

Figure 23-34. Total rectal excision. Rectal mobilization; a cylinder of tissue is removed.

pelvic floor musculature (Fig. 23-34). The rest of the rectal mobilization is therefore left to the perineal operator guided synchronously by the abdominal surgeon.

Perineal Dissection

An oval incision is made around the anus. The size of the resulting cutaneous island should be commensurate with the pathology. For example, it should be greater for an anal canal or margin tumor in order to achieve adequate local clearance.

The key to the perineal resection is exposure. The St. Mark's retractor is an ideal instrument for achieving this. It can be fixed to the drapes covering the legs by towel clips to retain it in position during the entire procedure (Fig. 23-35). Dissection using electrocoagulation minimizes blood loss.

The dissection is deepened to the ischiorectal fossa on each side and then posteriorly toward the coccyx, which can be palpated easily in most cases. Unless the tumor is locally extensive posteriorly, there is no need to excise the tip of the coccyx, a maneuver that can cause discomfort postoperatively. The dissection is continued beyond the tip of the coccyx and the posterior part of the wound is widened laterally. This will reveal the posterior surface of Waldeyer's fascia, which is then divided transversely (Fig. 23-36). At this point the perineal operator is guided by the abdominal surgeon in directing a pair of scissors from the perineum into the pelvis. The appropriate angulation

is gauged by the latter and the scissors are gently pushed proximally to enter the pelvis. They are splayed open to enlarge the incision; the perineal operator then inserts an index finger through the opening. It is then possible to sweep the finger round the upper surface of the levator on one side. With counterpressure by the thumb on the inferior surface of the levator, the muscle is freed laterally from its pelvic attachments by several cuts with strong scissors (Fig. 23-37). The procedure is repeated on the contralateral side, thereby freeing the rectum posteriorly and laterally. During this maneuver the finger and thumb are always held between the scissors and the rectum, to minimize the chance of perforation.

Female. The anterior dissection in the female is easier than in the male. The pelvis is entered through the posterior vaginal wall above the level of the anterior pelvic dissection (Fig. 23-38) This also is done with guidance by the perineal operator. Having entered the pelvis anteriorly from below, the tissues on each side, which mainly consist of the anterior trunks of the puborectalis, can be divided piecemeal. There is a danger of damaging the ureter during this maneuver and here again the abdominal surgeon can be helpful in advising on the direction of the dissection. After a certain amount of tissue has been divided, it will be possible to hook remaining tissue with the index finger and thus to cut it safely.

There may be considerable bleeding from the posterior vagi-

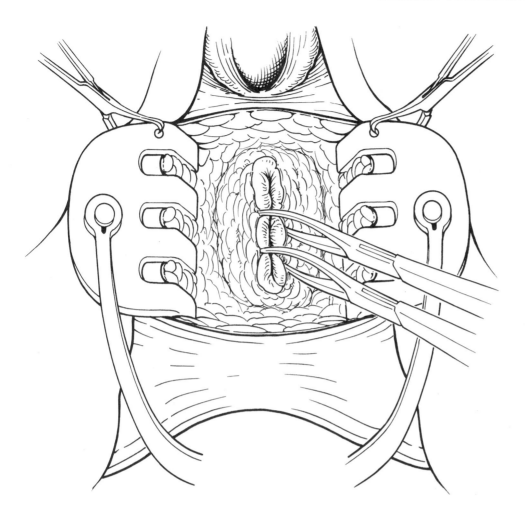

Figure 23-35. Perineal dissection. The general setup.

nal venous plexus and a running suture to establish hemostasis should be placed along the divided vaginal wall.

The skin is sutured and a corrugated or similar drain is left through the posterior vaginal wall into the pelvis. Such a wound is open and by definition will heal by secondary intention.

Male. In the male the procedure is identical up to the moment of the anterior dissection. This is among the most difficult in colorectal surgery. Perforation of the rectum will render the operation palliative and the responsibility on the part of the surgeon is great. The dissection should not be left to a trainee unless under direct supervision.

Having freed the rectum posteriorly and laterally, the recto-prostatic plane is developed. This may be difficult to enter but guided by the landmark of the posterior border of the superficial transverse perineal muscles, the plane will gradually become apparent (Fig. 23-39). The urinary catheter is in practice very difficult to feel and is therefore of little use as a landmark in this dissection. The rectoprostatic plane is more or less horizontal when the patient is in the Trendelenburg position with 20° of tilt (Fig. 23-40). This is extremely useful in the dissection. By a combination of sharp and blunt dissection, progress will be made upward in the rectoprostatic septum until the finger of the abdominal operator is clearly felt.

When the distance between the perineal and abdominal dissections is judged to be sufficiently close, scissors guided by the abdominal operator are insinuated by the perineal surgeon from below to enter the pelvis anterior to the rectum. The dissection then proceeds as in the female although it is more difficult owing to the greater bulk of the puborectalis muscles on each side anteriorly. Division of the puborectalis muscles is best made by electrocautery coagulating vessels as they appear.

Perineal Wound. In the male it is possible to close the perineal wound primarily and this should be done unless there has been contamination or excessive bleeding. In this circumstance the wound should be packed. A useful technique is to use a bowel bag placed from the perineum into which gauze packing is inserted. It may be possible to remove the pack subsequently on the ward under sedation rather than give the patient a general anesthetic. In a prospective nonrandomized study, Robles Campos et al.[179] compared open packing of the wound (34 patients), closure with perineal drainage (34 patients), and closure with abdominal irrigated drainage (34 patients). Primary healing occurred in 53% and 85% of the two respective closure groups and the mean duration of hospital stay was 36, 24, and 15 days, respectively. It appears, therefore, that primary perineal skin closure with the pelvis drained per abdomen is the method

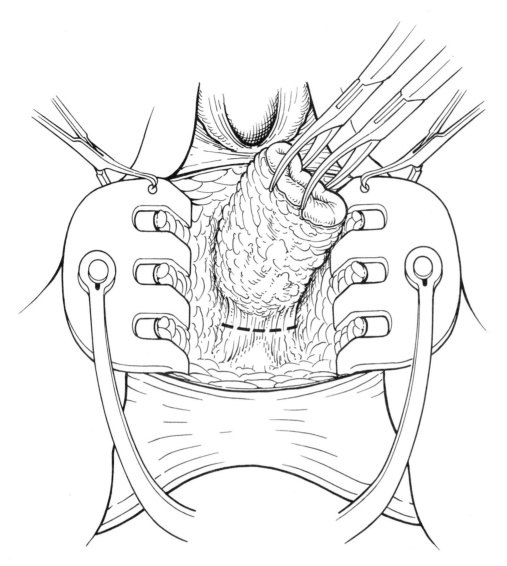

Figure 23-36. Perineal dissection. Division of fascia of Waldeyer.

of choice. It is not possible to suture the pelvic floor musculature because this has been completely removed as part of the surgical clearance.

Before closure of the abdomen, most surgeons will close the pelvic peritoneum. However, this is an optional maneuver and may not be necessary. It creates a dead space that may allow hematoma to form with subsequent breakdown of the wound.[180,181] Irvin and Goligher[182] found no difference in primary healing whether the peritoneum was closed or not. The mobilization of an omental pedicle to fill the pelvic dead space has been advocated as a means of diminishing the chance of breakdown of the perineal wound[183] by discouraging hematoma formation.

Local Excision

There are three techniques for surgical local excision of rectal tumors. These include conventional endoanal removal (Parks), transanal endoscopic microsurgery (TEM) developed by Buess,[150] and removal through a posterior approach.[31] Case

selection has already been discussed. Patients undergoing endoanal removal or TEM can be released from the hospital within 1 or 2 days.

Endoanal Technique (Parks)

Using a suitable anal retractor, the tumor is visualized and stay sutures are placed at about 10 mm distant from the accessible peripheral margins. This may be possible only inferiorly and laterally. A circumferential excision is made by electrocautery around the lower part of the tumor at a distance just outside the perimeter defined by the sutures (Fig. 23-41). The incision is continued through the whole thickness of the bowel wall until the perirectal fat is reached. The incision is gradually extended around the tumor, which can increasingly be displaced distally by gentle traction on the stay sutures. This greatly improves access to the upper margin. Following the removal of the specimen, the rectal wound is irrigated with povidone iodine solution and closed with interrupted sutures with the main purpose of achieving hemostasis.

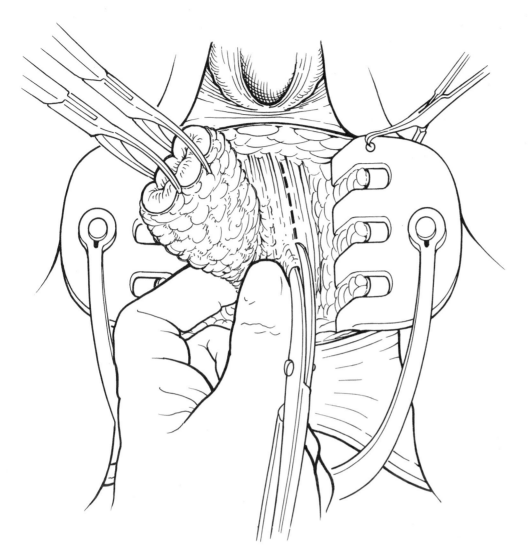

Figure 23-37. Perineal dissection. Division of levator ani.

A modification of this technique was described by Faivre[184] in which the dissection starts at the anal canal with the excision of a flap of anoderm including the underlying internal sphincter. The dissection is continued upward toward and then around the tumor. Creation of the flap allows the tumor to be displaced distally with great facility thereby allowing enhanced control of hemostasis and the margin of surgical excision.

Transanal Endoscopic Microsurgery

Transanal endoscopic microsurgery (TEM)[149,150] uses a sophisticated rigid endoscopic system having binocular optics, suction, and carbon dioxide insufflation with sealable ports on the instrument to enable the introduction of specially designed instruments (Fig. 23-42). The sigmoidoscope is 4 mm in diameter and is fixed to the operating table by a Martin arm, which can be adjusted to alter the position of the instrument. Setting up the apparatus and the execution of surgery requires formal training. The establishment of instruction courses as with laparoscopic work has been an important positive development of this innovative technique. Visualization of the operative field is excellent but manipulation of the long instruments requires practice. The instruments themselves include needle holders, tissue forceps, and scissors, all available in right- and left-handed versions. Cutting is by a high-frequency electrode coagulator also mounted on a long shaft.

The technique is identical in principle to conventional endo-anal excision. The margin of the tumor is identified by coagulation points placed circumferentially at a distance of 10 mm from the edge of the tumor. The incision is then made with the electrocutter and bleeding vessels are coagulated as necessary. The tumor is removed with a full thickness of rectal wall. The resulting defect is closed endoscopically using sutures with a short length of thread fixed by silver clips rather than knots.

Posterior Approach

From the time of Kraske[5] to the development of safer abdominal surgery, posterior removal was the most common method used for treatment of rectal carcinoma.[185] In recent years this ap-

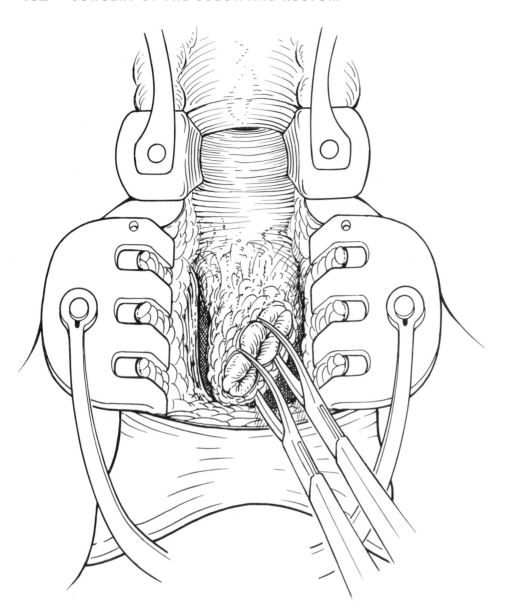

Figure 23-38. Perineal dissection (female). Removal of posterior vaginal wall in continuity with the anorectum.

proach has been advocated for local excision of benign sessile and selected malignant tumors.[31] With the patient in the jack-knife position, a longitudinal incision is made over the lower sacrum and coccyx and extended through the midline raphe in the pelvic floor posteriorly to expose the tumor. Mason modified the Kraske approach at this point by dividing anal sphincters to achieve greater exposure. The tumor is then excised with a 10-mm margin of surrounding normal rectum and the rectal wound is closed. The sphincter complex is then sutured in layers and the skin sutured.

Although sphincter function is usually satisfactory, the fear of implantation of viable tumor cells leading to local recurrence has deterred its use by most surgeons. Local recurrence under such circumstances crosses anatomic planes and renders salvage surgery less likely to achieve adequate clearance of the tumor.

Furthermore, recovery is longer than with the other techniques of local excision.

Operative Mortality

Elective operative mortality fell steadily during the first half of the century. Grinnell[55] reported a fall from 40.9% between 1916 and 1920 to 6.7% from 1946 to 1950 in a series of 1,026 patients treated during that time. Lockhart Mummery et al.[35] showed a similar trend with a reduction of 6.8% from 1948 to 1952 to 2.1% from 1968 to 1972 and others[146] have reported a similar diminution from 7.9% to 2.4% over a 20-year period. The reported operative mortality for total rectal excision and major restorative resection has varied from respective rates of 1.9% and 2.9%,[35] 8% and 7%,[75] and 12.5% and 6.8%.[51]

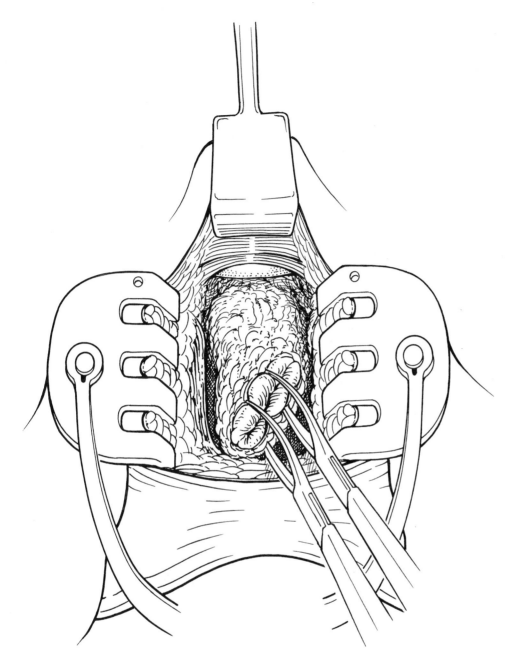

Figure 23-39. Perineal dissection (male). Entry into rectoprostatic septum. Superficial and deep transverse perineal muscles anterior.

Mortality is related to age[43] and stage of disease. In 1,766 cases operated on between 1946 and 1957, Vandertol and Beahrs[123] reported 74 (4.2%) deaths. The rate in patients undergoing palliative procedures was three times greater. Goligher[186] demonstrated an even more marked difference in his personal series of 896 total rectal excisions with operative death occurring in 21% of those having a palliative compared with 3% having a curative procedure. Mortality in palliative cases may be increased further by preoperative radiotherapy.[83]

Complications

Anastomotic Leakage

Anastomotic leakage is the most serious complication following anterior resection. In a series of 1,766 patients having anterior resection over a 10-year period to 1957, there were 74 deaths (4.2%). About one-third of these were due to anastomotic leakage.[128] In the personal series of 553 cases operated on by Goligher[186] there were 39 (7.3%) operative deaths. Most of these

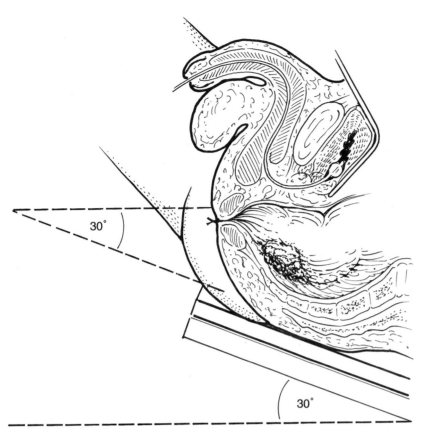

Figure 23-40. Perineal dissection (male). Rectoprostatic plane is parallel to the horizontal with 30° of headdown tilt.

Figure 23-41. Local excision of rectal tumor. Access enhanced by distal traction by stay sutures.

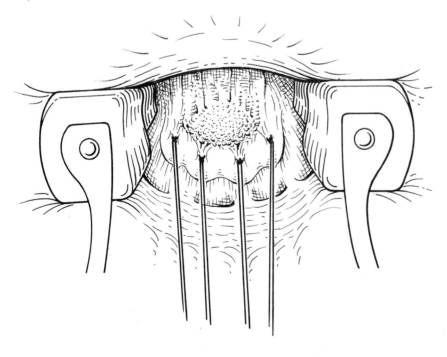

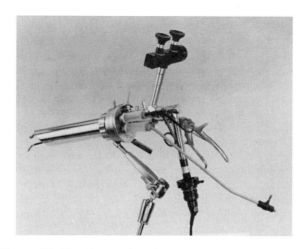

Figure 23-42. Transanal endoscopic microsurgery. General view of apparatus.

Table 23-5. Comparative Leak Rates, Stapled Versus Sutured Anastomoses—Retrospective Studies

Author	Sutured Anastomosis		Stapled Anastomosis	
	No.	Leaks	No.	Leaks
Goligher et al.[166]	135	48	62	6
Adloff et al.[223]	25	4	20	1
Bolton and Britton[234]	10	1	20	1
Cady et al.[190]	56	16	10	1
Killingback[153]	87	16	57	5
Total	313	85 (27.1%)	169	14 (8.2%)

were due to cardiorespiratory complications but 9, approximately one-quarter, were due to sepsis. There is some evidence that leakage may increase the chance of local recurrence.[187]

Prospective studies of anastomotic healing have shown the incidence of leakage to be higher than had previously been appreciated.[188] Examination by digital palpation, rigid sigmoidoscopy, and water-soluble contrast radiology of the anastomosis in the early postoperative period revealed evidence of anastomotic insufficiency in 35.6% of 135 cases having anterior resection. However, clinical leak rate in this group was only 6.6%. Of the 135 cases, 84 had a high and 51 a low anterior resection. In the former group clinical leakage occurred in 1.2% and radiologic in 18.8%. In the latter group of patients having a low anterior resection these respective rates were 16% and 49%.

This work showed that contrast radiology reveals a leak rate several times that of clinical leakage and that leakage is much more frequent after low than high anterior resection. Vandertoll and Beahrs[128] demonstrated that anastomotic leakage was three times more frequent in palliative than in curative cases.

It is clear that there is a surgeon-related variable in the causation of anastomotic leakage. The first indication of this resulted from an analysis of the results obtained by over 90 surgeons working in 23 hospitals participating in the Large Bowel Cancer Project. Fielding et al.[165] collected 1,466 such patients having a resection. The overall leak rate was 13% but this ranged from 0.5% to over 30% among the surgeons. The higher leak rate after anterior resection (18.7%) compared with intraperitoneal anastomosis (10.8%) was confirmed. The variation of surgical performance was not due to an uneven distribution of anterior resection cases nor was it related to the technique employed, the grade of the surgeon, the use of antibiotics, or whether the operation was an elective or emergency procedure. Mortality in patients who had leakage was 22% compared with 7.1% in those who did not. McArdle and Hole[54] reported similar results from a group of 13 surgeons working in one hospital over the same period. Anastomotic leak rates ranged from 0 to 25%.

Several trials have been carried out over the last 20 years comparing various anastomotic techniques. Caution should be exercised in interpreting results from series carried out by one surgeon and those that are multicentric. Nevertheless it is possi-

ble to draw useful conclusions from these studies. First there appears to be no great difference between a two-layer continous and a one-layer interrupted colorectal anatomosis.[188,189]

Of greater relevance today is the question whether stapled anastomoses are less likely to leak than hand-sutured anastomoses. The initial years of stapling were characterized by reports from single non-comparative series.[153,166,168,190] These suggested that leakage was less likely after stapled than hand-sutured anastomosis (Table 23-5). In a large multicenter analysis of the results obtained by the members of the American Society of Colon and Rectal Surgeons, anastomotic leakage using stapling techniques was less than 10%.[167] These early claims that dehiscence rates were less after stapling have not been substantiated by the few well-conducted prospective randomized clinical trials. One of the earliest[191] showed no difference between three anastomotic techniques including two hand-sutured and one stapled. Beart and Kelly[192] reported leak rates of less than 4% at both stapled and hand-sutured groups. They did not, however, carry out contrast radiology on the patients and the rates reported referred to clinical leakage. In a randomized controlled trial by one surgeon, McGinn et al.[193] reported a clinical leak rate of 3.3% in 60 patients undergoing hand suture and 12.1% in 58 having a stapled anastomosis. In a recent randomized trial of 1,004 patients having gastrointestinal anastomosis, the West of Scotland and Highland Anastomosis Study Group[194] reported five (4.5%) cases of clinical leakage in 113 patients having hand-sutured colorectal anastomosis and nine (8.1%) out of 111 having a stapled colorectal anastomosis. The conclusion from these studies is that there is no great difference between hand or stapled anastomosis with regard to leakage. Karanjia et al.[195] indicate that leakage may be higher after total mesorectal excision. Of 219 patients undergoing anterior resection, major leakage occurred in 24 (11%). Factors responsible include the level of the anastomosis and perhaps ischemia owing to the mesorectal excision.

Leakage after coloanal anastomosis was reported by Parks and Percy[170] to be 17%. Reports in the literature, however, indicate that here again there is a considerable range from less than 10%[196,197] to 30% or more.[198] It is not clear why this should be because in the last report the surgeons were all experienced. There is some indication that anastomotic failure of colonic pouch-anal anastomosis may be less frequent.[169,173,199] Seow Choen and Goh[175] reported no case of anastomotic complication in a randomized prospective trial of 40 patients undergoing coloanal anastomosis in which 20 were randomized to a straight reconstruction and 20 to a colonic pouch reconstruction.

Management

There is now less inclination by surgeons to use contrast radiology routinely to assess the anastomosis. Indeed this may be damaging particularly in cases where the anastomosis is low. If a contrast enema is carried out and shows a defect, then there is no indication for any special management if there are no associated clinical disturbances. A clinical leak is usually indicated by pyrexia a few days postoperatively. This may be associated with tachycardia and more profound systemic effects if the septic focus is large or if there is peritonitis. Assessment of the patient will therefore include a general examination looking for signs of septicemia and peritonitis and a local examination of the anastomosis itself. The latter may reveal a defect in the anastomosis on digital palpation where the anastomosis is accessible. In cases of doubt, a gentle contrast enema using a water-soluble medium is indicated. Sometimes this does not demonstrate a leak but it usually does. It may also show a widened presacral space indicating the presence of a collection. Further imaging by CT scanning is indicated where the diagnosis is not evident.

Management will depend on the degree of localization of the associated abscess and the size of the perianastomotic cavity. If there is general peritonitis, then resuscitation with urgent surgery is required. This will include the establishment of a defunctioning stoma if not already present and peritoneal lavage. Unless the anastomosis has completely disrupted, proximal defunctioning with drainage of the anastomosis itself should be the procedure of choice. However, where complete rupture has occurred, then exteriorization of the proximal component of the anastomosis should be undertaken. Where the anastomosis is defunctioned but otherwise left undisturbed, then the bowel distal to the stoma should be irrigated to clear it of feces. This can be done via a catheter placed down the distal limb of the stoma allowing the irrigant to escape per anum through a proctoscope.

A localized dehiscence if small is likely to resolve spontaneously. It may, however, be necessary to assist drainage and a formal examination under anesthetic will allow this to be done. Where the cavity is large, it will be necessary to establish a defunctioning stoma if this is not already present and to irrigate the cavity by a catheter introduced per anum. Experience and clinical judgment are required in deciding on the best management and this should be exercised in the light of circumstances in the individual case.

Where a perianastomotic cavity shows little or no evidence of closing down over a period of weeks or more, the possibility of local recurrence should be considered. Although this might seem early in the postoperative course, there may have been inadequate local clearance of the tumor.

Covering Stoma

The indications for a stoma are discussed in greater detail elsewhere. It is a matter of judgment by the surgeon as to whether the anastomosis in a particular case should be covered by a defunctioning stoma. The tendency over the last 10 to 20 years has been a fall in the number of patients so managed. The decision must be based on the surgeon's analysis of the likelihood of anastomotic failure occurring in the individual case. It is generally agreed that an intraperitoneal anastomosis does not need a stoma and many low anterior resections also. Risk factors for dehiscence include the general condition of the patient, whether the operation has been palliative or curative, the level of the anastomosis, and whether there are any particular intraoperative difficulties. In patients with a colon loaded with feces, an on-table lavage should be carried out, thus eliminating fecal loading as an indication for a stoma. Intraoperative factors such as contamination, difficulty in placing sutures, inadequate doughnuts, a positive air test, or tension, might lead the surgeon to perform a defunctioning stoma where otherwise this would not have been indicated.

Some authors have suggested that it is no longer necessary to cover a low anastomosis.[200] but others have strongly advocated fecal diversion of ultralow colorectal or coloanal anastomosis.[79,104,175] Grabham et al.[201] have suggested a selective approach to defunctioning in which this is carried out only where the surgeon feels particular concern about the anastomosis and where doughnuts are incomplete. Of 77 patients having low anterior resection, seven (9%) had a stoma with clinical leakage observed in two (3%) of the entire series, neither of which was present in the defunctioned group.

Urinary and Gynecologic

Urinary and gynecologic complications are described in Chapter 46.

Perineal Wound

In contaminated cases or where hemorrhage is considerable, the perineal wound should be packed. On removal of the pack 48 hours later, it is reasonable to consider delayed primary suture. If left open, the wound will take several weeks to months before it closes.

Breakdown of a perineal wound sutured primarily occurs in a up to 50% of cases.[180,182,183,202,203]. This is usually associated with hematoma or abscess formation. Drainage with subsequent management as for an open wound is the treatment of choice in such cases. Occasionally a chronic perineal sinus develops. This may be associated with a constriction of the wound creating an hourglass deformity. Persistence may be due to the presence of foreign material, for example nonabsorbable sutures. In such cases it may be worth exploring the wound to open the constriction and to search by curettage for foreign bodies. This approach has been reported to result in healing in 50% of cases operated on for ulcerative colitis.[204]

Where a chronic sinus is unresponsive to such measures, placement of a myocutaneous flap into the pelvic dead space should be considered with the involvement of a plastic surgeon. The rectus abdominus muscle is preferred over the gracilis because vascular perfusion appears to be better. A rectus abdominus flap skin paddle, taken from the contralateral side to the stoma, leaves remarkably little deformity.[205,206]

Function and Quality of Life

General

Devlin et al.[49] studied a group of 83 patients undergoing abdominoperineal excision with a permanent colostomy and demonstrated a high incidence of depression, social isolation, and poor quality of life. In a comparison of outcomes after abdominoperineal excision and anterior resection, Williams and Johnston[207] showed a marked difference in depression score after the former (4.6 ± 3.6) compared with the latter (2.8 ± 2.9). A perception of change of body image occurred in 66% of patients after total rectal excision compared with only 5% after anterior resection. There was no difference in anxiety score suggesting that this was more related to the original pathology than the functional outcome. Amelioration of the difficulty of a permanent colostomy can be achieved by appropriate stoma care including irrigation.

Bowel Function

Following anterior resection, there is no doubt that the loss of rectal reservoir and its replacement by colon can lead to frequency and urgency of defecation. Furthermore, an already impaired sphincter may contribute to this. Goligher and Hughes[208] indicated the importance of rectal sensibility and Goligher et al.[98] considered it important to retain 6 to 8 cm of rectum following anterior resection on functional grounds. Subsequently Lane and Parks[209] demonstrated that the rectum was not necessary for normal continence and showed that after coloanal anastomosis patients experienced a feeling of evacuation similar to the normal.

Function after a straight colorectal reconstruction is dependent on the length of the residual rectal stump.[210] Following low anterior resection about 20% of patients have some soiling postoperatively with a further 10% having difficulty in holding flatus. After pull-through operations in which the rectal stump is either very short or absent, function is less satisfactory. Fewer than 10% of patients had perfect control following the Bacon pull-through procedure and only 25% had normal continence after the Cutait-Turnbull operation.[211] Parks and Percy,[170] however, reported acceptable function in 90% of patients having straight coloanal anastomosis with continence being normal in 50% and nearly normal in 46%. All patients in the series of Localio et al.[212] had normal continence after abdominosacral resection.

Karanjia et al.[213] studied the influence of anastomotic level on function in 26 patients with an anastomosis 3 cm from the anal verge and 42 with it lying at 6 cm. In both groups, frequency of defecation postoperatively was increased from the preoperative value. There was a significant difference in urgency postoperatively whereby 17 of the 26 patients with the anastomosis at 3 cm experienced this form of dysfunction compared with 17 of the 42 patients with the anastomosis at 6 cm.

There are now several studies that show unequivocally that maximal tolerable volume of the rectum or neorectum is inversely related to frequency and urgency of defecation. Heppel et al.[214] demonstrated this relationship for straight ileoanal anastomosis, Nicholls and Pezim[199] for ileal reservoir-anal anastomosis, and Lazorthes et al.[172] for colonic pouch-anal anastomo-

sis. Lewis et al.[215] in a study of 73 patients having anterior resection with coloanal anastomosis reported a maximal tolerable volume in the neorectum of 73 ml (55 to 110) versus 120 ml (80 to 190) in patients having poor and satisfactory function, respectively.

Bennett[211] showed that function following anterior resection improves over a period of 6 months to 1 year or more postoperatively. Although this positive outcome in many patients is of obvious benefit, those who are destined to die of recurrent cancer may live a considerable proportion of their remaining life with poor function. The introduction of the colonic reservoir has undoubtedly been of great benefit in that function is better earlier following restoration of intestinal continuity. Lazorthes et al.[172] first described this technique and demonstrated in a noncontrolled fashion improved function with regard to frequency and urgency over the first year postoperatively. Similar results were obtained by Parc et al.[173] Nicholls et al.[174] demonstrated a difference in neorectal compliance and capacitance in patients having a colonic pouch compared with straight reconstruction. Pelissier et al.[216] compared 33 patients after coloanal pouch and 36 healthy controls and observed no difference in frequency of defecation, urgency, or continence between the two groups. They did, however, report poorer evacuation in patients having a pouch reconstruction. This observation had already been made by Parc et al.[173] and up to 25% in their series had some difficulty in expulsion of feces. In a recent controlled trial of 43 patients randomized to a colonic pouch (23 patients) and to straight coloanal reconstruction (20 patients), Seow-Choen and Goh[175] demonstrated improved function at 1, 6, and 12 months in the former group. At 1 year 19 of 19 evaluable pouch patients had normal continence compared with 14 of 20 following a straight reconstruction. Frequency of defecation of less than three times per 24 hours at 12 months was present in 95% of the pouch patients compared with 70% of those having a straight coloanal anastomosis. There was no evacuation difficulty in any of the patients. These data show unequivocally the advantages of a colonic pouch reconstruction.

Sphincter function is the second important factor determining function. Miller et al.[171] studied 30 patients after coloanal anastomosis. Postoperatively only 11 had normal continence and 19 suffered from some degree of soiling with or without urgency. They showed that continence difficulties were related to anal resting tone and voluntary contraction pressure. There was a marked gender difference. The male/female ratios in the continent patients (11 patients) and incontinent patients (19 patients) were 10:1 and 6:13, respectively. The authors ascribed this to occult sphincter damage. Kusonoki et al.[217,218] studied function in three groups of patients having a coloanal pouch reconstruction after no radiotherapy (8 patients), preoperative radiotherapy 30 Gy (8 patients), and preoperative radiotherapy 80 Gy (8 patients). They demonstrated poorer function in the group having high-dose radiotherapy and noted a diminution in anal resting tone in that group. The inference was that radiotherapy in high dose causes internal sphincter damage.

Sexual Function

There is an extensive literature on sexual function vitiated to some extent by the failure to establish the situation preoperatively. Obtaining the information itself can be difficult because patients may not be prepared to discuss these matters. End points of sexual function in males including impotence and failure of ejaculation are easier to ascertain than sexual dysfunction in females. In both sexes, however, there are important psychological aspects relating to loss of libido and depression.

Williams and Johnston[207] studied prospectively sexual function before and after major rectal surgery. Of 38 patients who underwent abdominoperineal excision of the rectum, only 20 had been sexually active preoperatively. Among this group there were 17 men of whom 8 (47%) had developed complete impotence. One patient who retained erection experienced failure of ejaculation. With three further patients experiencing partial erection, the total proportion of patients having sexual impairment was 67%. The authors compared this rate with the 40 patients having anterior resection of whom, 28 (including 20 males) were sexually active beforehand. Of the 20, 6 (30%) experienced impaired sexual function. The authors concluded that sexual impairment was more likely after abdominoperineal excision.

There is some evidence that the level of anterior resection may influence sexual function. In a study of 25 patients under the age of 60 undergoing abdomino perineal excision (9) and anterior resection (16), Santangelo et al.[219] reported four instances of impotence and three cases of failure of ejaculation in 12 patients having low anterior resection compared with no incidence of impotence in the four patients having a high anterior resection. Although these numbers are small, they suggest a difference according to level of resection, a result that might be expected on anatomic grounds. Cosimelli et al.[220] reported sexual function in 188 patients having radical rectal surgery including lumbo-aortic clearance and total mesorectal excision. An attempt was made to identify the presacral nerves and to preserve them. Nearly 50% of patients had chemotherapy and or radiotherapy. The authors reported that only 16.6% of sexually active males retained sexual function after abdominoperineal resection. This rate compared with 56.6% after anterior resection.

There is less information on females. This is due to the limited number of studies and also to the difficulty in assessing end points. Physical factors such as vaginal stenosis, urinary or fecal incontinence, and pain on intercourse are easier to assess[221] than psychological factors.[223]

REFERENCES

1. Faget J (1743) Remarques sur les abces qui arrivent au fondamont. Memories de l'Academie Royale de Chirurgie, pt 11, pp 257–267
2. Lisfranc J (1826) Observation sur une affection cancereuse du rectum guèrie par l'excision. Rev Med Franc Etrang 2: 380
3. Verneuil AA (1873) Quoted by Tuttle JP (1905) A Treatise on Diseases of the Anus, Rectum and Pelvic Colon. 2nd Ed. p. 963. Appleton, New York
4. Viso L, Uriach J (1995) The first twenty operations for rectal cancer. Int J Colorectal Dis 10:167–168
5. Kraske P (1885) Zur Exstirpation hochsitzender Mastdarmkrebse. Verhdt Chir 14:464
6. Hochenegg J (1888) Die sakrale methode der exstirpation von mast-darmkrebsen bach Prof. Kraske: Wien Klin Wschr 1: 272–354
7. Hochenegg J (1889) Beitrage zur Chirurgie des Rektums under der Beckenorgone. Wien Klin Wschr 2:578
8. Hochenegg J (1900) Mein Operation der Folge bei Rektumkarzinom. Wein Klin Wschr 13:399
9. Maunsell HW (1892) A new method of excising the two upper portions of the rectum and the lower segment of the sigmoid flexure of colon. Lancet 2:473–476
10. Weir RF (1901) An improved method of treating high-seated cancers of the rectum. Am J Surg Gynecol (St. Louis) 15: 134–135
11. Miles WE (1908) A method of performing abdomino-perineal excision for carcinoma of the rectum and of the terminal portion of the pelvic colon. Lancet 2:1812–1813
12. Dixon CF (1939) Surgical removal of lesions occurring in sigmoid rectosigmoid. Am J Surg 46:12–17
13. Babcock WW (1939) Experience with resection of the colon and the elimination of colostomy. Am J Surg 46:186–303
14. Bacon HE (1945) Evolution of sphincter muscle preservation and re-establishment of continuity in the operative treatment of rectal and sigmoid cancer. Surg Gynecol Obstet 81: 113–127
15. Goligher JC (1951) The functional results after sphincter saving resection of the rectum. Ann R Coll Surg Engl 8:421–439
16. Westhues A (1930) Uber die Entstehung und Vermeidung des lokalen Rektumcarcinom Rezidivs. Arch Klin Chir 161: 582–624
17. Westhues H (1934) Die Pathologisch-Anatomischen Grundlagen der Chirurgie des Rektum Karzinoms. p. 68. Georg Thieme, Leipzig
18. Dukes CE (1932) The classification of cancer of the rectum. J Pathol Bacteriol 35:323–332
19. Kirschner M (1934) Das synchrone kombinierete Verfahren bei der Radikalbehandlung des Masdarmkrebses. Langenbecks Arch Klin Chir 180:296–308
20. Lloyd-Davies OV (1939) Lithotomy-Trendelenberg position for resection of rectum and lower pelvic colon. Lancet 2:74
21. Lockhart-Mummery P (1914) Diseases of the Rectum and Anus. Ballière Tindall, London
22. Virchow RLK (1858) Cellular Pathologie
23. Willis RA (1960) Pathology of Tumours. 3rd Ed. Butterworths, London, pp. 148–193
24. D'Allaines F (1956) Die Chirurgische Behandlung des Rektumcarzinoms. Borth, Leipzig
25. Black BM (1952) Combined abdomino-endorectal resection: technical aspects and indications. Arch Surg (Chicago) 65: 406–416
26. Turnbull RB Jr, Cuthbertson FM (1961) Abdomino rectal pull-through resection for cancer and for Hirschprung's disease. Cleve Clin Q 28:109–115
27. Cutait DE, Figlioni FJ (1961) A new method of colorectal anastomosis in abdomino-perineal resection. Dis Colon Rectum 4:335–342
28. Cutait DE, Cutait R, Ioshimoto et al (1985) Abdomino-perineal endoanal pull-through resection. Dis Colon Rectum 28: 294

29. Parks AG (1972) Transanal technique in low rectal anastomoses. Proc R Soc Med 65:975–976

30. Localio SA, Eng K, Gouge TH, Ransome JHC (1978) Abdomino-sacral resection for carcinoma of the mid-rectum: 10 years experience. Ann Surg 188:745–780 31. Mason AY (1972) Trans-sphincteric exposure for low rectal anastomosis. Proc R Soc Med 65:974

32. Phillips RKS, Hittinger R, Fry JS, Fielding LP (1985) Malignant large bowel obstruction. Br J Surg 72:196–302

33. Minister JJ (1964) Comparison of obstructing and non-obstructing carcinoma of the colon. Cancer 17:242–247

34. Ohman V (1982) Prognosis in patients with obstructing colorectal carcinoma. Am J Surg 143:742–747

35. Lockhart-Mummery HE, Ritchie JK, Hawley PR (1976) The results of surgical treatment for carcinoma of the rectum at St Mark's Hospital from 1948–1972. Br J Surg 63:673–677

36. Finlay IG, McArdle CS (1986) Occult hepatic metastases in colorectal carcinoma. Br J Surg 73:732–735

37. Dukes CE, Bussey HJR (1958) The spread of rectal cancer and its effect on prognosis. Br J Cancer 12:209–220

38. Gilchrist RK, David VC (1947) A consideration of pathological factors influencing five year survival in radical resection of the large bowel and rectum for carcinoma. Ann Surg 126:421–438

39. Newstead RG, Chapuis PH, Pheils M, Macpherson JG (1981) The relationship of survival staging and grading of colorectal carcinoma. Cancer 47:1424–1429

40. Fielding LP (1988) Clinico-pathologic staging of large bowel cancer. A report of the ASCRS Committee. Dis Colon Rectum 31:204–209

41. Fielding LP, Arsenault PA, Chapuis PH et al (1991) Working Party. Report to the World Congress of Gastroenterology, Sydney 1990. Clinicopathological staging for colorectal cancer: an International Documentation System (IDC) and an International Comprehensive Anatomical Terminology (ICAT). J Gastroenterol Hepatol 6:325–344

42. Chapuis PH, Dent of Fisher R, Newland RC et al (1985) A multivariate analysis of clinical and pathological variables in prognosis after resection of large bowel cancer. Br J Surg 72:698–702

43. Fielding LP, Phillips RKS, Hittinger R (1989) Factors influencing mortality after curative resection for large bowel cancer in elderly patients. Lancet 1:595–596

44. Devlin HB, Plant JA, Griffen M (1971) Aftermath of surgery for anorectal cancer. BMJ 2:413

45. Kettlewell MGW (1988) Neoplasm: present surgical treatment. Curr Opin Gastroenterol 4:19–27

46. Bown SG, Barr H, Matthewson K et al (1986) Endoscopic treatment of inoperable, colorectal cancers with the Nd-YAG laser. Br J Surg 73:949–952

47. Symposium (1989). Lasers in the treatment of colorectal disease. Int J Colorectal Dis 4:1–29

48. Madden JL, Kandalaft S (1971) Clinical evaluation of electrocoagulation in the treatment of cancer of the rectum. Am J Surg 122:347

49. Bright N, Hale P, Mason R (1992) Poor palliation of colorectal malignancy with the neodymium, yttrium-aluminium-garnet laser. Br J Surg 79:308–309

50. Slaney G (1971) Results of treatment of carcinoma of the colon and rectum. In Irvine WT (ed): Modern Trends in Surgery. 3rd Ed. Butterworth, London

51. Whittaker M, Goligher JC (1976) The prognosis after surgical treatment for carcinoma of the rectum. Br J Surg 63:384–388

52. Nicholls RJ (1982) Surgery of colorectal cancer. pp. 101–112. In Duncan (ed): Recent Results in Cancer Research. Vol. 83, Springer-Verlag

53. Peloquin AS (1973) Cancer of the colon and rectum: comparison of the results of three groups of surgeons using different techniques. Can J Surg 16:28–34

54. McArdle CS, Hole D (1991) Impact of variability among surgeons on postoperative morbidity, mortality and ultimate survival. BMJ 302:1501–1505

55. Grinnell RS (1953) Results in the treatment of carcinoma of the colon and rectum. Surg Gynecol Obstet 96:31

56. Allen AW, Welch CE, Donaldson GA (1947) Carcinoma of the colon: effect of recent advances in the surgical management. Ann Surg 126:19

57. Dukes CE (1930) The spread of cancer of the rectum. Br J Surg 17:643–648

58. Astler VB, Coller FA (1954) The prognostic significance of direct extension of carcinoma of the colon and rectum. Ann Surg 139:846–853

59. Talbot IC, Ritchie S, Leighton MH et al (1980) The clinical significance of invasion of veins by rectal cancer. Br J Surg 67:439–442

60. Sauer I, Bacon HE (1952) A new approach for excision of carcinoma of the lower portion of the rectum and anal canal. Surg Gynecol Obstet 95:229–242

61. Deddish MR, Stearns MW (1961) Anterior resection for carcinoma of the rectum and rectosigmoid area. Ann Surg 154:961–966

62. Hojo K, Koyama Y, Moriya Y (1982) Lymphatic spread and its prognostic value in patients with rectal cancer. Am J Surg 144:350–354

63. Pezim ME, Nicholls RJ (1984) Survival after high or low ligation of the inferior mesenteric artery during curative surgery for rectal cancer. Ann Surg 200:729–733

64. Surtees P, Ritchie JK, Phillips RKS (1990) High versus low ligation of the inferior mesenteric artery in rectal cancer. Br J Surg 77:618–621

65. Turnbull RB, Kyle K, Watson FB, Spratt J (1967) Cancer of the colon: the influence of the no touch technique on survival rates. Ann Surg 166:420–429

66. Wiggers T, Jeekel J, Arends JW et al (1988) No touch isolation technique in colon cancer: a controlled prospective trial. Br J Surg 75:409–415

67. Deddish MR, Stearns MW (1960) Surgical procedures for carcinoma of the left colon and rectum with five year results following abdomino-pelvic dissection of lymph nodes. Am J Surg 99:188–192

68. Enker WI, Pilipshen SJ, Heilwell MI et al (1986) En bloc pelvic lymphadenectomy and sphincter preservation in the surgical management of rectal cancer. Ann Surg 293:426–433

69. Scholefield, Northover JMA (1995) Surgical management of rectal cancer. Br J Surg 82:745–748

70. Moriya Y, Hojo K, Sawada T, Doyama Y (1989) Significance of Lateral node dissection for advanced rectal carcinoma at

or below the peritoneal reflection. Dis Colon Rectum 32: 307–315

71. Hojo K, Sawada T, Moriya Y (1989) An analysis of survival, voiding and sexual function after wide iliopelvic lymphadenectomy in patients with carcinoma of the rectum, compared with conventional lymphadenectomy. Dis Colon Rectum 32: 128–133

72. Moreira LF, Hizuta A, Iwagajitt et al (1994) Lateral lymph node dissection for rectal carcinoma below the peritoneal reflection. Br J Surg 81:293–296

73. Berge T, Ekelund G, Mellner C et al (1973) Carcinoma of the colon and rectum in a defined population. Acta Chir Scand, suppl. 4:38

74. Phillips RKS, Hittinger R, Blesovsky L et al (1984) Local recurrence following curative surgery for large bowel cancer. I. The overall picture. Br J Surg 71:12–16

75. Phillips RKS, Hittinger R, Blesovsky L et al (1984) Local recurrence following curative surgery for large bowel cancer: II. The rectum and rectosigmoid. Br J Surg 71:17–20.

76. McCall JL, Cox MR, Wattchow DA (1995) Analysis of local recurrence rates after surgery alone for rectal cancer. Int J Colorectal Dis 10:126–132

77. Stearns MW, Deddish MR, Quan SHQ, Leaming RH (1974) Preoperative roentgentherapy for cancer of the rectum and rectosigmoid. Surg Gynecol Obstet 138:584–586

78. Roswit B, Higgins GA, Keehn RJ (1975) Preoperative irradiation for carcinoma of the rectum and rectosigmoid colon. Report of a national Veterans Administration randomized study. Cancer 35:1597–1602

79. Heald RJ, Ryall FDH (1986) Recurrence and survival after total mesorectal excision for rectal cancer. Lancet 1: 1479–1482

80. Stockholm Rectal Cancer Study Group (1987) Short-term preoperative radiotherapy for adenocarcinoma of the rectum. Am J Clin Oncol 10:369–375

81. Stockholm Rectal Cancer Study Group (1990) Preoperative short-term radiation therapy in operable rectal carcinoma. A prospective randomised trial. Cancer 66:49–55

82. Balslev I, Pedersen M, Teglbjaerg PS et al (1986) Postoperative radiotherapy in Dukes' B and C carcinoma of the rectum and rectosigmoid. A randomized multicentre study. Cancer 58:22–28

83. Goldberg PA, Nicholls RJ, Porter NH et al (1994) Long-term results of a randomised trial of short-course low-dose adjuvant preoperative radiotherapy for rectal cancer: reduction in local treatment failure. Eur J Cancer 30A:1602–1606

84. Gerard A, Buyse M, Nordlinger B et al (1988) Preoperative radiotherapy as adjuvant treatment in rectal cancer. Final results of a randomized study of the European Organization for Research and Treatment of Cancer (EORTC). Ann Surg 208: 606–614

85. Marsh PJ, James RD, Schofield PF (1995) Definition of local recurrence after surgery for rectal cancer. Br J Surg 82: 465–468

86. Goldberg PA, Nicholls RJ (1995) Prediction of local recurrence and survival of carcinoma of the rectum by surgical and histopathological assessment of local clearance. Br J Surg 82:1054–1056

87. Morson BC, Vaughan EG, Bussey HJR (1963) Pelvic recurrence after excision of rectum for carcinoma. BMJ 2:13–17

88. Hermanek P (1994) pp. 7–14. In Hermanek P, Marzoli GP (eds): Lokale Therapie des Rektumkarzinoms. Springer Verlag

89. Pollett WG, Nicholls RJ (1983) The relationship between the extent of distal clearance and survival and local recurrence rates after curative anterior resection for carcinoma of the rectum. Ann Surg 70:159–163

90. Heald RJ, Husband EM, Ryal RDH (1982) The mesorectum in rectal cancer surgery—the clue to pelvic recurrence. Br J Surg 69:613–616

91. Blenkinsopp WR, Stewart Brown S, Blesovsky L et al (1981) Histopathology reporting in large bowel cancer. J Clin Pathol 34:509–513

92. Elliot ME, Todd IP, Nicholls RJ (1982) Radical restorative surgery for poorly differentiated carcinoma of the mid rectum. Br J Surg 69:273–274

93. Quer EA, Dahlin DC, Mayo CW (1953) Retrograde intramural spread of carcinoma of the rectum and rectosigmoid. A microscopic study. Surg Gynecol Obstet 96:24–30

94. Grinnell RS (1954) Distal intramural spread of carcinoma of the rectum and rectosigmoid. Surg Gynecol Obstet 99: 421–429

95. Penfold JCB (1974) A comparison of restorative resection of carcinoma of the middle third of the rectum with abdominoperineal excision. Aust NZ J Surg 44:354–356

96. Quirke P, Durdey P, Dixon MF, Williams NS (1986) Local recurrence of rectal adenocarcinoma due to inadequate surgical resection. Histopathological study of lateral tumour spread and surgical excision. Lancet 2:996–999

97. Enker WE, Laffer UT, Block GE (1979) Enhanced survival of patients with colon and rectal cancer is based upon wide anatomic resection. Ann Surg 190:350–358

98. Goligher JC, Dukes CE, Bussey HJR (1951) Local recurrences after sphincter saving excisions for carcinoma of the rectum and rectosigmoid. Br J Surg 39:199–211

99. Wilson SM, Beahrs OH (1975) The curative treatment of carcinoma of the sigmoid, rectosigmoid and rectum. Ann Surg 183:556–565

100. Williams NS, Dixon MF, Johnston D (1983) Re-appraisal of the 5 cm rule of distal excision for carcinoma of the rectum: a study of distal intramural spread and of patients' survival. Br J Surg 70:150–154

101. Hurst PA, Prout WG, Kelly JM et al (1982) Local recurrence after low anterior resection using the staple gun. Br J Surg 69:275–276

102. Hermanek P (1991) Onkologische Chirurgie/Paathologisch—Anatomische Sicht. Langenbecks Arch Chir suppl: 277–281

103. Scott N, Jackson P, Al-Jaberi T et al PJ (1995) Total mesorectal excision and local recurrence: a study of tumour spread in the mesorectum distal to the tumour. Br J Surg 82:1031–1033

104. MacFarlane JK, Ryall RDH, Heald R (1993) Mesorectal excision for rectal cancer. Lancet 341:457–460

105. Jones PF, Thomson HJ (1982) Long term results of a consistent policy of sphincter preservation in the treatment of carcinoma of the rectum. Br J Surg 69:564–568

106. Williams NS, Johnston D (1984) Survival and recurrence after sphincter-saving resection and abdomino-perineal excision for carcinoma of the middle third of the rectum. Br J Surg 71:278–282

107. Nicholls RJ, Ritchie JK, Wadsworth J et al (1979) Total excision or restorative resection for carcinoma of the middle third of the rectum. Br J Surg 66:625–627

108. Akyol AM, Mc Gregor JR, Galloway DJ et al (1991) Recurrence of colorectal cancer after sutered and stapled large bowel anastomosis. Br J Surg 78:1297–1300

109. Umpleby HC, Williamson RCN (1987) Anastomotic recurrence in large bowel cancer. Br J Surg 74:873–878

110. Cole WH (1952) Recurrence in carcinoma of the colon and proximal rectum following resection for carcinoma. Arch Surg 65:264–270

111. Beal JM, Cornell GN (1956) A study of the problem of recurrence of carcinoma of the anastomotic site following resection of the colon for carcinoma. Ann Surg 143:1–7

112. Wright HK, Thomas WH, Cleveland JC (1969) The low recurrence rate of colonic carcinoma in ileo colic anastomosis. Surg Gynecol Obstet 129:960–962

113. Hojo K (1986) Anastomotic recurrence after sphincter saving resection for rectal cancer. Dis Colon Rectum 29:11–14

114. McDermott FT, Hughes ESR, Pihl E et al (1985) Local recurrence after potentially curative resection for rectal cancer in a series of 1008 patients. Br J Surg 72:34–37

115. Rosenberg IL, Russell CW, Giles GR (1978) Cell viability studies on the exfoliated colonic cancer cell. Br J Surg 65: 188

116. Umpleby HC, Fermor B, Symes MO, Williamson RCN (1984) Viability of exfoliated colorectal carcinoma cells. Br J Surg 71:659–663

117. Mayo WJ (1913) Grafting and traumatic dissemination of carcinoma in course of operations for malignant disease. JAMA 60:512–513

118. Killingback MJ, Wilson E, Hughes ESR (1965) Anal metastases from carcinoma of the rectum and colon. Aust NZ J Surg 34:178–187

119. Monson et al (1994)

120. Keynes WM (1961) Implantation from the bowel lumen in cancer of the large intestine. Ann Surg 153:357–364

121. Southwick HW, Harridge WH, Cole WH (1962) Recurrence at the suture line following resection for carcinoma of the colon. Incidence following preventative measures. Am J Surg 103:86–89

122. Phillips RKS, Cook HT (1986) Effect of steel wire sutures on the incidence of chemically induced rodent colonic tumours. Br J Surg 73:671–674

123. Umpleby HC, Williamson RCN (1984) The efficacy of agents employed to prevent anastomotic recurrence in colorectal carcinoma. Ann R Coll Surg Engl 66:192–194

124. Williams NS, Jass JR, Hardcastle JD (1988) Clinicopathological assessment and staging of colorectal cases. Br J Surg 75: 647–652

125. Hughes KS, Rosenstein RB, Songhorabodi S et al (1988) Resection of the liver for colorectal carcinoma metastases. Dis Colon Rectum 31:1–4

126. Adson MA, Van Heerden JA (1980) Major hepatic resections for metastatic colorectal cancer. Ann Surg 191:576–583

127. Wood CB, Gillis CR, Blumgort LH (1976) A retrospective study of the natural history of patients with liver metastases from colorectal cancer. Clin Oncol 2:285–288

128. Vandertoll DJ, Beahrs OM (1965) Carcinoma of the rectum and low sigmoid: evaluation of anterior resection in 1776 favourable lesions. Arch Surg 90:793–798

129. Wang CC, Schultz MD (1962) The role of radiation therapy in the management of carcinoma of the sigmoid, rectosigmoid and rectum. Radiology 79:1–5

130. Hildebrandt U, Boscaini M, Beynon J et al (1986) Symposium: endosonography of the rectum. Int J Colorectal Dis 1: 201–204

131. Beynon J, Foy DMA, Roe N et al (1986) Endoluminal ultrasound in the assessment of local invasion in rectal cancer. Br J Surg 73:474–478

132. Thaler W, Watzka S, Martin F et al (1994) Preoperative staging in rectal cancer by endoluminal ultrasound vs magnetic resonance imaging. Dis Colon Rectum 37:1189–1193

133. Nicholls RJ, Mason AY, Morson BC et al (1982) Clinical staging of the extent of rectal carcinoma. Br J Surg 69: 404–409

134. Chan TW, Kressel HY, Milestone B et al (1991) Rectal carcinoma: staging at MR imaging with endorectal surface coil. Radiology 181:461–467

135. Dworak O (1989) Number and size of lymph nodes and node metastases in rectal carcinomas. Surg Endosc 3:96–99

136. Mason AY (1976) Selective surgery for carcinoma of the rectum. Aust NZ J Surg 46:322

137. Nicholls RJ, Galloway RJ, York Mason A, Boyle P (1975) Clinical local staging of rectal cancer. Br J Surg 72:551–552

138. Higgins GA, Humphrey EW, Dwight RW et al (1986) Preoperative radiation and surgery for cancer of the rectum: VA Surgical Oncology Group Trial II: Cancer 58:352–359

139. Second Report of an M.R.C. Working Party (1984) The evaluation of low dose preoperative X-ray therapy in the management of operable rectal cancer: results of a randomly controlled trial. Br J Surg 71:21–25

140. Rider WD, Palmer JA, Mahoney LJ, Robertson CT (1977) Pre-operative irradiation in operable cancer of the rectum: report of the Toronto Trial. Can J Surg 20:335–338

141. GTSG (1985) Prolongation of the disease-free interval in surgically treated rectal carcinoma. N Engl J Med 312: 1465–1472

142. Stevens KR, Fletcher WS (1983) High dose preoperative pelvic irradiation for unresectable adenocarcinoma of the rectum and sigmoid. Int J Radiat Oncol Biol Phys, (suppl) 9:148

143. James RD, Schofield PF (1985) Resection of 'inoperable' rectal cancer following radiotherapy. Br J Surg 72:279–281

144. Dosoretz DE, Gunderson LL, Hedberg S et al (1983) Preoperative irradiation for unresectable rectal and rectosigmoid carcinoma. Cancer 52:814–818

145. Emami B, Bilepich M, Willet C (1982) Effect of preoperative irradiation on resectability of colorectal carcinomas. Int Radiat Oncol Biol Phys 8:1295–1297

146. Slanetz CA, Herter FP, Grinnell RS (1972) Anterior resection versus abdomino-perineal resection for cancer of the rectum and rectosigmoid. Am J Surg 123:110–115

147. Nicholls RJ, Hall C (1996) Treatment of non-disseminated cancer of the lower rectum. Br J Surg 83:15–18

148. Morson BC, Bussey HJR, Samoorian S (1977) Policy of local excision for early cancer of the colorectum. Gut 18: 1045–1050

149. Buess G, Hutterer F, Theiss J et al (1984) Das System für die transanale rektum operation. Chirurg 55:677–680

150. Buess G, Kipfmuller K, Heald R et al (1989) Transanale endoskopische Mikrochirurgie beim Rektum carcinom. Chirurg 60:901–904

151. Nicholls RJ (1994) Results at St Mark's Hospital. pp. 137–139. In Hermanek P, Marzoli GP (eds): Lokale Therapie des Rektumkarzinoms. Springer Verlag

152. Biggers OR, Beart RW, Ilstrup DM (1986) Local excision of rectal cancer. Dis Colon Rectum 29:374–377

153. Killingback MJ (1985) Indications for local excision of rectal cancer. Br J Surg, suppl. 72:554–556

154. Whiteway J, Nicholls RJ, Morson BC (1985) The role of surgical local excision in the treatment of rectal cancer. Br J Surg 72:694–697

155. Lock MR, Cairns DW, Ritchie JK, Lockhart Mummery HE (1978) The treatment of early colorectal cancer by local excision. Br J Surg 65:346–349

156. Lock MR, Ritchie JK, Hawley PR (1993) Reappraisal of radical local excision for carcinoma of the rectum. Br J Surg 80:928–929

157. Hager T, Gall FP, Hermneck P (1983) Local excision of cancer of the rectum. Dis Colon Rectum 26:149–151

158. Hermanek P, Gall FP (1986) Early (microinvasive) colorectal carcinoma. Pathology, diagnosis, surgical treatment. Int J Colrectal Dis 1:79–84

159. Buess G, Mentges B, Manncke K et al (1992) Technique and results of transanal endoscopic microsurgery in early rectal cancer. Am J Surg 163:63–70

160. Salm R, Lampe H, Bustos A, Matern U (1994) Experience with TEM in Germany. Endosc Surg Allied Techno 2:251–254

161. Said S, Huber P, Pichlmaier H (1993) Technique and clinical results of endorectal surgery. Surgery 113:65–75

162. Graham RA, Garnsey L, Jessup JM (1990) Local excision of rectal carcinoma. Am J Surg 160:306–312

163. Banerjee AK, Jehle EC, Shorthouse AJ, Buess G (1955) Local excision of rectal tumours. Br J Surg 82:1165–1173

164. Knight CD, Griffen FD (1980) An improved technique for low sphincter resection of the rectum using the EEA stapler. Surgery 88:710

165. Fielding LP, Stewart Brown S, Blesovsky L, Kearney G (1980) Anastomotic integrity after operations for large bowel cancer. A multicentre study. BMJ 281:411–414

166. Goligher JC, Lee PWR, Macfie J, Lintott DJ (1979) Experience with the Russian model 249 suture gun for anastomosis of the rectum. Surg Gynecol Obstet 148:517–524

167. Smith LE (1981) Anastomosis with EEA stapler after anterior colonic resection. Dis Colon Rectum 29:236–242

168. Heald RJ, Leicester RJ (1981) The low stapled anastomosis. Br J Surg 68:333–337

169. Lazorthes F, Chiotasso P (1986) Stapled colorectal anastomoses: preoperative integrity of the anastomosis and rate of post operative leakage. Int J Colorectal Dis 1:96–98

170. Parks AG, Percy JP (1982) Resection and sutured coloanal anastomosis for rectal carcinoma. Br J Surg 69:301–304

171. Miller AS, Lewis WG, Williamson MER et al (1995) Factors that influence functional outcome after coloanal anastomosis for carcinoma of the rectum. Br J Surg 82:1327–1330

172. Lazorthes F, Fages P, Chiotasso P et al (1986) Resection of the rectum with construction of a colonic reservoir and colo-anal anastomosis for carcinoma of the rectum. Br J Surg 73:136–138

173. Parc R, Tiret E, Frileux P et al (1986) Resection and colo-anal anastomosis with colonic reservoir for rectal carcinoma. Br J Surg 73:139–141

174. Nicholls RJ, Lubowski DZ, Donaldson DR (1988) Comparison of colonic reservoir and straight colo-anal reconstruction after rectal excision. Br J Surg 75:318–320

175. Seow Choen F, Goh HS (1995) Prospective randomised trial comparing J colonic pouch-anal anastomosis and straight coloanal reconstruction. Br J Surg 82:608–610

176. Koruth NM, Krukowski ZH, Youngson GG et al (1985) Intraoperative colonic irrigation in the management of left-sided large bowel emergencies. Br J Surg 72:708–709

177. Dudley HAF, Radcliffe AG, McGeechan D (1980) Intraoperative irrigation of the colon to permit primary anastomosis. Br J Surg 67:80–81

178. Thomson WHF, Carter SC (1986) On-table lavage to achieve safe restorative rectal and emergency left colonic resection without covering colostomy. Br J Surg 73:61–63

179. Robles Campos R, Garcia Ayllon J, Parrilla Daricio et al (1992) Management of perineal wound following abdomino-perineal resection: postoperative study of three methods. Br J Surg 79:29–31

180. Lieberman RC, Feldman S (1984) Primary closure of the perineal wound with closed continuous transabdominal pelvic irrigation after rectal excision. Dis Colon Rectum 27:526–528

181. Tompkins RG, Warshaw AL (1985) Improved management of the perineal wound after proctectomy. Ann Surg 202:760–765

182. Irvin TT, Goligher JC (1975) A controlled trial of three different methods of perineal wound management following excision of the rectum. Br J Surg 62:287–291

183. Page CP, Carlton PK, Becker DW (1990) Closure of the pelvic and perineal wounds after removal of the rectum and anus. Dis Colon Rectum 23:2–9

184. Faivre J, Weber F (1977) La place de l' électro résection dans le traitment du cancer du rectum. Bordeaux Med 10:2131–2136

185. Lockhart-Mummery P (1926) Two hundred cases of cancer of the rectum treated by perineal excision. Br J Surg 14:110–124

186. Goligher JC (1984) Surgery of the Anus, Rectum and Colon. Ballière Tindall, London

187. Akyol AM, Galloway DJ, Murray GD et al (1991) Anastomotic leaks and tumour recurrence. Eur J Surg Oncol 17:113–114

188. Goligher JC, Simpkins KC, Linlott DJ (1977) A controlled comparison of one and two-layer techniques of suture for high and low colorectal anastomoses. Br J Surg 64:609

189. Everett WG (1975) A comparison of one layer and two layer techniques for colorectal anastomosis. Br J Surg 62:135–140

190. Cady J, Godfroy J, Sibaud O et al (1980) La désunion anastomotique en chirurgie colique et rectale. Etude comparative des procédés de suture manuelle et mécanique á propos d'une serie de 149 resections. Ann Chir 34:350–356

191. Overy RD, Godfrey PJ, Evans M, Pollock AV (1980) Staples or sutures in the colon? A random controlled trial of three methods of colon anastomosis. Br J Surg 67:363–368

192. Beart RW, Kelly KA (1981) Randomised prospective evaluation of the EEA stapler for colo-rectal anastomoses. Am J Surg 141:143–147

193. McGinn FP, Gartell PC, Clifford PC, Brunton FJ (1985) Staples or sutures for low colorectal anastomoses: a prospective randomised trial. Br J Surg 72:603–605

194. West of Scotland and Highland Anastomosis Study Group (1991) Suturing or stapling in gastrointestinal surgery: a prospective randomised study. Br J Surg 78:337–341

195. Karanjia ND, Corder AP, Bearn P, Heald RJ (1994) Leakage from stapled low anastomosis after total mesorectal excision for carcinoma of the rectum. Br J Surg 81:1224–1226

196. Wunderlich M, Karner-Hariasch J, Schissel R (1986) Results of coloanal anastomosis. A prospective study. Int J Colorectal Dis 1:757–761

197. Hautefeuille P, Valleur P, Perniceni T et al (1988) Functional and oncologic results after coloanal anastomosis for low rectal carcinoma. Ann Surg 207:61–64

198. Sweeney JL, Ritchie JK, Hawley PR (1989) Resection and sutured per anal anastomosis for carcinoma of the rectum. Dis Colon Rectum 32:103–106

199. Nicholls RJ, Pezim ME (1985) Restorative proctocolectomy for ulcerative colitis and familial adenomatous polyposis: a comparison of three reservoir designs. Br J Surg 72:470–474

200. Fielding LP, Stewart Brown S, Hittinger R, Blesovsky L (1984) Covering stoma for elective anterior resection of the rectum: an outmoded operation. Am J Surg 147:524–530

201. Grabham JA, Moran BJ, Lane RHS (1995) Defunctioning colostomy for low anterior resection: a selective approach. Br J Surg 82:1331–1332

202. Broader JH, Marselink BA, Oates GD, Williams JA (1974) Management of the pelvic space after proctectomy. Br J Surg 61:94–97

203. Marks CG, Leighton M, Ritchie JK, Hawley PR (1976) Primary suture of the perineal wound following rectal excision for adenocarcinoma. Br J Surg 63:322–326

204. Oakley Jr, Fazio VW, Jagelman DG et al (1985) Management of the perineal wound after rectal excision for UC. Dis Colon Rectum 28:885–888

205. Skene AL, Gault DT, Woodhouse CRJ et al (1990) Perineal, vuval and vaginoperineal reconstruction using the rectus abdominis myocutaneous flap. Br J Surg 77:635–637

206. Brough WA, Schofield PF (1991) The value of the rectus abdominis myocutaneous flap in the treatment of complex perineal fistula. Dis Colon Rectum 34:148–150

207. Williams NS, Johnston D (1983) The quality of life after rectal excision for low rectal cancer. Br J Surg 70:460–462

208. Goligher JC, Hughes ESR (1951) Sensibility of the rectum and colon—its role in the mechanism of anal continence. Lancet 1:543–548

209. Lane RHS, Parks AG (1977) Function of the anal sphincters following colo-anal anastomosis. Br J Surg 64:596–599

210. Goligher JC, Duthie HC, de Dombal FT et al (1965) Abdomino-anal pull-through excision for tumours of the mid third of the rectum: a comparison with lower anterior resection. Br J Surg 52:323–335

211. Bennett RS (1976) The place of pull-through operations in treatment of carcinoma of the rectum. Dis Colon Rectum 19:420–424

212. Localio SA, Eng K, Coppa GF (1983) Abdominosacral resection for midrectal cancer. Ann Surg 198:320–324

213. Karanjia ND, Schache DJ, Heald RJ (1992) Function of the distal rectum after low anterior resection for carcinoma. Br J Surg 79:114–116

214. Heppel J, Kelly KA, Phillips SF et al (1982) Physiologic aspects of continence after colectomy, mucosal proctectomy and endorectal ileo-anal anastomosis. Ann Surg 195:435–443

215. Lewis WG, Martin IG, Williamson MER et al (1995) Why do some patients experience poor functional results after anterior resection of the rectum for carcinoma. Dis Colon Rectum 38:259–263

216. Pelissier EP, Blum D, Bachour A, Bosset JF (1992) Functional results of coloanal anastomosis with reservoir. Dis Colon Rectum 35:843–846

217. Kusunoki M, Shoji Y, Yahaji H et al (1991) Function after ano-abdominal rectal resection and colonic J pouch-anal anastomosis. Br J Surg 78:1434–1438

218. Kusunoki M, Shoji Y, Yanaji H et al (1993) Anorectal function after preoperative intraluminal brachytherapy and colonic J pouch—anal anastomosis for rectal carcinoma. Br J Surg 80:933–935

219. Santangelo ML, Romano G, Sassaroli C (1987) Sexual function after resection for rectal cancer. Am J Surg 154:502–504

220. Cosimelli M, Mannella E, Gianarelli D et al (1995) Nerve-sparing surgery in 302 resectable rectosigmoid cancer patients: genito-urinary morbidity and 10 year survival. Dis Colon Rectum, suppl. 37:542–546

221. Watts JM, De Dombal FT, Goligher JC (1966) Long-term complications and prognosis following major surgery for ulcerative colitis. Br J Surg 53:1014–1022

222. Petter O, Gruner N, Rerdar N et al (1977) Marital status and sexual adjustment after colectomy. Scand J Gastroenterol 12:193–197

223. Adloff M, Arnaud JP, Schoegel M, Thibaud D (1985) Factors influencing local recurrence after abdomino-perineal resection for cancer of the rectum. Dis Colon Rectum 28:413–415

224. Carlsson U, Lasson A, Ekelund G (1987) Recurrence rates after curative surgery for rectal carcinoma with special reference to their accuracy. Dis Colon Rectum 30:431–434

225. Cawthorn SJ, Parums DV, Gibbs NM et al (1990) Extent of mesorectal spread and involvement of lateral resection margin as prognostic factors after surgery for rectal cancer. Lancet 335:1055

226. Karanjia ND, Schache DJ, North WRS, Heald RJ (1990) 'Close shave' in anterior resection. Br J Surg 77:501–512

227. Lasson ALL, Ekielund GR, Lindstrom CG (1984) Recurrence risks after stapled anastomosis for rectal carcinoma. Acta Chir Scand 150:85–89

228. Pahlman L, Glimelius B (1984) Local recurrences after surgical treatment for rectal carcinoma. Acta Chir Sc and 150:513–516

229. Zirngibl H, Huse, amm B, Hermaneck P (1990) Intraoperative spillage of tumour cells in surgery for rectal cancer. Dis Colon Rectum 33:610–614

230. Stearns MW, Binkley GE (1953) The influence of location on prognosis in operable rectal cancer. Surg Gynecol Obstet 96:368–370

231. Gilbertson VA (1960) Adenocarcinoma of the rectum: incidence and locations of recurrent tumour following operations for cure. Ann Surg 151:340–348

232. Philipshen SJ, Heilweil M, Quan SHQ et al (1984) Patterns of pelvic recurrence following definitive resections of rectal cancer. Cancer 53:1354–1362

233. Luke M, Kirkegaard P, Lendorf A, Christiansen J (1983) Pelvic recurrence rate after abdominoperineal excision and low anterior resection for rectal cancer before and after introduction of stapling technique. World J Surg 7:616–619

234. Bolton RA, Britton DC (1980) Restorative surgery of the rectum with circumferential staple. Lancet 1:850–851

235. Radcliffe AG, Dudley HAF (1983) Intraoperative antegrade irrigation of the large intestine. Surg Gynecol Obstet 156: 721–723

236. Williams NS, Durdey P, Johnston D (1985) The outcome following sphincter saving resection and abdomino-perineal resection for low rectal cancer. Br J Surg 72:595–598

24

RADIOTHERAPY

Lars Påhlman
Bengt Glimelius

Both surgery and radiotherapy are forms of regional treatment. For this reason radiotherapy might not be expected to make a great impact on survival since it will not deal with metastatic disease. However, when local recurrence is the first sign of treatment failure and provided such an event can be prevented by radiotherapy, an effect on survival could be expected.

Radiotherapy aimed at controlling local disease has been applied to three broad clinicopathologic groups of patients with large bowel cancer. Thus it is given as treatment adjuvant to curative surgery, as the sole primary treatment for rectal cancer, and for surgically unresectable disease. The last group includes patients with unresectable disease at initial presentation, incompletely resected disease, and local recurrence some time after initial "curative" surgery (Fig. 24-1).

Shortly after the discovery of radium at the end of the 19th century, radiotherapy was applied to rectal cancer; due to the high local recurrence rates following perineal surgery, in 1908 Ernest Miles[1] proposed abdominal perineal excision, with the advice: "Perform the biggest possible operation for the earliest possible case." In the early decades of the 20th century, there were several reports of radium as a radiation source. At the International Conference of Cancer in London 1928, the combination of surgery and radiation was discussed.[2-4] At the time, very little therapeutic value was seen for this treatment, and it was more or less forgotten; severe toxicity caused by the lack of appropriate dosimetry resulted in radiation damage, particularly to the superficial tissues. The development of dose fractionation in the 1930s led to a significant improvement in radiotherapy in general: higher doses could be administered to a field of tissue over a longer period of time, thus reducing morbidity and improving effectiveness. The energy of the irradiation delivered during the 1930s and 1940s was within the kilovoltage range. Thus, it was still difficult to deliver high doses of irradiation to deeply placed structures. The lack of penetration of low-voltage irradiation resulted in greater dissipation of energy to superficial tissue than was desirable. In the 1950s, with the development of cobalt 70 sources, higher energy radiation became possible, and the era of modern radiotherapy began, whereby higher doses could be delivered to deeply placed structures.

This chapter discusses the place of radiotherapy in colorectal cancer, the rationale for combining surgery and radiotherapy, and how to select patients for adjuvant and supplementary treatment. It is divided into sections dealing with radiotherapy for resectable cancer (which chiefly means adjuvant treatment) and radiotherapy for nonresectable rectal cancer. Radiotherapy as the sole treatment for curative intent and its use in palliation of nonresectable or recurrent disease is discussed. Finally, the role of radiotherapy in colonic cancer is considered.

IS THERE A NEED FOR RADIOTHERAPY IN COLORECTAL CANCER?

Local Recurrence After Surgery

Surgery is the most important treatment modality for patients with colorectal cancer, but local failure is particularly common after surgery for rectal cancer. The proportion of patients who develop clinically relevant local failure after rectal cancer surgery has been variably reported to range from less than 5% to more than 50%.[5-15] There may be several reasons for these large differences, including patient selection, the definition of radicality, the accuracy and duration of follow-up, the definition of local failure, and the skill of the surgeon. In all controlled randomized trials reported during the last few decades in which radiotherapy (pre- or postoperative) has been compared with surgery alone, the surgery-alone group has shown a local recurrence rate that has always exceeded 20% (see below, and Table 24-1), with an average of about 30%. This figure probably represents the average rate worldwide after standard rectal cancer surgery. Lower rates reported in the literature always derive

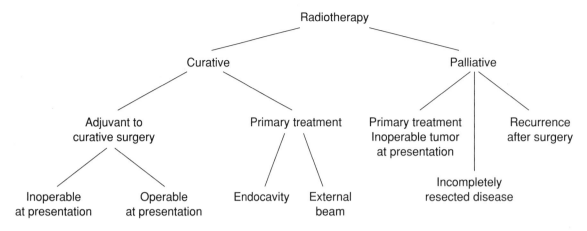

Figure 24-1. Clinicopathologic groups potentially suitable for radiotherapy.

Table 24-1. Pelvic Recurrence After a Combination of Surgery and Radiotherapy in Rectal Carcinoma (Controlled Trials With a Surgery Alone Group)

Study	Irradiation (Dose [Gy] Number of Fractions)	CRE Value	LQ Time	Surgery Alone (Number of Local Recurrences/Total [%])	Surgery + Radiotherapy (Number of Local Recurrences/Total [%])	P Value[a]	Percent Reduction in Local Failure Rates
Preoperative							
Rider et al., 1977[65]	5/1	5.0	7.5	[c]			
Duncan et al., 1984[63]	5/1	5.0	7.5	[d]			
	20/10	8.7	20.4	[d]			
Goldberg et al., 1994[82]	15/3	9.7	22.5	51/210[e] (24)	31/185[a] (17)	NS	29
Higgins et al., 1986[72]	31.5/18	11.1	26.8	[c]			
Horn et al., 1990[81]	31.5/18	11.1	26.8	31/131 (24)	24/138 (17)	NS	29
Roswit et al., 1975[66]	25/10	10.8	27.5	32/87[f] (37)	27/93[f] (22)	NS	22
James et al., 1991[83]	20/4	12.3	30.0	58/141 (41)	26/143 (18)	**	63
Gérard et al., 1988[80]	34.5/15	13.0	35.2	49/175 (28)	24/166 (14)	**	50
MRC2[g]	40/20	13.6	36.0	50/132 (38)	41/129 (32)	NS	16
SRCSG, 1990[84]	25/5	13.9	37.5	120/485 (28)	61/424 (14)	**	50
SRCT 1995[85]	25/5	13.9	37.5	131/557 (24)	51/553 (9)	**	63
Postoperative							
Balslev et al., 1986[86]	50/25	14.9	35.4	57/250 (23)	46/244 (19)	NS	17
MRC3[g]	40/20	13.6	36.0	69/235 (29)	46/234 (20)	**	31
GITSG 1985[87]	40–48/22	13.6	36.0	27/106 (25)	15/96 (16)	NS	36
Fisher et al., 1988[88]	46.5/26	14.9	39.3	45/184 (24)	30/184 (16)	NS	33
EORTC[h]	46/23	14.9	40.8	30/88 (34)	25/84 (30)	NS	13
Treuniet-Drukor and van Patten, 1991[89]	50/25	15.7	43.8	28/84 (33)	21/88 (24)	NS	41

[a] NS, $P > 0.05$; *, $P < 0.05$; **, $P < 0.01$; ***, $P < 0.001$.
[b] Only tethered tumors.
[c] Not reported.
[d] Only actuarial data reported, with no difference between groups.
[e] Outpatients only reported.
[f] Autopsy series only reported.
[g] MRC Trial Office, personal communication.
[h] EORTC Trial Office, personal communication.

from institutional series treated by well-trained surgeons with a special interest in the disease; they sometimes use more radical procedures than is usually the case.[7,10,17] Extensive surgery can increase morbidity through damage to neighboring organs and pelvic nerves, causing bladder and sexual dysfunction as well as hemorrhage.[19]

The relationship between the type of resection and local failure rates has been studied retrospectively. In comparing patients undergoing anterior resection or abdominoperineal excision, no difference was found by some authors,[9,14,19–22] whereas others have shown an increased incidence of local recurrence after the latter procedure.[23,24] One explanation for this finding is that small and locally nonadvanced tumors are more likely to be removed by a sphincter-saving procedure. However, some authors have reported the opposite outcome, namely, a higher local recurrence rate after an anterior resection.[12,13,25] These contradictory and inconclusive reports were common in the early 1980s, when sphincter-saving procedures were being increasingly performed after the introduction of the circular stapling instrument. Higher local recurrence rates after restorative surgery were explained by the "coning" effect, whereby the dissection on either side of the tumor converged, possibly prejudicing local clearance.[26]

Using the technique of total mesorectal excision popularized by Heald, the local recurrence rate has been reported to be very low.[15,27] With this technique a more complete resection of the whole rectum including the rectal fascia is performed. The posterior part of the mesorectum is dissected in the embryologic plane between the rectum surrounded by the fascia propia and Denonvilliers' fascia and adjacent structures. As the dissection continues downward within the same plane, good lateral margins are achieved, maintaining the same embryologic plane just outside Denonvilliers' fascia.

The importance of adequate surgical local clearance has recently been demonstrated by pathologic studies in which involvement of the lateral margin has been shown to be an important prognostic factor of local recurrence.[28,29] Moreover, the possibility of nests of malignant cells or deposits in lymph nodes distal to the tumor further indicates the importance of total mesorectal excision in rectal cancer surgery.[15,30]

In colonic cancer, clinically relevant local recurrences have been considered to be less common than in rectal cancer. There is evidence, however, that the true incidence of local recurrence after surgery for colonic cancer, especially in the retroperitoneal ascending and descending colon, is as high as in rectal cancer.[31,32] Such recurrences may not be clinically symptomatic, and their presence may be overshadowed by distant metastases.

In summary, while there is evidence, particularly for rectal cancer, that adequate local surgery through good technique can reduce local recurrence rates to a low level, globally the incidence of local failure is around 20 to 30%.

RESECTABLE RECTAL CANCER

Adjuvant Radiotherapy in Combination With Curative Surgery

Radiotherapy is suitable for patients with rectal cancer, since it can be delivered to a defined tissue volume with negligible damage to surrounding structures, particularly the small bowel.

With colonic cancer, however, it is more difficult to avoid irradiating surrounding vital and radiosensitive organs. The dose that can be given with sufficient safety is then mainly limited by small bowel tissue tolerance.

The possibility of achieving local tumor control and long-term survival by salvage surgery for local recurrence is less than 5% in most cases.[33,34] Such studies also show that other treatment modalities, for example radiotherapy and chemotherapy, have a very low chance of cure. The emphasis should therefore be on prevention. Unacceptably high local failure rates after standardized surgery for rectal cancer, together with the high morbidity associated with most local failures, indicate a need for either improvement in surgical technique or for additional treatment, or both.

The rationale for adjuvant radiotherapy is that the scope of surgery is limited by anatomic considerations, whereas radiotherapy rarely fails at the periphery of the tumor, where the number of tumor cells is limited and the area is well vascularized, giving good oxygenation to the cells. The radiation doses that can safely be given to the extrarectal tissues not able to be removed by surgery but at risk of harboring tumor deposits are sufficient to kill microscopic foci of tumor cells and are well tolerated.

Selection of Patients

Radiotherapy has an objective biologic effect on rectal carcinoma. It can cause the tumor to shrink and may sterilize involved lymph nodes.

It is important to determine resectability preoperatively rather than to discover during surgery that the tumor is too extensive to be excised with adequate margins. This can sometimes be difficult to assess, but if doubt exists regarding operability, an examination under anesthesia can help to judge the fixity of the tumor. Imaging, including computed tomography, magnetic resonance and ultrasonography, may also facilitate assessment, but these techniques are not always accurate, they are costly, and they may not always be conclusive. Clinical judgment has been considered the most important means of evaluation, but with further development of imaging the situation is changing.[22] Digital examination is still an essential part of assessment.

If a tumor is considered resectable, radiotherapy used preoperatively is aimed at eradicating presumed microscopic nests of tumor cells not removed by surgery (Figs. 24-2 to 24-5). It can do so without major risk of complications or poor function postoperatively. On the other hand, in the case of a fixed tumor, considered to be either inoperable or of dubious operability, the aim of radiotherapy is to achieve shrinkage of the tumor with consequent down-staging to render the growth operable by curative intent after a delay of a few weeks. In this situation the treatment is aimed at macroscopic disease, in contrast to adjuvant therapy for a resectable tumor, in which eradication of microscopic disease is the intention.

Technical Considerations

Dose

In adenocarcinoma such as rectal cancer, radiation has the ability to sterilize colonogenic tumor cells. Whether it will succeed is mainly dependent on the number of tumor cells to be killed

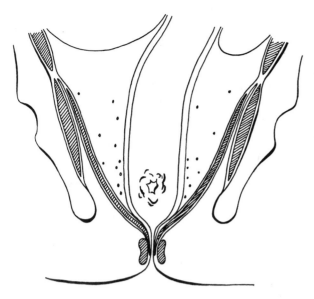

Figure 24-2. Rectal cancer with micrometastases.

and the radiosensitivity of the surrounding tissues. Despite the presence of relatively radioresistant normal tissue surrounding the rectum, radiation has a low probability of eradicating macroscopic deposits of more than 1 cm in diameter (or about 10^9 cells). The radiation dose required to achieve this would be

Figure 24-3. Rectal cancer after irradiation. Micrometastases are eradicated, but the primary tumor is still viable.

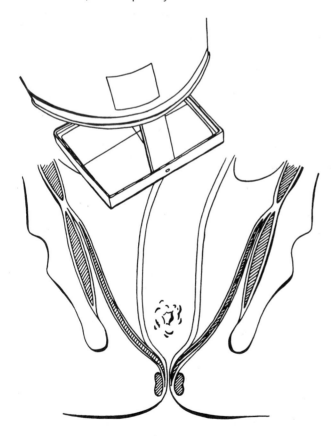

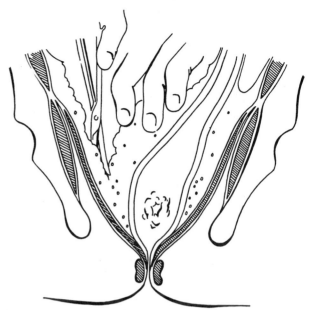

Figure 24-4. Surgery alone. The primary tumor is excised, but micrometastases are left along the pelvic wall.

around 60 to 70 Gy given over 6 to 7 weeks or a comparable dose with other fractionation schedules. By contrast, the minimum dose required to kill micrometastases (defined as being less than a few millimeters in diameter, at most 10^8 cells) is around 50 Gy given over 5 weeks. Although this information has mainly been obtained from studies on breast and head and neck cancer, it is likely to be valuable as a general guide in large bowel cancer.[35–38]

Data comparing pre- with postoperative radiography indicate that a higher dose (60 to 70 Gy) is required postoperatively to achieve similar effects on micrometastases.[37,39] Repopulation

Figure 24-5. Surgery after preoperative radiotherapy. The primary tumor is excised, and no micrometastases are left behind.

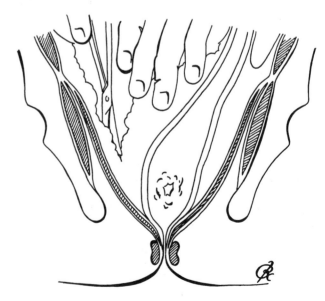

of cells in the time interval between surgery and the start of radiotherapy is probably the most important explanation for this finding,[38] but local hypoxia of tumor cells in the surgical bed is another likely factor contributing to the higher radioresistance occurring postoperatively.[40]

The effects of radiation on tissue are not only dependent on the total dose but also on factors such as the dose of each fraction and the overall treatment time. Since these three parameters have varied between trials and even occasionally within a single trial, it is often difficult to compare the results of different trials. Most authors give the dose simply in terms of rad or Gy, but a more useful way of comparing different regimens would be to estimate the biologic effect of the irradiation or to apply some of the other methods used to calculate the relative effectiveness of radiotherapy schedules. In this chapter, we have used both the linear-quadratic (LQ) formula with a time correction factor for immediate effects[41] and one of the older concepts, the cumulative radiation effect (CRE),[42] with corrections for late effects as described by Turesson.[43] In the LQ-time estimations, the common LQ quotient α/β was chosen as being 10 Gy for tumor and immediate effects and 3 Gy for late effects, the repair ratio α/β as being 0.6 Gy/day, and the initial delay time T_K as being 7 days.[41] The estimations are given in Table 24-2.

A dose fraction of 1.8 or 2 Gy given daily 5 days a week (8 to 10 Gy/week) is a regimen that has been arrived at empirically, but it is practical and at present appears to give the highest therapeutic ratio in the treatment of most malignant tumors. To achieve a dose of 50 Gy (i.e., the minimum dose required to kill micrometastases with high probability), the patient has to be treated for 5 weeks. To reduce the treatment time, the dose at each fraction has been increased to 5 Gy in several preoperative trials. According to the CRE concept and the LQ formula, 5 Gy/day for 5 days to a total dose of 25 Gy corresponds approximately to the biologic effect achieved when conventional irradiation (2 Gy fraction) in a dose of 40 to 50 Gy is given. If a high dose is delivered at each session, the duration of treatment will be shorter. This may have practical advantages, but the therapeutic ratio will probably be decreased. This decrease is

Table 24-2. Hypothetical Probability of Killing Micrometastases Using Different Dose Fractionation Schedules

Probability[a]	Total Dose (Gy)		LQ time[c]	CRE Value[c]
	2 Gy Fraction[b]	5 Gy Fraction[b]		
10	30	10	25–30	11–12
30		15	30–33	12–13
50	40	20	34–36	13–14
70		25	37–40	14–15
90	50		41–45	15–16

[a] Approximate figures owing to major uncertainties. All values refer to treatment in a surgically undisturbed area.

[b] All estimations are based on one fraction a day, 5 days a week, no split.

[c] Linear quadratic (LQ) and cumulative radiation effect (CRE) coefficients.

of major importance if the total dose is close to normal tissue tolerance but may be acceptable as a practical compromise if the dose is lower or if the only aim is to kill microscopic tumor cell deposits.

By using modern high-voltage radiotherapy equipment in combination with appropriate dose planning, it is possible to deliver doses of up to 60 to 70 Gy in 6 to 8 weeks to limited volumes of the abdomen. If the irradiated volume has to be larger because of the size of the tumor, the upper dose limit is lower, being of the order 45 to 55 Gy in 4 to 6 weeks.[44] This means that the likelihood of eradicating subclinical disease in surgically undisturbed areas can be high, whereas the likelihood of curing anything other than small clinical cancers in the abdomen is considerably lower.[37]

Target Volume

By definition, the clinical target volume in radiotherapy is the volume at risk of containing tumor cells.[45] The areas of failure after rectal cancer surgery often lie posteriorly to the bladder, prostate or vagina.[6,46–49] In addition, the lateral lymph nodes close to the pelvic wall, which are not always excised during surgery, as well as the lymph nodes along the internal iliac artery, are common areas of recurrences. Therefore, the entire dorsal part of the pelvic cavity should be included in the target volume when radiotherapy is carried out as an adjuvant to surgery. The posterior region of the prostate or the posterior of the vaginal wall and the posterior part of the urinary bladder constitute the anterior delineation of the target volume. Dorsally, the target must include the anterior part of the sacrum, and laterally the margins should extend to the bony pelvis.

An important but more difficult question is the extent of the target volume cranially and caudally. The justification of trying to eradicate tumor cells situated in the lymph nodes along the proximal part of the inferior mesenteric artery can be questioned. In cases with detectable tumor deposits in these areas, the chance of cure is almost nil or less than 2%.[50–53] In most patients tumor cells within pelvic nodes indicate disseminated disease. The purpose of irradiating lymph nodes above the pelvis is not to prevent local failure, but to improve survival. Such lymph nodes have been included in the field in several trials (see below). From these studies, we have learned that much of the morbidity associated with the additional radiotherapy can be ascribed to irradiation of tissues above the pelvic cavity.[46,54]

With regard to caudal extent, the question is raised of whether the anal sphincter region should be included or not. It is obvious that if the tumor is growing very low in close vicinity to the anal canal, the sphincter should be included. However, if an anterior resection is planned, it might be advisable in the case of preoperative radiotherapy not to include the sphincters in the field. Although no firm data are available in the literature, sphincter function can be damaged by radiation therapy, and if the surgeon is convinced that a sphincter-saving procedure can be undertaken without jeopardizing the outcome, the sphincters should not be irradiated.[55,56] Moreover, we know that rectal cancer rarely has intramural distal spread of more than a few millimeters.[51,57–59] Lymph node metastases and tumor nests in the mesorectum can, however, be identified at a distance more than 2 cm distal to the lower tumor margin.[15,30] This indicates that the lower border of the target should include the mesorectum, which would be at a level of about 4 cm from the anal verge.

Ideally, all volumes at risk of containing tumor cells should be included in the irradiated field, and all volumes not at risk should be excluded. Even in low rectal tumors, extension into the lower part of the anal canal is rarely seen, although superficial perineal recurrences may occur. With such a tumor it is probably advisable to include the anal canal in the target volume, whereas in tumors lying at more than 4 to 6 cm from the anorectal junction, this is probably unnecessary.

Timing

Besides the question of whether or not adjuvant radiotherapy should be offered routinely to patients with rectal cancer, the timing in relation to surgery is the second main concern. As seen in Table 24-3, there are advantages and disadvantages to pre- and postoperative treatment. The sandwich technique was offered as a compromise; patients received a low dose preoperatively and only those subsequently shown on histopathologic examination to have advanced disease (Dukes stage B or C) received further radiotherapy postoperatively. The rationale of this treatment is disputable, however, since the dose used preoperatively, 5 to 15 Gy, is not high enough to have any major impact on cancer cell sterilization.[60–62] Moreover, the dose given preoperatively actually limits the possibility of giving an appropriate postoperative dose according to the guidelines regarding dose and effects on subclinical disease.[37] The remaining two options are therefore either preoperative or postoperative irradiation.

Effect on Local Recurrence

It is important to remember that a dose corresponding to a CRE value of about 14.5 (LQ time$_{acute}$ about 40 Gy with the assumptions given above) is required to give a high probability of killing micrometastases. With these figures in mind, no major effect on local recurrence rates should be expected in trials in which considerably lower doses (CRE less than 11, LQ time less than 25) have been used. This has been the case in several of the early trials of preoperative radiotherapy.[63–66] Furthermore, these trials were carried out in an era in which the important end point of local recurrence was not considered in the protocol.

Table 24-3. Advantages and Disadvantages of Pre- and Postoperative Radiotherapy

Parameter	Preoperative Irradiation	Postoperative Irradiation
Compliance (%)	100	85
Tolerance to treatment	Good	Less good
Negative effect on surgery	Yes	No
Acute adverse effects	Similar	
Late adverse effects (%)	10	20
Effect on local recurrence rate	High	? Moderate
Effect on survival	Slight	None
Pathologic stage known before treatment	No	Yes

With higher doses corresponding approximately to a CRE of 11 to 14 or an LQ time of 25 to 40, a local recurrence rate of less than 10% has been reported in several uncontrolled trials using preoperative[67–73] or postoperative irradiation.[74–79] For details, see Table 24-4, where the studies are compiled according to the dose as evaluated by the LQ formula, and the CRE value is also given.

Pre- Versus Postoperative Radiotherapy

In Table 24-1 all controlled trials reported hitherto using pre- or postoperative radiotherapy are summarized. As in Table 24-4, the trials are compiled with regard to the LQ formula. There is clearly a dose-response relationship concerning reduction in local recurrence rates. It is also clear that this effect at any given dose was higher when irradiation was given before surgery.

In the European Organization for Research and Treatment in Cancer (EORTC) trial, which used preoperative irradiation to a moderate dose (34.5 Gy in 3 weeks, CRE 13.0, LQ time 35.2), a significant reduction in local recurrence rate was found.[80] A substantial although not statistically significant decrease in the local recurrence rate was also achieved in a Norwegian study in which 31.5 Gy was given in 3.5 weeks (CRE 11.1, LQ time 26.8) preoperatively.[81] Conventionally fractionated radiotherapy was used in these studies (i.e., a daily dose of about 2 Gy [1.8 to 2.3]). In four other trials, 5-Gy fractions were given 3 to 5 times a week.[82–85] Here a dose-response relationship was observed. The trial using 3 × 5 Gy carried out by the Imperial Cancer Research Fund[82] showed an effect on local recurrence rate but not of the same magnitude as trials using 4 × 5 Gy[83] or 5 × 5 Gy.[84,85] In the largest of these, the Swedish Rectal Cancer Trial, reduction in local recurrence rate was 63%.[85]

Radiotherapy given postoperatively has had less effect on local recurrence than preoperative irradiation (Table 24-4). It appears from the data in Table 24-4 that postoperative doses of about 15 to 20 Gy higher than preoperative are required to reach the same reduction in the local failure rate. With such high doses there is a substantially increased risk of damaging normal tissues, particularly the small bowel. In the Danish trial, in which postoperative radiotherapy to a dose of 50 Gy (CRE 14.9, LQ time 35.4) was delivered in 7 weeks and compared with surgery alone, no significant reduction in the local recurrence rate was found.[86] A slight but not statistically significant reduction in this rate was observed in the study by the Gastrointestinal Tumor Study Group (GITSG), in which 40 to 48 Gy in 4 to 5 weeks was given postoperatively.[87] In this trial radiotherapy was more effective when it was combined with chemotherapy (see below). A similarly modest reduction in local recurrence rate was found in the National Surgical Adjuvant Bowel Project (NSABP), whereas a greater reduction was observed in the third trial of the British Medical Research Council (MRC), in which 40 Gy was given in 4 weeks (MRC Trial Office, personal communication). In the Dutch trial, which used 50 Gy in 25 fractions, a tendency toward a reduced local recurrence rate was found in the irradiated group.[89]

In only one trial, the Uppsala (Sweden) trial, was preoperative and postoperative radiotherapy compared in a randomized manner.[44,71,9] Patients in the preoperative group received 25.5 Gy in five fractions of 5.1 Gy daily over 5 to 7 days (CRE 14.0, LQ time 38.0). Surgery was performed in the following

Table 24-4. Pelvic Recurrence After Surgery and Intermediate to High Dose Radiotherapy for Rectal Carcinoma (Uncontrolled Trials, Major Series Only)

Study	Dose (Gy)	CBE Value	LQ Time	No. of Patients	Local recurrences No.	Local recurrences %
Preoperative						
Friedman et al., 1985[67]	40–45	13.5–14.5	36.0–39.3	36	2	6
Mohuiddin and Marks, 1987[70]	40–45	13.5–14.5	36.0–39.3	43	6	14
Glimelius et al., 1982[68]	25.5	15.4	38.0	41	3	7
Påhlman and Glimelius, 1990[71,a]	25.5	15.4	38.0	209	26	12
Mendenhall et al., 1985[70]	35–50	12.5–15.5	38.0–39.3	64	5	8
Stevens et al., 1978[73]	50–60	15.0–17.5	43.8–47.4	45	1	2
Postoperative						
Romsdahl and Withers, 1978[75]	45	14.5	39.3	62	5	8
Tepper et al., 1987[76]	45–51	14.5–15.5	39.3–40.8	152	29	19
Påhlman and Glimelius, 1990[a 71]	60	17.0	47.4	204	43	21
Sandwich						
Mohuiddin et al., 1982[61]	5 + 45	—[b]	—[b]	31	2	7
Gunderson et al., 1983[60]	10 + 45–50	—[b]	—[b]	32	2	6
Shank et al., 1987[62]	15 + 41	—[b]	—[b]	47	1	2

[a] These two regimens were randomly compared with each other, but not with surgery alone.
[b] Could not be calculated appropriately because of the long delay between the two courses.

week. Among the patients allocated to the postoperative irradiation group, only patients with a Dukes B or C stage tumor received the radiotherapy. This trial used the highest dose ever in a postoperative setting. The postoperative treatment was planned to start within 6 weeks of surgery. Irradiation was given with 2 Gy fractions daily for 5 days a week over 4 weeks. After an interval of 10 to 14 days, further irradiation was given for a period of 2 weeks, up to a total dose of 60 Gy (CRE 16.9, LQ time 46.9). After a minimum of 5 years' follow-up, a statistically significantly reduced local recurrence rate was found in the preoperatively irradiated group (12%) compared with the postoperative group (21%) (P <0.02).[90]

As might be expected, the effect of radiotherapy on local recurrence is dose dependent. Preoperative irradiation is more dose effective than postoperative radiation. There are two possible explanations for this. First, cancer cells remaining after surgery will grow and become more numerous than the population outside the zone of removal before surgery, and second, cells in the infiltrating zones may be less well oxygenated than before surgery. If the preoperative dose is sufficiently high (i.e., corresponding to 40 to 50 Gy in 4.4 to 5 weeks), a decrease in the local recurrence rate by approximately 65% is to be expected.

Survival

Like surgery, radiotherapy to the primary tumor cannot affect occult metastases in distant organs such as liver and lung. However, if local recurrence is prevented and if it would have been the only form of treatment failure, radiotherapy should theoretically have an impact on survival. In a meta-analysis of adjuvant radiotherapy including all controlled trials published up to 1984, a slightly higher survival of 4.3% was noted in irradiated patients.[92] The authors concluded that the trials were too small to detect a statistically significant survival benefit, which probably existed. A new meta-analysis is in progress in which the more recently published trials using moderate to high doses are being included. These comprise the North-West trial in England,[83,92] the trial from the Imperial Cancer Research Fund in England,[82] and the Swedish Rectal Cancer Trial.[85] A subset analysis with respect to dose level will be performed, and the results are awaited (Gray et al., 1995, personal communication).

Table 24-5 shows survival data from the most recent trials with moderate to high doses. In the EORTC trial, the survival curves are diverging as the period of follow-up lengthens, but no statistically significant results have been obtained.[80] Similarly,

Table 24-5. Survival in Relation to Percentage Reduction in Local Recurrences Rates (Only High-Dose Controlled Trials Presented)

Trial	Dose (Gy)/LQ Time (No. of Fractions)	% Reduction in Local Recurrence	Improved Survival With Irradiation Overall	Improved Survival With Irradiation Cancer-specific
Goldberg et al., 1994[82]	15/3 (22.5)	29	No	Tendency
Marsh et al., 1994[90]	20/4 (30.0)	63	Tendency	Yes
Gérard et al., 1988[82]	46/23 (35.2)	50	No	Yes
Cedermark et al., 1995[93]	25/5 (37.5)	50	No	Yes
SRCT, 1995[85]	25/5 (37.5)	65	Yes	Yes

when the survival curves were corrected for postoperative deaths in the Stockholm/Malmö trial (see below), survival was increased in the group of patients who received preoperative radiotherapy.[85] In a recent report from the Stockholm group, an improvement in cancer-specific survival was noted in the so-called Stockholm II trial.[93] Patients randomized in this trial between 1987 and February 1990 are part of the Swedish Rectal Cancer Trial; subsequently the Stockholm II trial continued recruiting patients up to 1993. Superior cancer-specific survival was also noted in the combined treatment group in the North-West trial and in the Imperial Cancer Research Trial.[82,92]

In the Swedish Rectal Cancer Trial, patients were randomly allocated to receive 5×5 Gy preperatively in 1 week followed by surgery in the following week, or to undergo surgery alone. A total of 1,168 patients was included between 1987 and 1990. Survival data after a minimum of 5 years' follow-up have shown an increase in overall survival by 25% to 30% in the irradiated group (Swedish Rectal Cancer Trial).[93a]

In two early controlled trials with a low dose, an increase in the 5-year survival rate was observed after preoperative radiotherapy. In one of these trials, in which 20 Gy was given in 2 weeks (CRE 8.7, LQ time 20.4) the survival rate was increased from 31.5% to 39%, but this difference was only observed after abdominoperineal excision.[66] In the other trial, in which 5 Gy was given preoperatively on the day of surgery (CRE 5.0), a significantly increased 5-year survival rate was found among patients with Dukes C lesions; the number of patients was small, however, precluding any firm conclusions.[65] In the first MRC trial in England, these two regimens, one with a single dose of 5 Gy in 1 day just prior to surgery and the other with a total of 20 Gy in 2 weeks, were tested in a large number of patients against no radiotherapy.[63] Neither regimen had any impact on survival compared with the surgery-only arm. In the trials in which postoperative radiotherapy alone has been used, no effect on survival has been demonstrated.[86,81]

In the only trial in which preoperative has been tested against postoperative radiotherapy (the Uppsala trial), no survival difference between the two treatment groups was found.[71]

Combined Chemotherapy and Radiotherapy

Combinations of radiotherapy and chemotherapy should theoretically improve cancer-specific end points since the cell kill mechanisms differ between the two techniques, and synergistic effects may occur. The two treatments have different aims: chemotherapy against systemic disease, and radiotherapy to achieve local tumor control. It is also possible, however, that combined treatment might have an improved effect on local disease. The rationale of combining these two methods is to achieve therapeutic gain by increasing the effect on the tumor without simultaneously excerbating normal tissue reactions.[95,96] The knowledge of how to combine these two regimens in a preoperative setting is limited at present. The reason for caution against the use of modalities used simultaneously is the risk of more severe adverse effects. Combined adjuvant treatment given postoperatively was found in a Dutch trial to increase complications.[96] A Danish trial, although initiated with the aim of treating fixed (nonresectable) tumors, had to be closed because of adverse effects in the combined treatment arm.[99]

The effects on local recurrence rates appear to be slightly

Table 24-6. Pelvic Recurrence and Overall Survival After Surgery With or Without Postoperative Radiotherapy or Chemotherapy

Trial	Additional Treatment	No. of Local Recurrences Total (%)	5-Year Survival (%)	P Value
GITSG, 1985[87]	None	14/58 (24)	43	
	Chemo.	13/48 (27)	56	NS
	Irrad.	10/50 (20)	52	NS
	Chemo. + irrad.	5/46 (11)	59	
Fisher et al., 1988[88]	None	45/184 (24)	43	
	Irrad.	30/184 (16)	41	NS
	Chemo.	46/187 (25)	53	
Krook et al., 1991[98]	Irrad.	25/100 (25)	47	
	Chemo. + irrad.	14/104 (14)	58	

Abbreviation: GITSG, Gastrointestinal Tumor Study Group.

improved when chemotherapy is combined with postoperative radiotherapy, indicating that the former might have a potentiating or at least an additive effect on the latter (Table 24-5). In a Norwegian trial in which 46 Gy (CRE 14.9, LQ time 39.3) with 5-fluorouracil (5-FU) was compared with surgery alone, a reduction in the local recurrence rates by approximately 50% was found (i.e., a greater effect than would have been seen with radiotherapy alone) (Tveit et al.: personal communication).

In the GITSG trial, survival was improved in the group of patients that received both radiotherapy and chemotherapy, although the numbers in the treatment arms were small.[87] In a second American trial (NSABP), postoperative radiotherapy combined with chemotherapy gave a survival benefit compared with surgery alone.[90] In another randomized trial, the North Central Cancer Treatment Group (NCCTG), postoperative radiotherapy alone was compared with postoperative radiotherapy plus chemotherapy; improved survival was noted in the radiochemotherapy arm.[98] The drugs used in these three trials were 5-FU and methyl-CCNU (Table 24-6).

On the basis of these findings, the consensus conference sponsored by the National Institutes of Health in the United States recommended that all patients with a tumor of Dukes stage B or C should receive postoperative adjuvant radiotherapy (45 to 50 Gy in 4 to 6 weeks) together with chemotherapy (5-FU and methyl-CCNU).[99] This created a somewhat dogmatic framework, which was likely to inhibit rather than enhance progress. Thus in two subsequent trials in the United States, it was shown that the addition of methyl-CCNU to 5-FU was not required.[100,102] It was also found that continuous infusion of 5-FU rather than bolus 5-FU during the radiotherapy was more effective.[103] In contrast to the general opinion held in the United States, expressed by the NIH consensus statement in 1990 and the NCI clinical announcement,[99] no strong evidence shows that the improvement in survival is due to the combined treatment. It is possible, rather, that the survival benefit might be due solely to the chemotherapy, since patients allocated to the radiochemotherapy arm continued chemotherapy for 1 year in some trials.

The improvements in survival observed in the Swedish Rectal Cancer Trial are of the same magnitude as those reported from the American postoperative combined radio-chemotherapy trials. Since preoperative radiotherapy is more dose effective than postoperative, it seems logical to give preoperative radiotherapy and to add chemotherapy postoperatively in those patients with more advanced cancer (i.e., tumors of Dukes stages B and C). The main concern will then be the risk of overtreatment, which has been stated as an objection to this strategy. This is most obvious in patients with a Dukes stage A tumor, but it is also relevant in patients with disseminated disease found at surgery. It is here that improvements in preoperative staging will make a useful contribution. Expert clinical assessment of local disease with imaging (including endoluminal ultrasound, computed tomography, and magnetic resonance) will minimize this source of error.[22] With preoperative endoluminal ultrasound of the rectum it is possible to identify tumor penetration of the rectal wall in 95% of cases.[102–104]

Mortality

Adverse effects after radiotherapy are dependent on the total dose, the treatment time, and the irradiated volume. The irradiated volume is the volume of tissue that receives 95% or more of the prescribed dose. Ideally this should be the same or only marginally larger than the target volume (i.e., the volume of tissue at risk of containing tumor cells). In the Uppsala trial, in which the technique was designed to avoid irradiation of those parts of the pelvis and abdomen outside the target volume, no influence on postoperative mortality was noted, even though no upper age limit was used. Thus it is clear that preoperative radiotherapy in high doses (25.5 Gy in 1 week, giving a CRE of 14.5 and an LQ time of 38) can be delivered without affecting surgical mortality.[71] By contrast, however, in the parallel Stockholm-Malmö trial, postoperative mortality was significantly increased (2 versus 8% $P <0.001$) in the irradiated group, even though the doses used were similar to those in the Uppsala trial, (5 × 5 Gy for 1 week with surgery in the subsequent week.[93,10] In the Stockholm-Malmö trial, the patients were treated with one dorsal and one frontal portal, with the upper limit of the field placed at the level of the mid-second lumbar vertebra. Large volumes of the abdomen were thus unnecessarily irradiated, and it may be that such differences in field between the two trials were responsible for the differences in postoperative mortality.[46]

In the Stockholm-Malmö trial, mortality was predominantly found among the elderly and those with generalized disease. Another trial, also using a two-portal technique, similarly found an increased postoperative mortality rate among patients over 75 years of age and those with disseminated disease discovered at surgery.[85]

One deliberate end point of the Swedish Rectal Cancer Trial (5 × 5 Gy in 1 week) was to evaluate the question of postoperative mortality given the conflicting results from the Uppsala and Stockholm-Malmö trials. The protocol included the use of three or four portals, but for unexplained reasons four hospitals used the two-portal technique. In those centers mortality was significantly higher than in the others treated according to proto-

col.[106] In these the mortality was the same in each arm, surgery only versus surgery with radiotherapy (2.6% versus 2.6%). The results from this trial support the conclusion that a two-portal technique, a large treatment volume, and a high radiation dose before surgery may be too much of a burden for an elderly patient. Futhermore, the results show that radiotherapy, once decided on, should be properly planned and meticulously monitored during the treatment course.

Morbidity

In most early trials in which preoperative radiotherapy was used, breakdown of the perineal wound after abdominoperineal excision occurred in almost 20%. After surgery alone this figure is approximately 10%.[71,93,106] Perineal wound disruption is not a disaster for the patient, and the wound will usually heal within 1 or 2 months.[71] The rare complication of perineal sinus is no more common after radiotherapy.[44] No increase in abdominal wound infections has been seen in controlled trials after preoperative irradiation.

Another concern has been the safety of the anastomoses in irradiated tissues. In all controlled randomized trials, no increase in anastomotic dehiscence has been found after preoperative radiotherapy.[80,82,93,101,107] Moreover, experimental data indicate that preoperative irradiation does not affect anastomotic healing adversely.[108–110]

In one trial using 5-Gy fractions preoperatively (the Uppsala trial), acute neurogenic pain a few hours after irradiation of the lower lumbar region was reported.[71] This was usually of short duration, but it persisted for several months in a few patients. Occasionally acute neurogenic symptoms resulted in an inability to walk. In a review of the total experience in Uppsala from 1980 to 1994, it was found that of 550 patients treated with 5 × 5 Gy within prospective protocols, 19 (3%), reported pain. In six (1%) patients the pain lasted for more than a few days, and in four of these subacute neurogenic symptoms developed. An extensive enquiry did not reveal any technical or human error in treatment.

The origin of this acute, potentially dangerous adverse effect is unknown. The pain is more common in women than in men and also in obese patients and those with diabetes or a previous neurologic disorder. It may represent an extreme sensitivity to high radiation doses in a susceptible patient. A technique of avoiding hot spots in the region of the lower lumbar nerves is essential. Furthermore, this complication, although very rare, indicates that the target volume should not be unnecessarily large. For prevention of local failure it is not necessary to irradiate volumes above the sacral promontory.

Late Effects

Several references have been made to delayed intestinal obstruction after postoperative radiotherapy.[54,86,111] Chronic diarrhea is another late complication. Both occur when small bowel is included in the treatment volume. When postoperative radiotherapy is to be given, surgical techniques have been described to prevent the small bowel from falling into the pelvis, which would expose it to increased risk of damage from the radiotherapy.[113–115] The most common method is the use of a mesh or an omental flap.[115–119] If radiotherapy extends high up in the abdomen, the risk of small bowel obstruction is 30 to 40%, compared with 5 to 10% when only the dorsal part of the pelvic cavity is included.[55]

In the Uppsala trial all patients have been followed up extensively and re-examined with respect to late adverse effects of irradiation. The patients who received preoperative radiotherapy have not differed with respect to bowel obstruction or other possible late adverse effects from those having surgery alone. The number of patients at risk after 10 years of follow-up, however, was rather limited. In the group of patients given postoperative radiotherapy, a significantly higher incidence of late irradiation-related adverse effects was found despite the use of a technique that was intended to avoid irradiation to large volumes of small bowel.[44]

Another concern after adjuvant radiotherapy is sphincter function. There is very little information on this matter, but some indications show that postoperative radiotherapy will impair this function.[56] Almost no data are available regarding preoperative radiotherapy, but in a small study in the Uppsala area, patients irradiated preoperatively were followed up after anterior resection with a questionnaire regarding bowel function. There was some evidence that preoperative radiotherapy might have altered sphincter function.[55] The reasons for this are unclear, but irradiation might damage either the sphincters or the pudendal nerves.

Tolerance to Treatment

The acute adverse effects of pre- and postoperative radiotherapy have been studied prospectively in the Uppsala trial in which the preoperative treatment was well tolerated and only one patient allocated to preoperative irradiation did not receive treatment.[107] By contrast, postoperative irradiation was completed without any complication in only 9% of patients. In seven, the treatment was discontinued because of fatigue and infectious complications. Diarrhea, skin reactions, and urinary disorders occurred frequently during the treatment period. Most patients were managed as outpatients, but five had to be hospitalized for parenteral nutrition owing to diarrhea. According to the protocol, the prescribed treatment period, including the split, should have comprised 52 days (28 days plus 8 to 10 days split), but only 49% of the patients completed the postoperative irradiation within this period.

Similar difficulties were reported from the Danish trial using postoperative radiotherapy.[86] Only 85% of the patients who started the postoperative irradiation completed the treatment, even though a split was introduced to diminish the subjective toxicity. A split increases the compliance, but, as discussed above, it also diminishes the tumor cell kill effect and should be avoided whenever possible.

The adverse effects associated with postoperative chemoradiotherapy are often more pronounced. In all such trials an increase in dermatitis in the irradiated area has been observed, and several patients have had diarrhea. Chemotherapy-dependent side effects such as leukopenia occur in approximately 10% of patients.[87,88,120] If methyl-CCNU is used, an increased risk of secondary leukemia exists.[123]

Summary

It is clear from the collected international experience that if adjuvant radiotherapy is to be used, preoperative rather than postoperative treatment is to be preferred, since it is more dose effective. It is also clear that the field should be focused on the tissue at risk of containing tumor cells and that the dose should be sufficiently high.

The main objection to the preoperative approach is a concern for irradiating patients with Dukes stage A lesions, as well as patients with metastatic disease. With endoluminal ultrasonography, a Dukes A lesion can usually be identified.[102–104] It is possible to identify preoperatively most patients with generalized disease by computed tomography of the liver and lung, ultrasonography of the liver, and chest X-ray examination. It is established that patients with low rectal tumors have a higher risk of having local recurrence than those with tumors in the upper rectum. We therefore recommend that preoperative radiotherapy be given in all cases in which it is clear that the treatment of choice is an abdominoperineal excision. This is especially true for males, in whom the operation may be difficult, especially when the tumor is anterior.

In conclusion, preoperative radiotherapy has been convincingly shown to reduce local treatment failure by more than 50% when given in combination with standard surgery. Although not formally tested by a prospective randomized trial, much evidence indicates that this reduction must be at least of the same magnitude even if the surgery is performed at the most expert level possible. Since such so-called expert surgery results in fewer recurrences compared with standard surgery, the absolute number of patients who benefit will be reduced. This implies that radiotherapy has to be very safe. Large irradiated volumes and inappropriate radiation techniques have resulted in severe complications, but trials using appropriate techniques have convincingly shown that the treatment can be given safely.

Since postoperative radiotherapy is less effective, has more adverse effects, and is more resource demanding than preoperative schedules, it is difficult to understand why postoperative radiotherapy continues to be recommended. The most logical approach must be to use an appropriate surgical procedure with the most optimal radiotherapy. This should now include high-dose preoperative irradiation, with good surgery. Incorporating the possibility of adjuvant chemotherapy, the possibility exists that local treatment failure might be effectively eradicated (Table 24-7).

Other important aspects of adjuvant radiotherapy are compliance and economic considerations. In the Uppsala trial, all but one patient in the preoperatively treated group received the prescribed treatment, compared with only 85% in the postoperative group.[90] If the treatment is recommended, the compliance needs to be high. In this respect, the collected experience again indicates that preoperative treatment is to be preferred. The economic aspects can be summarized in practice by the number of treatments given. The short preoperative schedules that have proved to be effective and safe (provided the techniques are appropriate) must be more cost effective than postoperative courses, which at least so far have only been evaluated using conventional fractionation. In the long term, if all eligible patients are to be irradiated, this will have a substantial impact on the resources. Different aspects of the pros and cons of the

Table 24-7. Local Failure Rates After Rectal Cancer Surgery With and Without Preoperative Radiotherapy

	Additional Treatment	
	None (%)	Preoperative High-Dose Radiotherapy (%)
International standards[a]	24–41	9–18
Superspecialist[b]	5–6	0–2
Improved standards[c]	5–10	0–4

[a] The figures are a summary of all randomized trials using doses higher than those corresponding to an LQ time above 30.0.
[b] The figures are a summary of data presented by Heald and Ryall[28] and Enker et al.,[17] with estimated effects if preoperative radiotherapy had been used.
[c] The present authors' interpretation of current experience and clinical knowledge based on data from the Swedish Rectal Cancer Trial with figures from "excellent" centers.

two treatment options (pre- and postoperative radiotherapy) should be carefully weighed when the choice of treatment is considered (Table 24-7).

RESECTABLE COLONIC CANCER

Adjuvant radiotherapy has been used after curative colonic cancer surgery. The irradiated volume may, however, involve organs such as the kidney, spleen, and small bowel, which usually do not tolerate the high doses necessary for substantial effect on tumor cells. For this reason it has not been generally used and there are therefore few reports in the literature and none from randomized studies. Another reason is that distant metastases usually cause symptoms before local recurrence does. Most reported series have been compared with historic controls, which notoriously give false data.

Radiotherapy might have a rationale where by local recurrence is not uncommon after surgery, for example, in tumors situated in the retroperitoneal part of the colon (i.e., the ascending and descending colon).[31,32] In several studies, patients with tumors of Dukes stage B or C have received postoperative radiotherapy alone or in combination with 5-FU.[122-125] Most have been small, containing around 20 to 50 patients. In the series from Massachusetts General Hospital from 1976 to 1989, radiotherapy was given to patients with Dukes stage B and C tumors, to a total dose of 45 Gy delivered in 1.8 Gy fractions.[124] The findings were compared with those of 395 patients with tumors in the same Dukes stages undergoing surgery alone in 1970 to 1977. Local control and overall survival were significantly better in irradiated patients with tumors that had extensive pericolonic growth. Since, however, there have been no randomized controlled trials, the value of adjuvant radiotherapy in colonic cancer is far from established.

NONRESECTABLE RECTAL CANCER

Ten to 15% of rectal carcinomas are locally nonresectable at presentation, owing to extensive local spread that cannot be removed surgically. In this group 50% have distant metastases

at the time of diagnosis.[126-128] Untreated, this subgroup of patients has a median survival time of 6 to 8 months, often with severe symptoms including pain, hemorrhage, fecal incontinence, and urinary problems. Radiotherapy given as palliation can provide valuable symptomatic relief. It may also result in tumor regression to such an extent that resection becomes possible. The likelihood of this occurring is 40% to 70% A small proportion of the patients may also be cured in the long term.[129]

The judgment as to whether or not the tumor is fixed to another organ is usually made by palpation or by imaging. This assessment is uncertain even in experienced hands, since it is difficult to decide whether there actually is tumor overgrowth or only extensive fibrosis adjacent to the tumor.[22,127] In some studies, nonresectability has been verified by laparotomy before radiotherapy. When the fixation ultimately turns out to be the result of tumor infiltration, radiotherapy is essential. Using magnetic resonance imaging it has been shown in a high proportion of cases that fixation due to tumor or fibrosis can be distinguished.[130]

External Irradiation

In patients with nonresectable tumors there is no justification for giving high-dose short-term irradiation (dose fractions more than 2 Gy), as down-staging is essential and never occurs rapidly. Thus conventional irradiation with 1.8 to 2 Gy fractions is ideal. A prolonged course of preoperative radiotherapy to a dose of 45 to 50 Gy can be delivered without any substantial risk to the patient. The results from the major reported trials are given in Table 24-8. The great discrepancies in resectability rates are probably due to differences in the criteria for nonresectability, in the radiotherapy dose and technique, and in the surgical aggressiveness.[107,129,131-136]

The most commonly used dose has been between 40 and 50 Gy, with surgery usually 3 to 4 weeks later, to allow time for tumor regression. The optimal irradiation dose has not, however, been established. Fortier et al.[128] reported that the local control rate was 67% after 40 Gy and 91% after 50 Gy, but the number of patients was small and the design was not randomized, so no firm conclusions could be drawn. There are some indications that combined chemo- and radiotherapy increases resectability. The use of different cytostatic regimens, particularly those based on 5-FU, concomitantly with irradiation has been claimed to produce greater tumor shrinkage than irradiation alone.[94,95] In a few trials, a combination of radiotherapy and chemotherapy has been tested. The initial results have been promising regarding the effect on local tumor burden,[132,134,135] but morbidity is substantially increased with combined treatment.[132,136-138134,138-140] In two randomized trials such combined treatment was compared with radiotherapy alone, but no positive effects were detected.[97,138] Thus today it may be said that scientific evidence for superiority of the combined approach is virtually lacking. Nevertheless, combined therapy is considered to be the standard at several centers, particularly in the United States.[134,138-142]

Intraoperative Irradiation

In attempts to improve the treatment results even further in patients with nonresectable and residual rectal cancer, intraoperative irradiation with electrons alone or more often in combi-

Table 24-8. Resectability After Preoperative Radiotherapy in Patients With Locally Nonresectable Rectal Cancer (Uncontrolled Trials Only)

Study	Dose (Gy)	CRE Value	LQ Time	Additional Chemotherapy	No. of Patients	Resectable After Irradiation No.	%
Frykholm et al., 1989[132]	40	14.0	36.0	Yes	21	16	76
Bjerkeset and Dahl, 1980[126]	45	14.5	36.9	No	37	16	43
Dosoretz et al., 1989[131]	40–45	14.0–14.5	36.0–39.8	No	25	18	72
Wassif-Boulis, 1983[136]	34.5	13.0	35.2	Yes	25	40	40
Overgaard et al., 1989[87]	23–73	11.0–17.8	24–50	Yes	18	3	17
Påhlman et al., 1985[107]	46–60	14.8–17.6	40.8–47.4	No	44	17	39
Minsky et al., 1992[159]	50.4	15.7	43.8	Yes	20	17	85
Minsky et al., 1993[160]	50.4	15.7	43.8	Yes	12	9	75

nation with external irradiation has been used. The rationale of using intraoperative radiotherapy is the possibility of delivering a high dose to a small tumor-containing volume without damaging surrounding tissues. This technique would seem to be a tempting alternative to irradiation of areas in the pelvis when the surgeon has some doubt about radicality. The experience from this treatment is still limited. Although it has been available at several centers for more than a decade, no firm conclusions can yet be drawn.[141] Since facilities for intraoperative treatment are expensive and the treatment is time-consuming and available in only a few centers, there is an urgent need for randomized trials to compare preoperative external beam therapy with intraoperative radiotherapy in addition to preoperative external radiotherapy.

Summary

A fixed tumor must be regarded as a locally advanced lesion. With this assumption, such patients will run a high risk of local failure even if the tumor can be resected for cure. They will therefore probably benefit from preoperative irradiation. This is definitely true when fixation proves to be the result of tumor infiltration. Here radiotherapy is essential. In this group of patients a prolonged course of preoperative radiotherapy to doses of 45 to 50 Gy or probably a little higher can be delivered without any substantial risk to the patient. The question of whether or not irradiation should be combined with chemotherapy is not yet settled, since no radnomzied trial has shown any advantage for the combined approach. Even though some randomized trials for other gastrointestinal tumors such as gastric pancreatic cancer have shown some advantage by combining radiotherapy and chemotherapy, this approach should still be investigational.[145,146] The appropriateness of intraoperative radiotherapy should also be questioned, in view of the lack of positive results from properly designed clinical trials.

CURATIVE TREATMENT BY RADIOTHERAPY ALONE

External Beam

The classic work of Rider et al.[45] has established the effectiveness of radiotherapy given in moderate to high doses as a primary treatment. In a series of 123 patients without metastases considered inoperable, "radical" radiotherapy of 50 Gy or more without specified fractionation resulted in an overall 5-year survival rate of 21%. There was, however, a considerable difference between patients with tumours that were mobile before treatment (38% survival) and those with fixed tumors (2% survival). Failure to obtain local control was common, occurring in 96 (78%) of cases.[147] In the light of these results it is clear that radiotherapy is less effective as primary treatment than surgery.

Endocavity Irradiation

In very selected early cases, radiotherapy of rectal cancer as the only treatment modality has been used, leading to a high probability of cure. Here the treatment options will lie between local excision and radiotherapy. Surgery has the advantage of producing a specimen for histopathologic examination, although lymph nodes are not excised. Ultrasound imaging has permitted objective assessment of the tumor, facilitating case selection.

Selection of Patients

Curative treatment with radiotherapy alone is possible if the tumor is large (in a small minority of cases; see above). However, primary radiotherapy has mostly been applied to small mobile tumors, especially when the tumor is situated very distally and when an abdominoperineal excision would otherwise be necessary. With digital examination combined with endoluminal ultrasound, it is possible to identify suitable cases. Proposed criteria for local treatment by radiotherapy include a diameter of less than 3 cm, polypoid morphology, mobility, and a low grade of malignancy established on biopsy.

Technique

Endocavity radiotherapy uses low-voltage X-rays (50 kv) applied directly to the surface of the tumor by a probe introduced via a special rectal tube. Papillon[148] showed that a dose of 100 to 150 Gy can safely be given over a 6 to 7-week period. The treatment is delivered in four or five applications. Depending on the effect of the first two, further irradiation may be postponed and surgery proposed. The experience of this type of treatment is limited, since it has been used in only a few centers. The results show that local tumor control can be achieved in over 80% of cases. It is noteworthy that exophytic tumors are significantly more likely to respond than ulcerative tumors, with respective local failure rates of 9.5 and 26%.[149] With more refined patient selection, this can be even higher.[148,150–152]

Whether this treatment should still be recommended in selected cases is not certain. The long-term results are similar to those achieved by local surgical excision and probably less satisfactory than after total rectal excision. In our own hands, only patients with concurrent disease who are unable to undergo an abdominoperineal excision are considered for such local treatment.

RADIOTHERAPY FOR LOCALLY RECURRENT DISEASE

In the early days of megavoltage radiotherapy, series of patients with inoperable cancer or local recurrent cancer treated by radiotherapy were reported. Symptomatic relief of pain and bleeding was achieved in over 50% of patients.[129,135,153–155] This effect might last for a few weeks to months only,[156,157] and a dose-response relationship was shown to exist.[135] However, the median length of survival with a locally not curable rectal cancer, whether primary or recurrent, was 6 to 8 months.[33,34] In most of these reports a small but significant long-term survival of about 5% was seen at 5 years. These results demonstrated that radiotherapy could be curative even in patients with locally advanced tumors.

The question of whether radiotherapy should be combined with chemotherapy, preferably a 5-FU-based treatment, is not yet solved. Several reports using a historic control have indicated a superior result with combined treatment.[132,134,137,138,140] No randomized trial has been performed on recurrent colorectal cancer, but in a controlled trial in gastrointestinal malignancy, radiotherapy alone was tested against radiotherapy and 5-FU. This trial included patients with recurrent colorectal cancer and the combined treatment was superior to controls in terms of symptomatic relief and survival.[145]

REFERENCES

1. Miles WE (1908) A method of performing abdomino-perineal excision for carcinoma of the rectum and the terminal portion of the pelvic colon. Lancet 2:1812–1813
2. Gordon-Watson C (1928) Radiation in the treatment of cancer of the rectum. pp. 100–106. Report of the International Conference on Cancer.
3. Neuman F, Coryn C (1928) Report of the International Conference on Cancer pp. 128–130
4. Quick (1928) The combination of surgery and radiation in the treatment of cancer of the rectum. Report of the International Conference on Cancer, pp. 125–127
5. Berge T, Ekelund G, Mellner C et al (1973) Carcinoma of the colon and rectum in a defined population. Acta Chir Scand Suppl 438:174
6. Gunderson LL, Sosin H (1974) Areas of failure found at reoperation (second or symptomatic look) following "curative surgery" for adenocarcinoma of the rectum. Cancer 34: 1278–1292
7. MacFarlane JK, Ryall RD, Heald RJ (1993) Mesorectal excision for rectal cancer. Lancet 341:457–460
8. McCall JJ, Cox MR, Wattchow DA (1995) Analysis of local recurrence rates after surgery alone for rectal cancer. Int J Color Dis 10:126–132
9. McDermott FT, Hughes ESR, Pihl EA, Milne BJ (1985) Local recurrence after potentially curative resection for rectal cancer in a series of 1008 patients. Br J Surg 72:34–36
10. Morson BC, Bussey HJR (1967) Surgical pathology of rectal cancer in relation to adjuvant radiotherapy. Br J Radiol 40: 161–165
11. Påhlman L, Glimelius B (1984) Local recurrences after surgical treatment for rectal carcinoma. Acta Chir Scand 150: 331–335
12. Pheils MT, Chapuis PH, Newland RC, Colquhoun (1983) Local recurrence following curative resection for carcinoma of the rectum. Dis Colon Rectum 26:98–102
13. Phillips RKS, Hittinger R, Blesovsky L et al (1984) Local recurrence following "curative" surgery for large bowel cancer. I. The overall picture. Br J Surg 71:12–16
14. Williams NS, Johnston D (1984) Survival and recurrence after sphincter saving resection and abdominoperineal resection for carcinoma of the middle third of the rectum. Br J Surg 71:460–462
15. Heald RJ, Husband EM, Ryall RDH (1982) The mesorectum in rectal cancer surgery—the clue to pelvic recurrence? Br J Surg 69:613–616
16. Enker WE, Laffer UT, Block GE (1979) Enhanced survival of patients with colon and rectal cancer is based upon wide anatomic resection. Ann Surg 190:350–360
17. Moriya Y, Hojo K, Sawada T, Koyama Y (1989) Significance of lateral node dissection for advanced rectal carcinoma at or below the peritoneal reflection. Dis Colon Rectum 32: 307–315
18. Hojo K, Sawada T, Moroija Y (1989) An analysis of survival and voiding, sexual function after wide illiopelvic lymphadenectomy in patients with carcinoma of the rectum, compared with conventional lymphadenectomy. Dis Colon Rectum 32:128–133
19. Adloff M, Arnaud JP Schloegel M et al (1985) Factors influencing local recurrence after abdominoperineal resection of cancer of the rectum. Dis Colon Rectum 28:413–417
20. Holm T, Rutqvist L-E, Johansson H, Cedermark B (1995) Abdominoperineal resection and anterior resection in the treatment of rectal cancer: results in relation to adjuvant preoperative radiotherapy. Br J Surg 82:1213–1216
21. Slanetz C, Herter F, Grinnell R (1972) Anterior resection versus abdominoperineal resection for cancer of the rectum and rectosigmoid. Am J Surg 123:110–117
22. Nicholls RJ, York Mason A, Morson BC et al (1982) The clinical staging of rectal cancer. Br J Surg 69:404–409
23. Deddish M, Stern M (1961) Anterior resection for carcinoma of the rectum and rectosigmoid area. Ann Surg 154:961–966
24. Theile DE, Cohen JR, Evans EB et al (1982) Pelvic recurrence

after curative resection for carcinoma of the rectum. Australas NZ J Surg 52:391–394

25. Pilipshen SJ, Heilweil M, Quan SH et al (1984) Patterns of pelvic recurrence following definitive resections of rectal cancer. Cancer 53:1354–1356

26. Anderberg B, Enblad P, Sjödahl R, Wetterfors J (1983) Recurrent rectal carcinoma after anterior resection and rectal stapling. Br J Surg 70:1–4

27. Heald RJ, Ryall RDH (1986) Recurrence and survival after total mesorectal excision for rectal cancer. Lancet June 28: 1479–1482

28. Adam IJ, Mohamdee MO, Martin IG et al (1994) Role of circumferential margin involvement in the local recurrence of rectal cancer. Lancet 344:707–111

29. Quirke P, Durdey P, Dixon MF, Williams NS (1986) Local recurrence of rectal adenocarcinoma due to inadequate surgical resection. Histopathological study of lateral tumour spread and surgical excision. Lancet 2:996–999

30. Scott N, Jackson P, Al-Jaberi T et al (1995) Total mesorectal excision and local recurrence: a study of tumour spread in the mesorectum distal to rectal cancer. Br J Surg 82:1031–1033

31. Gunderson LL, Sosin H, Levitt S (1984) Extrapelvic colon areas of failure in a reoperation series: implications for adjuvant therapy. Int J Radiat Oncol Biol Phys 11:731–741

32. Willett CG, Tepper JE, Cohen A et al (1984) Failure patterns folowing curative resection of colonic carcinoma. Ann Surg 200:685–690

33. Holm T, Cedermark B, Rutqvist L-E (1994) Local recurrence of rectal adenocarcinoma after "curative" surgery with and without preoperative radiotherapy. Br J Surg 81:452–455

34. Jansson-Frykholm G, Påhlman L, Glimelius B (1995) Treatment of local recurrences of rectal carcinoma. Radiother Oncol 34:185–194

35. Denham JW (1986) The radiation dose-response relationship for control of primary breast cancer. Radiother Oncol 7: 107–123

36. Fletcher GH (1973) Clinical dose-response curves of human malignant epithelial tumours. Br J Radiol 46:1–12

37. Fletcher GH (1984) Subclinical disease. Cancer 53: 1274–1284

38. Withers HR, Peter LJ, Taylor JMG (1995) Dose-response relationship for radiation therapy of subclinical diseases. Int J Radiat Oncol Biol Phys 31:353–359

39. Gray LH, Conger AD, Ebert M et al (1953) The concentration of oxygen dissolved in tissue at the time of irradiation as a factor in radiotherapy. Br J Radiol 26:638–648

40. Trotti A, Klotch D, Endicott J et al (1993) A prospective trial of accelerated radiotherapy in the postoperative treatment of high risk squamous cell carcinoma of the head and neck. pp. 13–21. In Johnson JT, Didoklar MS (eds): Head and Neck Cancer. Vol. 26 Elsevier, Amsterdam

41. Fowler JF (1989) The linear-quadratic formula and progress in fractionated radiotherapy. Br J Radiol 62:679–694

42. Kirk J, Gray WM, Watson ER (1971) Cumulative radiation effect. Part I. Fractionated treatment regimes. Clin Radiol 22: 145–155

43. Turesson I (1978) Fractionation and dose rate in radiotherapy. An experimental and clinical study of cumulative radiation effect. Thesis, Gothenburg

44. Jansson-Frykholm G, Sintorn K, Montelius A et al (1997) Preoperative radiotherapy in rectal carcinoma—aspects of acute adverse effects and radiation technique. (ms. in preparation)

45. International Commission on Radiation Units and Measurements (1993) Report 50. Prescribing, Recording, and Reporting Photon Beam Therapy. International Commission on Radiation Units and Measurements, Washington, DC

46. Jansson-Frykholm G, Glimelius B, Påhlman L (1993) Preoperative or postoperative irradiation in adenocarcinoma of the rectum: final treatment results of a randomized trial and an evaluation of late secondary effects. Dis Colon Rectum 36: 564–572

47. Mendenhall WM, Million RR, Pfaff WW (1983) Patterns of recurrence in adenocarcinoma of the rectum and rectosigmoid treated with surgery alone: implications in treatment planning with adjuvant radiation therapy. Int J Radiat Oncol Biol Phys 9:977–985

48. Rao A, Kagan R, Chan P et al (1981) Patterns of recurrence following curative resection alone for adenocarcinoma of the rectum and sigmoid colon. Cancer 48:1492–1495

49. Rich T, Gundersson LL, Lew R et al (1983) Patterns of recurrence of rectal cancer after potentially curative surgery. Cancer 52:1317–1329

50. Grinell RS (1965) Results of ligation of inferior mesenteric artery at the aorta in resections of carcinoma of the descending and sigmoid colon and rectum. Surg Gynecol Obstet 120: 1031–1036

51. Hermanek P, Gall FP (1981) Der aborale Sicherheitsabstand bei der sphinctererhaltenden Rectumresektion. Chirurg 52: 25–29

52. Pezim ME, Nicholls RJ (1984) Survival after high or low ligation of the inferior mesenteric artery during curative surgery for rectal cancer. Ann Surg 200:729–733

53. Surtees P, Ritchie JK, Phillips RKS (1990) High versus low ligation of the inferior mesenteric artery during curative surgery for rectal cancer. Br J Surg 77:618–621

54. Letchert JGJ Lebesdue JV, de Boer RW et al (1990) Dose-volume correlation in radiation-induced late small-bowel complications: a clinical study. Radiother Oncol 18:307–320

55. Graf W, Ekström K, Glimelius B, Påhlman L (1995) Factors influencing bowel function after colorectal anastomosis. Dis Colon Rectum 34:744–749

56. Lewis WG, Williamson MER, Kuzu A et al (1995) Potential disadvantages of postoperative adjuvant radiotherapy after anterior resection for rectal cancer: a pilot study of sphincter function, rectal capacity and clinical outcome. Int J Color Dis 10:133–137

57. Grinell RS (1954) Distal intramural spread of carcinoma of the rectum and rectosigmoid. Surg Gynecol Obstet 99: 421–439

58. Sondenaa K, Kjellevold KH (1990) A prospective study of the length of the distal margin after low anterior resection for rectal cancer. Int J Color Dis 5:103–105

59. Williams NS, Dixon MF, Johnston D (1983) Reappraisal of the 5 centimetre rule of distal excision for carcinoma of the rectum: a study of distal intramural spread and of patients' survival. Br J Surg 70:150–154

60. Gunderson LL, Dosoretz DE, Hedberg SE et al (1983) Low-dose preoperative irradiation, surgery, and elective postopera-

tive radiation therapy for resectable rectum and rectosigmoid carcinoma. Cancer 52:446–451

61. Mohuiddin M, Kramer S, Marks G, Dobelbower RR (1982) Combined pre- and postoperative radiation for carcinoma of the rectum. Int J Radiat Oncol Biol Phys 8:133–136

62. Shank B, Enker W, Santa J et al (1987) Local control with preoperative radiotherapy alone versus "sandwich" radiotherapy for rectal carcinoma. Int J Radiat Oncol Bio Phys 13:111–115

63. Duncan W, Smith AN, Freedman LS et al (1984) The evaluation of low dose pre-operative X-ray therapy in the management of operable rectal cancer; results of a randomly controlled trial. Br J Surg 71:21–25

64. Kligerman MM, Urdaneta-Lafee N, Knowlton A (1972) Preoperative irradiation of rectosigmoid carcinoma including its regional lymph nodes. AJR 114:498–503

65. Rider WD, Palmer JA, Mahoney LJ, Robertson CI (1977) Preoperative irradiation in operable cancer of the rectum: report of the Toronto trial. Can J Surg 20:335–338

66. Roswit B, Higgins G, Keehn R (1975) Preoperative irradiation for carcinoma of the rectum and rectosigmoid colon: report of a National Veterans Administration randomized study. Cancer 35:1597–1602

67. Friedman P, Garb JL, Park W et al (1985) Survival following moderate-dose preoperative radiation therapy for carcinoma of the rectum. Cancer 55:967–973

68. Glimelius B, Graffman S, Påhlman L et al (1982) Preoperative irradiation with high-dose fractionation in adenocarcinoma of the rectum and rectosigmoid. Acta Radiol, Oncol 21:373–379

69. Mendenhall WM, Million RR, Bland KI et al (1985) Preoperative radiation therapy for clinically resectable adenocarcinoma of the rectum. Ann Surg 202:215–222

70. Mohuiddin M, Marks GJ (1987) High dose preoperative radiation and sphincter preservation in the treatment of rectal cancer. Int J Radiat Oncol Biol Phys 13:839–842

71. Påhlman L, Glimelius B (1990) Pre- and postoperative radiotherapy in rectal carcinoma: report from a randomized multicenter trial. Ann Surg 211:187–195

72. Higgins G, Humphrey E, Dwight R et al (1986) Preoperative radiation and surgery for cancer of the rectum. VASOG trial II. Cancer 58:352–359

73. Stevens K, Fletcher W, Allen C (1978) Anterior resection and primary anastomosis following high dose preoperative radiotherapy for adenocarcinoma of the rectosigmoid. Cancer 41:2065–2071

74. Hoskin B, Gunderson L, Dosoretz D et al (1985) Adjuvant postoperative radiotherapy in carcinoma of the rectum and rectosigmoid. Cancer 55:61–71

75. Romsdahl M, Withers R (1978) Radiotherapy combined with curative surgery. Arch Surg 113:446–453

76. Tepper JE, Cohen AM, Wood WC et al (1987) Postoperative radiation therapy of rectal cancer. Int J Radiat Oncol Biol Phys 13:5–10

77. Turner SS, Vieira EF, Ager PJ et al (1977) Elective postoperative radiotherapy for locally advanced colorectal cancer. Cancer 40:105–108

78. Wiggenraad R, Ravasz L, Probst-van Zylen F (1988) Adjuvant postoperative radiotherapy in carcinoma of the rectum and rectosigmoid. Int J Radiat Oncol Biol Phys 15:753–756

79. Zucali R, Gardani G, Volterani F (1980) Adjuvant postoperative radiotherapy in locally advanced rectal and rectosigmoidal cancer. Tumori 66:595–600

80. Gérard A, Buyse M, Nordlinger B et al (1988) Preoperative radiotherapy as adjuvant treatment in rectal cancer. Ann Surg 208:606–614

81. Horn A, Halvorsen JF, Dahl O (1990) Preoperative radiotherapy in operable rectal cancer. Dis Colon Rectum 33:823–828

82. Goldberg PA, Nicholls RJ, Porter NH, et al (1994) Long-term results of a randomised trial of short-course low-dose adjuvant pre-operative radiotherapy for rectal cancer. Reduction in local treatment failure. Eur J Cancer 30A;11:1602–1606

83. James RD, Haboubi N, Schofield PF (1991) Prognostic factors in colorectal carcinoma treated by preoperative radiotherapy and immediate surgery. Dis Colon Rectum 34:546–551

84. Stockholm Rectal Cancer Study Group (1990) Preoperative short-term radiation therapy in operable rectal carcinoma. Cancer 66:49–53

85. Swedish Rectal Cancer Trial (1996) Local recurrence rate in a randomized multicentre trial of preoperative radiotherapy compared to surgery alone in resectable rectal carcinoma. Eur J Surg 162:397–402

86. Balslev I, Pedersen M, Teglbjaerg PS et al (1986) Postoperative radiotherapy in Dukes' B and C carcinoma of the rectum and rectosigmoid. A randomized multicenter study. Cancer 58:22–28

87. Gastrointestinal Tumor Study Group (1985) Prolongation of the disease-free interval in surgically treated rectal carcinoma. N Engl J Med 312:1464–1472

88. Fisher B, Wolmark N, Rockette H et al (1988) Postoperative adjuvant chemotherapy or radiation therapy for rectal cancer: results from NSABP Protocol R-01. J Natl Cancer Inst 80:21–29

89. Treuniet-Donker AD, van Putten WLJ (1991) Postoperative radiation therapy for rectal cancer. Cancer 67:2042–2048

90. Påhlman L, Glimelius B, Graffman S (1985) Pre- versus postoperative radiotherapy in rectal carcinoma: an interim report from a randomized multicentre trial. Br J Surg 72:961–966

91. Buyse M, Zeleniuch-Jacquotte A, Chalmers TC (1988) Adjuvant therapy of colorectal cancer. Why we still don't know. JAMA 259:3571–3578

92. Marsh PJ, James RD, Schofield PF (1994) Adjuvant preoperative radiotherapy for locally advanced rectal carcinoma. Results of a prospective, randomized trial. Dis Colon Rectum 37:1205–1214

93. Cedermark B, Johansson H, Rutquist LE, Wilking N (1995) The Stockholm I trial of preoperative short term radiotherapy in operable rectal carcinoma. Cancer 75:2269–2275

93a. Swedish Rectal Cancer Trial (1997) Improved survival with preoperative radiotherapy in resectable rectal cancer. N Engl J Med 336

94. Byfield J, Calabro-Jones P, Klisak I, Kulhanian F (1982) Pharmacologic requirements for obtaining sensitization of human tumor cells in vitro to combined 5-fluorouracil or Ftorafur and X-rays. Int J Radiat Oncol Biol Phys 8:1923–1933

95. von der Maase H (1986) Experimental studies on interactions of radiation and cancer chemotherapeutic drugs in normal tissues and a solid tumour. Radiother Oncol 7:47–68

96. Wassif-Boulis S (1982) The role of preoperative adjuvant

therapy in management of borderline operability of rectal cancer. Clin Radiol 33:353–358

97. Overgaard M, Berthelsen K, Dahlmark M et al (1989) A randomized trial of radiotherapy alone or combined with 5-FU in the treatment of locally advanced colorectal carcinoma. ECCO 5, meeting abstract 0–0626

98. Krook JE, Moertel CG, Gunderson LL et al (1991) Effective surgical adjuvant therapy for high-risk rectal carcinoma. N Engl J Medi 324:709–715

99. National Cancer Institute (1991) Clinical announcement. Adjuvant therapy for rectal cancer. March 14

100. Gastrointestinal Tumor Study Group (1992) Radiation therapy and fluorouracil with or without semustine for the treatment of patients with surgical adjuvant adenocarcinoma of the rectum. J Clin Oncol 10:549–557

101. O'Connell MJ, Martenson JA, Wieand HS et al (1994) Improving adjuvant therapy for rectal cancer by combining protracted infusion fluorouracil with radiation therapy after curative surgery. N Engl J Med 331:502–507

102. Beynon J, Mortensen NJ McC, Foy DMA et al (1986) Preoperative assessment of local invasion in rectal cancer: digital examination, endoluminal sonography or computed tomography? Br J Surg 73:1015–1017

103. Hildebrant U, Fiefel G (1985) Pre-operative staging of rectal cancer by intrarectal ultrasound. Dis Colon Rectum 28:42–46

104. Lindmark G, Elvin A, Påhlman L, Glimelius B (1992) The value of endosonography in preoperative staging of rectal cancer. Int J Colon Dis 7:162

105. Stockholm Rectal Cancer Study Group (1987) Short-term preoperative radiotherapy for adenocarcinoma of the rectum. Am J Clin Oncol 10:369–375

106. Swedish Rectal Cancer Trial (1993) Preoperative irradiation followed by surgery vs surgery alone in resectable rectal carcinoma—postoperative morbidity and mortality in a Swedish multicenter trial. Br J Surg 80:1333–1336

107. Påhlman L, Glimelius B, Ginman C et al (1985) Preoperative irradiation of primary non-resectable adenocarcinoma of the rectum and rectosigmoid. Acta Radiol Oncol 24:35–39

108. Bubrik MP, Rolfmeyers ES, Schauer RM et al (1982) Effects of high-dose and low-dose preoperative irradiation on low anterior anastomosis in dogs. Dis Colon Rectum 25:406–415

109. Degges RD, Cannon DJ, Lang NP (1983) The effects of preoperative radiation on healing of rat colonic anastomosis. Dis Colon Rectum 26:598–600

110. Schauer RM, Bubrick MP, Feeney DA et al (1982) Effects of low-dose preoperative irradiation on low anterior anastomosis in dogs. Dis Colon Rectum 25:401–405

111. Mak AC, Rich TA, Schulthesis TE (1994) Late complications of postoperative radiation therapy for cancer of the rectum and rectosigmoid. Int J Radiat Oncol Biol Phys 28:597–603

112. Feldman MI, Kavanah MT, Devereux DF, Choe S (1988) New surgical method to prevent pelvic radiation enteropathy. Am J Clin Oncol 11:25–33

113. Gunderson LL, Russell AH, Llewellyn HJ et al (1985) Treatment planning for colorectal cancer: radiation and surgical techniques and value of small-bowel films. Int J Radia Oncol Biol Phys 11:1379–1393

114. Kumar PP, Good RR, Plantz SH, Hynes PR (1987) Technique of postoperative pelvic radiation in the management of rectal and rectosigmoid carcinoma. J Natl Med Assoc 6:609–615

115. Dasmahapatra KS, Swaminatha AP (1991) The use of biodegradable mesh to prevent radiation-associated small bowel injury. Archi Surg 126:366–369

116. Deluca FR, Ragins H (1985) Construction of an omental envelope as a method of excluding the small intestine from the field of postoperative irradiation of the pelvis. Surg Gynecol Obstet 160:365–370

117. Gallagher MJ, Brereton HD, Rostock RA et al (1986) A prospective study of treatment techniques to minimize the volume of pelvic small bowel with reduction of acute and late effects associated with pelvic irradiation. Int J Radiat Oncol Bio Phy 12:1565–1573

118. Russ JE, Smoron GL, Gagnon JD (1984) Omental transposition flap incolorectal carcinoma: Adjunctive use in prevention and treatment of radiation complications. Int J Radiat Oncol Biol Phys 10:55–62

119. Trimbos JB, Snijders A, Keilhold T, Petes AA (1991) Feasibility of application of a resorbable polyglycolic-acid mesh (Dexon mesh) to prevent complications of radiotherapy following gynecological surgery. Eur J Surg 157:281–284

120. Cafiero F, Gipponi M, Di Somma C et al (1995) Adjuvant postoperative radiotherapy vs radiotherapy plus 5-FU and levamisole in patients with TNM stage II–III resectable rectal cancer. A phase III randomized clinical trial. Eur J Surg Oncol 21:391–392

121. Boice JD Jr, Greene MH, Killen JY (1983) Leukemia and preleukemia after adjuvant treatment of gastrointestinal cancer with semustine (methyl-CCNU). N Engl J Med 309:1079–1084

122. Duttenhaver JR, Hoskins RB, Gunderson LL, Tepper JE (1986) Adjuvant postoperative radiation therapy in the management of adenocarcinoma of the colon. Cancer 57:955–963

123. Loeffler RK (1984) Postoperative radiation therapy for Dukes' C adenocarcinoma of the caecum using two fractions per day. Int J Radiat Oncol Biol Phys 10:1881–1884

124. Willett CG, Tepper JE, Skates SJ et al (1987) Adjuvant postoperative radiation therapy for colonic carcinoma. Ann Surg 206:694–698

125. Wong CS, Harwood AR, Cummings BJ et al (1985) Postoperative local abdominal irradiation for cancer of the colon above the peritoneal reflection. Int J Radiat Oncol Biol Phys 11:2067–2071

126. Bjerkeset T, Dahl O (1980) Irradiation and surgery for primarily inoperable rectal adenocarcinoma. Dis Colon Rectum 23:298–303

127. Durdey P, Williams NS (1984) The effect of malignant and inflammatory fixation of rectal carcinoma on prognosis after rectal excision. Br J Surg 71:787–790

128. Fortier GA, Krochak RJ Kim JA, Constable WC (1986) Dose response to preoperative irradiation in rectal cancer: implications for local control and complications associated with sphincter sparing surgery and abdominoperineal resection. Int J Radiat Oncol Biol Phys 12:1559–1563

129. Wang CC, Schultz MD (1962) The role of radiation therapy in the management of carcinoma of the sigmoid, rectosigmoid and rectum. Radiology 79:1–5

130. Frykholm G, Hemmingsson A, Nyman R (1992) Non-resectable adenocarcinoma of the rectum assessed by MR imaging before and after chemotherapy and irradiation. Acta Radiol 33:447–452

131. Dosoretz DE, Gunderson LL, Hedberg S et al (1989) Preoperative irradiation for unresectable rectal and rectosigmoid carcinomas. Cancer 52:814–818

132. Frykholm G, Påhlman L, Glimelius B (1989) Preoperative irradiation with and without chemotherapy (MFL) in the treatment of primarily nonresectable adenocarcinoma of the rectum. Results from two consecutive studies. Eur J Cancer Clin Oncol 25:1535–1541

133. Minsky BD, Cohen AM, Kemeny N et al (1993) Preoperative 5-FU, and low dose leucovorin and sequential radiation therapy for unresectable rectal cancer. Int J Radiat Oncol Biol Phys 25:821–827

134. Minsky BD, Cohen AM, Kemeny N, Enker WE (1992) Enhancement of radiation-induced downstaging of rectal cancer by fluorouracil and high-dose leucovorin chemotherapy. J Clin Oncol 10:79–84

135. Overgaard M, Overgaard J, Sell A (1984) Dose-response relationship for radiation therapy of recurrent, residual, and primarily inoperable colorectal cancer. Radiother Oncol 1: 217–222

136. Wassif-Boulis S (1983) Ten years' experience with a multimodality treatment of advanced stages of rectal cancer. Cancer 52:2017–2024

137. Danjoux CE, Gelber RD, Catton GE, Klaassen DJ (1985) Combination chemoradiotherapy for residual recurrent or inoperable carcinoma of the rectum: E.C.O.G. study (EST 3276). Int J Radiat Oncol Biol Phys 11:765–771

138. Rominger CJ, Gelber RD, Gunderson LL, Conner N (1985) Radiation therapy alone or in combination with chemotherapy in the treatment of residual or inoperable carcinoma of the rectum and rectosigmoid or pelvic recurrence following colorectal surgery. Radiation Therapy Oncology Group study (76–16). Am J Clin Oncol 8:118–27

139. Poon MA, O'Conell MJ, Moertel CG et al (1989) Biochemical modulation of fluorouracil: evidence of significant improvement of survival and quality of life in patients with advanced colorectal carcinoma. J Clin Oncol 7:1407–1418

140. Wong CS, Cummings BJ, Keane TJ et al (1991) Combined radiation therapy, mitomycin C, and 5-fluorouracil for locally recurrent rectal cancer: results of a pilot study. Int J Radiat Oncol Biol Phys 21:1291–1296

141. Gunderson LL, Martin JK, Beart RW et al (1988) Intraoperative and external beam irradiation for locally advanced colorectal cancer. Ann Surg 207:52–60

142. Kallinowski F, Elbe MJ, Buhr HJ et al (1995) Intraoperative radiotherapy for primary and recurrent rectal cancer. Eur J Surg Oncol 21:191–194

143. Sichy B (1986) Intraoperative electron beam radiation therapy with particular reference to the treatment of rectal carcinomas—primary and recurrent. Dis Colon Rectum 29:714–718

144. Willet CG, Shellito PC, Tepper JE et al (1991) Intraoperative electron beam radiation therapy for primary, locally advanced rectal and rectosigmoid carcinoma. J Clin Oncol 9:843–847

145. Moertel CG, Childs DS, Reitemeier RJ et al (1969) Combined 5-fluorouracil and supervoltage radiation therapy of locally unresectable gastrointestinal carcinoma. Lancet 2:865–867

146. Moertel CG, Frytak S, Hahn RG et al (1981) Therapy of locally unresectable pancreatic carcinoma: a randomized comparison of high dose (6000 rads) radiation alone, moderate dose radiation (4000 rads + 5-fluorouracil), and high dose radiation + 5-fluorouracil. Cancer 48:1705–1710

147. Cummings BJ, Rider WD, Harwood AR (1983) Radical external beam radiation therapy for adenocarcinoma of the rectum. Dis Colon Rectum 26:30–36

148. Papillon J (1982) Conservative treatment by irradiation—an alternative to radical surgery. pp. 66–95. In Papillon J (ed): Rectal and Anal Cancer: Springer-Verlag, New York

149. Papillon J (1975) Intracavitory irradiation of early rectal cancer for cure. Cancer 36:696–701

150. Lavery IC, Jones IT, Weakley FL et al (1987) Definitive management of rectal cancer by contact (endocavitary) irradiation. Dis Colon Rectum 30:835–838

151. Roth SL, Horiot JC, Calais G et al (1989) Prognostic factors in limited rectal cancer treated with intracavitary irradiation. Int J Radiat Oncol Biol Phy 16:1445–1451

152. Sichy B, Granery MJ, Hinson EJ (1984) Endocavitary irradiation for adenocarcinoma of the rectum. Cancer 34:333–339

153. Williams IG, Horvitz H (1956) The primary treatment of adenocarcinoma of the rectum by high voltage roentgen rays (1000 Kv). AJR 76:919–928

154. Whiteley HW, Stearns MW, Leaming RH et al (1970) Palliative radiation therapy in patients with cancer of the colon and rectum. Cancer 25:343–346

155. Uradenata-Lafee N, Kligerman MM, Knowlton AH (1972) Evaluation of palliative irradiation in rectal carcinoma. Radiology 104:673–677

156. Ciatto S, Pacini P (1982) Radiation therapy of recurrences of carcinoma of the rectum and sigmoid after surgery. Acta Radiol Oncol 21:105–109

157. Allum WH, Mach P, Priestman TJ et al (1987) Radiotherapy for pain relief in locally recurrent colorectal cancer. Ann of R Coll Surg 69:220–221

158. Minsky BD, Cohen AM, Enker WE (1992) Combined modality therapy of rectal cancer: decreased acute toxicity with the preoperative approach. J Clin Oncol 10:1218–1224

25

CHEMOTHERAPY

U. Metzger
Th. Gross
H. P. Honegger

Colorectal cancer is a major public health problem in Western industrialized countries. In the United States and western Europe more than a quarter of a million people are newly affected each year. Over the past 30 years, the population-adjusted incidence has remained constant at 45 to 50 cases per 100,000 and thus the increasing number of cases must be due to growth and aging of the population. About three-quarters of patients will have a primary surgical resection but, despite the high resectability rate and a general improvement in surgical therapy, nearly half of all patients with colorectal cancer die from metastatic tumor. Nonsurgical treatment has been used as an adjuvant to resection in the treatment of advanced surgically incurable disease. Options include chemotherapy, radiation therapy, and immunotherapy.

ADJUVANT CHEMOTHERAPY

Over the past three decades, many studies have failed to demonstrate benefits from adjuvant chemotherapy. Claims of efficacy have been viewed with skepticism. Only in the last 5 to 8 years have trials yielded reproducible positive results. New data have demonstrated delays in recurrence and increases in survival for specific groups of patients.

WHO IS AT RISK OF RECURRENCE?

Clarification of the role of adjuvant therapy for colon and rectal cancer and maximization of the benefit of adjuvant regimens require identification of those individuals most likely to develop recurrent disease. TNM staging should be carried out in all cases.[1] Patients should undergo examination of the remainder of the large bowel for synchronous lesions. The presence of inflammatory bowel disease, familial adenomatous polyposis, hereditary nonpolyposis colorectal cancer, or more subtle famil-

ial associations should be determined. Abdominal computed tomography (CT) or ultrasound for liver metastases should be done and carcinoembryonic antigen (CEA) should be measured preoperatively.

At laparotomy complete surgical exploration is mandatory. Subsequent recurrence is related to the extensiveness of resection, colonic lesions should be removed with an anatomically complete lymphovascular pedicle. Adequate radial margins must be obtained to minimize local recurrence and the pathologist should examine the specimen particularly to assess the adequacy of surgical margins in all planes and the depth of penetration. The number of nodes removed should be stated and the number involved with tumor determined, particularly whether the apical node is positive. Characteristics such as venous or lymphatic invasion, perineural invasion, histologic subtype, and grade should be documented. The presence of a lymphatic reaction around the tumor and the nature of the advancing margin are further histopathologic features that can be related to ultimate treatment failure.[2]

Although there are several possible prognostic factors in defining subgroups of patients at risk for recurrence, pathologic stage is the most important. The degree of penetration of the primary lesion, lymph node involvement, and the number of involved nodes are all significant risk factors. There are differences in the natural history and patterns of failure between colon and rectal cancer that require the testing of distinct adjuvant strategies for lesions in the two sites. Elevation of CEA preoperatively indicates increased rate of recurrence and correlates with stage and histologic grade. A normal CEA does not obviate the need for adjuvant therapy in node-positive patients and it may indicate a high-risk subset of patients with node-negative colon cancer. It is premature to use certain cellular or molecular characteristics as standard determinants of risk of recurrence. Ploidy status and S-phase fraction are not significantly correlated with overall recurrence and survival. With refinement and standardization of the methodology, these factors may perhaps in the future help to delineate high-risk subjects.

At the molecular level, gene mutation and allele loss have been documented in many colorectal cancers and may be critical in mechanisms of tumor progression. Data from colorectal tumor cell lines that are characterized as poorly, moderately, or well differentiated suggest that production and interaction of growth factors correlate with degree of differentiation. The clinical significance of these findings remains to be elucidated. At the present time adjuvant chemotherapy should be considered for tumors with nodal or venous involvement or with moderate or extensive extrarectal local spread. Wherever possible, patients should be entered into prospective trials of adjuvant treatment.

COLON CANCER

When colon cancer recurs it tends to do so in the peritoneal cavity, the liver, or other distant sites with only a small proportion of patients developing isolated local failure. Thus systemic chemotherapy or immunotherapy are the most rational adjuvant modalities. In the 1960s 5-fluorouracil (5-FU) and FUDR were given as adjuvants for varying periods postoperatively in a wide range of dosage schedules. Activity was demonstrable but in individual trials this was not convincing statistically.

5-Fluorouracil in Combination With Levamisole

A meta-analysis suggested some benefit with 5-FU.[3] Levamisole with 5-FU was first demonstrated to be effective in 1987.[3,4] The Mayo Clinic and the North Central Cancer Treatment Group (NCCTG) used this combination for stage II and III resectable colorectal cancer.[5] Quality control and analysis in this study were excellent with a median follow-up of 7 years. The combination significantly reduced recurrence and subset analysis of stage III patients showed significant improvement in overall survival. In the light of these positive results, the Intergroup confirmatory trial for patients with Dukes' stage B and C colon carcinoma was initiated.[6] Patients were stratified for tumor stage and randomly allocated to the treatment schedules used in the preceding trial. Based on the treatment results of 971 patients with Dukes' stage C cancer, 5-FU plus levamisole is now recommended as standard therapy for such patients who are otherwise not in a clinical trial.[7] The combination increased the recurrence-free survival and overall survival significantly. The recurrence rate itself was reduced at all sites but most strikingly those outside the peritoneal cavity including lung, retroperitoneal nodes, peripheral nodes, and abdominal wall. In a recent update of The Intergroup Study after a median follow-up period of 5 years, the earlier results were confirmed with a reduction in the recurrence rate by 39% ($P < .0001$). The observed respective recurrence rates for patients having surgical resection only, surgical resection with levamisole, or 5-FU/levamisole were 53%, 52%, and 37%. The cancer-related death rate was also significantly reduced by 32% ($P < .004$) (surgery only 45%, levamisole 44%, 5-FU/levamisole 33%). These results were obtained despite some difficulty with patient compliance, with as many as 30% having interrupted the weekly chemotherapy within the 12-month treatment period.[8]

The results of the intergroup study raised the question as to

whether levamisole was contributing to the beneficial effect of the regimen and at present the data available leave it unanswered. EORTC trial No. 40781 found no difference in terms of disease-free and overall survival for node-positive colon cancer after adjuvant levamisole versus placebo.[9] Unfortunately the only investigation in which adjuvant 5-FU was randomly compared with fluorouracil plus levamisole is compromised by the small number of patients with stage C disease (only 41 of 141).[4] Nevertheless, there was an indication of a survival advantage for 5-FU only when given with levamisole.

Levamisole does not add to the antitumor activity of 5-FU patients with advanced disease.[10] In view of the results obtained in adjuvant trials, 5-FU plus levamisole is currently being randomly compared with 5-FU alone in advanced disease. If levamisole is active in the adjuvant setting, its effect on the immune system may be more important than its antitumor or synergistic properties.[11]

5-Fluorouracil in Combination With Folinic Acid

In 1977, the National Surgical Adjuvant Breast and Bowel Projects (NSABP) initiated a randomized three-arm comparison of postoperative chemotherapy using methyl-CCNU, vincristine, and 5-FU (MOF); the nonspecific immunostimulant Bacillus Calmette-Guerin (BCG), and surgery only.[12] The particular chemotherapy regimen was chosen because studies in advanced disease had suggested it to be superior when compared with 5-FU alone. Patients with colonic cancer of stages B2 and C (Astler Coller) were included. This large study, which included 1,166 patients, demonstrated an improvement in disease-free survival ($P < .02$) and overall survival ($P < .05$) in patients in the combined chemotherapy arm. BCG was ineffective.

Subsequently, the NSABP CO3 protocol compared the MOF regimen with 5-FU and folinic acid.[13] Stage II and III patients were randomly allocated to receive folinic acid 500 mg/m^2 weekly for six cycles repeated every 8 weeks or MOF therapy. At a three-year follow-up assessment preliminary data on 1,081 patients indicated an improvement in disease-free and overall survival for 5-FU and folinic acid compared with MOF therapy (73% versus 64%, $P = .0004$ and 84% versus 77%, $P = .003$, respectively). The advantage was seen equally in stage II and III patient groups.

The NIH Consensus Conference (1993) defined 5-FU plus levamisole as the current standard adjuvant chemotherapy for stage III disease. As a result protocols that included an untreated control arm were closed prematurely. Some preliminary data of these trials are, however, now available. In the most recent trial of the NCCTG and Mayo Clinic, 309 stage II and III patients were randomized to a surgery-only group or to surgery plus six cycles of 5-FU (425 mg/m^2/day) with folinic acid (20 mg/m^2/day) with the first five cycles repeated at 4-week intervals.[14] At a median follow-up of 3 1/2 years, a significant reduction in the recurrence rate (77% versus 64%, $P \leq .004$) and a significant improvement of the overall survival ($P \leq .04$) was seen. The treatment was associated with acceptable toxicity.

Italian, Canadian, and French investigators pooled data of national randomized trials for stage II and III patients.[15] Patients received either 5-FU (375 to 400 mg/m^2) with folinic acid (200 mg/m^2) for five consecutive days for 6 months, or surgical resection only. Overall 1,493 patients were evaluated. The dis-

Table 25-1. Disease-Free Survival After 5-Fluorouracil (5-FU)/Folinic Acid at 3 to 5 Years Compared With 5-FU/Levamisole Treatment at 5 Years Given as Adjuvant Treatment

Study	Stage	Surgery Only	MOF	FU/Lev	FU/FA
Intergroup 1993 (Moertel et al.[8])	III	47%	—	63%	—
NCCTG 1993 (O'Connell et al.[14])	II/III	64%	—	—	77%
NASBP 1993 (Wolmark et al.[13])	II/III	—	64%	—	73%
French/Italian Canadian 1994 (Erlichman et al.[15])	II/III	63%	—	—	72%

ease-free survival was consistently reduced in every country and the difference was highly significant at 3 years (72% versus 63%, $P < .001$) in favor of the fluorouracil/folinic acid adjuvant treatment. Respective overall rates were 83% versus 78% ($P < .03$).

5-Fluorouracil/Levamisole or 5-Fluorouracil/Folinic Acid?

The three adjuvant trials containing a 5-FU/folinic acid arm show similar results (Table 25-1). Disease-free survival rates at 3 years in the surgery-only control groups were 64% in the NCCTG study,[14] and 63% in the pooled Italian, French, and Canadian trial.[15] 5-FU and folinic acid treatment resulted in disease-free survival of 77% (NCCTG), 74% (pooled trial) and 73% (NSABP). The Intergroup trial,[8] which was responsible for 5-FU/levamisole being adopted as standard treatment, reported a disease-free survival of 63% at 5 years but it should be appreciated that this trial included only stage III patients whereas 5-FU/folinic acid trials had recruited stage II and III patients, making it impossible to compare these trials.

Preliminary survival data are given in Table 25-2, again demonstrating an advantage for chemotherapy. Before accepting 5-FU/folinic acid as the new standard adjuvant regimen for stage II and III disease, longer term follow-up of the Intergroup trial is required and comparison with the other trials is essential. Cost ($1,565 for 5-FU/levamisole, $545 for fluorouracil/folinic acid [NCCTG], $4,110 for fluorouracil/folinic acid [French/Italian/Canadian trial], and $13,540 for 5-FU/folinic acid [NSABP]) should be taken into consideration.[16] At present both 5-FU/levamisole and 5-FU/folinic acid are commonly used regimens.

Adjuvant Intraportal Chemotherapy

The liver is a major site of metastasis in colon adenocarcinoma. Tumor invasion into the mesenteric veins causes spread of malignant cells along the portal vein, which may result in microscopic metastasis formation.[17] Regional adjuvant chemotherapy

is based on the rationale that tumor cells might be disseminated into the portal circulation at the time of surgery. Thus it is generally recommended that the treatment should start immediately postoperatively. The patient selection for trials of regional adjuvant treatment has been to some extent compromised by the histopathologic stage not being available in the early postoperative period. Some patients may therefore be overtreated. Table 25-3 summarizes the results of eight published studies although not all are yet available in detail. The results are still inconclusive and unfortunately data on the site and timing and the rate of recurrence are not uniformly available.

The first trial carried out by Taylor et al.[18] reported a decrease in the incidence of liver metastasis and overall recurrence rate and a survival advantage in the chemotherapy arm. The large NSABP CO2 trial, which included 1,152 patients, did not demonstrate a reduction in the incidence of liver metastasis initially but on a longer follow-up of minimum 7.5 years, this study has now shown an improved survival for regional therapy ($P = .03$).[19] Some investigators provide information on subgroup analysis suggesting improvement in survival for stage III patients, but these results are still conflicting and it is doubtful that this information on stage III patients will be clinically relevant. Results of pathologic staging need to be available within hours of surgery to allow proper stratification with immediate randomization to regional therapy. Despite these methodologic difficulties meta-analysis of regional adjuvant chemotherapy has indicated that this approach might be as effective as systemic adjuvant treatment.[20] In the most recent meta-analysis based on 3,824 individual patient files and analyzed according to intent to treat, a reduced risk of recurrence of 14% ± 5% ($P < .007$) and for death of 13% ± 6% ($P < .007$) after a median follow-up time of 5 years was reported. It also appeared that liver infusion resulted in an increased interval between surgery and the occurrence of metastases (risk reduction: 27% ± 8%; $P < .008$).[21]

The indication from these studies that regional adjuvant treatment might improve overall survival without reducing the inci-

Table 25-2. Overall Survival After 5-Fluorouracil (5-FU)/Folinic Acid at 3 to 3.5 Years Compared With 5-FU/Levamisole Treatment at 5 Years Given as Adjuvant Treatment

Study	Stage	Surgery Only	MOF	FU/Lev	FU/FA
Intergroup 1993 (Moertel et al.[8])	III	55%	—	67% ($P = .004$)	—
NCCTG 1993 (Wolmark et al.[13])	II/III	?	—	—	? ($P = .04$)
NSABP 1993 (Wolmark et al.[13])	II/III	—	77%	—	84% ($P = .003$)
French/Italian Canadian 1994 (Erlichman et al.[15])	II/III	78%	—	—	83% ($P = .03$)

Abbreviations: MOF, methyl-CCNU, vincristine, 5-fluorouracil; FU: 5-fluorouracil; LEV, levamisole; FA, folinic acid.

Table 25-3.   Randomized Trials of Adjuvant Regional Chemotherapy

Author	Tumor-Site, Stage	Regimen	Median Follow-up (years)	No. of Patients	% Recurrences		DFS	% Survival
					All Sites	Liver Only		
Taylor[18]	Colon-rectum Dukes' A/B/C	Control FU/heparin 1 g ci days 1–7	5	127 117	33 18	17.3 4.3	n.a.	50 69 P = .002
Wereldsma[75]	Colon-rectum Dukes' A/B/C	Control urokinase FU/heparin 1 g ci days 1–7	3–5	102 103 99	37 30 19	23 18 7	n.s.	64 n.s. 69 74
NCCTG[76]	Colon-rectum Dukes' B2 + C	Control FU 0.5 g/m² × 7 days	5.5	109 110	n.a. n.a.	13 15	n.s.	68 68
NSABP CO2[19]	Colon Dukes' A/B/C	Control FU 0.6 g/m² × 7 days	7.5	459 422	40 32	n.s. n.s.	60 68 P = .01	71 76 P = .03
SAKK[77]	Colon-rectum Dukes' A/B/C	Control FU 0.5 g/m² × 7 days MMC 10 mg/m² dl	8	253 252	45 40	21 18	48 57 P = .051	55 66 P = .026
Ryan[78]	Colon-rectum Dukes' A/B/C	Control Heparin FU 1 g/m² days 1–5 MMC 12 mg/m² dl	2.5	232	n.a.	n.a.	n.s.	n.s.
Gray[79]	Colon Dukes' B/C	Control FU 0.6 g/m² × 7 IP FU 0.6 g/m² × 7		232	n.a.	n.a.	n.a.	61 P < .04 54 [Dukes' C 81 P = .006]
Fielding[80]	Colon-rectum Dukes' A/B/C	Control FU/heparin 1 g ci days 1–7 Heparin	5	145 130 123	n.s.	n.s.	n.s.	n.s. [Dukes' C P < .03]

Abbreviations: n.a., not available; n.s., difference not statistically significant; DFS, disease-free survival.

dence of liver metastasis probably indicates that the systemic effect of regionally applied 5-FU is more important than the drug concentration achieved in the liver. Regional adjuvant trials differ in the timing of chemotherapy compared with systemic treatment, which usually does not start until about 3 weeks after surgery. The concept of early regional therapy is attractive; chemotherapy over the shorter period of 7 days improves patient compliance because they are in the hospital and also reduces toxicity and cost compared with conventional systemic adjuvant therapy, which is given over a far longer period of up to 12 months.

The EORTC (protocol No. 40911) has launched an interesting trial to compare regional and systemic therapy. Patients with colorectal cancer are being randomized to receive either early regional postoperative therapy plus systemic chemotherapy or systemic chemotherapy alone. A choice of regional therapy is available including intraportal application (5-FU mg/m²/24 hour and heparin 5,000 IU/24 hour for 7 days) or intraperitoneal infusion (5-FU mg/m² in 1.5 L of dialysis fluid instilled over 3 hours from the 4th to the 9th day) postoperatively.

Immunotherapy

Nonspecific immunotherapy has been utilized as adjuvant therapy since the 1970s.[22] BCG has been the most frequently used agent but has failed to demonstrate any superiority over surgery only control or surgery plus chemotherapy groups. Autologous tumor cell-BCG treatment has recently been reported to prolong survival in patients with colon cancer after curative surgical

resection compared with a surgery-only control group,[23] but the methodology of this study has been criticized.[24] German investigators have used monoclonal antibodies with specificity for colorectal cancer as adjuvant treatment. Initial results appear to be promising, demonstrating improved survival for patients treated with the monoclonal antibody 17-A,[25] but further work and longer follow-up are needed. So far immunotherapy has been disappointing with no firm evidence of useful activity. Furthermore, it is not without risk.

Recommendations for Adjuvant Therapy of Colon Cancer

Based on current data, patients with stage III colon cancer unable to enter a clinical trial should be offered 5-FU and levamisole (administered as in an intergroup study) or 5-FU with folinic acid unless there are medical or psychological contraindications. At the present time the data available do not allow a recommendation of any specific adjuvant therapy for patients with stage II colon cancer outside clinical trials. The situation is only likely to improve with the development of new drugs that prove to be more active against colorectal carcinoma. Rigorous assessment by prospective randomized trial will continue to be essential.

RECTAL CANCER

In contrast to colon cancer, there is a significant risk of symptomatic locoregional failure as the first or sometimes the only manifestation of recurrence in patients with rectal cancer curatively resected. Local recurrence is related to several factors including the pathology of the tumor (see Ch. 19), the quality of surgery, and anatomic constraints in obtaining wide margins of resection (see Ch. 4). Over the past 10 to 15 years, adjuvant radiation therapy has been evaluated when used either preoperatively or postoperatively. The data show that local recurrence rates are significantly decreased when radiotherapy is given preoperatively and with an adequate dose but almost all studies have shown no significant benefit in disease-free or overall survival rates.[26] In the first GITSG trial (No. 7175), the combination of 5-FU and methyl-CCNU with postoperative radiotherapy showed initially a significant improvement in local control and this has been maintained after 10 years of follow-up when compared with surgery alone or with radiotherapy or chemotherapy on its own.[27] In the NCCTG study, (No. 794751) at a median follow-up of 6 years, the same combination was superior to radiotherapy alone.[28] In the NSABP study (No. R-01) a combination of 5-FU methyl-CCNU, and vincristine was significantly better than surgery alone but the local failure rate (23%) remained high.[29] There is thus some evidence to indicate that combined adjuvant treatment for rectal cancer is more effective than single modality use, but toxicity is increased.[30]

When considered to be clinically indicated, the best combination for rectal cancer is probably chemotherapy plus radiotherapy, preferably preoperative. Incorporation of semustine in combined modality regimens caused concern because of the associated risk of acute leukemia.[31] More recent trials have shown that semustine does not contribute to the therapeutic effect of the combined approaches.[32,33] The regimen without semustine therefore seems more appropriate.

The addition of fluorouracil to radiation therapy appears to be crucial for the reduction in local recurrence seen in these two trials. In vitro studies of tumor cell lines indicate that a continuous infusion of fluorouracil may provide more effective radiosensitization than short courses of bolus administration.[34] The early results at a median follow-up of 4 years of the NCCTG study No. 864751, comparing continuous infusion with bolus administration of fluorouracil during radiation, showed that the former resulted in significantly lower rates of recurrence and higher survival with a rate of local recurrence of 8%. If these results are sustained, they will serve as a new standard for adjuvant treatment of patients with rectal carcinoma.[35]

Local treatment failure is highly related to the quality of surgery and yet this factor is rarely referred to in most reports of outcome. This is true especially for lymphadenopathy and the extent of free margins around the tumor. Reports of local recurrence rates and survival after surgery alone are available that compare favorably with these most recent NCCTG data.[36,37] The extent of surgical excision is difficult to quantify but a description of the surgical procedure with a subsequent histopathologic statement giving the number of dissected and invaded lymph nodes might help to allow comparison between studies. It is essential that a clear distinction between surgical resection in which no residual tumor is present (R0) and those in which microscopic (R1) and macroscopic (R2) residual disease is left after surgery should be made. The last two categories correspond to noncurative resection[1] and should therefore never be included in trials of adjuvant treatment.

Adjuvant therapy must be balanced against possible side effects. Chronic radiation damage can be severe (see Ch. 24).

When postoperative radiotherapy is to be used, surgical attention should be directed toward preventing small intestine loops from entering the pelvis, with either natural structures or a synthetic mesh. Chemotherapy should be administered by trained oncologists.

Adjuvant therapy is most conclusively established for patients with stage III disease. However, newer prognostic markers such as DNA content, proliferative activity, surface glycoprotein, gastrin receptor, oncogenes/tumor-suppressor genes, and allelic deletions may allow the refinement of prognostic groups. Although local relapse is not common in colon cancer, there are certain groups, for example T4 N1/N2 stage, that have high local failure rates. These patients should be included in trials of radiotherapy combined with chemotherapy.

Because combined therapy can significantly reduce symptomatic local recurrence in rectal cancer, the next series of trials must define the proper dose, sequence, and integration of these modalities. The impact on local recurrence and disease-free and overall survival must be measured against any increased toxicity resulting from the combined approach. Quality of life and the cost benefit ratio of adjuvant therapy should also be assessed.

ADVANCED DISEASE

Approximately one-third of patients presenting with colorectal cancer already have distant metastases. Of patients treated surgically for cure, failure occurs in 50% with the development of local recurrence or metastatic disease or both simultaneously. With distant failure, the most common site is the liver, followed by the lung. Other sites of distant metastasis are rare and include the skeleton, ovaries, adrenals, and retroperitoneal.[38] Transcolonic spread within the peritoneal cavity may occur. Ovarian involvement may give rise to large ovarian tumors. Taking the limited data available from adjuvant studies, the pattern of failure has remained unchanged over the years. Local recurrence is a major problem and liver metastasis is the most common distant manifestation[39–41] (Table 25-4).

Treatment of disseminated colorectal cancer is palliative and basically consists of chemotherapy. The rare patient with a solitary metastasis in the liver or even more rarely in the lung, can be salvaged by resection. Surgery for limited hepatic or pulmonary metastases results in a 5-year survival rate of 20% to 30% and 13% to 36%, respectively.[42–45] Painful inoperable recurrent colorectal lesions or painful metastatic bone deposits are amenable to radiation therapy, achieving palliation in 80% of patients.

PALLIATIVE CHEMOTHERAPY

The median survival for patients with disseminated colon cancer is only 6 to 10 months, reflecting the natural course of disease. Chemotherapy is the only available means to control advanced, multiorgan disease. Due to the fact that the number of marginally effective drugs is limited, careful judgment is needed concerning when to start palliative chemotherapy. For decades only 5-FU was available and over many years the decision to start with palliative chemotherapy was not based on objective information but was the result of subjective judgment.

Some data are now available on the effectiveness of palliative chemotherapy. In a useful study comparing chemotherapy with

Table 25-4. Sites of Local and Distant Treatment Failure After Surgery Plus Adjuvant Chemotherapy

| | Surgery Only | | Surgery and Chemotherapy | | | |
	1965–1978	1984–1987	L	5-FU + L	MOF	5-FU + FA
Lung	6%	13%	12%	7%	9%	21%
Liver	39%	27%	25%	20%	39%	31%
Abdominal	21%	14%	13%	11%	22%	24%
Locoregional	6%	9%	10%	8%	b	b
Retroperitoneal	a	9%	7%	6%	b	b
Other	6%	9%	8%	7%	17%	15%
No. of patients		302	310	302	524	521
Ref.	Minsky et al.[40]	Moertel et al.[39]	Moertel et al.[39]	Moertel et al.[39]	Wolmark et al.[41]	Wolmark et al.[41]

Abbreviations: MOF, MeCCNU (lomustin), vincristine, 5-fluorouracil; 5-FU, 5-fluorouracil; L, levamisole; FA, folinic acid.
[a] Not given.
[b] Included in "abdominal."

supportive care against supportive care alone, a difference in survival was observed. Median survival in the two groups was 11 months and 5 months, respectively. This was despite the fact that the chemotherapy included 5-FU, folinic acid, and cisplatinum at a time before the effective antiemetic Ondansetron became available. The quality of life during the "additional" 6 months was at least as good as for patients receiving supportive care only.[46] In another randomized study of chemotherapy versus supportive treatment in asymptomatic patients, early chemotherapy was shown significantly to prolong survival and the duration of the asymptomatic period compared with best supportive care alone. Time to disease progression was approximately 6 months longer in the treated group.[47] Both of these studies used quality of life assessments, which showed an advantage for early active treatment.

Single-Agent Chemotherapy With 5-Fluorouracil

Reported response rates to 5-FU alone differ considerably. Several factors including patient selection, the site of disease and dose and mode of administration of the drug are likely to be responsible for this variability. The ideal single-agent schedule for 5-FU remains to be determined. Most of the "standard" 5-FU treatment arms in randomized studies include a loading phase followed by weekly bolus injections (Table 25-5). Prolonged infusions over 5 to 7 days yield a higher response rate than when given as a bolus. This difference is significant in some studies but not in all.[48–50] However, no difference in survival was demonstrated. Oral administration of 5-FU has been abandoned due to erratic absorption of the drug.

Side effects of 5-FU given according to standard therapy include leukopenia, diarrhea, and stomatitis. Prolonged infusions cause more stomatitis and the so-called hand-foot syndrome (palmar-plantar erythrodysthesia), amenable to treatment with vitamin B_6. In higher doses and when given by continuous infusion cardiac toxicity can occur.[51] Advanced age is significantly associated with more severe toxicity. Elderly women seem particularly at risk, probably because they metabolize the drug at a lower rate.[52]

Biomodulation of 5-Fluorouracil by Folinic Acid (Leucovorin)

A meta-analysis was performed including more than 1,500 patients from nine randomized trials, comparing 5-FU to 5-FU/folinic acid. Folinic acid was given either weekly or monthly in combination with 5-FU and produced a significantly higher tumor response rate of 23% over single-agent 5-FU, which had a response rate of 11%. Overall survival was, however, not different with a median survival of 11 months for 5-FU alone and 11.5 months for the combination.[53]

In a study by the North Central Cancer Treatment Group, weekly 5-FU and folinic acid (500 mg/m² high dose) was compared with folinic acid (20 mg low dose) followed by 5-FU (425 mg/m²) bolus for 5 consecutive days repeated at 4 and 8 weeks and every 5 weeks thereafter.[54] Objective tumor response was 35% and 31% and median survival 9.3 and 10.7 months. There was, however, a significant difference in toxicity with the intensive course regimen associated with more leukopenia and stomatitis. The weekly regimen, on the other hand, caused more diarrhea and hospitalization. The intensive 5-day course bolus 5-FU plus low-dose folinic acid regimen had the advantage of lower cost and less need for hospitalization than the weekly regimen.

Biochemical Modulation of 5-Fluorouracil by Methotrexate

A meta-analysis of eight randomized trials comparing 5-FU with 5-FU and methotrexate included 564 patients allocated to the former and 604 patients to the latter treatment. Respective tumor responses were 10% and 19%, a significant difference. There was also a small difference in median overall survival of 9.1 months and 10.7 months.[55] Thus, modulation of 5-FU by methotrexate doubles the response rate although it yields no discernible improvement in survival after fluorouracil.

The NCCTG-Mayo Clinic trial compared 5-FU and methotrexate with 5-FU and folinic acid within a six-arm study.[56] The tumor response rate was 42% for 5-FU and low-dose folinic acid, 31% for 5-FU with high-dose folinic acid, and 14% for 5-FU and methotrexate. Three of eight studies included in a

Table 25-5. 5-Fluorouracil Used as a Single Agent: Dosage and Mode of Administration in Advanced Disease (Early Studies)

Ref.	Starting	Maintenance	Response	Overall Survival (Median), Weeks
Ansfield et al.[81]	12 mg/kg 5 days Bolus IV Then 50% dose Alternate day × 11	Weekly 15 mg/kg Bolus IV	33	52
	15 mg/kg once weekly Bolus IV	Weekly 15 mg/kg Bolus IV	13	40
	500 mg for 4 days Bolus IV	Weekly 500 mg	14	40
	Oral 15 mg/kg for 6 days	Weekly 15 mg/kg orally	13	28
Seifert et al.[82]	12.0 mg/kg 5 days Bolus IV	Repeated every 4 weeks	22	8
	30 mg/kg per 24 hr Contin. infusion for 5 days	Repeated every 4 weeks	44	32
				Duration of Response (Median) Weeks
Hahn et al.[83]	Oral 20 mg/kg 5 days	Repeated every 5 weeks	19	11
	13.5 mg/kg 5 days Bolus IV	Repeated every 5 weeks	26	20

fluorouracil meta-analysis contained a direct comparison between 5-FU and folinic acid and 5-FU and methotrexate. Data from these showed no difference for either chemotherapy regime.[55]

5-Fluorouracil With Interferon

The cytotoxic effect of 5-FU can be modulated by interferon. In the phase II study of Wadler et al.,[57] 42% of 32 patients with metastatic colon cancer responded.

5-FU was given by a 5-day continuous infusion loading dose and thereafter by weekly bolus injections. Interferon was applied three times weekly by subcutaneous injection. Toxicity was considerable including mainly leukopenia and severe diarrhea. Recently published randomized trials of 5-FU/interferon modulation are summarized in Table 25-6 with response rates ranging between 19% and 38%.[58–60] The general impression from these trials is that the addition of interferon-α does not improve response rates or survival compared with 5-FU alone or with folinic acid. Fewer patients were generally able to tolerate the 5-FU/interferon combination. Interferon-α significantly increased toxicity and led to an unacceptable mortality of 10% with the high-dose 5-FU regimen.[58]

In summary, fluorouracil modulation by interferon has shown no significant clinical benefit in metastatic colorectal cancer so far, neither in response rate nor survival despite appreciable mortality and morbidity.

NEW DRUGS

New drugs for the treatment of colorectal cancer include more potent thymidylate synthase inhibitors such as ZD 1694 (Tomudex). In a large phase II study Tomudex produced a response rate of 26% and was considered to be acceptably safe and con-

venient to administer.[61] A randomized phase III trial comparing 5-FU and folinic acid with Tomudex has been completed in Europe and a similar trial in the United States is still ongoing. The results are not yet available. Other thymidylate synthase inhibitors tested in phase I trial studies include LY 231514[62] and AG 331.[63] Useful data on these are not yet available. The topoisomerase I inhibitors are another class of compounds with promising activity against colorectal cancer. In a French phase II study, CPT 11 (Irinotecan) has shown activity with a response rate of 20% in patients with metastatic colon cancer.[64] Most interesting is the fact that Irinotecan yielded a response rate of 16% in patients with metastatic colorectal cancer refractory to 5-FU-based chemotherapy.[65] Confirmatory trials are in progress. A randomized study of Irinotecan versus 5-FU and folinic acid is ongoing in Europe and will help to clarify the future role of Irinotecan in colon cancer.

Doxetacel (Taxotere), a compound related to Paclitaxel (taxol), has not demonstrated any useful activity against metastatic colorectal carcinoma.[66]

FUTURE DIRECTIONS OF CHEMOTHERAPY

Long-term protracted infusions of 5-FU over 10 weeks have been shown in a phase II study to yield a response rate of 30%, similar to that reported with bolus 5-FU and folinic acid but without the gastrointestinal toxicity.[67] The addition of folinic acid to prolonged fluorouracil infusion produced a response rate of 46%.[68] A similar rate was observed with interferon modulation.[69] There is evidence from in vitro data that prolonged low-dose folinic acid given simultaneously with continuous 5-FU administration may minimize the cytotoxic effect.[70]

In metastatic colorectal cancer phase II studies with the doubled modulation of 5-FU by folinic acid and interferon yielded response rates of 54% and 58%, respectively.[71,72] A randomized

Table 25-6. Recent Randomized Trials of 5-Fluorouracil (5-FU) With Interferon in Advanced Disease

	Starting	Maintenance	Response (%)	Survival (%)
Köhne et al.[58]	FU 2,600 mg/m² contin. infusion IV for 1 day + FA 500 mg/m²	Weekly 6×	39	Not given
	FU 2,600 mg/m² contin. infusion IV for 1 day + Inf-α 3 Mio. SC 3 × weekly	Weekly 6×	Not given	Not given
	FU 2,600 mg/m² contin. infusion IV for 1 day + Inf-α 3 Mio. FA 500 mg/m² IV	Weekly 6×	38	Not given
Hill et al.[84]	FU 750 mg/m² contin. infusion IV day 1–5	FU 750 mg/m² bolus IV weekly	30	39
	FU 750 mg/m² contin. infusion IV + Inf-α 10 Mio. SC weekly 3×	FU 750 mg/m² bolus IV + Inf-α 10 Mio. SC weekly 3×	19	29
Hill et al.[84]	FU 300 mg/m²/day contin. infusion IV 10 weeks	None	33	43
	FU 300 mg/m²/day contin. infusion IV + Inf-α 5 Mio. SC weekly 3×	None	22	48
Corfu-A[60]	FU 750 mg/m²/day contin. infusion IV for 5 days + Inf-α 9 Mio. SC weekly 3×	FU 750 mg/m² bolus IV + Inf-α 9 Mio. SC weekly 3×	21	44
	FU 370 mg/m²/day bolus IV for 5 days + FA 200 mg/m² IV for 5 days	Every 4 weeks	18	44

Abbreviations: Inf, interferon; FA, folinic acid.

trial comparing 5-FU with folinic acid with this combination plus interferon was completed in early 1994[73]; results are not yet available.

Modulation of 5-FU with methotrexate and leucovorin was no more effective in terms of response and overall survival than modulation with 5-FU by folinic acid alone.[74] Furthermore, a combination of Irinothecan (CPT 11) with 5-FU or 5-FU and folinic acid may be promising, provided that the gastrointestinal toxicity can be minimized.

SUMMARY

The literature on chemotherapy for advanced disease is voluminous and often conflicting. Studies vary in their quality including sample size and duration of follow-up. However, the data available allow several useful conclusions.

Palliative chemotherapy should start as soon as metastatic disease is diagnosed even if the patient is asymptomatic. With this strategy, a gain of some 6 months of good quality of life may be achieved.

Palliative chemotherapy should at the least include 5-FU with a loading dose either bolus intravenous or continuous infusion to give optimal response. Response is most important in symptomatic patients and a significant higher response rate is achievable by using bolus 5-FU and folinic acid in low dose. The high-dose folinic acid regimens have no added advantage and are not cost effective.

Higher doses of 5-FU may be more toxic especially in elderly patients and those with pre-existing heart disease should in particular be carefully assessed.

Modulation of 5-FU by agents other than low-dose folinic acid is no more effective in terms of response rate.

Overall survival is not prolonged by 5-FU modulation with interferon or other agents compared with 5-FU bolus alone.

REFERENCES

1. Union International Contre Le Cancer (1987) In Hermanek P, Sobin LH (eds): TNM, Classification of Malignant Tumors, 4th Ed. Springer Berlin
2. Jass JR, Love SB, Northover JMA (1987) A new prognostic classification of rectal cancer. Lancet 1:1303–1306
3. Buyse M, Zeleniuch A, Chalmers TC (1988) Adjuvant therapy of colorectal cancer. JAMA, 259:3571–3578
4. Windle R, Bell PRF, Shaw D (1987) Five year results of a randomized trial of adjuvant 5-fluorouracil and levamisole in colorectal cancer. Br J Surg 74:569–572
5. Laurie JA, Moertel CG, Fleming TR et al for the North Central Cancer Treatment Group and the Mayo Clinic (1989) Surgical adjuvant therapy of large-bowel carcinoma: an evaluation of levamisole and the combination of levamisole and fluorouracil. J Clin Oncol 7:1447–1456
6. Moertel CG, Fleming TR, Macdonald JS et al (1990) Levamisole and fluorouracil for adjuvant therapy of resected colon carcinoma. N Engl J Med 322:352–358
7. NIH Consensus Conference (1990) Adjuvant therapy for patients with colon and rectal cancer. JAMA 264:1444–1450
8. Moertel C, Fleming T, Macdonald J et al (1993) The Intergroup study of fluorouracil (5-FU) plus levamisole (LEV) and levamisole alone as adjuvant therapy for stage C colon cancer, abstracted. Proc Am Soc Clin Oncol 11:161
9. Arnaud JP, Buyse M, Nordlinger B et al (1989) Adjuvant therapy of poor prognosis colon cancer with levamisole: results of an EORTC double-blind randomized clinical trial. Br J Surg 76:284–289
10. Buroker TR, Moertel CG, Fleming TR et al (1985) A controlled evaluation of recent approaches to biochemical modulation or

enhancement of 5-fluorouracil therapy in colorectal carcinoma. J Clin Oncol 3:1624–1631

11. Stevenson HC, Green I, Hamilton JM et al (1991) Levamisole: known effects on the immune system, clinical results, and future applications to the treatment of cancer. J Clin Oncol 9: 2052–2066

12. Wolmark N, Fisher B, Rockette H et al (1988) Postoperative adjuvant chemotherapy or BCG for colon cancer: results from NSABP protocol C-01. J Natl Cancer Inst 80:30–36

13. Wolmark N, Rockette H, Fisher B et al (1993) Leucovorin-modulated 5-FU (LV-FU) as adjuvant therapy for primary colon cancer: NSABP C-03, abstracted. Proc Am Soc Clin Oncol 12:197

14. O'Connell M, Mailliard J, Macdonald J et al (1993) An Intergroup Trial of Intensive Course %-FU and low dose leucovorin as surgical adjuvant therapy for high risk colon cancer, abstracted Proc Am Soc Clin Oncol 12:190

15. Erlichman C, Marsoni S, Seitz JF et al (1994) Event free and overall survival is increased by FUFA in resected B and C Colon cancer: a prospective pooled analysis of 3 randomized trials (RCTS). Proc Am Soc Clin Oncol 13:194

16. Moertel G (1994) Chemotherapy for colorectal cancer. N Engl J Med 330:1136–1142

17. Fisher ER, Turnbull RB (1995) The cytological demonstration and significance of tumour cells in the mesenteric blood in patients with colorectal cancer. Surg Gynecol Obstet 100: 102–107

18. Taylor I, Machin D, Mullee M et al (1985) A randomized controlled trial of adjuvant portal vein cytotoxic perfusion in colorectal cancer. Br J Surg 72:359–363

19. Wolmark N, Rockette H, Petrelli N et al (1994) Long-term results of the efficacy of perioperative portal vein infusion of 5-FU for treatment of colon cancer: NSABP C-02, abstracted. Proc Am Soc Clin Oncol 13:561

20. Gray R, James R, Mossman J et al (1991) AXIS—suitable case for treatment. UK Coordinating Committee on Cancer Research (UKCCCR) Colorectal Cancer Subcommittee, editorial. Br J Cancer 8:1466–1475

21. Piedbois P, Buyse M, Gray R et al (1995) Portal vein infusion is an effective adjuvant treatment for patients with colorectal cancer, abstracted. Proc ASCO 14:192

22. Friedman MA, Hamilton JM (1988) Progress in the adjuvant therapy of large bowel cancer. Important Adv Oncol 273–296

23. Hoover HC, Brandhorst JS, Peters LC et al (1993) Adjuvant active specific immunotherapy for human colorectal cancer: 6.5-year median follow-up of a phase III prospectively randomized trial. J Clin Oncol 390–399

24. Moertel CG (1993) Vaccine adjuvant therapy for colorectal cancer: "very dramatic" or ho-hum? J Clin Oncol 11:385–386

25. Riethmüller G, Schneider E, Schlimock G et al (1993) Effective adjuvant treatment of resected colorectal cancer Dukes C with murine monoclonal antibody. Ann Hematol, Suppl. 67: A102

26. Molls M, Fink U (1994) Perioperative radiotherapy +/– chemotherapy in rectal cancer. Ann Oncol, 5, suppl. 3:105–113

27. Douglass HO Jr, Moertel CG, Mayer RJ et al (1986) Survival after postoperative combination treatment of rectal cancer. N Engl J Med 315:1294–1295

28. Krook JE, Moertel CG, Gunderson LL et al (1991) Effective surgical adjuvant therapy for high-risk rectal carcinoma. N Engl J Med 324:709–715

29. Fisher B, Wolmark N, Rockette H et al (1988) Postoperative adjuvant chemotherapy or radiation therapy for rectal cancer: result from NSABP protocol R-01. J Natl Cancer Inst 80:21–29

30. Thomas PRM, Stablein DM, Luidblad AM et al (1983) Toxicity associated with adjuvant postoperative therapy for adenocarcinoma of the rectum. Int J Radiat Oncol Biol Phys, 9, suppl. 1:137

31. Boice JD Jr, Greene MH, Killen JY Jr et al (1983) Leukemia and preleukemia after adjuvant treatment of gastrointestinal cancer with semustine (methyl-CCNU). N Engl J Med 309: 1079–1084

32. The Gastrointestinal Tumor Study Group (1992) Radiation therapy and fluorouracil with or without semustine for the treatment of patients with surgical adjuvant adenocarcinoma of the rectum. J Clin Oncol 10:549–557

33. O'Connell M, Wieand H, Krook J et al (1991) Lack of value for methyl-CCNU as a component of effective rectal cancer surgical adjuvant therapy, abstracted. Proc Am Soc Clin Oncol 10:134

34. Byfield JE, Calabro-Jones P, Klisak I, Kulhanian F (1982) Pharmacologic requirements for obtaining sensitization of human tumour cells in vitro to combined 5-fluorouracil or florafur and X rays. Int J Radiat Oncol Biol Phys 8:1923–1933

35. O'Connell MJ, Martenson JA, Wieand HS et al (1994) Improving adjuvant therapy for rectal cancer by combining protracted-infusion fluorouracil with radiation therapy after curative surgery. N Engl J Med 331:502–507

36. Macfarlane JK, Ryall RDH, Heald RJ (1993) Mesorectal excision for rectal cancer. Lancet 341:457–460

37. Hermanek P (1991) Data collection aspects for the design of adjuvant treatment protocols in colorectal carcinoma. Onkologie 14:491

38. Berge T, E Kelund G, Mellner C et al (1973) Carcinoma of the colon and rectum in a defined population. Acta Chir-Scand, 4, suppl.:38

39. Moertel Ch. G, Fleming TR, Macdonald JS et al (1995) Fluorouracil plus levamisole as effective adjuvant therapy after resection of stage III colon carcinoma: a final report. Ann Intern Med 122:321–326

40. Minsky D, Mies C, Rich TA et al (1988) Potentially curative surgery of colon cancer: patterns of failure and survival. J Clin Oncol 6:106–118

41. Woolmark N, Rockette H, Fisher B et al (1993) The benefit of leucovorin-modulated fluorouracil as postoperative adjuvant therapy for primary colon cancer: results from National Surgical Adjuvant Breast and Bowel Project Protocol C-03. J Clin Oncol 11:1879–1887

42. Scheele J, Stang R, Altendorf-Hofmann A, Paul M (1995) Resection of colorectal liver metastases. World J Surg 19:59–71

43. Nordlinger B, Vaillant JC, Guiget M et al (1994) Survival benefit of repeat liver resections for recurrent colorectal metastases: 143 cases. J Clin Oncol 12:1491–1496

44. Shironzu K, Isomoto H, Hagashi A et al (1995) Surgical treatment for patients with pulmonary metastases after resection of primary colorectal carcinoma. Cancer 76:393–398

45. McCormack PM, Burt ME, Bain MS et al (1992) Lung resection for colorectal metastases. Arch Surg 127:1403–1406

46. Scheithauer W, Rosen H, Kornek G-V et al (1993) Randomised

comparison of combination chemotherapy plus supportive care with supportive care alone in patients with metastatic colorectal cancer. BMJ 306:752–755

47. Nordic Gastrointestinal Tumour Adjuvant Therapy Group (1992) Expectancy or primary chemotherapy in patients with advanced asymptomatic colorectal cancer: a randomised trial. J Clin Oncol 10:904–911

48. Rougier P, Paillot B, La planche A et al (1992) End results of a multicentric randomized trial comparing 5-FU in a continuous systemic infusion to bolus administration in measurable colorectal cancer. Proc Am Soc Clin Oncol 11:465

49. Hansen R, Ryant, Anderson T et al (1992) A phase III trial of bolus 5-FU versus protracted infusion 5-FU +/– cisplatin in metastatic colorectal cancer. An Eastern Cooperative Oncology Group study. Proc Am Soc Clin Oncol 11:499

50. Schöber C, Papageorgiou E, Harstrick A et al (1993) Cardiotoxicity of 5-fluorouracil in combination with folinic acid in patients with gastrointestinal cancer. Cancer 72:2242–2247

51. Gradishar WJ, Vokes EE (1990) 5-Fluorouracil cardiotoxicity: a critical review. Ann Oncol 1:409–414

52. Stein BN, Petrelli NJ, Douglass HO et al (1995) Age and sex are independent predictors of 5-fluorouracil toxicity. Cancer 75:11–17

53. Advanced Colorectal Cancer Meta Analysis Project (1992) Modulation of fluorouracil by leucovorin in patients with advanced colorectal cancer: evidence in terms of response rate. J Clin Oncol 10:896–903

54. Buroker TR, O'Connell MJ, Wiland HS et al (1994) Randomised comparison of two schedules of fluorouracil and leucovorin in the treatment of advanced colorectal cancer. J Clin Oncol 12:14–20

55. Advanced Colorectal Cancer Meta-Analysis Project (1994) Meta-analysis of randomized trials testing the biochemical modulation of 5-fluorouracil by methotrexate in metastatic colorectal cancer. J Clin Oncol 12:960–969

56. Poon MA, O'Connell MJ, Moertel CG et al (1989) Biochemical modulation of fluorouracil. Evidence of significant improvement of survival and quality of life in patients with advanced colorectal cancer. J Clin Oncol 7:1407–1417

57. Wadler S, Lembersky B, Atkins M et al (1991) Phase II trial of fluorouracil and recombinant interferon-alfa-2a in patients with advanced colorectal carcinoma: an Eastern Cooperative Oncology Group study. J Clin Oncol 9:1806–1810

58. Köhne CH, Wilke H, Hecker H et al (1995) Interferon-alpha does not improve the antineoplastic efficacy of high-dose infusional 5-fluorouracil plus folinic acid in advanced colorectal cancer. Ann Oncol 6:461–466

59. Hill M, Norman A, Cunningham D et al (1995) Royal Marsden phase III trial of fluorouracil with or without interferon alfa-2b in advanced colorectal cancer. J Clin Oncol 13:1297–1302

60. Corfu-A Study Group (1995) Phase III randomised study of two fluorouracil combinations with either interferon alpha 2b or leucovorin for advanced colorectal cancer. J Clin Oncol 13:921–928

61. Zalchberg J, Cunningham D, Green M et al (1995) The final result of a large phase II study of the potent thymidylate synthese inhibitor TOMUDEX (ZD 1694) in advanced colorectal cancer. Proc Am Soc Clin Oncol 14:204

62. Rinaldi DA, Burris HA, Dorr FA et al (1994) A phase I evaluation of the novel thymidylate synthase inhibitor LY 231514 in patients with advanced solid tumours. Proc Am Soc Clin Oncol 13:159

63. Clendeninn NJ, Peterkin JJ, Jeffers CJ et al (1994) AG 331, a non classical, lipophilic thymidylate synthase inhibitor for the treatment of solid tumours. Ann Oncol 5:133

64. Rougier Ph, Culine S, Bougat R et al (1994) Multicentric phase II study of first line CPT 11 (linotecan) in advanced colorectal cancer: preliminary results. Proc Am Soc Clin Oncol 13:585

65. Bougat R, Rougier, Douillard JY et al (1995) Efficacy of irinotecan HCL (CPT 11) in patients with metastatic colorectal cancer after progression while receiving a 5-FU based chemotherapy. Proc Am Soc Clin Oncol 14:222

66. Pazdur R, Lassere Y, Soh LT et al (1994) Phase II trial of docetaxel (Taxotere) in metastatic colorectal carcinoma. Ann Oncol 5:468–470

67. Lokich JJ, Ahlgren J, Gullo J et al (1989) A prospective randomized comparison of continuous infusion fluorouracil with a conventional bolus schedule in metastatic colorectal carcinoma: a mid-Atlantic oncology program study. J Clin Oncol 7:425–432

68. Leichmann CG, Leichman L, Spears P et al (1993) Prolonged continuous infusion of fluorouracil with weekly bolus leucovorin: a phase II study in patients with disseminated colorectal cancer. J Natl Cancer Inst 85:41–44

69. Findlay M, Hill A, Cunningham D et al (1994) Protracted venous infusion 5-fluorouracil and interferon-α in advanced and refractory colorectal cancer. Ann Oncol 5:239–243

70. Jolivet J (1995) Role of leucovorin dosing and administration schedule. Eur J Cancer 31 A:1311–1315

71. Buter J, Harm A, Sinnige M et al (1995) 5-fluorouracil/leucovorin/interferon alpha in patients with advanced colorectal cancer. Cancer 75:1072–1076

72. Grem JL, Jordan E, Robson ME et al (1993) Phase II study of fluorouracil, leucovorin and interferon alpha in metastatic colorectal carcinoma. J Clin Oncol 11:1737–1745

73. Grem J, van Groeningen, Ismail A et al (1994) The role of interferon alpha as a modulator of fluorouracil and leucovorin. Eur J Cancer 31A:1316–1320

74. Abad A, Garcia P, Gravalos C et al (1995) Sequential methotrexate, 5-fluorouracil and high dose leucovorin versus 5-FU alone for advanced colorectal cancer. Cancer 75:1238–1244

75. Wereldsma JC, Bruggink ED, Meijer WS et al (1990) Adjuvant portal liver infusion in colorectal cancer with 5-fluorouracil/heparin versus urokinase versus control. Results of a prospective randomized clinical trial (colorectal adenocarcinoma trial I). Cancer 65:425–432

76. Beart RW Jr, Moertel CG, Wienand HS et al (1990) Adjuvant therapy for resectable colorectal carcinoma with fluorouracil administered by portal vein infusion. Arch Surg 125:897

77. Laffer U, Metzger U and Swiss Group for Clinical Cancer Research (SAKK) (1995) Long-term results of single course of adjuvant intraportal chemotherapy for colorectal cancer. Lancet 345:349–353

78. Ryan J, Heiden P, Crowley J, Bloch K (1988) Adjuvant portal vein infusion for colorectal cancer: a 3-arm randomized trial. Proc ASCO 7:361

79. Gray BN, DeZwart J, Fisher R et al (1987) The Australia and New Zealand trial of adjuvant chemotherapy in cancer. S. 537.

In Salmon SE (Hrsg.): Adjuvant therapy of cancer V. Grune & Stratton, New York

80. Fielding LP, Hittinger R, Grace RH, Fry JS (1992) Randomised controlled trial of adjuvant chemotherapy by portal-vein perfusion after curative resection for colorectal adenocarcinoma. Lancet 340:502

81. Ansfield F, Klotz J, Nealon T et al (1977) A phase III study comparing the clinical utility of four regimens of 5-fluorouracil. Cancer 39:34–40

82. Seifert P, Baker LH, Reed MD et al (1975) Comparison of continuously infused 5-fluorouracil with bolus injection in the treatment of patients with colorectal adenocarcinoma. Cancer 36:123–128

83. Hahn G, Moertel CG, Schutt AJ et al (1975) A double-blind comparison of intensive course of 5-fluorouracil by oral versus intravenous route in the treatment of colorectal cancer. Cancer 35:1031–1035

84. Hill M, Norman A, Cunningham D et al (1995) Impact of protracted venous infusion fluorouracil with or without interferon alfa-2b in tumour response, survival and quality of life in advanced colorectal cancer. J Clin Oncol 13:2317–2323

26

RECURRENT COLORECTAL CANCER

Denis C.N.K. Nyam
Heidi Nelson

Despite significant advances in postoperative adjuvant therapies, many patients still suffer from recurrent disease following bowel resection.[1,2] Although the primary goal for treating colorectal cancer should always be to reduce the risk of recurrence, using proper surgical techniques and appropriate adjuvant therapies, the curative potential for recurrent disease must also be recognized. Using postoperative surveillance programs several sites of recurrence can be detected early and treated with intent to cure. Lungs, liver, and locoregional sites are most frequently involved with recurrent disease and have the greatest potential for cure. Although much has been established regarding the potential to cure isolated hepatic and pulmonary lesions, less is known about locoregional recurrences, such as in the pelvis following treatment of rectal cancer primaries. Accordingly, although all three sites of recurrence are reviewed, a more probing discussion of locoregional recurrences is detailed below.

TUMOR RECURRENCE

Incidence

The incidence of overall recurrences for colorectal cancer is variably reported as between 25% and 50%, depending in part on the length and intensity of follow-up. Furthermore, rates of recurrence based on sites can vary depending on whether early, first sites of recurrence, or late, all sites of recurrence are reported. On the premise that salvage therapy for early recurrence favorably influences disease progression, it is logical to focus salvage efforts on first sites of recurrence. First sites of recurrence most often involve the liver, locoregional sites, or lungs (Fig. 26-1), all of which can be targeted for resective surgery. Only rarely are sites such as the ovaries, bone, anastomosis, or brain affected.

Risk Factors

A large number of factors have been associated with recurrence of colorectal cancer, including tumor-related and technical factors. Knowing the risk of recurrence presumably heightens

awareness, focuses surveillance efforts, and increases detection of early curable disease.

Tumor-Related Factors

Tumor-related factors can be considered as biologic factors, such as standard histologic features that predict tumor behavior, or as more mechanical factors, such as the local extent of disease that predicts risk of local recurrence. It has long been recognized that tumor behavior correlates with certain features of histology. Aggressive behavior is anticipated for tumors that are high grade, mucin producing, or demonstrate venous or lymphatic invasion and diminished lymphatic stromal reaction.[3] More recently molecular markers, including aneuploidy[4,5] and the presence of mutant p53[6,7] have also been found to predict aggressive tumor behavior. Extent of disease, or stage, the single most important predictive factor, indicates risk of recurrence in several ways, including the risk of systemic spread when tumor cells have been identified in regional lymph nodes, and risk of local spread when tumor cells penetrate beyond the confines of the bowel.[8] Additional indicators of risk include the presence of bowel obstruction[9] or perforation[10] and tumor perforation or local organ adherence.[11]

Technical Factors

As much as tumor location within the large bowel influences rates of recurrence for biologic reasons, it may also affect rates of recurrence for technical reasons. Tumors in the distal rectum, being more difficult to resect, typically are more often associated with local recurrences (26%) than tumors of the middle and proximal rectum (21 and 14%, respectively).[12] Further illustrating the influence of technical factors is the fact that results from rectal cancer resections are highly variable and surgeon

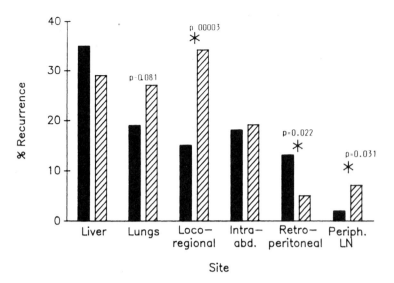

Figure 26-1. Site of first recurrence in colon (solid bars) and rectal cancer (dashed bars). (From Galandiuk et al.,[92] with permission.)

dependent, with recurrence rates ranging from a low of 4% to a high of 40%.[13–15] Although it is clear that surgical variability is important, it is not entirely clear which techniques are key determinants of outcome. It has been proposed that adequacy of excision, including mesorectal, lateral, distal, and proximal mesenteric margins, is critical.

Although all margins of excision may be important, greatest emphasis recently has been focused on mesorectal margins. Heald, who reports recurrence rates as low as 2.6% attributes

---

Factors Associated With High Risk of Recurrence for Resected Rectal Cancer

Tumor Factors

Advanced stage of disease

High grade of tumor (poorly differentiated)

Mucin production

Obstruction/perforation

Tumor location

Adjacent organ involvement

Venous invasion

Perineural invasion

Diminished lymphatic stromal reaction

Aneuploidy

Mutant p53 gene expression

Technical Factors

Incomplete excision of primary—lateral, distal, and mesorectal margins

Implantation of exfoliated cells

Tumor location (pelvis being technically more challenging)

---

his success to the technique of complete mesorectal resection.[16] The concept of reducing local recurrences using total mesorectal excision is based on the premise that microscopic tumor deposits are present within the mesorectum. Completely removing the mesorectum all the way to the pelvic floor removes the risk that residual tumor deposits can give rise to subsequent tumor nodules. That complete mesorectal resection devascularizes the distal rectum and requires distal rectal anastomosis in all cases probably accounts for the high leak rate reported by Heald and raises concern regarding functional outcomes.

Compared with mesorectal excision, less controversy has been generated in recent years on the importance of distal, lateral, and proximal mesenteric resection margins. The introduction of circular staplers and sphincter-preserving procedures caused great scrutiny of distal margins,[17,18] and now a number of clinical studies support the efficacy of 2-cm margins.[19–21] Radical lateral and proximal mesenteric margins, aimed at reducing lymphatic spread using surgical means, do not convincingly affect survival. Enthusiasm for high ligation of the inferior mesenteric vessels waned when even large series of high-risk patients could not demonstrate survival advantage for a high versus low level of inferior mesenteric ligation. The increased frequency of complications from high ligation was not balanced by cancer-related advantages.[22] Regarding radical pelvic lymphadenectomy, similar results are reported, namely, that morbidities are not balanced by measurable survival benefits.[23] Increasingly, nodal disease is being viewed as systemic disease, less in the realm of surgical treatment and more in the realm of adjuvant therapies.[1,2]

DETECTION OF RECURRENCES

Surveillance

The primary aim of postoperative surveillance, and key to improved survival in the treatment of recurrent colorectal cancers, is early detection. Although diagnosis is usually easy when

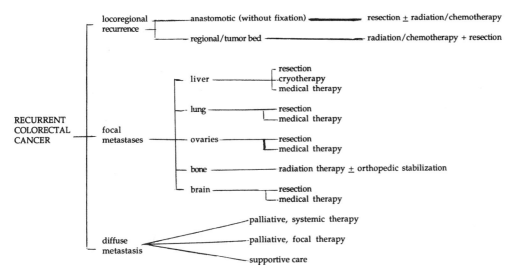

Figure 26-2. Flow chart of therapeutic options for recurrent colorectal cancer. (From Wexner and Vernava,[93] with permission.)

lesions are advanced, the challenge is to detect recurrent lesions at an early stage, when they have the greatest possible chance of cure. There are usually two stages in the evaluation of recurrent disease, namely, that of routine surveillance when disease is not clinically suspected, and assessment or confirmation of recurrent disease, when it is suspected based on symptoms or laboratory abnormalities. When surveillance detects the presence of disease, confirmatory tests should delineate the extent of disease and should differentiate between single-site locoregional or focal metastatic (resectable) and diffuse (nonresectable) disease (Fig. 26-2). This algorithm summarizes our clinical approach to recurrent disease, the details of which are described below.

A number of surveillance programs aimed at detecting early recurrence have been described[24–26]; unfortunately, no general agreement exists on which program is the least costly and most effective. The accompanying box outlines surveillance studies most commonly performed. Although it is beyond the scope of this text to debate the merits of different surveillance programs, the authors suggest that surveillance efforts should be focused on those sites that are most frequently affected and amenable to curative resection. With the rationale outlined below, sites that should be targeted for detection of asymptomatic lesions include liver, lung, and locoregional sites.

History and Physical Examination

As is true for most patient contacts, the surveillance evaluation should start with identification of symptoms. Symptoms that might suggest recurrence include abdominal, pelvic, perineal, or sciatic pain, change in bowel habits, obstruction, anorexia, weight loss, malaise, and rectal bleeding or discharge. It is unfortunate that many of these symptoms indicate late-stage disease, beyond hope of cure. It is also discouraging to note that these symptoms often develop between routine cancer checks. In a follow-up of 180 patients over 15 years, involving 2,319 visits, only 42% of recurrences were detected during visits, and the rest were detected in between visits, as a result of new

symptoms.[27] Since results for salvage surgery are generally better for patients who are symptom free, detecting recurrent disease prior to symptom development is considered ideal. Physical examination, which is of limited value in most asymptomatic patients, may in rare cases be revealing for advanced disease, such as node-positive disease or the presence of a mass in the abdomen, rectum, vagina, or perineum. Even if the examination does not detect recurrence, it always provides valuable information regarding the overall health status of the patient, a key determining factor for selecting candidates for resective surgery.

Laboratory Studies

Routine blood counts, blood chemistries, and chest x-rays are low in cost but also low in yield. Rarely anemia will indicate bleeding from a new primary or recurrent lesion. Liver function tests are rarely elevated; such elevations are often indicative of extensive hepatic metastases.[28,29] The chest x-ray is the most logical of the group since it potentially detects asymptomatic, but resectable lesions.

Endoscopy

Endoscopy provides the opportunity to detect metachronous lesions[30,31] and anastomotic recurrences.[14,15] It is generally not practical or cost effective to perform colonoscopy more often than once a year for proximal bowel resections, but it is reasonable to perform frequent proctosigmoidoscopic examinations for rectal resection cases. The mucosal aspect of the anastomosis may be abnormal, or there may be a suggestion of an underlying, extraluminal recurrence. As is discussed below, pelvic recurrences following rectal resection frequently occur outside the lumen of the bowel since the mesorectum rather than the bowel is the origin of the recurrence.

Carcinoembryonic Antigen

With the intent of simplifying surveillance, the carcinoembryonic antigen (CEA) test was introduced long ago as a serologic marker, an acclaimed indicator of disease. It was proposed that

---

Detection and Evaluation of Recurrence in Colorectal Cancer

Currently Recommended Surveillance Studies

History

Physical examination (abdomen, nodes, rectum, and vagina)

Complete blood count

Chemistries (liver function tests)

Endoscopy

± CEA

± CT scan

Site-Directed Surveillance Studies (under consideration)

History

Physical examination

Chest x-ray

Endoscopy

Hepatic ultrasound

Confirmation Studies

Locoregional Recurrence

CT scan pelvis

Biopsy—CT-guided or endoscopic or transrectal/transvaginal

± Endorectal ultrasound

± Magnetic resonance imaging

Hepatic Metastases

CT scan abdomen

Hepatic ultrasound

± Hepatic angiogram (not routine)

Intraoperative ultrasound

Pulmonary Metastases

CT chest

Under Investigation

Radiolabeled anti-tumor antibody scan

Endorectal coil

Magnetic resonance imaging

Abbreviations: CEA, carcinoembryonic antigen; CT, computed tomography.

---

frequent CEA monitoring, every 4 to 6 weeks for the first 2 years and every 8 to 10 weeks for the next 3 years, would indicate the presence of recurrence before it was otherwise clinically detected.[32] In fact, rising CEA levels do indicate the presence of local and hepatic recurrence before they are otherwise clinically apparent, with median lead times of 6 and 3.5 months, respectively.[32–34] It was also proposed that CEA levels would provide information on sites of recurrence that are not readily examined with standard imaging modalities, such as local recurrences. In fact, serial elevations of CEA levels indicate abdominal recurrence of large bowel carcinoma in 85 to 90% of cases.[34] Although CEA monitoring has some clinical merit, a number of limitations deserve discussion.

As is true for all tests, clinical utility is determined by sensitivity, specificity, practicality, and impact on outcome. Although rising CEA levels generally indicate the presence of recurrent disease, with a sensitivity of between 86 and 94%,[35,36] normal CEA values are not reassuring since the specificity of CEA is only between 58 and 66%.[33,35] Furthermore, whether CEA monitoring significantly impacts survival is subject to debate. Advocates report that CEA-directed second-look surgery detects recurrence in 95% of cases with resection for cure in 81% of cases[32] and 5-year survival rates of 31%.[37] By contrast, others have reported that CEA monitoring detected disseminated disease but was of little value in detecting locally recurrent disease.[38] Although early detection using CEA levels is established for some centers, none have yet convincingly demonstrated survival advantage for CEA-based surveillance.[39] In a limited retrospective evaluation comparing standard oncologic follow-up with and without CEA monitoring, Moertel and colleagues[40] demonstrated no survival advantage for those in the CEA follow-up group. Results from a multicenter trial in the United Kingdom should be available soon to resolve this issue.[34]

In conclusion, the goal for any surveillance program should be early detection of resectable disease. It is the opinion of the authors that surveillance efforts should be focused on (1) patients who are suitable surgical candidates; (2) tumors of favorable prognosis (i.e., slow-growing, presenting at least 1 year after primary resection); and (3) sites of disease amenable to resection for cure — hepatic, pulmonary, and locoregional sites.

LOCOREGIONAL RECURRENCE

Local recurrence, for reasons outlined above, is most likely to occur following rectal rather than colon cancer resection. This section of the text addresses diagnostic and therapeutic strategies for locally recurrent rectal cancer, recognizing that these principles can be applied as well to recurrent colon cancer.

Isolated locoregional disease accounts for 5% to 19% of colon recurrences and 7% to 33% of rectal recurrences, with between 7% and 20% considered resectable for curative intent.[12,41,42] According to the natural history, patients with locally recurrent rectal cancer live a median of 7 months, with only rare patients (less than 4%) living for 5 years.[43] The use of radiation therapy alone in this setting provides temporary relief of symptoms of approximately 6 months duration.[44] Although radiation alone prolongs survival (for a median of 10 to 17 months), it offers no chance for cure.[45,46] By contrast, when complete resection of locally recurrent disease is possible, mean survivals of 33 to 59 months and long-term 5-year survival rates of about 30% can be expected.[47,48] The opportunity to provide effective palliation and the possibility of cure in patients with locally recurrent rectal cancer deserve further discussion.

Patients with locally recurrent rectal cancer without gross evidence of extrapelvic cancer represent a complex challenge. Locoregional recurrences are often technically difficult to access, involve multiple organs or structures, and consequently require extensive resection to accomplish negative margins. Whereas it is often possible to effect palliation with these surgeries, this should not be the primary goal of surgery. Only rarely is palliative surgery indicated for control of refractory bleeding or sepsis. In all other cases, it should be the intent of surgery to accomplish gross and microscopic total resection. Whether total resection can be achieved with acceptable morbidity and mortality is determined by several factors, including the patient's overall fitness, the status of extrapelvic sites of disease, and finally the extent of local disease. Each of these aspects must be investigated before resection is considered.

Preoperative Evaluation and Patient Selection

General Health

When salvage surgery is contemplated, the patient should be in good general health, have technically resectable disease, have no extrapelvic disease, and have expressed willingness and interest in pursuing aggressive therapy. At the start, the patient should undergo a general health assessment. Such extensive treatment with preoperative radiation therapy and chemotherapy followed by extensive reresective surgery is not appropriate for patients who are in poor health (American Society of Anesthesiology classification IV–V).[49,50] The magnitude of the undertaking for reresection should be thoroughly understood by patient and physician alike. Appropriately, all patients do not desire such aggressive therapies.

Excluding Extrapelvic Disease

Once the patient is considered fit for surgery, it should further be established, by physical examination and laboratory tests, whether the patient has isolated locoregional disease. Extrapelvic disease can be assessed by performing computed tomography (CT) of the abdomen and pelvis in addition to standard surveillance tests, as described above. For an equivocal chest x-ray or abdominal CT scan, a chest CT or liver ultrasound, respectively, can be obtained. These tests are not, however, routine. The evaluation for extrapelvic disease is usually performed twice, once at the initiation of preoperative radiation and chemotherapy and again just prior to resective surgery. This strategy provides some measure of assurance that patients with aggressive metastasizing tumors will be identified preoperatively and therefore not be subjected to surgery.

Confirming Local Disease

It is usually straightforward to establish that the patient is fit for surgery and free of extrapelvic disease. By contrast, it is often challenging to establish that the pelvic lesion is present and resectable for cure. Confirming the diagnosis with biopsies and determining the extent of disease requires a careful physical examination of the rectum and vagina, supplemented with endoscopy and radiologic studies, including at least a pelvic CT scan and occasionally a magnetic resonance image. Since alterations in pelvic anatomy are commonplace following rectal surgery, it is often difficult to differentiate postoperative change from tumor. There are basically three ways postoperative

change can be distinguished from tumor. The first is to notice change, such as enlargement, over time; the second is to note invasion of local organs; and the third is to perform CT-guided biopsies of suspicious tissues, which is especially useful when the patient has new-onset pelvic symptoms. CT-guided biopsy may not be required if there is a luminal or mucosal component, in which case the lesion can be biopsied endoscopically. For extraluminal lesions that are palpable per rectum or vagina, biopsies can be obtained using a transrectal or transvaginal needle biopsy technique.

We have generally had the good fortune of being able to document the presence of disease histologically using one of these three methods. Despite these approaches it is still possible to miss the diagnosis. If pelvic disease is suspected, because of rising CEA or worsening symptoms, histologic proof should be sought, but exploratory pelvic surgery should be discouraged. Confidently excluding the possibility of pelvic recurrence using exploratory surgery requires that the entire pelvis be explored to the level of the levators. Risks of such surgery are prohibitive due to scarring and the close proximity to other organs. Also, it is often quite difficult to distinguish scar from tumor even at surgery. Whereas some tumors produce nodular recurrences with defined anatomic limits, others produce more infiltrative sheets, with tumor cells distributed within fibrous tissue.

Determining Extent of Disease/Resectability

Locoregional recurrences of rectal tumors can include anterior, posterior, and/or lateral pelvic recurrences and due to location can involve intestinal, urologic, gynecologic, bone, or vascular structures. Since any of these pelvic structures alone, or in combination, can be involved, it is nearly impossible to discuss such cases and compare results without having some defined classification scheme. Several schema have been described, including one proposed by Philipsen[51] whereby tumors are categorized according to whether they are (1) anastomotic, arising in and contained within the bowel; (2) perianastomotic, in proximity or involving anastomosis by extension of disease with inward invasion; (3) perineal, in the perineal scar following abdominoperineal resection; (4) on the pelvic wall, fixed to bone, major blood vessels, and/or nerves, usually precluding resection for cure; or (5) in the anterior genitourinary region,

---

Resection of Locally Recurrent Rectal Cancer: Contraindications

Extrapelvic disease

Sciatic pain

Bilateral ureteral obstruction

Circumferential or extensive pelvic side-wall involvement

S1 or S2 involvement (bony or neural)

Poor general condition and surgical risk (ASA IV–V and rare ASA III)

requiring anterior exenteration. Unfortunately, local recurrences generally defy such clean and singularly distinct categories.

Another classification schema, proposed by Suzuki, and colleagues,[47] categorizes extent of disease based on degree of fixation: F0 indicates no sites of fixation, and F1 to F3 indicates one to three sites of fixation, respectively. To our way of thinking, two factors are important; fixation, which indicates resectability, and anatomic location, which indicates organs/structures requiring resection (Fig. 26-3). We have chosen, therefore, to modify the fixation schema of Suzuki to indicate whether

the disease is not fixed (F0), fixed but resectable (FR), or fixed and not resectable (FNR). Further noting anatomic sites of fixation allows for determination of the extent of resection. Whereas lesions without fixation can be simply resected, fixed, resectable lesions may require partial or complete cystectomy or hysterectomy (in the case of anterior fixation) or sacrectomy (in the case of posterior fixation) (Fig. 26-3).

With or without a classification schema, it is not always possible to determine resectability prior to surgery. However, a few findings reliably predict that curative resection is not possible. Bilateral ureteral obstruction is one such finding. Unless a dis-

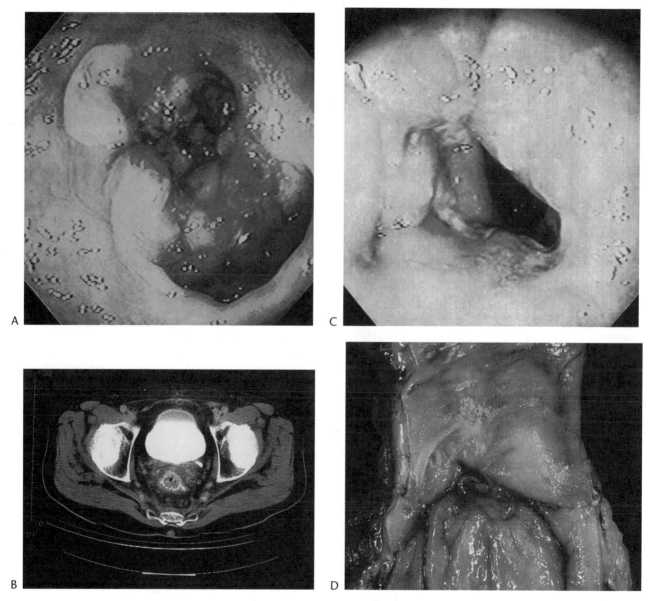

Figure 26-3. Classification of Recurrent Rectal Cancers. FO: Primary T3N1M0 rectal cancer treated with a low anterior resection without adjuvant therapy. (**A**) An anastomotic recurrence with no external fixation was found (CT scan) (**B**) on follow-up proctoscopy examination (left endoscopy plate). (**C**) Following a course of external beam and chemotherapy (right endoscopy plate), (**D**) a completion abdominoperineal resection and IOERT were performed. *(Figure continues.)*

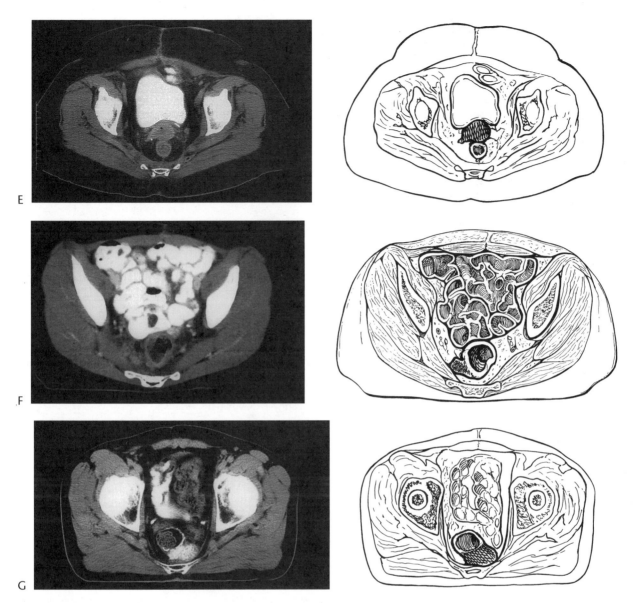

Figure 26-3. *(Continued)* **(E) FR (anterior):** A primary T3N0M0 rectal cancer was treated with low anterior resection without adjuvant therapy. The anterior recurrent tumor fixed at the base of the bladder was treated with preoperative chemoirradiation and then resection with IOERT. **(F) FR (lateral):** Following a primary low anterior resection for T2N0M0 rectal adenocarcinoma without adjuvant therapy this patient developed a lateral pelvic recurrence. After receiving a full course of external beam plus chemotherapy she underwent completion abdominal perineal resection with negative margins. **(G) F-R (posterior):** Recurrence after a T3N0M0 lesion with postoperative chemoradiation therapy, now invading the sacrum. After a course of external beam plus chemotherapy, IOERT was given after an en bloc resection of the tumor and distal sacrum was accomplished with negative margins. *(Figure continues.)*

tal, central lesion near the trigone is blocking both ureters, bilateral obstruction is usually indicative of bulky, unresectable disease at the level of the pelvic inlet. Any evidence of circumferential tumor or extensive pelvic side-wall tumor indicates unresectable disease. Finally, sciatic, S1, or S2 nerve root involvement or S1 or S2 sacral bone involvement is not resectable. Sciatic pain, typically unilateral, indicates sciatic nerve involvement. Occasionally this pain results from nerve

compression rather than nerve invasion, and complete resolution may follow initiation of treatment with radiation and chemotherapy. Wide resection is rarely possible for lesions associated with persistent sciatic pain. Perineal and buttock pain are less ominous symptoms. Sacrectomy proximal to S2 results in sacroiliac joint instability. Whereas stabilization with internal fixation is technically feasible, it is not warranted in cases of locally recurrent rectal cancer.

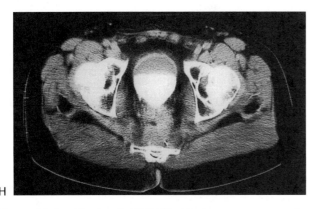
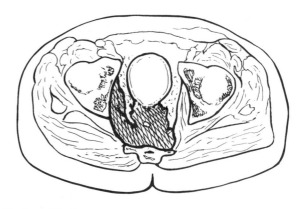

H

Figure 26-3. *(Continued).* **(H) F-NR:** Massive recurrent cancer found in the pelvis after an abdominoperineal resection for a T3N1M0 tumor with a full course of postoperative chemoirradiation. The tumor was fixed to vital pelvic organs and was unresectable.

Multimodality Therapy for Locally Recurrent Rectal Cancer

For locally recurrent rectal cancer, the mainstay of treatment with curative intent is surgery. Having stated that, local and systemic failure rates are high with surgery alone, suggesting a role for radiation therapy and chemotherapy, respectively.[52]

Preoperative Radiation Therapy and Chemotherapy

As stated above, radiation therapy when administered alone provides temporary relief of symptoms but does not offer a chance of cure. However, when radiation therapy is combined with surgery for locally advanced primary rectal tumors, local recurrence rates are reduced and resectability rates increased.[53–56] In the same manner, radiation therapy can be employed in the setting of locally recurrent rectal cancer. The recent demonstration of added benefit from combined radiation therapy and fluorouracil chemotherapy prompts us to use the same basic regimen to reduce local and systemic failures.[1,56] To reduce the risk of local recurrence further while avoiding dose-related toxicities, we combine external beam radiation preoperative radiation therapy plus chemotherapy with intraoperative electron radiation therapy (IOERT), the results of which are discussed below. IOERT offers the advantages of localized tumor-directed therapy, limited normal tissue exposure, single-fraction high biologic equivalence, and improved control for high-risk sites.

Patients with local recurrence who have not undergone previous pelvic radiation therapy receive a full course of external beam radiotherapy (5,040 cGy) in conjunction with 5-fluorouracil (5-FU). Since maximum synergy between external and intraoperative radiation therapy is accomplished within an 8-week period, patients are restaged and taken for surgery and IOERT within 4 to 8 weeks following completion of external beam and chemotherapy treatments. Patients with local recurrence who received adjuvant postoperative radiation therapy as part of their primary tumor treatment are treated with low-dose (2,000 cGy) preoperative radiation plus 5-FU-based chemotherapy, when possible. When low-dose radiation therapy is used, surgery can be scheduled within 1 to 2 weeks.

Multimodality Therapy for Locally Recurrent Cancers

General Evaluation

Healthy (ASA I–III)

Disease-Specific Evaluation: Initial Staging

Exclude extrapelvic disease or contraindications

Confirm local disease (histology)

Determine extent of disease
  F0: Not fixed
  FR: Fixed resectable, indicate anatomic site
  FNR: Fixed nonresectable

Multimodality Preoperative Therapies

No previous radiation—5,040 cGy external beam + 5-fluorouracil intravenous

Previous radiation—2,000 cGy external beam + 5-fluorouracil intravenous

Restaging

Reevaluate after chemoradiation for metastases

Surgery

Ureteral stents

Laparotomy

Mobilization, colectomy, colostomy

± Hysterectomy

± Cystectomy, partial or complete

± Sacrectomy

Frozen section margins

Intraoperative electron radiation therapy

Pelvic reconstruction
  Omentum
  Rectus abdominus flap

Surgery

Before embarking on reresective pelvic surgery, it is essential that the patient and family members understand the magnitude of the planned procedure. In our practice, sphincter-preserving surgery is not indicated in cases of local failure; therefore, patients must be willing to accept a permanent colostomy. Those with anterior or posterior fixation must understand the consequences of an ileal conduit or sacrectomy, respectively. Patients are admitted the night before surgery for mechanical and antibiotic bowel preparation, intravenous hydration, and preoperative pulmonary teaching.

At our institution essentially all cases of locally recurrent rectal cancer are scheduled in a dedicated IOERT suite. This suite, within operative room facilities, houses a linear accelerator, standard operating room equipment, and special anesthesia equipment that facilitates moving from operating to radiating positions (Fig. 26-4). For pelvic cases, patients are placed in the legs-up position. Special care must be taken to ensure that the lower extremities are not resting on the stirrups since compartment syndrome can occur during these long procedures.[57] Under cystoscopic guidance, bilateral ureteral stents are placed at the beginning of the case. Abnormalities of the bladder may be appreciated at the time of cystoscopic stent placement.

The abdomen is opened using a lower midline incision. If a rectus abdominus flap is anticipated, care must be taken to preserve epigastric vessels during the celiotomy. Adhesions are typically present and must be lysed to allow full abdominal exploration. Careful examination of the liver, peritoneal surfaces, retroperitoneum, and wound should be performed to establish the absence of extrapelvic disease, which would contraindicate radical resection. Rarely, in very young patients with limited pelvic disease, liver metastases and pelvic recurrence have simultaneously been resected, but this is the exception rather than the rule.

A self-retaining oval or circular retractor is used to retract the wound edges laterally and the bladder inferiorly; then the small bowel is packed into the upper abdomen to facilitate pelvic exposure. It is typical to find pelvic fibrosis, and for this reason the pelvic dissection is commenced at the level of the aortic bifurcation. Ureters and iliac vessels are dissected from the level of the pelvic brim to the side-walls; this allows safe dissection in the posterior pelvis along the sacrum. It is generally necessary to trace the ureters all the way to their insertion into the bladder, which allows safe lateral dissection in a reoperative pelvis. When sacrectomy or cystectomy is required, the ureters are actually dissected for their entire pelvic length, to prevent injury from the posterior dissection, or to allow insertion into an ileal conduit, respectively.

Nonfixed Lesions

Completion abdominoperineal resection, for F0 lesions following low anterior resection, is performed in a manner nearly identical to standard abdominoperineal resection. The only difference typically is the ease of dissection, which is more difficult due to fibrosis and alterations in anatomic relations. As is true for all locally recurrent rectal cancer cases, it is often difficult to distinguish between normal scar and tumor-infiltrated scar. When fibrosis is encountered, particularly in areas that are outside the realm of possible resection, such as along the sacral promontory or high along the lateral side-walls, frozen section should be obtained. If diffuse, dense pelvic fibrosis is present within the pelvis and tumor cells are identified within samples of the fibrosis by frozen section, complete resection is not feasible.

Fixed-Resectable, Posterior Lesions

Posterior fixation (FR) is best managed by distal sacrectomy. As discussed above, the proximal limit of sacral resection is around the S2–3 junction. Removing portions of sacrum proxi-

Figure 26-4. The IOERT suite, showing the equipment, operating room table, and linear accelerator.

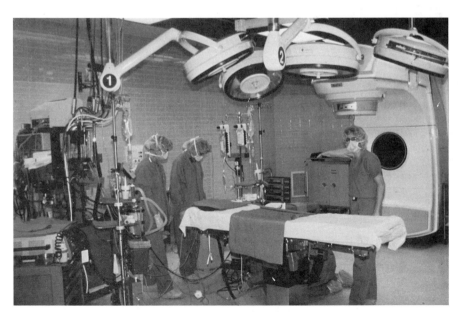

mal to S2 requires elaborate internal fixation and reconstructive procedures for sacroiliac stability; this is beyond what is reasonable for locally recurrent rectal cancer. Furthermore, preserving one S3 nerve root is generally sufficient to preserve bladder function.

Distal sacrectomy, performed in four consecutive stages, includes anterior procedures, posterior procedures, IOERT, and pelvic reconstruction. As described above, anterior procedures are performed using the legs-up position. The exploration is completed before the pelvis is entered. To avoid inadvertent injury from anatomic displacement, the ureters and iliac vessels are dissected starting at the level of the aortic bifurcation (Fig. 26-5A) and extending deep into the pelvis. Anterior and lateral

lines of resection are delineated, and adherent organs or structures are dissected and removed en bloc with the posterior-based tumor. The posterior dissection stops just proximal to the level of fixation. Frozen section biopsies, at this point, will help to determine whether the lesion is resectable and will establish the site at which a negative sacral margin can be accomplished. This maneuver facilitates ease of completing the posterior sacral transsection.

Once resectability is established, the anterior and lateral pelvic dissections are completed, so that only the posterior tumor-sacral attachments remain. Next, internal iliac artery and vein ligation is performed to reduce blood loss when sacral transection proximal to the S3–S4 junction is anticipated (Fig. 26-5B).

Figure 26-5. Pelvic dissection of iliac vessels. (**A**) Broad view of dissected iliac vessels. (**B**) Vein dissection and ligation are accomplished prior to S3 sacral transection to minimize blood loss.

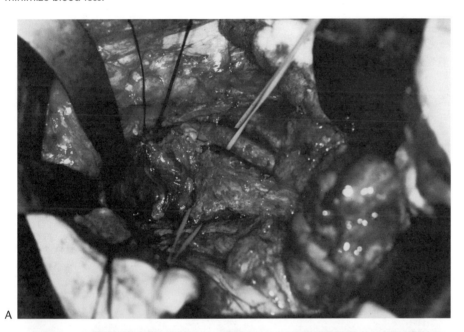

A

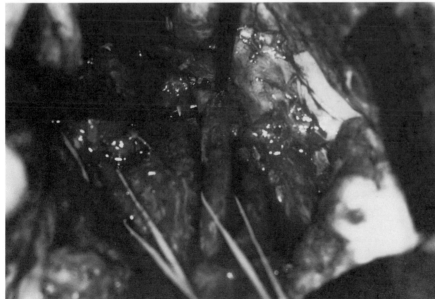

B

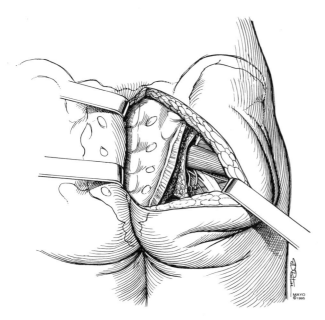

Figure 26-6. Posterior sacrectomy exposure. (From Magrini et al.,[59] by permission of Mayo Foundation).

Finally, before closing the abdomen, gastrointestinal and/or urinary stomas are fashioned, as required, and either the omentum or rectus abdominus flap are mobilized and placed in the pelvis for subsequent pelvic reconstruction.

The patient is repositioned flex-prone, and a posterior midline incision is made. The gluteus is dissected from the sacrum to facilitate exposure and allow for division of the sacrotuberous and sacrospinous ligaments (Fig. 26-6). The pyriformis muscle is divided while the sciatic and pudendal nerves are protected. At this time the endopelvic fascia is entered, and, by palpation from behind, the level of sacral transection can be identified. While the orthopedic surgeon performs the laminectomy, dural sac ligation, and bony transsection, the pelvic surgeon assists in the final dissection of the lateral pelvic side-walls to protect the ureters, bladder, urethra, and sciatic nerve from injury. It is occasionally necessary to sacrifice lateral sacrospinous ligament attachments to accomplish clear lateral margins. Intraoperative radiation therapy and closure are performed as described below.

Fixed-Resectable, Anterior Lesions

The extent of resection required for anterior fixation depends on whether the patient has a uterus or a rectum, or both. Usually the presence of a uterus ensures that the bladder will not be tumor adherent. By contrast, when there is no uterus or rectum, such as in the male who has previously undergone abdomino-perineal resection, there is a much greater likelihood that the bladder will be involved with tumor. If the tumor is confined to a portion of the bladder that can be sacrificed and primarily repaired, then partial cystectomy will suffice. Having said that, caution should be exercised when primary repair of a radiated bladder is being considered. If the tissues are poor, it may be safer to remove the entire bladder. When the trigone or prostate

are tumor involved, cystectomy and an ileal conduit are required.

Intraoperative Electron Radiation Therapy

The resected specimen and additional patient-side biopsies, as required, are reviewed with the pathologist and radiation oncologist to determine margins and the need for IOERT. When IOERT is required, a lucite cylinder is placed into the pelvis to expose tissues at risk, and the patient is repositioned beneath the linear accelerator (Fig. 26-7). Doses of between 1,000 and 2,000 cGy to one or more fields are delivered, depending on the extent of margin involvement. Typically, a dose of 1,000 cGy is recommended for minimal residual disease, 1,500 cGy for gross residual disease of 2 cm or less, and 2,000 cGy for unresected or gross residual disease of 2 cm or more. These single-dose radiation treatments are biologically equivalent to two to three times the same quantity delivered as external beam fractions. As an example, when combined with an external beam dose of 4,500 to 5,000 cGy delivered in 18 fractions over 5 weeks, single IOERT boost doses of 1,000 cGy, 1,500 cGy, and 2,000 cGy produce effective combined doses of 6,500 to 8,000 cGy, 7,500 to 9,500 cGy, and 8,500 to 11,000 cGy, respectively.[44]

Perineal Wound Closure

Finally, each procedure is completed by closing the perineal wound over drains. Since residual pelvic defects are often quite sizable and are tissues of poor quality due to radiation therapy, some type of flap should be used to partition the pelvis separate from the perineum. If the omentum is not of suitable size or consistency, the rectus abdominus flap should be used. The rectus is especially preferred for sacrectomy wounds, since it not only fills the pelvic dead space, but it also provides a fresh, nonradiated, vascularized skin paddle for closing the perineum (Fig. 26-8). The rectus abdominus can also be used to enlarge the vagina, when narrowing or shortening occurs as a result of extensive resection.

Results

Results from the multimodality approach to locally recurrent rectal cancer have recently been published for 224 patients treated at the Mayo Clinic from 1981 to 1988.[58] Forty-eight of these patients were found to have extrapelvic disease before or during surgery for local recurrence. An additional 106 patients underwent surgery with intent to cure, but due to the presence of residual tumor were designated as "palliative" resections. Finally, 70 patients had potentially "curative" resections, with tumor-free histopathologic margins. Results from palliative and curative resections were reported independently.[47,58]

When the palliative (n = 106) and curative (n = 70) groups are compared, it is perhaps not surprising that patients in the curative group presented sooner and less often with symptoms and fixation.[47] The interval from primary surgery to surgery for recurrence was 18.9 months in the curative group and 29.4 months in the palliative group. Patients in the curative group were more likely to be asymptomatic (36%) or symptomatic

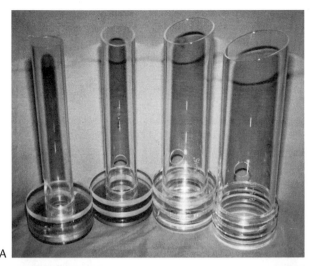

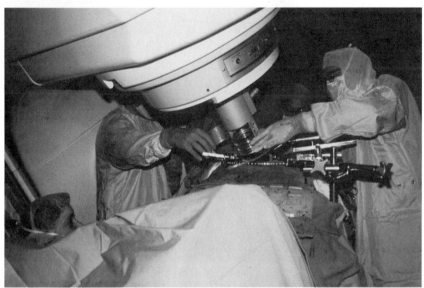

Figure 26-7. Intraoperative electron beam radiation therapy is accomplished (**A**) using lucite cylinders of differnt sizes and bevels to (**B**) focus the electron beam from the linear accelerator.

without pain (36%) than symptomatic with pain (29%). Conversely, patients in the palliative group were less likely to be asymptomatic (11%) or symptomatic without pain (13%) and more likely to be symptomatic with pain (75%). Fixation showed the same trend: no or single-site fixation was present in 65 and 20%, respectively, of curative patients and only 3 and 40%, respectively, of palliative patients. Consequently, intraoperative radiation therapy was more often delivered in the palliative group (40%) than in the curative group (7%).

Morbidity

Although operative deaths are rare (1%), complications are not uncommon following multimodality therapy, with a total of 38 palliative patients (36%) and 14 curative patients (22%) suffering severe complications.[47] Frequently occurring complications included pelvic abscess, small bowel obstruction, fistula formation, perineal wound problems, and ureteral obstruction. That extent of resection generally correlates with rate and severity of complications was observed in the curative group (30% for extended versus 17% for limited resections). Similarly, in the palliative group, the rate of severe complications was higher for those receiving intraoperative radiation therapy and highest for those with two or three sites of fixation. When patients undergoing sacrectomy (n = 16) were analyzed and reported separately, the complication rate was as high as 50%, with most morbidities related to the posterior wound.[59]

Cancer Outcomes

As might be anticipated, patients with disease amenable to curative resection have better cancer outcomes (34% 5-year survival) than patients with residual disease (12% 5-year survival).[58] Five-year survival was further influenced by the extent of residual disease, with rates of 33% for minimal residual versus 9% for gross residual. In addition to extent of resection, factors associated with improved 5-year survival figures in univariate analysis included the use of intraoperative radiation therapy, asymptomatic patient status, lack of fixation, and favorable preoperative Eastern Cooperative Oncology Group status.[47,58]

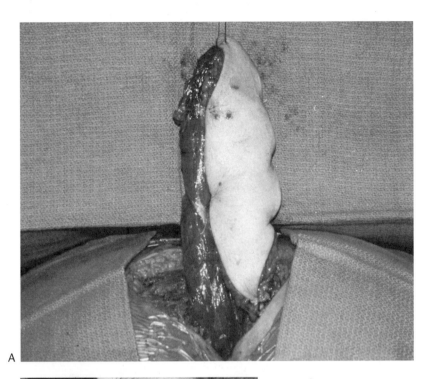

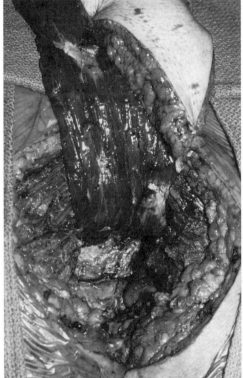

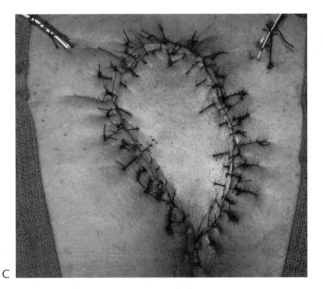

Figure 26-8.   The rectus abdominis flap (**A**) including muscle and skin paddle (**B**) fills the pelvic defect and (**C**) provides well-vascularized, nonradiated skin to ensure perineal healing. (From Magrini et al.,[59] with permission.)

Even though the use of intraoperative radiation therapy was associated with a lower rate of local progression in patients with gross residual disease, this component of multimodality therapy has not been tested in a controlled, prospective manner. However, based on retrospective studies, it appears that intraoperative radiation therapy does provide good local control, with failure rates as low as 2% within the IOERT field compared with 17% within the external field.[60] That many patients eventually fail due to distant metastases (39%) raises concern that new adjuvants are essential.[60] Since these tumors often recur during or following standard adjuvant chemotherapy, new reagents with different mechanisms of activity should be considered.

Finally, patients with local tumor recurrence often have disabling symptoms of pain, bleeding, and/or tenesmus, and the role of multimodality therapy and reresective surgery in controlling or relieving these symptoms should not be disregarded. Although we do not recommend palliative surgery for lesions that are considered unresectable preoperatively, except in rare cases of refractory bleeding or sepsis, it is evident from the reports described above that curative intent surgery is often in fact palliative. Although median survivals are longer with multimodality therapy, those patients left with gross residual disease still have a low probability of long-term survival benefit. Whether multimodality therapy provides effective palliation in such patients is difficult to know, but evidence shows that, at least in the sacrectomy group, patients benefit from relief of symptoms. When surveyed with questionnaire follow-up, eight of nine alive patients in the sacrectomy series reported reduction in pain and improved quality of life; six of these patients returned to work.[59] More rigid quality of life evaluations are warranted before definitive statements can be made regarding the value of multimodality therapy in long-term palliation.

Summary

Patients in generally good health who are found to have isolated locally recurrent tumors, may be candidates for multimodality therapy with external beam radiation therapy, chemotherapy, reresection, and IOERT. Degree of tumor fixation and anatomic location determine not only the extent of resection, including the necessity for anterior or posterior exenteration, but also the possibility of cure. Resections with negative margins or microscopic residual disease treated with IOERT are associated with acceptable 5-year survival rates.

DISTANT, RESECTABLE METASTASES

Hepatic Metastases

The liver is the most common site of recurrence following large bowel resection for malignancy. Untreated liver metastases from primary colorectal cancer are associated with a poor prognosis, with a median survival of 6 months to a year.[28,61] That there are occasional 5-year survivors, however, indicates that survival may be influenced by a number of factors. Indeed, length of survival appears to be influenced by both tumor and patient factors. Tumors that are poorly differentiated, extensive within the liver, or involve extrahepatic sites are associated with a worse prognosis.[28,62] In the same manner, patient factors that adversely affect outcome include hepatomegaly, liver dysfunc-

tion, abnormal performance status, and weight loss of greater than 10%.[63] Certainly patients presenting late, with extensive disease and in poor health, are likely not to benefit from aggressive therapeutic interventions. By contrast, many therapeutic options have been described for the more salvageable patients, those with limited hepatic disease.

The only therapy that has produced meaningful long-term survivors is that of hepatic resection. Fluorouracil-based chemotherapy regimens have prolonged median survival and improved quality of life but rarely produced 5-year survivors.[64] It is unfortunate that most patients with hepatic metastases have widespread disease, but it is fortunate that those who have resectable disease can expect a 25 to 37% chance of 5-year survival.

Patient Evaluation and Selection for Resection

In general, potential candidates for hepatic resection should have a good clinical performance, nearly normal liver function, and metastatic disease confined to the liver. As described above, imaging studies can be used to exclude the presence of extrahepatic disease and to determine the extent of liver metastases. Although interinstitutional variability exists as far as imaging preferences for hepatic disease, most would agree that both abdominal CT and ultrasound are useful for delineating the number and location of lesions and their proximity to vital structures. At the Mayo Clinic, angiography is rarely indicated; by contrast, intraoperative ultrasound is routinely employed.

In the initial experience with liver resection for colorectal secondaries, there was controversy over how the number and location of lesions affected prognosis and resectability. It is now becoming clear that resection is indicated if imaging confirms isolated hepatic lesions that are potentially resectable with tumor-free resection margins (1 to 2 cm). The type of resection is dictated by the site, size, and number of metastases.

Timing of Resection—Immediate Versus Delayed

Hepatic metastases can present during the management of the primary tumor or during the surveillance period. Metastases detected pre- or intraoperatively should be assessed before resection is performed, since the operative risk is increased when colectomy is combined with a major hepatic resection. Synchronous hepatic resection should only be done if the primary disease and any regional disease is completely resected and no residual extrahepatic disease is present. A small peripheral solitary metastasis that can be safely and simply excised should be resected at the time of colectomy, to spare the patient a second surgery. More complex disease, detected intraoperatively, should be subjected to a formal postoperative assessment. Treatment is deferred in this case until full recovery from colectomy is accomplished. The timing of hepatic resection should be individualized according to the patient and tumor status. In some cases the waiting period (up to 3 months) is revealing for disease progression or other features of unresectability.

Results of Surgical Resection

Surgery for isolated hepatic metastases remains the only treatment modality with the potential for cure. With better knowledge of liver anatomy and improved surgical techniques and

Table 26-1. Results of Hepatic Resection for Colorectal Metastases

Author	No. of Patients	Operative Mortality (%)	5-Year Survival (%)	Median Survival (months)
Hughes et al., 1988[66]	859	—	33	—
Stephenson et al., 1988[84]	55	0	30	40
Schlag et al., 1990[85]	122	4	30	32
Doci et al., 1991[86]	100	5	30	28
Petrelli et al., 1991[87]	62	8	27	25
Scheele et al., 1991[61]	219	6	37	—
Vogt et al., 1991[88]	36	0	20	29
Lind et al., 1992[89]	50	9	28	26
Nakamura et al., 1992[90]	31	3	45	28
Nordlinger et al., 1992[91]	1818	2.4	25	—
Rosen et al., 1992[65]	280	4	25	34

perioperative care, hepatic resection can be accomplished with low mortality and measurable cancer success with 5-year survival rates ranging from a low of 20% to a high of 45% (Table 26-1). Such favorable results are reported not only for single institution experiences, but also for multicenter collective experiences. That long-term survival can only be achieved with resection, not systemic therapies, has led to the progressive expansion of surgical indications to include multiple and bilateral metastases.[65] The ultimate outcome following hepatic resection depends on many variables. Tumor variables influencing survival are number (three or less) and size of metastases, type of hepatic resection, stage of the primary carcinoma, disease-free interval, and distribution of metastases.[66,67] The most important determinants of long-term outcome include the absence of extrahepatic disease and the ability to accomplish complete resection, with greater than 1-cm margins. As stated previously, if complete resection is not anticipated or if extrahepatic disease is identified based on preoperative studies, hepatic resection is contraindicated. Finally, high CEA levels and aneuploid DNA status correlate with poor survival, whereas normal clinical performance correlates with prolonged survival.

Adjuvant Chemotherapy After Hepatic Resection

Even though a number of patients will live beyond 5 years following hepatic resection, many patients will fail due to systemic or hepatic recurrence. Although rare patients will be given a second chance with reresection for hepatic metastases, this is not feasible for most patients.[68,69] Ideally, in this high-risk setting, adjuvant systemic therapy should follow surgery, but unfortunately prospective studies have not shown that such therapies impact survival. This lack of effect may be due to chemotherapy resistance. Perhaps newer agents with different mechanisms of action would provide effective ''secondary'' adjuvant therapy.

Other Therapeutic Options for Hepatic Metastases

Even when the extent of hepatic disease is limited, hepatic resection may not be feasible or advised for technical or patient-related reasons. In such cases, cryosurgery using a freezing probe under ultrasound guidance offers an alternate operative approach for palliating pain and bleeding.[70] Cryoablation can be used alone or in combination with resective surgery. Although long-term results are sparse, disease-free survivals of 25% at a median follow-up of 2 to 3 years have been reported.[71] Nonsurgical therapies principally involve systemic or intrahepatic administration of fluorouracil-based chemotherapy with modulators such as leucovorin.[72] A full review of chemotherapy can be found in Chapter 25.

Summary

The liver is a frequent site of metastatic spread from colorectal primaries. Whereas patients with untreated hepatic lesions rarely live for 5 years, between 20% and 45% of patients treated with resection for isolated lesions can expect to live for 5 years. As is true for any resective approach to recurrent cancer, favorable results can be anticipated for healthy patients who have disease amenable to wide resection.

Pulmonary Metastases

Even though pulmonary metastases are less common than hepatic metastases, the therapeutic approaches, outcomes, and controversial issues are nearly identical. In general, favorable results can be expected when isolated lesions can be completely resected in healthy patients.

Patient Evaluation and Selection for Resection

Most pulmonary lesions will be detected on radiographs of the chest. Once pulmonary lesions are detected, a CT scan of the thorax is indicated to pursue the possibility that they are resectable. Extrathoracic lesions can be excluded according to the diagnostic strategies described above. Although optimal selection criteria are not as well defined for pulmonary resection as they are for hepatic resection, general guidelines are the same. All disease must be amenable to resection, and patients must be in good health and have good pulmonary function.

Results of Surgical Resection

According to current reports, pulmonary resection for metastases can be performed safely, with low mortality rates and high success rates (Table 26-2). Five-year survival rates vary from

Table 26-2. Results After Pulmonary Resection for Colorectal Secondaries

Author	No. of Patients	Operative Mortality (%)	5-Year Survival (%)
McAfee et al., 1992 (Mayo)[76]	139	1.4	30.5
Goya et al., 1989[75]	65	4	42
Sauter et al., 1990[73]	18	4	47
Brister et al., 1988[74]	27	0	21
McCormack et al., 1992[77]	144	0	40

a low of 21% to a high of 47%.[73,74] As was true for hepatic lesions, the number of lesions influences outcome. Five-year survival rates for resected solitary metastases (36.9%) are significantly better than for two or more lesions (19.3% and 7.7%, respectively).[75] Furthermore, size is important, with solitary lesions less than 3 cm associated with more favorable post-thoracotomy outcome.[75] In the Mayo Clinic series of 139 patients, 71% had solitary lesions. These authors reported an operative mortality of 1.4%, a 5-year survival of 31%, and a 20-year survival of 16%.[76] Interestingly, neither the disease-free interval nor the state of the primary colorectal cancer significantly influence survival rates following thoracotomy.[77] By contrast, incomplete resection was associated with low survival rates.[77] The role for post-thoracotomy adjuvant therapy has not been established. No evidence shows that systemic therapies reduce the high risk of recurrence in these patients. Recurrent pulmonary metastases can be reresected, as described for liver metastases. Survival following reresection is similar to that reported for first resections.[77]

Summary

Although the lungs are a less common site of metastases, it is rewarding to identify individuals with isolated pulmonary lesions amenable to resection. Not only are first resections associated with reasonable 5-year survival rates, but reresections for recurrent lesions are as well associated with reasonable chance for cure. The most important criteria for patient selection are resectability, good health, and good pulmonary function.

Other Sites of Focal Metastases

The ovaries, bone, and brain are much less frequently involved with isolated metastases. Ovarian recurrences typically indicate a peritoneal process, and bone and brain lesions are typically manifestations of widespread disease. Since the chance of cure

at the time of ovarian recurrence is low, prophylactic oophorectomy has been recommended, although supportive data are lacking.[78,79] Bone metastases are usually treated with radiation therapy, with internal fixation as required for stabilization purposes.[80] In rare cases of isolated brain metastases, craniotomy and resection may be reasonable; more often steroids and radiation therapy are palliative.[81]

Diffuse Metastases

Even though curative options are not available for patients with diffuse disease, the complexity and importance of treatment options (i.e., palliative therapies) should not be underestimated. Although such a discussion is beyond the scope of this chapter, a few words on palliation are indicated, particularly since a practice that includes focal metastatic disease will unfortunately automatically include diffuse metastatic disease.

Palliation begins with refocusing the goals of therapy. Pursuit of a cure is replaced by short-term goals of prolonging life and improving quality of life. Resources and referrals should be available to facilitate coping with chronic illness and the concept of death and to alleviate disabling symptoms. Palliation may require tumor-reducing therapies, such as radiation or chemotherapy, both of which can minimally prolong life and provide improved quality of life.[72,82] Alternatively, palliation may be entirely focused on relieving symptoms, either through the use of surgical or medical means. Surgery is most typically employed to relieve bowel obstruction. Endoscopic laser ablation may be used to relieve obstruction or bleeding for low-lying rectal lesions, with an endoluminal component.[83] Medical therapies, including narcotics, antidepressants, and local nerve blocks, can be used to reduce pain and improve coping abilities. Finally, patients and families typically need reassurance and assistance. They must not feel abandoned by their medical support system.

CONCLUSIONS

Recurrent colorectal cancer, although often complex in presentation, can readily be stratified according to whether it is resectable or not for possible cure. That long-term survival is possible for isolated metastatic disease, particularly involving the liver, lungs, and locoregional sites, is encouraging. Further gains may be witnessed when new secondary adjuvants with different mechanisms of action are made available to reduce the risk of systemic failure. Meanwhile, focusing surveillance efforts on the goal of early detection of high-risk but resectable sites may improve results with recurrent disease. When diffuse disease is present, clinical efforts should not be abandoned, but rather refocused on quality of life issues.

REFERENCES

1. Krook JE, Moertel CG, Gunderson LL et al (1991) Effective surgical adjuvant therapy for high-risk rectal carcinoma. N Eng J Med 324:709–715
2. Moertel CG, Fleming TR, MacDonald JS et al (1990) Levamisole and fluorouracil for adjuvant therapy of resected colon carcinoma. N Engl J Med 322:352–358
3. Feil W, Wunderlich M, Kovatz E et al (1988) Rectal cancer: factors influencing the development of local recurrence after radical anterior resection. Int J Colon Dis 3:195–200
4. Witzig TE, Loprinzi CL, Gonchoroff NJ et al (1991) DNA ploidy and cell kinetic measurements as predictors of recurrence and survival in stages B2 and C colorectal adenocarcinoma. Cancer 68:879–888
5. Albe X, Vassilakos P, Helfer-Guarnori K et al (1990) Indepen-

dent prognostic value of ploidy in colorectal cancer. Cancer 66:1168–1175

6. Hamelin R, Laurent-Puig P, Olschwang S et al (1994) Association of p53 mutations with short survival in colorectal cancer. Gastroenterology 106:42–48

7. Sun X-F, Carstensen JM, Stal O et al (1993) Prognostic significance of p53 expression in relation to DNA ploidy in colorectal adenocarcinoma. Virchows Arch [A] 423:443–448

8. Manson PN, Corman ML, Coller JA et al (1976) Anterior resection for adenocarcinoma: Lahey Clinic experience from 1963 through 1969. Am J Surg 131:431–441

9. Wolmark N, NSABP Investigators (1983) The prognostic significance of tumor location and bowel perforation in Dukes' B and C colorectal cancer. Ann Surg 198:743–750

10. Ranbarger KR, Johnston WD, Chang JC (1982) Prognostic significance of surgical perforation of the rectum during abdominoperineal resection for rectal carcinoma. Am J Surg 143: 186–188

11. Durdey P, Williams NS (1984) The effect of malignant and inflammatory fixation of rectal carcinoma as prognosis after rectal excision. Br J Surg 71:787–790

12. McDermott FT, Hughes ESR, Pihl E et al (1985) Local recurrence after potentially curative resection for rectal cancer in a series of 1008 patients. Br J Surg 72:34–37

13. Quirke P, Durdey P, Dixon MF et al (1986) Local recurrence of rectal adenocarcinoma due to inadequate surgical resection: histologic study of lateral tumour spread and surgical excision. Lancet 2:996–999

14. Philips RKS, Hittinger R, Blesovsky L et al (1984) Local recurrence following curative surgery for large bowel cancer. II. The rectum and rectosigmoid. Br J Surg 71:17–20

15. Phillips RKS, Hittinger R, Blesovsky L et al (1984) Local recurrence following 'curative' surgery for large bowel cancer: I. The overall picture. Br J Surg 71:12–16

16. Heald RJ, Ryall RD (1986) Recurrence and survival after total mesorectal excision for rectal cancer. Lancet 1:1479–1482

17. Wolmark N, Fisher B (1986) An analysis of survival and treatment failure following abdominoperineal resection and sphincter saving resection in Dukes' B and C rectal carcinoma. Ann Surg 204:480–487

18. Williams NS, Durdey P, Johnston D (1985) The outcome following sphincter saving resection and abdominoperineal resection for low rectal cancer. Br J Surg 72:595–598

19. Pollet WG, Nicholls RJ (1984) The relationship between the extent of distal clearance and survival and local recurrence rates after curative anterior resection for carcinoma of the rectum. Ann Surg 198:159–163

20. Williams NS, Dixon ME, Johnson D (1983) Reappraisal of the 5 cm rule of distal excision for carcinoma of the rectum: a study of distal intramural spread and of patients' survival. Br J Surg 70:150–154

21. Madsen PM, Christiansen J (1986) Distal intramural spread of rectal carcinoma. Dis Colon Rectum 29:279–282

22. Pezim ME, Nicholls RJ (1984) Survival after high or low ligation of the inferior mesenteric artery during curative surgery for rectal cancer. Ann Surg 200:729–733

23. Hojo K, Sawada T, Moriya Y (1989) An analysis of survival and voiding, sexual function after wide ileopelvic lymphadenectomy in patients with carcinoma of the rectum compared to conventional abdominosacral lymphadenectomy. Dis Colon Rectum 32:128–133

24. Vernava AM, Longo WE, Virgo KS (1994) Current follow-up strategies after resection of colon cancer: results of a survey of ASCRS. Dis Colon Rectum 37:573–583

25. Bruinvels DJ, Stiggelbout AM, Kievit J et al (1994) Follow-up of patients with colorectal cancer: a metaanalysis. Ann Surg 219:174–182

26. Buhler H, Seefeld U, Deyhle P et al (1984) Endoscopic follow-up after colorectal cancer surgery: early detection of local recurrence? Cancer 54:791–793

27. Cochrane JPS, Williams JT, Faber RG, Slack WW (1980) Value of outpatient follow-up after curative surgery for carcinoma of the large bowel. BMJ 280:593–595

28. Bengtsson G, Carlsson G, Hafstrom L, Jonsson PE (1981) Natural history of patients with untreated liver metastases from colorectal cancer. Am J Surg 141:586–589

29. Kim NK, Yasmmeh WG, Freler EF et al (1977) Value of alkaline phosphatase, 5-nucleotidase gamma-glutamyl transferase and glutamic dehydrogenase activity measurements (single and combined) in serums in diagnosis of metastases to the liver. Clin Chem 23:2034–2038

30. Bussey HJR Wallace MH, Morson BC (1967) Metachronous carcinoma of the large intestine and intestinal polyps. Proc R Soc Med 60:208–210

31. Olsen HW, Lawrence WA, Snook CW, Mutch WM (1988) Review of recurrent polyps and cancer in 500 patients with initial colonoscopy for polyps. Dis Colon Rectum 31:222–227

32. Martin EW Jr, Minton JP, Carey LC (1985) CEA-directed second-look surgery in the asymptomatic patient after primary resection of colorectal carcinoma. Ann Surg 202:310–316

33. McCall JL, Black RB, Rich CA et al (1994) The value of serum carcinoembryonic antigen in predicting recurrent disease following curative resection of colorectal cancer. Dis Colon Rectum 37:875–881

34. Northover JMA (1985) Carcinoembryonic antigen and recurrent colorectal cancer. Br J Surg, suppl. 72:S44–46

35. Wang JY, Tang R, Chiang JM (1994) Value of carcinoembryonic antigen in the management of colorectal cancer. Dis Colon Rectum 37:272–277

36. Hall NR, Finan PJ, Stephenson BM et al (1994) The role of CA-242 and CEA in surveillance following curative resection for colorectal cancer. Br J Cancer 70:549–553

37. Orefice S, Gennari L, Mor L, Costa D (1981) The value of the CEA test in the diagnosis of metastases of adenocarcinoma of the gastroenteric tract. Tumori 67:109

38. Beart RW Jr, Metzger PP, O'Connell MJ, Schutt AJ (1981) Postoperative screening of patients with carcinoma of the colon. Dis Colon Rectum 24:585–588

39. Stock W, Thielman-Jonen, Muller J, Wintzer G (1980) Follow-up of colorectal carcinoma. Therapie-woche 30:8595–8599

40. Moertel CG, Flemming TR, Macdonald JS et al (1993) An evaluation of the carcinoembryonic antigen (CEA) test for monitoring patients with resected colon cancer. JAMA 270: 943–947

41. Rich T, Gunderson LL, Lew R (1983) Patterns of recurrence of rectal cancer after potentially curative surgery. Cancer 52: 1317–1329

42. Philpshen SJ, Heilweil M, Quan SHQ S et al (1984) Patterns of pelvic recurrence following definitive resections of rectal cancer. Cancer 53:1354–1362

43. Gunderson LL, Sosin H (1974) Areas of failure found at reoperation following curative surgery for adenocarcinoma of the rectum. Cancer 34:1278–1292

44. Gunderson LL, O'Connell MJ, Dozois RR (1992) The role of intra-operative irradiation in locally advanced primary and recurrent rectal adenocarcinoma. World J Surg 16:52–60

45. Gunderson LL, Martenson JA (1988) Irradiation of adenocarcinoma of the gastrointestinal tract. Frontiers Radiat Ther Oncol 22:127–148

46. O'Connell MJ, Childs DS, Moertel CG et al (1982) A prospective controlled evaluation of combined pelvic radiotherapy and methanol extraction residue of BCG (MER) for locally unresectable or recurrent rectal carcinoma. Int J Radiat Oncol Biol Phys 8:1115–1119

47. Suzuki K, Gunderson LL, Devine RM et al (1995) Intraoperative irradiation after palliative surgery for locally recurrent rectal cancer. Cancer 75:939–952

48. Martin EW Jr, Carey LC (1991) Second-look surgery for colorectal cancer: the second time around. Ann Surg 214:321–327

49. Beecher HK, Todd DP (1954) A study of the deaths associated with anesthesia and surgery. Ann Surg 140:2–34

50. Dripps RD, Lamont A, Eckenhoff JE (1961) The role of anesthesia in surgical mortality. JAMA 178:261–266

51. Pilipshen S (1990) Cancer of the rectum: local recurrence. pp. 137–149. In Fazio VW (ed): Current Therapy in Colon and Rectal Surgery. Brain C Decker, Toronto

52. Kramer T, Share R, Kiel K, Roseman D (1991) Intraoperative radiation therapy of colorectal cancer. pp. 308–310. In Abe M (ed): Intraoperative Radiation Therapy. Pergamon Press, New York

53. Wassif SB, Langenhorst BL, Hop CJ (1974) The contribution of preoperative radiotherapy in the management of borderline operability rectal cancer. pp. 612–626 In Salmon SE, Jones SE (eds): Adjuvant Therapy of Cancer II. Grune & Stratton, New York

54. Gerard A, Buyse M, Nordlinger B et al (1988) Preoperative radiotherapy as adjuvant treatment in rectal cancer: final results of a randomized study (EORTC). Ann Surg 208:606–614

55. Pahlman L, Glimelius B (1990) Pre- or postoperative radiotherapy in rectal and rectosigmoid carcinoma. Ann Surg 211:187–195

56. Boulis-Wassif S, Gerard A, Loygue J et al (1984) Final results of a randomized trial on the treatment of rectal cancer with preoperative radiotherapy alone or in combination with 5-fluorouracil followed by radical surgery. Trial of European Organization on Research and Treatment of Cancer Gastrointestinal Tract Cancer Cooperative Group. Cancer 53:1811–1818

57. Neagle CE, Schaffer JL, Heppenstall RB (1991) Compartment syndrome complicating prolonged use of the lithotomy position. Surgery 110:566–569

58. Suzuki K, Dozois RR, Devine RM et al (1996) Curative reoperations for locally recurrent rectal cancer. Dis Colon Rectum 39:730–736

59. Magrini S, Nelson H, Gunderson LL, Sim FH (1996) Sacropelvic resection and intraoperative electron irradiation in the management of recurrent anorectal cancer. Dis Colon Rectum 39:1–9

60. Gunderson LL, Martin JK, Beart RW Jr et al (1988) Intraoperative and external beam irradiation for locally advanced colorectal cancer. Ann Surg 207:52–60

61. Scheele J, Stangl R, Altendorf-Hofmann A (1990) Hepatic metastases from colorectal carcinoma: impact of surgical resection on the natural history. Br J Surg 77:1241–1246

62. Wood CB, Gillis CR, Blumgart LH (1976) A retrospective study of the natural history of patients with liver metastases from colorectal cancer. Clin Oncol 2:285–288

63. Goslin R, Steele G Jr, Zamcheck N et al (1982) Factors influencing survival in patients with hepatic metastases from adenocarcinoma of the colon and rectum. Dis Colon Rectum 25:749–754

64. Allen-Marsh TG, Earlam S, Fordy C et al (1994) Quality of life and survival with continuous hepatic-artery floxuridine infusion for colorectal liver metastases. Lancet 344:1255–1260

65. Rosen CB, Nagorney DM, Taswell HF et al (1992) Perioperative blood transfusion and determinants of survival after liver resection for metastatic colorectal carcinoma. Ann Surg 216:493–505

66. Hughes KS, Simon R, Songhorabodi S et al (1988) Resection of the liver for colorectal carcinoma metastases: a multiinstitutional study of indications for resection. Surgery 103:278–288

67. Cobourn CS, Makowka L, Langer B et al (1987) Examination of patient selection and outcome for hepatic resection for metastatic disease. Surg Gynecol Obstet 165:239–246

68. Hemming AW, Langer B (1994) Repeat resection of recurrent hepatic colorectal metastases. Br J Surg 81:1553–1554

69. Fong Y, Blumgart LH, Cohen A et al (1994) Repeat hepatic resections for metastatic colorectal cancer. Ann Surg 220:657–662

70. Gage AA (1992) Cryosurgery in the treatment of cancer. Surg Gynecol Obstet 174:73–92

71. Ravikumar TS, Steele G Jr, Kane R et al (1991) Experimental and clinical observations on hepatic cryosurgery for colorectal metastases. Cancer Res 51:6323–6327

72. Nagorney DM (1987) Hepatic resection for metastases from colorectal cancer. Prob Gen Surg 4:83–92

73. Sauter ER, Bolton JS, Willis GW (1990) Improved survival after pulmonary resection of metastatic colorectal carcinoma. J Surg Oncol 43:135–138

74. Brister SJ, de Varennes B, Gordon PH et al (1988) Contemporary operative management of pulmonary metastases of colorectal origin. Dis Colon Rectum 31:786–792

75. Goya T, Miyazawas N, Kondo H et al (1989) Surgical resection of pulmonary metastases from colorectal cancer. 10 year follow-up. Cancer 64:1418–1421

76. McAfee MK, Allen MS, Trastek VF et al (1992) Colorectal lung metastases: results of surgical excision. Ann Thorac Surg 53:780–786

77. McCormack PM, Burt ME, Bains MS et al (1992) Lung resection for colorectal metastases. 10 year results. Arch Surg 127:1403–1406

78. Mackeigan JM, Ferguson JA (1979) Prophylactic oophorectomy and colorectal cancer in premenopausal patients. Dis Colon Rectum 22:401–405

79. Morrow M, Enker WE (1984) Late ovarian metastases in carcinoma of the colon and rectum. Arch Surg 119:1385–1388

80. Nielsen OS, Munro AJ, Tannock IF (1991) Bone metastases:

pathophysiology and management policy. J Clin Oncol 9: 509–524

81. Fadul C, Misulis KE, Wiley RG (1987) Cerebellar metastases: diagnostic and management considerations. J Clin Oncol 5: 1107–1115

82. Rhomberg W, Eiter H, Hergan K, Schneider B (1994) Inoperable recurrent rectal cancer: results of a prospective trial with radiation therapy and razoxane. Int J Radiat Oncol Biol Phys 30:419–425

83. Rantala A, Ovaska J (1995) Palliative laser treatment of rectal cancer. Scand J Gasteroenterol 30:177–179

84. Stephenson KR, Steinberg SM, Hughes KS et al (1988) Perioperative blood transfusions are associated with decreased time to recurrence and decreased survival after resection of colorectal liver metastasis. Ann Surg 208:679–687

85. Schlag P, Hohenberger P, Herfath C (1990) Resection of liver metastases in colorectal cancer—competitive analysis of treatment results in synchronous versus metachronous metastases. Eur J Surg Oncol 16:360–365

86. Doci R, Gennari L, Bignami P et al (1991) One hundred patients with hepatic metastases from colorectal cancer treated by resection: analysis of prognostic determinants. Br J Surg 78:797–801

87. Pitrelli NJ, Nambisan RN, Herrera L, Mittelman A (1985) Hepatic resection for isolated metastases from colorectal carcinoma. Am J Surg 149:205–209

88. Vogt P, Raab R, Ringe B et al (1991) Resection of synchronous liver metastases from colorectal cancer. World J Surg 15: 62–67

89. Lind DS, Parker GA, Horsely JS et al (1992) Formal hepatic resection of colorectal liver metastases. Ann Surg 215: 677–684

90. Nakamura S, Yoloi Y, Suzuki S et al (1992) Results of extensive surgery for liver metastases in colorectal carcinoma. Br J Surg 79:35–38

91. Nordlinger B, Jaeck D, Guiget M et al (1992) Multicentric retrospective study by the French Surgical Association. pp. 129–146. In Nordlinger B, Jaeck D (eds): Treatment of Hepatic Metastases of Colorectal Cancer. Springler-Verlag, Paris

92. Galandiuk (1992) Surg Gynecol Obstet 174:27–32

93. Wexner SD, Vernava AM (1995) Clinical Decision Making in Colorectal Surgery. Igaka-Shoin, New York

94. Scheele J, Stangl R, Altendor-Hofmann A et al (1991) Indicators of prognosis after hepatic resection for colorectal secondaries. Surgery 110:13–29

27

RARE TUMORS

Joe J. Tjandra

Over 98% of tumors of the large bowel are derived from glandular epithelium, being either benign (adenoma) or malignant (adenocarcinoma). Anal carcinoma and retrorectal tumors are discussed elsewhere. This chapter therefore deals with those tumors that are only occasionally seen in practice but when identified may pose particular problems. Owing to their rarity, it may be difficult in some cases to set useful guidelines for treatment. Management is often based on individual case reports rather than consensus derived from experience with large series.

CLASSIFICATION

It is helpful to classify such tumors, and a general plan is given in Table 27-1. Rare tumors can be primary or secondary (see Ch. 19) and can be of epithelial or mesodermal origin. Neuronal tumors or those arising from a neural crest origin (carcinoid or melanoma, for example) are examples of the former. Tumors of intestinal smooth muscle are the commonest type derived from mesoderm. The distinction between benign and malignant is not clear cut. Pathologists now look on leiomyoma as a tumor with varying degrees of malignant potential. The picture is complicated further by the presence of non-smooth muscle elements, including cells derived from neural epithelium. The term *gastrointestinal stromal tumor* is now used by many pathologists to describe such tumors. Other mesodermal tumors include those arising from fat, vascular tissue, and white cell clones.

SMOOTH MUSCLE TUMORS (GASTROINTESTINAL STROMAL TUMOR)

Smooth muscle tumors are rather less common in the large bowel than in the stomach but there may be a higher tendency toward malignant behavior.[1] They usually arise from the muscularis propria, occasionally from the muscularis mucosae. They can rarely occur in the anal canal within the internal anal sphincter.[2] They are composed of smooth muscle with other stromal tissues; neural elements may also be present.[3] The lesion may remain intramural, but it often expands outside the profile of the bowel wall and can assume a dumbbell shape affecting the bowel itself and also resulting in extramural compression of other structures. Microscopically it may appear well circumscribed, but on microscopic examination a definite capsule is not always present. For this reason histologic examination to determine the potential malignancy of the lesion is essential. This can, however, be difficult.[2]

Morson and Dawson[4] distinguish leiomyomas arising from the muscularis mucosa from those originating from the muscularis propria. The former present as small nodules rarely more than 1 cm in diameter and are usually an incidental finding. The latter can be very extensive and may produce ulceration of the overlying mucosa. They may grow to 20 cm or more in diameter. Of the 48 patients described by Walsh and Mann,[2] 26 had tumors arising from the muscularis mucosae and 18 from the muscularis propria.

Histologically the lesion is composed of spindle-shaped cells arranged in interlacing bundles and whorls. In difficult cases minimum histochemical staining can help to demonstrate the presence of vimentin and desmin, proteins that are associated with smooth muscle cells.

The criteria for assessing malignancy are based on the size of the lesion, the presence of nuclear pleiomorphism, and particularly the mitotic rate.[5] Using the index of mitotic figures per high power field, it is possible to gauge the degree of malignancy that can be shown to relate to prognosis. Metastases to regional lymph nodes may occur with anaplastic tumors, and distant metastases can also be related to degree of histologic agressiveness. It is very difficult for the pathologist to distinguish between a benign leiomyoma and a leiomyosarcoma of low-grade malignancy. Furthermore, a degree of pleiomorphism exists within these tumors.[6] Today all such tumors are considered to have malignant potential to a greater or lesser degree.

Leiomyomas are more common in males, with a male/female ratio of 1.8:1.[2] While rare in the large bowel, they are more frequently seen in the rectum than the colon. Carlier and Vander

Table 27-1. Classification of Rare Tumors of the Large Bowel

Primary
  Ectodermal
    Neuroendocrine
      Carcinoid
      Neurilemma
      Neurofibroma
      Melanoma (gastrointestinal stromal tumor)
Connective tissue
Smooth muscle
  (Gastrointestinal stromal tumor)
  (Leioma; leiosarcoma)
Fat
  Lipoma
  Liposarcoma
Blood vessel
  Hemangiosarcoma
  Kaposi's sarcoma
Lymphoid
  Non-Hodgkin's B cell
    High grade
    Low grade
Leukemic infiltration
Secondary
  Breast
  Malignant melanoma
  Other

Espt[7] were the first to report a smooth muscle tumor from the rectum that was removed surgically and characterized histopathologically. The condition has been estimated to comprise less than 0.1% of all tumors of the rectum and anus.[8] Over a 35-year period at the Mayo Clinic, only 10 cases were found.[9] Tjandra et al.[10] found only about 250 cases of rectal and 10 cases of anal leiomyosarcoma in the literature. Most were isolated case reports.

Clinical Features

As with lipoma (see below), leiomyoma may be asymptomatic and may be discovered incidentally on physical examination or at laparotomy. In the rectum leiomyoma most commonly presents as a mass noted incidentally, but it may cause obstruction to defecation with tenesmus and the sensation of impending or incomplete evacuation. Colonic leiomyomas if symptomatic may present with abdominal pain or mass. Of 18 cases with adequate documentation of symptoms, tenesmus occurred in 10 and bleeding in 7. Only three were asymptomatic.[2]

The size of the lesion will depend on its site of origin (muscularis mucosae or muscularis propria) as well as the degree of malignancy. Where ulceration of the mucosa has occurred, bleeding may be noticed by the patient. Often, even in large lesions, the mucosa is intact, however (Fig. 27-2).

The diagnosis is made on histologic examination (Fig. 27-2). In the case of a large lesion in the rectum, a needle biopsy carried out endoluminally may be justified. In small lesions or

those in the colon, histologic examination should follow surgical excision. Even on a biopsy, pathologists may have difficulty in making the diagnosis and, as emphasized above, in deciding on the degree of malignancy. Prognostic factors including tumor size, cellularity, number of mitoses, and presence of necrosis and anaplasia may be difficult to define.[11]

Treatment

Treatment is controversial, as the experience in most centers is limited. Clinical assessment of rectal leiomyomas should be augmented by computed tomography (CT) scanning of the pelvis, abdomen, and chest to detect distant spread in the liver or lung. Pelvic CT will demonstrate the extent of the lesion and its relationship to surrounding structures.

Endorectal ultrasound may help in preoperative staging by defining the depth of local invasion. It is a useful adjunct to clinical examination when conservative local excision is contemplated (Fig. 27-3).

Radical surgical excision offers the best chance of cure.[2] In an early series from the Mayo Clinic, overall only 48% of patients underwent resection with curative intent.[12] Since 80% of these

Figure 27-1. A large leiomyosarcoma containing fleshy areas with hemorrhage and necrosis. Despite its large size, the mucosa (M) overlying the tumor (T) is intact. (From Tjandra et al.,[10] with permission.)

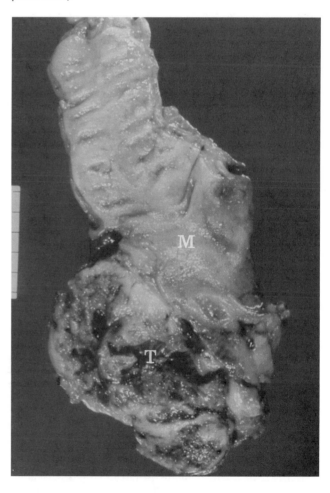

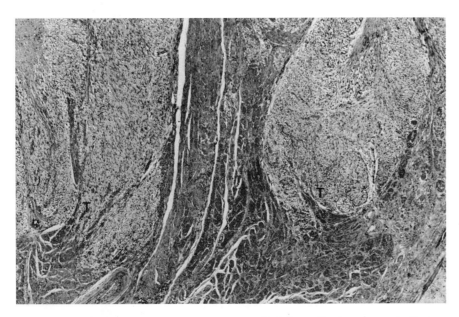

Figure 27-2. A leiomyosarcoma may appear well circumscribed macroscopically, but microscopic invasion may be present. Here two fascicles of sarcoma (T) infiltrate areas of the internal anal sphincter. (From Tjandra et al.,[10] with permission.)

tumors are in the lower rectum and anal canal, abdominoperineal excision is the operation most frequently performed. With mid- and proximal rectal lesions, restorative resection should be undertaken.

Average 5-year survival rates range from 20 to 50% after radical surgery, and reported median survival is around 2 years.[10,13,14] Death is usually due to metastases in the liver or lung.[13] Patients with high grade or large tumors greater than 6 cm tend to have a worse prognosis.[10,15]

Smaller tumors of 1 to 2 cm in diameter are likely to have arisen from the muscularis mucosae. In this group the prognosis after local excision is good, indicating their essentially benign

Figure 27-3. Endorectal ultrasound image showing a hypoechoic well-defined tumor (T) in the submucosa separate from the internal anal sphincter (S).

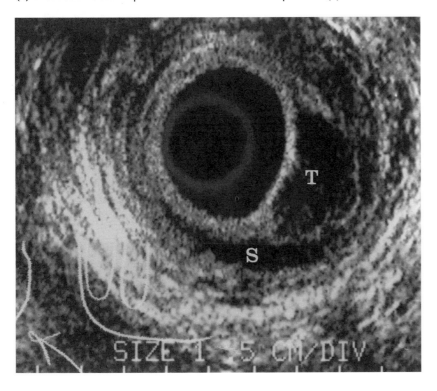

condition. Endoanal removal, provided the tumors are adequately distal for sufficient access, is the treatment of choice.

In a more recent series of 22 patients treated at the Mayo Clinic between 1950 and 1985, the resectability rate was 95%. Surgical procedures used included wide local excision (10 cases), abdominoperineal excision (8 cases), pelvic excision (2 cases), and low anterior resection (1 case). Six of the tumors were confined to the mucosa, and five further lesions did not penetrate the muscularis propria. Lymph node involvement was absent in all patients in whom this assessment could be made. Overall survival at 10 years was 51%, with a disease-free survival at the same time of 40%. Pathologic heterogeneity, with at least six in the good prognostic group of mucosal confinement, was reflected in the outcome after local excision (54% 10-year survival) compared with major surgery (36% 10-year survival). There was a progressive rise in mortality in the patients undergoing radical surgery: the 5-year survival rate of 70% fell to 36% at 10 years.[13] Walsh and Mann[2] reported a similar experience at St. Mark's Hospital. In the 18 patients in whom the tumor arose from the muscularis propria, local excision was carried out in 10 and radical excision in 8. In the former group, there were six local recurrences at a mean follow-up of 88 months, and five of the patients had died. Metastatic disease was responsible for death in three cases. In the eight patients who had radical excision (followed for 99 months), there were no recorded local recurrences, but five patients had died, four of whom had metastatic disease. Of the 18 patients, 4 had a poorly differentiated tumor and all died of the disease. Of the 10 with a well-differentiated tumor, there were 4 recorded local recurrences and 3 patients died. Follow-up information on the 26 patients with tumors arising from the muscularis mucosae was not adequate to determine prognosis after surgery. Twenty-two were treated by local excision; in the four remaining cases the tumor was found coincidentally in the operative specimen of the rectum removed for adenocarcinoma.

The evidence at present indicates that small tumors should be treated by local excision and large tumors by radical resection. There is a place for the posterior approach for local excision in the lower rectum. This was originally described by Kraske[16] in 1886, and with subsequent modifications[17] permits excellent exposure for wide local excision.

No evidence shows that adjuvant radiotherapy or chemotherapy are beneficial. In the series from the Mayo Clinic,[13] three patients had undergone chemotherapy and four irradiation. In a further patient, both modalities were combined. The numbers treated were too small to allow for comparison with patients who did not have adjuvant treatment, but 64% of cases had developed recurrence at 5 years and all had done so at 10 years. Of the eight patients who had adjuvant treatment, only two were alive at 10 years.

LIPOMA

Lipoma is the second most common nonepithelial benign tumor of the large bowel and is the commonest neoplasm to cause intussusception in adults. About 90% are located in the submucosa and 10% in the subserosal layer.[18] The most common sites are in the cecum, right colon, and rectum, in that order.[19] Most lipomas occur singly and probably never turn malignant. Multiple lipomatosis has been reported rarely.[20]

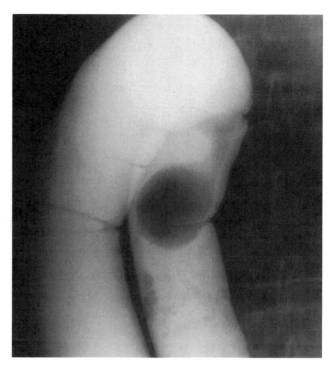

Figure 27-4. A lipoma of the large bowel appearing as a smooth pedunculated lesion on barium enema.

Clinical Features

Most lipomas are asymptomatic, particularly if they are less than 2 cm in diameter. Patients are usually aged between 50 and 70 years. When symptoms occur they are often due to partial large bowel obstruction from intermittent intussusception. Bleeding develops rarely if the overlying mucosa becomes ulcerated. The diagnosis is usually made incidentally on barium enema examination, on colonoscopy, or by histopathologic examination of biopsy specimens removed for other reasons. In a historic series 11% were resected on the basis of contrast radiology to exclude a carcinoma.[20] Barium enema shows the lesion as a smooth curved filling defect (Fig. 27-4). CT will show an encapsulated submucosal mass. Colonoscopy is diagnostic in most cases. It shows a characteristic yellow and soft submucosal swelling readily indented with the biopsy forceps. If doubt exists, a biopsy including the submucosa is diagnostic. It may be difficult to differentiate an ulcerated lipoma from an adenocarcinoma; in this circumstance biopsy is essential.

Treatment

Small and asymptomatic lipomas may be safely left alone if the diagnosis is certain. They can, however, be removed endoscopically. Colonoscopic snare removal of a large lipoma is not recommended because of the risk of perforation and bleeding. A great amount of diathermic current is required to incise the lipoma. A symptomatic lipoma should be removed by partial colectomy. Occasionally an asymptomatic lesion is encountered at laparotomy, and the diagnosis may not be obvious. Here again colectomy should be performed to establish a diagnosis and exclude a cancer.

CARCINOID TUMORS

Carcinoid tumors arise from the enterochromaffin cells in the crypts of Lieberkuhn. These cells are of endodermal origin and have an affinity for silver stains, hence the common alternative name of *argentaffinoma*.[21] The cells may secrete serotonin, which is responsible for the carcinoid syndrome including flushing, bronchoconstriction, increased bowel peristalsis, diarrhea, and tachycardia. This syndrome is usually a sign of metastatic disease and occurs only when serotonin is secreted into the hepatic vein or systemic circulation. Carcinoid syndrome is very rare.[22]

Carcinoid tumors may be found in various locations, but most occur within the gastrointestinal tract. Depending on their site of origin, the tumors are different in the histochemical, chemical, and clinical properties. Carcinoids of the large bowel are rare, constituting 2.5% of all gastrointestinal carcinoid tumors. Most are in the rectum, and only 12% of rectal carcinoids are malignant.[23]

Carcinoid tumors are classified according to their anatomic site and their reactivity to silver incorporation by cytoplasmic granules. A positive argentaffin reaction indicates that the cytoplasmic granules can reduce ionic silver to metallic silver.[24] The tumor cells may be argentaffin positive, or argyrophilic, or both.

Midgut carcinoids tend to contain argyrophil and argentaffin-positive cells that are multicentric. They are thus more likely to be associated with the carcinoid syndrome owing to their capacity to secrete polypeptides.[24,25] Hindgut carcinoids contain unicentric cells that are argyrophilic rather than argentaffin positive.[24] They are rarely associated with the carcinoid syndrome.[26]

The histologic diagnosis of carcinoid tumor is usually straightforward. Microscopically they consist of rosettes, ribbons, or masses of uniform small, round, or polygonal cells with prominent nuclei and acidophilic cytoplasmic granules. Differentiation between a benign and malignant lesion is difficult in biopsy specimens. The arrangement of cells in columns may be a useful indicator of malignancy. Cytologic evidence of malignancy such as brisk mitotic activity or cellular atypia is often lacking.[25] The diagnosis of malignancy is, however, often made based on local or distant invasion. Indeed, the only consistent microscopic feature of malignancy is invasion of the muscularis propria. However, the risk of malignancy increases with the size of tumor. When the lesion is less than 2 cm, only 7% are malignant, whereas when the lesion is larger, only 4% are benign.[25]

Clinical Features

Carcinoid tumors of the large bowel tend to remain asymptomatic until they reach a large size. Sometimes the diagnosis is made incidentally during a routine endoscopic examination, as a single firm nodule in the mucosa and submucosa, similar in appearance to an adenoma. Submucosal carcinoids are seen on ultrasound examination and are amenable to deep biopsy. Preoperative staging with CT scan of the liver is important. If no metastases are seen, a radical resection offers the best chance of cure. If metastases are present, a more limited resection offers good palliation.

Treatment

Management of rectal carcinoids depends on the tumor size and the extent of invasion. Endorectal ultrasound helps to stage the rectal disease locally. A lesion of less than 2 cm in the mid- or low rectum can be safely treated by transanal local excision. For larger or more proximal carcinoids, a more radical resection is required by restorative resection whenever possible.

The criteria for anterior resection or total rectal excision are similar to those used for adenocarcinoma. After resection of tumours larger than 2 cm, the median survival is 10 months.[27] A small early lesion may be cured by local excision or resection. Lymph node metastases have not been shown in tumors of less than 2 cm in diameter.[28] In a report on 595 rectal carcinoids, the 5-year survival rate for patients without regional lymph node metastases was 92%, whereas for patients with nodal involvement it was 44%.[29] Patients with distant metastases have a poor prognosis, with a 5-year survival rate of 7%. The role of adjuvant chemotherapy or radiotherapy is not clear, nor is optimal management of hepatic metastases. In contrast to small bowel carcinoids, those arising in the large bowel do not usually cause carcinoid syndrome. Single and combination chemotherapy with streptozotocin, fluorouracil, and cyclophosphamide has been disappointing. The response rate averages 25% for a duration of 7 months, and the median survival is around 20 months.[27] Alternative treatment strategies including hepatic artery ligation or liver resection are equally disappointing and have a high morbidity.[30]

LYMPHOMA

The gastrointestinal tract is the most common site for extranodal lymphoma. Colorectal lymphoma comprises 10% of all primary gastrointestinal lymphomas. The cecum is the most common site, followed by the rectum.[31,32] Although malignant lymphoma is the third most common malignancy of the large bowel after adenocarcinoma and carcinoid tumor, it is still rare, comprising 0.1% of rectal and 0.5% of colonic neoplasms.[33]

Pathology

The tumor may be polypoid or ulcerated and may be diffuse, causing thickening of a long segment of the colon. Multiple lesions with malignant lymphomatous polyposis have also been described. Large bowel lymphomas are classified according to cellular morphology and immunologic surface markers. Most are T- or B-cell non-Hodgkin's lymphomas, although typical Hodgkin's disease may occur.[34] Non-Hodgkin's lymphomas tend to be highly malignant. They invade locally, and about half the patients have lymph node metastases at operation. The prognosis is related more to the stage of the disease than to cell type and is generally poor.[35] Malignant lymphoma is associated with lymphocytic leukemia.[36] An association exists among lymphoma, inflammatory bowel disease, and celiac disease.[35]

Clinical Features

The tumors usually present in patients over 50 years old, although they may occur at any age. This is a difficult tumor to diagnose and may present very similarly to adenocarcinoma. A lymphoma of the rectum often appears as a submucosal tumor with intact mucosa. When it is more locally advanced, mucosal ulceration develops, and the lesion may mimic a carcinoma. Biopsy and histologic examination should be diagnostic. Staining for cell surface antigens will further differentiate lymphoma from an anaplastic carcinoma.

Staging will involve examination for lymphadenopathy and splenomegaly, a chest x-ray, CT scan of the abdomen, and hematologic examination of peripheral blood and bone marrow.[37] A number of patients with the acquired immunodeficiency syndrome (AIDS) develop colorectal lymphoma.[38]

Treatment

Surgical resection offers the best method of treatment for localized primary lymphoma. Adjuvant chemotherapy is generally given, especially if regional lymph nodes are involved. The role of radiotherapy is not clear, but it should be considered after resection of a locally advanced lymphoma. The overall 5-year survival is 55%, but it declines sharply to 12% if regional lymph nodes are involved.[39] Advanced-stage, high-grade, and unresectable lymphoma may benefit from combined radiation and chemotherapy. A case may be made for preoperative radiotherapy in cases of rectal lymphoma, followed postoperatively by chemotherapy.

AIDS-RELATED TUMORS

Immunosuppression associated with AIDS predisposes patients to the development of unusual malignancies. Fifty percent of patients with AIDS and Kaposi's sarcoma of the skin and lymph nodes also have a tumor of the gastrointestinal tract.[40] Surgical excision is not recommended except for histologic diagnosis. Systemic azidothymidine may have a therapeutic effect on the disease.

Other tumors arising from immunocytes such as small cell cancer of the rectum or large bowel lymphoma have been reported.[38,41] A higher incidence of smooth muscle tumors has also been noted.[42] Other large bowel malignant tumors described include malignant melanoma, adenocarcinoma, and anal squamous carcinoma.[43] Careful evaluation of anorectal symptoms in patients in high-risk groups for AIDS is important.

ANORECTAL MALIGNANT MELANOMA

Primary malignant melanoma of the rectum anus is rare, consisting of less than 1% of all anorectal malignancies and only 0.2% of all melanomas seen in population-based registries.[44,45] Consequently, the experience with this disease is limited, even in major centers. Anorectal melanoma arises from melanocytes in the nonkeratinizing squamous epithelium below the dentate line or the mucosa of the anal transitional zone above the dentate line. It rarely arises from the true rectal mucosa.[46]

The prognosis in most reports is poor, with less than 10% of patients surviving beyond 5 years.[44,47] This is much worse than with the cutaneous melanomas. In the Cleveland Clinic experience of 15 patients, none survived beyond 7 years.[44] Others have noted that longer term survivors tend to be women.[47] Similarly, female gender is associated with a more favorable

outcome in cutaneous melanoma, although the reasons for this are unclear.[48]

Delays in diagnosis are common because of the rarity of these tumors. Pigmentation is absent in up to 25% of cases, and the diagnosis may be confused with hemorrhoids or adenoma.[44] Most anorectal melanomas are thicker than 1.7 mm at diagnosis, a thickness known to be associated with a poor prognosis.[44,47] In one study, median size of the primary tumor in survivors following surgery was 2.5 cm compared with 4.0 cm for patients who did not survive long term.[47] A high proportion of patients already have distant and pelvic metastases at presentation. Endoluminal ultrasound may facilitate clinical assessment of tumor thickness and possible nodal metastases, and CT scan will document distant and regional metastases.

Controversy surrounds the optimal surgical treatment. Whereas radical abdominoperineal excision of the rectum, with or without block dissection of the inguinal lymph nodes, would provide the most radical locoregional clearance, most patients have a dismal outcome and will die of their disease regardless of therapy. In a small subset, probably less than 10%, the disease is truly localized and is curable by radical surgery.[44,48] One of our patients with a small (8 mm) and thin (0.9 mm) melanoma had extensive liver metastases at presentation.[44] Local transanal excision may be associated with a higher local recurrence rate because of submucosal spread. However, most patients succumb from systemic disease before local recurrence becomes symptomatic.[44]

In most patients, a wide transanal local excision provides as good a survival as total rectal excision.[48]

With little prospect of data from prospective randomized trials on surgical treatments becoming available, a local excision to achieve wide margins of clearance appears to be the treatment of choice for most cases. Endoluminal ultrasound provides a useful evaluation of tumor thickness. Abdominoperineal excision should be reserved for the very large tumors that are still resectable. Chemotherapy or radiotherapy is generally ineffective.

OTHER MALIGNANT TUMORS

Squamous Cell Carcinoma

Squamous cell carcinoma of the large bowel is very rare, with fewer than 60 cases reported. The lesion is associated with radiotherapy, schistosomiasis, and long-standing ulcerative colitis.[44] It should be treated in the same way as adenocarcinoma. When total rectal excision is felt to be necessary, a preoperative course of combined radiation and chemotherapy similar to that used for anal carcinoma should be considered.

Fibrosarcoma

Fibrosarcomas are very rare in the large bowel, and most arise in the rectum. The lesion is resected as for an adenocarcinoma. The role of radiation or chemotherapy is not clear.

Hemangiopericytoma

Hemangiopericytoma is a rare vascular tumor of mesenchymal cell origin arising from pericytes of blood vessels. It occurs most commonly in the fifth and sixth decades, with an equal sex distribution. The diagnosis is difficult because of the morphologic appearance of pericytes, which may look like endothelial cells on light microscopy. Immunohistochemical or electron microscopy is usually required for diagnosis and differentiation from other highly vascular tumors.

Hemangiopericytoma can occur at any site where capillaries are present. It appears as a well-circumscribed mass with a thin vascular pseudocapsule. On microscopy, endothelium-lined vascular channels are seen.[49] The cells stain positive for vimentin, owing to their mesenchymal origin, and negative for cytokeratin, ruling out an epithelial origin. They are also negative for desmin and actin, which are of muscle origin.[50]

If the diagnosis is made preoperatively, wide local excision for a hemangiopericytoma with few mitoses, necrosis, or hemorrhage, should suffice. With less well differentiated tumors, a more aggressive resection is performed. The effect of radiation is said to be variable,[51] but combination chemotherapy including Adriamycin has been reported to produce complete or partial response in at least 50% of patients.[52]

The recurrence rate is high, occurring in more than 50% of patients within 5 years.[53] It occurs either locally or at distant sites. Metastasis to regional lymph nodes is rare.

Hemangioma

Hemangioma is a rare and congenital hamartomatous vascular lesion that is therefore pathologically different from the degenerative condition of angiodysplasia. The lesion arises from embryonic sequestration of mesodermal tissue and is commonest in the rectum.

OTHER BENIGN TUMORS

Fibroma

Fibroma is very rare and affects the colon more often than the rectum. It consists of numerous spindle cells and may arise from any layer of the large bowel. It is readily differentiated from a leiomyoma by differential tissue staining.[54]

Neurofibroma

Neurofibroma may occur in the large bowel as a solitary lesion or as part of neurofibromatosis (von Recklinghausen's disease).[55] It arises in the submucosa or muscularis propria. Common presentations include bleeding or intussusception. Malignant change may occur, and surgical resection is recommended.

REFERENCES

1. Willis RA (1960) Pathology of Tumours. 3rd Ed. p. 738. Butterworth Medical Publications, London
2. Walsh TH, Mann CV (1984) Smooth muscle neoplasm of the rectum and anal canal. Br J Surg 71:597–959
3. Newman PL, Wadham C, Fletcher CD (1991) Gastrointestinal stromal tumours: correlation of immunophenotype with clinicopathological features. J Pathol 164:107–117
4. Morson B, Dawson J (1960) Gastrointestinal Pathology. 3rd Ed. p. 634. Blackwell Scientific Publications, Oxford
5. Evans HL (1985) Smooth muscle tumours of the gastrointestinal tract. The study of fifty-six cases followed through a minimum of ten years. Cancer 56:2242
6. Ranchod M, Kempson RL (1977) Smooth muscle tumours of the gastrointestinal Tract and retroperitoneum. Cancer 39:255
7. Carlier E, Vander Espt V (1881) Myoide du rectum: extraction, guerison. J Med Chir Pharmacol 72:140–143
8. Somervell JL, Mayer PF (1971) Leiomyosarcoma of the rectum. Br J Surg 58:144–146
9. Anderson PA, Dockerty MB, Buiela DA (1950) Myomatous tumours of the rectum (leiomyomas and myosarcomas). Surgery 28:642–650
10. Tjandra JJ, Antoniuk PM, Webb B et al (1993) Leiomyosarcoma of the rectum and anal canal. Aust NZ J Surg 63:703–709
11. Vandoni RE, Givel JC, Essinger AR (1992) Rectal leiomyosarcoma: acute presentation after local injury. Eur J Surg 158:383–386
12. Akwari OE, Dozois RR, Weiland LH, Bearhs OH (1978) Leiomyosarcoma of the small and large bowel. Cancer 42:1375–1384
13. Randleman CD Jr, Wolff BG, Dozois RR et al, (1989) Leiomyosarcoma of the rectum and anus. Int J Color Dis 4:91–96
14. Ng EH, Pollock RE, Munsell MF et al (1992) Prognostic factors influencing survival in gastrointestinal leiomyosarcomas. Ann Surg 215:68–77
15. Moyana TN, Friesen R, Tan LK (1991) Colorectal smooth muscle tumors. Arch Pathol Lab Med 115:1016–1021
16. Kraske P (1886) Extirpation of high carcinoma of the large bowel, Arch F Klin Chir (Berl) 33:563–595. (Translated in Dis Colon Rectum (1984) 27:499–501.)
17. Mason AY (1980) The trans-sphinctoric approach. pp. 271–272. In Welyaart K (ed): Colorectal Cancer. Martinus Nijhoff, Boston
18. Gordon RT, Beal JM (1978) Lipoma of the colon. Arch Surg 113:897–899
19. Taylor B, Wolff BG (1987) Colonic lipomas. Report of two unusual cases and review of the Mayo Clinic experience, 1976–1985. Dis Colon Rectum 30:888–893
20. Mayo CW, Pagtalunan RJG, Brown DJ (1963) Lipoma of the alimentary tract. Surgery 53:598
21. Williams CJ, Krikorian JG, Green MR, Raghavan E (eds) (1988) Textbook of Uncommon Cancer. pp. 512–514. John Wiley & Sons, New York
22. Cheek RC, Wilson H (1970) Carcinoid tumours. Curr Probl Surg 1:4–31
23. Burke M, Shepherd N, Mann CV (1978) Carcinoid tumours of the rectum and anus. Br J Surg 74:358–361
24. Taxy JB, Mendelsohn G, Gupta PK (1980) Carcinoid tumours of the rectum. Silver reactions, fluorescence and serotonin content of the cytoplasmic granules. Am J Clin Pathol 74:791–795
25. Orloff MJ (1971) Carcinoid tumours of the rectum. Cancer 28:175–180
26. Black WC III (1968) Enterochromaffin cell types and corresponding carcinoid tumours. Lab Invest 19:473–486
27. Thompson GB, van Heerden JA, Martin JK et al (1985) Carcinoid tumours of the gastrointestinal tract: presentation, management and prognosis. Surgery 98:1054–1063
28. Sauven P, Ridge JA, Quan SH, Sigurdson ER (1990) Anorectal

carcinoid tumours. Is aggressive surgery warranted? Ann Surg 211:67–71

29. Nauneim KS, Zeitels J, Kaplan EL et al (1983) Rectal carcinoid tumours: treatment and prognosis. Surgery 94:670–676

30. Bengmark, Ericsson M, Lundquist A et al (1982) Temporary liver deterioralisation in patients with metastatic carcinoid disease. World J Surg 6:46–53

31. Dragosics B, Bauer P, Radaszkiewicz T (1985) Primary gastro-intestinal non-Hodgkin's lymphomas. A retrospective clinico-pathologic study of 150 cases. Cancer 55:1060–1073

32. Jinnai D, Iwasa Z, Watanuki T (1983) Malignant lymphoma of the large intestine: operative results in Japan. Jpn J Surg 13:331–336

33. Sherlock P, Winawer SJ, Goldstein MJ et al. Malignant lymphoma of the gastrointestinal tract. pp. 367–391. In Glass GB (ed): Progress in Gastroenterology. Vol. 2. Grune & Stratton, New York

34. Issacson PG, Wright DH (1984) Immunocytochemistry of lymphoreticular tumours. In Poluk N, van Noorden S (eds): Immunocytochemistry. Modern Methods and Applications. 2nd Ed. Wright, Bristol

35. Lewin KJ, Ranchod M, Dorfman RF (1978) Lymphomas of the gastrointestinal tract. A study of 117 cases presenting with gastrointestinal disease. Cancer 42:693–707

36. Waldenstrom JG (1960) Studies on conditions associated with disturbed gamma globulin formation (gammopathies) Harvey Lect 56:211–231

37. Dawson IMP, Cornes JS, Morson BC (1961) Primary malignant lymphoid tumours of the gastrointestinal tract. Br J Surg 49:80–89

38. Levine AM, Gill PS, Meyer PR et al (1985) Primary malignant lymphoid tumours of the gastrointestinal tract. Br J Surg 49:80–89

39. Contreary K, Nance FC, Becker WF (1980) Primary lymphoma of the gastrointestinal tract. Ann Surg 191:593–598

40. Friedman SL (1988) Gastrointestinal and hepatobiliary neoplasms in AIDS. Gastrointest Clin North Am 17:465–486

41. Smitherman MH, Morris LE Jr, Chang BK et al (1990) Rectal small cell cancer in an HIV-positive man. Am J Med 89:239–240

42. Chadwick EG, Connor EJ, Hanson IC et al (1990) Tumours of smooth muscle origin in HIV-infected children. JAMA 263:3182–3184

43. Rabkin CS, Blattner WA (1991) HIV infective and cancers other than non-Hodgkin lymphoma and Kaposi's sarcoma. Cancer Surg. 10:151–160

44. Antoniuk PM, Tjandra JJ, Webb BW et al (1993) Anorectal malignant melanoma has a poor prognosis. Int J Color Dis 8:81–86

45. Weinstock MA (1993) Epidemiology and prognosis of anorectal melanoma. Gastroenterology 104:174–178

46. Werdin C, Limas C, Knodell RG (1988) Primary malignant melanoma of the rectum: evidence for origination from the rectal mucosal melanocytes. Cancer 61:1364–1370

47. Brady MS, Kabolius JP, Quan SH (1995) Anorectal melanoma. A 64-year experience at Memorial Sloan-Kettering Cancer Center. Dis Colon Rectum 38:146–1451

48. Ward MWN, Romano G, Nicholls RJ (1986) The surgical treatment of anorectal malignant melanoma. Br J Surg 73:68–69

49. Enzinger FM, Weiss SW (1983) Soft Tissue Tumors. CV Mosby, St. Louis

50. Lo YM, Gillett MB, Vina M et al (1989) Haemangiosarcoma of the rectum after chronic anorectal ulceration. U Clin Gastroenterol 11:77–81

51. Graham WJ, Bogardus CR Jr (1981) Angiosarcoma treated with radiation therapy alone. Cancer 48:912–914

52. Wong PP, Yagoda A (1978) Chemotherapy of malignant haemangiopericytoma. Cancer 41:1256–1260

53. Felix EL, Wood DK, Dasgupta TK (1981) Tumors of the retroperitoneum. pp. 1–47. In Hickey RC, Clark RL, Benfield JR et al (eds). Current Problems in Cancer. Year Book, Chicago

54. Rose TF (1972) True fibrome of the caecum. Med J Aust 1:532–533

55. Manley KA, Skyring AP (1961) Some heritable causes of gastrointestinal disease: special reference to haemorrhage. Arch Intern Med 107:182–203

28

RETRORECTAL TUMORS

Roger R. Dozois
Leo Kai-Ming Chiu

The retrorectal or presacral space can be the site of heterogeneous and rare tumors that are often silent or may produce ill-defined symptoms, at times for prolonged periods; thus their presence may be difficult to detect. For all of these reasons, the diagnosis is not infrequently delayed until the tumors reach considerable size, which may in turn complicate their management. Better awareness of their existence and clinical course may lead to earlier diagnosis and may optimize their management and outcome.

ANATOMIC CONSIDERATIONS

The boundaries of the retrorectal region include the posterior wall of the rectum anteriorly and the sacrum posteriorly. This space extends superiorly to the peritoneal reflection and inferiorly to the rectosacral fascia.[1] The space immediately below is the horseshoe-shaped supralevator space (Fig. 28-1). Laterally, the area is bordered by the lateral ligaments, the ureters, and the iliac vessels.

Important vascular and neural structures are located in this area, where they either originate or traverse, and their sacrifice may have important neurologic and musculoskeletal consequences. Also, some of the vascular structures may need to be ligated at the time of operation to reduce bleeding. It is important to be aware that if all sacral roots on one side of the sacrum are sacrificed, patients will continue to have normal anorectal function. Indeed, if the upper three sacral(s) roots are left intact on either side of the sacrum, the patient's ability to defecate spontaneously and to control anorectal contents will remain essentially intact (Fig. 28-2). If, however, both S3 roots are destroyed, the external sphincter will no longer contract in response to gradual balloon dilation of the rectum (Fig. 28-2) and this will translate clinically into anorectal incontinence and difficult defecation.[2]

PRESACRAL CYSTS AND TUMORS

Presacral lesions are rare. Reports from various large referral centers would indicate that their incidence may be as low as 1 in 40,000 hospital admissions, and it is likely that their true incidence is even lower.[3] Two-thirds of the lesions are of congenital origin, and of these two-thirds are developmental whereas the remainder are neoplastic.[3,4]

Presacral lesions may be either cystic or solid, benign or malignant (Tables 28-1 and 28-2). Most cystic lesions are seen in women, and most solid lesions are chordomas. Developmental cysts can originate from any of the three germ layers (Table 28-3) and can include epidermoid and dermoid cysts, enterogenous cysts, tailgut cysts, and teratomatous tumors.[5] In the pediatric age group, teratomas are the most common tumors encountered.

Although rare, sacrococcygeal chordoma is the most common malignancy of this region. These tumors are believed to originate from the primitive notochordal tissue, either from normal nuclei pulposi or from so-called abnormal rests. They can be located anywhere along the spinal column, but have a prediliction for its two extremities; namely, the spheno-occipital region at the base of the skull or the sacrococcygeal region (Fig. 28-3). Approximately one-half of the lesions are located in the sacral area.[6] They predominate in men and are encountered rarely in patients younger than 30 years of age. Depending on their mucin content, they may be soft, gelatinous, or firm.

Benign neurogenic tumors may include neurilemoma (Fig. 28-4) and ganglioneuromas; their malignant counterparts include neuroblastomas, schwannomas, and ganglioneuroblastomas. Neurogenic tumors grow slowly and may become quite large before their detection, a factor that, combined with their location, may result in catastrophic sequelae. Primary osseous neoplasms are rare and can originate from fibrous tissue, cartilage, bone, or marrow. A wide en bloc excision is ideal, but recurrences are not uncommon. Overall, malignancy is most

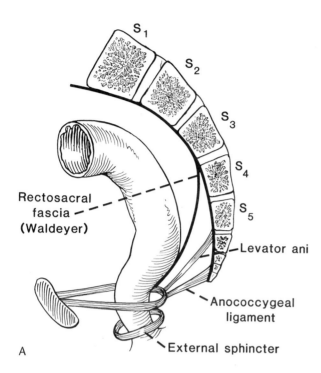

A

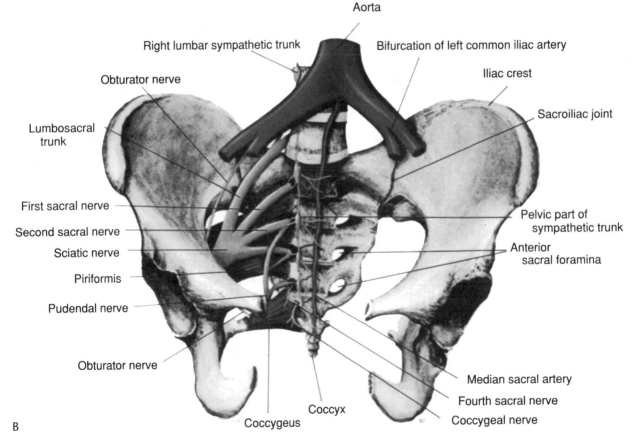

B

Figure 28-1. (A) The retrorectal space and its anterior, posterior, superior, and inferior boundaries. **(B)** Relationships among pelvis, sacrum, and neural and vascular structures. (From Dozois,[18] with permission.)

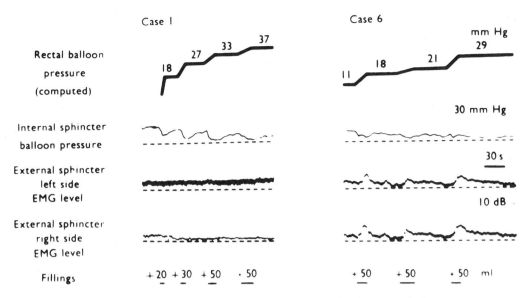

Figure 28-2. Pressure tracings and electromyogram (EMG) results during gradual filling of the rectal balloon. The case 1 patient is without any S3 roots, and the case 6 patient is without S1 through S5 roots on the left side. The rectoinhibitory reflex is seen in both patients, but external sphincter activity is noted in the case 6 patient only. (From Gunterberg et al.,[2] with permission.)

common in men even though most presacral tumors occur in women. This may be because benign lesions are frequently asymptomatic and are often discovered incidentally and earlier at the time of a routine gynecologic examination. By contrast, malignant tumors are more often symptomatic and are found at a later stage of their evolution. Other lesions may include metastatic tumors or infectious processes.

DIAGNOSIS

History and Physical Examination

Not uncommonly, retrorectal tumors are silent and are found incidentally at the time of a periodic pelvic examination. They may indeed remain asymptomatic for prolonged periods of time. Symptomatic patients typically complain of vague, long-standing pain in the perineal or low back area, or both. Such pain is often aggravated by sitting and ameliorated by standing or walking. In our own experience, pain is more common when the tumor is malignant rather than benign (88% versus 39%).[3] Patients with cystic lesions are almost always women (15:1);

occasionally, patients may complain of long-standing perianal discharge, and their symptoms may be confused with those of an anal fistula or pilonidal disease. Several conditions may alert the clinician to the possibility of a retrorectal cystic lesion, including repeated operations for "anal fistula," the inability of the examiner to uncover a primary source of infection at the level of the dentate line, recurrent infection of the retrorectal space without any obvious cause, the presence of a postanal dimple, and fullness and fixation of the precoccygeal area.[1] Teratoma can occur equally in adults and children, and a teratocarcinoma has been seen in our institution in a patient as young as 9 months. By contrast, epidermoid and mucus-secreting cysts can be encountered in adolescents as well as in the elderly. All patients with osseous tumors complained of low back or perineal pain, or both.[3] Patients may have been previously referred to a psychiatrist because of the clinician's inability to ascertain the origin of the chronic, ill-defined pain in patients who appear otherwise healthy. In the presence of large, advanced tumors,

Table 28-1. Classification of Retrorectal Tumors Seen at the Mayo Clinic Between 1960 and 1979

Classification	No. of Patients	%
Congenital	79	65
Neurogenic	14	12
Osseous	13	11
Miscellaneous	14	12
Total	120	100

(From Jao et al.,[3] with permission.)

Table 28-2. Congenital Retrorectal Tumors Seen at the Mayo Clinic Between 1960 and 1979

Type of Tumor	No. of Patients
Epidermoid	15
Mucus-secreting cysts	16
Teratoma	15
Teratocarcinoma	3
Chordoma	30
Meningocele[a]	2

[a] One associated with lipoma and another with epidermoid cyst; counted as lipoma and epidermoid cyst, respectively.
(From Jao et al.,[3] with permission.)

Table 28-3.   Germ Layer Origin of Developmental Cysts

	Epidermoid	Dermoid	Enterogenous	Teratomatous
Tissue of origin	Ectoderm	Ectoderm	Endoderm	All three layers
Histologic characteristics	Stratified squamous	Stratified squamous with skin appendages (sweat glands, sebaceous glands, hair follicles)	Columnar or cuboidal lining; may have secretary function	Various degrees of differentiation between cysts and cell layers of single cysts
General state	Benign[a]	Benign[a]	Benign	Benign or malignant

[a] Malignant variant is rare.
(From Goldberg et al.,[5] with permission.)

patients may complain of constipation, rectal as well as urinary incontinence, and sexual dysfunction. In almost all patients, a rectal digital examination will typically reveal the presence of an extrarectal mass dysplacing the rectum anteriorly with a smooth, overlying intact mucosa.[1]

Radiography

The diagnosis of a presacral tumor can be established by simple x-ray films of the sacrum, computed tomography (CT), or magnetic resonance imaging (MRI). Simple anteroposterior and lateral views of the sacrum may help to identify bone expansion with destruction, calcification, and soft tissue-occupying masses, all characteristic of chordoma (Fig. 28-5). Bone destruction may be present in one-third of such patients, and in more than two-thirds of them the lesion is malignant. Rare benign tumors such as giant cell tumors, neurilemoma, aneurysmal bone cysts, and osteochondroma can also cause bone destruction.[3] The characteristic scimitar sign denotes the presence of an anterior sacral meningocele (Fig. 28-6), a diagnosis that can be confirmed by myelography.

Imaging of the sacral area with CT or MRI has become the most important means of establishing the diagnosis of these tumors. These imaging techniques can distinguish between cystic, solid, or mixed tumors (Fig. 28-7) and thus help clarify the diagnosis based on the appearance of the lesion. Moreover, imaging by CT or MRI clearly delineates the upper extension of the tumor, which in turn helps to determine the best surgical approach. On occasion, a sinogram may be performed to delineate chronically suppurating sinuses.

Role of Preoperative Biopsy

Some clinicians feel that all solid tumors should be sampled preoperatively by biopsy.[7] Indeed, some presacral tumors will benefit from preoperative chemotherapy or radiation therapy, or both. This approach would be particularly applicable to osseous tumors such as Ewing's sarcoma and osteogenic sarcoma, malignant neurofibrosarcoma (Fig. 28-8), or very large tumors such as a desmoid (Fig. 28-9) that can be removed more easily by reducing their size.

Transrectal biopsy of lesions of any type should be avoided. Indeed, in the presence of a cystic lesion, such an approach is likely to result in infection, rendering its future complete ex-

Figure 28-3.   Distribution of chordomas seen at Mayo Medical Center prior to 1986. Note the predilection for the sacrococcygeal (n = 133) and spheno-occipital (n = 97) regions.

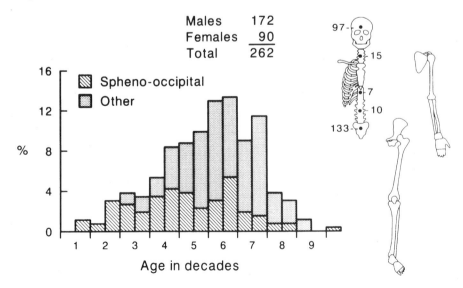

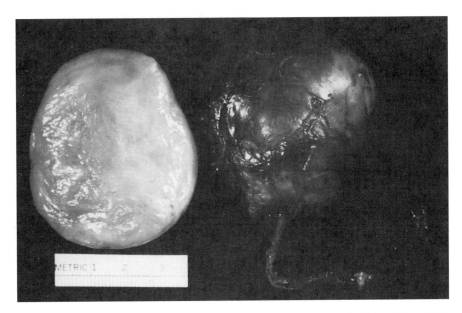

Figure 28-4. Neurilemoma (schwannoma) (5.5 × 4.5 × 4.5 cm), with unilateral S2 nerve root tumor involvement in 35-year-old man with an asymptomatic mass. (From Dozois,[18] with permission.)

Figure 28-5. Anteroposterior (**A**) and lateral (**B**) views of the sacrum with characteristic midline lytic defect and erosion of the middle and lower parts of the sacrum. (From Dozois,[1] with permission.)

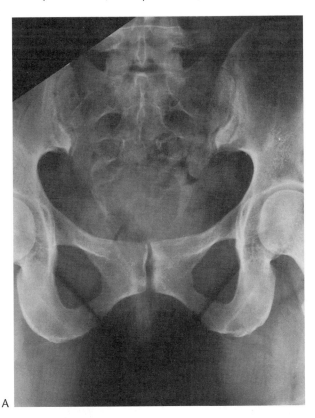

A

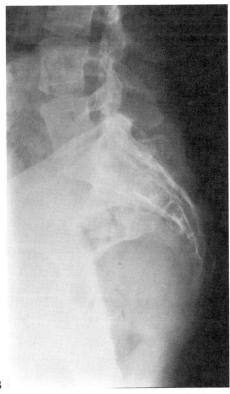

B

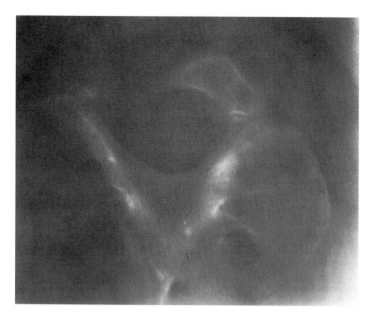

Figure 28-6. Typical computed tomographic (CT) appearance of an anterior sacral meningocele with a scimitar-shaped defect. (From Jao et al.,[3] with permission.)

cision more difficult and increasing the likelihood of postoperative complications and recurrence. More importantly, inadvertent transrectal needling of a meningocele may lead to disastrous sequelae such as meningitis and even death. Finally, chordomas which usually have a very characteristic appearance on plain films of the sacrum and CT scan and represent the most common solid tumor of this region, do not, in our view, require biopsy unless the diagnosis is uncertain. Violation of the tumor capsule may jeopardize curability and require proctectomy to enable excision of the biopsy tract. If soft tissue

Figure 28-7. CT (**A**) and magnetic resonance image (**B**) of a cystic teratoma of the presacral space. The mass to the right of the midline is filled with fat, calcium, and mixed, isodense soft tissue. (Fig. 7A from Dozois,[1] with permission; Fig. 7B from Dozois,[18] with permission.)

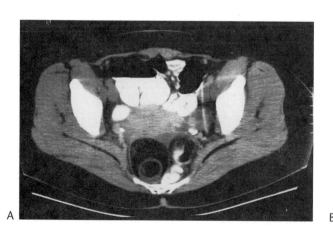

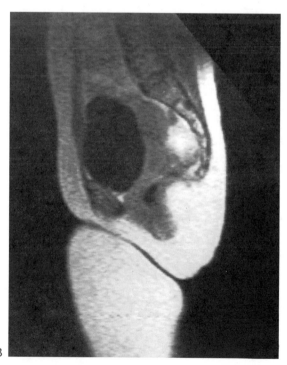

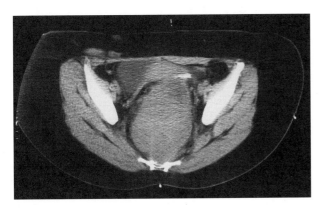

Figure 28-8. Fibrosarcoma in a woman with unexplained perineal pain for 2 years. Tumor was radiated prior to surgical excision of mass.

tumors are suspected or if the diagnosis remains unclear despite exhaustive evaluation, a transperineal or parasacral needle biopsy within the field of an impending surgical resection is preferable to the transrectal route.

SURGICAL TREATMENT

Current Rationale

Once the diagnosis of a retrorectal tumor is established, surgical therapy should be initiated immediately. This approach is based on several arguments:

1. The lesion may already be malignant.
2. In patients with teratomas, especially those in the pediatric age group, the risk of malignant transformation is considerable and continues to increase dramatically if their removal is delayed.[8,9]
3. Untreated anterior sacral meningocele may become infected

Figure 28-9. Desmoid tumor in 18-year-old man. Note large, mixed density, predominantly solid mass displacing rectum and bladder.

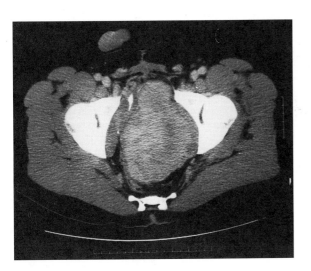

and may lead to meningitis, which is associated with a high mortality.[10]
4. Cystic lesions may become infected, especially with transrectal biopsy, making their excision difficult and increasing the probability of postoperative infection and later recurrence.
5. A presacral mass in a young woman may cause dystocia at the time of vaginal delivery.

Also, in the past, many surgeons had adopted a rather defeatist attitude toward sacrococcygeal chordomas and other tumors of this area based on a number of erroneous misconceptions. Chordomas are slow-growing tumors producing vague symptoms, often resulting in a diagnosis delayed for months and even years. Thus patients may seek treatment late in the course of their disease, and the presence of a large mass in this less familiar anatomic area may make some surgeons reluctant to consider an aggressive surgical approach for fear of serious postoperative complications. The same reluctance to operate would apply to other types of lesions. Moreover, chordomas have all too often been considered to have a benign clinical behavior characterized by slow local growth. We now know, however, that these tumors will metastasize distally and that the longer the diagnosis is delayed the greater the risk of distant spread. Finally, and most importantly, tumors of this area have all too often been treated inadequately in the past because of tumor violations, their large size and location, and fear of neurologic compromise or musculoskeletal instability. Tumor violation can take place preoperatively when such tumors are biopsied transrectally or intraoperatively, when margins of resection are inadequate or tumor cells are spilled in an effort to be too conservative, or when the lesion is rather soft and gelatinous and is disrupted, or when the surgeon is attempting to avoid injury to the rectal wall or important neurologic structures or restrict excision. Kaiser and his colleagues[11] have found that the local recurrence rate increased from 28% to 64% when chordomas were violated perioperatively. One can therefore argue that the cure rate could be improved if the diagnosis was secured earlier through increased awareness and better imaging technique, and if tumor violation was avoided. Such an aggressive approach may comprise wide en bloc resection of portions of the sacrum, sacral nerve roots, and at times the rectum itself. Indeed, if the lesion is quite large and the risk of entering the tumor capsule and spilling malignant cells is a significant concern, it might be preferable to excise the rectum en bloc with the tumor and involved segment of sacrum, especially if it is also obvious that both third sacral roots will need to be sacrificed, rendering the rectum nonfunctional. This is the exception rather than the rule, however, and if it is safe to remove the lesion without removing the rectum the latter should be retained even if both S3 roots are to be sacrificed.

Surgical Approach

It is of great importance that an experienced team consisting of a colorectal surgeon, an orthopedic surgeon, and a neurosurgeon be available to evaluate and surgically treat such tumors, especially those that are large and extend in the vicinity of the upper half of the sacrum.

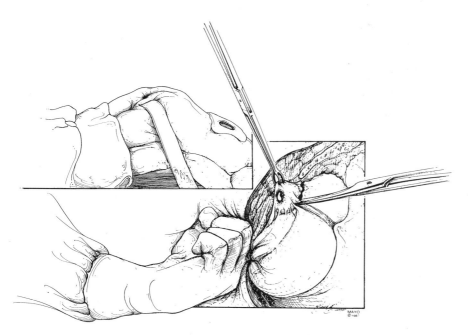

Figure 28-10. Patient in the prone jackknife position with the buttocks spread with tape (inset); the surgeon's left index finger is in the rectum propping the retrorectal tumor for easier dissection. (From Dozois,[1] with permission.)

Figure 28-11. Posterior surgical approach for a low-lying retrorectal tumor, with a vertical incision over the lower sacrum and coccyx extending to the anus. Retraction of the levator ani muscles and division of the anococcygeal ligament help to expose the tumor. (From Dozois,[1] with permission.)

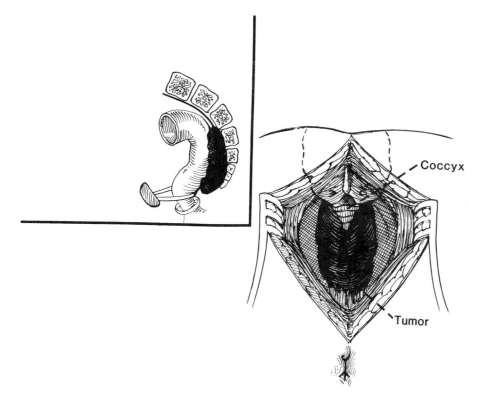

Again, CT scan or MRI may be helpful in trying to define the best possible surgical approach to a given presacral lesion. Small and low-lying (below the level of S3) cystic as well as solid lesions can be removed transperineally through a parasacral incision, whereas tumors extending above the S3 level, especially if quite large, may require a combined anterior and posterior approach. For low-lying tumors, the patient is placed in the prone-jackknife position with the buttocks spread with tape (Fig. 28-10). An incision is made over the lower portion of the sacrum and coccyx down to the anus, taking care to avoid damage to the external sphincter (Fig. 28-11). Resection of the tumor is facilitated by transsection of the anococcygeal ligament. The lesion can then be dissected from the surrounding tissues, including the rectal wall, in a plane between the retrorectal fat and the tumor mass itself (Fig. 28-12). In the case of very small lesions, especially if cystic, the surgeon may double-glove the left hand and, with the index finger in the anal canal and lower rectum, push the lesion outward, away from the depths of the wound (Fig. 28-8). This technique facilitates dissection of the lesion off the wall of the rectum without injury to the latter. If necessary, the lower sacrum or coccyx or both can be excised en bloc with the lesion to facilitate its excision.

If the upper pole of the tumor extends clearly above the S3 level (Fig. 28-13), an anterior-posterior approach is usually preferable. Patients may be placed in the supine[1] or the lateral position,[12] depending on the surgeon's preference and previous experience. Through a lower midline incision, the abdomen should be carefully examined to rule out the possibility of unsuspected distant metastasis or other important pathology. After the lateral attachments of the sigmoid have been mobilized, the presacral space is entered just below the promontory and the posterior rectum can be dissected from the upper sacrum down to the level of the upper extension of the tumor (Fig. 28-14). The rectum can then be mobilized laterally and, if necessary, anteriorly.

If it seems likely that at least one S3 root can be preserved or that the malignant tumor can be safely separated from the posterior wall of the rectum without risk of entering the tumor capsule, the lesion can be dissected in a plane between its capsule and the mesorectal fat and the rectum can be retained. If the tumor is extremely large, markedly compressing and displacing the rectum and making dissection between the rectal wall and the tumor hazardous, and if it is obvious that both S3 roots will need to be sacrificed, one may elect to remove the rectum en bloc with the tumor and the involved segment of the sacrum. In this situation, the upper rectum is transected with a stapling device at about the level of the promontory. Under those circumstances, it is imperative that the anterior wall of the rectum be completely freed from the seminal vesicle and prostate in men and the upper two-thirds of the vagina in women. The pelvic floor can then be reconstructed over the rectal remnant and the attached tumor, and a sigmoid colostomy established in the left lower abdominal wall. Also, in the presence of large tumors, blood loss during the later perineal phase of the operation may be minimized by ligating the middle sacral vessels and even the internal iliac vessels and their branches on the side of greatest extension of the tumor (Fig. 28-14).

When the presacral tumor is extremely large, most of the sacrum will need to be excised, and it is likely that the patient will need postoperative radiation. The internal iliac vessels will need to be tied bilaterally. In this situation one may wish to mobilize one rectus muscle on its vascular pedicle and place it in to the presacral area, where it can later be used in the closure of the perineal wound.[13] After the abdominal incision is closed and the colostomy is matured, the anesthetized patient can be moved from the supine to the prone position. The perineal approach is similar to that used for benign low-lying cystic or solid tumors, except that a wider and more proximal dissection will be necessary. After an incision has been made over the sacrum and coccyx down to the anus, the anococcygeal ligament is transected and the levator ani muscles are retracted laterally. If the rectum is to be preserved, the tumor can be separated from the rectum by careful dissection in the plane between the rectum and the tumor (Fig. 28-12). The orthopedic surgeon can then proceed with separation of the gluteus maximus muscles on both sides, detachment of the sacrospinous and sacrotuberous ligaments (Fig. 28-15), and division of the piriformis muscles bilaterally exposing the sciatic nerves. An osteotomy at the level of S3 or higher is performed after exposing and protecting, if at all possible, at least one S3 root (Fig. 28-16). The neural sac may need to be ligated. In this manner the lesion can be removed en bloc with the lower sacrum, coccyx, and involved sacral roots. If the surgeon previously elected to excise the rectum en bloc with the tumor, it is preferable to remove the anus and anal canal with the rectal specimen. The wound is then closed over suction Silastic drains.

RESULTS

The results of surgical treatment of retrorectal neoplasms and cysts depend on the natural behavior of the lesion being treated and the adequacy of the resection. Most malignant tumors have had a rather poor prognosis. In our experience, the 5-year survival for patients with tumors other than chordomas has been 17%.[3] Only one patient with a neuroblastoma, one with a neurofibrosarcoma, and one with Ewing's sarcoma were alive without recurrence after 3, 5, and 7 years, respectively.[3] Patients with lymphoma may fare well if they respond favorably to adjuvant therapy.

In the literature, the prognosis for patients with chordomas has been variable, ranging from 15 to 76% at 10 years after surgical therapy.[3,14–17] Gray and his coworkers[15] have reported an almost inevitable risk of local recurrence and a 10% incidence of distal metastases. At the Mayo Clinic, the 5-year survival rate in 1985 was reported to be 75%,[3] and more recently we have found the 5- and 10-year survivals to be 80% and 56%, respectively (Chiu et al., unpublished data). Of 16 patients with a chordoma that was completely resected, 9 had no clinical or radiologic evidence of recurrence 4 to 14 years later.[3] Isolated metastatic lesions to the lungs, ribs, spine, and long bones can sometimes be excised successfully and provide patients with symptomatic relief and substantial prolongation of life.

Benign tumors and cysts can be treated adequately by complete excision via a posterior approach and by avoiding contamination by transrectal biopsy. Larger cystic lesions, such as teratoma, extending high in the pelvis can be excised entirely

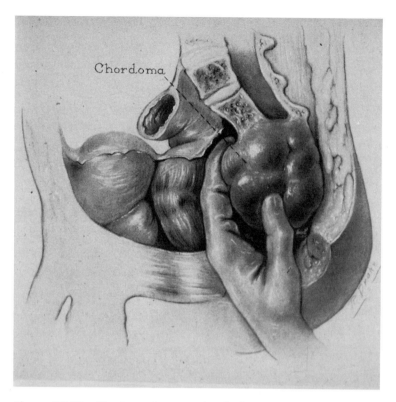

Figure 28-12. The tumor incorporating the lower sacrum and coccyx is separated from the lower rectum. (From MacCarthy et al.,[19] with permission.)

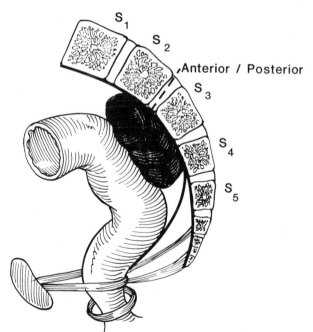

Figure 28-13. Anterior/posterior approach used for high-lying (above S3) tumors. (From Dozois,[1] with permission.)

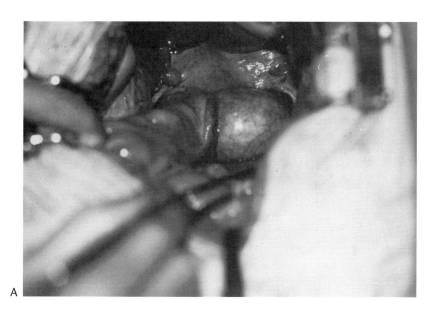

A

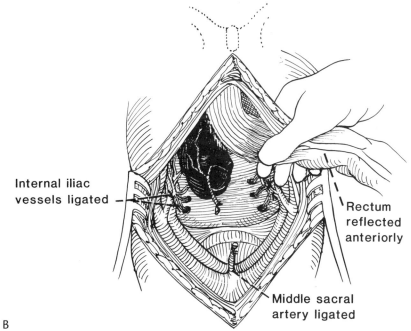

Internal iliac
vessels ligated —

Rectum
reflected
anteriorly

Middle sacral
artery ligated

B

Figure 28-14. (**A**) The tumor is exposed through a lower midline abdominal incision and mobilization of the rectum. (**B**) The middle sacral artery has been transected and tied to reduce bleeding (Fig. 14A from Dozois,[18] with permission; Fig. 14B from Dozois,[1] with permission.)

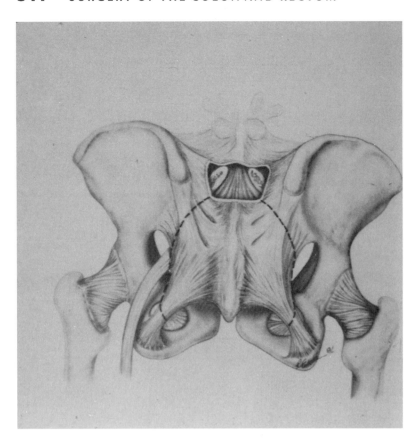

Figure 28-15. Division of the sacrospinous and sacrotuberous ligaments (posterior view). (From Dozois,[18] with permission.)

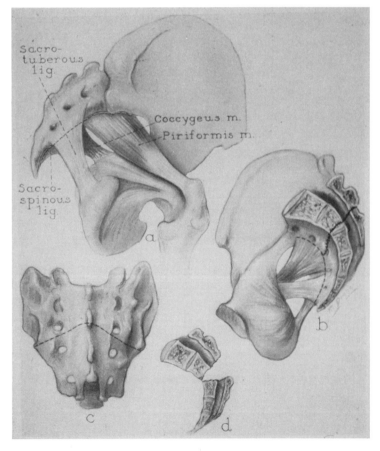

Figure 28-16. Division of the sacrospinous and sacrotuberous ligaments (lateral view) with osteostomy at the S2–S3 level and distal sacrectomy. (From MacCarthy et al.,[19] with permission.)

transabdominally. We have had no experience with transrectal or intersphincteric approaches for these types of lesions.

CONCLUDING REMARKS

Presacral tumors are rare, and their diagnosis is notoriously difficult and late; their treatment requires an experienced team of surgeons. A higher index of suspicion and the availability of better imaging techniques may reverse this situation. Once the diagnosis is established, surgical treatment is mandatory, even in asymptomatic patients. Retrorectal tumors do not necessarily need to be biopsied except under specific circumstances and never through the transrectal route. Moreover, a more aggressive approach with avoidance of tumor violation and wide en bloc resection should improve suvivorship and decrease the risk of local recurrence.

REFERENCES

1. Dozois RR (1990) Retrorectal tumors: spectrum of disease, diagnosis, and surgical management. Perspect Colon Rectal Surg 3:241–255
2. Gunterberg B, kewenter J, Petersen I, Stener B (1976) Anorectal function after major resections of the sacrum with bilateral or unilateral sacrifice of sacral nerves. Br J Surg 63:546–554
3. Jao SW, Beart RW Jr, Spencer RJ et al (1985) Retrorectal tumors: Mayo Clinic experience. Dis Colon Rectum 28:644–652
4. Stewart RJ, Humphreys WG, Parks TG (1986) The presentation and management of presacral tumours. Br J Surg 73:153–155
5. Goldberg SM, Gordon PH, Nivatvongs S (1980) Essentials of Anorectal Surgery. Lippincott-Raven, Philadelphia
6. Dahlin DC (1978) Bone Tumors: General Aspects and Data on 6,221 Cases. 3rd Ed. Charles C Thomas, Springfield, IL
7. Eilber FR (1990) Expert commentary on Dozois RR. Retrorectal tumors: spectrum of disease, diagnosis, and surgical management. Perspect Colon Rectal Surg 3:241–255
8. Waldhausen JA, Kolman JW, Vellios F, Battersby JS (1963) Sacrococcygeal teratoma. Surgery 54:933–939
9. Altman RP, Randolph JG, Lilly JR (1974) Saccrococcygeal teratoma: American Academy of Pediatrics Surgical Section Survey—1973. Pediatr Surg 9:933–949
10. Amacher AL, Drake CG, McLachlin AD (1968) Anterior sacral meningocele. Surg Gynecol Obstet 126:986–994
11. Kaiser TE, Pritchard DJ, Unni KK (1984) Clinicopathologic study of sacrococcygeal chordoma. Cancer 53:2574–2578
12. Localio SA, Francis KL, Rossano PG (1967) Abdominosacral resection of sacrococcygeal chordoma. Ann Surg 166:394–402
13. Bostwick J III, Hill HL, Nahai F (1979) Repairs in the lower abdomen, groin, or perineum with myocutaneous or omental flaps. Plast Reconst Surg 63:186–194
14. Finne CO (1989) Presacral tumors and cysts. In: Current Surgical Therapy. 3rd Ed. Marcel Decker, Toronto
15. Grundfest-Broniatowski S, Marks K, Fazio VW (1990) Sacral and retrosacral tumors. In: Current Therapy in Colon and Rectal Surgery, Marcel Decker, Toronto
16. Gray SW, Singhabhandu B, Smith RA, Skandalakis JE (1975) Sacrococcygeal chordoma: report of a case and review of the literature. Surgery 78:573–682
17. Perlman AW, Friedman M (1970) Radical radiation therapy of chordoma. Am J Roentgenol Radium Ther Nucl Med 108:332–341
18. Dozois RR (1995) Retrorectal tumors. In Mazier WP, Levien DH, Luchtefeld MA, Senagore AJ (eds): Surgery of the Colon, Rectum, and Anus. WB Saunders, Philadelphia
19. MacCarthy CS, Waugh JH, Mayo CW, Coventry MB (1952) The surgical treatment of presacral tumors: a combined problem. Proc Staff Meet Mayo Clin 27:73–84

29

ETIOLOGY

Judy Cho
Stephen B. Hanauer

The idiopathic inflammatory bowel diseases (IBD; ulcerative colitis and Crohn's disease), like other chronic inflammatory diseases such as rheumatoid arthritis, lupus, and multiple sclerosis, share many epidemiologic features. The concepts of etiopathogenesis are also similar, with evidence for both genetic predisposition and triggering by environmental factors. Elucidation of specific genes and environmental factors in IBD is hampered by the absence of subclinical markers of disease presence or susceptibility (e.g., rheumatoid factor or antinuclear antigens) and the increasing evidence that considerable phenotypic and genotypic heterogeneity exists in ulcerative colitis and Crohn's disease. Indeed, the eventual elucidation of etiopathogenesis will require a better classification of these disorders into a series of ulcerative colitides and Crohn's diseases. Meanwhile, we present evidence in favor of the genetic predisposition and potential environmental factors associated with the development of ulcerative colitis and Crohn's disease.

GENETICS

The specific molecular mechanisms of Crohn's disease and ulcerative colitis are unknown. It has long been observed that cases of IBD tend to cluster within families, and multiple lines of evidence suggest that both diseases have a significant genetic component to their pathogenesis. As opposed to simple genetic diseases, which follow a straightforward mendelian pattern of inheritance, Crohn's disease and ulcerative colitis are complex genetic disorders; disease expression results not from a single gene mutation, but from a complex interplay of multiple disease susceptibility loci interacting with myriad environmental factors.[1] While only 10 to 20% of all patients with IBD have a similarly affected relative, previous experience with other genetic disorders such as colon cancer have demonstrated that molecular mechanisms initially defined in familial cases often apply in nonfamilial cases as well.[2,3] We shall proceed by reviewing (1) the evidence that IBD is a genetic disorder, (2) the

complexity of IBD inheritance, (3) the definitions of specific subsets of IBD patients that may be genetically more similar, and (4) candidate genes that have been suggested to contribute to a picture of chronic intestinal inflammation.

One index of the heritability of a disease is obtained through relative risk data. In various studies, the disease prevalence in first-degree relatives divided by the prevalence in the general population is between 10 and 20 for both ulcerative colitis and Crohn's disease, indicating that both diseases have a significant tendency to cluster within families.[4–7]

Relative risk data do not, however, distinguish between genetic and environmental factors; increased relative risk within families could reflect shared environmental factors as opposed to genetic susceptibility. Comparing concordance rates between dizygotic and monozygotic twins is one method of dissecting these factors. A Swedish twin registry study demonstrated a concordance rate for Crohn's disease of 3.8% in dizygotic twins and 58.3% in monozygotic twins, indicating the presence of a genetic component. By contrast, the concordance rate for ulcerative colitis was zero (no concordance in 20 twins) in dizygotic twins and 4% (1 of 26 twin pairs were concordant) in monozygotic twins, indicating that while ulcerative colitis also has a genetic contribution, it may be less significant than that present with Crohn's disease.[8]

The mode of inheritance of IBD does not follow a simple monogenic mendelian pattern of inheritance and therefore represents a complex genetic disorder. The possible contribution of major gene effects for both Crohn's disease and ulcerative colitis has been established through complex segregation analyses. These studies suggest an autosomal recessive pattern for Crohn's disease and either an autosomal dominant pattern with low penetrance or multifactorial inheritance for ulcerative colitis.[9,10]

Whereas complex segregation analyses such as these are useful in establishing the contribution of a major gene effect with a dominant or recessive type of pattern, neither Crohn's disease nor ulcerative colitis follow a simple mendelian pattern of inheritance. Proof of the complexity of IBD inheritance is provided by comparing prevalence rates in white non-Jewish compared with white Jewish populations. It is well established that the prevalence of IBD is increased in Jewish populations.[11] A number of rare autosomal recessive disorders with high penetrance, such as Tay-Sachs disease, are more common in Ashkenazi Jewish populations. However, within affected non-Jewish families, the prevalence of Tay-Sachs disease in subsequent family members is the same as that observed in affected Jewish families.[12] By contrast, in families affected by Crohn's disease, the risk to additional family members is higher in Jewish families than in non-Jewish families, suggesting the influence of modifier or additional genes, more prevalent in Jewish populations.[11]

Identification of a Susceptibility Locus for Crohn's Disease

A whole genome search of sibling pairs affected by Crohn's disease has recently implicated a susceptibility locus, *IBD1*, on chromosome 16.[13] The potential significance of this finding is that a gene contributing to the pathogenesis of Crohn's disease resides in this genomic region. The relative risk attributed to *IBD1* is relatively modest (1.3) compared with the overall disease relative risk to siblings of 10. Shared environmental factors as well as additional susceptibility loci account for the remaining current risk. As more genome searches are completed, additional susceptibility loci for Crohn's disease (and presumably ulcerative colitis) will be identified. The occurrence of mixed families having members with both Crohn's disease and ulcerative colitis suggests that some common loci will contribute to the pathogenesis of both diseases.

Complexity

By definition, a complex genetic disorder does not follow simple mendelian pattern of inheritance. This complexity can result from a number of factors, of which we will discuss two: (1) variable penetrance, and (2) genetic heterogeneity.

Variable Penetrance

The degree of penetrance refers to the fraction of patients who manifest disease among all those who have inherited a given genetic predisposition. Variable penetrance can result from the influence of modifier or additional genes, as discussed in the previous section. In addition, a number of known environmental factors affect disease expression and activity in IBD (see below).

Genetic Heterogeneity

Genetic heterogeneity refers to the likelihood that different sets of genes may contribute to similar disease expression in different groups of patients. For example, in the case of diabetes mellitus, it is known that the clinical expression of glucose intolerance encompasses several distinct genetic syndromes including insulin-dependent diabetes mellitus, non-insulin-depen-

dent diabetes mellitus, and maturity onset diabetes of the young. A key to understanding the pathogenesis of IBD, then, involves identifying possible sources of genetic heterogeneity with the goal of defining subgroups sharing more similar disease courses, therapeutic responses, and genetic backgrounds. This section reviews evidence for genetic heterogeneity in IBD with respect to (1) variation in clinical characteristics, (2) perinuclear anti-neutrophil cytoplasmic antibodies (pANCA) studies, and (3) variable age of onset.

Clinical Characteristics and Genetic Heterogeneity

How Many Diseases Are There?

Ulcerative colitis and Crohn's disease are typically thought of as separate entities, but in approximately 10 to 15% of patients with inflammation confined to the large intestine, a definitive distinction cannot be made between the two conditions. These cases are termed indeterminate colitis.[14] Furthermore, in an additional 10% of patients, the diagnosis is changed between ulcerative colitis and Crohn's disease.

It is more likely for affected relatives to have the same disease as the proband, but it is quite common for both diseases to be unequivocally present in a given family. Specifically, given a proband with Crohn's disease, a 3.85-fold increased risk exists of a first-degree relative having ulcerative colitis.[5] Conversely, with ulcerative colitis probands, a 1.72-fold increased risk exists that first-degree relatives will have Crohn's disease. One explanation for these observations is that contributions from multiple genetic loci are required for the phenotypic expression of Crohn's disease or ulcerative colitis and that some of these loci are shared in the two disorders. These shared loci could account for the similar clinical characteristics seen with ulcerative colitis and Crohn's disease, as well as for the increased familial risk observed between the two disorders.

Many monozygotic twins sharing the diagnosis of ulcerative colitis or Crohn's disease have been reported, but no cases to date of one twin having ulcerative colitis and the other Crohn's disease. As the molecular basis for the IBDs is elucidated, reclassification of disease categories will evolve based on inheritance of various patterns of myriad "IBD susceptibility loci."

Heterogeneity Within Crohn's Disease: Penetrating Versus Nonpenetrating Disease

In some instances the inflammatory process affecting the intestinal wall in Crohn's disease may result in penetrating complications such as bowel perforation, fistulization, or abscess formation.[15] In these cases, the inflammation has extended through the intestinal wall and represents a more aggressive form. Patients undergoing an intestinal resection for penetrating complications required reoperation earlier (4.7 years) than patients operated on for nonpenetrating indications (average of 8.8 years). Furthermore, patients tend to follow their own disease course with regard to inflammatory type.[16]

In addition to clinical differences, molecular evidence exists for two forms of Crohn's disease based on the presence or absence of penetrating complications. The cytokine profile observed in resection specimens from Crohn's patients is distinctly different in the two inflammatory types. Intestinal mucosa demonstrate decreased levels of interleukin-1β (IL-1β) in penetrating specimens compared with nonpenetrating specimens, suggesting that IL-1β protects against penetration.[17]

Heterogeneity Within Ulcerative Colitis: Studies on Perinuclear Antineutrophil Cytoplasmic Antibodies

Indirect immunofluorescence studies on fixed neutrophils demonstrates the presence of pANCA in most patients with ulcerative colitis, significantly more frequently than is observed in patients with Crohn's disease or healthy controls.[11,18–20] Although the epitope for pANCA has not been defined, it is not believed to play a pathogenic role, as pANCA status has not been found to correlate with disease severity or extent.[21]

It has been hypothesized that the presence or absence of pANCA in patients with ulcerative colitis may be genetically determined and may represent fundamental genetic heterogeneity within ulcerative colitis. pANCA positivity is associated with the HLA-DR2 subtype, whereas pANCA-negative patients have an increase in the HLA-DR4 subtype.[18] In North American and German studies, an increased prevalence of pANCA positivity in healthy first-degree relatives of pANCA-positive probands was observed.[22,23] These findings have not been duplicated in other populations.[24–26] Furthermore, in families with multiple siblings affected with ulcerative colitis, there was no concordance of pANCA status within families.[27] Finally, in monozygotic twin pairs having one member affected by ulcerative colitis, there was not a significant increase in the incidence of pANCA positivity in the healthy twins compared with unrelated healthy controls.[21] Taken together, there is insufficient evidence at present to conclude that pANCA status can be used to define genetic heterogeneity in ulcerative colitis.

Age of Onset

Variable age of onset is often used to delineate genetic heterogeneity. In heritable cases of colon[28] and breast cancer,[29] early age of onset was used to define a more homogeneous subgroup. The bimodal distribution of age of onset (the larger peak occurs between 15 and 35 years of age and a second peak occurs in the sixth to seventh decade) has been used to infer genetic heterogeneity.[30] The concept that ''genetic anticipation'' may exist in IBD has been recently supported by evidence that in parent-child pairs with Crohn's disease, the child more often develops the disease at a younger age than the parent.[31,32]

As with many other genetic disorders, there is some suggestion that familial cases of IBD tend to be characterized by an earlier age of onset as well as a more severe course.[33] However, as opposed to heritable cases of cancer, in which a characteristic mutation often predictably results in disease at an earlier age after a period of accumulated, neoplastic transformation, it is not clearly established at present that families characterized by an early age of onset represent a separate, unique subtype of IBD.

SUBSETS

Racial and Ethnic Classification

The racial prevalence rates for ulcerative colitis and Crohn's disease can be inferred from population-based incidence rates of various countries. Both disorders are more prevalent in English

stock, U.S. whites and Northern Europeans, less frequent in Central Europe and the Middle East, and infrequent in South America, Asia, and Africa.[24] A survey from a California-based health maintenance organization estimated that the prevalence (in 100,000) of Crohn's disease was 43.6 among whites, 29.8 among blacks, 4.1 among Hispanics, and 5.6 among Asians.[34]

Within the white population, a three- to fivefold increased rate is seen among Jewish populations.[11,35,36] Interestingly, the prevalence of Crohn's disease among Jews in Israel, while increasing, is lower than that found in Europe or the United States, again emphasizing the role of environmental factors.[37] The relatively high prevalence of IBD in Jewish populations, combined with the relative homogeneity observed genetically, suggests that this group may be an important subset to study.[38]

Ankylosing Spondylitis and Primary Sclerosing Cholangitis

Both ankylosing spondylitis (AS) and primary sclerosing cholangitis (PSC) are present more frequently in patients with IBD and their first-degree relatives. In addition, both diseases are associated with specific HLA subtypes (HLA-B27 for AS and HLA-B8 DR3 for PSC). In patients with IBD but not AS or PSC, however, these HLA subtypes are not present more frequently.[7,39,40]

CANDIDATE GENES

HLA and IBD

Crohn's Disease

Evidence for HLA associations in Crohn's disease by association studies have yielded inconsistent results with no clear associations.[6] More recently, linkage analysis in familial aggregations of Crohn's disease involving genotyping of HLA-DRB1 and 16 other loci on chromosome 6 was performed using the lod score method. This study, while not excluding the HLA region as a minor contributing locus, suggests that the major autosomal recessive locus suggested by segregation analyses[9] does not reside on chromosome 6.[41]

Ulcerative Colitis

There are clearer HLA associations in ulcerative colitis, with multiple studies revealing association of ulcerative colitis with HLA-DR2.[42,43] Furthermore, ulcerative colitis patients can be classified as ANCA positive or negative. Correlations between ANCA positivity and HLA-DR2 as well as ANCA negativity and HLA-DR4 have been used as further evidence for genetic heterogeneity in ulcerative colitis.[18]

The Interleukin-1 Gene Family

IL-1 is a major proinflammatory cytokine with two secreted forms, IL-1a and IL-1b, the latter being the major agonist. In addition, an IL receptor antagonist, (RA) competes with IL-1 for binding to the receptor. Whereas IL-1 is increased in various forms of colitis reflecting nonspecific activation of the immune system, the ratio of IL-RA to IL-1 as measured by immunoassay is decreased in patients with IBD compared with healthy controls and, importantly, controls with self-limited colitis. Furthermore, the IL-RA/IL-1 ratio is inversely correlated with disease severity.[44]

HOST FACTORS

The highest incidence of ulcerative colitis and Crohn's disease is seen in Europe and North America, but these diseases are increasing worldwide in an intriguing pattern: ulcerative colitis is described first, followed by Crohn's disease almost a decade later.[45] The most consistent finding is the association of IBD with improved sanitation, suggesting either exposure to an environmental trigger unique to ''developed'' countries or the loss of protective exposures. The (relative) contributions of genetically determined host factors versus environmental triggers initiating disease in a population ''at risk'' need to be separated.[46]

Defective Mucosal Barrier Function

A major function of the intestine is antigen sampling from the environment, hence aberrant sampling of dietary or ingested agents is a primary candidate for the initiation of an overly exuberant mucosal immune response leading to chronic IBD. The gastrointestinal mucosa is normally impermeable to macromolecules, which, in the case of nutritional products, are routinely absorbed across the columnar epithelium. Macromolecules are transported across microfold cells (M cells) that are in direct contact with underlying antigen sampling macrophages and lymphocytes.[47] The antigen sampling in normal individuals induces a general state of immune tolerance to most foreign molecules within the gut; however, evidence in patients with IBD shows that there is aberrant processing of antigens by epithelial cells with preferential delivery to CD4+ rather than CD8+ lymphocytes, leading to immune activation rather than tolerance.[48] Further immunoregulator dysfunction has been postulated by the demonstration of defective immunosuppressive response to IL-4 in peripheral blood monnuclear cells, including defective IL-1RA secretion.[49] This observation is supportive of the possible imbalance between IL-1 and IL-1RA noted in patients with IBD compared with normal controls.[50] Recent immunologic paradigms analogize T-cell immune dysregulation to models of immune processing in mice in which specific antigens induce differential cytokine profiles according to the induction of T-cell subtypes categorized as T helper$_1$ (T$_{H1}$) or T helper$_2$ (T$_{H2}$).[51] Ulcerative colitis is hypothesized to mimic the T$_{H2}$ profile, whereas in Crohn's disease the cytokines released parallel the mouse T$_{H1}$ mediators.

Additional mucosal factors that may lead to IBD include an increase in membrane receptors and response to chemotactic oligopeptides and endotoxin,[52,53] leading to increased production of toxic oxygen metabolites and nitric oxide synthesis that are well recognized to contribute to the inflammatory process in IBD.[54] Mucosal epithelial defects have also been postulated in IBD, more often in ulcerative colitis, including alterations in colonic mucin[40] and defective metabolism of short chain fatty acids.[55] These abnormalities may lead to breakdown of the epithelial surface barrier and allow the transgression of luminal antigens into the mucosa, inducing a proinflammatory rather than downregulatory response of typical intestinal tolerance.

Enhanced intestinal permeability to macromolecules has been demonstrated in inflamed and uninflamed intestine in Crohn's disease and remains a controversial arena of investigation into possible pathogenic proclivity.[51,56] Altered small bowel permeability has been observed in patients with Crohn's disease in remission and in "unaffected" relatives.[57]

Environmental Factors

Nonsteroidal Anti-inflammatory Agents

Nonsteroidal anti-inflammatory agents (NSAIDs) present a potential link between intestinal permeability and clinical disease initiation or perpetuation.[52] NSAIDs have multiple potential actions on the intestinal mucosa including direct cellular toxicity, increasing mucosal permeability, and alteration of eicosanoid profiles in favor of proinflammatory events by preferential inhibition of cyclooxygenase compared with the lipoxygenase pathway, leading to increased concentrations of leukotriene metabolites. NSAIDs in animal models also demonstrate the genetic disposition to develop IBD and the role for luminal antigens (primarily bacterial) in developing acute and chronic inflammation.[51] NSAIDs have been demonstrated to exacerbate human IBD and should be proscribed for patients to avoid recurrence.[58–60]

Cigarette Smoking

The role of cigarette smoking in the epidemiology of IBD has produced the most consistent and intriguing results. In adults, cigarette smoking has a protective effect against the development of ulcerative colitis but is an aggressive factor in Crohn's disease. Cessation of smoking is associated with a risk of developing ulcerative colitis,[61,62] but, conversely, continuation of smoking in Crohn's disease makes the condition more refractory to medical therapy and is associated with an increased risk of recurrence after surgery.[61–64] The mechanism(s) by which smoking influences the occurrence of IBD remains undefined. Cigarette smoking has multiple physiologic effects, including direct morphologic injury to endothelial cells associated with the formation of microthrombi and elevated fibrinogen, plasminogen activator, and enhanced platelet aggregation; influence on colonic mucus; impact on both humoral and cellular immunity; and alterations in arachidonic acid metabolism.[65] The beneficial effects of smoking in ulcerative colitis have begun to translate into therapeutic advances using nicotine, but the opposite effects of smoking on the course of ulcerative colitis and Crohn's disease remains enigmatic. Furthermore, although passive smoking has been associated with the development of both ulcerative colitis and Crohn's disease in children, the overall impact of smoking on IBD must be kept in perspective since the diseases often have their onset in childhood prior to exposure.

Oral Contraceptives

Like other possible etiologic factors, the role of oral contraceptives on the development of IBD is controversial, with conflicting data from case-control and observational series.[66–68] The possible minor increase in the relative risk of women developing Crohn's disease related to oral contraceptives must also be distinguished from the risk related to cigarette smoking.[68] The possible pathogenic mechanisms for the risk in Crohn's disease include increased levels of fibrinogen, prothrombin, and factors VII, VIII, and X.[69] Additional procoagulant effects include reduced levels of tissue plasminogen activator and antithrombin III, which contribute to the increased risk of thromboembolism and vascular damage that have been noted in Crohn's disease.[70]

The recent "vasculitis" hypothesis regarding the development of Crohn's disease due to multifocal gastrointestinal (mesenteric) infarction and granulomatous vasculitis is consistent with the prothrombotic effect of oral contraceptives[71]; however, these observations still do not account for the lack of gender differences in the incidence of Crohn's disease nor the development of Crohn's disease in children.

Dietary Factors

Over time, many dietary constituents have been implicated in the development of IBD. To date, no factor has been reproducibly associated with the development of either ulcerative colitis or Crohn's disease. Associations have been sought for the ingestion of breakfast cereal, fiber, protein, fat, cow's milk, meat products, and total calories.[72] The possibility that increased intake of refined sugar is a risk factor for Crohn's disease has not been confirmed, and the implicating studies have serious design flaws.[46,72]

The ingestion of foreign substances has been an obvious source of speculation regarding the cause of IBD for many decades.[46] Granuloma-inducing agents such as beryllium, zirconium, silica, and wood particles have, at one time or another,

been proposed as etiologic agents and have led to speculation regarding components of toothpaste or abrasives in processed foods, which are more common in industrialized nations, as possible correlates to the epidemiologic patterns of disease. Recent hypotheses have also speculated on genetically influenced metabolism of xenobiotics and interaction with gut microflora as initiating factors.[73]

SUMMARY

Current theories on the etiopathogenesis of IBD must account for the recognized epidemiologic patterns of disease as well as the spectrum of illness observed in families and individual patients. Environmental influences such as cigarette smoking are useful clues due to the differential effect on ulcerative colitis and Crohn's disease. Current paradigms from animal models suggest that the IBDs are due to an abnormal host response to a ubiquitous (normally nonpathogenic) organism or luminal agent rather than a specific pathogen, although the recent elucidation of *Helicobacter pylori* as a causative agent in peptic ulcer disease is a humbling insight with immediate implications for IBD. Nevertheless, (current) conventional wisdom proposes that these diseases are due to aberrant host responses to (enteric) environmental antigens in genetically susceptible individuals. To date, neither the genetic susceptibility nor the environmental agents have been elucidated, hence the persistence of the term *idiopathic* IBD. The future is bright, however, with the potential for further defining clinical disease subsets, subclinical markers, and specific genetic patterns so that the etiologies will soon be clarified.

REFERENCES

1. Duerr RH (1996) Genetics of inflammatory bowel disease. Inflammatory Bowel Dis 2:48–60
2. Calkins BM, Mendeloff AI (1986) Epidemiology of inflammatory bowel disease. Epidemiol Rev 8:60–91
3. Monsen U, Bernell O, Johansson C, Hellers G (1991) Prevalence of inflammatory bowel disease among relatives of patients with Crohn's disease. Scand J Gastroenterol 26:302–306
4. Lashner BA, Evans AA, Kirsner JB, Hanauer SB (1986) Prevalence and incidence of inflammatory bowel disease in family members. Gastroenterology 91:1396–1400
5. Orholm M, Munkholm P, Langholz E (1991) Familial occurrence of inflammatory bowel disease. N Engl J Med 324:84–88
6. McConnell RB (1990) Genetics of inflammatory bowel disease. pp. 11–23. In Allan RN, Keighley MRB, Alexander-Williams J, Hawkins C (eds): Inflammatory Bowel Disease. 2nd Ed. Churchill-Livingstone, Edinburgh
7. Satsangi J, Jewell DP, Rosenberg WMC, Bell JI (1994) Genetics of inflammatory bowel disease. Gut 35:696–700
8. Tysk C, Linkberg E, Jarnerot G, Floderus-Myrhed B (1988) Ulcerative colitis and Crohn's disease in an unselected population of monozygotic and dizygotic twins: a study of heritability and the influence of smoking Gut 29:990–996
9. Orholm M, Iselius L, Sorensen TIA (1993) Investigation of inheritance of chronic inflammatory bowel diseases by complex segregation analysis. BMJ 306:20–24
10. Kuster W, Pascoe L, Purrmann J (1989) The genetics of Crohn's disease: complex segregation analysis of a family

study with 265 patients with Crohn's disease and 5,387 relatives. Am J Med Genet 32:105–108
11. Yang H, McElree C, Roth MP (1993) Familial empirical risks for inflammatory bowel disease: differences between Jews and non-Jews. Gut 34:517–524
12. Kaback MM, Rimoin DL, O'Brien JS (eds) (1977) Tay-Sachs Disease: Screening and Prevention. Alan R Liss, New York
13. Hugot MP, Laurent-Puig P, Gower-Rousseau C et al (1996) Mapping of a susceptibility locus for Crohn's disease on chromosome 16. Nature 379:821–823
14. Targan SR, Shanahan F (eds) (1994) Inflammatory Bowel Disease: From Bench to Bedside. Williams & Wilkins, Baltimore
15. Sachar DB, Andrews HA, Farmer RG et al (1992) Proposed classification of patient subgroups in Crohn's disease. Gastroenterol Intern 5:141–54
16. Greenstein AJ, Lachman P, Sachar DB et al (1988) Perforating and non-perforating indications for repeated operations in Crohn's disease: evidence for two clinical forms. Gut 29:588–592
17. Gilberts ECAM, Greenstein AJ, Katsel P et al (1994) Molecular evidence for two forms of Crohn disease. Proc Natl Acad Sci USA 91:12721–12724
18. Yang H, Rotter JI, Toyoda H et al (1993) Ulcerative colitis; a genetically heterogeneous disorder defined by genetic (HLA class II) and subclinical (antineutrophil cytoplasmic antibodies) markers. J Clin Invest 92:1080–1084
19. Seibold F, Welber P, Klein R (1992) Clinical significance of

antibodies against neutrophils in patients with inflammatory bowel disease and primary sclerosing cholangitis. Gut 33: 657–662

20. Cambridge G, Rampton DS, Stevens TRJ (1992) Anti-neutrophil antibodies in inflammatory bowel disease: prevalence and diagnostic role. Gut 33:668–674

21. Yang P, Jarnerot G, Danielsson D (1995) P-ANCA in monozygotic twins with inflammatory bowel disease. Gut 36:887–890

22. Shanahan F, Duerr RH, Rotter JI et al (1992) Neutrophil autoantibodies in ulcerative colitis: familial aggregation and genetic heterogeneity. Gastroenterology 103:456–461

23. Seibold F, Klein R, Slametschka D (1993) p-ANCA in family members of patients with ulcerative colitis and PSC. Gastroenterology 104:A778

24. Reumaux D, Delecourt L, Colombel JF (1992) Anti-neutrophil cytoplasmic autoantibodies in relatives of patients with ulcerative colitis Qobletter Qcb. Gastroenterology 103:1706

25. Lee JCW, Cambridge G, Lennard-Jones JE (1994) Prevalence of anti-neutrophil antibodies in familial inflammatory bowel disease: specificity for ulcerative colitis in genetically related individuals. Gastroenterology 106:A718

26. Monteleone G, Doldo P, Marasco R et al (1994) Perinuclear neutrophil autoantibodies (p-ANCA) in affected relative of patients with ulcerative colitis (UC). Suggestions against familial aggregation. Gut, suppl. 4, 35:S31

27. Lee JCW, Lennard-Jones JE, Cambridge G (1995) Antineutrophil antibodies in familial inflammatory bowel disease. Gastroenterology 108:428–433

28. Peltomaki P, Aaltonen LA, Sistonen P et al (1993) Genetic mapping of a locus predisposing to human colorectal cancer. Science 260:810–812

29. Hall JM, Lee MK, Newman B (1990) Linkage of early-onset familial breast cancer to chromosome 17q21. Science 250: 1684–1689

30. Evans JG, Acheson DE (1965) An epidemiological study of ulcerative colitis and regional enteritis in the Oxford area. Gut 6:311–324

31. Burress GC, Barclay SK, Kirschner (1994) Parents developing IBD after their children—clinical features and implications for family studies. Gastroenterology 106:A658

32. Polito JM 2d, Rees RC, Childs B (1996) Preliminary evidence for genetic anticipation in Crohn's disease. Lancet 347: 798–800

33. Farmer RG, Michener WM, Mortimer EA (1980) Studies of family history among patients with inflammatory bowel disease. Clin Gastroenterol 9:271–277

34. Kurata JH, Kantor-Fish S, Frankl H (1992) Crohn's disease among ethnic groups in a large health maintenance organization. Gastroenterology 102:1940–1948

35. Acheson ED (1960) The distribution of ulcerative colitis and regional enteritis in United States veterans with particular reference to the Jewish religion. Gut 1:91–93

36. Monk M, Mendeloff AI, Siegel CI (1969) An epidemiological study of ulcerative colitis and regional enteritis among adults in Baltimore. Gastroenterology 56:847–857

37. Shapira M, Tamir A (1994) Crohn's disease in the Kinneret sub-district, Israel, 1960–1990. Incidence and prevalence in different ethnic subgroups. Eur J Epidemiol 10:231–233

38. Motulsky AG (1995) Jewish diseases and origins. Nature Genet 9:99–101

39. Russell AS (1977) Arthritis, inflammatory bowel disease, and histocompatibility antigens. Ann Intern Med 86:820–821

40. Chapman MA, Grahn MF, Boyle MA et al (1994) Butyrate oxidation is impaired in the colonic mucosa of sufferers of quiescent ulcerative colitis. Gut 35:73–76

41. Hugot JP, Laurent-Puig P, Gower-Rousseau C et al (1994) Linkage analyses of chromosome 6 loci, including HLA, in familial aggregations of Crohn disease. Am J Med Genet 52: 207–213

42. Smolen JS, Gangl A, Polterauer P (1982) HLA antigens in inflammatory bowel disease. Gastroenterology 82:34–38

43. Asakura H, Tsuchiya M, Aiso S et al (1982) Association of human lymphocyte-DR2 antigen with Japanese ulcerative colitis. Gastroenterology 82:413–418

44. Casini-Raggi V, Kam L, Chong YJ et al (1995) Mucosal imbalance of IL-1 and IL-1 receptor antagonist in inflammatory bowel disease. A novel mechanism of chronic intestinal inflammation. J Immunol 154:2434–2440

45. Calkins BM, Mendeloff AI (1995) The epidemiology of idiopathic inflammatory bowel disease. p. 31. In Kirsner JB, Shorter RG (eds): Inflammatory Bowel Disease. 4th Ed. Williams & Wilkins, Baltimore

46. Levine J (1992) Exogenous factors in Crohn's disease. A critical review. J Clinil Gastroenterol 14:216–26

47. Elson CO, McCabe RP Jr (1995) The immunology of inflammatory bowel disease. p. 203. In Kirsner JB, Shorter RG (eds): Inflammatory Bowel Disease, 4th Ed. Williams & Wilkins, Baltimore

48. Mayer L, Eisenhardt D (1990) Lack of induction of suppressor T cells by intestinal epithelial cells from patients with inflammatory bowel disease. J Clin Invest 86:1255–1260

49. Schreiber S, Heinig T, Panzer U et al (1995) Impaired response of activated mononuclear phagocytes to interleukin-4 in inflammatory bowel disease. Gastroenterology 108:21–33

50. Isaacs KL, Sartor RB, Haskill S (1992) Cytokine messenger RNA profiles in inflammatory bowel disease mucosa detected by polymerase chain reaction amplification. Gastroenterology 103:1587–1595

51. Sartor RB (1995) Current concepts of the etiology and pathogenesis of ulcerative colitis and Crohn's disease. Gastroenterol Clin North Am 24:p475

52. Anton PA, Targan SR, Shanahan F (1989) Increased neutrophil receptors for and response to the proinflammatory bacterial peptide formyl-methionyl-leucyl-phenylalanine in Crohn's disease. Gastroenterology 97:20–28

53. Baldassano RN, Schreiber S, Johnston RBJ et al (1993) Crohn's disease monocytes are primed for accentuated release of toxic oxygen metabolites. Gastroenterology 105:50–66

54. Conner EM, Brand SJ, Davis JM (1996) Role of reactive metabolites of oxygen and nitrogen in inflammatory bowel disease: toxins, mediators, and modulators of gene expression. Inflammatory Bowel Dis 2:133–147

55. Roediger WE, Duncan A, Kapaniris O et al (1993) Reducing sulfur compounds of the colon impairs colonocyte nutrition: implications for ulcerative colitis. Gastroenterology 104: 802–809

56. May GR, Sutherland LR, Meddings JB (1993) Is small intestinal permeability really increased in relatives of patients with Crohn's disease? Gastroenterology 104:1627–1632

57. Peeters M (1995) Familial aggregation and the importance of increased small intestinal permeability in the pathogenesis of Crohn's disease. Thesis, Katholieke Universiteit Leuven, Leuven

58. Bjarnason I, Macpherson AJS, Teahon K (1993) Nonsteroidal anti-inflammatory drugs and inflammatory bowel disease. Cancer J Gastroenterol 7:160–169

59. Bjarnason I, Zanelli G, Smith T et al (1987) Nonsteroidal anti-inflammatory drug-induced intestinal inflammation in humans. Gastroenterology 93:480–489

60. Gibson GR, Whitacre EB, Ricotti CA (1992) Colitis induced by nonsteroidal anti-inflammatory drugs. Report of four cases and review of the literature. Arch Intern Med 152:625–632

61. Calkins BM (1989) A meta-analysis of the role of smoking in inflammatory bowel disease. Dig Dis Sci 34:1841–1854

62. Sutherland LR, Ramcharan S, Bryant H, Fick G (1990) Effect of cigarette smoking on recurrence of Crohn's disease. Gastroenterology 98:1123–1128

63. Duffy LC, Zielezny MA, Marshall JR et al (1990) Cigarette smoking and risk of clinical relapse in patients with Crohn's disease. Am J Prevent Med 6:161–166

64. Lindberg E, Jarnerot G, Huitfeldt B (1992) Smoking in Crohn's disease: effect on localisation and clinical course. Gut 33: 779–782

65. Cohen RD, Hanauer SB (1996) Nicotine in ulcerative colitis: has the smoke cleared? Clin Immunother 5:169–174

66. Sandler RS, Wurzelmann JI, Lyles CM (1992) Oral contraceptive use and the risk of inflammatory bowel disease. Epidemiology 3:374–378

67. Boyko EJ, Theis MK, Vaughan TL, Nicol-Blades B (1994) Increased risk of inflammatory bowel disease associated with oral contraceptive use. Am J Epidemiol 140:268–278

68. Katschinski B, Fingerle D, Scherbaum B, Goebell H (1993) Oral conceptive use and cigarette smoking in Crohn's disease. Dig Dis Sci 38:1596–1600

69. Beller FK, Ebert C (1985) Effects of oral contraceptives on blood coagulation. A review. Obstet Gynecol Surv 40:425–436

70. de Bruin PA, Crama-Bohbouth G, Verspaget HW et al (1988) Plasminogen activators in the intestine of patients with inflammatory bowel disease. Thromb Haemost 60:262–266

71. Wakefield AJ, Sawyer AM, Dillon AP et al (1989) Pathogenesis of Crohn's disease: multifocal gastrointestinal infarction. Lancet 2:1057–1062

72. Kelly DG, Fleming CR (1995) Nutritional considerations in inflammatory bowel diseases. Gastroenterol Clin North Am 24:597–611

73. Crotty B (1994) Ulcerative colitis and xenobiotic metabolism. Lancet 343:35–38

30

PATHOLOGY

Ian C. Talbot

The etiology of this group of conditions is unknown, hence the term "idiopathic inflammatory bowel disease." It is nevertheless entirely possible that, despite the title of this section, infective agent(s) may play a part in their causation. Conventionally, the group has been subdivided into ulcerative colitis and Crohn's disease, but it is now clear that the term "inflammatory bowel disease" also embraces the microscopic colitis group.

Resected specimens are best sent directly to the laboratory unopened and unfixed, so that they can be handled in controlled conditions by the pathologist.[1] The bowel should be opened along its anterior aspect and then slightly stretched and pinned in the correct anatomic position onto a board of cork, to be floated upside down, overnight, in a tank of 4% formalin. By following such a procedure it is possible to achieve both adequate preservation of the pathologic anatomy and good fixation of the delicate and diagnostically critical mucosa.

ULCERATIVE COLITIS

Ulcerative colitis begins in the rectum, but spreads proximally to involve the colon in two-thirds of cases. In one-third there is total involvement of the entire colon at presentation. The disease undergoes dynamic evolution, with periods of exacerbation and of remission and by the time of surgical intervention the rectum may have passed into a healing phase, even appearing relatively normal.

Macroscopic Appearances

Externally the serosa is typically congested but otherwise may appear and feel normal, unless there is fulminant disease. Again, unless there is fulminant disease, the unopened bowel is typically contracted and shortened and narrowed, particularly distally, with obliteration of the sigmoid loop (Fig. 30-1; see also Plate 30-1). There is muscular contraction and edema of the mesentery, which in the rectum is associated with an increase in the sacrorectal distance, seen radiologically. A short length of the terminal ileum can be involved, but this is not usually apparent on the external surface.

On opening the bowel, blood oozes from the mucosal surface. In active but nonfulminant ulcerative colitis the disease is limited to the mucosa, which is congested, hemorrhagic, and friable. Ulcers vary from superficial erosions to full thickness loss of mucosa. The latter may be patchy but are frequently linear, along the line of the taenia coli. Between areas of ulceration islands of mucosa are often swollen by acute inflammation, particularly with edema and congestion. At the edges of ulcers the mucosa is frequently undermined, forming mucosal islands, tags, or inflammatory polyps,[2] commonly referred to as *pseudopolyps*. Healed ulcers tend to appear flat and depressed below the surrounding residual inflamed mucosa, but fibrosis is relatively slight and the bowel does not become severely deformed. Healing of inflammatory polyps and mucosal tags may result in elongated strands of mucosa, forming *postinflammatory polyps*. These polyps, also called "filiform" polyps, may be present in large numbers and show bizarre appearances, like coral or pasta, with bridges due to adhesions between tags. When numerous, the terms *colitis polyposa* or *bizarre polyposis* are appropriate (Fig. 30-2; see also Plate 30-2). Postinflammatory polyps are markers of healing and rarely have any neoplastic significance.

The ileum may be affected in 10% of cases for a distance of up to 25 cm proximal to the ileocecal valve.[3] Because in these cases the ileocecal valve is usually dilated and incompetent, the term *backwash ileitis* is appropriate. Inflammation is limited to the mucosa and resembles colorectal disease, although frank ulceration is unusual.

In about one-half of all cases of ulcerative colitis there is inflammation of the appendix confined to the mucosa, similar to that seen in the colon, without progression to suppurative appendicitis. This can occur even when there is only distal ulcerative colitis.[4]

Microscopic Appearances

The histologic features of ulcerative colitis vary, depending on whether the disease is active, resolving, or in remission. Except in fulminant colitis, only the mucosa is affected.

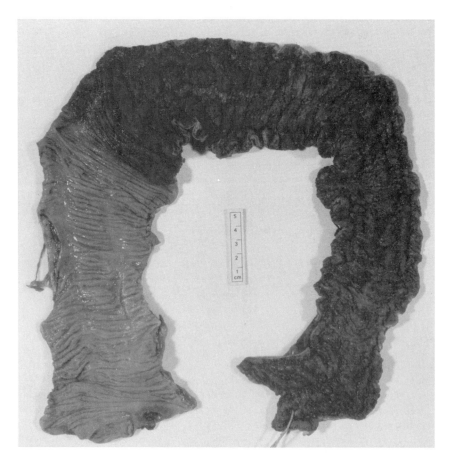

Figure 30-1. Opened specimen of colon from a patient with extensive active ulcerative colitis, showing swollen, granular, friable, bleeding mucosa. There is contraction and shortening of the left colon.

Figure 30-2. Multiple postinflammatory polyps in ulcerative colitis ("colitis polyposa").

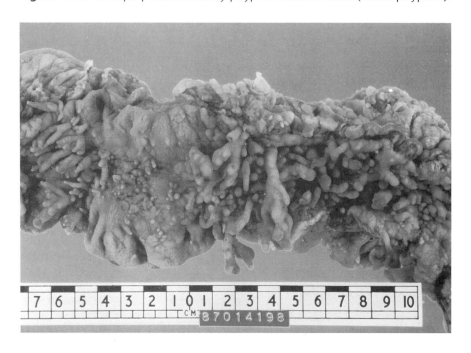

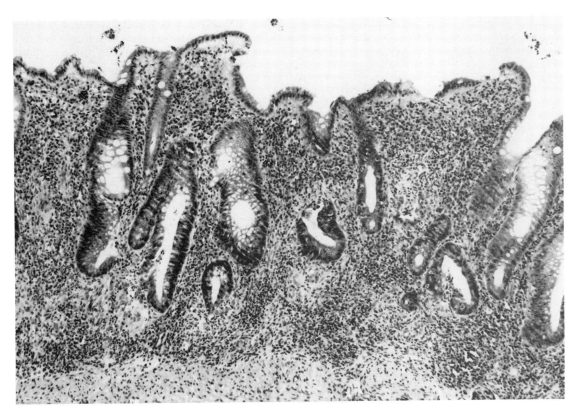

Figure 30-3. Histologic appearance of rectal mucosa in active ulcerative colitis, with a villiform configuration and distortion of crypt pattern. There is a heavy diffuse chronic inflammatory cell infiltrate. Goblet cells are inconspicuous and there is active inflammation shown by cryptitis and crypt abscesses. Giant cells are present in association with destruction of crypt bases but this is not granuloma formation as seen in Crohn's disease.

Active Disease

In early active disease the mucosa is thickened, with a villiform surface (Fig. 30-3). The lamina propria is heavily and diffusely infiltrated by plasma cells and lymphocytes, together with neutrophils, eosinophils, and mast cells. Capillaries are engorged with blood, so that the surface bleeds at the slightest touch. Goblet cells discharge their mucin, so that in active colitis they are less conspicuous or even absent. Infiltration by neutrophil polymorphs is the most important marker of activity; when neutrophils are present only within the crypt epithelium ("cryptitis") activity is said to be mild; when there is an occasional crypt abscess (polymorph exudate into the crypt lumen), activity is moderate; when there are numerous crypt abscesses activity is severe. Bursting of crypt abscesses, either onto the surface or into the submucosa, is responsible for much of the ulceration and inflammatory polyp formation by disrupting the surface or undermining the adjacent mucosa, respectively. Very quickly, there is damage to crypt base epithelium with destruction and loss of crypts. The epithelium of those crypts that remain is required to proliferate at an increased rate to make up the deficit left by crypt loss. The nuclei of the regenerating epithelial cells are enlarged and hyperchromatic and the cytoplasm is also more darkly stained than normal, giving the epithelium an atypical appearance that can be distinguished from dysplasia by the way the "atypical" features give way to more

normal cells as the more mature cells approach the luminal surface (Fig. 30-4). Crypt epithelial damage results in deformation of the crypt architecture, with distortion and branching. The latter are the most specific features of ulcerative colitis.

Fulminant Colitis

When ulceration is extensive, large areas of submucosa and muscularis propria are exposed to the bowel lumen and become covered by a layer of granulation tissue. Granulation tissue and edema extend into the muscularis propria and the muscle loses its contractility, dilates, and becomes thinned, leading to the state of acute toxic dilatation. Stretching of the friable granulation tissue leads to splitting, with acute fissure formation.

Resolving Colitis

Crypt abscesses run their course and are not renewed. Inflammatory cells of all types are diminished and their density becomes patchy. Goblet cells return to normal but architectural distortion remains (Fig. 30-5). When ulcerative colitis has been in remission for a considerable time, the chronic inflammatory cell infiltrate may be so inconspicuous that the mucosa may appear almost normal. However, there is almost invariably some degree of distortion of architecture to indicate previous disease,

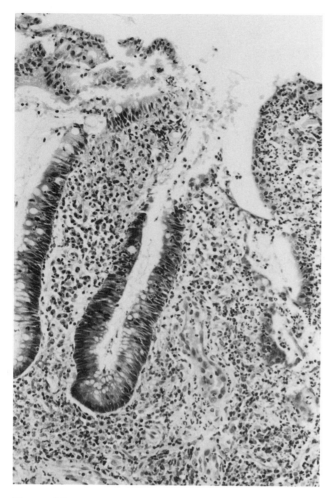

Figure 30-4. Regenerating crypt epithelium in active ulcerative colitis. Note the prominent enlarged nuclei with pseudostratification, giving an atypical appearance that must be distinguished from dysplasia by the way the epithelial cells regain their mature features as the top of the crypt is approached.

including atrophy of crypts, which are shortened and irregular in shape. The presence of Paneth cells at the bases of the crypts (Paneth cell metaplasia) is also a marker of previous colitis.

Cancer and Dysplasia

Only 3% to 5% of all colitics develop bowel cancer and colitic patients account for less than 1% of fatal colorectal cancers.[5] The increased risk applies to those who have had extensive disease for at least 8 years. Colorectal cancers are often multiple in colitis and differ from sporadic colorectal cancers in usually being flat and plaquelike. The proportion of mucinous carcinomas is higher among the adenocarcinomas that arise in colitic patients than in other colorectal carcinomas, but the prognosis is no worse and, among patients on a surveillance program, may be better.[6] There is therefore a rational basis for surveillance colonoscopy of those patients with extensive ulcerative colitis with a history of over 8 years. Despite evidence that technologies such as DNA flow cytometry.[7,8] and immunocytochemistry for expression of the oncogene $p53$[9,10] are more sensitive in

detecting precancerous states, the histologic assessment of colonoscopic biopsies for dysplasia remains the most practical method of identifying patients at high risk of cancer in colitis. As with colitis it takes the form of flat plaques or sessile nodules or there may be a velvety mucosal surface. However, sometimes the dysplastic mucosa is thickened sufficiently to produce a lesion easily visible endoscopically (a "dysplasia-associated lesion or mass [DALM]") (Fig. 30-6).

Histologic Features of Dysplasia

In most instances dysplastic mucosa is thickened due to proliferation of epithelium to give an adenomalike pattern, either with a villous configuration (Fig. 30-7A) or, due to glandular budding, with a more tubular structure (Fig. 30-7B). The appearances differ from adenomas in general in lacking discrete structure and covering a larger ill-defined area without polyp formation. Adenomatous polyps of ordinary type with classic adenomatous features do occur in colitic patients. The patients are usually older. Their diagnosis should only be made after extensive biopsy sampling of the mucosa throughout the colon and rectum has excluded the presence of nonpolypoid colitis-associated dysplasia, because an apparent solitary adenomatous polyp may be a marker for the more clinically sinister precancerous sign of nonpolypoid dysplasia.

The features of dysplasia can be mimicked by regenerating epithelium in active ulcerative colitis (Fig. 30-4) and in resolving disease. The latter is the most common reason for erroneously overdiagnosing dysplasia. For this reason, the classification of dysplasia proposed by Riddell and colleagues[12] is useful and has stood the test of time.

The classification reflects the subjectivity inherent in an appraisal of such complex and subtle histologic features. The indefinite categories are necessary as signals indicating that the pathologist thinks that although there is epithelial atypia, it may be related to active inflammatory damage of epithelium and the clinical response should be weighted accordingly. After a period of medical treatment the uncertainty will be resolved one way or another in at least one-half of these cases.[13] Dysplasia, when confidently diagnosed, amounts to intramucosal neoplasia. Observer variation studies have shown that high-grade dysplasia is the least difficult category to diagnose because it incorporates those cases in which there are severe architectural and/ or cyto-

---

Classification of Dysplasia

Negative
Indefinite
    Probably negative
    Equivocal
    Probably positive
Positive
    Low grade
    High grade

(Modified from Riddell et al.,[12] with permission.)

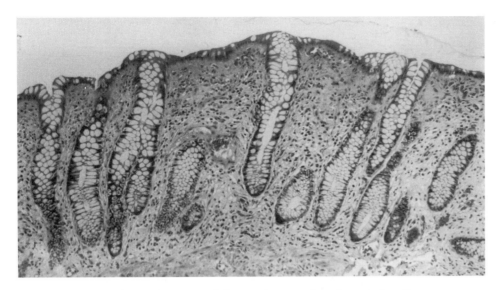

Figure 30-5. Histologic appearance of the rectal mucosa in quiescent ulcerative colitis. There are no infiltrating neutrophil polymorphs and there is very little chronic inflammatory cell infiltration. Distortion of the crypt pattern with atrophy remains.

Figure 30-6. Dysplasia-associated lesion (DALM) in the colonic mucosa of a patient with many years' history of ulcerative colitis. There was invasive adenocarcinoma adjacent to this lesion, part of which can be seen permeating a submucosal vein beneath the DALM.

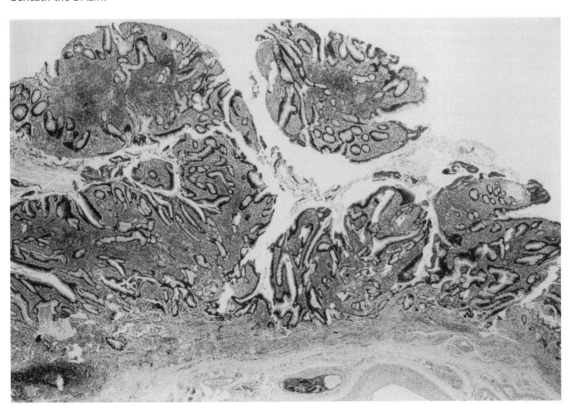

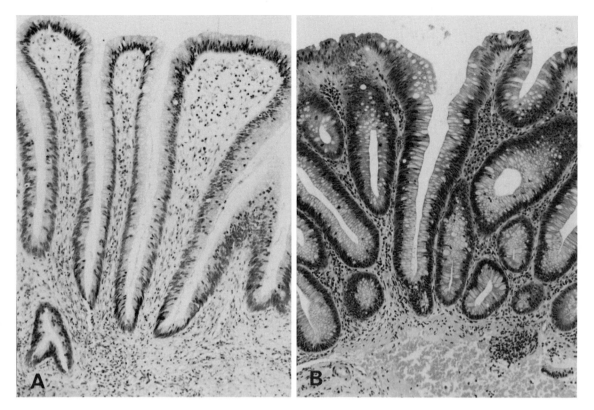

Figure 30-7. Low-grade dysplasia in ulcerative colitis with (**A**) villous architecture and (**B**) tubular architecture.

logic abnormalities (Fig. 30-8). Low-grade dysplasia shows definite but less severe changes of intramucosal neoplasia (Fig. 30-7). Observer variation studies have shown considerable overlap between low-grade dysplasia and indefinite for dysplasia.[6]

As a result of an intensive study of 50 colitic specimens removed at surgery for colorectal cancer, dysplasia was found in 41 (82%). Of the 37 cases in which dysplasia was found at a distance from the tumor, two were classified as indefinite probably positive, 19 were low grade, and 16 were high grade.[14] This suggests that surveillance by examination of colonoscopic biopsies for dysplasia is a valuable tool for cancer detection and prevention with a potential sensitivity of 82%. The other study by the same group showed that by applying strict criteria for the diagnosis of dysplasia, some cases formerly labeled low-grade dysplasia were reclassified as indefinite or negative, resulting in increased specificity for the finding of dysplasia.[6] The results of this study suggest that surgical intervention should not await the appearance of high-grade dysplasia and should be entertained even when only low-grade dysplasia is found. This new concept is being incorporated into the surveillance policy at St. Mark's Hospital.

Total proctocolectomy is the correct treatment for cancer or dysplasia in colitis, unless distant spread dictates that surgery can only be palliative. It is important to remember that up to 50% of patients with dysplasia will not have cancer and to regard a colectomy "negative" for cancer in such cases as a successful cancer prevention procedure.

CROHN'S DISEASE

The large bowel is involved in approximately one-third of patients with Crohn's disease. Of these, approximately one-half also have small intestinal disease, most frequently involving the terminal ileum.

Macroscopic Appearances

In the patient having an elective investigation, Crohn's disease differs in many respects from ulcerative colitis. The features, compared and contrasted with ulcerative colitis, are shown in Table 30-1.

Microscopic Appearances

Referring to the macroscopic appearances given in Table 30-1, the histologic features of Crohn's disease include the following:

1. The distribution of Crohn's disease is characteristically patchy. This is seen at a naked eye level and also microscopically. The grossly uninvolved rectum or the bowel between skip lesions can be histologically entirely normal. In a section of bowel there may be almost normal mucosa immediately next to a severely inflamed area and within a single biopsy there is often patchy inflammation or lymphoid aggregates in the presence of otherwise normal mucosa.

2. A feature in approximately two-thirds of cases of Crohn's disease is the presence of noncaseating granulomas, composed

of ill-defined collections of epithelioid macrophages (Fig. 30-9). These can be found anywhere in the mucosa or wall of the bowel or within lymph nodes. When present on the serosal surface they can be visible to the naked eye as a "rosary" of tubercles. They are less frequently found in long-established cases in which there can often be relatively little mucosal inflammation despite stricturing, fistula, and abscess formation.

3. Transmural chronic inflammation and all its consequences are what makes Crohn's disease so different from ulcerative colitis in clinical significance. Foci of chronic inflammatory cell infiltration (lymphoid aggregates) develop in the submucosa. There is a tendency for these foci to be centered on lymphatic channels and to spread along the course of the lymphatics through the bowel wall (Fig. 30-10; see also Plate 30-3). Together with granulomas, these foci result in lymphatic obstruction, with lymphangiectasia and lymphedema. There is progressive fibrosis of the chronically edematous tissues. The result is as if there were elephantiasis of the bowel, with thickening of the wall and fibrous stricturing. The affected areas are typically pale and relatively bloodless, compared with the congested and hemorrhagic bowel of ulcerative colitis.

4. The serositis, which is part of the phenomenon of transmural inflammation, is accompanied by the formation of fibrous adhesions and extension of mesenteric adipose tissue with "wrapping" of mesentery around the bowel.

5. Another feature related to the transmural distribution of inflammation is the way in which ulcers in Crohn's disease extend deep into the submucosa and often beyond into the muscle layers (Fig. 30-10), forming characteristic fissuring ulcers and leading to sinus, abscess, and fistula formation to adherent loops of bowel or bladder or female genitalia.

6. Anal lesions are found in 75% of patients with colorectal Crohn's disease and in 25% of patients with intestinal disease confined to the small bowel. In 5% of cases Crohn's disease affects only the anus.[15] However, patients with latent intestinal Crohn's disease may present with anal lesions or intestinal disease may only become manifest many years after the development of an anal lesion. Edematous and cyanosed tags at the anal verge are the feature most frequently encountered. More

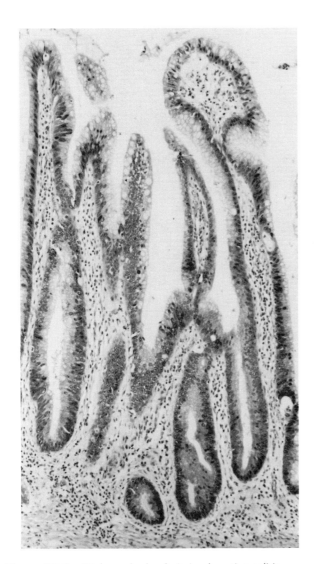

Figure 30-8. High-grade dysplasia in ulcerative colitis.

Table 30-1. Gross Appearance of Crohn's Disease Contrasted With Ulcerative Colitis

Ulcerative Colitis	Crohn's Disease
Rectum usually abnormal	Rectum normal in 50%
Bowel affected in continuity	Disease usually discontinuous, "skip lesions," segmental colitis
Terminal ileum dilated and incompetent in 10%	Terminal ileum stenosed and wall thickened in 30%
Bowel uniformly shortened (strictures only in malignancy)	Bowel length normal or shortened irregularly due to stricturing
Anal lesions in <25% (acute fissures, excoriation, rectovaginal fistula)	Anal lesions in 75% (chronic fissuring, ulceration, edema and cyanosis, tags, fistulas)
Serosa unremarkable	Serositis, adhesions, tubercles, wrapping of mesenteric fat, abscesses
Bowel wall not thickened	Wall irregularly thickened
Fistulas only following intervention (e.g., rectovaginal)	Internal or enterocutaneous fistulas in 10%
Mucosa diffusely congested, granular, ulcers shallow, undermining islands of surviving mucosa	Ulcers discrete, early ones being small pinheadlike erosions (aphthoid ulcers), when more developed being serpiginous and fissuring, intervening mucosa unremarkable or swollen and cobblestoned

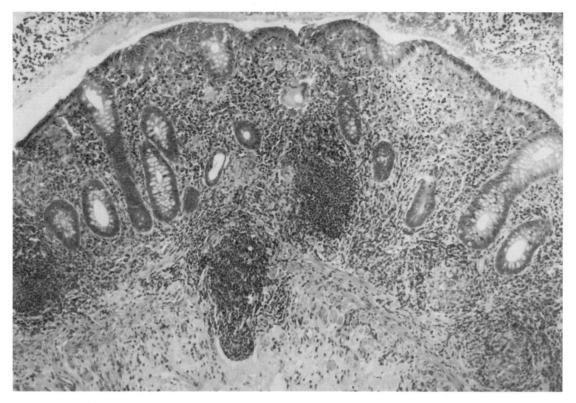

Figure 30-9.   Crohn's disease of colon with mucosal granulomas and patchy chronic inflammation with lymphoid aggregates. There is mild activity with cryptitis but the architecture is only mildly distorted.

severe lesions are chronic fissures and ulcers and complex fistulas. Granulomas are frequently present in biopsies of suspected anal lesions.

7. Rectal or colonic mucosal biopsies in Crohn's disease are much more variable in diagnostic value than in ulcerative colitis. This is understandable because ulcerative colitis affects principally the mucosa and is diffuse in distribution, whereas Crohn's disease extends deep into the bowel wall and is patchy. In one series, only one-third of rectal biopsies was useful in contributing to a diagnosis of Crohn's disease. The clinician is likely to take a colorectal biopsy in four circumstances: (1) from a small or aphthoid ulcer, (2) from a focus of overtly abnormal, often deeply ulcerated mucosa, (3) from intact mucosa between obvious lesions, or (4) from endoscopically normal bowel. In case (1), aphthoid ulcers are small shallow erosions overlying lymphoid follicles and sometimes include a granuloma, the features being diagnostic of Crohn's. In case (2), when there is ulceration, the biopsy may consist only of granulation tissue and, unless granulomas are found there may be no specific features. The mucosa adjacent to an ulcer may show focal inflammation with lymphoid aggregates or with isolated crypt abscesses (Fig. 30-9) or with neutrophil infiltration of isolated crypts (focal cryptitis). However, the mucosal architecture in Crohn's disease is characteristically undisturbed, with long, straight, unbranched crypts. In case (3), endoscopically normal mucosa in Crohn's disease will also show normal architecture but often shows infiltration by excess chronic inflammatory cells and there may also be lymphoid aggregates and even an occasional isolated crypt abscess or cryptitis (Fig. 30-9). These features will often be reported as "nonspecific inflammation."

Cancer and Dysplasia

There is undoubtedly an increased risk of colorectal adenocarcinoma in long-standing Crohn's disease, but its incidence varies, depending on the clinical management of patients with Crohn's disease and the frequency with which colectomy is undertaken. Neoplasia tends to occur in chronic lesions such as fistulas, particularly around the anus[16] and biopsy examination of the luminal mucosa for dysplasia in such cases is not rewarding. This is probably why endoscopic surveillance programs based on biopsy detection of precancerous changes have not been introduced on the scale of those for ulcerative colitic patients.[17]

FULMINANT COLITIS AND ACUTE TOXIC MEGACOLON

Up to 13% of patients develop a fulminant attack, either at the onset of ulcerative colitis or as an acute relapse in established disease. In such cases a segment of colon, frequently the transverse colon, becomes severely dilated (so-called toxic megacolon or acute toxic dilatation). This is characterized by extensive and confluent ulceration, with exposure of the submucosa and muscle of the bowel wall to the potentially infective bowel contents. Acute inflammation and edema extend into the muscle layers, resulting in loss of function. The smooth muscle bundles

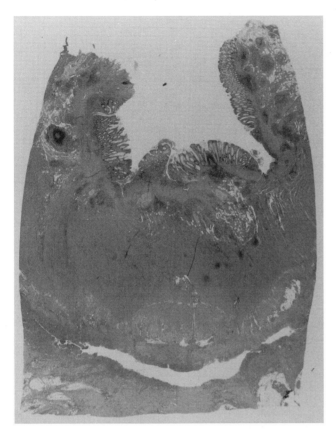

Figure 30-10. Crohn's disease with transmural chronic inflammation, fibrosis, and pericolic abscess formation.

become separated and undergo acute atrophy. Muscle tone is lost and the bowel rapidly dilates to form an inert infected hemorrhagic bag; the patient meanwhile becomes severely ill due to toxemia and bacteremia (the clinical picture of fulminant colitis with acute toxic dilatation or toxic megacolon). The bowel wall is hemorrhagic, paper-thin, and frequently perforates, either spontaneously or as a result of handling. Histologically, granulation tissue lines the ulcerated surface and because of the friability of granulation tissue and of the damaged muscle, in the face of the colonic dilatation, acute clefting or fissuring into the bowel wall develops (Fig. 30-11; see also Plate 30-4). This picture should not be confused histologically with the fissuring of Crohn's disease, which is a more chronic process and is usually associated with more chronic inflammatory cell infiltration and fibrosis. The transverse colon is the most frequently affected by acute toxic dilatation, followed by the descending colon, possibly due to the relative distensibility of these parts of the colon, with their extensive peritoneal surfaces.

INDETERMINATE COLITIS

Frequently, in colons resected in the above circumstances, the nonulcerated mucosa, including that of the distal colon, will show surprisingly little that is abnormal and features diagnostic of either ulcerative colitis or Crohn's disease will not be evident. Diagnosis of the nature of the inflammatory bowel disease underlying the fulminant colitis cannot then be made and the pa-

thologist may have to return a verdict of "colitis indeterminate." The situation often arises because intensive medical therapy has been given in the period leading up to surgery, usually with topical and/or systemic steroids. Steroids have the dual effect of bringing about resolution of active colitis while at the same time rendering ulcerated tissues more vulnerable to infection and further damage. More useful diagnostic information can often be gained by review of any biopsies taken before the patient became severely ill. Despite all efforts, the diagnosis will remain unclassified in 5% to 10% of patients. In these circumstances, a specific diagnosis can only emerge from the subsequent clinical course.[18]

The diagnostic difficulty between the two forms of inflammatory bowel disease has been recognized for many years.[19] The pathologic criteria for distinguishing between them were defined by Lockhart-Mummery and Morson,[20] Cook and Dixon,[21] and Schachter and Kirsner.[22] The macroscopic and microscopic features were summarized by Lennard-Jones et al.[23] (Table 30-1). Confusion can arise if there are insufficient numbers of characteristic attributes of either disorder, or if there is considerable overlapping of features of either. In addition, atypical appearances can be seen, making it impossible to arrive at a confident diagnosis. Histologically these patients have been labeled as having "colitis unclassified" or "colitis unclassified possibly/probably Crohn's disease or ulcerative colitis." In this circumstance, the pathologist might lean in one direction or another, but still be unprepared to come down firmly on either side of the fence.

The term "indeterminate colitis" was introduced by Price[24] to describe operation specimens from cases with inflammatory bowel disease in which histologic appearances were typical neither of ulcerative colitis nor Crohn's disease. The diagnostic label is essentially histopathologic. It has no further meaning than that the histopathologist cannot distinguish between the two. About 10% of all resection specimens fall into this category. Usually the dilemma arises in specimens removed during an acute phase of the disease. In Price's original series of 30 operative specimens, 27 were from patients with a severe acute colitis often with megacolon. This may lead to the occurrence of features atypical of ulcerative colitis. For example, the severity of inflammation may be most marked in the transverse colon where maximal dilatation has occurred. Previous treatment of the rectum by local steroids may give the impression of rectal sparing. Severe ulceration may be irregular in its distribution, spuriously suggesting skip lesions. At a microscopic level the severity of acute inflammation may obscure histologic features more specific for either condition. Fissuring can occur in acute severe ulcerative colitis and even transmural inflammation may be present. Thus the diagnosis of indeterminate colitis is more likely to follow examination of a severely diseased operative specimen.

In practical terms diagnostic error in patients having pouch surgery has been responsible for the large bulk of patients with Crohn's disease treated by this procedure. Six (3%) out of 210 patients operated on at St. Mark's Hospital were found to have Crohn's disease.[25] Fleshman et al.[26] reported that 5 (3%) out of 179 patients had Crohn's disease and Hyman et al.[27] found a somewhat higher incidence of 25 (7%) out of 362 patients. In these series Crohn's disease was in most cases not suspected before the pouch operation.

How can the diagnostic accuracy become more refined? Fur-

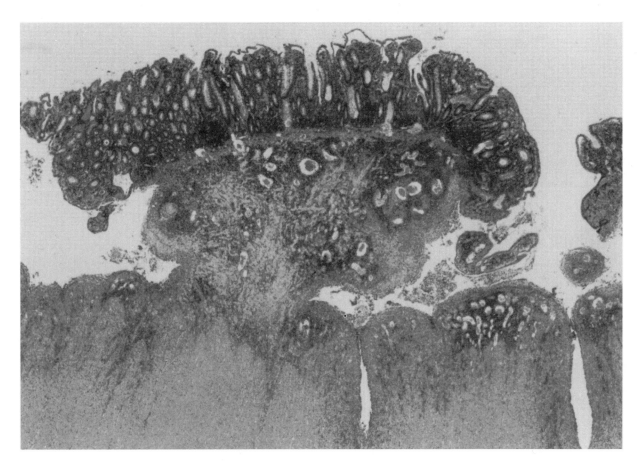

Figure 30-11. Acute toxic megacolon in fulminant ulcerative colitis. This histologic section shows an island of mucosa undermined by deep ulceration. Granulation tissue and fissures extend deeply into the muscularis propria, which is undergoing destruction ("myocytolysis").

thermore, what is the fate of patients with a histologic diagnosis of indeterminate colitis? In both circumstances the combination of clinical and radiologic features along with the histopathology is essential. The cardinal feature of Crohn's disease is patchiness. This word implies disconnected lesions and is applicable both macroscopically and microscopically. Endoscopic features that show areas of vascular pattern separated by areas of inflammation or radiologic evidence of skip lesions are almost diagnostic of Crohn's disease. The presence of small bowel disease should exclude ulcerative colitis. An anal lesion is less diagnostic. Approximately 10% of patients with ulcerative colitis having a proctocolectomy have an anal lesion. Of 112 such patients with ulcerative colitis proven histologically at one hospital, 12 (10%) had an anal lesion.[23] These were, however, minor, including low fistula-in-ano and fissure. Although rectovaginal fistula does occur in ulcerative colitis, its presence is more likely to indicate Crohn's disease.[29] High or complex fistula-in-ano or anal ulceration should be regarded as more likely to be Crohn's disease rather than ulcerative colitis.[30]

The most reliable histologic features that distinguish the two diseases include crypt distortion and the distribution of inflammatory cells within a biopsy. Crypt distortion is characteristic of ulcerative colitis and much less obvious in Crohn's disease. Within the lamina propria, inflammatory cell infiltrate is diffuse

in ulcerative colitis. In Crohn's disease it is patchy within an individual biopsy and often varies markedly from biopsy to biopsy. Indeed, single crypts can have surrounding inflammation adjacent to normal crypts. Granulomas are less specific. They can occur in ulcerative colitis in response to mucin release from ruptured crypts (Fig. 30-3) and they may also be seen in mucosa from ileal reservoirs in patients unequivocally having originally had ulcerative colitis. Their presence may well lean the diagnosis toward Crohn's disease, but is not necessarily diagnostic.[31]

The pathologic features of Crohn's colitis or ulcerative colitis are more usually seen in the chronic stages of disease. This is typified by the granulomas in up to 60% of cases with chronic Crohn's colitis, but in only 25% of those in the acute phase.[24,32] The features of myocytolysis, capillary engorgement, and acute V-shaped clefts described by Price[24] in many of his cases of indeterminate colitis are merely indicators of fulminant disease. The same can be said of muscle dissolution and disintegration where toxic dilatation is present whatever the cause.[33,34]

DIVERSION PROCTOCOLITIS

Following a defunctioning colostomy or ileostomy, any large bowel distal to the stoma no longer exposed to the fecal stream usually undergoes chronic inflammatory changes, labeled ''diversion colitis.''[35,36] The mucosa is commonly infiltrated to a variable degree by chronic inflammatory cells. Sometimes the infiltration is intense, with lymphoid follicle formation. Occasional scattered crypt abscesses are frequently present and there may be mild distortion of architecture. This seems to be a mucosal response to withdrawal from the milieu of short chain fatty acids, from which the epithelium normally derives nourishment.[37] The picture can resemble a mild form of ulcerative colitis. This renders it very difficult to make a definitive diagnosis of inflammatory bowel disease from rectal biopsies taken from a defunctioned rectum, perhaps after a colectomy. Examination of the resected colon or of preoperative biopsies will be more productive. The picture can be still more confusing in the defunctioned rectum of a patient with previous inflammatory bowel disease. If the patient has Crohn's disease, there may be superimposed ulcerative-colitis–like features in a defunctioned rectum. If the patient previously had ulcerative colitis, there is a tendency for chronic inflammation, with fibrosis, to extend through the wall of a defunctioned rectum.[38] In both circumstances, the unwary may question the original diagnosis or even suggest that the patient has both ulcerative colitis and Crohn's disease.

PRESTOMAL ILEITIS

After colectomy, whether accompanied by ileostomy, ileorectal anastomosis, or ileal pouch procedure, in a small but significant proportion of patients, a troublesome chronic inflammatory process can develop in the terminal ileal mucosa, with ulceration and bleeding.[39,40] Histologically, biopsies show chronic active inflammation without granulomas or other specific features. There may occasionally be pseudo-obstruction in these circumstances, but fibrous stricture formation is rare. The etiology is obscure, although ischemia has been suggested.

ILEAL POUCHES

Following ileal pouch construction with anastomosis to the anus, the pouch mucosa undergoes changes depending on the circumstances. In the absence of inflammatory bowel disease, for example when the surgery has been undertaken in the treatment of familial adenomatous polyposis, there is frequently no significant change in the ileal mucosal features although some degree of villous atrophy occurs in most cases.

Pouch inflammation was first recognized in continent ileostomies by Kock[41] and subsequently in ileoanal ileal reservoirs by Handelsman et al.[42] Histologic changes in ileal reservoirs of a chronic inflammatory or atrophic type had been reported in both types of reconstruction by Philipson et al.[43] and by Nicholls et al.[44] It was subsequently appreciated that pouchitis occurs predominantly in ulcerative colitis and only rarely in familial adenomatous polyposis. Various possible causes, including stasis, bacterial flora, and biochemical factors, for example short chain fatty acids or bile salts, have been studied. Various treatments from antibiotics to bile salt binding agents, short chain fatty acids, xanthene oxidase inhibitors, and conventional anti-inflammatory medication have been tried.

The picture is somewhat confused, owing to ignorance of the etiology of inflammatory bowel disease, differing diagnostic criteria, and the possibility that acute inflammation may be due

to various agents.[45,46] Pouchitis implies inflammation and it cannot therefore be diagnosed solely by the presence of symptoms or abnormal endoscopic appearances. Histopathologic evidence of acute inflammation must be present.

Histopathology of the Reservoir

General Changes

Almost all functioning pouches show some mucosal abnormality. These occur in patients with both ulcerative colitis and familial adenomatous polyposis. They may vary in their severity but are qualitatively similar.[47] The changes are characterized by an increase in the presence of chronic inflammatory cells within the lamina propria including lymphocytes, plasma cells, and eosinophils.[48] In addition, there is villous atrophy to a varying degree from individual to individual and also within the same pouch. The degree of villous atrophy is associated with crypt hyperplasia.[49]

These changes appear to occur early after restoration of the fecal stream[43,50] (Setti-Carraro et al., unpublished observations). They are almost always confined to the reservoir and only rarely extend into the proximal ileum.[47] The same authors have demonstrated more severe changes in the posterior than the anterior aspect of the lower part of the reservoir. In patients with previous ulcerative colitis, after the pouch becomes functional and exposed to the new fecal environment, the mucosa usually becomes thickened and infiltrated by plasma cells and lymphocytes, the crypts become lengthened, and the villi become shortened. The small bowel mucosa resembles colon in most respects except its retention of disaccharidase activity and the ability to absorb vitamin B_{12}, xylose, and bile acids.[51] This reaction of ''colonic metaplasia'' is seen in other circumstances of environmental stress, such as celiac disease or bacterial overgrowth and can take place within a few weeks.[52]

Active inflammation rapidly accompanies the chronic inflammatory changes in a high proportion of cases to a variable degree, with the appearance of neutrophil polymorphs migrating through surface and crypt epithelium.[53] In more severe activity, crypt abscesses form and there may be surface erosion or ulceration. The picture resembles ulcerative colitis.[51,54] This active inflammation seems to be a reflection of the ulcerative colitis that previously affected the large bowel and is sometimes accompanied by clinical symptoms of discharge of mucus and blood with the stool and by pain and frequency of defecation (the clinical picture of pouchitis). There is no direct relationship between the severity of any pouchitis, the extent or activity of the previous colitis, or previous backwash ileitis.[55] Pouchoscopy and biopsy soon after the pouch becomes functional may be predictive of the subsequent course in the majority of patients.[56] The grade of severity of inflammation in the pouch is best documented by a scoring system so that progress can be monitored. The scheme of Shepherd and colleagues, shown in Table 30-2, is simple, reproducible, and widely used.[54] The scores are intended to be considered separately, without being summated, as acute inflammation greatly outweighs chronic inflammation in clinical significance.

Setti-Carraro et al. (unpublished observations) in a study of 57 patients having four biopsies taken from the pouch at 5-cm intervals from distal to proximal, identified three groups of

Table 30-2. A Scoring System for Pouch Inflammation

Acute
  Cells (neutrophil infiltrate) in epithelium   1
    Few crypt abscesses   2
    Many crypt abscesses   3
  Ulceration
    Mild   1
    Moderate   2
    Severe   3
Chronic
  Cells (lymphocyte and plasma cell infiltrate)
    Mild   1
    Moderate   2
    Severe   3
  Villous atrophy
    Mild distortion   1
    Partial   2
    Subtotal   3

(From Shepherd et al.,[54] with permission.)

patients. These included 8 patients in which none of the biopsies showed any acute inflammation, 25 in which all biopsies showed acute inflammation, and 26 in which there was a gradient of decreasing inflammation always from distal to proximal.

It has been suggested that these changes may be the result of an alteration in milieu due to the presence of increased numbers of fecal bacteria compared with the normal ileostomy effluent. Bacterial colonization may lead to changes in colonic intraluminal carbohydrate fermentation of dietary fiber with altered production of short chain fatty acid and changes in bile salt concentration and type. We do not yet know what the mucosal dynamics are in response to this alteration in microenvironment, nor do we know the factors responsible. Nasmyth et al.[52] have, however, presented data suggesting that the degree of villous atrophy is inversely related to the concentration of butyrate in the pouch feces. The degree of villous atrophy is also related to crypt cell turnover as determined immunohistochemically using the monoclonal antibody Ki-67.[57] A similar result was obtained by Goldberg et al.[58] who demonstrated an increase in labeling index within the ileal mucosa in patients with ulcerative colitis after pouch construction. There was no change in patients with familial adenomatous polyposis.

Colonic Metaplasia

Histologically the presence of severe villous atrophy and crypt hyperplasia resembles colonic mucosa. When inflammation is present the picture looks like ulcerative colitis.[50,54] Studies have shown colonic-type mucin in ileal pouches irrespective of the original diagnosis. Using Alcian blue staining techniques and the monoclonal antibody PR3A5, which is thought to be specific for colon-type mucin, the presence of sulfated mucin has been demonstrated in ileal pouch mucosa.[51,54] A similar result has been reported using an S_{35}-H_3 glucosamine labeling technique.[59]

These changes are, however, not complete. For example, the pouch mucosa retains certain properties of small intestinal en-

terocytes with preservation of disaccharidase activity and the activity to absorb B_{12}, xylose, and bile acids.[51] It is not known whether colonic metaplasia is a prerequisite for pouchitis.[47]

"Diversion" Changes

In defunctioned pouches (i.e., before closure of the ileostomy), histologic abnormalities have been reported in a proportion of patients.[60] These include villous atrophy, chronic inflammation with eosinophil predominance, and acute inflammation. The changes are not typical of ischemia or Crohn's disease and the author speculated on the possibility that they may represent a form of diversion ileitis analogous to that described in the rectum.[36,61]

Acute Inflammation

Acute inflammatory changes have been reported in 20% to over 50% of patients. Pouchitis is characterized by the presence of acute inflammation. This is correlated with the severity of chronic inflammation.[51,53,54,56] The appearance is similar to ulcerative colitis in an active phase. Polymorphs appear to be located predominantly throughout the epithelium with crypt abscess formation. Aggregates are seen in the lamina propria but are often focal. Ulceration is present. There may be evidence of colonic metaplasia but sometimes small intestinal sialomucins predominate.[54] Perhaps this is similar to the appearance of sialomucins in cases of acute ulcerative colitis.[62] In contrast with celiac disease, intraepithelial lymphocyte counts in ileal pouches are low and do not increase in pouchitis.[63] De Silva et al[51] reported low intraepithelial lymphocytes in cases with pouchitis, but Goldberg et al.[58] showed counts to be similar in ulcerative colitis and familial adenomatous polyposis.

Pouchitis is mostly confined to patients with ulcerative colitis. Although case reports of its occurrence in familial adenomatosis have been reported, it is rare and histologic confirmation is not always obtained. In 37 polyposis patients followed for a mean of 5 years, there was not a single case[64] and Lohmuller et al.[65] reported relative incidences of 6% for polyposis and 31% for ulcerative colitis.

Evolution

The timing of these morphologic changes is unknown in detail. Apel et al.[48] studied biopsies taken at 6 weeks and 6 months from 22 patients with ulcerative colitis. At 6 weeks partial villous atrophy was present in 12 out of 22 with polymorphoneutrophil infiltration and partial transition to colonic-type mucin. A slight but not significant increase in crypt cell proliferation was observed. These changes were very similar at 6 months with a greater degree of mononuclear cell infiltration. There was a striking increase in eosinophils in the lamina propria at both 6 weeks and 6 months, suggesting the existence of a hypersensitivity response.

In a study of 60 pouch patients with an original diagnosis of ulcerative colitis biopsied over a median period of 97 months (range 90 to 173 months), patients could be divided into three groups. In group A (45%) chronic changes were minor with acute changes never seen. In group B (42%) chronic changes were more severe and there were transient episodes of acute inflammation. In group C (13%) severe chronic and severe acute inflammation were constantly present. Pouchitis never occurred in group A and was constantly present in group C. Most significantly, patients were identified to their group within 6 months of closure of the ileostomy and remained in that group indefinitely. If these data are true, patients at risk of developing pouchitis can be identified on biopsy at an early stage in the postoperative course.[56] Verres et al.[66] have made similar observations. They have furthermore reported dysplasia, albeit rarely, but exclusively in group C. So far no case of carcinoma has been described.

Although adenomatous polyp formation in pouches is frequent in familial adenomatous polyposis patients, very few patients with ulcerative colitis and chronic pouchitis have been documented with dysplasia and none with primary adenocarcinoma.[56]

Pouch Mucosa in Crohn's Disease

Despite the best efforts of the clinicopathologic team, patients undergoing pouch surgery sometimes prove to have Crohn's disease. In these cases, there can be problems with patchy fissuring ulceration and peripouch abscess formation, or there may be a more diffuse severe pouchitis, which on histologic examination will be seen to show features of Crohn's disease, with lymphoid aggregates, granulomas, and submucosal chronic inflammation. Sometimes there may be surprisingly mild active inflammation by the above criteria of pouchitis scoring, which is of limited value in these circumstances. It is of interest that in one series, only 30% of pouches in patients with Crohn's disease failed.[67]

In a recent report indicating that pouch survival in patients with Crohn's disease is high, many of the patients could well have had ''indeterminate colitis'' of the ulcerative colitis type and these should be reviewed by second histopathologic opinion because true rectal Crohn's disease without an anal lesion is very uncommon.[68]

MICROSCOPIC COLITIS

Patients presenting with troublesome chronic high volume watery diarrhea, in whom no radiologic or endoscopic abnormality is demonstrable, sometimes nevertheless have an inflammatory condition involving the whole of the colorectal mucosa, when biopsies are examined.[69] The inflammation is diffuse and chronic, consisting of infiltration of the lamina propria by plasma cells, lymphocytes, and eosinophils. The crypt and surface epithelium is infiltrated by lymphocytes but the goblet cell population and architecture are normal. When the intraepithelial lymphocytes are conspicuous the picture has been descriptively labeled *lymphocytic colitis*. When there is, in addition, a prominent layer of collagen beneath the surface epithelium, with polymorph infiltration of the surface epithelium and surface epithelial degenerative changes, the picture is known as *collagenous colitis*. It is not known whether these are variants of the same condition or two separate conditions. Patients with this problem do not usually require surgery but the author knows of one patient who presented in this way and had such severe and persistent diarrhea that emergency colectomy was performed.[69a]

DIVERTICULAR DISEASE

Most cases of diverticular disease, even when there is pericolic abscess formation, are not accompanied by inflammation of the mucosa apart from the diverticula. However, occasionally there can be features of mucosal prolapse in the redundant mucosal folds of the contracted segment of bowel, with crypt elongation and irregularity and with edema, fibrosis, and smooth muscle in the lamina propria. Some patients can also have a granulomatous inflammatory reaction with a transmural distribution, resembling Crohn's disease. These patients may have no clinical stigmata of Crohn's disease or develop any further clinical features of it and it is uncertain whether they should be categorized as having Crohn's disease or not.[70]

Biopsy interpretation by the pathologist uses knowledge of the features described above in the context of the site of biopsy (for colonoscopic biopsies) and the clinical and endoscopic features of the particular patient. In addition to an adequate history and endoscopy report, the site of every biopsy should be identified to the pathologist. It is helpful for orientation in the laboratory that rectal biopsies are mounted on thin card or ground glass. Colonoscopic biopsies should be so mounted or alternatively on cellulose acetate strip, a method preferred by the author.[1] At the very least, colonoscopic biopsies should be submitted to the pathologist in a way that permits identification of the location in the colon of each one, because the distribution of inflammation is one of the most important criteria for diagnosis of inflammatory bowel disease. It is also necessary to localize any focus of dysplasia that is present, so that further biopsies can be correctly targeted.

When interpreting colorectal biopsies, the most specific feature of ulcerative colitis, crypt distortion, if present, will permit a specific diagnosis to be made. However, in between 33% and 66% of cases it may be impossible to be more precise than confirming inflammatory bowel disease. In the absence of distortion of architecture and of chronic inflammation, infective colitis can be suggested if there is a neutrophil polymorph infiltrate. In cases of doubt, it can be useful to examine further biopsies taken after an interval, because ulcerative colitis tends to develop whereas an infection tends to resolve and Crohn's disease and microscopic colitis remain more constant.

REFERENCES

1. Sheffield JP, Talbot IC (1992) ACP Broadsheet 132. Gross examination of the large intestine. J Clin Pathol 45:751–755
2. Kelly JK, Gabos S (1987) The pathogenesis of inflammatory polyps. Dis Colon Rectum 30:251–254
3. Morson BC, Dawson IMP, Day DW et al (1990) Ileal involvement in ulcerative colitis. p. 497. In Morson BC, Dawson IMP (eds): Morson and Dawson's Gastrointestinal Pathology. 3rd Ed. Blackwell, Oxford
4. Davison AM, Dixon MF (1990) The appendix as a 'skip lesion' in ulcerative colitis. Histopathology 16:93–95
5. Morson BC, Dawson IMP, Day DW et al (1990) Cancer in ulcerative colitis. p. 505. In Morson BC, Dawson IMP (eds):

Morson and Dawson's Gastrointestinal Pathology. 3rd Ed. Blackwell, Oxford

6. Connell WR, Lennard-Jones JE, Williams CB et al (1994) Factors affecting the outcome of endoscopic surveillance for cancer in ulcerative colitis. Gastroenterology 107:934–944

7. Meling GI, Clausen OP, Bergan A et al (1991) Flow cytometric DNA ploidy pattern in dysplastic mucosa, and in primary and metastatic carcinomas in patients with longstanding ulcerative colitis. Br J Cancer 64:339–344

8. Porschen R, Robin U, Schumacher A et al (1992) DNA aneuploidy in Crohn's disease and ulcerative colitis: results of a comparative flow cytometric study. Gut 33:663–667

9. Yin J, Harpaz N, Tong Y et al (1993) p53 point mutations in dysplastic and cancerous ulcerative colitis lesions. Gastroenterology 104:1633–1639

10. Ilyas M, Talbot IC (1995) p53 expression in ulcerative colitis: a longitudinal study. Gut 37:802–804

11. Blackstone M, Riddell RH, Rodgers B, Lewis B (1981) Dysplasia-associated lesion or mass (DALM) detected by colonoscopy in long-standing ulcerative colitis: an indication for colectomy. Gastroenterology 80:366–374

12. Riddell RH, Goldman H, Ransohoff DF et al (1983) Dysplasia in inflammatory bowel disease: standardized classification with provisional clinical applications. Hum Pathol 14:931–968

13. Morson BC, Dawson IMP, Day DW et al (1990) Implications of reporting dysplasia. p. 505. In Morson BC, Dawson IMP (eds): Morson and Dawson's Gastrointestinal Pathology. 3rd Ed. Blackwell, Oxford

14. Connell WR, Talbot IC, Harpaz N et al (1994) Clinicopathological characteristics of colorectal carcinoma complicating ulcerative colitis. Gut 35:1419–1423

15. Lockhart-Mummery HE (1975) Crohn's disease: anal lesions. Dis Colon Rectum 18:200–202

16. Connell WR, Sheffield JP, Kamm MA et al (1994) Lower gastrointestinal malignancy in Crohn's disease. Gut 35:347–352

17. Sachar DB (1994) Cancer in Crohn's disease: dispelling the myths. Gut 35:1507–1508

18. Wells AD, McMillan I, Price AB et al (1991) Natural history of indeterminate colitis. Br J Surg 78:179–181

19. Kent TH, Ammon RK, DenBesten L (1970) Differentiation of ulcerative colitis and regional enteritis of colon. Arch Pathol 89:20–29

20. Lockhart-Mummery HE, Morson BC (1960) Crohn's disease (regional enteritis) of the large intestine and its distribution from ulcerative colitis. Gut 1:87–105

21. Cook MG, Dixon MF (1973) An analysis of the reliability of detection and diagnostic value of various pathological features in Crohn's disease and ulcerative colitis. Gut 14:255–262

22. Schacter H, Kirsner JB (1975) Definition of inflammatory bowel disease of unknown aetiology. Gastroenterology 68:591–600

23. Lennard-Jones JE, Lockhart-Mummery HE, Morson BC (1968) Clinical and pathological differentiation of Crohn's disease and proctocolitis. Gastroenterology 54:1162–1170

24. Price AB (1978) Overlap in the spectrum of non-spectrum inflammatory bowel disease—'colitis-indeterminate.' J Clin Pathol 31:567–577

25. Nicholls RJ (1987) Restorative proctocolectomy with various types of reservoir. World J Surg 11:751–762

26. Fleshman JW, Cohen Z, McLeod RS et al (1988) The ileal reservoir and ileoanal anastomotic procedure: factors affecting technical and functional outcome. Dis Colon Rectum 31:10–16

27. Hyman NH, Fazio VW, Tuckson WB, Lavery IC (1991) The consequence of ileal pouch-anal-anastomosis for Crohn's colitis. Dis Colon Rectum 34:653–657

28. Mortensen NJMcC (1992) p. 11. In Nicholls RJ, Bartolo DCC, Mortensen NJMcC (eds): Restorative Proctocolectomy. Blackwell Scientific Publications, Oxford,

29. Radcliffe AG, Ritchie JK, Hawley PR et al (1988) Anovaginal and rectovaginal fistula in Crohn's disease. Dis Colon Rectum 31:94–99

30. Morson BC, Dawson IMP, Day DR et al (1990) pp 265–266. Inflammatory disorders. In Morson DC, Dawson IMP, Day DR et al (eds): Morson and Dawson's Gastrointestinal Pathology. 3rd Ed. Blackwell Scientific Publications, Oxford

31. Warren BF, Shepherd NA (1992) The role of pathology in pelvic ileal reservoir surgery. Int J Colorect Dis 7:68–75

32. Lennard-Jones JE (1992) Definition and Diagnosis. pp. 105–112. In Engel A, Larsson T (eds): Regional Enteritis (Crohn's Disease). Skandia International Symposia, Nordiska Bokhandelns Forlag, Stockholm

33. Roth JCA, Valdes Dapena A, Stein GN, Bockus HL (1959) Toxic megacolon in ulcerative colitis. Gastroenterology 37:239–255

34. Lumb G, Protheroe RHB, Ramsey GS (1975) Ulcerative colitis with dilatation of the colon. Br J Surg 43:182–188

35. Geraghty JM, Talbot IC (1991) Diversion colitis: histological features in the colon and rectum after defunctioning colostomy. Gut 32:1020–1023

36. Harig JM, Soergel KH, Komorowski RA, Wood CM (1989) Treatment of diversion colitis with short chain fatty acid irrigation. N Engl J Med 320:23–38

37. Haque S, West AB (1992) Diversion colitis—20 years a-growing, editorial. J Clin Gastroenterol 15:281–283

38. Warren BF, Shepherd NA, Bartolo DC, Bradfield JW (1993) Pathology of the defunctioned rectum in ulcerative colitis. Gut 34:514–516

39. Knill-Jones RP, Morson BC, Williams R (1970) Prestomal ileitis: clinical and pathological findings in five cases. Quart J Med 154:287–297

40. Hallak A, Baratz M, Santo M et al (1994) Ileitis after colectomy for ulcerative colitis or carcinoma. Gut 35:373–376

41. Kock NG, Darle N, Hulten L et al (1977) Ileostomy. Curr Probl Surg 14:36–38

42. Handelsman JC, Fishbein RH, Hoover HE et al (1983) Endorectal pull-through operation in adults after colectomy and excision of rectal mucosa. Surgery 93:247–253

43. Philipson B, Brandberg A, Jagenburg R et al (1975) Mucosal morphology, bacteriology and absorption in intra-abdominal ileostomy reservoir. Scand J Gastroenterol 10:145–153

44. Nicholls RJ, Belleveau P, Neill M et al (1981) Restorative proctocolectomy with ileal reservoir: a patho-physiological assessment. Gut 22:462–468

45. Tytgat GNJ, van Deventer SJH (1989) Pouchitis. Int J Colorect Dis 3:226–228

46. Madden MV, Farthing MJG, Nicholls RJ (1990) Inflammation in ileal reservoirs—'pouchitis.' Gut 31:247–249

47. Shepherd NA, Healey CJ, Warren BF (1993) Distribution of

mucosal pathology and an assessment of colonic phenotypic change in the pelvic ileal reservoir. Gut 34:101–105

48. Apel R, Cohen Z, Andrews CW et al (1994) Prospective evaluation of early morphological changes in pelvic pouches. Gastroenterology 107:435–443

49. Warren BF, Shepherd NA (1993). Pouch Pathology. pp. 147–162. In Nicholls RJ, Bartolo DCC, Mortensen NJMcC (eds): Restorative Proctocolectomy. Blackwell Scientific Publications, Oxford

50. De Silva HJ, Millard PR, Prince C et al (1990) Serial observations of the mucosal changes in ileoanal pouches. Gut 31: A1168–1169

51. de Silva HJ, Millard PR, Kettlewell M et al (1991) Mucosal characteristics of pelvic ileal pouches. Gut 32:61–65

52. Nasmyth DG, Godwin PG, Dixon MF et al (1989) Ileal ecology after pouch-anal anastomosis or ileostomy. A study of mucosal morphology, fecal bacteriology, fecal volatile fatty acids, and their interrelationship. Gastroenterology 96:817–824

53. Moskowitz RL, Shepherd NA, Nicholls RJ (1986) An assessment of inflammation in the reservoir after restorative proctocolectomy with ileoanal ileal reservoir. Int J Colorect Dis 1: 167–174

54. Shepherd NA, Jass JR, Duval I et al (1987) Restorative proctocolectomy with ileal reservoir: pathological and histochemical study of mucosal biopsy specimens. J Clin Pathol 40:601–607

55. Gustavsson S, Weiland LH, Kelly KA (1987) Relationship of backwash ileitis to ileal pouchitis after ileal pouch-anal anastomosis. Dis Colon Rectum 30:25–28

56. Setti-Carraro P, Talbot IC, Nicholls RJ (1994) Longterm appraisal of the histological appearances of the ileal reservoir mucosa after restorative proctocolectomy for ulcerative colitis. Gut 35:1721–1727

57. De Silva HJ, Gatter KC, Millard PR et al (1990) Crypt cell proliferation and HLA-DR expression in pelvic ileal pouches. J Clin Pathol 43:824–849

58. Goldberg PA, Herbst F, Beekett CG et al (1996) Leucocyte typing, cytokine expression and epithelial turnover in the ileal pouch in patients with ulcerative colitis and familial adenomatous polyposis. Gut 38:549–553

59. Corfield AP, Warren BF, Bartolo DCC (1990) Colonic metaplasia following restorative proctocolectomy monitored using a new metabolic labelling technique for mucin. J Pathol 160: 170A

60. Warren BF, Bartolo DCC, Collins CMP (1990) Preclosure pouchitis—a new entity. J Pathol 160:170A

61. Editorial (1989) Diversion colitis. Lancet 764

62. Jass JR, England J, Miller K (1986) Value of mucin histochemistry in follow up surveillance of patients with long-standing ulcerative colitis. J Clin Pathol 39:393–398

63. Shepherd NA (1989) Pouchitis workshop: the pathology of the ileal reservoir. Int J Colorectal Dis 4:206–208

64. Madden MV, Neale KF, Nicholls RJ et al (1991) Comparison of morbidity and function after colectomy with ileorectal anastomosis or restorative proctocolectomy for familial adenomatous polyposis. Br J Surg 78:789–792

65. Lohmuller JL, Pemberton JH, Dozois RR et al (1990) Pouchitis and extraintestinal manifestations of inflammatory bowel disease after ileal pouch-anal anastomosis. Ann Surg 211: 622–629

66. Veress B, Reinholt FP, Lindquist K, Liljeqvist L (1992) Mucosal adaptation in the ileal reservoir after restorative proctocolectomy. A long term follow up study. Ann Chir 46:10–18

67. Grobler SP, Hosie KB, Affie E et al (1993) Outcome of restorative proctocolectomy when the diagnosis is suggestive of Crohn's disease. Gut 34:1384–1388

68. Panis Y, Poupard B, Nemith J et al (1996) Ileal pouch/anal anastomosis for Crohn's disease. Lancet 347:854–857

69. Jawhari, Talbot (1996) Microscopic, lymphocytic and collagenous colitis. Histopathology 29:101–110

69a. Bowling TE, Price AB, al-Adnani M et al (1996) Interchange between collagenous and lymphocytic colitis in severe disease with autoimmune associations requiring colectomy: a case report. Gut 38:788–791

70. Makapugay LM, Dean PJ (1996) Diverticular disease-associated chronic colitis. Am J Surg Pathol 20:94–102

31

MEDICAL TREATMENT

DRUG THERAPY

Alastair Forbes

The medical management of inflammatory bowel disease (IBD) is poised to enter a new era if the early promise shown by immunomodulatory regimens results in confirmed effective therapy. At present, however, there are only a few firmly established routes to pharmacologic success. Corticosteroids and the 5-aminosalicylate (5-ASA) drugs (sulfasalazine and its successors) form the mainstays of therapy, with azathioprine and mercaptopurine established second-line agents for resistant disease. Cyclosporine and methotrexate are now also finding their own niches in the therapeutic armory.

This chapter explores the role of the above agents and, where possible, of the newer agents, in current management. Treatment of acute and more chronic disease is included with some attention to the special case of fulminant ulcerative colitis. The place of nutritional therapy is considered briefly.

CORTICOSTEROIDS

Corticosteroids, given mostly as various forms of prednisolone and hydrocortisone, remain a cornerstone in the medical management of patients with inflammatory bowel disease. They provide rapid and effective relief of symptoms in acute exacerbations, although this is not always accompanied by full endoscopic remission. There is little difference between the response to hydrocortisone and to prednisolone in equivalent doses (4 mg methylprednisolone:5 mg prednisolone:25 mg hydrocortisone), although there are some differences in their mineralocorticoid effects, which can occasionally be important. Although intravenous therapy can certainly be demonstrated to be more efficacious than oral administration in resistant cases, this is an effect of the more direct route (and usually also a higher dose) and not because of a switch from one formulation to another, for example, prednisolone to hydrocortisone.

The therapeutic effects of steroids are mediated by inhibition of several inflammatory pathways including direct suppression of the 5-lipoxygenase mediated metabolism of arachidonic acid, modulated mRNA transcription of glucocorticoid-sensitive pro-

teins, and suppression of mRNA for most of the interleukins.[1] Typical regimens comprise prednisolone 0.5 to 1.0 mg/kg body weight, with a rapid reduction once response begins in order to avoid unnecessary steroid toxicity. As steroids have been shown in all but one study to be largely ineffective in maintaining remission, but contribute significantly to long-term morbidity via their side effects, they should be withdrawn once the acute episode has settled. Growth suppression in children, osteoporosis, and suppression of the hypothalamic pituitary axis have been of particular concern, especially with high doses and prolonged treatment. Even topical steroids have the potential for toxicity when used for prolonged periods, as up to 80% of the applied dose may be absorbed systemically. More recent data suggest, however, that much of the apparent toxicity of steroids on bone mass (and growth) is actually a reflection of greater disease activity in patients treated with steroids, and that it is the active disease (and the need for steroids) that is the prime determinant of tissue damage.[2] It is appropriate nonetheless that attention has centered on newer corticosteroids, which are poorly absorbed or extensively inactivated by the liver, and on new delivery systems that limit steroid absorption. Steroid-sparing immunomodulatory drugs should continue to be considered in patients who remain apparently steroid dependent.

Topically Active Corticosteroids

Prednisolone metasulfobenzoate, which is available in enema form, is relatively poorly absorbed, yielding systemic levels significantly lower than those from a dose of prednisolone phosphate achieving equivalent rectal tissue levels.[3] Therapeutic efficacy is similar, but measurable adrenal suppression can still be shown and it should be noted that the degree of systemic absorption is directly related to the degree of inflammation.[4] Tixocortol pivalate,[5] budesonide,[6] and beclomethasone[7] are all rapidly metabolized in the liver and red blood cells. Budesonide has the additional advantages that it is poorly absorbed from the intestine and is highly protein bound in circulation permitting little "free hormone" action. Trials of topical administration have demonstrated at least equal efficacy to hydrocortisone and mesalamine in the treatment of acute distal ulcerative colitis. Each of the newer steroids has low systemic bioavailability and causes less suppression of endogenous cortisol secretion than prednisolone or hydrocortisone. Whether this is of major clinical advantage is, however, questionable given the general intention to confine topical steroid usage to the short-term management of the acute relapse.[4,8]

The use of new orally administered corticosteroids is showing some promise in Crohn's disease. Although trials using fluticasone propionate have been disappointing, the results obtained with budesonide are more encouraging. This agent, which is quite widely used as a topical steroid in treatment of asthma, has very high affinity for the glucocorticoid receptor, and is rapidly metabolized in the liver. Accordingly only about 10% of the absorbed drug reaches the systemic circulation. To aid maximal efficacy in the terminal ileum and in extensive colitis, it has been coated with Eudragit, an acrylic resin familiar to users of mesalamine, which dissolves at pH 6 (Eudragit L), or pH 7 (Eudragit S). Initial pilot studies have now been followed by two careful multicenter trials in the treatment of ileocecal Crohn's disease. In the first, which was essentially a dose-ranging study in active disease, doses between 3 and 15 mg daily were compared with placebo.[9] A 9-mg dose appeared optimal, there being no therapeutic gain, but an appreciable increase in adrenal suppression with 15 mg. In the European study 9 mg of budesonide daily was compared with a tapering dose of prednisolone (starting at 40 mg daily).[10] The results indicate similar efficacy for the two agents. It should be noted, however, that although there were no statistically significant differences in any of the measures of efficacy, in each case the numeric advantage lay with prednisolone. Adrenal toxicity was certainly less with budesonide but far from absent in this study, which was too short term to provide information on other toxicologic concerns. Abstract data from the German budesonide study group are very similar,[11] and only a single study so far points to better clinical results with the new agent.[12] To date there are no reports on the use of oral budesonide in ulcerative colitis, but it would be reasonable to assume that similar advantages and disadvantages will apply.

The full potential of budesonide is likely to be compromised in Crohn's disease (and to a lesser extent in ulcerative colitis), given the variable distribution of the disease, an often shortened gut with rapid transit, and altered intraluminal pH, as these may result in unreliable delivery of the drug to sites of active disease. In some patients with extraintestinal manifestations it may in any event be necessary to administer systemically active steroids. Further studies will no doubt clarify the most appropriate uses of the new agents in the overall management of inflammatory bowel disease.

AMINOSALICYLATES

Oral Aminosalicylates

Sulfasalazine has been used effectively in the treatment of ulcerative colitis since the early 1950s, when controlled trials demonstrated efficacy in treatment of acute colitis and maintenance of remission; reductions in relapse rates of up to fourfold are

typical. Early studies showed no benefit in Crohn's disease, but recent studies using newer formulations of 5-ASA, which has been shown to be the principal active ingredient, have shown considerable promise. The mechanisms of action of 5-ASA in reducing intestinal inflammation are not entirely clear, but include inhibition of 5-lipoxygenase metabolism and the production of interleukins and inflammatory leukotrienes, suppression of platelet-activating factor, of chemotaxis of neutrophils and monocytes, normalization of intestinal permeability, reduction of epithelial HLA DR expression, stimulation of cytoprotective prostaglandins, and scavenging of free radicals. All are documented (some only in vitro) and are potentially relevant.[13]

Targeted Delivery

Up to 15% of individuals are intolerant of the sulfapyridine moiety of sulfasalazine, but although (most of) its therapeutic benefit results from the 5-ASA molecule, oral administration of 5-ASA is ineffective because of proximal absorption and metabolism. Alternative formulations of 5-ASA have therefore been developed. In each case it proves possible to use larger equivalent doses than has usually been the case with sulfasalazine, as few patients develop upper gastrointestinal intolerance. There is also no problem with oligospermia with the newer agents. In 1996, five 5-ASA preparations were commercially available in Europe. "Asacol" is 5-ASA coated with an acrylic-based resin (Eudragit-S), which dissolves rapidly above pH 7.0; this typically occurs in the region of the cecum and ascending colon. Eudragit-L dissolves at pH 6.0 and is used to coat "Claversal" and "Salofalk," with which release in the terminal ileum is to be expected. "Pentasa" consists of microgranules of 5-ASA coated by a semipermeable ethyl cellulose membrane that releases 5-ASA steadily after tablet disintegration in the stomach, with enhanced release above pH 6.0; 5-ASA is made available throughout the small and large intestine. Olsalazine is a 5-ASA dimer, the two molecules linked by an azo bond, which is broken by the same azo-reductase of colonic bacterial flora that degrades sulfasalazine. Potential advantage for olsalazine shown over other 5-ASA preparations is limited by an osmotic diarrhea provoked by the drug, which affects up to 10% of patients, but may be minimized by taking the drug with food. Balsalazide has a 5-azo bond linking 5-ASA to an inert amino acid carrier; early studies indicate comparable activity to other 5-ASAs and it will soon be generally available. Other formulations are also being developed. It is clearly evident, but surprisingly often neglected, that all of the 5-ASA preparations that depend on colonic bacteria for degradation of the azo bond cannot be effective in patients with colectomy and ileostomy. Too often sulfasalazine and olsalazine are prescribed inappropriately and uselessly in this context.

Ulcerative Colitis

It is widely accepted, when equivalent doses are given, that the oral 5-ASA preparations are therapeutically equipotent to sulfasalazine. Olsalazine and mesalamine have been shown to be similarly efficacious in maintenance of remission and in treating mildly to moderately severe active ulcerative colitis, with only one major study significantly favoring olsalazine in the latter context.[14] In this study in which olsalazine and mesalamine as Asacol were compared, Courtney et al.[14] demonstrated a lower relapse rate with olsalazine in left-sided ulcerative colitis, presumed to be due to relatively enhanced delivery of 5-ASA to the left side of the colon. This study has, however, been criticized for its overreliance on patient assessment and absence of sigmoidoscopic review. It is possible also that olsalazine was unduly favored by the dosage schedule employed (1.0 g olsalazine versus 1.2 g Asacol).

Given the continuing uncertainty as to the clinical relevance or otherwise of a dose response to 5-ASA and some concern about nephrotoxicity, the Dutch Pentasa Study Group[15] have recently reported on both the efficacy and safety of daily doses of 1.5 g and 3 g of 5-ASA in the maintenance of remission in ulcerative colitis. More than 150 patients with ulcerative colitis in remission were randomized to one of the two doses and monitored to 12 months or to earlier relapse. The higher dose of 5-ASA achieved a better 12-month remission rate on intention to treat, 67% versus 50%. This difference just failed to reach statistical significance.

Crohn's Disease

Early studies failed to show worthwhile benefit from sulfasalazine in Crohn's disease, but Prantera et al.[16] have recently demonstrated efficacy of Asacol 2.4 g/day in the prevention of clinical relapse. These results are further supported by a meta-analysis of all the completed studies of 5-ASA therapy in maintenance of remission.[17] More encouraging still are the results of two recent randomized controlled trials. Caprilli et al.[18] showed that administration of Asacol 2.4 g/day beginning within 6 weeks of surgery was effective in preventing postoperative recurrence, as judged endoscopically. There was a 39% reduction of all endoscopic recurrences and a 55% reduction of severe endoscopic recurrence at 2 years, with an accompanying reduction in symptomatic recurrence. Similar results come from a North American study of 163 patients,[19] reporting a clinical recurrence rate (symptomatic and endoscopic) of 31% on 3 g of 5-ASA daily (as Rowasa or Salofalk) compared with 41% on placebo. These results are of great clinical importance in view of the high rate of early postoperative endoscopic recurrence (29% at 6 months, 56% at 1 year, and 85% at 2 years), and the development of recurrent symptoms in these patients in approximately 90% by 3 years.[20] Longer follow-up of the various trial patients is required to determine whether the endoscopic advantages will be associated with a prolonged decrease in morbidity. Although Singleton et al.[21] in a 16-week study, have shown substantial benefit from mesalamine in active Crohn's disease, currently it appears that prevention rather than treatment of relapse is a better strategy in the postoperative management of patients with Crohn's disease.[22]

A relatively large dose of 5-ASA seems to be required in Crohn's disease, there being a more obvious dose response effect[17] than in ulcerative colitis (see above). At least 2 g daily, and perhaps as much as 4 g daily, may be necessary to yield therapeutic or prophylactic benefit in Crohn's.

Renal Toxicity

Increased use of any drug, whether by increased numbers of recipients or by higher dose, is likely to cause toxicity, and 5-ASA is no exception. Since the late 1980s there has been concern that the upper gastrointestinal side effects, reversible oligospermia, and occasional anaphylaxis from sulfasalazine were being succeeded by renal toxicity related to treatment with 5-ASA, which was sometimes responsible for end-stage renal failure requiring renal dialysis or transplantation.[23,29] Debate continues as to the relative importance in such cases of idiosyncracy, and/or the very rare dose-independent nephritis, versus dose-dependent renal toxicity in which direct renal exposure to 5-ASA is the likely cause.

Although there is a substantial literature and much clinical experience supporting the renal safety of the pH-dependent delivery systems, with the increased use of 5-ASA,[25] renal failure is recorded more often with these agents.[24] This excess renal risk probably remains when corrected for the relative frequency of use of the different products, but is not of sufficient magnitude to be a major influence on choice of agent.

Toxicity was actively sought throughout the Dutch Pentasa study[15] and a probable or definite drug-related adverse event affected seven patients (4%) with no difference in the toxicity profile for the two doses used, nor in the dropout rate attributable to poor compliance. Pentasa yields a high total circulatory 5-ASA concentration compared with other 5-ASA preparations, but relatively low levels of free nonacetylated 5-ASA.[25] Two (1.3%) patients developed modest and reversible renal impairment (one with mesalamine-related interstitial nephritis).

Prescribers of other 5-ASA preparations, worried that they are responsible for excessive or avoidable renal toxicity, will be somewhat comforted to note that Pentasa is also associated with renal problems quite frequently. If irreversible toxicity is, however, the result of sustained high, or peak, concentrations of free 5-ASA, then the results for Pentasa (or indeed those for the agents dependent on colonic bacteria for 5-ASA release) are not necessarily wisely extrapolated to all pharmaceutical formulations. The particular concern with pH release systems is that there is the potential for release of a sufficiently large "bolus" in the small intestine to overwhelm mucosal acetylation and thereby lead to a transient but very high-dose 5-ASA challenge to the kidney.

Whichever 5-ASA preparation is chosen, it must be remembered that it is likely to be employed in the very long term, and the clinician must remain alert to the possibility of insidious nephrotoxicity developing after some years of treatment. As for phenacetin there may be a rising incidence of late renal impairment with very prolonged use, for example, 10 years or more. Data on this are not yet available. It is important that prescribers audit their practice carefully, taking account of the renal dysfunction that may complicate the disease itself, quite independently of any drug used.[26,27]

Topical Aminosalicylates

5-ASA

Topical mesalamine is firmly established as an effective agent in the treatment of active proctitis and (as enemas generally reach to the splenic flexure) also in distal colitis. The usual response rate is in excess of 70% over 3 to 6 weeks. These results are comparable to those of topical steroids[28] and of oral 5-ASA.[29] Topical 5-ASA has also been shown to achieve remission in some patients who have previously been resistant to oral 5-ASA or to topical steroids.[4] It is also effective in the maintenance of remission, administered daily as a liquid enema, foam, or suppository. There is little gained from dose escalation,[30] and 1 g daily is not obviously inferior to 2 g or 4 g. When enemas are employed there is no difference in efficacy between foam and liquid preparation. Patients, however, tend to prefer the foam formulation and long-term compliance may therefore be improved should the drug be used for maintenance. Little 5-ASA is absorbed when it is administered rectally and it may therefore be inferred that the above results generally reflect a topical effect. No controlled data yet exist for the use of topical 5-ASAs in distal Crohn's disease, but personal experience suggests that some patients with otherwise resistant disease will respond.

4-ASA

Distal ulcerative colitis will also respond to topical 4-ASA (also known as para-amino-salicylic acid [PAS]) with comparable results to topical prednisolone.[31] Clinical experience suggests, as for 5-ASA, that although the overall proportion of responsive patients is virtually identical, the particular patients who respond may differ, making a switch to an alternative topical regimen worthwhile in those who do not initially achieve remission.

IMMUNOSUPPRESSANT THERAPY

Immunosuppressant drugs are valuable in refractory disease where they help to achieve and maintain clinical remission, reduce steroid use, and avoid surgery. Their usefulness has, however, been vitiated by limited efficacy, lack of selectivity, and significant toxicity. An increasing understanding of the mucosal immune response in inflammatory bowel disease should allow future agents to be targeted at particular, critical steps in immune activation. The central role of T-cell activation and involvement of associated proinflammatory cytokines in pathogenesis is increasingly established.[32] This was illustrated by an inverse relationship, in one study, between the activity of Crohn's disease and the level of T-helper cells in superadded human immunodeficiency virus (HIV) infection.[33] Trials of cyclosporine, which is mainly active against the CD4 cell, have therefore been conducted, and newer therapeutic approaches based on "blocking" monoclonal antibodies, for example, against tumor necrosis factor-α, are beginning to emerge in the literature.

Azathioprine and 6-Mercaptopurine

Azathioprine and 6-mercaptopurine (6-MP) are purine analogs that competitively inhibit the biosynthesis of purine nucleotides. Their mode of action is poorly understood but they are known to have selective suppressant effects on T cells. Azathioprine is metabolized to 6-MP in vivo, and subsequently to the inactive 6-thiouric acid by xanthine oxidase. Congenital deficiency of this enzyme or its inhibition by allopurinol predispose to accumulation of 6-MP with the potential for severe bone marrow suppression.[32] Myelosuppression can occur in the normal population, especially when high doses (>2 mg/kg azathioprine) are employed but more so in heterozygotes for enzyme deficiency,

and is almost the rule in homozygotes who have almost undetectable enzyme concentrations.

Persuasive evidence for a role for azathioprine or 6-MP in the management of refractory Crohn's disease dates from the study of Present et al.[34] in which induction of remission, and reduction of steroid requirement has been demonstrated. Supportive data come from studies that have confirmed benefit in the maintenance of remission.[35,36] Whereas steroids and 5-ASA preparations seem to have no specific role in the treatment of Crohn's-related enterocutaneous fistulae, 6-MP appears more effective than placebo (31% versus 6%).[34] A subsequent uncontrolled 6-month trial in 34 patients from the same center has reported a 39% fistula closure rate, with worthwhile improvement in another 26%. Most of the patients had not previously been treated surgically for the fistulae.[37] The mean time to respond was over 3 months, so this cannot be considered a panacea, and many patients will still require surgery.

Purine analogs have also been shown to be effective in the induction and maintenance of remission in refractory ulcerative colitis,[38,39] with significantly greater relapse rates in patients in whom the drug is subsequently withdrawn.[35,40]

Approximately two-thirds of patients selected for purine analog therapy in the management of problematic disease will both tolerate and respond to it. The onset of action is slow, however, as it depends on effects on newly dividing cells, a phenomenon that necessitates treatment for at least 3 months before judging the treatment to have failed. Many patients are, however, not prepared to accept the long duration of this treatment. The usual dose of 6-MP is 1.5 mg/kg and 2.0 mg/kg for azathioprine. Approximately 10% of patients are intolerant to these agents with serious but idiosyncratic toxicities including pancreatitis, hepatitis, and hypersensitivity reactions, all of which recur on repeated administration. Bone marrow suppression is dose related and reversible. It usually occurs in the first 6 months of treatment but can do so much later.[41,42] This therefore necessitates regular monitoring of the white blood cell count every 4 to 6 weeks while therapy continues. If myelosuppression develops, it may be possible to retain therapeutic efficacy safely by reduction of dosage. It has even been proposed that efficacy is dependent on the development of some degree of leukopenia.[43] A prospective study to clarify this is in progress in North America.

Concern that the increased incidence of malignancy (particularly lymphomas) seen in transplant patients treated with azathioprine might occur in inflammatory bowel disease has not been borne out. Recent data from St. Mark's Hospital based on a prospective follow-up of 755 patients for a median of 9 years from the time of introduction of azathioprine[44] demonstrated a small overall increase in malignancy. Thirty-one malignancies occurred compared with a figure of 24.3 predicted from national mortality rates for the same age and sex distribution, a difference that was not statistically significant ($P = .186$). There were no lymphomas among the patients, but there was a significant excess of colorectal and anal tumors (15 observed versus 2.27 expected: $P < .00001$). This was attributed to the underlying disease rather than to any complication of treatment. This conclusion was supported by comparison of azathioprine-treated patients with ulcerative colitis, to patients matched for the nature of their disease but who had never received azathioprine. A modest difference in relative risk (30.8 versus 23.8) was not statistically significant ($P = .54$). It is reasonable to conclude that any increase in neoplasia in patients with inflammatory bowel disease treated with azathioprine/6-MP can be explained by the disease itself. A note of caution must remain, however. Although the period of follow-up was substantial, few patients had received azathioprine for more than 2 years and the median duration was only 12.5 months. Thus there could be an increased risk of neoplasia with greater duration of immunosuppression and these reassuring data from a relatively brief treatment should not be accepted to indicate that there is no risk.

CYCLOSPORINE

Cyclosporine is a lipid-soluble fungal derivative with potent immunosuppressive effects. It acts primarily on T-cell function and proliferation, mainly by inhibition of interleukin-2 gene transcription. There is consequent loss of recruitment of cytotoxic cells and inhibition of cytotoxic lymphokines.[45] There is therefore considerable logic in its application to the treatment of inflammatory bowel disease. Cyclosporine has not yet been very widely used but this can be expected to change with the positive results reported for its use in fulminant ulcerative colitis.[46]

Crohn's Disease

Early uncontrolled studies of cyclosporine in Crohn's disease and ulcerative colitis claimed impressive response rates within 5 to 10 days, followed then by a high late failure rate. There are currently four published, randomized, double-blind, placebo-controlled trials of oral cyclosporine in refractory Crohn's disease, which have been critically reviewed.[47] Brynskov et al.[48] reported improvement in 50% compared with only 32% in controls. Although this was significant, only 19% of the responding patients retained the improvement up to 6 months after gradually discontinuing the drug. The study by Jewell et al.[49] was more disappointing, even when continuing maintenance therapy was used. The Canadian Crohn's Relapse Prevention Trial Investigators[50] have since reported a multicenter, double-blind, placebo-controlled trial of low-dose cyclosporine in which a total of 305 patients were entered. Actively treated patients had a worse symptomatic outcome than the placebo group, and there was no reduction in requirement for other medication. Very similar conclusions come from the fourth study.[51] Although it is possible that a better response might be obtained with higher doses, renal toxicity precludes this as a long-term measure. Most workers in the field have, however, seen a few responses to cyclosporine when all other options have failed and this may reflect high-dose therapy, as in the study of Brynskov et al.[48] A role may also exist for the patient with fistulating disease, to judge from an uncontrolled study of 16 such patients.[52] All had failed on standard therapies, and were started on cyclosporine 4 mg/kg by continuous intravenous infusion. Fourteen patients showed some response, and seven fistulae closed. However, there was substantial toxicity, and a high relapse rate when parenteral therapy was discontinued. The authors concluded that intravenous cyclosporine was effective in fistulating Crohn's disease, but that its future role in this respect should be determined by controlled trial. The use of cyclosporine in Crohn's disease, despite the occasional apparently dramatic response, can only be justified by entry of patients into formal clinical trials.

Ulcerative Colitis

The initial promising results from an open pilot study of intravenous cyclosporine in fulminant ulcerative colitis have subsequently been vindicated by the same group. A dual-center randomized study was set up to include 40 patients who failed to respond to 5 days of high-dose intravenous steroids.[46] Fulminant colitis was defined from the revised Oxford criteria.[53] The patients were randomized to receive either intravenous cyclosporine (4 mg/kg) as a continuous infusion together with continued high-dose steroids, or to continue conventional therapy alone. The study was stopped prematurely on statistical and ethical grounds after only 20 patients had been entered. Nine of 11 patients given cyclosporine responded as compared with none of the nine continuing conventional therapy alone. This improvement was maintained in 60% of patients at 6 months after discharge from the hospital. These results still require verification from other centers, but indicate a place for the drug in selected patients with severe acute or refractory ulcerative colitis.

All patients with severe colitis have a potentially life-threatening condition and are best managed jointly by physician and surgeon. The use of cyclosporine is a short-term measure aimed at avoiding surgery. This pharmacologic intervention must not be permitted to delay surgery in the patient who continues to deteriorate or who shows no obvious response to medical therapy over a period of a few days, for example, 5 to 7 days up to a maximum of 12 days depending on clinical circumstances. In the opinion of the author there is no place for medical management of patients with complications such as megacolon, perforation, or major life-threatening hemorrhage.

Monitoring Potential Long-Term Use

To date there are no controlled data to determine whether cyclosporine has a role in maintenance or in the chronically active steroid-dependent patient. Most specialist centers are avoiding such use, preferring to transfer patients who have responded to the drug in fulminant disease onto more established maintenance regimens including azathioprine or 6-MP. Cyclosporine enemas have been properly assessed in refractory ulcerative proctitis, however, and here prove no better than placebo.[54]

Toxicity is relatively frequent even on short-term use and is mainly dose related, there being a narrow therapeutic index. Reversible nephrotoxicity, hyperkalemia, hyperuricemia, hepatotoxicity, hypertension, and seizures are relatively unusual with careful use, but hypertrichosis, gingival hyperplasia, tremor, and paresthesiae are all common and of great concern to patients. Whole blood (not plasma) levels measured by high-performance liquid chromatography, or monoclonal antibody radioimmunoassay should be adjusted to 100 to 200 ng/ml in chronic low-dose oral therapy and to 200 to 400 ng/ml in high-dose intravenous therapy. Intestinal absorption of the drug is affected by active intestinal disease and short bowel, and by cholestasis. Dietary factors such as grapefruit juice but not other fruit juices can significantly affect blood levels.[55] These factors may account in part for the poor results reported in Crohn's disease if an insufficient dose of the active agent has been prescribed.

There is concern that cyclosporine may increase the incidence of lymphoproliferative disorders, but experience in patients after organ transplantation shows that it probably does so less than other immunosuppressive agents.[56] There are no data available for IBD. Continued monitoring will therefore be needed in patients with IBD treated with long-term cyclosporine, not only for lymphoproliferative disorders but also for skin cancers, which are increased in transplantation series.[57] It is disturbing[58] that an 11.1% rate of colorectal carcinoma has been described among 27 patients with ulcerative colitis within the first 14 months after liver transplantation for primary sclerosing cholangitis. These patients were immunosuppressed conventionally with prednisolone, azathioprine, and cyclosporine, and clearly represent a highly selected group, not least since sclerosing cholangitis is probably itself a risk factor for colonic neoplasia.[59] It seems wise to enter such patients into an accelerated colonoscopic screening program, but whether the risk is primarily related to the drug, the transplant, or the disease remains unclear. Cyclosporine does not appear to be mutagenic.[60]

METHOTREXATE

Methotrexate is a dihydrofolate reductase inhibitor that interferes with normal DNA synthesis. It has immunosuppressive and anti-inflammatory properties, and has accordingly been widely used in conditions such as psoriasis and rheumatoid arthritis, as well as in oncologic practice. Kozarek et al.[61] reported the results of an open trial of 12 weeks of methotrexate in patients with refractory Crohn's disease ($n = 14$) and ulcerative colitis ($n = 7$). There was an apparent short-term response in the majority of both groups allowing significant reduction in steroid dosage, which was then sustained by maintenance therapy in two-thirds of the responders to 72 weeks. Previous failure to respond to azathioprine or 6-MP did not preclude a response to methotrexate.[62]

Controlled data have now been published by the North American Crohn's Study Group Investigators.[63] In a study of 141 patients with active Crohn's disease, all were brought to a common daily dosage of 20 mg prednisolone, either by being able to wean down a higher dose or by increasing a lower maintenance dose. A steroid-weaning protocol was then followed for the study period. Half were randomized to receive intramuscular methotrexate (25 mg) each week for 16 weeks. This was a relatively large dose by comparison with its use in other nonmalignant conditions. The end points comprised an assessment of Crohn's disease activity and the extent to which reduction of steroids was possible. Remission was achieved in 39.4% of those given methotrexate compared with only 19.1% in those given placebo. The overall rather poor results are accounted for by the initial severity of disease (all patients requiring prednisolone at a dose of at least 10 mg/day). Methotrexate was not associated with substantial toxicity in this relatively short-term study, although there was a deterioration in the parameters of liver function in 7%, and nausea led to withdrawal from the drug in 6%. A longer term continuation of the study in the same group of patients, using 15 mg/week, is in progress to determine whether the apparent advantage from methotrexate is main-

tained without development of hepatic fibrosis, myelosuppression, or other problems.

The risk of malignancy complicating long-term therapy is thought to be less than that from azathioprine. It may perhaps be negligible because methotrexate does not react with, or become incorporated into, host nucleic acid.[64] To date, no carcinogenic effect of the low doses of methotrexate typically used for nonmalignant indications has been demonstrated,[65] and background incidence rates of malignancy are apparently unaltered (see, e.g., Tishler et al.[66]).

OTHER IMMUNOSUPPRESSIVE AGENTS

Tacrolimus (previously FK506) is a macrolide with potent immunosuppressive activity. It has similar mechanisms of action to cyclosporine and has gained a major role in solid organ transplantation. Extrapolation from its use in patients undergoing small bowel transplant suggests that it may have a role in IBD and preliminary results suggest some benefit in chronic Crohn's fistulae and pyoderma gangrenosum.[67] Animal data suggest that the drug may be acting in part as a suppressor of superoxide radical formation by neutrophils.[68]

K-76 is a fungal derivative of *Stachybotrys complementi*. It has been shown to have potentially beneficial immunomodulatory effects in inflammation, prompting a Japanese group to examine its effects in IBD.[69] They reported a good response in four of five patients when used alone. Seven of 21 patients with refractory disease unresponsive to steroids responded to the addition of K-76. Further assessment is necessary.

ANTIBIOTICS

Metronidazole

Antibiotics have a clear role in the management of complications of inflammatory bowel disease such as abscess and toxic dilatation. Their role in primary therapy is less certain. Metronidazole is licensed as an antimicrobial with action against anerobes and protozoa but it is probable that it also has independent anti-inflammatory actions. It is frequently used for management of perianal Crohn's disease given an expected benefit in two-thirds of recipients.[70] An earlier study in the UK was less enthusiastic. Despite doubling the response rate at 2 weeks for placebo from 35% to 67% or 71% depending on whether cotrimoxazole was also used, this effect was not sustained at 4 weeks.[71] Toxicity, particularly peripheral neuropathy, is a concern. Nerve conduction studies showed that 85% of treated patients had abnormalities, 46% were symptomatic, and in 11% the neuropathy was not reversible on discontinuing the drug.[72]

Some benefit from metronidazole has also been demonstrated in ileocolonic Crohn's disease but not in disease affecting the small bowel alone.[73] A controlled trial of 60 patients undergoing terminal ileal resection randomized to a 3-month course of metronidazole (20 mg/kg) or placebo starting within 1 week of surgery showed a statistically significant reduction in clinically apparent recurrence at 1 year of 4% versus 25%. This marked difference was, however, not maintained at 2 or 3 years.[74]

Antituberculous Therapy

A variety of antimycobacterial regimens have been evaluated in the treatment of Crohn's disease; some of these trials were in part an attempt to test the hypothesis that *Mycobacterium paratuberculosis* is of etiologic relevance.[75] The published results have been disappointing, with no study yet demonstrating significant benefit. Trials using newer drugs and regimens continue.

Other Antibiotics

A number of broad-spectrum antibiotics have been evaluated in Crohn's disease. There is evidence, mostly from small uncontrolled studies, demonstrating some efficacy. One study[76] using a variety of broad-spectrum antibiotics given continuously for 6 months reported symptomatic improvement in 93% of patients with refractory Crohn's disease. Radiologic improvement was seen in 57%, and 40% were able to discontinue steroids. Burke et al.[77] reported long-term symptomatic and histologic improvement in patients with refractory extensive colitis treated with a 1-week course of oral tobramycin. Some 90% of their patients were able to discontinue steroids, but subsequent trials have not proved supportive. A more recent study[78] comprising a 6-month double-blind placebo-controlled trial of ciprofloxacin given in addition to conventional therapy in 83 patients with moderate to severe ulcerative colitis, has, however, demonstrated a reduction in treatment failures from 56% in the placebo group to 21% in the ciprofloxacin group ($P < .03$). There was also an associated reduction in the need for colectomy from 40% to 16%. Corroborative data are needed.

NUTRITIONAL THERAPY

Nutritional intervention is crucial in all malnourished patients, but particularly so in children, where permanent growth retardation will result if it is neglected. The patient with Crohn's disease of the small bowel is particularly at risk. Nutrition used as primary therapy should be distinguished from providing nutritional support in malnutrition. Primary nutritional therapy has not been shown to have any place in ulcerative colitis, but there is an expanding literature indicating a limited role in selected patients with Crohn's disease.[79,80]

Dietary antigens have been thought to contribute to the pathogenesis of IBD and it is therefore logical to test exclusive parenteral nutrition with "bowel rest." Early studies have indicated a 65% to 95% response rate in patients with refractory Crohn's disease. However, it has subsequently been realized that elemental, "predigested," and polymeric liquid formula diets can appear to have similar efficacy to exclusive parenteral feeding and indeed to systemic steroids in inducing remission.[79,80] It remains unclear whether nutritional repletion, relative bowel rest, or other factors explain these improvements. It is recognized that much of the supportive literature for nutritional therapy comes from a small number of enthusiastic centers and that when analysis of results by strict "intention to treat" is performed, steroids are found to be more effective in inducing remission. The greater commitment required of the patient for nutritional therapy reflected by these analyses, coupled with a tendency for a slower induction of remission, lead most gastro-enterologists to continue to favor systemic steroids as first-line treatment for acute relapses of Crohn's disease. There should be no doubt, however, that they can be effective in some patients who have failed on steroids, in those in whom steroids are strongly contraindicated, and when they are refused by the patient. Whether there is a place for exclusion diets, with systematic slow reintroduction of foods once remission has been achieved, remains ill-defined. Such diets are difficult to implement even in patients brought to remission by nutritional therapy but this approach has been advocated as maintenance treatment.[81]

Fatty Acids

Although controversial,[80] it is possible that a component of the therapeutic response to nutritional therapy in Crohn's disease is from a reduced intestinal exposure to fat. Linoleic acid appears particularly disadvantageous presumably because it is a key precursor of arachidonic acid and thus of the inflammatory eicosanoids leukotriene B4, thromboxane, A2, and prostaglandin E2.[82] Various dietary methods of reducing eicosanoid synthesis have been considered. Fish oils, which contain large amounts of eicosapentanoic acid, divert eicosanoid metabolism toward leukotriene B5 and prostaglandin E3, which are much less inflammatory than leukotriene B4 and prostaglandin E2.[83] In a multicenter double-blind, crossover trial of eicosapentanoic acid in active ulcerative colitis, there was a significant reduction in rectal dialysate leukotriene B4 levels, associated with clinical and histologic improvement in the treatment period.[84] The Nottingham group also showed modest benefit from fish oil supplementation in active colitis but no advantage in maintenance.[85]

Short chain fatty acids are released from dietary fats by anerobic bacteria and, particularly in the case of butyrate, they are physiologically important colonocyte nutrients.[86] Good evidence now exists that their absence in the defunctioned colon is an important factor in the development of diversion colitis, a condition that can be reversed by short chain fatty acid enemas.[87] Short chain fatty acids or butyrate alone in the form of an enema have also been used in idiopathic distal colitis given the observation of reduced fecal concentrations of these acids in some patients. In a randomized trial in patients with acute distal colitis Senagore et al.[88] demonstrated a remission rate equivalent to that for topical steroids or mesalamine, with an overall 80% response rate. It is speculated that this benefit derived from restoration of a free fatty acid deficiency itself the result of functionally abnormal anerobic bacteria that produce excess sulfur mercaptides.[89] The attraction of using a natural agent with low toxicity is offset by the current high cost of fatty acid preparations, the pharmaceutical difficulties resulting from their volatility, and unpleasant smell. In the face of these difficulties and another similar trial that has shown no benefit,[90] this is not a regimen currently to be recommended.

Similar mechanisms to those of the free fatty acids may also underlie the effect of topical arsenicals in the form of acetarsol, an agent of proven similar efficacy to steroids.[91] There should be a degree of caution in using an arsenical but the short- and medium-term risks are low.[92] There is uncertainty concerning the long-term cancer risk, and the drug cannot be generally recommended.

EICOSANOIDS AND THEIR INHIBITORS

Leukotriene B4, which is generated by the action of 5-lipoxygenase on arachidonic acid, has been shown to play a central role in the inflammatory cascade. Elevated levels are detected in the colonic mucosa of patients with active ulcerative colitis, but not in steroid-treated quiescent disease.[93,94] Several 5-lipoxygenase inhibitors now exist and early data both in vitro and in vivo using zileuton were promising.[94,95] Unfortunately an 8-week randomized, double-blind, controlled trial has shown poorer results than placebo in ulcerative colitis.[96] In maintenance of remission, zileuton is better than placebo but no more effective than 5-ASA.[97]

A leukotriene receptor antagonist appears effective in a rabbit immune colitis model, but human studies are still in their earliest stages.[75] Verapamil, a calcium channel blocker, has been shown to reduce leukotriene B4 release and accelerate healing in experimental colitis in the rat. This is probably because 5-lipoxygenase is calcium dependent. The use of calcium channel blockers warrants study in humans.[98]

Prostaglandins in the normal gastrointestinal tract appear to have a protective role, contributing (for example) to microvascular integrity and mucus production. It is tempting to associate their inhibition with the general tendency of nonsteroidal anti-inflammatory agents to worsen the disease. It was thus logical to explore the therapeutic use of prostaglandin analogs. Unfortunately misoprostol, one such agent, exacerbated proctitis (unpublished data). This is paradoxic given the undoubted efficacy of the 5-ASA drugs, which act against the cyclooxygenase pathway. A possible differing influence on expression of the two main classes of cyclooxygenase may provide the explanation. In the normal intestine, protective eicosanoids are synthesized by a constitutively expressed cyclooxygenase, but in inflammatory states an inducible cyclooxygenase (Cox-2) predominates, with uncoupling of oxidative phosphorylation and inhibition of prostaglandin synthesis.[99]

THROMBOXANE SYNTHESIS INHIBITORS AND ANTAGONISTS

Thromboxanes are produced in excess in both ulcerative colitis and Crohn's disease[100,101] by activated neutrophils, mononuclear cells, and platelets. Increased mucosal permeability may be the trigger to their release through allowing entry of bacterial antigens (such as lipopolysaccharides), which induce neutrophil activation. Ridogrel and picotamide both inhibit thromboxane A2 synthesis and competitively block its receptors, and may be useful in IBD. Picotamide also has important effects on platelet function and a fibrinolytic effect, and both agents stimulate production of prostacyclin. They are effective in experimental models of colitis, and preliminary studies in humans are encouraging.[101] The eicosanoids and their effects in the normal and diseased intestine have recently been comprehensively reviewed.[102]

TUMOR NECROSIS FACTOR AND OTHER CYTOKINES

The etiopathogenic role of proinflammatory cytokines in IBD is discussed elsewhere. They are abnormally represented and contribute to the inflammatory response.[103,104] Accordingly a variety of means of their selective inhibition by reduced synthesis, impaired release, or by inhibited action, are under investigation. A preliminary report of the use of anti–tumor necrosis factor-α (TNF-α) monoclonal antibodies in refractory Crohn's disease has given encouraging results. A chimeric neutralizing antibody to TNF-α was used in an open study in 10 Crohn's patients with intractable disease.[105] One patient was unassessable because of an iatrogenic colonic perforation, but eight of the remainder had significant improvements in the Crohn's Disease Activity Index and endoscopic healing by 4 weeks. The clinical responses were on average of 4 months' duration. A multicenter controlled trial has now finished recruiting patients and results are expected soon. The response to further doses and the incidence of neutralizing antibody formation is not yet known.

There are reports indicating a useful therapeutic effect for thalidomide in a variety of inflammatory conditions. An impressive account of its value in two patients with HIV-related aphthi[106] has been critically discussed with reference to potential mechanisms of the drug.[107] Thalidomide is a specific inhibitor of TNF-α through enhanced degradation of TNF-α mRNA, which is probably how it exerts its activity in inflammatory conditions (immunomodulation without immunosuppression).[108] Only anecdotal data exist for thalidomide therapy but a formal trial is perhaps now warranted. Clearly the risk of phocomelia will always preclude its use in all but the most carefully selected female patients.

Interleukin-10 (IL-10) is an immunoregulatory cytokine produced by Th2 (helper) T cells that has predominantly inhibitory effects on other T cells and on antigen presentation, with downregulation of class II major histocompatibility complex (MHC) antigens. The production and release of a variety of proinflammatory cytokines are suppressed by IL-10 both in vitro and in vivo.[109] Although IL-10 levels are well preserved or high in IBD[110] there is evidence that the concentrations are inadequate to the demand and that supplementary therapeutic IL-10 may be beneficial. An open study of topical IL-10 therapy in resistant distal colitis showed promise[111] and larger trials are planned both in ulcerative colitis and Crohn's disease.

INTRAVENOUS IMMUNOGLOBULIN, T-CELL APHERESIS, AND MONOCLONAL ANTIBODIES TO CD4 CELLS

Intravenous immunoglobulin (IVIG) has been used successfully in a number of autoimmune diseases. Given that inflammatory bowel disease may be mediated by an abnormal immune response to an unidentified infectious agent, a gut-associated antigen, or an autoimmune disorder, assessment of IVIG has seemed reasonable. Preliminary open-label pilot studies in refractory disease have been encouraging,[112] but the uncertain risks of transmission of viral infections and the considerable expense require it to be very carefully assessed before sanctioning wider use.

On similar grounds, T-cell apheresis and the use of anti-CD4 monoclonal antibodies have been proposed. T-cell apheresis using differential centrifugation has been assessed in patients with chronic resistant Crohn's disease in an open trial.[113,114] Interpretation of the results is complicated by the simultaneous administration of parenteral nutrition. However, long-term remission with steroid withdrawal in 64 of 72 patients is recorded. The French GETAID group has reported similarly good results from a controlled study of T-cell apheresis in 28 Crohn's patients recently brought to remission by steroids.[115] The study group received lymphopheresis (nine procedures within 4 to 5 weeks) and all 12 achieved full weaning from steroids compared with only 5 of 12 controls, although this was not significant. No adverse effects were seen but there was a high rate of relapse over 18 months of follow-up occurring in 83% in the lymphopheresis and in 62% in the control group. A Japanese group has examined a similar technique in an open study of 30 patients with active ulcerative colitis.[116] The Plasauto 1000 apheresis unit equipped with a Cellsorba leukocyte removal filter was administered weekly during 5 weeks of intensive therapy and at approximately 1-month intervals during 5 months of maintenance therapy. Approximately 95% of all passaged white cells were removed. There were no side effects, and clinical improvement was claimed in 24 patients. Heparin was thought unlikely to have contributed to the effect. Abnormalities of polymorphonuclear leukocyte function is well established in IBD[117] and the more global effect on white cells with the Japanese device may act partly through this route. Despite these early results, only prolonged remission would justify the invasiveness and costs of such regimens, and it is unlikely that apheresis will ever have more than a peripheral place in management.

It may be hoped that similar results can be obtained from the use of monoclonal antibodies to CD4 cells.[118,119] Humanized mouse antibodies have been synthesized to overcome the problem of human anti-mouse antibodies developing.[120] Chimeric antibodies containing mouse antigen binding sites are transplanted onto human antibodies. This reduces immunogenicity and increases the half-life. Initial studies using chimeric anti-CD4 antibodies in patients with active Crohn's disease yielded clinical remission in 10 (83%) of 12 patients with complete steroid withdrawal in two-thirds. Remissions, however, were not long lasting, and the long-term effects of iatrogenic chronic CD4 cell suppression are a cause for concern.

REACTIVE OXYGEN METABOLITES

Oxygen free radical production by neutrophils and granulocytes is increased in patients with IBD, both in the peripheral circulation and in the intestinal mucosa. This almost certainly contributes to the inflammatory process.[121] Inhibition of oxygen free radical production reduces inflammation in animal models of colitis,[122] and this may be an important mechanism of action of the 5-ASA derivatives. Millar et al.[123] indicate that this may prove a promising direction of research in humans also.

Iron in its ferric state is known to contribute to oxygen free radical generation. This prompted a trial of the value of chelation by desferrioxamine in pouchitis.[124] This possibility has not yet been assessed in other forms of IBD but the addition of allopurinol, a xanthine oxidase inhibitor, or dimethyl sulfoxide, hydroxyl radical scavenger, to sulfasalazine maintenance has been shown to improve symptoms and prolong remission in ulcerative colitis.[125] Finally Emerit et al.[126] reported good long-term results in an open study of 334 patients with refractory Crohn's disease using copper zinc superoxide dismutase. This enzyme accelerates the clearance of O_2^-. Again controlled trials are awaited.

LIGNOCAINE

There is evidence that there is an abnormal innervation of the submucosa, muscularis mucosae, and mucosa in ulcerative colitis. This is supported by immunohistochemical staining demonstrating increased numbers of mucosal nerve fibres and expression of neuropeptide Y and tyrosine hydroxylase.[127] The same authors obtained good results in all of 21 patients from topical lignocaine therapy in distal colitis. There are, however, no controlled data nor support from other centers for this observation, there being only a very modest clinical response in the author's experience using the same dose of topical lignocaine gel in British colitic patients.

HEPARIN

Heparin is best known as an anticoagulant but, like its endogenous equivalent, it has important anti-inflammatory properties. The anticoagulant effects on thrombin themselves produce secondary inhibition of neutrophil activation and pathologic increases in endothelial permeability. There is also inhibition of neutrophil elastase, which reduces the ability of these cells to penetrate endothelium, associated with inactivation of a range of cytokines and binding of lactoferrin. In a case report, the Liverpool group[128] postulated that these effects of heparin may have contributed to its apparent therapeutic role in a patient with arthropathy and pyoderma gangrenosum. It is suggested that margination of neutrophils, that is, the degree to which the cells "roll" along the endothelium, may be of key importance. This analysis lends scientific credibility for the impressive results reported from Eire,[129] in which it was found that heparin, given for an incidental deep venous thrombosis, was apparently effective in problematic ulcerative colitis. This case and a further nine patients treated by full heparinization have now been reported. Nine of the 10 entered remission, rectal bleeding being the first symptom to resolve. Controlled data are as yet lacking.

SMOKING AND NICOTINE PATCHES

Epidemiologic studies reveal a significant association between nonsmoking and ulcerative colitis, which is not completely explained. Decreased production of arachidonic acid metabolites, disruption of mucus-producing capacity, and protective barrier function of the colon are probably important.[130] Thus a possible beneficial effect of nicotine is plausible and a double-blind placebo-controlled trial of nicotine patches in active ulcerative colitis has now been reported.[131]

Encouraging results were reported that reached significance, but there were irregularities in the study that have been criticized in an accompanying editorial.[132] The case for nicotine was further weakened by data from the original unit on the use of nicotine patches in maintenance of remission.[133] This was a well-designed study and addressed most of the shortcomings of the methodology of the initial investigation. No difference between nicotine and placebo was demonstrable. The ethics of a placebo-controlled trial in maintenance of ulcerative colitis may also be questioned given the established value of 5-ASA drugs for this indication.

CONCLUSIONS

There have been several important recent advances in the treatment of inflammatory bowel disease that should lead to the development of new therapeutic strategies. The selective use of intravenous cyclosporine in acute severe colitis, methotrexate in resistant Crohn's disease, and 5-ASA derivatives for maintenance of remission and prevention of postoperative recurrence in Crohn's disease are already becoming widely accepted. However, all currently available therapies have limited efficacy. Incomplete responses and the potential for short- and long-term toxicity leave a continuing need for pharmacologic development. Although the medical portents are good, surgical intervention will continue to be necessary for a substantial minority of patients for the foreseeable future.

REFERENCES

1. Fahey JV, Guyre PM, Munck A (1981) Mechanisms of anti-inflammatory actions of glucocorticoids. pp. 21–51. In Weissman G (ed): Advances in Inflammation Research. Vol. 2. Lippincott-Raven, Philadelphia
2. Polk DB, Hattner JA, Kerner JA Jr (1992) Improved growth and disease activity after intermittent administration of a defined formula diet in children with Crohn's disease. J Parent Enter Nutr 16:499–504
3. McIntyre PB, Macrea FA, Berghouse L et al (1985) Therapeutic benefits from a poorly absorbed prednisolone enema in distal colitis. Gut 6:822–824
4. Anderson FH (1995) The rectal approach to treatment in distal ulcerative colitis. Lancet 346:520–521
5. Levinsson RA (1986) Intrarectal treatment of ulcerative colitis with tixocortol pivalate, a topical, nonsystemic antinflammatory steriod, comparison with hydrocortisone enema. Gastroenterology 90:1449A
6. Matzen P and the Danish Budesonide Group (1991) Budesonide enema in ulcerative colitis. A randomised dose-response trial with prednisolone enema as a positive control. Scand J Gastroenterol 26:1225–1230
7. Mulder CJJ, Endert E, Van der Heyde H et al (1989) Comparison of beclomethasone dipropionate (2 and 3 mg) and prednisolone sodium phosphate enemas (30 mg), in the treatment of distal ulcerative colitis. Neth J Med 35:18–24
8. Mulder CJJ, Tytgat GNJ (1993) Review article: topical corticosteroids in inflammatory bowel disease. Aliment Pharmacol Ther 7:125–130
9. Greenberg GR, Feagon BG, Martin F et al (1994) Oral budesonide for active Crohn's disease. N Engl J Med 331:836–841
10. Rutgeerts P, Lofberg R, Malchow H et al (1994) A comparison of budesonide with prednisolone for active Crohn's disease. N Engl J Med 331:842–845
11. Gross V, Andus T, Caesar l et al (1995) Oral pH-modified release budesonide vs 6-methyl-prednisolone in active Crohn's disease. Gut, 37, suppl. 2:A104
12. Campieri M, Ferguson A, Doe W et al (1995) Oral budesonide competes favourably with prednisolone in active Crohn's disease. Gut, 37, suppl. 2:A64
13. Greenfield SM, Punchard NA, Teare JP, Thompson PH (1993) Review article: the mode of action of aminosalicylates in inflammatory bowel disease. Aliment Pharmacol Ther 7:369–383
14. Courtney M, Nunes D, Bergin C et al (1992) Randomised comparison of olsalazine and mesalazine in prevention of relapses in ulcerative colitis. Lancet 339:1279–1281
15. Fockens P, Mulder CJJ, Tytgat GNJ et al (1995) Comparison of the efficacy and safety of 1.5 vs 3.0g oral slow-release mesalazine (Pentasa) in the maintenance treatment of ulcerative colitis. Eur J Gastroenterol Hepatol 7:1025–1030
16. Prantera C, Pallone F, Brunetti G et al (1992) Oral 5-amino-salicylic acid (Asacol) in the maintenance treatment of Crohn's disease. Gastroenterology 103:363–368
17. Messori A, Brignola C, Trallori G et al (1994) Effectiveness of 5-aminosalicylic acid for maintaining remission in patients with Crohn's disease: a meta-analysis. Am J Gastroenterol 89:692–698
18. Caprilli R, Andreoli A, Capurso L et al (1994) Oral mesalazine (5-aminosalicylic acid; Asacol) for the prevention of post-operative recurrence of Crohn's disease. Aliment Pharmacol Ther 8:35–43
19. McLeod RS, Wolff BG, Steinhart AH et al (1995) Prophylactic mesalamine treatment decreases postoperative recurrence of Crohn's disease. Gastroenterology 109:404–413
20. Rutgeerts P, Heboes K, Vantrappen G et al (1990) Predictability of the postoperative course of Crohn's disease. Gastroenterology 99:956–963
21. Singleton JW, Hanauer SB, Gitnick GL et al (1993) Mesalamine capsules for the treatment of active Crohn's disease: results of a 16-week trial. Gastroenterology 104:1293–1301
22. Tremaine W (1992) Maintenance of remission in Crohn's disease: is 5-aminosalicylic acid the answer? Gastroenterology 103:694–704
23. Anonymous (1990) Nephrotoxicity associated with mesalazine. Curr Probl (Committee on Safety of Medicines) 30:2
24. Thuluvath PJ, Ninkovic M, Calam J, Anderson M (1994) Mesalazine induced interstitial nephritis. Gut 35:1493–1496
25. Laursen LS, Stokholm M, Bukhave K et al (1990) Disposition of 5-aminosalicylic acid by olsalazine and three mesalazine preparations in patients with ulcerative colitis: comparison of intra-luminal colonic concentrations, serum values, and urinary excretion. Gut 31:1271–1276
26. Asacol Study Group (1995) Sensitive markers of renal dysfunction are elevated in chronic ulcerative colitis. Gastroenterology 108:A919
27. Bonnet J, Lemann M, Prunat A et al (1995) Renal function in patients with inflammatory bowel disease on long-term mesalazine or olsalazine. Gastroenterology 108:A786
28. Danish 5-ASA Group (1987) Topical 5-aminosalicylic acid versus prednisolone in ulcerative proctosigmoiditis. A randomized, double-blind multicenter trial. Dig Dis Sci 32:598–602
29. Rowasa Study Group (1995) A double-blind comparison of oral versus rectal mesalamine versus combination therapy in the treatment of distal ulcerative colitis. Gastroenterology 108:A909

30. Campieri M, Gionchetti P, Belluzi A et al (1991) Optimum dosage of 5-aminosalicylic acid as rectal enemas in patients with active ulcerative colitis. Gut 32:929–931

31. O'Donnell LJ, Arvind AS, Hoang P et al (1992) Double blind, controlled trial of 4-aminosalicylic acid and prednisolone enemas in distal ulcerative colitis. Gut 33:947–949

32. Kozarek RA (1993) Review article: immunosuppressive therapy for inflammatory bowel disease. Aliment Pharmacol Ther 7:117–123

33. James S (1988) Remission of Crohn's disease after human immunodeficiency virus infection. Gastroenterology 95:1667–1669

34. Present DH, Korelitz BI, Wisch N et al (1980) Treatment of Crohn's disease with 6-mercaptopurine. A long-term randomized double-blind study. N Engl J Med 402:981–987

35. O'Donoghue DP, Dawson AM, Powell-Tuck J et al (1978) Double blind withdrawal trial of azathioprine as maintenance treatment for Crohn's disease. Lancet 2:955–957

36. Markowitz J, Rosa J, Grancher K et al (1990) Long term 6-mercaptopurine treatment in adolescents with Crohn's disease. Gastroenterology 99:1347–1351

37. Korelitz B, Present DH (1985) Favorable effect of 6-mercaptopurine on fistulae of Crohn's disease. Dig Dis Sci 30:58–64

38. Present DH, Chapman ML, Rubin PH (1988) Efficacy of 6-mercaptopurine in refractory ulcerative colitis. Gastroenterology 94:359A

39. Adler DJ, Korelitz Bl (1990) The therapeutic efficacy of 6-mercaptopurine in refractory ulcerative colitis. Am J Gastroenterol 85:717–722

40. Hawthorne AB, Logan RFA, Hawkey CJ et al (1992) Randomised controlled trial of azathioprine withdrawal in ulcerative colitis. Br Med J 305:20–22

41. Connell WR, Kamm MA, Ritchie JK, Lennard-Jones JE (1993) Bone marrow toxicity caused by azathioprine in inflammatory bowel disease: 27 years of experience. Gut 34:1081–1085

42. Present DH, Meltzer ST, Krumholz MP et al (1989) 6-Mercaptopurine in the management of inflammatory bowel disease: short- and long-term toxicity. Ann Intern Med 111:641–649

43. Colonna T, Korelitz BI (1994) The role of leukopenia in the 6-mercaptopurine induced remission of refractory Crohn's disease. Am J Gastroenterol 89:362–366

44. Connell WR, Kamm MA, Dickson M et al (1994) Long-term neoplasia risk after azathioprine treatment in inflammatory bowel disease. Lancet 343:1249–1252

45. Hodgson H (1991) Cyclosporin in inflammatory bowel disease. Aliment Pharmacol Ther 5:343–350

46. Lichtiger S, Present DH, Kornbluth A et al (1994) Cyclosporine in severe ulcerative colitis refractory to steroid therapy. N Engl J Med 330:1841–1845

47. Sandborn WJ (1995) Cyclosporine therapy for inflammatory bowel disease: definitive answers and remaining questions. Gastroenterology 106:1001–1003

48. Brynskov J, Freund L, Rasmussen S et al (1989) A placebo controlled, double blind randomized trial of cyclosporin therapy in active chronic Crohn's disease. N Engl J Med 321:845–850

49. Jewell DP, Lennard-Jones JE, and the Cyclosporin Study Group of Great Britain and Ireland (1994) Oral cyclosporin for chronic active Crohn's disease. Eur J Gastroenterol Hepatol 6:499–505

50. Feagan BG, McDonald JWD, Rochon J et al (1994) Low-dose cyclosporine for the treatment of Crohn's disease. N Engl J Med 330:1846–1851

51. Stange EF, Modigliani R, Pena AS et al (1995) European trial of cyclosporine in chronic active Crohn's disease: a 12 month study. Gastroenterology 109:774–782

52. Present DH, Lichtiger S (1994) Efficacy of cyclosporine in treatment of fistula of Crohn's disease. Dig Dis Sci 39:374–380

53. Chapman RW, Selby WS, Jewell DP (1986) Controlled trial of intravenous metronidazole as an adjunct to corticosteroids in severe ulcerative colitis. Gut 27:1210–1212

54. Sandborn WJ, Tremaine WJ, Schroeder KW et al (1994) A placebo-controlled trial of cyclosporine enemas for mildly to moderately active left-sided ulcerative colitis. Gastroenterology 106:1429–1435

55. Yee GC, Stanley DL, Pessa LJ (1995) Effect of grapefruit juice on blood cyclosporin concentration. Lancet 345:955–956

56. von Graffenried B (1989) Sandimmun (ciclosporin) in autoimmune disease: overview on early clinical experience. Am J Nephrol 9:51–56

57. Kurki PT (1992) Safety aspects of long term cyclosporin A therapy. Scand J Rheumatol 95:35–38

58. Bleday R, Lee E, Jessurun J et al (1993) Increased risk of early colorectal neoplasms after hepatic transplant in patients with inflammatory bowel disease. Dis Colon Rectum 36:908–912

59. Ahnen DJ, McHugh JBD, Arsenault LL, Warren G (1993) Does primary sclerosing cholangitis increase the risk of colon cancer in patients with chronic ulcerative colitis? Gastroenterology 104:A658

60. Olshan AF, Mattison DR, Zwanenburg TS (1994) Cyclosporine A: review of genotoxicity and potential for adverse human reproductive and developmental effects. Muta Res 317:163–173

61. Kozarek R, Patterson D, Gelfand M et al (1989) Methotrexate induces clinical and histologic remission in patients with refractory inflammatory bowel disease. Ann Intern Medi 110:353–356

62. Kozarek R, Patterson D, Botoman V et al (1991) Methotrexate use in inflammatory bowel disease patients who have failed azathioprine or 6-mercaptopurine. Gastroenterology 100:A222

63. Feagan BG, Rochon J, Fedorak RN, Irvine EJ (1995) Methotrexate for the treatment of Crohn's disease. N Engl J Med 332:292–297

64. Turnbull C, Roach M (1980) Is methotrexate carcinogenic? BMJ 281:808

65. Weinblatt ME (1995) Methotrexate for chronic diseases in adults. N Engl J Med 332:330–331

66. Tishler M, Caspi D, Yaron M (1993) Long-term experience with low dose methotrexate in rheumatoid arthritis. Rheumatol Int 13:103–106

67. Reynolds J, Trellis D, Abu-Elmagd K, Fung J (1993) The rationale for FK506 in inflammatory bowel disease. Can J Gastroenterol 7:208–210

68. Hoshino H, Goto H, Sugiyama S et al (1995) Effects of FK506

on an experimental model of colitis in rats. Aliment Pharmacol Ther 9:301–307

69. Kitano A, Matsumoto T, Nakamura S et al (1992) New treatment of ulcerative colitis with K-76. Dis Colon Rectum 35: 560–567

70. Sartor RB (1993) Antimicrobial therapy of inflammatory bowel disease: implications for pathogenesis and management. Can J Gastroenterol 7:132–138

71. Ambrose NS, Allan RN, Keighley MR et al (1985) Antibiotic therapy for treatment in relapse of intestinal Crohn's disease. A prospective randomized study. Dis Colon Rectum 28: 81–85

72. Duffy LF, Daum F, Fisher SE et al (1985) Peripheral neuropathy in Crohn's disease patients treated with metronidazole. Gastroenterology 88:681–684

73. Sutherland L, Singleton J, Session J et al (1991) Double blind placebo-controlled trial of metronidazole in Crohn's disease. Gut 32:1071–1075

74. Rutgeerts P, Hiele M, Geboes K et al (1995) Controlled trial of metronidazide treatment for prevention of Crohn's recurrence after ileal resection. Gastroenterology 108:1617–1621

75. Lichtenstein G (1993) Medical therapies for inflammatory bowel disease. Curr Opin Gastroenterol 9:588–599

76. Moss A, Carbone J, Kressel H (1978) Radiologic and clinical assessment of broad-spectrum antibiotic therapy in Crohn's disease. Am J Roentgenol 131:787–790

77. Burke DA, Axon AT, Clayden SA et al (1990) The efficacy of tobramycin in the treatment of ulcerative colitis. Aliment Pharmacol Ther 4:123–129

78. Turunen U, Farkkila M, Hakala K et al (1994) A double-blind, placebo controlled six-month ciprofloxacin treatment improves prognosis in ulcerative colitis. Gastroenterology 106:A786

79. Fernandez-Banares F, Cabre E, Esteve-Comas M, Gassuli MA (1995) How effective is enteral nutrition in inducing clinical remission in active Crohn's disease? A meta-analysis of the randomized clinical trials. J Parenter Enteral Nutr 19: 356–364

80. Griffiths AM, Ohlsson A, Sherman PM, Sutherland LR (1995) Meta-analysis of enteral nutrition as a primary treatment of active Crohn's disease. Gastroenterology 108: 1056–1067

81. Alun Jones V, Dickinson R, Workman E et al (1985) Crohn's disease: maintenance of remission by diet. Lancet 2:177–180.

82. Greenberg G (1992) Nutritional support in inflammatory bowel disease: current status and future directions. Scand J Gastroenterol 27, suppl. 192:117–122

83. Norday A (1991) Is there a rational role for N-3 fatty acids (fish oil) in clinical medicine? Drugs 42:331

84. Stenson W, Cort D, Rodgers J et al (1992) Dietary supplementation with fish oil in ulcerative colitis. Ann Intern Med 87: 609–614

85. Hawthorne AB, Daneshmend TK, Hawkey CJ et al (1992) Treatment of ulcerative colitis with fish oil supplementation: a prospective 12 month randomised controlled trial. Gut 33: 922–928

86. Roediger WEW (1980) The colonic epithelium in ulcerative colitis: an energy deficiency disease? Lancet 2:712–715

87. Harig JM, Soergel KH, Komorowski RA, Wood CM (1989) Treatment of diversion colitis with short chain fatty acid irrigation. N Engl J Med 320:23–28

88. Senagore A, MacKeigan J, Scheider M, Ebrom S (1992) Short chain fatty acid enemas: a cost effective alternative in the treatment of nonspecific proctosigmoiditis. Dis Colon Rectum 35:923–927

89. Florin THJ, Gibson GR, Neal G et al (1990) A role for sulfate reducing bacteria in ulcerative colitis. Gastroenterology 98: A170

90. Nightingale JMD, Rathbone BJ, West et al (1995) Butyrate enemas are less effective than prednisolone enemas in treating distal or left sided ulcerative colitis. Gut, 37, suppl. 2:A41

91. Connell AM, Lennard-Jones JE, Misiewicz JJ et al (1965) Comparison of acetarsol and prednisolone-21-phosphate suppositories in the treatment of idiopathic proctitis. Lancet 1: 238–239

92. Forbes A, Britton TC, House IM, Gazzard BG (1989) Safety and efficacy of acetarsol suppositories in unresponsive proctitis. Aliment Pharmacol Ther 3:553–556

93. Wardle TD, Hall L, Turnberg LA (1993) Inter-relationships between inflammatory mediators released from colonic mucosa in ulcerative colitis and their effects on colonic secretion. Gut 34:503–508

94. Hawthorne AB, Boughton-Smith NK, Whittle BJ, Hawkey CJ (1992) Colorectal leukotriene B4 synthesis in vitro in inflammatory bowel disease: inhibition by the selective 5-lipoxygenase inhibitor BWA4C. Gut 33:513–517

95. Collawn C, Rubin P, Perez N et al (1992) Phase II study of the safety and efficacy of a 5-lipoxygenase inhibitor in patients with ulcerative colitis. Am J Gastroenterol 87:342–346

96. Peppercorn M, Das K, Elson C et al (1994) Zileuton, a 5-lipoxygenase inhibitor, in the treatment of active ulcerative colitis: a double blind placebo controlled trial. Gastroenterology 106:A751

97. Hawkey C, Gassull M, Lauritsen K et al (1994) Efficacy of Zileuton, a 5-lipoxygenase inhibitor, in the maintenance of remission in patients with ulcerative colitis. Gastroenterology 106:A697

98. Gertner D, Rampton D, Stevens T, Lennard-Jones J (1992) Verapamil inhibits in-vitro leucotriene B4 release by rectal mucosa in active ulcerative colitis. Aliment Pharmacol Ther 6:163–168

99. Hayllar J, Bjarnason I (1995) NSAIDs, Cox-2 inhibitors and the gut. Lancet 346:521–522

100. Hawkey C, Rampton D (1985) Prostaglandins and the gastrointestinal mucosa: are they important in its function, disease or treatment? Gastroenterology 89:1462–1488

101. Rampton D, Collins C (1993) Review article: thromboxanes in inflammatory bowel disease—pathogenic and therapeutic implications. Aliment Pharmacol Ther 7:357–367

102. Eberhart CE, Dubois RN (1995) Eicosanoids and the gastrointestinal tract. Gastroenterology 109:285–301

103. Beagley K, Elson C (1992) Cells and cytokines in mucosal immunity and inflammation. Gastroenterol Clin North Am 21:347–366

104. Murch S, Lamkin V, Savage M et al (1991) Serum concentration of tumour necrosis factor in childhood chronic inflammatory bowel disease. Gut 32:913–917

105. Van Dullemen HM, Van Deventer SJH, Hommes DW et al (1995) Treatment of Crohn's disease with anti-tumor necrosis

factor chimeric monoclonal antibody (cA2). Gastroenterology 109:129–135

106. Ghigliotti G, Repetto T, Farris A et al (1993) Thalidomide: treatment of choice for aphthous ulcers in patients seropositive for human immunodeficiency virus. J Am Acad Dermatol 28:271–272

107. Oldfield EC (1994) Thalidomide for severe aphthous ulceration in patients with human immonodeficiency virus (HIV) infection. Am J Gastroenterol 89:2276–2279

108. Moreria A, Sampaio E, Zmuidzinas A et al (1993) Thalidomide exerts its inhibitory action on tumor necrosis factor alpha by enhancing mRNA degradation. J Exp Med 177: 1675–1680

109. Moore KW, O'Garra A, de Waal Malefyt R et al (1993) Interleukin-10. Ann Rev Immunol 11:165–190

110. Kucharzik T, Stoll R, Lugering N et al (1995) Antiinflammatory cytokine interleukin-10 in patients with inflammatory bowel disease. Gut, 27, suppl. 2:A65

111. Schreiber S, Koop I, Heinig T et al (1995) Downregulation of IBD mononulcear phagocyte activation in vitro and in vivo by interleukin 10. Gut, 37, suppl. 2:A112

112. Levin S, Fischer S, Christie D et al (1992) Intravenous immunoglobulin therapy for active extensive and medically refractory idiopathic ulcerative or Crohn's colitis. Am J Gastroenterol 87:91–100

113. Bicks RO, Groshart KD (1989) The current status of T-lymphocyte apheresis (TLA) treatment of Crohn's disease. J Clin Gastroenterol 11:136–138

114. Bicks R, Groshart K, Luther R (1988) Total parenteral nutrition plus T-lymphocyte apheresis in the treatment of severe chronic active Crohn's disease. Gastroenterology 94:A34

115. Lerebours E, Bussel A, Modigliani R et al (1994) Treatment of Crohn's disease by lymphocyte apheresis: a randomized controlled trial. Gastroenterology 107:357–361

116. Sawada K, Ohnishi K, Kosaka T et al (1995) Leukocytapheresis as new therapy for ulcerative colitis. Gut, 37, suppl. 2: A153

117. Kirk AP, Cason J, Fordham JN et al (1983) Polymorphonuclear leukocyte function in ulcerative colitis and Crohn's disease. Dig Dis Sci 28:236–248

118. Emmrich J, Seyfarth M, Fleig W, Emmrich F (1991) Treatment of inflammatory bowel disease with anti-CD4 monclonal antibody. Lancet 338:570–571

119. Keusch K, Mauthe B, Reither C et al (1993) CD4-antibody treatment of inflammatory bowel disease. Gastroenterology 104:691A

120. Winter G, Harris W (1993) Humanized antibodies. Immunol Today 14:243–246

121. Verspaget H, Mulder T, Van der Sluys Veer A et al (1991) Reactive oxygen metabolites and colitis: a disturbed balance between damage and protection: a selective review. Scand J Gastroenterol 26:44–51

122. Kesharvarzian A, Hatdeck J, Zahibi R et al (1992) Agents capable of eliminating reactive oxygen species: catalase, WR-272, or Cu(II)2(2,3DIPS)4 decrease experimental colitis. Dig Dis Sci 37:1866–1873

123. Millar AD, Blake DR, Rampton DS (1994) An open trial of antioxidant nutrient therapy in active ulcerative colitis. Gut, 35, suppl. 5:S29.40

124. Levin K, Pemberton J, Phillips S et al (1992) Role of oxygen free radicals in the aetiology of pouchitis. Dis Colon Rectum 35:452–456

125. Salim A (1992) Role of oxygen derived free radical scavengers in the management of recurrent attacks of ulcerative colitis: a new approach. J Lab Clin Med 119:710–717

126. Emerit J, Pelletier S, Likforman J et al (1991) Phase II trial of copper zinc superoxide dismutase in the treatment of Crohn's disease. Free Radic Res 12–13:563–569

127. Bjorck S, Dahlstrom A, Ahlman H (1989) Topical treatment of ulcerative proctitis with lidocaine. Scand J Gastroenterol 24:1061–1072

128. Dwarakanath AD, Yu LG, Brookes C et al (1995) "Sticky" neutrophils pathergic arthritis and response to heparin in pyoderma gangrenosum complicating ulcerative colitis. Gut 37: 585–588

129. Gaffney PR, Doyle CT, Gaffney A et al (1995). Paradoxical response to heparin in 10 patients with ulcerative colitis. Am J Gastroenterol 90:220–223

130. Cope G, Heatley R (1992) Cigarette smoking and intestinal defences. Gut 32:721–723

131. Pullan RD, Rhodes J, Ganesh S et al (1994) Transdermal nicotine for active ulcerative colitis. N Engl J Med 330: 811–815

132. Hanauer SB (1994) Nicotine for colitis—the smoke has not yet cleared. N Engl J Med 330:856–857

133. Thomas GAO, Rhodes J, Mani V et al (1995) Transdermal nicotine as maintenance therapy for ulcerative colitis. N Engl J Med 332:988–992.21

NUTRITION

Vandana Nehra
Darlene G. Kelly

Nutritional support (total parenteral and enteral nutrition) in the management of inflammatory bowel disease (IBD) has emerged with considerable interest over the past two decades, not only as a primary therapeutic modality, but also as an adjunct for improving nutritional status. Despite several initial encouraging reports the role of nutritional support for achieving and maintaining clinical remission continues to be compared with conventional treatment with drugs. However, the optimal route, composition of nutrient delivery, and precise mechanisms whereby nutritional therapy contributes to clinical improvement are not entirely defined. The objective of this review is to place into perspective the role of nutritional therapy in IBD and highlight areas currently under clinical investigation.

MALNUTRITION IN INFLAMMATORY BOWEL DISEASE

Malnutrition is a major complication afflicting most patients with IBD. It is recognized that patients with Crohn's disease are at greater risk for nutritional deficiencies than patients with ulcerative colitis. In addition, it has been reported that up to 75% of hospitalized Crohn's disease patients are malnourished, as documented by weight loss, hypoalbuminemia, anemia, negative nitrogen balance, or vitamin D deficit.[1] The mechanisms contributing to chronic malnutrition are usually multifactorial and secondary to the following factors: (1) decreased oral intake, (2) increased gastrointestinal losses, (3) malabsorption, (4) increased nutritional requirements, and (5) drug–nutrient interactions.

Decreased Oral Intake

To avoid pain, diarrhea, and nausea associated with eating or painful oral lesions patients restrict their total oral intake. Additionally, many patients avoid specific foods or have been given restricted diets for IBD.

Increased Gastrointestinal Losses

In addition to inadequate intake patients may suffer excessive gastrointestinal losses, thus contributing to their poor nutritional status. The main factors resulting in increased loss of nutrients include diarrhea; fluid, electrolyte, and trace element losses from fistulae protein exudation from the inflamed gut; and iron losses secondary to intestinal blood loss.

Malabsorption

Extensive mucosal disease, bacterial overgrowth, and surgical resection all contribute to inadequate absorption of nutrients resulting in malabsorption, particularly involving depletion of the bile acid pool and consequent fat and fat-soluble vitamin malabsorption.

Increased Nutritional Requirements

Increased metabolic requirements may also exacerbate the preexisting poor nutritional state. Although energy expenditure in these patients appears to be normal, requirements will be increased if fever, abscess, or sepsis develop.[2–4]

Drug–Nutrient Interactions

Drugs used for IBD, such as sulfasalazine (folate), steroids (calcium), and cholestyramine (fat and fat-soluble vitamins), may bind nutrients or alter their absorption.

CLINICAL PRESENTATION OF MALNUTRITION

The most prominent symptom of malnutrition in Crohn's patients is weight loss, which has been reported in 65% to 80% of patients.[1,5–7] Even in the absence of active disease, 20% of patients were observed to be greater than 10% below their ideal body weight.[8]

Following weight loss the next most common nutritionally related finding in Crohn's disease is anemia (iron, folate, vitamin B_{12}). Iron deficiency has been reported with an incidence of 20% to 40% resulting from poor intake, blood loss from the gastrointestinal tract, and malabsorption of iron.[6] It is more common in patients with colonic involvement than in patients whose disease is limited to the small bowel. Approximately 33% of Crohn's patients have been found to have low serum folate levels due to malabsorption of folate secondary to gastrointestinal mucosal involvement or related to the use of sulfasalazine, which interferes with folate absorption.[9,10] Patients with Crohn's disease may also develop anemia as a result of vitamin B_{12} malabsorption due to loss of ileal mucosa associated with inflammation, and bowel resection. Finally, 30% of Crohn's patients experience bacterial overgrowth, and bacteria in the small intestine compete for vitamin B_{12} and thus affect absorption.[11]

Hypoalbuminemia, a common finding in patients with active Crohn's disease, has been observed in 25% to 80% of adults[6] and in 59% of children.[1] The etiology of Crohn's-related hypoalbuminemia is multifactorial and includes intestinal protein loss, reduced hepatic protein synthesis, malabsorption, anorexia, and increased metabolism. In general, serum albumin levels reflect disease activity rather than the nutritional status.[4]

The importance of magnesium deficiency in Crohn's patients has been reported by Hessov and colleagues.[12] This results from poor intake, increased intestinal losses, and malabsorption.

Serum levels are poor indicators of magnesium status, while urinary excretion during an intravenous loading dose is a sensitive index of deficiency in IBD.[13] Zinc deficiency has been reported in about 40% of patients with Crohn's disease,[14,15] and is particularly prevalent in patients with severe diarrhea or enteric fistulae.[16] Serum zinc levels can be misleading, in part owing to the binding of zinc by serum proteins and subnormal protein concentrations in IBD.[14] A combination of low serum and urinary zinc levels is highly suggestive of zinc deficiency.

The most common trace element deficiency reported is that of selenium with resultant clinical manifestations of myopathy and cardiomyopathy. Deficiencies of copper, manganese, or molybdenum have rarely been reported and occur primarily in IBD patients on long-term total parenteral nutrition (TPN) with inadequate supplementation.[17] Deficiencies of water-soluble vitamins, other than vitamin B_{12} and folate, although rare, have been reported in IBD and include scurvy (ascorbic acid), Wernickes encephalopathy (thiamine), photophobia with dermatologic changes (riboflavin), and pellagra (niacin).[18] Fat-soluble vitamin deficiency results from maldigestion caused by a decreased bile salt pool because of terminal ileal disease or resection. Malabsorption may occur because of extensive mucosal inflammation, loss of absorptive surface secondary to scarring or resection, or bacterial overgrowth.[18] Osteomalacia from vitamin D deficiency is the most common presentation of fat-soluble vitamin deficiency. In addition, corticosteroids can contribute to metabolic bone disease in those with IBD.[19]

Malnutrition in ulcerative colitis is a less common problem than in patients with Crohn's disease. During an acute exacerbation of ulcerative colitis, nausea, vomiting, and fever may contribute to poor oral intake and increased nutritional requirements. Weight loss has been reported in 18% to 62% of patients with ulcerative colitis usually associated with acute exacerbation of the disease.[20] Nearly 40% of these patients suffer from iron deficiency related to blood loss.[21]

METABOLIC RATE AND NUTRITIONAL REQUIREMENTS

A number of studies have investigated energy expenditure and nitrogen excretion rates in patients with both active and inactive IBD. In general, metabolic rates do not differ from normal in patients with inactive disease, but may exceed predicted rates during acute inflammatory attacks. Utilizing indirect calorimetry, Chan et al.[22] demonstrated that in patients with inactive Crohn's disease, resting energy expenditure was equivalent to predicted energy expenditure for healthy subjects. Stokes and Hill,[23] utilizing dual energy x-ray absorptiometry, neutron activation analysis, and tritiated water dilution methodology confirmed that total energy expenditure was the same for quiescent Crohn's disease and active disease. In addition, they showed that as Crohn's disease activity increases, the active energy expenditure decreases, thus tending to offset any increases in resting energy expenditure, yet maintaining total energy expenditure at a constant level. In patients with inactive IBD, energy expenditure is estimated at 30 to 40 kilocalories/kg ideal body weight per day while protein requirements are 1 to 1.5 g/kg ideal body weight.[23] In critically ill IBD patients, energy requirements may be difficult to predict, and indirect calorimetry may be the most reliable method by which to avoid under- or overfeeding.

NUTRITIONAL SUPPORT IN CROHN'S DISEASE

Total Parenteral Nutrition in Crohn's Disease

In patients with IBD, nutritional support may be provided as adjunctive therapy to correct malnutrition or primary therapy to facilitate remission. Unlike ulcerative colitis where nutritional support is limited to an adjunctive role, in Crohn's disease TPN may be used both as primary therapy to facilitate remission or as adjunctive therapy for nutritional repletion. It is well recognized that protein calorie malnutrition interferes with wound healing, and is associated with impaired immunocompetence and an increased risk of infection. Nutritional repletion results in stimulation of protein synthesis, at both the systemic and intestinal level.

Total Parenteral Nutrition as Adjunctive Therapy and Perioperative Nutritional Support

Simi and co-workers[24] utilized a prognostic index to identify the increased risk of postoperative morbidity in the presence of a nutritional deficit in patients with Crohn's disease. All deaths reported in this series were in patients who had diffuse, severe lesions and preoperative malnutrition. Many studies have examined the effect of perioperative nutrition support, particularly with TPN, on the surgical outcome of malnourished patients with Crohn's disease. These are summarized in Table 31-1. Rombeau and colleagues[25] retrospectively reviewed records of consecutive patients with IBD who underwent surgical procedures and stated that the use of preoperative TPN was associated with significantly fewer postoperative complications. The presence of albumin levels less than 3.5 g/dl or transferrin levels of less than 150 mg/dl was indicative of significant complications. Lashner et al.[26] compared the effect of TPN on the outcome of surgical intervention in patients with Crohn's disease and historic controls and reported that although TPN did significantly decrease the length of small bowel resected, the total duration of the hospital stay was prolonged in the TPN group, whereas there was no significant difference in the postoperative complications. In another retrospective series[27,28] 88% ($n = 51$) were considered to have had their clinical course improved by the administration of TPN, but the incidence of postoperative complications was not stated, suggesting that various other factors besides malnutrition correlate with surgical outcome in patients with Crohn's disease. The extent of the operative procedure, the number of previous operations, and the necessity for ileostomy all play major roles in determining postoperative complication rates, particularly those that include sepsis.[29]

Analysis of cited reports revealed positive changes in the nutritional parameters with preoperative nutrition, but this was not accompanied by reduced rate of postoperative complications. A 7- to 14-day course of TPN in the malnourished patients with IBD improved respiratory and skeletal muscle strength, as well as demonstrated a trend toward improvement in levels of transferrin and prealbumin.[30] However, the use of preoperative TPN in Crohn's disease should be restricted to seriously malnourished patients who are not candidates for enteral nutrition and who are scheduled to undergo elective or semielective operations.

Table 31-1. Preoperative Total Parenteral Nutrition (TPN) in Crohn's Disease

Author/Year	Number of Patients	Duration of Preoperative TPN (Days)	Number of Complications	Remarks
Vogel et al., 1974[78]	6	14	1	
Eisenberg et al., 1974[27]	25	21	2	
Fazio et al., 1976[28]	48	20	n/r	30 postoperative courses improved
				12 patients avoided surgery
Allardyce, 1978[79]	7	49.5		Improved nutritional parameters
Bos & Weterman, 1980[80]	25	41	2	
Rombeau et al., 1982[25]	30	10 < 5 days	5	
		20 > 5 days	1	
Gouma et al., 1988[81]	35	33	5	
Lashner et al., 1989[26]				
TPN	49			
no TPN	54			Significant reduction of resected small bowel in TPN group

Abbreviation: n/r, Data not reported.
(From Afonso and Rombeau,[64] with permission.)

Total Parenteral Nutrition Primary Therapy in Crohn's Disease

A number of studies have similar conclusions concerning the role of TPN as primary therapy. In a large retrospective series of patients with Crohn's disease who were refractory to conventional medical management, Ostro and associates[31] achieved remission rates of 63% to 89% using TPN, regardless of the intestinal segment that was involved.

Similarly, a prospective controlled trial by Dickinson et al.[32] randomized patients with Crohn's disease to receive TPN or normal hospital diet (control group). Long-term follow-up (15 months) revealed all control group patients had relapsed while a single patient was symptom free in the TPN group. McIntyre et al.,[33] in a multicenter controlled trial of bowel rest for the treatment of acute Crohn's colitis, stated that after a median of 43 months of follow-up, 69% (n = 11) patients with Crohn's disease had relapsed.

Utilizing TPN as the only form of therapy, Muller et al.[34] reported that although 83% (n = 25) responded promptly to TPN and surgery was avoided, the cumulative recurrence rate in the TPN group after 4 years of follow-up was about four times that of the surgical group. These authors concluded that TPN as a form of primary therapy was not a reasonable alternative when compared to surgery for patients with Crohn's disease resistant to medical therapy.

Matuchansky[35] emphasized the high recurrence rate of 40% to 62% at 2 years, and urged consideration of the costs and risk of TPN before use of this therapy. Recognition of the importance of luminal nutrients for bowel integrity prompted Payne-James and Silk[36] to recommend that TPN be used only in supportive roles (rather than the primary therapy). This recommendation is further substantiated by data from Shiloni and colleagues[37] indicating that the use of TPN during severe Crohn's disease may only delay an inevitable operation while increasing the risk and cost of therapy.

In summary, TPN appears to induce remission during acute attacks of Crohn's disease, but sustained long-term remission is less frequent. Hence use of TPN in Crohn's disease should be restricted to patients in whom enteral diets have failed, or the use of the enteral route is not feasible.

Role of Bowel Rest

Although bowel rest has been suggested as one of the major mechanisms whereby TPN or elemental diets contribute to improvement in patients with Crohn's disease, there is no statistically confirmed benefit. A prospective trial by Lochs et al.[38] randomized patients to be maintained on complete bowel rest or a low residue oral diet ad libitum. At the end of the 4 weeks of therapy, not only was there improvement in nutritional status observed in both groups, but also a similar decrease in disease activity. Although parenteral nutrition provides nutritional repletion and reduces disease activity, these data suggest that bowel rest is not a prerequisite for clinical improvement. Subsequently, Greenberg and colleagues[39] assessed the role of bowel rest in a prospective trial (n = 51) with patients with active Crohn's disease who were resistant to other medical management including corticosteroids. Patients were randomly assigned to three groups receiving different levels of nutritional support (i.e., TPN and nothing by mouth, a defined formula diet via a nasogastric tube, or oral diet ad libitum with partial parenteral nutrition) for 21 days. The clinical remission rates were similar in the three groups, thus providing evidence that bowel rest achieved with parenteral nutrition has no distinct advantage in the management of patients with active Crohn's disease.

Enteral Nutrition in Crohn's Disease

In recent years there has been an increased interest in the use of elemental diets in the management of patients with Crohn's disease. Several mechanisms have been proposed to explain the apparent benefit of these diets including the concept of providing bowel rest; reducing the antigenic stimulus to the gut, possibly by altering the bowel flora; and decreasing intestinal permeability and protein loss from the inflamed mucosa.[40] Total enteral nutrition (TEN) provided as amino acid, peptide, or protein hydrolysate-based composition has been utilized as an alternative to TPN for primary therapy of Crohn's disease. Potential advantages of this approach when compared to TPN include lower cost, simpler administration, and fewer complications as well as the potential negative effects of TPN on the intestinal mucosal barrier. Among the issues related to TEN that are not entirely resolved include the clinical efficacy of enteral diets when compared with TPN, the potential influence of enteral diet composition on clinical outcome, and the efficacy of enteral diets versus drug therapy or in combination with drugs.

In examining the role of enteral nutrition as a therapeutic modality in Crohn's disease, it is important to differentiate between trials using the various types of diet. After more than 10 years of investigations on the effect of TEN as primary treatment of active Crohn's disease, there are no clear conclusions. Enteral diets have been characterized as elemental, oligomeric and polymeric. Elemental diets (EDs) contain free l-amino-acids, glucose, and low fat (providing 1% to 2% of the total calories) as long chain triglycerides, with minerals and other micronutrients. EDs do not require intestinal enzymes for digestion and assimilation. The main disadvantages of EDs are their unpalatability, lack of compliance, and high cost. They are non-allergenic, and glutamine constitutes about 17% of the total amino acid content. Oligomeric diets consist of partial protein hydrolysates with variable peptide chain lengths, short chain maltodextrins, and a higher fat content (10% to 35% of the total calories) as long chain and medium chain triglycerides. These diets can be allergenic, and glutamine content is less than 10% of the total amino acid content. Polymeric diets are composed of whole protein (soy, whey, or casein), carbohydrates, and maltodextrins. The fat, composed of long chain and medium-chain triglycerides, contributes 30% to 40% of the calories. As with oligomeric diets, glutamine content is less than 10% of the total amino acids, and they are often considered to be allergenic.

Total Enteral Nutrition Versus Total Parenteral Nutrition

The efficacy of TEN against TPN as a primary therapeutic modality in Crohn's disease has been compared in one prospective controlled trial that found equivalent short-term remission rate as well as long-term outcome.[39] Review of the published data indicates that in acute Crohn's disease, patients receiving enteral nutrition for 3 to 6 weeks will achieve an average remission rate of 67% at 3 months and in 49% of patients this remission will be sustained at the 12-month follow-up.[41] Hence, given the advantages of TEN and observations indicating remission rate comparable to those achieved with the use of TPN, it appears that TEN is the preferred form of nutritional support for patients with acute Crohn's disease.

Total Enteral Nutrition Versus Drugs

Elemental Diet Compared With Standard Medical Therapy

Randomized, prospective trials of ED versus steroids as primary treatment for active Crohn's disease described equal clinical response for the two regimens.[42–45] However, when Okada et al.[46] compared the use of ED with steroids in newly diagnosed patients with Crohn's disease, they found the remission rate with ED to be 80% at 6 weeks versus 11% in the group treated with steroids.

Oligomeric Diet Compared With Standard Medical Therapy

The European cooperative trial[47] demonstrated a 79% remission rate at 6 weeks in the group treated with steroids and 53% in those randomized to diet only. A subsequent trial by Malchow et al.[48] using a defined formula diet found similar response rates favoring standard medical therapy with steroids and sulfasalazine over oligomeric diets.

Polymeric Diet Compared with Standard Medical Therapy

Only one trial[49] has compared the use of steroids with polymeric diet in management of acute Crohn's disease. This demonstrated no difference between the beneficial effects of a polymeric diet over standard medical therapy.

Elemental Diet Compared With Oligomeric Diet

No difference in efficacy has been demonstrated between elemental and oligomeric diets.[50–52]

Elemental Diet Compared With Polymeric Diet

A randomized prospective trial of elemental versus polymeric formula by Giaffer and colleagues[53] showed elemental formula to be better in achieving remission. Other trials led to the conclusion that there was an equal response of Crohn's to either diet, but the long-term outcome of the disease was not influenced by the treatment.[54–56]

Fernandez-Banares et al.[57] recently published a meta-analysis of enteral nutrition as primary treatment of Crohn's, which examined 16 randomized trials that used enteral nutrition to treat acute Crohn's disease. These trials clarified that steroids are superior in inducing remission in active Crohn's disease when compared to enteral nutrition where the probability of achieving remission was lower than with steroids. These results were more evident with oligomeric than polymeric or elemental diets, thus raising the possibility that certain components of these diets may be of greater therapeutic benefit.

Fernandez-Banares and colleagues[58] also suggested that the clinical outcome of treatment of acute Crohn's disease with enteral diets may be related to their fat content, especially linoleic acid, and that diets containing large amounts of linoleic were associated with poor clinical outcome. Linoleic acid, the precursor of arachidonic acid is a substrate for the synthesis of the proinflammatory eicosanoids (leukotriene B4, thromboxane A2, and prostaglandin E2). Other investigators demonstrated improved outcome with very low fat content of diets (0.6% to 1.3% of the total calories).[43,51] Lee and colleagues[59] showed that diets with a low content of essential fatty acids were immunomodulatory and demonstrated a diminished inflammatory response.

NUTRITIONAL SUPPORT IN ULCERATIVE COLITIS

Although high-dose corticosteroids remain the mainstay of medical management in patients with acute exacerbation of ulcerative colitis, 25% to 50% with severe acute colitis will require urgent surgery that may be associated with mortality rates ranging from 20% to 25%. The role of TPN and bowel rest in this clinical setting has been evaluated by two prospective controlled trials. In the trial by Dickinson et al.[32] patients with acute ulcerative colitis all receiving prednisone were randomized to receive either TPN or only fluid, electrolytes, and blood products. The clinical remission rates and the requirements for surgery were equivalent in the two groups. McIntyre and co-workers[33] also showed that the outcome after a program of bowel rest and TPN was no different than with an oral diet. Hence it appears that given the high cost and the risk of complications, TPN does not have a primary therapeutic role in the management of acute ulcerative colitis.

Two studies have retrospectively assessed the role of elemental diets in the management of ulcerative colitis. Rocchio and colleagues[60] reported clinical remission in 33% ($n = 3$), while Axelsson and Jarnum[61] observed improvement in 35% ($n = 8$) in whom other medical therapy was considered failure. Although the numbers of patients are small, the published data indicate that nutritional support and bowel rest are of little value in the primary management of patients with acute ulcerative colitis.

NUTRITIONAL MANAGEMENT OF COMPLICATIONS OF INFLAMMATORY BOWEL DISEASE

Enteric Fistula and Nutrition

The prevalence of fistula in Crohn's disease ranges from 20% to 40%.[62] Although the majority of fistulae develop when the disease is active, reports have noted that they persist subsequently. The mechanism of fistula formation involves a deep abscess that penetrates through the intestinal wall and into the adjacent organs or the skin. Asymptomatic fistulae require no treatment, but high-output fistulae may result in alteration of nutritional status, and loss of fluid, electrolytes, and other nutrients, especially zinc.[15] Although some fistulae that evolve from sites of active Crohn's disease do respond to management with bowel rest and TPN, they often recur when a normal diet is reinstituted.[63] A review by Afonso and Rombeau[64] determined a 38% closure rate of Crohn's disease-related fistulae after TPN, and in the few studies that included long-term follow-up (3 to 120 months), the success rate was even less (Table 31-2). Hence, nutritional and medical therapy is a reasonable initial approach in management of fistulae in patient's with Crohn's disease and if closure cannot be achieved with the use of short-term trial of TPN, surgical management is recommended.

Growth and Development

Growth failure with shortened stature and delayed sexual development has been described in as many as 36% of adolescents and children with Crohn's disease.[65] This often antedates the clinical presentation of Crohn's disease. Weight loss is a common presenting sign, as well as a long-term manifestation, in pediatric patients with Crohn's disease. This may be the result of decreased food intake, as well as prolonged use of steroids.[66–68]

Nutritional support using oral diet,[69] parenteral nutrition,[70] elemental diet by tube feeding[71] or by mouth,[72] and nocturnal tube feedings using polymeric formula[66] has been shown to reverse growth failure in pediatric patients with Crohn's disease. The use of night-time feedings has been especially successful in teenagers who place their own feeding tubes on a nightly basis.

Short Bowel Syndrome

Home parenteral nutrition remains the mainstay in the management of patients with short bowel syndrome, in cases of diffuse Crohn's disease that preclude adequate absorption, or in complicated fistulous disease. Using this therapy, the majority of patients are able to return to a productive life as a student, worker, or homemaker.[73] Complications, including catheter sepsis, cen-

Table 31-2. Crohn's Disease Fistulae and Total Parenteral Nutrition (TPN)

Author/Year	No. of Patients	Duration of TPN (Days)	Short-Term Closures	Long-Term Closures	Length of Follow-Up (Months)
Eisenberg et al., 1974[29]	18	n/r	5 (27%)	4	3
Greenberg et al., 1976[82]					
TPN	7	21	1 (14%)	n/r	n/r
TPN + Pred	7		6 (85%)		
Mullen et al., 1978[83]	20	26	12 (60%)	10	120
Driscoll & Rosenberg, 1978[6]	6	n/r	0 (0%)	n/r	n/r
Elson et al., 1980[84]	4	36	1 (25%)	n/r	n/r
Holm, 1981[85]	3	71	3 (100%)	3	60
Muller et al., 1983[34]	3	84	2 (66%)	n/r	n/r
Ostro et al., 1985[31]	24	n/r	15 (62%)	8	12
Gouma et al., 1988[81]	22	33	13 (59%)	n/r	n/r

Abbreviations: n/r, Data not reported; Pred, prednisone.
(From Afonso and Rombeau,[64] with permission.)

Table 31-3. Role of Nutritional Support in Inflammatory Bowel Disease

Delivery	Disease	Therapeutic Goal	Outcome
Parenteral	CD	Primary therapy	Achieves remission, but disease recurs with oral diet
		Closure of Crohn's fistulae	Closure occurs, but recurrence with oral diet
		Preoperative rehabilitation	Corrects malnutrition
			May decrease complications in severely malnourished patients
		Reversal of growth failure	Achieves growth in children and adolescents
	UC	Primary therapy	No more effective than oral food in preventing surgery or achieving clinical remission
Enteral	CD	Primary therapy	Achieves remission, but disease recurs with oral diet
			Poor patient compliance
		Reversal of growth failure	Achieves growth in children and adolescents
	UC	Primary therapy	No therapeutic benefit as adjunct to steroid therapy
			Improvement of nutritional status
Oral diets	CD	Primary therapy	Very high calorie diet achieves remission, but relapse occurs
			Variable outcomes with elimination diets
			Special diet may restrict nutrient intake
	UC	Primary therapy	No data available

Abbreviations: CD, Crohn's disease; UC, ulcerative colitis.
(From Kelly and Fleming,[86] with permission.)

tral venous thrombosis, and liver disease, are relatively common, and TPN-related complications are responsible for death in about 6% of patients.[74] Consequently, this therapy should be reserved for those who have gut failure severe enough to exclude the use of the intestine as the route for alimentation. Recently published data on home elemental enteral nutrition in induction, as well as maintenance, of remission in Crohn's disease is promising and warrants consideration for future studies.[75]

EICOSANOIDS AS IMMUNOMODULATORS IN INFLAMMATORY BOWEL DISEASE

Recent interest in the role of eicosanoids as immunomodulators has prompted investigation of the role of fish oil in the treatment of IBD. Initial studies with fish oil supplemented in patients with ulcerative colitis showed decreased disease activity, but no such beneficial result on disease activity was evident in randomized trials using fish oil in patients with Crohn's disease.[76,77]

SUMMARY

Malnutrition is commonly observed in patients with active IBD. The main roles for nutritional support are in Crohn's disease. TPN remains a valuable adjunctive therapy in malnourished patients with Crohn's disease but has limited use as primary therapy (Table 31-3). Bowel rest is not a prerequisite to achieving remission in acute IBD. Enteral nutrition with defined formula is not as effective as standard medical therapy in inducing clinical remission in most situations. Intact protein diets appear to be as effective as elemental diets. Although closure of fistulae often occurs with bowel rest and the use of TPN, recurrence is common when oral diets are resumed. Nutritional support is particularly helpful in providing preoperative rehabilitation in cases of significant malnutrition complicating Crohn's disease, but it should be reserved for patients undergoing elective or semielective operations. Growth failure in pediatric patients with Crohn's disease can be reversed with nutritional support provided as parenteral, enteral, or enhanced oral diets. Nutritional support is also essential to the long-term management of short bowel syndrome. Current areas of investigation include the role of optimal nutrient composition and immunomodulation in achieving and maintaining remission.

REFERENCES

1. Seidman EG (1989) Nutritional management of inflammatory bowel disease. Gastroenterol Clin North Am 18:129–155
2. Barot LR, Rombeau JL, Steinberg JJ et al (1981) Energy expenditure in patients with inflammatory bowel disease. Arch Surg 116:460–462
3. Rosenberg IH, Bengoa JM, Sitrin MD (1985) Nutritional aspects of inflammatory bowel disease. Ann Rev Nutr 5:463–484
4. Stokes MA (1992) Crohn's disease and nutrition. Br J Surg 79:391–394
5. Crohn BB, Ginzburg L, Oppenheimer GD (1932) Regional ileitis. A pathologic and clinical entity. JAMA 99:1323–1329
6. Driscoll RH, Rosenberg IH (1978) Total parenteral nutrition in inflammatory bowel disease. Med Clin North Am 61:185–201
7. VanPatter WN, Bargen JA, Dockerty MB et al (1954) Regional enteritis. Gastroenterology 26:347–450
8. Harries AD, Jones LA, Heatley RV, Rhodes J (1982) Malnutrition in inflammatory bowel disease: an anthropometric study. Hum Nutr Clin Nutr 36:307–313

9. Franklin JL, Rosenberg IH (1973) Impaired folic acid absorption in inflammatory bowel disease: effects of salicylazosulfapyridine (Azulfidine). Gastroenterology 64:517–525

10. Selhub J, Dhar GJ, Rosenberg IH (1978) Inhibition of folate enzymes by sulfasalazine. J Clin Invest 61:221–224

11. Beeken W, Kanich RE (1973) Microbial flora of the upper small bowel in Crohn's disease. Gastroenterology 65:390–397

12. Hessov I, Hasselbad C, Fasth S, Hulten L (1983) Magnesium deficiency after ileal resections for Crohn's disease. Scand J Gastroenterol 18:643–649

13. Galland L (1988) Magnesium and inflammatory bowel disease. Magnesium 7:78–83

14. Fleming CR, Huizenga KA, McCall JT et al (1981) Zinc nutrition in Crohn's disease. Dig Dis Sci 26:865–870

15. McClain C, Soutour C, Zieve L (1980) Zinc deficiency: a complication of Crohn's disease. Gastroenterology 78:272–279

16. Valberg LS, Flanagan PR, Kertesz A, Bondy DC (1986) Zinc absorption in inflammatory bowel disease. Dig Dis Sci 31:724–731

17. Goldschmid S, Graham M (1989) Trace element deficiencies in inflammatory bowel disease. Gastroenterol Clin North Am 18:579–587

18. Gerson CD, Cohen N, Janowitz HD (1973) Small intestinal absorptive function in regional enteritis. Gastroenterology 64:907–912

19. Greenberg GR (1993) Nutritional management of inflammatory bowel disease. Semin Gastrointest Dis 4:69–86

20. Fleming CR (1990) Enteral and parenteral nutrition. pp. 145–157. In Peppercorn MA (ed): Therapy of Inflammatory Bowel Disease. New Medical and Surgical Approaches. Marcel Dekker, New York

21. Thomson ABR, Brust R, Ali MAM et al (1978) Iron deficiency in inflammatory bowel disease: diagnostic efficacy of serum ferritin. Am J Dig Dis 23:705–709

22. Chan ATH, Fleming CR, O'Fallon WM, Huizenga KA (1986) Estimated versus measured basal energy requirements in patients with Crohn's disease. Gastroenterology 91:75–78

23. Stokes MA, Hill GL (1993) Total energy expenditure in patients with Crohn's disease: measurement by the combined body scan technique. J Parenter Enter Nutr 17:3–7

24. Simi M, Leardi S, Minervini S et al (1990) Early complications after surgery for Crohn's disease. Neth J Surg 42:195–109

25. Rombeau JL, Barot LR, Williamson CE, Mullen JL (1982) Preoperative total parenteral nutrition and surgical outcome in patients with inflammatory bowel disease. Am J Surg 143:139–143

26. Lashner BA, Evans AA, Hanauer SB (1989) Preoperative total parenteral nutrition for bowel resection in Crohn's disease. Dig Dis Sci 34:741–746

27. Eisenberg HW, Turnbull RB, Weakley FL (1974) Hyperalimentation as preparation for surgery in transmural colitis (Crohn's disease). Dis Colon Rectum 19:469–475

28. Fazio VW, Kodner I, Jagelman DG et al (1976) Inflammatory bowel disease of the bowel: parenteral nutrition as primary or adjunctive treatment. Dis Colon Rectum 19:574–578

29. Heimann TM, Greenstein AJ, Mechanic L, Aufses AH Jr (1985) Early complications following surgical treatment for Crohn's disease. Ann Surg 201:494–498

30. Christie PM, Hill GL (1990) Effect of intravenous nutrition on nutrition and function in acute attacks of inflammatory bowel disease. Gastroenterology 99:730–736

31. Ostro MJ, Greenberg GR, Jeejeebhoy KN (1985) Total parenteral nutrition and complete bowel rest in the management of Crohn's disease. J Parenter Enter Nutr 9:280–287

32. Dickinson RJ, Ashton MG, Axon ATR et al (1980) Controlled trial of intravenous hyperalimentation and total bowel rest as an adjunct to the routine therapy of acute colitis. Gastroenterology 79:1199–1204

33. McIntyre PB, Powell-Tuck J, Wood SR et al (1986) Controlled trial of bowel rest in the treatment of severe acute colitis. Gut 27:481–485

34. Muller JM, Keller HW, Erasmi H, Pichlmaier H (1983) Total parenteral nutrition as the sole therapy in Crohn's disease: a prospective study. Br J Surg 70:40–43

35. Matuchansky C (1986) Parenteral nutrition in inflammatory bowel disease. Gut 27:81–84

36. Payne-James JJ, Silk DBA (1988) Total parenteral nutrition as primary treatment in Crohn's disease—RIP? Gut 29:1304–1308

37. Shiloni E, Coronado E, Freund HR (1989) Role of total parenteral nutrition in the treatment of Crohn's disease. Am J Surg 157:180–185

38. Lochs H, Meryn S, Marosi L et al (1983) Has total bowel rest a beneficial effect in treatment of Crohn's disease? Clin Nutr 2:61–64

39. Greenberg GR, Fleming CR, Jeejeebhoy JN et al (1988) Controlled trial of bowel rest and nutrition support in the management of Crohn's disease. Gut 29:1309–1315

40. Bernstein C, Shananhan F (1992) Braving the elements in Crohn's disease. Gastroenterology 103:1363–1364

41. Greenberg GR (1992) Nutritional support in inflammatory bowel disease: current status and future directions. Scand J Gastroenterol Suppl 192:117–122

42. Gorard DA, Hunt JB, Payne-James JJ et al (1993) Initial response and subsequent course of Crohn's disease treated with elemental diet or prednisolone. Gut 34:1198–1202

43. O'Moráin C, Segal AW, Levi AJ (1984) Elemental diet as primary treatment of acute Crohn's disease: a controlled trial. BMJ 288:1859–1862

44. Saverymuttu S, Hodgson HJF, Chadwick VS (1985) Controlled trial comparing prednisolone with an elemental diet plus non-absorbable antibiotics in active Crohn's disease. Gut 26:994–998

45. Seidman EG, Bouthillier L, Weber AM et al (1986) Elemental diet versus prednisone as primary treatment of Crohn's disease, abstracted. Gastroenterology 90:1625A

46. Okada M, Yao T, Yamamoto T et al (1990) Controlled trial comparing an elemental diet with prednisolone in the treatment of active Crohn's disease. Hepatogastroenterology 37:72–80

47. Lochs H, Steinhardt HJ, Klaus-Wentz B et al (1991) Comparison of enteral nutrition and drug treatment in active Crohn's disease. Results of the European Cooperative Crohn's Disease Study IV. Gastroenterology 101:881–888

48. Malchow H, Steinhardt HJ, Lorenz-Meyer H et al (1990) Feasibility and effectiveness of a defined-formula diet regimen in treating active Crohn's disease. European Cooperative Crohn's Disease Study III. Scand J Gastroenterol 25:235–244

49. González-Huix F, de León R, Fernández-Bañares F et al (1993) Polymeric enteral diets as primary treatment of active Crohn's disease: a prospective steroid controlled trial. Gut 34:778–782

50. Mansfield JC, Giaffer MH, Holsworth CD (1990) Controlled

trial of oligopeptide versus amino-acid diet in treatment of active Crohn's disease. Gut 36:60–66

51. Middleton SJ, Riordan AM, Hunter JO (1991) Peptide based diet: an alternative to elemental diet in the treatment of acute Crohn's disease, abstracted. Gut 32:A578

52. Royall D, Jeejeebhoy KN, Baker JP et al (1994) Comparison of amino acid versus peptide based enteral diets in active Crohn's disease: Clin Nutr Outcome. Gut 35:783–787

53. Giaffer MH, North G, Holdsworth CD (1990) Controlled trial of polymeric versus elemental diet in treatment of active Crohn's disease. Lancet 335:815–819

54. Park RHR, Galloway A, Danesh BSZ, Russel RI (1991) Double blinded controlled trial of elemental and polymeric diets as primary therapy in active Crohn's disease. Eur J Gastroenterol Hepatol 3:483–490

55. Raouf AH, Hildrey V, Daniel J et al (1991) Enteral feeding as sole treatment for Crohn's disease: controlled trial of whole protein v amino acid based feed and a case study of dietary challenge. Gut 32:702–707

56. Rigaud D, Cosnes J, LeQuintrec Y et al (1991) Controlled trial comparing two types of enteral nutrition in treatment of active Crohn's disease: elemental v polymeric diet. Gut 32:1492–1497

57. Fernandez-Barares F, Cabre E, Esteve-Comas M, Gassull MA (1995) How effective is enteral nutrition in inducing clinical remission in active Crohn's disease? A meta-analysis of the randomized controlled trials. J Parenter Enter Nutr 19:356–362

58. Fernandez-Barares F, Cabre E, GonSálex-Huix F, Gassull MA (1994) Enteral nutrition as a primary therapy in Crohn's disease. Gut 35:S55–S59

59. Lee TH, Hoover RL, Williams JD et al (1985) Effect of dietary enrichment with eicosapentanoic and docosahescaenoic acids on in-vitro neutrophil and monocyte leukotriene generation and neutrophil function. N Engl J Med 312:1217–1224

60. Rocchio MA, Cha CJ, Haas KF, Randall HT (1974) Use of chemically defined diets in the management of patients with acute inflammatory bowel disease. Am J Surg 127:469–475

61. Axelsson C, Jarnum S (1977) Assessment of the therapeutic value of an elemental diet in chronic inflammatory bowel disease. Scan J Gastroenter 12:89–95

62. Steinberg DM, Cook WT, Alexander-Williams J (1973) Abscess and fistulae in Crohn's disease. Gut 14:865–869

63. Yamazaki Y, Fukushima T, Sugita A et al (1990) The medical, nutritional and surgical treatment of fistulas in Crohn's disease. Jpn J Surg 20:376–383

64. Afonso JJ, Rombeau JL (1990) Nutritional care for patients with Crohn's disease. Hepatogastroenterology 37:32–41

65. Booth IW (1991) The nutritional consequences of gastrointestinal disease in adolescence. Acta Paediatr Scand Suppl 373:91–102

66. Aiges H, Markowitz J, Rosa J, Daum F (1989) Home nocturnal supplemental nasogastric feedings in growth-retarded adolescents with Crohn's disease. Gastroenterology 97:905–910

67. Kelts DG, Grand RJ, Shen G et al (1979) Nutritional basis of growth failure in children and adolescents with Crohn's disease. Gastroenterology 76:720–727

68. Markowitz J, Grancher K, Rosa J et al (1993) Growth failure in pediatric inflammatory bowel disease. J Pediatr Gastroenterol Nutri 16:373–380

69. Kirschner BS, Klich JR, Kalman SS et al (1981) Reversal of growth retardation in Crohn's disease with therapy emphasizing oral nutritional restitution. Gastroenterology 80:10–15

70. Layder T, Rosenberg J, Nemchausky B et al (1976) Reversal of growth arrest in adolescents with Crohn's disease after parenteral alimentation. Gastroenterology 70:1017–1021

71. Belli DC, Seidman E, Bouthillier L et al (1988) Chronic intermittent elemental diet improves growth failure in children with Crohn's disease. Gastroenterology 94:603–610

72. Thomas AG, Taylor F, Miller V (1993) Dietary intake and nutritional treatment in childhood Crohn's disease. J Pediatr Gastroenterol Nutr 17:75–81

73. Burnes JU, O'Keefe SJD, Fleming CR et al (1992) Home parenteral nutrition—a 3-year analysis of clinical and laboratory monitoring. J Parenter Enter Nutr 16:327–332

74. Fleming CR (1986) Comprehensive care of the gut failure patient: present and future. Trans Am Clin Climatol Assoc 98:197–207

75. Hirakawa H, Fukuda YU, Tanida N et al (1993) Home elemental enteral hyperalimentation (HEEH) for the maintenance of remission in patients with Crohn's disease. Gastroenterol Jpn 28:379–384

76. Aslan A, Triadafilopoulos G (1992) Fish oil fatty acid supplementation in active ulcerative colitis: a double-blind, placebo-controlled, crossover study. Am J Gastroenterol 87:432–437

77. Lorenz R, Weber PC, Szimnau P et al (1989) Supplementation with n-3 fatty acids from fish oil in chronic inflammatory bowel disease—a randomized, placebo-controlled, double-blind cross-over trial. J Intern Med 225:225–232

78. Vogel CM, Corwin TR, Baue AE (1974) Intravenous hyperalimentation in the treatment of inflammatory bowel disease. Arch Surg 108:460–467

79. Allardyce DB (1978) Preoperative parenteral feeding in Crohn's disease: preoperatively, to induce remission, and at home. Am Surg 44:510–516

80. Bos LP, Weterman I (1980) Total parenteral nutrition in Crohn's disease. World J Surg 4:163–166

81. Gouma DJ, von Meyenfeldt MF, Rouflart M, Soeters PB (1988) Preoperative total parenteral nutrition (TPN) in severe Crohn's disease. Surgery 103:648–652

82. Greenberg GL, Haber HB, Jeejeebhoy KN (1976) Total parenteral nutrition (TPN) and bowel rest in the management of Crohn's disease. Gut 12:828

83. Mullen JL, Hargrove C, Dudrick SJ et al (1978) Ten years experience with intravenous hyperalimentation and inflammatory bowel disease. Ann Surg 187:523–529

84. Elson CO, Layden TJ, Nemchausky BA et al (1980) An evaluation of total parenteral nutrition in the management of inflammatory bowel disease. Dig Dis Sci 25:42–48

85. Holm I (1981) Benefits of total parenteral nutrition (TPN) in the treatment of Crohn's disease and ulcerative colitis. Acta Chir Scand 147:271–276

86. Kelly D, Fleming C (1995) Nutritional considerations in inflammatory bowel diseases. Gastroenterol Clin North Am 24:597–611

32

SURGERY FOR ULCERATIVE COLITIS

Jacques Heppell
Keith A. Kelly
Roger R. Dozois

Chronic ulcerative colitis was first described over 135 years ago,[1] but its exact cause is still unknown. Medical treatment, therefore, is largely nonspecific and directed toward symptoms. Approximately 20% to 45% of patients with the disease eventually undergo surgery.[2] The operations used have evolved considerably over the past century as surgeons gradually recognized the need for removal of the inflamed large intestine and the establishment of an ileostomy (Table 32-1). In recent years, however, surgeons have aimed at complete excision of the disease with preservation of transanal defecation and avoidance of an ileostomy. These aims have been achieved using a newly devised operation, proctocolectomy with ileal pouch-anal canal anastomosis. In this procedure, the entire diseased large intestine is excised, but the anal sphincters are preserved. An ileal pouch is constructed from the terminal ileum and anastomosed to the anal canal, thus preserving transanal defecation. Because the anal sphincters remain intact and because the ileal pouch provides a reservoir for feces, reasonable fecal continence is maintained.

INDICATIONS FOR SURGERY

The indications for surgery among patients with chronic ulcerative colitis have changed little with the advent of the ileal pouch-anal canal anastomosis. They can still be divided into two major types: those requiring elective operation and those requiring emergency surgery.

Indications for Elective Surgery

Intractability to Medical Therapy

Patients who have debilitating symptoms, poor nutrition, and an impaired quality of life in spite of adequate medical therapy, should be considered for an elective ileal pouch-anal canal oper-

ation. Anemia, hypoproteinemia, giant inflammatory polyposis with protein-losing enteropathy,[3] and, in children, failure to grow,[4] provide further impetus for operation.

The need and timing of surgery are best determined by consultation among patient, gastroenterologist, and surgeon.[5] Some have suggested that prolonged medical therapy for drug-resistant ulcerative colitis increases the need for urgent operation, with a resulting increase in morbidity, hospital stay, and cost.[6] Others have found that a patient may maintain a satisfactory lifestyle on medical therapy but only when taking an excess of medication that, in itself, produces symptoms and has risks. Side effects, such as psychosis, hypertension, cataracts, and osteoporosis, appear with medical therapy, causing patient and physician to lean toward surgery. Still others believe that the quality of life after proctocolectomy with an ileal pouch-anal canal anastomosis compares favorably to that of patients with medically treated colitis.[7] These points favor early surgery.

Nonetheless, before advising surgery, careful consideration should be given as to whether an adequate trial of medical therapy has occurred.[5] Criteria of intractability are often difficult to define.[8] The degree of symptomatology that one is willing to label debilitating will vary from patient to patient and from physician to physician. Much depends on the patient's tolerance to the disease and the influence of the disease on the person's lifestyle. It is also important to remember that the patient intolerant to medical therapy may be the one least able to cope with an unexpected complication of an operation or the ultimate need for a permanent stoma.

Presence and Risk of Cancer

The presence of cancer in the large intestine is a strong indication for surgery. An increased risk of colorectal cancer occurring in those with extensive and long-standing ulcerative colitis

Table 32-1. History of Surgery for Chronic Ulcerative Colitis

1893	Mayo Robson, A.R. (Leeds)[202]	Sigmoid colostomy for colonic irrigation
1895	Keetley, C.B. (London)[203]	Appendicostomy for irrigation
1903	Lilienthal, H. (New York)[204]	Ileosigmoidostomy
1913	Brown, J.Y. (St. Louis)[205]	Ileostomy for complete physiologic rest of the colon
1933	Nissen, R. (Basel)[206]	Proctocolectomy and straight ileoanal anastomosis
1944	Koenig-Rutzen (Chicago)[207]	Design of bag to collect ileostomy effluent
1944	Strauss, A.A. (Chicago)[208]	Use of an adherent appliance
1947	Ravitch, M. and Sabiston, D. (Baltimore)[209]	Anal ileostomy with preservation of sphincter
1951	Goligher, J.C. (Leeds)[210]	Loop ileostomy to protect ileoanal anastomosis
1953	Aylett, S.O. (Sydney)[200]	Colectomy with ileorectal anastomosis
1958	Gill N., Turnbull R.B. (Cleveland)[211]	Enterostomal therapy
1969	Kock N.G. (Göteborg)[212]	Intra-abdominal ileal reservoir
1977	Martin, L.W. (Cincinnati)[213]	Renewed interest in anorectal mucosal stripping with ileoanal anastomosis
1978	Parks, A.G. & Nicholls, J. (London)[214]	Construction of S-shaped ileal pouch with pouch-anal anastomosis
1980	Utsunomiya, J. (Japan)[75]	Use of J-shaped ileal pouch

has been recognized in the past.[9–12] Nonetheless, studies in controlled populations suggest that the true risk of carcinoma is less[13,14] than that previously reported from referral centers.[15] In fact, in one recent study,[16] no increased risk of cancer in colitis was shown. Also, the risk of cancer in a given population may be lessened by the long-term treatment of quiescent colitis with mesalamine, by the rapid treatment of acute attacks with corticosteroids, and by the early surgical treatment of fulminant colitis unresponsive to medical therapy. Even so, among patients who had the onset of their colitis as children or teenagers, who have generalized colitis, and who have had their disease 10 years or more, 2% will develop cancer each year.[15] Such patients should be considered either for prophylactic proctocolectomy or at least should enter a close surveillance program. Patients with sclerosing cholangitis complicating their colitis

also are reported to have an especially increased risk of colorectal cancer.[17–19] In contrast, prophylactic proctocolectomy in adults with left-sided disease of short duration is usually not indicated. Surveillance, however, should be done.

Surveillance, while recommended, does have limitations. When patients have quiescent or mild disease, they often are reluctant to undergo biannual colonoscopy. If colonoscopy is performed, areas of abnormality may not be recognized. Dysplasia does not always precede carcinoma,[20] and a carcinoma may be flat or mainly submucosal and fail detection. Finally, all too often, carcinoma is already present in patients before dysplasia is found.[21,22] Patients continue to develop carcinomas while in surveillance programs, and such carcinomas are not uncommonly advanced. If a surveyed patient develops an obstructive lesion,[23] dysplasia, or a dysplasia-associated mass, surgery should be performed. These patients have a greater than 50% chance of having invasive cancer.[24]

For most patients, however, the choice of surveillance versus surgery is not clear. No controlled trials compare surveillance with prophylactic proctocolectomy. Decision analysis shows that endoscopic surveillance of patients with long-standing colitis does appear to improve survival, but prophylactic proctocolectomy seems to improve survival even more.[25] Nonetheless, most patients with mild or quiescent colitis choose colonoscopic surveillance and opt for surgery only if their symptoms get worse, if cancer develops, or if they are advised that a great risk of cancer is present based on the presence of high-grade dysplasia.[26]

Debilitating Extraintestinal Manifestations

Approximately 30% of patients with ulcerative colitis will have at least one extraintestinal manifestation of their disease that may contribute to the decision for surgery.[27–29] These manifestations, however, are seldom the sole indication for operation. Cutaneous, peripheral articular, ocular, hematologic, and vascular extraintestinal manifestations may improve after surgery.[5] However, healing of pyoderma gangrenosum after intestinal resection is uncertain,[30] while ankylosing spondylitis and rheumatoid arthritis[31] will not regress after surgery. Moreover, sclerosing cholangitis may progress to cirrhosis or cholangiocarci-

Indications for Surgery in Ulcerative Colitis

Elective Indications

Failure of Medical Treatment

Fulminant/unresponsive nature of first attack

Inadequate response to medical therapy

Excessive steroid dose required

Side effects/intolerance/complications related to medications

Noncompliance with medication

Chronic Complications of the Disease

Recurrent hemorrhage

Carcinoma, or the risk thereof

Growth retardation in children

Extraintestinal manifestations of ulcerative colitis

Emergent Indications

Fulminant colitis

Toxic megacolon

Perforation, hemorrhage, obstruction

noma after surgery.[32] The presence of hepatobiliary and thromboembolic extraintestinal manifestations of colitis increases the risk of perioperative complications.[5]

Indications for Emergency Surgery

Fulminant Colitis

Definitions of fulminant colitis lack uniformity. One authority[33] considers a patient to have fulminant colitis when evidence of at least two of the following exist: tachycardia, fever, leukocytosis greater than 10,500 cells/mm, and hypoalbuminemia. Severe ulceration and inflammation at endoscopy support the need for surgery.[34] Severe attacks may be the first manifestation of the disease.

Patients with fulminant colitis should first be managed aggressively with medication, but failure of their clinical status to improve or continued deterioration is an indication for emergency surgery. Indeed, although fulminant colitis has carried a high mortality in the past, the mortality has now fallen to less than 3%[35] due to prompt surgery when medical management fails. The goal is to operate before colonic perforation occurs.

Medical management of fulminant colitis does seem to be improving in recent years. In one study, 70% of patients with fulminant colitis not responding to intravenous steroids responded to intravenous cyclosporine to the degree that the patients could be discharged from the hospital and prepared for surgery on an elective basis.[36]

Toxic Megacolon

Toxic megacolon may require emergency surgery. Toxic megacolon is diagnosed when pain, fever, toxicity, and abdominal tenderness and distension are accompanied by a transverse colon whose diameter exceeds 7 cm on abdominal roentgenogram. The colonic dilatation can lead to perforation. Although megacolon has been reported to occur in 6% of hospitalized patients with colitis in the past,[37] its current incidence may be decreasing. Like fulminant colitis, it may be the initial manifestation of the disease. Because toxic megacolon with perforation is associated with an appreciable mortality (20% to 40% with perforation as compared to 4% with no perforation),[38] patients with megacolon should be operated on before perforation occurs. Surgery for toxic megacolon is indicated if no clinical improvement occurs within 24 hours of initiation of medical treatment or if deterioration occurs. Even those patients who respond to medical treatment have a high probability of a second attack of toxic megacolon (30%) and subsequent colonic resection (50%), often as an emergency.[39] Thus, medical management in this subset of patients is often a prelude to surgery.

Perforation, Hemorrhage, and Obstruction

Perforation of the colon with ulcerative colitis is a clear indication for surgery. Perforation is rare in the absence of toxic megacolon. Its occurrence without megacolon should raise a concern that the patient may have Crohn's disease and not ulcerative colitis. Large doses of steroids may mask symptoms. A high index of suspicion of perforation must be maintained in patients with severe colitis on steroids, especially when they develop pain after colonoscopy. The high mortality associated with perforation can only be decreased by early surgery.[40]

Massive bleeding from ulcerative colitis mandates emergency surgery. Such bleeding occurs infrequently in patients with ulcerative colitis, but it accounts for 10% of emergency colectomies. It is often associated with concomitant toxic megacolon.[41] Strictures causing colonic obstruction are rare with ulcerative colitis but, if present, may require emergency surgery. Usually, however, the obstruction is only partial, and the patient can be prepared for an elective procedure.

PREOPERATIVE MANAGEMENT

Once the decision is made to operate, the patient should be carefully prepared for the operation.[5] Hypovolemia and electrolyte disturbances should be corrected with intravenous infusion of crystalloid solutions, and blood should be given to treat anemia. When sepsis is suggested by the presence of fever, tachycardia, leukocytosis, or abdominal tenderness, blood cultures should be obtained, and broad-spectrum parenteral antibiotics administered. Patients who have received prior steroid therapy should be given 100 mg of hydrocortisone intravenously every 8 hours immediately before, during, and for 2 days after surgery, after which the dose can be tapered.

For elective procedures, the preparation of a patient with ulcerative colitis includes counseling and education on the expected outcome. The various surgical and nonsurgical options should be reviewed (Table 32-2) and the short- and long-term complications discussed. Patients should understand that the separation of ulcerative colitis from Crohn's disease is inexact and that about 10% of such patients may eventually be shown to have Crohn's disease. For patients who will receive an ileostomy, the participation of a qualified enterostomal therapist is helpful in selecting the ostomy site and in dispelling the patient's fears about the stoma.

Bedside assessment using clinical information will provide an accurate estimation of the nutritional status of most patients.[42] A weight loss of 5% of body weight in the past month or greater than 10% in the past 6 months, and a decreased serum albumin, total lymphocyte count, and transferrin are indicative of malnutrition.[43]

Little evidence exists to support the use of preoperative nutritional therapy in patients with mild or moderate malnutrition from their colitis.[44,45] In fact, such therapy may be harmful to patients who are relatively well nourished. The use of total parenteral nutrition (TPN) to avoid or circumvent surgery in patients with severe ulcerative colitis is also not beneficial.[46] However, among patients with severe malnutrition, attempts should be made to improve patient's nutritional status with parenteral replacement of protein, calories, specific vitamins, and minerals.[47] At least 10 to 14 days of preoperative TPN is needed to improve postsurgical healing and reduce postoperative complications[48] in malnourished patients. After surgery, parenteral nutrition should be continued until the patient is able to eat well.

Most elective operations for ulcerative colitis are "clean-contaminated" operations, with entrance into the gastrointestinal tract but no gross contamination of the surgical field. A combination of oral and intravenous preoperative antibiotics with gentle mechanical cleansing of the bowel will reduce the incidence of postoperative wound infection and pelvic sepsis.[49] Vigorous bowel preparation should not be done, especially in patients with toxic megacolon, high-grade obstruction, or suspected perforation.

Table 32-2. Choice of Operation for Ulcerative Colitis

Procedure	Advantages	Disadvantages
Proctocolectomy, ileal pouch-anal canal anastomosis	Complete excision of large intestinal disease Transanal defecation and fecal continence preserved No ileostomy	Two operations required At risk for pouchitis Nocturnal fecal spotting present
Proctocolectomy, ileal pouch-distal rectal anastomosis	Transanal defecation and excellent fecal continence preserved No ileostomy Ease of performance	At risk for pouchitis and symptoms of cancer from residual rectal mucosa
Proctocolectomy, continent ileostomy	Complete excision of large intestinal disease Fecal continence preserved No external appliance	Stoma present Intubation of pouch required At risk for pouchitis and need for valve revision
Proctocolectomy, Brooke ileostomy	Complete excision of large intestinal disease	Stoma present Incontinent for feces Need for external appliance
Cecal-colectomy, ileorectal anastomosis	Transanal defecation and fecal continence preserved No ileostomy	Diseased rectum remains to produce symptoms, require treatment, and predispose to cancer

The morbidity and mortality of anesthesia and surgery is increased in patients with significant liver disease associated with ulcerative colitis.[50,51] Poor hepatic function is a predictor of poor outcome.[52,53] Clotting abnormalities, electrolyte disturbances, hepatic encephalopathy, and ascites should be corrected preoperatively.

Thomboembolic complications are related to the hypercoagulability associated with colitis and major abdominopelvic surgery. Deep vein thrombosis and pulmonary embolism are the most common types of thromboembolic events; arterial thrombi are unusual and occur mostly in the postoperative period.[54] Prophylactic therapy with intermittent pneumatic compression of the legs combined with early postoperative mobilization and elastic compression stockings should be provided.[55]

PROCTOCOLECTOMY WITH ILEAL POUCH-ANAL CANAL ANASTOMOSIS

Selection of Patients for Surgery

Proctocolectomy with ileal pouch-anal canal anastomosis has been selected as the operation of choice for ulcerative colitis with greater frequency in recent years at St. Mark's Hospital, London, England,[56] at the Mayo Clinic in the United States (Fig. 32-1), and elsewhere. Fewer proctocolectomies with Brooke ileostomy, continent ileostomies, and ileorectal anastomoses are currently being done. Most patients wish to rid themselves of their disease and yet avoid an ileostomy. Surgeons should respect these wishes and honor them, recognizing that the pouch procedure may carry greater risks than some other operations and that the gain for some patients may be small.[57]

Most colitic patients who are candidates for elective operation are suitable for proctocolectomy with ileal pouch-anal canal anastomosis, but there are exceptions. Patients with Crohn's disease and those with an incompetent anal sphincter or cancer in the distal rectum are not candidates for the ileal pouch-anal canal anastomosis. The operation should not be performed in patients who have had their anal sphincter excised.

Advanced age is a relative contraindication to the operation, because of the greater risk of fecal incontinence in the elderly. The clinical results in fit patients over the age of 50, however, are as good as those in younger patients.[58] Nonetheless, anal sphincteric strength does decline after age 70.[59] Few patients beyond this age will be candidates for this operation. Among patients with preoperative fecal urgency and incontinence, anorectal manometry should be done to determine if their incontinence is caused by the disease-induced loss of the reservoir function of the rectum (microrectum) or by an impaired anal sphincter.[60] Adequate postoperative continence can be expected when a microrectum is replaced by a well-functioning ileal pouch, providing a competent anal sphincter is present. Patients with a damaged anal sphincter, such as those whose sphincter was injured at childbirth, may have their sphincter repaired operatively,[61] and then be candidates for the ileoanal procedure, but this is unusual.

The operation is technically more difficult in tall, muscular males with narrow pelves. In such patients, the ileal pouch will sometimes not reach the anal canal in spite of operative techniques designed to lengthen the mesentery.[62] In these patients, the anastomosis cannot be done.[63] Obesity is also a relative contraindication. A fatty ileal mesentery also may not allow the ileal pouch to reach the anal canal. Intraoperative reasons for abandoning the procedure should be discussed in the preoperative counseling.

Patients with indeterminant colitis,[64–66] colitis that has features of both chronic ulcerative colitis and Crohn's colitis, are considered by most surgeons to still be candidates for the ileoanal operation. These patients, however, must recognize that they are subject to a greater postoperative risk of anal strictures, fistulaes, and abscesses than are patients with conventional ulcerative colitis. The presence of coexisting cancer of the colon or proximal rectum does not rule out the ileoanal procedure, provided the cancer can be completely resected during the operation.[67–69] In patients with aggressive, locally invasive cancers or those with metastases to regional lymph nodes, it may be

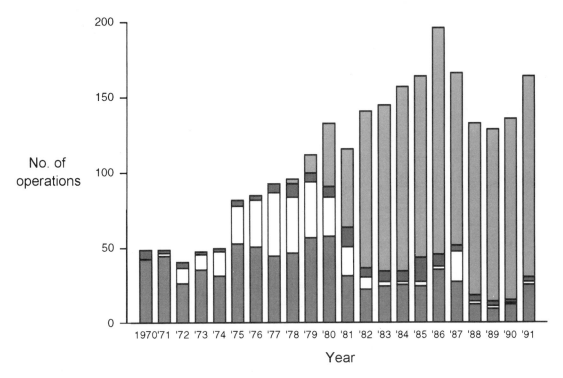

Figure 32-1. Use of operations for ulcerative colitis at Mayo Clinic Rochester over a 22-year period. Open, continent ileostomy; light stipple, Brodse ileostomy; medium stipple ileoanal operation; dark stipple, ileorectal anastomosis.

best to perform colectomy, closure of the rectum, and ileostomy, performing the ileal pouch-anal canal anastomosis later after adjuvant therapy for the cancer has been given.[68] In contrast, most patients with widespread metastatic cancer, such as those with metastatic deposits in the liver, should undergo colectomy and ileorectal anastomosis or Brooke ileostomy rather than the ileoanal procedure. Previous abdominal or anal operations[70] increase the difficulty of the ileoanal operation, but, again, do not rule it out. Previous resections of the small bowel, by resulting in an increased watery output from the gastrointestinal tract, pose a relative counterindication to surgery. Patients with sclerosing cholangitis and cirrhosis are at increased risk of complications after the ileoanal operation, but the operation can usually be performed successfully on them and has the advantage that it is not followed by peristomal varices, which may appear should a Brooke ileostomy be done.[71]

In contrast to patients with elective indications for surgery, most patients with emergent indications are not candidates for the ileal pouch-anal canal anastomosis.[72,73] These patients are too ill for the ileoanal procedure; the operation is too risky for them. They should have, instead, removal of the cecum and colon, closure of the divided proximal end of the rectum, and construction of an end ileostomy. Once these patients have recovered from their emergency operation and are restored to better health, the ileostomy can be taken down, the rectum and columnar anal mucosa can be removed, and the ileal pouch-anal canal anastomosis accomplished. An occasional exception to not doing an emergency ileoanal operation is the patient with severe hemorrhage from the rectum. That person may need to have the entire rectal and proximal anal mucosa removed at the

time of the emergent operation to control the bleeding. Under these circumstances, the ileoanal procedure must be done at that time.

Operative Management

The technique in most patients consists of excision of the cecum, colon, and proximal rectum, distal mucosal rectectomy, construction of an ileal pouch, and ileal pouch-anal anastomosis. The two-stage operative approach is used, protecting the pouch-anal anastomosis with a diverting loop ileostomy at the first operation and closing the loop ileostomy at a second operation about 2 months later.

The anesthetized patient is positioned on the operating table in the modified lithotomy Trendelenburg position, providing access to both abdomen and perineum. A vertical midline incision is made. The abdomen is explored and the presence of ulcerative colitis ascertained. The cecum and colon are mobilized, preserving the greater omentum. The rectum is freed down to the pelvic floor, keeping as close to the rectal wall as possible, thereby avoiding damage to the pelvic autonomic nerves.[74] The mobilized rectum is then divided at its midlevel using a stapling device. The cecum, colon, and proximal rectum are removed and sent for pathologic examination to confirm the diagnosis.

The ileal pouch is next constructed from the distal 30 to 35 cm of ileum. Several types of ileal reservoirs are currently being employed, including the J-shaped,[75] S-shaped,[76] W-shaped,[77] and the lateral-lateral pouch.[78] Thus far, we have preferred the modified J-shaped reservoir of Utsunomiya,[75] which is simpler to construct, uses less intestine, and can be done more rapidly than other more complex types of reservoirs, thus decreasing the chance of contamination and infection. Moreover, the J-pouch gives clinical results comparable to those obtained with the other reservoirs. Also, from a physiologic point of view, the J-pouch will ultimately accommodate nearly 400 ml of content, preserve the anorectal angle by fitting the concavity of the sacrum, generate low but coordinated propulsive contractions, and, most important, empty spontaneously.[79]

Pouch construction is begun by mobilizing the small intestinal mesentery from the retroperitoneum to allow the distal ileum to reach to the level of the dentate line. Dividing the visceral peritoneum along the right side of the superior mesenteric artery allows the mesentery to stretch and increases its length. If additional length is required, the ileocolic vessels or branches of the superior mesenteric vessels or both can be transected. When it is clear that the ileum will reach the dentate

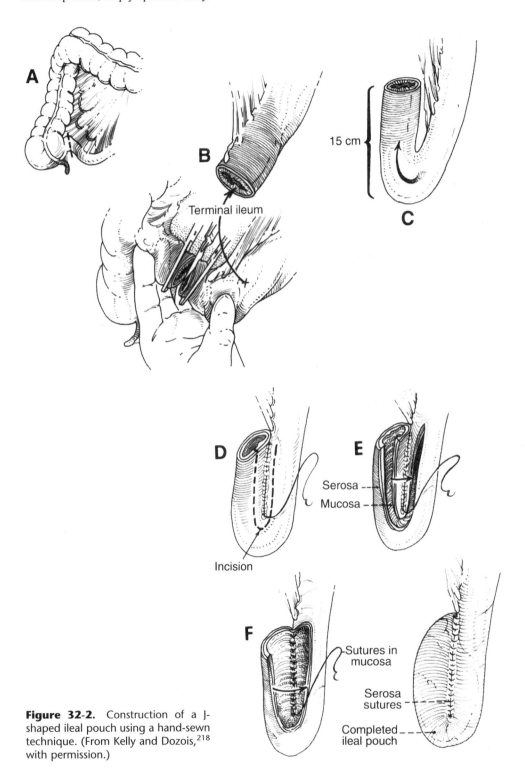

Figure 32-2. Construction of a J-shaped ileal pouch using a hand-sewn technique. (From Kelly and Dozois,[218] with permission.)

line, construction of the J-pouch is begun using the terminal 30 to 35 cm of the ileum. The ileum is folded into a shape of a ''J'' and its limbs approximated using continuous 2–0 chromic catgut or 2–0 polyglycolic acid sutures in the seromuscular layer of the two 15-cm limbs (Fig. 32-2). The antimesenteric border of the limbs is incised and the mucosal surface of the newly formed pouch exposed. A second row of sutures is used on the mucosal layer of the posterior wall. The anterior wall is then completed in the same two-layer fashion. Alternatively, the pouch may be constructed using several applications of a stapling device.

The surgeon then moves to the perineum to perform the distal mucosal rectectomy. The anus is effaced and dilated slightly by placing and opening two Gelpi self-retaining retractors at the anal verge (Fig. 32-3) or using a Lone Star retractor (Houston, Texas). A dilute (1:100,000) solution of epinephrine is injected into the submucosa at the dentate line to aid separation of the mucosa from the underlying muscularis and to reduce bleeding. Dissection of the diseased rectal mucosa using cautery or scissors in the submucosal plane begins at the dentate line and extends proximally and circumferentially a distance of 3 to 4 cm (Fig. 32-3). After the first 2 cm of mucosa are mobilized, the dissection can be completed either endoanally or extra-anally by everting the distal rectum onto the perineum. The dissection is extended to the row of staples, at which level the rectum is transected. We currently favor a short 3- to 4-cm muscular cuff, which reduces operating time, bleeding, and contamination (and thus the risk of pelvic sepsis), allows for better expansion of the neorectum, and decreases the chance of leaving behind potentially premalignant mucosal cells.

The previously constructed ileal J-pouch is then pulled endorectally through the muscular cuff and its most distal portion anastomosed to the anoderm of the dentate line, working intraluminally and using 3–0 adsorbable sutures (Fig. 32-4). A soft silastic drainage catheter is placed in the presacral space behind the pouch and brought to the surface through a left abdominal wall stab wound to drain the space in the postoperative period.

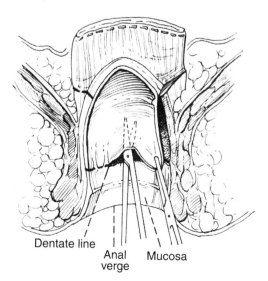

Figure 32-3. Technique of rectal mucosectomy. Gelpi retractors are used to efface anus and expose dentate line. (From Dozois,[219] with permission.)

Dentate line
Anal verge
Mucosa

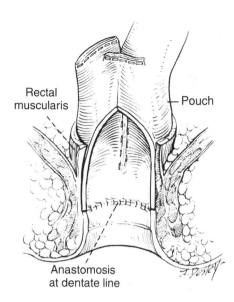

Figure 32-4. Anastomosis of stapled J-shaped reservoir to dentate line. (From Dozois,[219] with permission.)

Rectal muscularis
Pouch
Anastomosis at dentate line

A loop ileostomy is then established through an opening made in the right lower, anterior, abdominal wall (Fig. 32-5).

The patient is then allowed 2 or 3 months to recover from the first operation, after which the second operation is performed after ensuring that complete healing of the pouch and the anastomosis has occurred as demonstrated radiographically. The loop ileostomy is mobilized through a small transveres, biconvex incision that encompasses the stoma. The defect in the bowel is closed using sutures. The repair can be done with or without performing bowel resection including the old stoma.

A number of surgeons have performed ileal pouch anal anastomosis without a diverting ileostomy, as have we.[80–85] In one recent report, patients who were taking less than 20 mg of prednisone a day, who were on no other immunosuppressives, who had a tension-free anastomosis of the pouch to the anal canal, and who had an excellent blood supply to the pouch healed their anastomosis well without a diverting ileostomy.[86] Moreover, these patients without a diverting ileostomy had less small bowel obstruction and a shorter hospital stay than those with a diverting ileostomy. Thus, in selected patients, a diverting ileostomy is not always needed.

Early Clinical Results

The early clinical results are exemplified by our own series at Mayo. Over 1,700 patients have undergone the operation at our hospitals since January 1981. Approximately equal numbers of men and women were operated on. The mean age of the patients was 32 years; the ages ranged from 17 to 64 years.

A detailed analysis of patients showed a mean hospital stay of 10 days after the first stage of the operation and 7 days after the second.[87] Three patients died postoperatively (0.2%), one from a massive pulmonary embolism 3 weeks after dismissal from the hospital, one from complications of a perforated, steroid-induced gastric ulcer that led to fatal sepsis, and one from a subarachnoid hemorrhage. Thus, our experience, and that of others,[72,88–90] indicate that the operation can be done safely.

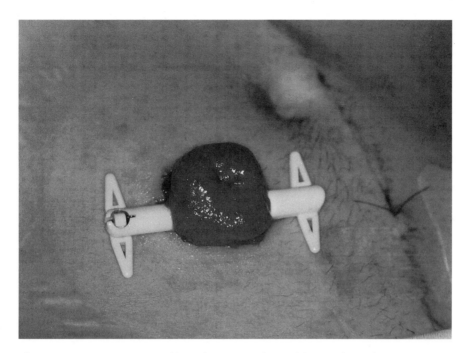

Figure 32-5. Construction of loop ileostomy. A loop of ileum is brought out through a defect in the right lower abdominal wall and the distal limb is opened flush with and sutured to skin with interrupted 3-0 chromic catgut. The proximal limb is everted and also sutured to skin. Final appearance with silastic loop ileostomy rod (Convatec, New Jersey.)

Early Complications

Postoperative morbidity, however, is not uncommon. The overall complication rate varies between 13% and 54%.[87,91] The most common early complications are bowel obstruction and sepsis.

Bowel Obstruction

Small bowel obstruction occurred in 13% of our patients after the first stage of the operation. About one-half of the patients required reoperation, while the other half resolved with nonoperative measures. This rate of small bowel obstruction is similar to that reported for other types of operation for ulcerative colitis.[92,93]

Pelvic and Wound Sepsis

Pelvic sepsis, manifesting itself as either a pelvic phlegmon or a frank abscess, occurred in 5% of our patients. The symptoms and signs included fever, leukocytosis, and pelvic or perineal pain with fullness and tenderness. Computed tomography (CT) helped to confirm the diagnosis. Patients with phlegmons were treated successfully by antibiotics alone, whereas those with frank abscesses underwent either CT-guided transperineal or transabdominal drainage or surgical drainage. Of those patients who required celiotomy for control of sepsis, 41% lost their pouch and only 29% eventually had satisfactory pouch-anal function. However, if no reoperation was required, 92% of patients with sepsis went on to satisfactory pouch-anal function. Persistent pelvic sepsis led to an indurated chronically inflamed

pelvis that resulted in a poor functional result.[94] Fortunately, the incidence of pelvic sepsis has diminished recently, as expertise in performing the operation has been gained.[87]

Water-soluble contrast "pouchogram" should be done prior to closure of the diverting ileostomy[95] to look for leaks at the ileoanal anastomosis or a space greater than 4 cm between the sacrum and the pouch on lateral view. Patients with a normal preclosure "pouchogram" show fewer long-term complications related to the pouch than those with sinuses and an expanded presacral space.[96]

In contrast to pelvic sepsis, wound infections were less common, occurring in only 3% of patients.

Pouch Bleeding

Clinically significant bleeding from the pouch can occur. It can be treated with local irrigation of diluted adrenaline solution or with a transanal suture.[89] Pouch infarction[89] has not been observed in our series.

Urinary Dysfunction

Urinary dysfunction is also uncommon. It occurred transiently in 5% of patients, with 2% requiring intermittent catheterization on dismissal from the hospital. None of the patients, however, have had to use a catheter over the long term. All patients were eventually able to void spontaneously.

Enteric Losses From Loop Ileostomy

Because of its more proximal location, the temporary loop ileostomy has a greater output than a terminal ileostomy.[97] Salt depletion and dehydration can occur. Patients will then present with weakness, tachycardia, and hypotension. To avoid this complication, patients should not leave the hospital until the ileostomy output is less than 1.5 L/day. To control ileostomy losses, loperamide hydrochloride, NaCl tablets, and a low-fat diet can be helpful. If losses persist, consideration should be given to early closure of the loop ileostomy.

Loop Ileostomy Complications

Complications from the loop ileostomy can occur. In one series among 296 patients with a diverting ileostomy, ileostomy-related complications occurred in 17 patients (5.7%).[98] These included obstruction requiring reoperation (2.4%), retraction requiring revision (1%), abscess behind the stoma (0.3%), and appliance problems (2.4%).

Complications After Ileostomy Closure

Small bowel obstruction was the most common complication after ileostomy closure, just as after the initial operation. In our series, it occurred in 9% of patients, with about one-half of them requiring reoperation. When these obstructions were added to those after the first stage of the operation, 22% of our patients had early small bowel obstruction after ileoanal anastomosis. Anastomotic leakage at the site of closure of the loop ileostomy occurred in 2% of our patients after surgery.[99] Bowel resection, including the stoma itself, and performance of an end-to-end or side-to-side anastomosis may reduce the likelihood of this complication.[100] In the St. Mark's series, 59 patients (22.4%) developed complications after closure of the ileostomy. Small bowel obstruction occurred in 30 patients; it was treated without surgery in 19 (7.2%) and by surgery in 11 (4.2%). Peritonitis occurred in 3 patients (1.1%) and enterocutaneous fistula in 2 (0.8%). Wound infection occurred in 14 patients (5.3%) and other miscellaneous problems in 14 (6.1%).

Late Clinical Results

Enteric Function

The ileoanal operation is effective in restoring acceptable anorectal function over the long term. Stool frequency, pattern of continence, ability to discriminate gas from stool, and the use

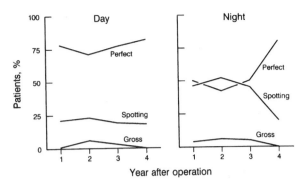

Figure 32-6. Daytime and nighttime continence after ileal pouch-anal operation against the years after operation. Perfect = no fecal leakage; spotting = fecal spotting of underclothes, 3 cm or less in diameter, two times or less per week; gross = gross fecal incontinence more than two times per week. Data points are connected for illustrative purposes only. (From Pemberton,[87] with permission.)

of medication after ileoanal anastomosis have been investigated extensively by us and by many others.[101] About six small, semi-solid stools are passed per day. Stool frequency is greater in older patients than in younger patients (older than 50 years, 8 ± 4 stools per day; 50 years or younger 6 ± 3 stools per day; $P = 0.05$), but women have the same number of stools each day as men. The frequency of stooling does not change appreciably over a period of 5 years (Table 32-3).

Fecal continence is usually acceptable after ileoanal anastomosis (Fig. 32-6). Frank incontinence is uncommon (less than 4% of patients), while fecal spotting is more frequent. It occurs in about 25% of patients during the day and in about 40% of the patients at night at 12 months after surgery. Women have more episodes of fecal spotting than men, both during the day (33% of women vs. 14% of men) and during the night (56% of women vs. 44% of men).[87] Older patients also have more spotting than younger patients. Of interest is the finding that the frequency of fecal spotting after ileoanal anastomosis seems to be affected by the preoperative stool frequency. The greater the number of stools before operation, the more likely are patients to have spotting after operation.[87] Fecal spotting can lead to perianal soreness and skin irritation. Fortunately, the inci-

Table 32-3. Functional Results of Ileal Pouch-Anal Anastomosis From 6 Months to 5 Years Postoperatively in 389 Patients

Parameter	Follow-Up					
	6 months	1 year	2 years	3 years	4 years	5 years
No. of stools (mean ± SD)						
Day	5 ± 2	5 ± 3	6 ± 3	6 ± 2	6 ± 3	6 ± 2
Night	1 ± 1	1 ± 1	2 ± 2	2 ± 1	1 ± 1	2 ± 1
Able to discriminate gas from stool (% of patients)	69	77	73	84	77	86
Lomotil (% of patients)	26	19	17	25	6	4
Metamucil (% of patients)	43	36	40	38	30	27

(From Pemberton,[215] with permission.)

dence of nocturnal spotting and the dependence on medications such as loperamide hydrochloride to control it decline considerably after the first 3 years after the operation (Fig. 32-6). Moreover, an assessment of fecal continence at 10 years after surgery shows that overall continence does not deteriorate with time.[102]

Sexual Function, Pregnancy, and Delivery

Postoperative sexual dysfunction occurred in 11% of men and 12% of women overall. Impotence and retrograde ejaculation or lack of ejaculation were noted in 1.5% and 4% of men, respectively. The remainder reported that ''lack of motivation'' or fatigue were the principal causes of sexual dysfunction. In women, dyspareunia was the primary complaint in 7% of patients after surgery whereas 3% feared leakage of stool during intercourse. Nonetheless, complaints of postoperative sexual dysfunction have been fewer in women with pelvic ileal pouches than in those with an ileostomy or after ileorectostomy.[103,104] It is important to remember that 49% of patients stated that they were sexually dysfunctional before the operation. Overall, sexual activity was increased after surgery compared to before surgery. The increase was attributed by most patients to an improvement in general health.[104]

Pelvic adhesions may form after the ileoanal operation and potentially could cause infertility. The incidence of this problem has not been addressed in detail, but we have found that 80% of ileoanal patients desirous of becoming pregnant were successful in doing so.

Pregnancy and delivery are well tolerated after ileal pouch-anal canal anastomosis. Among 40 women in our series who had at least one successful pregnancy post-ileoanal operation, no maternal deaths occurred, and only one child died soon after birth. The death was due to pulmonary hyaline membrane disease. Pouch function was minimally altered during and immediately after pregnancy. Moreover, the type of delivery, whether vaginal or by cesarean section, did not greatly alter postpartum pouch-anal function. We suggest that the use of vaginal delivery or cesarean section should be dictated primarily by obstetric reasons. If a vaginal delivery is contemplated, a mediolateral episiotomy is preferred to avoid damage to the ileal pouch and the anal sphincter. If the pelvic floor is scarred and not supple, however, vaginal delivery even with an episiotomy may pose a risk of perineal tear. In these patients, a cesarean section is preferred.

In spite of these encouraging early results, the long-term effects of pregnancy and delivery on pelvic ileal reservoir function are unknown. Future results could prompt greater use of cesarean section.

Quality of Life

The ileoanal anastomosis has replaced the once widely performed Brooke ileostomy at most medical centers because it provides an improved quality of life over that of the ileostomy. In a study at Mayo comparing performance among patients with Brooke ileostomy (n = 406) to that among ileoanal patients (n = 298), ileoanal patients outperformed the Brooke ileostomy patients in all key areas, including sexual activities, sports, social life, recreational activities, family relationships, work

around the house, and travel[105] (Tables 32-4 and 32-5). These results have been supported by those of others[99] and clearly indicate that patients not only regain their health, but also a satisfactory lifestyle. Generally speaking, the more the symptoms and restrictions before the operation, the greater the degree of satisfaction after the operation.[57]

Late Complications

Strictures

Strictures at the ileoanal anastomosis are usually caused by sepsis, undue tension at the anastomosis, and ischemia. The pouch may pull away from its anchoring to the dentate line leaving the underlying internal anal sphincter exposed to the anal content. Local sepsis and subsequent scarring may ensue, leading to the formation of a dense anal stricture of variable length. The anal stricture may also be associated with scarring of the pelvic floor itself.

Most strictures can be treated successfully with dilatation per anum.[106] Long, dense strictures, however, are difficult to treat by dilatation alone, although in some patients repeated dilatations may offer reasonable relief. Most often such strictures need operative therapy, either via a perineal approach, excising the stricture and advancing the pouch distally, or via an abdominal approach, elevating the pouch out of the pelvis, repairing it or constructing a new one, incising the scarred pelvic floor, and reanastomosing the apex of the pouch to the distal anal canal.[107] Occasionally, excision of the reservoir with establishment of a permanent ileostomy may be needed.

Fistulae and Abscesses

Pouch-perineal fistulae presenting early after surgery are usually associated with poor healing at the anastomosis. Fistulae presenting late after surgery, especially if originating from the dentate line, usually are the result of cryptoglandular infection. They can be treated by anal fistulotomy when they are superficial to the anal sphincter. Should the fistula lie deep to the sphincter, the use of a noncutting seton is recommended in order to avoid permanent damage to the anal sphincter. A seton is a suture or drain of nonabsorbable material that is passed from the cutaneous opening of the fistula, through the fistula into the lumen of the anal canal, and then back out to the skin surface where it is tied to itself. The seton can be gradually tightened to cut slowly through the sphincter over a period of days or it can simply be left in place where it acts as a drain. These ''noncutting'' setons are currently frequently used, because they preserve the anal sphincter and decrease the risk of postoperative incontinence.[108] In contrast, fistulae that do not arise from the dentate line should raise the suspicion of Crohn's disease. They often are best managed nonoperatively.

In males, chronic sinuses and abscesses can appear anteriorly at the anastomosis and lead to symptoms mimicking prostatitis. Incision and drainage of the infected sinuses should be done. In females, pouch-vaginal fistulae may appear in the early postoperative period, but they have been reported as late as 13 years after surgery.[109] They will often resolve in the early postoperative period by simply deferring closure of the diverting loop ileostomy for several months. If the fistula does not heal, local

Table 32-4. Patient Satisfaction After Creation of Brooke Ileostomy, Kock Pouch, or Ileal Pouch-Anal Anastomosis

Categories	% Responding		
	Brooke Ileostomy (n = 406)	Kock Pouch (n = 313)	Ileal Pouch-Anal Anastomosis (n = 298)
Diet restricted	28	46	22
Satisfied with diet	97	96	95
Returned to work or school	98	96	94
Desired change but satisfied	33	11	3
Definitely desired change	6	3	1
Overall satisfaction	93	98	96
Attitude since operation			
Improved	60	60	62
No change	35	36	34
Deteriorated	5	4	4

(From Pemberton,[215] with permission.)

Table 32-5. Patient Performance Responses After Creation of Brooke Ileostomy, Kock Pouch, or Ileal Pouch-Anal Anastomosis

Categories and Responses	% Responding		
	Brooke Ileostomy (n = 406)	Kock Pouch (n = 313)	Ileal Pouch-Anal Anastomosis (n = 298)
Social activity			
Restricted	21	22	14
No change	51	41	42
Improved	28	38	44
Sports			
Restricted	42	30	17
No change	42	44	43
Improved	15	26	40
Housework			
Restricted	14	8	9
No change	68	70	52
Improved	19	22	39
Recreation			
Restricted	30	24	17
No change	42	43	42
Improved	22	33	41
Family relationships			
Restricted	8	6	8
No change	68	64	51
Improved	24	30	41
Sexual activity			
Restricted	29	17	14
No change	56	52	42
Improved	15	30	45
Travel			
Restricted	26	32	20
No change	48	35	37
Improved	26	33	42

(From Köhler et al.,[216] with permission.)

repair, preferably under the continued cover of the ileostomy, may be required. The optimal management of pouch vaginal fistula is not yet established.[110]

Pelvic abscesses are now less common than in earlier years because of improved operative technique. Initial treatment usually entails prolonged fecal diversion with an ileostomy, but mobilization of the pouch, repair of any defects in the wall of the pouch or at the anastomosis, and reanastomosis of the pouch to the anal canal may be required. In some patients, especially those with a low-lying retropouch abscess, percutaneous CT-guided drainage may be feasible and successful.

Poor Anorectal Function

Another group of patients that may require reoperation are those with unsatisfactory postoperative anorectal function. These patients have sluggish or incomplete pouch emptying due to the presence of an efferent ileal limb between the pouch and the anal canal, incontinence related to a reservoir that is too small or too large, outlet obstruction due to mucosal prolapse,[111] or a mucosal septum.[104,112] Some of these patients will require shortening or, better, elimination of the efferent limb, revision or even excision of the existing reservoir with reconstruction of a new reservoir, or division of the mucosal septum. Although a transperineal approach may be used, we have found the transabdominal approach facilitates the reconstructive operation. None of the patients upon whom we have reoperated for these complications have died, and the reoperations have restored pouch function in two-thirds of patients. In them, stooling frequency and fecal continence were comparable to those found in patients who have not had postoperative complications.

Pouchitis

Pouchitis is the most frequent long-term complication of the ileoanal operation. Pouchitis is diagnosed when patients develop abdominal cramps; frequent watery stools, sometimes with blood, urgency, incontinence, malaise, and fever. In a recent evaluation at Mayo, the risk of pouchitis among 734 patients in whom ileoanal anastomosis was performed was 31%,[107] Pouchitis recurred in about one-half the patients with it, and required long-term treatment in about 10% of patients with it.[99]

The etiology of pouchitis remains unknown. It may be caused by anastomotic stenosis,[113] abnormal pouch motility leading to stasis,[114] bacterial overgrowth[115] or imbalance,[116–118] an immunologic reaction to bacterial products,[119] ischemia and reperfusion injury,[120] chemical injury,[121] or it may be a novel manifestation of idiopathic chronic ulcerative colitis.[122,123] Patients who are antineutrophil cytoplasmic antibodies (ANCA) positive are more likely to get pouchitis than those who are not.[124] "Backwash" ileitis, however, does not predispose to pouchitis.[125] It is of interest that pouchitis is rare in polyposis patients,[108,126,127] in whom the presence of fecal stagnation, overgrowth of bacteria, and ischemia of the pouch should not differ from those present after surgery in colitis patients. The rarity of pouchitis in polyposis patients suggests that whatever causes colitis may predispose to pouchitis. Leukotriene B_4 release from ileal pouch mucosa in ulcerative colitis is increased as compared with familial

adenomatous polyposis,[128] showing a difference in eicosanoid metabolism between the two diseases. This difference may explain a predisposition to pouchitis in ulcerative colitis patients. Interestingly, pouchitis may occur before closure of a loop ileostomy.[129]

Patients with sclerosing cholangitis are at greater risk of pouchitis than those without this extraintestinal manifestation.[71] In these patients, the pouchitis is chronic in nearly all. In fact, patients with extraintestinal manifestations of ulcerative colitis in general are also at greater risk of developing pouchitis. When extraintestinal manifestations were present preoperatively in our series, pouchitis occurred in 39 percent of patients, whereas it occurred in only 26% of our patients when no extraintestinal manifestations were present ($P < .001$).[130] In seven patients, extraintestinal manifestations recurred when pouchitis occurred and abated when the pouchitis was treated. Apparently, pouchitis can trigger an inflammatory response at distant sites similar to that which occurs in response to chronic ulcerative colitis itself. On the contrary, we have found that the incidence of pouchitis is not influenced by the type of pouch constructed, by the presence or absence of pelvic sepsis, or by the age and sex of the patient.

Pouchitis is a clinical syndrome, the activity of which has been graded using a "Pouchitis Activity Index."[131] The index employs clinical, histologic, and endoscopic criteria. The major problem with histologic criteria, however, is that biopsy specimens from the pouch are heterogeneous. A biopsy specimen from one part of the pouch may be read as normal "colon," from another as normal ileum, from another as chronic inflammation, and, finally, from another as acute inflammation. Although histologic criteria may be helpful in the diagnosis,[132,133] patients with classic signs and symptoms of pouchitis may not have such histologic changes and vice versa. Nonetheless, patients with severe acute and chronic pouchitis on endoscopy are at greater risk of developing chronic symptomatic pouchitis.[134]

Most patients with pouchitis can be treated successfully with metronidazole, ciprofloxacin, or other antibiotics with anti-anaerobic bacterial activity.[87,88,90,107,135,136] Recurrent episodes have also been treated successfully with the same medications. In chronic, unremitting pouchitis, metronidazole has been shown to be superior to placebo in reducing the median number of bowel motions per day.[137] However, the medicine does not alter the endoscopic or histologic grade of inflammation in the pouch, the serum c-reactive protein level, or symptomatic scores of the patients. Interestingly, metronidazole does not alter stool frequency in asymptomatic patients without pouchitis. Topical application of small doses of metronidazole does relieve symptoms of pouchitis[138] and is well tolerated as a long-term treatment. The effects of glutamine[139] and short chain fatty acids[140,141] are under investigation. Patients intractable to antibiotics require anti-inflammatory therapy similar to that directed at ulcerative colitis. Refractory pouchitis does not seem to reflect underlying Crohn's disease.[142]

Risk of Cancer

No reports have appeared describing the development of carcinoma in the mucosa of a pelvic pouch. However, changes are present in the mucosa. Quenu[143] demonstrated that the mucosa of a segment of ileum used in continuity with the colon was transformed into a colonic type of mucosa. An increased number of mucus-producing glands occurs in the pouch mucosa, along with a chronic inflammation of the mucosa and the lamina propria.[144] In fact, most authors have found inflammation to be present in almost every patient by 6 months after surgery.[145] The inflammation is associated with villous atrophy and crypt hyperplasia. The continual contact with a noxious medium and changes in bacterial flora are hypothesized as a cause of this phenomenon. The large number of proliferating cells and the frequent presence of inflammation may provide fertile ground for carcinogenesis.[146] Epithelial dysplasia associated with nuclear aneuploidy has been described in ileal pouches.[147] Experimentally, however, carcinoma failed to develop preferentially in ileal pouches of rats even when they were also given dimethylhydrazine.[148]

Clearly, an adaptive response of the ileal pouch mucosa to its new luminal environment is present. Long-term follow-up is needed to determine if the changes are reversible or progressive. The follow-up should include endoscopic and histopathologic surveillance of the pouch mucosa.[132,149] When subtotal or total villous atrophy accompanies severe pouchitis, mucosal biopsies should be performed, because low-grade dysplasia has been observed in patients in this setting.[150] The presence of high-grade dysplasia may be an indication for excision of the pouch. Certainly, patients with high-grade dysplasia and pathologic changes and pouchitis should receive surveillance.

Two cases of adenocarcinoma developing from remnants of dysplastic rectal epithelium left in the rectal cuff following excision of the rectal mucosa have been reported.[151,152] Studies[153,154] of specimens of excised ileoanal anastomoses have shown that small islands of residual rectal mucosa are present in the specimen. Although re-epithelialization with rectal mucosa does not occur, these two cases with cancer illustrate that incomplete mucosal excision can lead to the development of carcinoma at this site. "Cuff-cancer" must be considered in patients who develop late, nonspecific symptoms of pouch dysfunction.[152]

Rarer Complications

Unusual complications reported after the ileoanal operation include the superior mesenteric artery syndrome,[155] solitary ileal ulcer,[156] traumatic ileal perforation,[157] perforation of the ileal appendage of the pelvic ileal reservoir,[158] fibroid polyps of the ileal pouch,[159] puborectalis spasm, prolapse of the pouch with outlet obstruction,[111] and polypoid mucosal prolapse.[160]

Failure

In our experience, ileoanal anastomosis ultimately failed in 10% of patients by 10 years after surgery. Excision of the pouch and/or construction of a permanent abdominal ileostomy was then required. The most frequent causes of failure, occurring alone or in combination, were pelvic sepsis, gross fecal incontinence at night, multiple stools, and inadvertent operation for Crohn's colitis.[99] In Martin's experience[161] with a largely pediatric population, a postoperative diagnosis of Crohn's disease was eventually made in most of the patients whose postoperative course was unsatisfactory. This underscores the need for a more accurate means of distinguishing ulcerative colitis from Crohn's colitis before advising surgery. Only 2% of failures were due to pouchitis in our series, but others have found refractory pouchitis to be a major cause of pouch excision. Of all the failures, 76% occurred within 1 year of surgery. The incidence of failure likely will increase as the length of follow-up increases. In the St. Mark's experience, the cumulative probability of pouch failure was 12% at 5 years, with half of the failures occurring within 1 year. The most common reasons were perianal, pelvic sepsis, and probable Crohn's disease.[162]

Present Status

Quality of life after the ileoanal operation exceeds that of earlier operations like the Brooke ileostomy, the continent ileostomy, and ileorectostomy. Consequently, it has been the operation of choice in recent years (Fig. 32-1). Nonetheless, the frequent stools, the nocturnal fecal spotting, and the risk of pouchitis mandate that the quest for better operations be continued. A suggested alternative, the ileal pouch-distal rectal anastomosis, has recently emerged.

ILEAL POUCH-DISTAL RECTAL ANASTOMOSIS

The ileal pouch-distal rectal anastomosis is being used by some surgeons today as an alternative to the ileal pouch-anal canal anastomosis.[83,89,163,164] In this operation, the ileal pouch is sewn or stapled to the distal rectum or proximal anal canal instead of to the dentate line, as it is in the ileal pouch-anal canal anastomosis (Fig. 32-7). The rationale is that the operation is easier to perform than the ileal pouch-anal canal anastomosis; that the preservation of the anal transitional mucosa will maintain anal sensation, anal sphincter function, and postoperative continence, especially at night; and that the transitional mucosa left behind is not involved or is minimally involved with colitis and can safely be left. Some authors have also postulated that inflammation in the transitional mucosa, even if present, will subside after surgery.[165]

Figure 32-7. Diagram of ileal pouch-distal rectal anastomosis. (From Kelly,[220] with permission.)

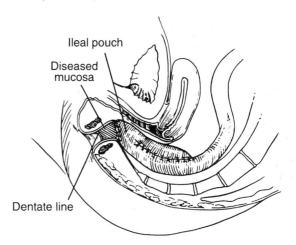

Ileal pouch

Diseased mucosa

Dentate line

Selection of Patients

Most patients who are suitable for the ileal pouch-anal canal anastomosis are suitable for the ileal pouch-distal rectal anastomosis. The distal rectal anastomosis should not be performed, however, in patients with cancer or severe dysplasia in the colonic mucosa[166] or in those with severe extraintestinal manifestations of colitis. It should be strongly considered in cases where mobilization of the pouch to perform a tension-free anastomosis is difficult and when extensive scarring from previous anal surgery is present.

Early Clinical Results

Early results suggest that the operation is faster than the ileal pouch-anal canal anastomosis and that anal sensation and anal sphincter strength are usually, although not always, better preserved.[83,136,164] Improved fecal continence, especially at night, has also been reported.[167–169] Those favorable results, however, have been based on data collected in retrospective studies. In contrast, three recent prospective randomized trials have shown little difference in function between the outcome of the ileal pouch-anal canal anastomosis and the outcome of the ileal pouch-distal rectal anastomosis.[170–172]

Late Clinical Results

A concern with the ileal pouch-distal rectal anastomosis is that the operation does leave diseased mucosa behind. Histologic re-examination of 50 colitis specimens removed by conventional proctocolectomy at the Mayo Clinic in past years showed that ulcerative colitis was present in the anal transitional mucosa within 1 cm of the dentate line in 90% of the specimens.[173] Moreover, Sugerman and associates[83] have also noted that 19 of 20 distal ''donuts'' of the rectum removed at the time of the stapled ileal pouch-distal rectal anastomosis harbored inflammatory mucosa. Finally, others have also shown that dysplasia/neoplasia can be present or develop in the transitional mucosa of patients with ulcerative colitis.[174–176] Resection of the dysplastic mucosa then needs to be performed.[166]

A technique of resection of the dysplasia mucosa via a perianal approach has been described.[177] This technique obviates the need for a complex abdominal perineal reoperation.

Long-term, prospective, randomized clinical trials comparing ileal pouch-distal rectal operation to ileal pouch-anal canal operations are needed. Until that time, our preference will continue to be the ileal pouch-anal canal operation.

Although the ileal pouch-anal canal anastomosis and the ileal pouch-distal rectal anastomosis are most often chosen when operating for ulcerative colitis today, other operations are still sometimes indicated. The most common of these alternatives are proctocolectomy with continent ileostomy, proctocolectomy with Brooke ileostomy, and cecal-colectomy with ileorectostomy.

PROCTOCOLECTOMY WITH CONTINENT ILEOSTOMY (KOCK POUCH)

The continent ileostomy (Kock pouch) also offers an alternative to an ileal pouch-anal canal anastomosis for certain patients with ulcerative colitis. In this operation, after excision of the

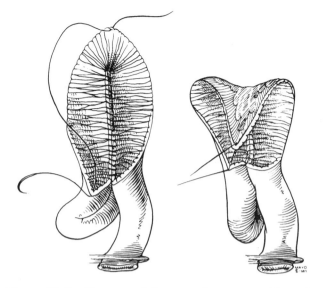

Figure 32-8. The reservoir ileostomy is constructed from the distal 45 cm of ileum. The reservoir is made from two 15-cm limbs of ileum opened on the antimesenteric side, sutured together and folded over to form the anterior and posterior walls. (From Dozois et al.,[179] with permission.)

large intestine, a pouch is made from 45 cm of the distal ileum (Fig. 32-8). A valve that prevents distal outflow from the pouch is created by intussuscepting the terminal ileum backward into the pouch and anchoring the intussusceptum in place with stainless steel staples (Fig. 32-9). The end of the terminal ileum is brought to the skin surface as a stoma. Once healed, the patient empties the pouch intermittently by passing a catheter through the stoma and valve into the pouch and draining the content of the pouch directly into the toilet through the tube. In between intubations, the pouch is continent for both gas and stool.

Selection of Patients

The continent ileostomy is indicated in patients who already have a conventional Brooke ileostomy, who have lost their anal

Figure 32-9. Stainless staples and interrupted sutures of 2-0 polyglycolic acid between the base of reservoir and efferent ileal limb anchor the intussuscepted segment within the pouch and so form the valve. (From Dozois et al.,[179] with permission.)

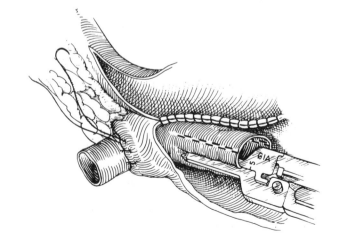

sphincter, and who wish to improve their quality of life. Patients needing a proctocolectomy who wish to preserve continence but are not candidates for an ileoanal anastomosis, usually due to poor sphincter function, are also candidates, as are patients who prefer a continent ileostomy to an ileoanal anastomosis. The latter are usually patients whose daily work takes them away from toilet facilities for prolonged periods of time. Lastly, patients who have a failed ileoanal anastomosis but who prefer a continence-preserving procedure to a Brooke ileostomy and the wearing of an external appliance are also candidates.

The operation should be discouraged in patients older than 65 years, in patients with Crohn's disease, and in obese patients. A continent ileostomy should also not be performed on critically ill patients, such as those plagued by toxic megacolon. The psychologically unfit patient is unsuitable because of the inability to intubate properly and to tolerate reoperation should it be required. We have not performed this operation on children, although we believe children who are responsible and who could be taught to intubate and care for the pouch would be suitable candidates.

Early Clinical Results

Continent ileal reservoirs were constructed in 460 patients at the two Mayo-affiliated hospitals during the years between November 1, 1971 and January 1, 1982. There were nearly equal numbers of men and women in this series, their ages ranging from 16 to 67 years and their mean age 32 years. Since 1982, fewer continent ileostomies have been performed, because the great majority of patients selected the ileal pouch-anal canal anastomosis.

Most of our patients had chronic ulcerative colitis (92%), as did those in Kock's series.[178] The remainder had familial adenomatous polyposis (7%) or Crohn's disease of the large intestine (less than 1%). About two-thirds of our patients had the pouch constructed in conjunction with proctocolectomy and chose a continent ileostomy to avoid a conventional ileostomy. Three-tenths were dissatisfied with their incontinent Brooke ileostomy and sought change to an ileal pouch.

No pouch-related deaths occurred intraoperatively or postoperatively, and patients generally convalesced satisfactorily. The mean postoperative stay in the hospital was about 10 days. Compared to patients with conventional ileostomy, the patients with ileal reservoirs experienced more abdominal cramps and distension in the postoperative period and returned to a general diet more slowly, a reflection of the intestinal obstruction produced by the pouch and its valve. The symptoms gradually disappeared as the pouch dilated in the postoperative period.

Late Clinical Results

Long-term follow-up (up to 6 years) has shown excellent results in the series. Most of the patient's pouches have remained continent, with almost no peristomal irritation of the skin or unpleasant odors from the stoma. At the time of follow-up, 75% of patients stated they had always been continent for gas and stool, and, ultimately, 95% of the entire group have never had to wear an appliance.[179] In general, the patients have gained weight, returned to good health, and taken up their former employment or occupation.

Social, sexual, and psychologic disability have been absent or minimal. When quality of life after continent ileostomy was compared to that after Brooke ileostomy, satisfaction was greater and the desire for change less in Kock pouch patients than in Brooke ileostomy patients.[180] Also, more patients with continent ileostomy improved in their daily activities than patients with Brooke ileostomy. The need for excision of the reservoir has decreased from about 10% in our early experience to about 3% more recently.[179,181,182] This was accomplished by avoiding use of the continent ileostomy in patients with Crohn's colitis and by favoring revision over excision when reoperation for complications took place.

Late Complications

Malfunction of the Nipple Valve

The major technical problem has been maintaining competence of the nipple valve and continence of the pouch. Incontinence and difficult intubation of the pouch due to malfunction of the nipple valve resulted in reoperation in about 20% of our patients.[179] The malfunction has appeared between 1 month and 10 or more years after construction of the pouch. However, all but four instances occurred within the first year (Fig. 32-10). The risk of malfunction, necessitating revision or excision of the pouch, decreases with time. Reoperation is required when malfunction of the valve occurs. Valve revision has been successful, in that ultimately 95% of patients never have to wear an appliance. Nonetheless, in some centers with a high reoperation rate (up to 50%) because of nipple valve insufficiency, this operation is no longer recommended.[57]

Several factors would appear to influence the risk of valve revision[179,181,182] (Table 32-6). Younger patients (less than 40 years) require fewer revisions than older patients (40 years or older); the older the patient, the greater is the probability of revision. Fewer revisions are also required in women, in those patients who had their continent reservoirs constructed at the

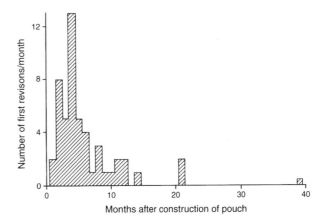

Figure 32-10. The number of patients requiring revision of the nipple valve is greatest 2 to 6 months after construction of the pouch. Only four patients in a series of 129 patients required revision after 1 year. (From Dozois and Kelly,[221] with permission.)

Table 32-6. Factors Influencing Valve Revision in Continent Ileostomies

Factors	Revision, %	P value[a]
Age		<.05
<40 years	20	
≥40 years	35	
Sex		<.05
Women	17	
Men	28	
Operation		<.05
Colectomy and pouch	16	
Conversion of ileostomy	30	
Obesity[b]		
Yes	75	
No	23	

[a] Estimates of cumulative probability were based on multivariate analysis.
[b] From Schrock,[217] with permission.

same time as the colectomy, and in nonobese patients than in men, in patients who had a previously constructed Brooke ileostomy converted to a continent ileostomy, and in obese patients. Still, about 20% of patients need revisional surgery of the valve at some point in their postoperative course. With radiologic examination, the correct diagnosis of valve malfunction can be made in 96% of patients.[183]

Pouchitis and Diarrhea

About 30% of patients develop episodes of watery diarrhea in the late postoperative period. *Staphylococcus aureus*, *Campylobacter*, or other pathogens have been cultured from the ileal content in some of the patients, and the diarrhea subsided when appropriate antibiotic therapy was given. Other patients have had diarrhea secondary to a mechanical obstruction of the small intestine. Lysis of adhesions resolved the diarrhea. Still other patients had nonspecific pouchitis with reddened, friable, edematous mucosa in the pouch without evidence of abnormal fecal flora or mechanical obstruction of the small intestine proximal to the nipple valve. In fact, the incidence of pouchitis in Kock pouches is nearly identical to that after ileal pouch-anal canal anastomosis. Management is also similar. These patients usually respond to metronidazole per os, suggesting that overgrowth of anaerobic bacteria in the pouch[184] or in the jejunoileum proximal to the pouch[185] might be responsible for the pouchitis.

Overall Evaluation

As yet, metabolic, nutritional, hepatic, renal, or oncologic complications have not appeared in our patients, but the long-term consequences of chronic ileal stasis are unknown.

PROCTOCOLECTOMY WITH BROOKE ILEOSTOMY

Proctocolectomy with Brooke ileostomy has been the "gold standard" to which other operations for ulcerative colitis have been compared for many years. Although its role is now more limited, it still has a place in certain categories of patients.

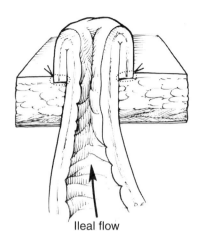

Figure 32-11. Diagram of a Brooke ileostomy. (From Kelly,[222] with permission.)

The advantages of the operation are that it is relatively easy to perform, that it is followed by few postoperative complications, and, most important, that it removes all of the diseased large intestine. The major disadvantage is that the patient is left with a permanent incontinent stoma requiring the wearing of an external appliance at all times (Fig. 32-11). Also, the perineal wound created by the rectal excision may be slow to heal and cause discomfort and inconvenience. The intersphincteric approach to rectal excision, however, causes little discomfort, heals well, and seldom results in urinary or sexual dysfunction.[186–188]

Selection for Surgery

This operation may be preferable in patients who are not candidates for a sphincter-saving ileoanal procedure or a continent ileostomy, either because of age (greater than 65 years), the presence of an incompetent or absent anal sphincter, or obesity. The operation may also be indicated when malignancy has supervened in the distal rectum or if other medical problems are of such severity that a more complex, longer operation is too risky. The operation may also be used in patients whose work makes it easier for them to handle an appliance as opposed to a pelvic ileal reservoir or a continent ileostomy. In a recent study,[36] 20% of patients requiring surgical treatment for ulcerative colitis chose a permanent ileostomy over an ileal pouch-anal canal anastomosis. These patients were generally older and eager to return to good health and work in the shortest possible time.

Clinical Results

Complications from this operation are infrequent but not negligible. Intestinal obstruction, infection, bleeding, and failure of the perineal wound to heal are the most common early complications. Late complications largely relate to the stoma and include stomal retraction, prolapse, hernia, bleeding, stenosis, varices, and obstruction. In a prospective study to evaluate the frequency and severity of complications after ileostomy for ulcerative colitis, a reoperation rate of 44% at 8 years was found.[189] The most frequent indications for reoperation were stenosis and retraction of the stoma. Revision of the stoma was performed under local anesthesia without the need for laparotomy in 83% of patients. Parastomal ulcers can occur late after ileostomy.[190] They can be the result of dermatologic conditions (e.g., contact dermatitis, bullous pemphigoid, lichen sclerosis, eczema, or psoriasis) or contact ulcers from faceplate pressure. Peristomal pyogangrenosum can also occur.[191,192] Other late complications are intestinal obstruction, urinary stone formation, gallstone formation,[193] adenocarcinoma of the ileostomy,[194] and urinary and sexual dysfunction. The latter arise from damage to innervation of these organs during the removal of the rectum and from psychological factors. Impotence may occur in 0 to 3% of male patients,[89,195] but is more likely in older patients. Women may be troubled by dyspareunia and episodic vaginal discharge as a result of pelvic floor disruption.[104] Involuntary sterility is also a common complaint.[196] These complications can be minimized by meticulous dissection in close proximity to the rectum and by excising the rectum and anus in the intersphincteric plane.[197]

Quality of life of patients undergoing proctocolectomy and Brooke ileostomy is usually greatly improved after operation, owing to the eradication of the disease and to the restoration of the general health of the patient. The presence of the stoma, however, may limit social, sexual, and sporting activities. Nonetheless, over 90% of patients adapt to these limitations, have a nearly normal lifestyle, and are satisfied with the results.

CECAL-COLECTOMY WITH ILEORECTAL ANASTOMOSIS

Cecal-colectomy with ileorectostomy are rarely used today in the treatment of ulcerative colitis. The reason is that this operation does not excise the diseased rectum, which continues to cause symptoms such as bleeding, pain, and diarrhea, which may require treatment. The diseased rectum also carries a risk of carcinoma. Nonetheless, some patients, especially those with minimal rectal involvement by the disease, may be candidates for this procedure. Points in favor of the operation are its lack of complexity and the fact that other surgical alternatives are usually still available if ileorectostomy is unsuccessful.

The obvious advantage is maintenance of the anal route of defecation and reasonable fecal continence. It is also a relatively safe operation associated with few immediate complications. Comparative studies, however, have shown no major benefit of cecal-colectomy with ileorectal anastomosis over the ileoanal anastomosis in terms of postoperative morbidity, mortality, stool frequency, and continence.[126,187,198]

Selection for Surgery

The operation may be indicated in patients who are not suitable candidates for an ileoanal operation, but wish to maintain the anal route of defecation. It may also serve a useful role in young males who are anxious to avoid any type of ileostomy and its disabilities or any risk of sexual or urinary dysfunction occasioned by proctectomy. Importantly, the disease should have been of short duration because of the increased risk of carcinoma. Relative sparing of the rectum and of its reservoir capacity and distensibility help to provide the best possible postopera-

tive functional results. This can be documented by anorectal manometry and rectal compliance studies. The operation may also be a good choice among patients in whom Crohn's disease cannot be excluded and among patients with ulcerative colitis complicated by advanced malignancy of the colon, especially if the rectum is relatively spared.

The operation should also be avoided in patients with severe rectal disease, especially those with a rigid, noncompliant "microrectum." It should be avoided when dysplastic changes are present in the rectum. The operation should not be performed in emergency situations due to the increased risk of anastomotic breakdown. Finally, uncontrollable rectal bleeding, an incompetent anal sphincter, and a stenotic rectum are also contraindications. In this situation, the cut end of the proximal rectum should be sutured or stapled closed and a Brooke ileostomy constructed. At Mayo, the procedure was performed in less than 10% of patients requiring operation for ulcerative colitis[199] even in an era when ileal pouch-anal canal anastomosis was not available. Patients should be informed preoperatively that the anastomosis may have to be taken down later either because of poor function or the development of rectal dysplasia or cancer.

Operative Management

Cecal-colectomy with ileorectal anastomosis may be performed as a one-stage procedure in those undergoing elective operation or as a two-stage procedure in those requiring emergency surgery. In the latter instance, the first stage should comprise colectomy with ileostomy and either mucous fistula or oversewing of the rectal stump. The second stage consists of restoring bowel continuity with ileorectal anastomosis.

The ileorectostomy is created at the level of the sacral promontory, leaving 12 to 15 cm of rectum as a reservoir (Fig. 32-12). A temporary loop ileostomy is not necessary on a routine basis. As much ileum as possible should be preserved. Aylett[200] suggested ligation of the superior hemorrhoidal artery to decrease subsequent rectal inflammation. This recommendation, however, has not been followed by most surgeons.[186]

Figure 32-12. Diagram of an ileorectostomy. (From Kelly,[220] with permission.)

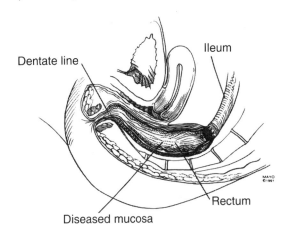

Clinical Results

Of 63 patients who had ileorectostomy at Mayo, two died post-operatively (3.2%) and one suffered an anastomotic leak (1.6%). In the long term, only 55% of the patients had satisfactory functional results.[199] Impotence and urinary dysfunction were rare, although retrograde ejaculation was found.[126] Many patients passed more than eight stools per day, had the continued need for steroids, and experienced incontinence and poor health. Eventually, 30% of the patients required proctectomy within a few years. Other centers have reported a similar spectrum of results,[198] with perioperative mortality ranging from 0 to 7%, an anastomotic leak rate ranging from 0 to 11%, and eventual proctectomy in 4% to 37% of patients. Satisfactory rectal function has also varied, being reported in 32% to 96% of patients. These varied results reflect the selection of patients for the procedure, the varying length of follow-up, and the degree of individual enthusiasm for the procedure.

The risk of cancer in the residual rectum has been reported at 6% after 20 years of disease and 15% after 30 years.[201] The risk, therefore, is considerable, recognizing that most patients operated upon are young and have many years yet to live. Regular follow-up by annual proctoscopy and biopsy is required. A registry for all patients with ileorectal anastomosis may help to ensure that patients comply with the follow-up.[186]

REFERENCES

1. Wilks S (1859) The morbid appearances in the intestines of Miss Banbes. Medical Times Gazette 2:264
2. Leijonmarck CE, Liljeqvist L, Poppen B, Hellers G (1992) Surgery after colectomy for ulcerative colitis. Dis Colon Rectum 35:495–502
3. Koga H, Iida M, Aoyagi K et al (1995) Generalized giant inflammatory polyposis in a patient with ulcerative colitis presenting with protein-losing enteropathy. Am J Gastroenterol 90:829–831
4. Berger M, Gribetz D, Korelitz BI (1975) Growth retardation in children with ulcerative colitis: the effects of medical and surgical therapy. Pediatrics 55:549
5. Stark ME, Tremaine WJ (1994) Medical care of the inflammatory bowel disease patient. pp. 411–449. In Quigley EMM, Sorrell MF (eds): The Gastrointestinal Surgical Patient. Williams & Wilkins, Baltimore
6. Ferzoco SJ, Becker JM (1994) Does aggressive medical therapy for acute ulcerative colitis result in a higher incidence of staged colectomy? Arch Surg 129:420–423
7. Sagar PM, Lewis W, Holdsworth PJ et al (1993) Quality of life after restorative proctocolectomy with a pelvic ileal reservoir compares favorably with that of patients with medically treated colitis. Dis Colon Rectum 36:584–592
8. Beart RW Jr, McIlrath DC, Kelly KA et al (1980) Surgical management of inflammatory bowel disease. Curr Probl Surg 12:534–584
9. Ekbom A, Helmick C, Zack M, Adami HO (1990) Ulcerative colitis and colorectal cancer. A population-based study. N Engl J Med 323:1228–1233
10. Katzka I, Brody RS, Morris E, Katz S (1983) Assessment of colorectal cancer risk in patients with ulcerative colitis: experience from a private practice. Gastroenterology 85:22–29
11. Kewenter J, Ahlman H, Hultén L (1978) Cancer risk in extensive colitis. Ann Surg 188:824–828
12. Mellemkjaer L, Olsen JH, Frisch M et al (1995) Cancer in patients with ulcerative colitis. Int J Cancer 60:330–333
13. Hendriksen C, Kreiner S, Binder V (1985) Long term prognosis in ulcerative colitis—based on results from a regional patient group from the country of Copenhagen. Gut 26:158–163
14. Prior P, Gyde SN, Macartney JC et al (1982) Cancer morbidity in ulcerative colitis. Gut 23:490–497
15. Devroede G (1980) Risk of cancer in inflammatory bowel disease. In Winawer SJ, Schottenfeld R, Sherlock R (eds): Colorectal Cancer: Prevention, Epidemiology, and Screening. Lippincott-Raven, Philadelphia
16. Langholz E, Munkholm P, Davidsen M, Binder V (1992) Colorectal cancer risk and mortality in patients with ulcerative colitis. Gastroenterology 103:1444–1451
17. Brentnall TA, Haggitt RC, Rabinovitch PS et al (1995) Risk and natural history of colonic neoplastic progression in patients with primary sclerosing cholangitis and ulcerative colitis, abstracted. Gastroenterology 108:A452
18. Gurbuz AK, Giardello FM, Bayless TM (1995) Colorectal neoplasia in patients with ulcerative colitis and primary schlerosing cholangitis. Dis Colon Rectum 37:1281–1285
19. Pincowsky D, Ekbom A (1995) Is there an increased risk of colorectal cancer among ulcerative colitis patients with primary sclerosing cholangitis. Gastroenterology 108:Abstract 29
20. Ransohoff DF, Riddell RH, Levin B (1985) Ulcerative colitis and colonic cancer. Problems in assessing the diagnostic usefulness of mucosal dysplasia. Dis Colon Rectum 28:383–388
21. Lennard-Jones JE, Morson BC, Ritchie JK, Williams CB (1983) Cancer surveillance in ulcerative colitis. Experience over 15 years. Lancet 2:149–152
22. Morson BC, Pang LS (1967) Rectal biopsy as an aid to cancer control in ulcerative colitis. Gut 8:423–434
23. Reiser JR, Waye JD, Janowitz HD, Harpaz N (1994) Adenocarcinoma in strictures of ulcerative colitis without antecedent dysplasia by colonoscopy. Am J Gastroenterol 89:119–122
24. Blackstone MO, Riddle RH, Rogers BH, Levin B (1981) Dysplasia-associated lesion or mass (DALM) detected by colonoscopy in long-standing ulcerative colitis: an indication for colectomy. Gastroenterology 80:366–374
25. Provenzale D, Kowdley KV, Arora S, Wong JB (1995) Prophylactic colectomy or surveillance for chronic ulcerative colitis? A decision analysis. Gastroenterology 109:1188–1196
26. Lennard-Jones JE (1995) Colitic cancer: supervision, surveillance, or surgery? Gastroenterology 109:1388–1391
27. Britton A, Peppercorn MA (1995) Emergencies in inflammatory bowel diseases. Crit Care Clin 11:513–529
28. Greenstein AJ, Janowitz HD, Sachar DB (1976) The extraintestinal complications of Crohn's disease and ulcerative colitis: a study of 700 patients. Medicine 55:401

29. Kochlar R, Mehta SK, Nagi B et al (1991) Extra intestinal manifestations of idiopathic ulcerative colitis. In J Gastroenterol 10:88–89

30. Levitt MD, Ritchie JR, Lennard-Jones JE, Phillips RKS (1991) Pyoderma gangrenosum in inflammatory bowel disease. Br J Surg 78:676–678

31. Gravallese EM, Kantrowitz FG (1988) Arthritic manifestations of inflammatory bowel disease. Am J Gastroenterol 83:703–709

32. Cangemi JR, Wiesner RH, Beaver SJ et al (1989) Effect of proctocolectomy for chronic ulcerative colitis on the natural history of primary sclerosing cholangitis. Gastroenterology 96:790–794

33. Fazio VW (1980) Toxic megacolon in ulcerative colitis and Crohn's colitis. Gastroenterol 9:389–407

34. Modigliani R (1993) Indications for surgery in ulcerative colitis: European view. Ann Chir 47:943–945

35. Hawley PR (1988) Emergency surgery for ulcerative colitis. World J Surg 12:169–173

36. Hurst RD, Finco C, Rubin M, Michelassi F (1995) Prospective analysis of perioperative morbidity in one hundred consecutive colectomies for ulcerative colitis. Surgery 118:748–755

37. Greenstein AJ, Sachar DB, Gibas A et al (1985) Outcome of toxic dilatation in ulcerative and Crohn's colitis. J Clin Gastroenterol 7:137–143

38. Heppell J, Farkouh E, Dube S et al (1986) Toxic megacolon. An analysis of 70 cases. Dis Colon Rectum 29:789–792

39. Grant CS, Dozois RR (1984) Toxic megacolon: ultimate fate of patients after successful medical management. Am J Surg 147:106–110

40. Korelitz BI, Dyck WP, Klion FM (1968) Fate of the rectum and distal colon after subtotal colectomy for ulcerative colitis. Gut 10:198–201

41. Robert JH, Sachar DB, Aufses AH Jr, Greenstein AJ (1990) Management of severe hemorrhage in ulcerative colitis. Am J Surg 159:550–555

42. Baker JP, Detsky AS, Wesson DE et al (1982) Nutritional assessment: a comparison of clinical judgement and objective measurements. N Engl J Med 306:969–972

43. Blackburn GL, Bistrian BR, Maini BS et al (1977) Nutritional and metabolic assessment of the hospitalized patient. J Parenter Enter Nutr 1:11–22

44. Detsky AS, Baker JP, O'Rourke K, Goel V (1987) Perioperative parenteral nutrition: a meta-analysis. Ann Intern Med 107:195–203

45. The Veterans Affairs Total Parenteral Nutrition Cooperative Study Group (1991) Perioperative total parenteral nutrition in surgical patients. N Engl J Med 325:525–532

46. Jacobs DO, Becker JM (1994) Surgical management of ulcerative colitis. pp. 567–581. In Targan SR, Shanahan F (eds): Inflammatory Bowel Disease from Bench to Bedside. Williams & Wilkins, Baltimore

47. American Society of Parenteral and Enteral Nutrition Board of Directors (1986) Guidelines for the use of total parenteral nutrition in the hospitalized patients. J Parenter Nutr 10:441–445

48. Rombeau JL, Barot LR, Williamson CE, Mullen JL (1982) Preoperative total parenteral nutrition and surgical outcome in patients with inflammatory bowel disease. Am J Surg 143:139–143

49. Becker JM, Alexander DP (1991) Colectomy, mucosal proctectomy, and ileal pouch-anal anastomosis. A prospective trial of optimal antibiotic management. Ann Surg 213:242–247

50. Christophi C, Hughes ER (1985) Hepatobiliary disorders in inflammatory bowel disease. Surg Gynecol Obstet 160:187–193

51. Martin FM, Rossi RL, Nugent FW et al (1990) Surgical aspects of sclerosing cholangitis. Results in 178 patients. Ann Surg 212:551–556

52. Pugh RN, Murray-Lyon IM, Dawson JL et al (1973) Transection of the oesophagus for bleeding oesophageal varices. Br J Surg 60:646–649

53. Wirthlin LS, Van Urk H, Malt RB, Malt RA (1974) Predictors of surgical mortality in patients with cirrhosis and nonvariceal gastroduodenal bleeding. Surg Gynecol Obstet 139:65–68

54. Talbot RW, Heppell J, Dozois RR, Beart RW Jr (1986) Vascular complications of inflammatory bowel disease. Mayo Clin Proc 61:140–145

55. Hull RD, Raskob GE, Hirsh J (1986) Prophylaxis of venous thromboembolism. An overview. Chest 89:374S–383S

56. Melville DM, Ritchie JK, Nicholls RJ, Hawley PR (1994) Surgery for ulcerative colitis in the era of the pouch: the St Mark's Hospital experience. Gut 35:1076–1080

57. Köhler L, Troidl H (1995) The ileoanal pouch: a risk-benefit analysis. Br J Surg 82:443–447

58. Lewis WG, Sagar PM, Holdsworth PJ et al (1993) Restorative proctocolectomy with end to end pouch-anal anastomosis in patients over the age of fifty. Gut 34:948–952

59. McHugh SM, Diamant NE (1987) Effect of age, gender, and parity on anal canal pressures. Contribution of impaired anal sphincter function to fecal incontinence. Dig Dis Sci 32:726–736

60. Cohen Z (1993) Contra-indications of ileal pouch-anal anastomosis. Ann Chir 47:946–947

61. Thompson JS, Quigley EMM (1995) Anal sphincteroplasty for incontinence after ileal pouch-anal anastomosis. Dis Colon Rectum 38:215–218

62. Thirlby RC (1995) Optimizing results and techniques of mesenteric lengthening in ileal pouch-anal anastomosis. Am J Surg 169:499–502

63. Chun HK, Smith LE, Orkin BA (1995) Intraoperative reasons for abandoning ileal pouch-anal anastomosis procedures. Dis Colon Rectum 38:273–275

64. Nicholls RJ, Wells AD (1992) Undeterminate colitis. Baillieres Clin Gastroenterol 6:105–112

65. Pezim ME, Pemberton JH, Beart RW et al (1989) Outcome of indeterminant colitis. Dis Colon Rectum 32:653–658

66. Wells AD, McMillan I, Price AB et al (1991) Natural history of indeterminate colitis. Br J Surg 78:179–181

67. Taylor BA, Wolff BG, Dozois RR et al (1988) Ileal pouch anal anastomosis for ulcerative colitis and familial polyposis complicated by adenocarcinoma. Dis Colon Rectum 31:358–362

68. Wiltz O, Hashmi HF, Schoetz DJ Jr et al (1991) Carcinoma and the ileal pouch-anal anastomosis. Dis Colon Rectum 34:805–809

69. Ziv Y, Fazio VW, Strong SA et al (1994) Ulcerative colitis and coexisting colorectal cancer: recurrence rate after restorative proctocolectomy. Ann Surg Oncol 1:512–515

70. Parker MC, Nicholls RJ (1992) Restorative proctocolectomy

in patients after previous intestinal or anal surgery. Dis Colon Rectum 35:681–684

71. Kartheuser AH, Dozois RR, Wiesner RH et al (1993) Complications and risk factors after ileal pouch-anal anastomosis for ulcerative colitis associated with primary sclerosing cholangitis. Ann Surg 217:314–320

72. Heyvaert G, Penninckx F, Filez L et al (1994) Restorative protocolectomy in elective and emergency cases of ulcerative colitis. Int J Colorectal Dis 9:73–76

73. Ziv Y, Fazio VW, Church JM et al (1995) Safety of urgent restorative proctocolectomy with ileal pouch-anal anastomosis for fulminant colitis. Dis Colon Rectum 38:345–349

74. Lee JF, Maurer VM, Block GE (1973) Anatomic relations of pelvic autonomic nerves to pelvic operations. Arch Surg 107:324–328

75. Utsunomiya J, Iwama T, Imajo M et al (1980) Total colectomy, mucosal proctectomy, and ileoanal anastomosis. Dis Colon Rectum 23:459–466

76. Parks AG, Nicholls RJ, Belliveau P (1980) Proctocolectomy with ileal reservoir and anal anastomosis. Br J Surg 67:533–538

77. Nicholls RJ, Pezim ME (1985) Restorative proctocolectomy with ileal reservoir for ulcerative colitis and familial adenomatous polyposis: a comparison of three reservoir designs. Br J Surg 72:470–474

78. Fonkalsrud EW (1980) Total colectomy and endorectal ileal pull-through with internal ileal reservoir for ulcerative colitis. Surg Gynecol Obstet 150:1–8

79. Kelly KA, Pemberton JH (1987). Mechanisms of fecal continence: alterations with ileal pouch-anal anastomosis. pp. 399–418. In Szurszewski JH (ed): Cellular Physiology and Clinical Studies of Gastrointestinal Smooth Muscle. Elsevier, Amsterdam

80. Cohen Z, McLeod RS, Stephen W et al (1992) Continuing evolution of the pelvic pouch procedure. Ann Surg 216:506–511

81. Galandiuk S, Wolff BG, Dozois RR, Beart RWJ (1991) Ileal pouch-anal anastomosis without ileostomy. Dis Colon Rectum 34:870–873

82. Sagar PM, Lewis W, Holdsworth PJ, Johnston D (1992) One stage restorative proctocolectomy without temporary defunctioning ileostomy. Dis Colon Rectum 35:582–588

83. Sugerman HJ, Newsome HH, Decosta G, Zfass AM (1991) Stapled ileoanal anastomosis for ulcerative colitis and familial polyposis without a temporary diverting ileostomy. Ann Surg 213:606–617

84. Tjandra JJ, Fazio VW, Milsom JW et al (1993) Omission of temporary diversion in restorative proctocolectomy—is it safe? Dis Colon Rectum 36:1007–1014

85. Williams N, Scott NA, Watson JS, Irving MH (1993) Surgical management of perianal and metatastic cutaneous Crohn's disease. Br Surg 80:1596

86. Gorfine SR, Galernt IM, Bauer JJ et al (1995) Restorative proctocolectomy without diverting ileostomy. Dis Colon Rectum 38:188–194

87. Pemberton JH, Kelly KA, Beart RW Jr et al (1987) Ileal pouch-anal anastomosis for chronic ulcerative colitis. Long-term results. Ann Surg 206:504–513

88. Cohen Z, McLeod RS, Stern H et al (1985) The pelvic pouch and ileoanal anastomosis procedure. Surgical technique and initial results. Am J Surg 150: 601–607

89. Fazio VW, Ziv Y, Church J-M et al (1995) Ileal pouch-anal in 1005 patients. Ann Surg 222:120–127

90. Schoetz DJ Jr, Coller JA, Veidenheimer MC (1986) Ileoanal reservoir for ulcerative colitis and familial polyposis. Arch Surg 121:404–409

91. Harms BA, Hamilton JW, Yamamoto DT, Starling JR (1987) Quadruple-loop (W) ileal pouch reconstruction after proctocolectomy: analysis and functional results. Surgery 102:561–567

92. Francois Y, Dozois RR, Kelly KA et al (1989) Small intestinal obstruction complicating ileal pouch-anal anastomosis. Ann Surg 209:46–50

93. Roy PH, Sauer WG, Beahrs OH, Farrow GM (1970) Experience with ileostomies: evaluation of long-term rehabilitation in 497 patients. Am J Surg 119:77–86

94. Scott NA, Dozois RR, Beart RW Jr et al (1988) Postoperative intra-abdominal and pelvic sepsis complicating ileal pouch-anal anastomosis. Int J Colorectal Dis 3:149–152

95. Kelly IM, Bartram CI, Nicholls RJ (1994) Water-soluble contrast pouchography—technique and findings in 85 patients. Clin Radiol 49:612–616

96. Grossman E, Svendsen LB, Wettergren A et al (1994) Radiological findings in patients with a J-shaped ileal reservoir. Ugeskr Laeger 156:2893–2897

97. Feinberg SM, McLeod RS, Cohen Z (1987) Complications of Surg 153:102–107

98. Senapati A, Nicholls RJ, Ritchie JK et al (1993) Temporary loop ileostomy for restorative protocolectomy. Br J Surg 80:628–630

99. Kelly KA, Pemberton JH, Wolff BG, Dozois RR (1992) Ileal pouch-anal anastomosis. Curr Probl Surg 29:57–131

100. Kestenberg A, Becker JM (1985) A new technique of ileostomy closure after endorectal ileoanal anastomosis. Surgery 98:109–111

101. Wexner SD, Wong WD, Rothenberger DA, Goldberg SM (1990) The ileoanal reservoir. Am J Surg 159:178–183

102. McIntyre PB, Pemberton JH, Wolff BG et al (1994) Comparing functional results one year and ten years after ileal pouch-anal anastomosis for chronic ulcerative colitis. Dis Colon Rectum 37:303–307

103. Grüner OPN, Naas R, Fretheim B, Gjone E (1977) Martial status and sexual adjustment after colectomy: results in 178 patients operated on for ulcerative colitis. Scand J Gastroenterol 12:193–197

104. Metcalf AM, Dozois RR, Kelly KA (1986) Sexual function in women after proctocolectomy. Ann Surg 204:624–627

105. Pemberton JH, Phillips SF, Ready RR et al (1989) Quality of life after Brooke ileostomy and ileal pouch-anal anastomosis. Comparison of performance status. Ann Surg 209:620–626

106. Lewis WG, Kuzv A, Sagar PM et al (1994) Stricture at the pouch-anal anastomosis after restorative proctocolectomy. Dis Colon Rectum 37:120–125

107. Galandiuk S, Scott NA, Dozois RR et al (1990) Ileal pouch-anal anastomosis. Reoperation for pouch-related complications. Ann Surg 212:446–452

108. White RA, Eisenstat TE, Rubin RJ, Salvati EP (1990) Seton management of complex anorectal fistulas in patients with Crohn's disease. Dis Colon Rectum 33:587–589

109. Carraro PS, Nicholls RJ, Groom J (1992) Pouch-vaginal fistula occuring 13 years after restorative protocolectomy. Br J Surg 79:716–717

110. Groom JS, Nicholls RJ, Hawley PR, Philips RK (1993) Pouch-vaginal fistula. Br J Surg 80:936–940

111. Pena JP, Gemlo BT, Rothenberger DA (1992) Ileal pouch-anal anastomosis: state of the art. Baillieres Clin Gastroenterol 6:113–127

112. Sakanoue Y, Shoji Y, Kusunoki M, Utsunomiya J (1993) Transanal division of an apical pouch bridge after restorative proctocolectomy with a J shaped reservoir. Br J Surg 80:248

113. Fleshman JW, Cohen Z, McLeod RS et al (1988) The ileal reservoir and ileoanal anastomosis procedure. Factors affecting technical and functional outcome. Dis Colon Rectum 31:10–16

114. Campbell AP, Merrett MN, Kettlewell M et al (1994) Expression of colonic antigens by goblet and columnar epithelial cells in ileal pouch mucosa: their association with inflammatory change and faecal stasis. J Clin Pathol 47:834–838

115. O'Connell PR, Rankin DR, Weiland LH, Kelly KA (1986) Enteric bacteriology, absorption, morphology and emptying after ileal pouch-anal anastomosis. Br J Surg 73:909–914

116. Luukkonen P, Valtonen V, Sivonen A et al (1988) Fecal bacteriology and reservoir ileitis in patients operated on for ulcerative colitis. Dis Colon Rectum 31:864–867

117. Nasmyth DG, Godwin PG, Dixon MF et al (1989) Ileal ecology after pouch-anal anastomosis or ileostomy. A study of mucosal morphology, fecal bacteriology, fecal volatile fatty acids, and their interrelationship. Gastroenterology 96:817–824

118. Ruseler-van Embden JG, Schouten WR, van Lieshout LM (1994) Pouchitis: result of microbial imbalance? Gut 35:658–664

119. de Silva HJ, Gatter KC, Millard PR et al (1990) Crypt cell proliferation and HLA-DR expression in pelvic ileal pouches. J Clin Pathol 43:824–828

120. Levin KE, Pemberton JH, Phillips SF et al (1992) Role of oxygen free radicals in the etiology of pouchitis. Dis Colon Rectum 35:452–456

121. Breuer NF, Rampton DS, Tammar A et al (1983) Effect of colonic perfusion with sulfated and non-sulfated bile acids on mucosal structure and function in the rat. Gastroenterology 84:869–977

122. Knobler H, Ligumsky M, Okon E et al (1986) Pouch ileitis—recurrence of the inflammatory bowel disease in the ileal reservoir. Am J Gastroenterol 81:199–201

123. Sandborn WJ (1994) Pouchitis following ileal pouch-anal anastomosis: definition, pathogenesis, and treatment. Gastroenterology 107:1856–1860

124. Sandborn WJ, Landers CJ, Tremaine WJ et al (1995) Antineutrophil cytoplasmic antibody correlates with chronic pouchitis after ileal pouch–anal anastomosis. Am J Gastroenterol 90:740–747

125. Gostafsson S, Weiland LH, Kelly KA (1987) Relationship of backwash ileitis to iliac pouchitis after ileal pouch–anal anastomosis. Dis Colon Rectum 30:25–28

126. Ambroze WL Jr, Dozois RR, Pemberton JH et al (1992) Familial adenomatous polyposis: results following ileal pouch-anal anastomosis and ileorectostomy. Dis Colon Rectum 35:12–15

127. Kmiot WA, Williams MR, Keighley MR (1990) Pouchitis following colectomy and ileal reservoir construction for familial adenomatous polyposis. Br J Surg 77:1283

128. Gertner DJ, Rampton DS, Madden MV et al (1994) Increased leukotriene B4 release from ileal pouch mucosa in ulcerative colitis compared with familial adenomatous polyposis. Gut 35:1429–1432

129. Trabucchi E, Doldi SB, Foschi D et al (1988) Pouch ileitis in excluded reservoir: an unusual complication of restorative proctocolectomy for ulcerative colitis. Int Surg 73:187–189

130. Lohmuller JL, Pemberton JH, Dozois RR et al (1990) Pouchitis and extraintestinal manifestations of inflammatory bowel disease after ileal pouch-anal anastomosis. Ann Surg 211:622–627

131. Sandborn WJ, Tremaine WJ, Batts KP et al (1994) Pouchitis after ileal pouch-anal anastomosis: a pouchitis disease activity index. Mayo Clin Proc 69:409–415

132. Shepherd NA, Jass JR, Duval I et al (1987) Restorative proctocolectomy with ileal reservoir: pathological and histochemical study of mucosal biopsy specimens. J Clin Pathol 40:601–607

133. Tytgat GNJ, van Deventer SJH (1988) Pouchitis. Int J Colorectal Dis 3:226–228

134. Setti-Carraro P, Talbot IC, Nicholls RJ (1994) Long-term appraisal of the histological appearances of the ileal reservoir mucosa after restorative proctocolectomy for ulcerative colitis. Gut 35:1721–1727

135. Becker JM, Raymond JL (1986) Ileal pouch-anal anastomosis. A single surgeon's experience with 100 consecutive cases. Ann Surg 204:375–383

136. Nasmyth DG, Williams NS, Johnston D (1986) Comparison of the function of triplicated and duplicated pelvic ileal reservoirs after mucosal proctectomy and ileo-anal anastomosis for ulcerative colitis and adenomatous polyposis. Br J Surg 73:361–366

137. Madden MV, McIntyre AS, Nicholls RJ (1994) Double-blind crossover trial of metronidazole versus placebo in chronic unremitting pouchitis. Dig Dis Sci 39:1193–1196

138. Nygaard K, Bergan T, Bjornek-Lett A et al (1994) Topical metronidazole treatment of pouchitis. Scand J Gastroenterol 29:462–467

139. Wischmeyer P, Grotz RL, Pemberton JH, Phillips SF (1992) Treatment of pouchitis after ileo-anal anastomosis with gurtamine and butyric acid, abstracted. Gastroenterology 102:A947

140. de Silva HJ, Ireland A, Kettlewell M et al (1989) Short-chain fatty acid irrigation in severe pouchitis. N Engl J Med 321:1416–1417

141. Wischmeyer PE, Tremaine WJ, Haddad AC et al (1991) Fecal short chain fatty acids in patients with pouchitis after ileal pouch-anal anastomosis, abstracted. Gastroenterology 100:A848

142. Subramani K, Harpaz N, Bilotta J et al (1993) Refractory pouchitis: does it reflect underlying Crohn's disease. Gut 34:1539–1542

143. Quenu J (1933) L'ileocoloplastie. J Chir 42:15

144. Heppell J, Kelly KA, Phillips SF et al (1982) Physiologic aspects of continence after total colectomy, mucosal proctectomy and endorectal ileo anal anastomosis. Ann Surg 195:435–443

145. Moskowitz RL, Shepherd NA, Nicholls RJ (1986) An assessment of inflammation in the reservoir after restorative proctocolectomy with ileo-anal ileal reservoir. Int J Colorectal Dis 1:167–174

146. Apel R, Cohen Z, Andrews W et al (1994) Prospective evalua-

tion of early morphological changes in pelvic ileal pouches. Gastroenterology 107:435–443

147. Lofberg R, Liljeqvist L, Lindquist K et al (1991) Dysplasia and DNA aneuploidy in a pelvic pouch. Report of a case. Dis Colon Rectum 34:280–284

148. Heppell J, De Zubiria M, Brais MF et al (1990) An assessment of the risk of neoplasia in long-term ileal reservoirs using the DMH rodent model. Dis Colon Rectum 33:26–31

149. Mignon M, Settler C, Phillips SF (1995) Pouchitis—a poorly understood entity. Dis Colon Rectum 38:100–103

150. Veress B, Reinholt FP, Lindquist K et al (1995) Long-term histomorphological surveillance of the pelvic ileal pouch: dysplasia develops in a subgroup of patients. Gastroenterology 109:1090–1097

151. Puthu D, Rajan N, Rao R et al (1992) Carcinoma of the rectal pouch following restorative proctocolectomy. Report of a case. Dis Colon Rectum 35:257–260

152. Stern H, Walfisch S, Mullen B et al (1990) Cancer in an ileoanal reservoir: a new late complication? Gut 31:473–475

153. Heppell J, Weiland LH, Perrault J et al (1983) Fate of rectal mucosa after rectal mucostectomy and ileo-anal anastomosis. Dis Colon Rectum 26:768–771

154. O'Connell PR, Pemberton JH, Weiland LH et al (1987) Does rectal mucosa regenerate after ileoanal anastomosis? Dis Colon Rectum 30:1–5

155. Ballantyne GH, Graham SM, Hammers L, Modlin IM (1987) Superior mesenteric artery syndrome following ileal J-pouch anal anastomosis. An iatrogenic cause of early postoperative obstruction. Dis Colon Rectum 30:472–474

156. Franceschi D, Chen PF, Yuh JN (1986) Solitary J-pouch ulcer causing pouchitis-like syndrome. Dis Colon Rectum 29:515–517

157. Hsu TC (1989) Traumatic perforation of ileal pouch. Report of a case. Dis Colon Rectum 32:64–66

158. Pezim ME, Taylor BA, Davis CJ, Beart RW Jr (1987) Perforation of terminal ileal appendage of J-pelvic ileal reservoir. Dis Colon Rectum 30:161–163

159. Tysk C, Schnurer LB, Wickbom G (1994) Obstructing inflammatory fibroid polyp in pelvic ileal reservoir after restorative proctocolectomy in ulcerative colitis. Report of a case. Dis Colon Rectum 37:1034–1037

160. Blazeby JM, Durdey P, Warren BF (1994) Polypoid mucosal prolapse in pelvic ileal reservoir. Gut 35:1668–1669

161. Martin LW (1993) Current surgical management of patients with ulcerative colitis. J Pediatr Gastroenterol Nutr 17:121–131

162. Setti-Carraro P, Ritchie JK, Wilkinson KH et al (1994) The first 10 years' experience of restorative proctocolectomy for ulcerative colitis. Gut 35:1070–1075

163. Heald RJ, Allen DR (1986) Stapled ileo-anal anastomosis: a technique to avoid mucosal proctectomy in the ileal pouch operation. Br J Surg 73:571–572

164. Tuckson W, Lavery I, Fazio V et al (1991) Manometric and functional comparison of ileal pouch anal anastomosis with and without anal manipulation. Am J Surg 161:90–95

165. O'Connell PR, Williams NS (1991) Mucosectomy in restorative proctocolectomy. Br J Surg 78:129–130

166. Ziv Y, Fazio VW, Sirimarco MT et al (1994) Incidence, risk factors, and treatment of dysplasia in the anal transitional zone after ileal pouch-anal anastomosis. Dis Colon Rectum 37:1281–1285

167. Johnston D, Holdsworth PJ, Nasmyth DG et al (1987) Preservation of the entire anal canal in conservative protocolectomy for ulcerative colitis: a pilot study comparing end-to-end ileoanal anastomosis without mucosal resection with mucosal proctectomy and endo-anal anastomosis. Br J Surg 74:940–944

168. Lavery IC, Tuckson WB, Fazio VW et al (1990) Pouch surgery—the importance of the transitional zone. Can J Gastroenterol 4:428–431

169. Martin LW, Torres AM, Fischer JE, Alexander F (1985) The critical level for preservation of continence in the ileoanal anastomosis. J Pediatr Surg 20:664–667

170. Choen S, Tsunoda A, Nicholls RJ (1991) Prospective randomized trial comparing anal function after hand sewn ileoanal anastomosis with mucosectomy versus stapled ileoanal anastomosis without mucosectomy in restorative proctocolectomy. Br J Surg 78:430–434

171. Kmiot WA, Keighley MRB (1989) Totally stapled abdominal restorative proctocolectomy. Br J Surg 76:961–964

172. Luukkonen P, Jarvinen H (1993) Stapled vs hand-sutured ileoanal anastomosis in restorative proctocolectomy. A prospective, randomized study. Arch Surg 128:437–440

173. Ambroze WL, Pemberton JH, Dozois RR, Carpenter HA (1991) Does retaining the anal transition zone (ATZ) fail to extirpate chronic ulcerative colitis (CUC) after ileal pouch-anal anastomosis (IPAA)? Dis Colon Rectum 35:P20

174. Emblem R, Bergan A, Larsen S (1988) Straight ileoanal anastomosis with preserved anal mucosa for ulcerative colitis and familial polyposis. Scand J Gastroenterol 23:913–919

175. King DW, Lubowski DZ, Cook TA (1989) Anal canal mucosa in restorative proctocolectomy for ulcerative colitis. Br J Surg 76:970–972

176. Tsunoda A, Talbot IC, Nicholls RJ (1990) Incidence of dysplasia in the anorectal mucosa in patients have restorative proctocolectomy. Br J Surg 77:506–508

177. Fazio VW, Tjandra JJ (1994) Transanal mucosectomy. Ileal pouch advancement for anorectal dysplasia or inflammation after restorative proctocolectomy. Dis Colon Rectum 37:1008–1011

178. Kock NG (1976) A new look at ileostomy. Surg Ann 8:241–256

179. Dozois RR, Kelly KA, Beart RW Jr, Beahrs OH (1985) pp. 180–195. Continent ileostomy: the Mayo Clinic experience. In Dozois RR (ed): Alternatives to Conventional Ileostomy. Year Book Medical Publishers, Chicago

180. Pemberton JH, Phillips SF, Dozois RR, Wendorf LJ (1985) pp. 40–50. Conventional ileostomy: current clinical results. In Dozois RR (ed): Alternatives to Conventional Ileostomy. Year Book Medical Publishers, Chicago

181. Dozois RR, Kelly KA, Beart RW Jr, Beahrs OH (1980) Improved results with continent ileostomy. Ann Surg 192:319–324

182. Dozois RR, Kelly KA, Ilstrup D et al (1981) Factors affecting revision rate after continent ileostomy. Arch Surg 116:610–613

183. Lycke KG, Gothlin JH, Jensen JR et al (1994) Radiology of the continent ileostomy reservoir. Abdom Imaging 19:124–131

184. Schjønsby H, Halvorsen JF, Hofstad T, Hovdenak N (1977) Stagnant loop syndrome in patients with continent ileostomy (intra-abdominal ileal reservoir). Gut 18:795–799

185. Kelly DG, Phillips SF, Kelly KA et al (1983) Dysfunction of the continent ileostomy: clinical features and bacteriology. Gut 24:193–201

186. Jagelman DG (1986) Ileorectal anastomosis for mucosal ulcerative colitis. pp. 211–225. In Jagelman DG (ed): Mucosal Ulcerative Colitis. Futura Publishing Company, Mount Kisco, New York

187. Oakley JR, Jagelman DG, Fazio VW et al (1985) Complications and quality of life after ileorectal anastomosis for ulcerative colitis. Am J Surg 149:23

188. Painter TA, Oakley J (1986) Intersphincteric proctocolectomy and ileostomy. pp. 189–210. In Jagelman DG (ed): Mucosal Ulcerative Colitis. Futura Publishing Company, Mount Kisco, New York

189. Scaglia M, Delaini GG, Hulten L (1992) The long-term complications from ileostomy in patients with Crohn's disease and ulcerative colitis. Chir Ital 44:211–212

190. Ng CS, Wolfsen HC, Kozarek RA et al (1992) Chronic parastomal ulcers: spectrum of dermatoses. J ET Nursing 19:85–90

191. Cairns BA, Herbst CA, Sartor BR et al (1994) Peristomal pyodermal gangrenosum and inflammatory bowel disease. Arch Surg 129:769–772

192. Giroux JM, Ouellet Y, Heppell J, Lacrois M (1987) Pyoderma gangrenosum piri stomall chez un patient atteint de rectocolite ulcero hemorragique. Ann Dermatol Venereol 114:935–939

193. Waits JO, Dozois RR, Kelly KA (1982) Primary closure and continuous irrigation of the perineal wound after proctectomy. Proc Mayo Clinic 57:185–188

194. Carey PD, Suvarna SK, Baloch KG et al (1993) Primary adenocarcinoma in an ileostomy: a late complication of surgery for ulcerative colitis. Surgery 113:712–715

195. Bauer JJ, Gelernt IM, Salky B, Kreel I (1983) Sexual dysfunction following proctocolectomy for benign diseases of the colon and rectum. Ann Surg 197:363–367

196. Aaztely M, Palmblad S, Wikland M, Hulten L (1991) Radiological study of changes in the pelvis in women following proctocolectomy. Int J Colorectal Dis 6:103–107

197. Leicester RJ, Ritchie JK, Wadsworth J et al (1984) Sexual function and perineal wound healing after intersphincteric excision of the rectum for inflammatory bowel disease. Dis Colon Rectum 27:244–248

198. Parc R, Legrand M, Frileux P et al (1989) Comparative clinical results of ileal-pouch anal anastomosis and ileorectal anastomosis in ulcerative colitis. Hepatogastroenterology 36:235–239

199. Farnell MB, Adson MA (1985) Ileorectostomy: current results: the Mayo Clinic experience. pp. 100–121. In Dozois RR (ed): Alternatives to Conventional Ileostomy. Year Book Medical Publishers, Chicago

200. Aylett SO (1953) Conservative surgery in the treatment of ulcerative colitis. BMJ 2:1348–1351

201. Baker WN, Glass RE, Ritchie JK, Aylett SO (1978) Cancer of the rectum following colectomy and ileorectal anastomosis for ulcerative colitis. Br J Surg 65:862–868

202. Mayo Robson AR (1893) Case of colitis with ulceration treated by injuenal colostomy. Trans Clini Soc London 26:213–215

203. Keetley CB (1895) Quoted by Corbett RS (1945) Proc R Soc Med 38:277–290

204. Lilienthal H (1903) Extirpation of the entire colon, the upper portion of the sigmoid fixture and four inches of the ileum for hyperplastic colitis. Ann Surg 37:616

205. Brown N (1913) The value of complete physiological rest of the large bowel in the treatment of certain ulcerative and obstruction lesions of this organ with description of operative technique and report of cases. Surg Gynecol Obstet 16:610–613

206. Nissen R (1933) Demonstrationen aus der operatinen chirurgie zunächst einige Beobach tungen aus der plastidun chirurgie. Zentralbl Chiru 60:88

207. Koenig-Rutzen R (1944) Quoted by Strauss AA, Strauss SF (1944) Surg Clin Nor Am 24:211–214

208. Strauss AA, Strauss SF (1944) Surgical treatment of ulcerative colitis. Surg Clin North Am 24:211–214

209. Ravitch MM, Sabiston DC (1947) Anal ileostomy with preservation of the sphincter. Surg Gynecol Obstet 84:1095–1099

210. Goligher JC (1951) The functional results after sphincter-saving resection of the rectum. Ann R Coll Surg Engl 8:421–439

211. Van Niel J (1986) Enterostomal therapy. pp. 277–296. In Jagelman DG (ed): Mucosal Ulcerative Colitis. Futura Publishing Company, Mount Kisko, New York

212. Kock NG (1969) Intra-abdominal "reservoir" in patients with permanent ileostomy: preliminary observations on a procedure resulting in fecal "continence" in five ileostomy patients. Arch Surg 99:223–231

213. Martin LW, LeCoultre C, Schubert WK (1977) Total colectomy and mucosal proctectomy with preservation of continence in ulcerative colitis. Ann Surg 186:477–480

214. Parks AG, Nicholls RJ (1978) Proctocolectomy without ileostomy for ulcerative colitis. BMJ 2:85–88

215. Pemberton JH (1991) Surgical approaches to proctocotectomy for inflammatory bowel disease. pp. 629–655. In Phillips SF, Pemberton JH, Shorter RG (eds): The Large Intestine: Physiology, Pathophysiology, and Diseases. Lippincott-Raven, Philadelphia

216. Köhler LW, Pemberton JH, Zinsmeister AR, Kelly KA (1991) Quality of life after proctocolectomy: a comparison of Brooke ileostomy, Kock pouch, and ileal pouch-anal anastomosis. Gastroenterology 101:679

217. Schrock TR (1979) Complications of continent ileostomy. Am J Surg 138:162

218. Kelly KA, Dozois RR (1990) Chronic ulcerative colitis. In Moody F (ed): Surgical Treatment of Digestive Diseases. 2nd Ed. Year Book Medical Publishers, Chicago

219. Dozois RR (1985) The ileal "J" pouch anastomosis. Br J Surg (suppl) 72:S80

220. Kelly KA (1992) Anal sphincter-saving operations for chronic ulcerative colitis. Am J Surg 163:5

221. Dozois RR, Kelly KA (1988) Newer operations for ulcerative colitis and Crohn's disease. pp. 655–683. In Kirsner JB, Shorter RG (eds): Inflammatory Bowel Disease. Lea & Febiger, Philadelphia

222. Kelly KA (1991) Approach to the patient with ileostomy and ileal pouch. pp. 796–809. In Yamada T et al (eds): Text book of Gastroenterology. Vol. 1. Lippincott-Raven, Philadelphia

33

CROHN'S DISEASE

Scott A. Strong

Crohn's disease is a chronic inflammatory condition of unknown etiology that can affect the entire intestinal tract. Typical presenting symptoms include abdominal pain, diarrhea, and weight loss. Although the terminal ileum and cecum are most often affected, the other common anatomic patterns include disease confined to the small bowel and disease limited to the large intestine. Rarely, Crohn's disease will primarily manifest itself with duodenal or, less rarely, anorectal symptoms. No medical or surgical therapy has yet been developed that will uniformly and reliably effect a cure. In general, operative treatment is reserved for patients whose quality of life is significantly impaired despite appropriate medical therapy or after disease-associated complications develop.

OPERATIVE INDICATIONS

Any review of the natural history of Crohn's disease reveals that most patients will ultimately require operative treatment of their disease. The National Cooperative Crohn's Disease Study reported the probability of undergoing an operation to be 78% and 90% after 20 years and 30 years of disease symptoms, respectively.[1] The indications for this surgical intervention can be subgrouped into one of two primary groups: elective indications and emergent indications. The incidence of these indications varies according to anatomic location of disease, disease extent, and behavioral pattern; however, fistula, abscess, and obstruction tend to be the most common reasons for operation in Crohn's disease patients with perforation and massive hemorrhage rarely occurring.

Elective Indications

Fistula With or Without Abscess

Fistula and abscess are the most common indications for the operative treatment of Crohn's disease according to Farmer et al.[2] Of the 482 patients treated by operation for intestinal disease

in this study from the Cleveland Clinic, 169 (35%) had a fistula with or without a concomitant abscess. More specifically, this complication occurred in 32% of 130 patients with small bowel Crohn's disease, 44% of 225 patients with ileocolitis, and 23% of 127 patients with Crohn's colitis.

Several different types of fistula can develop, including enteroenteric, enterovesical, enterovaginal, enterocutaneous, perianal, and perirectal. Similarly, abscesses can occur in various sites: enteroparietal, interloop, intramesenteric, and retroperitoneal. The diagnosis and management of these fistulae and abscesses are individually discussed later. In general, fistulae rarely heal with corticosteroid therapy. However, 6-mercaptopurine will promote fistula closure in 30% to 40% of cases, especially if obstruction and active disease are absent.[3,4] Abscesses generally require drainage and antibiotic therapy followed by resection of the associated segment of diseased bowel.

Obstruction

Bowel obstruction can be chronic or acute and can arise from single or multiple sites of stricturing. Although obstructive symptoms may improve with high-dose corticosteroids, the response is often temporary and symptoms typically recur as the medication is tapered. Moreover, high-grade obstructive lesions usually do not respond to medical therapy and early operative intervention is recommended before symptoms worsen or perforation occurs.

Obstruction was the second most common indication in Farmer et al.'s[2] study, accounting for 34% of the operations for Crohn's disease. The incidence based on intestinal disease location was 55% for small bowel disease, 35% for ileocolic involvement, and 12% for Crohn's colitis.

Failed Medical Therapy

The initial treatment of any patient with symptomatic Crohn's disease not complicated by high-grade obstruction, uncontrolled sepsis, malignancy, massive hemorrhage, or perforation is med-

---

Indications for the Operative Treatment of Crohn's Disease

Elective Indications

> Fistula with or without abscess
> Obstruction
> Failed medical therapy
> Malignancy
> Growth retardation

Emergent Indications

> Toxic colitis or megacolon
> Hemorrhage
> Perforation

---

ical therapy. Although the location, extent, and nature of the disease influence response to particular medications, a few principles of management are generally accepted. The majority of Crohn's disease patients fail initial medical treatment or respond and require maintenance therapy with antibiotics, sulfasalazine, 5-aminosalicylate (5-ASA) compounds, steroids, or immunosuppressants. If the response to medical treatment is incomplete, maintenance medications cannot be discontinued in a predetermined time period, or significant side effects develop, the patient has failed medical therapy, and operative treatment is indicated.

Carcinoma

The association between carcinoma of the intestine and Crohn's disease has been extensively reported. Although Crohn's disease is relatively easy to diagnose, carcinoma complicating the inflammatory state can be difficult to recognize. Crohn's disease and Crohn's disease complicated by adenocarcinoma are rarely distinguished by contrast roentgenogram and intraoperative examination. The diagnosis is most commonly established after histopathologic inspection of the specimen.

Obviously, a malignancy arising on a background of Crohn's disease mandates operative resection to accomplish cure. Unfortunately, Michelassi et al.[5] found the outcome with such treatment rather dismal. Of 11 Crohn's disease patients, the mean survival was only 6 months for small bowel cancers and 65 months for large bowel carcinomas.

Growth Retardation

Significant growth retardation has been well documented in 15% to 30% of children with Crohn's disease. This retardation can be related to malabsorption, nutritional deficits, secondary hypopituitarism, and corticosteroid therapy. Homer et al.[6] reported on 37 children and adolescents who underwent operative treatment of their symptomatic Crohn's disease. Catch-up growth occurred only in those children operated on before puberty who did not suffer early (2 years) recurrence. Therefore, growth failure is considered an important operative indication only in the prepubertal child and is not an indication after the onset of puberty.

Emergent

Toxic Colitis and Megacolon

Toxic colitis is a potentially fatal complication of Crohn's disease that warrants emergent treatment, especially if associated with megacolon. Although several definitions of toxic colitis have been proposed, the author prefers the description that includes both a subjective and objective component. Accordingly, toxic colitis is characterized as an acute ''flare'' of the disease accompanied by at least two of the following criteria: fever (greater than 38.6°C); hypoalbuminemia (less than 3.0 g/dL); leukocytosis (greater than 10.5×10^9 cells/L); tachycardia (greater than 100 beats/min). Toxic megacolon is toxic colitis with colonic dilatation exceeding 5 cm or dilatation less than 5 cm that persists on serial abdominal roentgenograms. The diagnosis and care of these extremely ill patients can be improved by recognizing the objective signs of toxic colitis in a patient who appears only mildly sick because of the masking nature of corticosteroids and immunosuppressants.

The initial treatment of toxic colitis is intended to reverse any physiologic deficits with intravenous hydration, correction of electrolyte abnormalities, and transfusion of blood products. Free perforation, massive hemorrhage, peritonitis, and septic shock are indications for emergent operative intervention after adequate resuscitation. Otherwise, medical therapy is initiated with high-dose corticosteroids or immunosuppressants, bowel rest, and broad-spectrum antibiotics; anticholinergics, antidiarrheals, and narcotics are avoided because they may conceal ominous symptoms or aggravate impaired colonic motility. Serial abdominal examinations and roentgenograms are performed to detect peritonitis or increasing colonic dilatation, respectively.

Any worsening of the clinical course or increasing megacolon during the initial 48 hours warrants emergent surgical treatment. Furthermore, if the patient improves minimally after 5 to 7 days of conventional therapy, the colitis is considered refractory to nonoperative therapy and urgent surgery is recommended.

Perforation

Free perforation, albeit rare, usually occurs during an acute exacerbation of chronic disease, particularly in the presence of distal obstruction, or during a bout of toxic colitis when transmural ulceration has developed. Perforation of small bowel Crohn's disease occurs in less than 2% of patients[7] with a similar incidence in large bowel Crohn's disease at 1% to 3%.[8,9] Bundred et al.[8] reported that only one of six colon perforations was associated with toxic dilatation of the diseased large bowel.

The transmural nature of Crohn's disease more typically results in the formation of inflammatory adhesions between the diseased segment and surrounding structures that seal most perforations. However, the resultant abscess may subsequently rupture, spill its contents, and create a communication between the bowel lumen and the peritoneal cavity.

Hemorrhage

Homan et al.[10] reported massive intestinal hemorrhage in 7 of 503 (1.4%) patients with Crohn's disease. The likelihood of bleeding did not correlate with patient age, duration of disease, use of corticosteroids, or disease activity. More likely, the hemorrhage is secondary to deep ulcerations eroding into moderate-sized blood vessels of the mucosa or submucosa.

Emergent operative treatment of hemorrhage from Crohn's disease should be individualized but must be considered in patients with no other obvious sources of bleeding (e.g., peptic ulcer disease, gastritis); life-threatening hemorrhage; failure to attain stabilization after initial transfusion with 4 to 6 units of packed red blood cells; significant rebleed during hospitalization; or coexisting indication for resection of the diseased bowel.

PRINCIPLES OF OPERATIVE TREATMENT

Disease-Related Axioms

Any physician or health care professional assisting in the care of patients with Crohn's disease must understand several characteristics that are unique to this inflammatory disorder of the gut. First, Crohn's disease is panintestinal, affecting the alimentary tract from the mouth to the anus. Second, the etiology of Crohn's disease remains elusive but appears linked to genetic predisposition, dietary factors, infectious agents, and immunologic disorders. This enigmatic nature makes the disease incurable by medical or operative measures. Third, Crohn's disease tends to follow a lifelong course that is typified by episodes of symptom flares that are interspersed between remissions induced by medical therapy or surgical intervention.

Considering these disease features, the goals of treatment for patients with Crohn's disease should be focused on long-term control of the patient's symptoms with a minimum of morbidity while maintaining the function and continuity of the gastrointestinal tract. These goals are best realized by close communication between the patient, gastroenterologist, and surgeon. As discussed earlier, most operations are for elective indications that afford the physicians an opportunity to decide on the appropriateness and timing of the procedure while the patient contemplates their recommendations without feeling coerced.

Patient Preparation

Mechanical and Antibiotic Preparation

If obstructive symptoms are absent or minimal, patients undergo a mechanical bowel preparation the day prior to surgery using a clear liquid diet and polyethylene glycol (4 L) or Fleet phospho-soda (90 ml). However, many patients will exhibit obstructive symptoms that necessitate omission or modification of this mechanical preparation. The modified preparation consists of a clear liquid diet and nutritional supplements for 3 to 5 days before surgery; magnesium citrate is occasionally added to gently purge the gastrointestinal tract. If colonic obstruction is part of the disease process, enemas from below can usually eliminate any stool harbored below the site of narrowing.

Antibiotic preparation can be oral or parenteral but should be directed against gram-negative rods and anaerobes. The author's preference is to parenterally deliver a third-generation cephalosporin and metronidazole on-call to the operating suite and during the first 24 hours postoperatively. If significant intraoperative contamination occurs, the antibiotics are continued for 5 days and their further use reassessed. Any abscesses that are encountered intraoperatively are cultured and antibiotic therapy adjusted to the appropriate antimicrobials as suggested by gram stains and sensitivity studies.

Steroids and Immunosuppressants

Stress dosing of corticosteroids is necessary if the patient has been treated with corticosteroids or adrenocorticotropic hormone (ACTH) within the previous 6 months. Stress dosing usually consists of 100 mg of parenteral hydrocortisone prior to induction of anesthesia, every 8 hours for 48 hours, and then each morning thereafter. Further tapering depends on the patient's clinical course, the dosage of preoperative corticosteroids, and the duration of this preoperative therapy. Most patients are weaned from corticosteroids within 3 months of their operation unless symptomatic disease mandates their continuation.

If the clinical scenario allows, immunosuppressants such as 6-mercaptopurine, azathioprine, and cyclosporine should be discontinued at least 2 weeks prior to operative intervention due to concerns of their potential negative impact on anastomotic and wound healing.

Correction of Deficits

Patients with symptomatic Crohn's disease commonly suffer from malnutrition and micronutrient deficiencies. Mechanisms responsible for these deficits include decreased nutrient intake secondary to anorexia or postprandial abdominal pain, malabsorption from inadequate small bowel absorptive surface after resection, or protein-losing enteropathy. Malnutrition usually manifests itself in a patient with Crohn's disease by weight loss (65% to 75%), hypoalbuminemia (25% to 80%), negative nitrogen balance (69%), and anemia (60% to 80%).[11] Deficiencies in trace minerals, essential vitamins, and minerals are common among Crohn's disease patients. More specifically, body stores of zinc, selenium, and iron are relatively depleted as are levels of vitamin D, vitamin A, and folic acid.

In Crohn's disease, the ability to correct malnutrition prior to operative intervention and the benefits derived from this correction are controversial issues. Lashner et al.[12] studied 103 patients referred for operative treatment of their Crohn's disease; 49 received total parenteral nutrition (TPN) prior to resection with the remaining 64 taken directly to surgery without nutritional supplementation. In the subgroup of patients undergoing small bowel resection, the length of small bowel resected was significantly less in the TPN group. Of the subgroup with large bowel disease, no benefits were noted in the TPN group. In a comprehensive literature review, postoperative complications were not significantly reduced by preoperative TPN in Crohn's disease although measured nutritional parameters did improve.

Other deficiencies such as anemia, electrolyte disturbances, dehydration, or coagulation defects should be readily corrected in elective and emergent situations.

Stoma Marking

Whether an ileostomy or a colostomy is intended to be temporary or permanent, correct siting of the stoma is paramount to patient satisfaction. Ideally, the stoma should be sited within the rectus abdominis muscle, remote from skin creases, scars, and bony prominences, readily visible to the patient, and situated at the peak of the infraumbilical fat mound. Therefore, it is imperative that the patient be marked preoperatively with inspection of the abdomen and potential stoma sites while the patient is standing, sitting, and lying supine.

Equally important in preparing the patient for a stoma is discussing the care and function of an ileostomy or colostomy and its impact on the patient's lifestyle. Enterostomal therapy nurses and lay ostomates can provide pertinent information and counseling that may help allay some of the patient's anxiety.

Operative Options

Regardless of disease location, a variety of operative procedures are appropriate in the management of Crohn's disease. These options include internal or external bypass, intestinal resection with or without anastomosis, and strictureplasty.

Bypass

Among the initial procedures described for the operative treatment of Crohn's disease was bypass. These bypass procedures divert bowel contents to an internal destination (e.g., gastrojejunostomy) or an external site (i.e., stoma). Due to relatively high recurrence rates and risk of malignancy, internal bypass of the small bowel or colon is rarely recommended. Homan and Dineen[13] reported that the 15-year recurrence rates of Crohn's disease initially treated by exclusion bypass, bypass in continuity, or resection were 82%, 94%, and 65%, respectively. As for small bowel carcinomas complicating pre-existing Crohn's disease, Faintunch et al.'s[14] review of the literature revealed that 30% of the adenocarcinomas developed in bypassed segments of jejunum or ileum.

However, in select situations, internal bypass is still considered acceptable, or preferred, therapy. If an ileocecal phlegmon is densely adherent to the retroperitoneum such that resection would risk damage to the iliac vessels or other retroperitoneal structures with resection, exclusion bypass with definitive resection and anastomosis planned 6 months later is acceptable therapy. In this instance, the ileal stump should be matured as a mucous fistula to avoid the accumulation of secretions and stump rupture. In the case of symptomatic gastroduodenal Crohn's disease, internal bypass and highly selective vagotomy is usually the preferred operative procedure.

External bypass without resection is also rarely practiced. Although fecal diversion for Crohn's disease of the colon and perianum is associated with a high incidence of sustained remission, restoration of intestinal continuity is unlikely in the majority of patients.

The blow-hole colostomy with ileostomy for toxic colitis and toxic megacolon is an external bypass procedure that was popularized at the Cleveland Clinic by Turnbull et al.[15] during the 1960s. Fortunately, the procedure is infrequently necessary these days as physician awareness and access to medical care have improved such that far fewer patients progress to severe toxic megacolon.

Resection With or Without Anastomosis

As indicated by Alexander-Williams et al.,[16] resection is typically the procedure of choice for Crohn's disease of the small and large bowel, especially when it is the patient's first operation. At this initial resection, the procedure provides ample tissue for certainty of histologic diagnosis. With scattered proximal small bowel lesions that may be amenable to strictureplasty, the distal ileal segment is usually the most inflamed site and generally warrants resection. For Crohn's disease of the colon, segmental resection with colocolic or colorectal anastomosis provides many Crohn's colitics quality years of life without a stoma.

Resection Margins

The length of "normal" bowel that should be removed proximal and distal to a segment affected by Crohn's disease is less controversial than previously argued.

Many authors, such as Berman and Krause,[17] favored extensive resection. In an uncontrolled trial with 7.5 to 9.5 years of follow-up, they noted a recurrence rate of 29% after radical resection compared with 84% after conservative procedures. In a study of 54 patients by Karesan et al.,[18] crude recurrence occurred in 8 of 12 patients with microscopic evidence of disease at the resection margins whereas only 14% of the 42 patients with normal margins suffered recurrence. Lindhager et al.[18] divided 110 patients into three pathologic subgroups described as normal histology, minor inflammatory changes, and major inflammatory changes at the resection margins. At 10 years, the cumulative recurrence rates were 37%, 44%, and 73%, respectively.

However, most series have subsequently found no relationship between microscopic inflammation of the resection margins and recurrence rates.[20-24] Moreover, Heuman et al.[25] found no value in the use of frozen sections to assess the status of margins as recurrence rates were not influenced by the margins' appearance. Hamilton et al.[26] compared 38 patients who underwent frozen section evaluation of their resection margins and 41 patients whose margins were chosen after gross visual inspection; clinical recurrence rates in the frozen section and non-frozen section groups were 60% and 66%, respectively, at 10 years of follow-up. Reoperation rates at 5 years were identical (18%) and at 10 years were similar (36% and 32%). Thus, the practice of frozen sections was not recommended.

The Cleveland Clinic reviewed a cohort of patients who fulfilled the following criteria: no prior surgery for Crohn's disease; all patients underwent small bowel resection with anastomosis; all surgeries were performed at the Cleveland Clinic; and resection margins were reviewed in all cases.[27] Of 100 patients studied, no significant differences in recurrence rates were found among four groups categorized according to the degree of inflammatory change at the margins. In a recent randomized, prospective study from the Cleveland Clinic[27a] comparing 131 patients with macroscopically free margins of 2 or 12 cm, the clinical and operative recurrence rates were not significantly different between these "conservative" and "radical" resection margin groups after an average follow-up of almost 5 years. Moreover, histologic evidence of inflammation at the resection margin did not adversely influence recurrence.

In summary, the use of frozen section analysis or extended resection margins does not lessen the likelihood of recurrence following the operative resection of Crohn's disease.

Disease Recognition

In its classic form, Crohn's disease of the small bowel is easily recognized. The involved segment is characteristically indurated, thick-walled, and constricted with omentum or adjacent bowel loops commonly adherent to the inflamed area. Skip lesions affecting short or long segments of small bowel occur in about 20% of cases. Ileal disease is typified by a fierce serositis or ''corkscrew'' appearance of the serosal vessels, thickening of the mesenteric margin of the bowel, and fat encroachment or wrapping on the sides of the intestinal wall. The scalloped appearance of the normal terminal ileal mesentery is lost by excess fat deposited between the terminal branches of the marginal vessels. The proximal bowel above the strictured segment is commonly dilated and, in the presence of chronic obstruction, this ''normal'' bowel may be quite thickened due to muscular hypertrophy. The mesentery of the involved small bowel is quite thickened, especially due to lymph node enlargement along the ileocolic and superior mesenteric vessels. Approximately 30% of these nodes contain enteric organisms, and in a few, active suppuration is present.

In some cases of small bowel Crohn's disease, these findings are absent. In this instance, if Crohn's disease is suspected and the external findings are not impressive, the best guide to operative disease location is palpation along the mesenteric margin of the bowel (Fig. 33-1). The margin of a diseased segment is invariably thickened, which often indicates an associated mesenteric ulcer. The surgeon can use this subtle abnormality as a guide to resection.

In Crohn's colitis, patchy or uniform thickening of the bowel wall may be seen with varying degrees of fat wrapping. However, this is not always the case and the distribution of disease, especially significant disease, may be best determined by intraoperative colonoscopy, particularly if preoperative endoscopy was not performed or does not correlate with the external appearance of the colon. In toxic colitis, it is often impossible to macroscopically distinguish Crohn's disease from ulcerative colitis unless there is concomitant small bowel disease.

Mesentery and Lymph Nodes

One of the most difficult problems associated with resection of ileal Crohn's disease is dividing the mesentery. This mesentery is usually thick due to fat deposition and enlarged mesenteric lymph nodes that straddle the ileocolic and superior mesenteric vessels. Attempts to perform conventional mesenteric division and ligature, as with operations for cancer or chronic diverticulitis, can injure the pedicle vessels and create a rapidly spreading hematoma. Controlling this hematoma can lead to prolonged surgery and, even worse, further vascular injury with distal bowel ischemia. Thus, the preferred technique is to use serial overlapping clamps on both sides of the intended line of transection (Fig. 33-2). The mesentery is divided so as to leave a margin

or cuff of tissue. Suture ligatures of heavy chromic catgut are used to underrun each pedicle secured by the clamp, eliminating the risk of spreading hematoma.

Enlarged mesenteric lymph nodes are not intentionally excised because this does not reduce the risk of recurrent disease. Contrarily, it is usually desirable to divide the mesentery remote from the bowel margin as this approach makes retrograde bleeding less troublesome. Furthermore, if a thick mesenteric cuff is left behind, there can be excessive tension on an anastomosis or ileostomy. The exception to this principle is when treating recurrent disease near the superior mesenteric vessels, especially if associated with a fistula. In this instance, these major vessels are best avoided by excising the diseased segment through the vascular plane between the mesentery and bowel wall. In general, the enlarged mesenteric nodes, especially along the ileocolic lymphovascular chain, should be excised assuming this does not mandate excision of ''normal'' small bowel.

Anastomosis Technique and Orientation

Whether the anastomosis is stapled or handsewn, the principles of safe technique include adequate blood supply to bowel ends, assurance of no tension or torsion to the bowel ends, equilibration of lumen size, and closure of the mesenteric defect. In particular for Crohn's disease, the mucosa of the bowel limbs must be inspected. An anastomosis should not be formed with strictured bowel and rarely with bowel that contains a deep, longitudinal ulcer. Contrarily, further resection is not necessary for aphthous ulcers found in soft, supple, otherwise healthy bowel.

In patients operated on for obstructive Crohn's disease, the distended proximal bowel can make abdominal closure difficult. In this instance, the bowel may be decompressed by retrograde massage of the luminal contents into the stomach for aspiration through an indwelling nasogastric tube. Alternatively, two linen tapes are passed through the bowel mesentery approximately 15 and 30 cm from the cut end of the proximal limb; a sterile nasogastric tube is then passed through the open end of the proximal bowel and secured in place by tightening the linen tapes. The luminal gas and succus are aspirated by advancing the tube while applying intermittent suction.

Although surgeons vary in their preferred technique, the anastomotic configuration does not seem to influence recurrence of symptomatic Crohn's disease. Scott et al.[28] compared 92 patients treated by ileocolic resection with anastomosis for Crohn's disease. Over a 20-year period, the annual rate of recurrence was nearly identical for side-to-side and end-to-side anastomoses.

Anastomosis With Proximal Diversion

A temporary ileostomy may be prudent in a variety of situations when operating for Crohn's disease. The principal intent for a diverting stoma is to decrease operative morbidity when bowel resection is indicated in the face of concomitant factors that could adversely affect anastomotic healing. The situations where a temporary stoma should be considered include the presence of incompletely drained sepsis, excessive blood loss, prolonged operation, and severe hypoalbuminemia. Contrarily, a

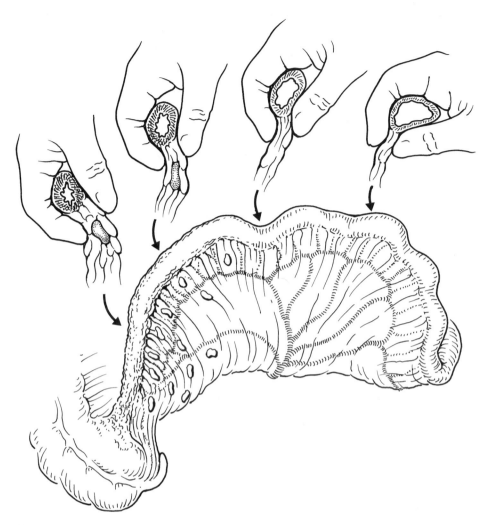

Figure 33-1. Intraoperative detection of disease limits by palpation of the terminal ileum. Nondiseased bowel proximal to the strictured segment may appear dilated with muscular hypertrophy, but mesenteric thickening is absent. A segment with mucosal disease will demonstrate thickening of the mesenteric margin: lymphadenopathy is pronounced in more inflamed portions with transmural involvement. The strictured bowel will feel firm and indurated with significant creeping fat, adenopathy, and mesenteric thickening.

history of recent steroid use does not necessarily indicate a need for temporary diversion.

Strictureplasty

Strictureplasty is intended to conserve small bowel while safely eliminating symptomatic strictures. Although the procedure was initially described for the treatment of tubercular strictures,[29] Lee and Papaioannou[30] pioneered this procedure for use in strictures secondary to Crohn's disease. Subsequently, many centers have conducted comprehensive studies and determined the procedure to be effective in relieving obstructive symptoms with weight gain and improved food tolerance. Although these diseased segments are left unresected and in continuity, steroid usage can usually be discontinued or lessened. Paramount to the safety of the procedure is appropriate patient selection. Although strictureplasty may be used for strictures of the small

bowel or for fibrotic recurrence at ileocolic or ileorectal anastomoses, colonic narrowing should not be treated by strictureplasty.

Strictureplasty is indicated for diffuse involvement of the small bowel with multiple strictures, strictures in a patient who has undergone previous major resections of small bowel (greater than 100 cm), rapid recurrence of Crohn's disease manifested as obstruction, stricture in a patient with short bowel syndrome, and nonphlegmonous, fibrotic stricture.

The contraindications to strictureplasty are free or contained perforation of the small bowel; phlegmonous inflammation, internal fistula, or external fistula involving the affected site; multiple strictures within a short segment; stricture in close proximity to a site chosen for resection; colonic strictures; and hypoalbuminemia (less than 2.0 g/dl). Occasionally, multiple strictures in a patient with an albumin value less than 2.5 g/dl might be regarded as a contraindication to performing a stric-

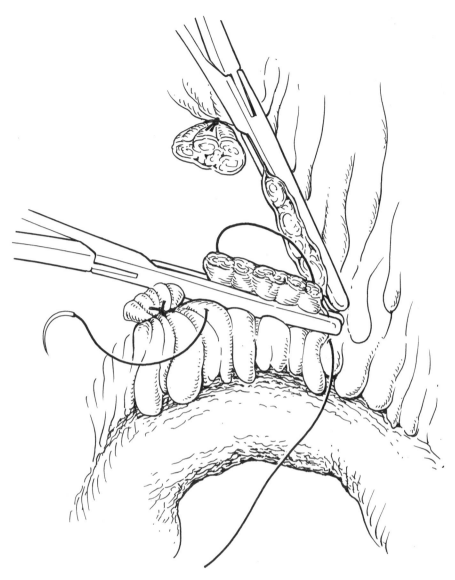

Figure 33-2. Suture ligature (no. 1 chromic catgut) technique for the thickened mesentery of Crohn's disease. Serfat Kocher clamps are applied in an overlapping manner that minimizes the risk of hematoma within the mesentery and maximizes hemostasis.

tureplasty. In this instance, a proximal diverting stoma should accompany the strictureplasties.

The operation has proven to be quite safe with no mortality reported from the major series. In the experience at the Cleveland Clinic, septic complications occurred in 5% of patients.[31] Of the parameters studied (i.e., hypoalbuminemia, steroid dosage, perforative or phlegmonous disease remote from the strictureplasty site, synchronous resection, number of strictureplasties, length of stricture), only hypoalbuminemia (less than 3.0 g/dl) was associated with an increased incidence of sepsis. Postoperative hemorrhage, although uncommon, can be particularly challenging to manage; if reoperation is necessary, one cannot be certain of the bleeding site without opening the several strictureplasties. Laparotomy to control hemorrhage can usually be avoided by selective mesenteric angiography with intra-arterial infusion of a vasoconstricting agent.

In addition to a low operative morbidity, the long-term results of strictureplasty for Crohn's disease are encouraging. Of 162 patients undergoing 698 strictureplasties and followed for a median of 42 months, 98% were relieved of obstructive symptoms; moreover, symptomatic recurrence affected only 22% of the patients.[31]

At operation, the stomach, duodenum, small intestine, and large bowel are examined. As the small bowel is traced from the duodenojejunal junction distally, suture tags are placed on segments affected by disease with normal and diseased sites measured in relationship to the ligament of Treitz. With experience, the subtle strictured segments can be readily recognized by the marginal thickening of the mesenteric angle discussed earlier.

For short strictures (less than 10 cm) (Fig. 33-3A), a linear incision is made along the antimesenteric aspect of the stricture,

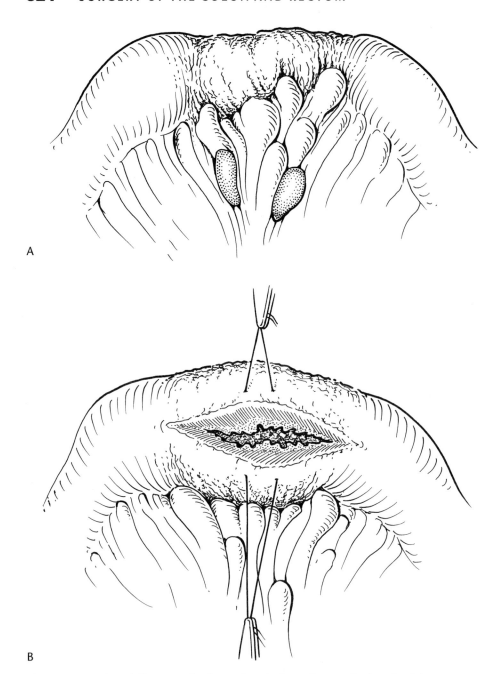

A

B

Figure 33-3. **(A–D)** The type of strictureplasty is dependent on the length of the stenotic segment. For strictures less than 10 cm in length, a Weinberg/Mikulicz (one-layer) technique of strictureplasty is used. A longitudinal enterotomy is made over the antimesenteric aspect of the stricture, and the defect then is closed transversely with polyglycolic acid sutures. It is important to biopsy any suspicious areas of mucosal ulceration, as well as to mark the mesentery adjacent to the strictureplasty with a titanium clip for future roentgenographic identification. *(Figure continues.)*

extending the incision for 3 cm beyond the stricture on either side.[32] Stay sutures are placed at both edges of the enterotomy site in its midpoint (Fig. 33-3B) and lateral traction applied to convert the longitudinal defect into a transverse one (Fig. 33-3C). A biopsy of any suspiciously ulcerated mucosa is performed to exclude carcinoma. Hemostasis of the wound edges may be time consuming, but is mandatory. The wound is then closed transversely using an interrupted single layer of 000 polyglycolic acid sutures (Fig. 33-3D). At the completion of the strictureplasty, a radiopaque titanium clip is applied to the mesenteric fat adjacent to the closure site. This marker allows for subsequent identification of strictureplasty sites during future contrast radiography of the small bowel.

Longer strictures may provide technical difficulties in per-

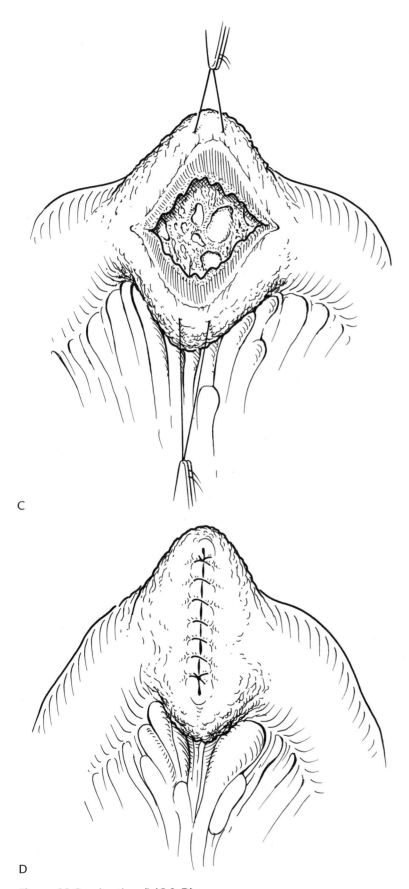

C

D

Figure 33-3.   *(continued)* **(C & D).**

forming a long side-to-side (Finney) strictureplasty unless the bowel is supple enough to bend into a U-shape and still allow for a tension-free anastomosis. If possible, the posterior portion of these strictureplasties is closed with a continuous 00 polyglycolic acid suture, taking all layers of the bowel wall. Interrupted sutures are added at 1.5-cm intervals. The anterior layer is closed in a similar fashion.

Incisions and Drains

When considering the type of incision to use, it is important to recall the recurrent nature of the disease and the possibility that fecal diversion may be necessary. Specifically, Post et al.[33] reported that 30% of patients undergoing operative treatment of Crohn's disease required temporary or permanent fecal diversion. Therefore, a vertical midline incision is preferred as it allows adequate operative exposure and preserves all abdominal quadrants for future stomas.

Drains are used if a pyogenic membrane remains, when an infected retroperitoneal space is present, or if presacral mobilization of the rectum has been performed. In the case of sepsis, multiple latex rubber drains are sutured over the residual septic focus to permit egress of infection and prevent drain migration. The drains are removed from such foci 2 weeks after surgery. Alternatively, if the site is remote from the skin surface and a residual cavity is possible, a small mushroom catheter is substituted for an additional 3 to 6 weeks. The additional drainage time is intended to prevent premature healing of the skin defect that can allow an abscess to re-form. Prior to removal of such catheters, sinography is recommended to assure collapse of the cavity and confirm absence of a fistula. For presacral mobilization of the rectum, large sump-suction drainage catheters are used to minimize the amount of blood that can collect in the pelvis and act as a culture medium for abscess-forming bacteria. In all situations, the drains are brought out remote from the main incision and near the area to be drained.

SITE-SPECIFIC MANAGEMENT

Gastroduodenal

Among patients with Crohn's disease, 0.5 to 4% will manifest primary gastro-duodenal disease. Although bleeding and anemia may occur, the most common presenting complaints are nonspecific and indistinguishable from peptic ulcer disease of the duodenum. As the disease progresses, symptoms of duodenal obstruction develop in the majority of patients. Radiologic investigation will reveal abnormal findings in 90% of patients.[34] Endoscopy will demonstrate macroscopic abnormalities in most affected patients with nodularity (93%), aphthous ulcers (64%), serpiginous ulcers (55%), and stricturing (50%).[35] At a microscopic level, granulomas suggestive of Crohn's disease, are present in 15% to 68% of patients undergoing biopsy.

Crohn's disease of the stomach is a rare entity usually associated with disease elsewhere in the intestinal tract. Typical findings on endoscopy include gastric dilatation and antral involvement with multiple superficial ulcerations. Because differentiation from gastric carcinoma may be difficult, many of the reported cases underwent total or subtotal gastrectomy. Fre-

quently, the diagnosis of Crohn's disease was made only after microscopic tissue review.

Most patients with nonobstructing duodenal disease will respond to antacids, hydrogen ion antagonists, and corticosteroids. However, Nugent and Roy[34] reported an operative rate of 37% (33 of 89 patients) with reoperation necessary in 8 of these 33 cases after a median follow-up of 9.7 years. Although few surgeons will argue that gastrojejunostomy is the operation of choice for obstructing duodenal Crohn's disease, past debate centered on the use of concomitant truncal vagotomy. Advocates cited the high incidence of marginal ulceration and protagonists were concerned about postvagotomy diarrhea. However, with the recent acceptance of highly selective vagotomy, most surgeons now feel the procedure of choice is gastrojejunostomy and highly selective vagotomy as this procedure adequately treats symptoms and avoids both complications.

An attractive alternative to gastrojejunostomy for duodenal obstruction is duodenal strictureplasty. By avoiding bypass of the pylorus, many of the sequelae associated with gastrojejunostomy are obviated. However, even among the groups who have an extensive experience with small bowel strictureplasty, very few operations of this kind have been performed. Such a procedure requires full mobilization of a sometimes brittle duodenum that is not as supple as the small bowel because of mesenteric tethering by the biliary ducts and pancreas. As well, a significant segment of the duodenal wall may have been destroyed by penetrating ulceration that precludes strictureplasty. In that case, duodenojejunostomy is required.

An alternative to the Heineke-Mikulicz (two-layer transverse closure) strictureplasty is the Finney procedure in which the antrum, pylorus, and duodenum are opened with a long enterotomy and a side-to-side antroduodenostomy is performed

The normal duodenum and gastric antrum of a patient with Crohn's disease may be secondarily affected by fistulae arising from primarily involved segments of ileum or colon. These complex fistulae are discussed later in detail.

Jejunoileal

Small bowel Crohn's disease can present with varying degrees of intestinal involvement. Among the variations seen is the scenario of isolated distal disease. Provided there is sufficient length (5 to 7 cm) of normal-appearing distal ileum after definitive ileal resection, the ileocecal valve should be preserved to minimize postoperative diarrhea and a hand-sewn anastomosis created using the distal ileal segment.

A second situation involves distal ileal disease separated from a more proximal skip lesion by a short segment that appears normal. When there is no threat of short bowel syndrome, as in most patients undergoing initial operation, the entire segment is resected and a single anastomosis is performed.

A third variation is typified by several stenotic segments separated from one another by noninvolved bowel. These stenoses range in length from a few centimeters to more than 50 cm. In this situation, the surgeon can resect the distal disease and ignore the more proximal diseased segments. This is a possible alternative if the proximal segments are not obstructing nor affected by a perforative process. However, any degree of bowel dilatation proximal to involved segments is indicative of an obstructive process and treatment is warranted. In practice, this

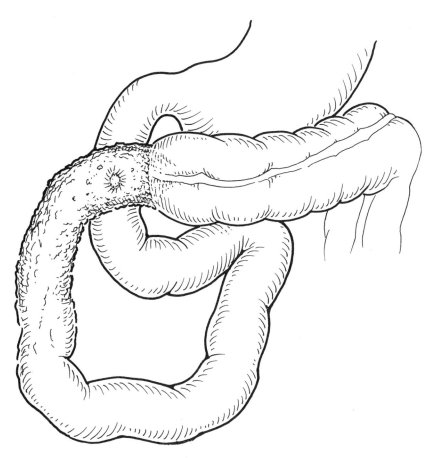

Figure 33-4. Schematic of duodenal fistula arising from recurrent Crohn's disease at an ileocolic anastomosis.

option of leaving proximal diseased segments undisturbed is rarely done and only for diffuse jejunoileitis uncomplicated by strictures. More likely, the multiple stenotic lesions are treated by strictureplasty.

Ileocecal

Ileocecal disease is the most common anatomic site of involvement accounting for 40% of all cases undergoing surgery. The typical presentations are perforative and obstructive disease. In the majority of cases, resection is possible with ileo-ascending colon anastomosis. Preservation of as much of the normal right colon as possible is desirable, to provide greater surface area for water absorption and to avoid the potential complication of ileocoloduodenal fistula associated with anastomotic recurrence when the anastomosis is located more distally in the transverse colon (Fig. 33-4).

Unilateral exclusion bypass was mentioned earlier for the apparently fixed ileocecal mass. This is a reasonable alternative in such circumstances provided any associated sepsis is drained and resection is later performed when the process has settled. In this case, even if such a patient was operated on years earlier, it is still usually possible to resect the terminal ileum and cecum, disconnect the ileo-transverse anastomosis, close the transverse colotomy, and anastomose ileum to nondiseased ascending colon.

Colonic

Nearly 25% of patients with Crohn's disease will demonstrate disease limited to the large intestine. Of these patients with large bowel disease, 25% will have disease confined to the colon with relative rectal or rectosigmoid sparing.[36] Only 10% of these patients will have segmental involvement of the colon.[37] The choice of operation for Crohn's disease affecting the large bowel depends on multiple variables including patient age, disease distribution, extent of involvement, previous resections, rectal compliance, and adequacy of fecal continence (Tables 33-1 and 33-2).

Segmental Colitis

Although the use of limited resection for Crohn's disease of the small intestine is widely accepted, the value of segmental resection in colonic Crohn's disease is more controversial. Among the large intestine's physiologic roles, the absorption of water and salt, particularly in the right colon, acts to protect against systemic dehydration and electrolyte imbalance. Therefore, although the large bowel is an expendable organ, attempts at its preservation are justified. Despite a high incidence of recurrence, the reoperative rate associated with segmental resection for Crohn's colitis or ileocolitis should not relegate the patient with focal colonic disease to a total proctocolectomy

Table 33-1.   Elective Surgery for Crohn's Disease of the Large Bowel

Site	Indication or Comment	Procedure
Right colon	Anastomosis overlying duodenum risks complex fistula with recurrence	Right colectomy, ileodistal transverse colostomy, wrap anastomosis with omentum
Right and transverse colon	Ileodescending colostomy has a large mesenteric defect	Extended colectomy with ileosigmoid colostomy
Segmental colon (transverse, descending, or sigmoid)	Older (>50 years) patients; previous enterectomy (>30 cm). High recurrence rate	Segmental resection, colocolic or cecocolic anastomosis
	Younger (<50 years) patients; minimal or no previous enterectomy	Resect diseased segment *plus* proximal colon with ileocolostomy
Rectum with colon sparing	Older (>50 years) patients; previous enterectomy (>30 cm)	Proctosigmoidectomy and colostomy
	Younger (<50 years) patients; minimal or no previous enterectomy	Proctocolectomy and ileostomy
Total colon disease	Rectum essentially normal; good rectal compliance; good continence; no perianal sepsis	Total colectomy and ileorectal anastomosis
	Above *plus* proximal rectal disease. High recurrence rate	Total colectomy, partial proctectomy, ileal (10 cm) pouch-rectal anastomosis

with end ileostomy. Although this operation may be eventually realized, the patient may be adequately palliated for a number of years by a segmental resection, thereby lessening the portion of the patient's life that is burdened with an ileostomy. In the younger patient especially, a sphincter-preserving operation may prevent the psychological and social heartache that occasionally accompanies a stoma during the formative years.

In patients with disease limited to the ascending colon, with or without ileal disease, resection of the involved bowel can leave the anastomosis overlying the second portion of the duodenum. Given the disease nature, an anastomotic recurrence may result in a complex fistula involving the duodenum and retroperitoneum. To obviate this disastrous outcome, the transverse colon is divided at the level of the middle colic vessels so the root of the mesentery is interposed between the retroperitoneal structures and the ileocolic anastomosis. Alternately, a more proximal anastomosis may be wrapped by a pedicle of omentum, thereby preventing the anastomosis from lying in direct contact with the duodenum.

Disease involving the ascending and transverse colons is treated in a similar manner. In this instance, however, resection limited to the diseased segment will result in an anastomosis between the ileum and descending colon with a mesenteric defect that is difficult to close. Therefore, an extended right colectomy is recommended as the mesenteric leaves of the ileum and sigmoid colon are more easily approximated. Resection of the additional colonic segment prevents the development of an internal hernia and does not appear to adversely affect the patient's functional outcome.

Crohn's disease of the transverse, descending, and sigmoid colons presents a situation where segmental resection and colocolic or colorectal anastomosis is most commonly employed. Segmental resection is particularly ideal for the older individual (greater than 50 years) and colitics who have previously undergone significant small bowel resection (greater than 30 cm). In both instances, maximal preservation of the colonic absorptive surface may dramatically improve the patients' functional results. In addition, maintenance of the ileocecal valve may afford some protective effect against diarrheal stools. Resection with coloproctostomy is used for these select patients with left-sided disease, whereas a cecorectal anastomosis is created if the transverse colon is additionally involved. In the younger patient and

Table 33-2.   Nonelective Surgery for Crohn's Disease of the Large Bowel

Right or segmental colitis	Toxic or severely malnourished patient with perforation and peritonitis	Resect disease, exclude distal bowel, proximal diversion
Rectal disease	Perforation or abscess with signs of sepsis	Drain abscess, colostomy; staged resection 6 months later
Total colon disease	Toxic megacolon with perforation; toxic colitis	Subtotal colectomy with ileostomy and extraperitoneal rectosigmoid stump or mucus fistula
	Toxic megacolon with contained perforation; dangerous colectomy due to high splenic flexure, pregnancy, or comorbid disease	Ileostomy and blow-hole colostomy; staged resection 6 months later
	Colonic hemorrhage	Subtotal colectomy with ileostomy and extraperitoneal rectosigmoid stump or mucus fistula
	Rectal hemorrhage	Proctocolectomy and ileostomy
	Colonoscopic perforation with quiescent colitis	Oversew or resect perforation with ileostomy

those without prior small bowel resection, the diseased segment and uninvolved proximal colon are resected with the construction of an ileosigmoid or ileorectal anastomosis.

As previously discussed, the abdomen is entered through a midline incision to provide adequate exposure without compromising potential ostomy sites. The abdomen is explored and the entire gastrointestinal tract inspected for evidence of disease involvement. The retroperitoneum and adjacent viscera are examined for possible fistulae and abscesses. If the preoperative and intraoperative evaluations are conducive, segmental resection with primary anastomosis is performed.

Our general approach is to recommend conservative resection margins of 5 cm for reasons mentioned earlier. Lymphadenectomy is not routinely performed; however, any suppurative nodes, which can be safely included without vascular compromise of the remaining bowel, are excised. Unless a malignancy is suspected, a high ligation of the mesenteric vessels is unnecessary. Instead, in order to prevent injury to the retroperitoneal organs and remaining bowel, the named vessels may be divided distal to their branching. Following resection of the diseased intestine, the open limbs of bowel are inspected and an anastomosis is subsequently constructed, avoiding any overtly diseased intestine.

Pancolitis

A population of patients with symptomatic Crohn's colitis exists where segmental resection is not feasible because of extensive colonic involvement. However, a subgroup of this population demonstrates relative rectal sparing, adequate fecal continence, and absence of active perianal sepsis; these individuals are considered candidates for colectomy with ileoproctostomy.

In an effort to better select individuals suitable for an ileoproctostomy, Keighley et al.[38] analyzed the physiologic function of these Crohn's colitics. Although quantitation of anal canal pressures was of no value in predicting functional outcome, patients whose maximum tolerated rectal volume measured less than 150 ml did poorly. Other surgeons rely merely on subjective evidence of rectal compliance as witnessed by distension with proctoscopic air insufflation.

Total colectomy and ileoproctostomy is done with the patient placed in a modified lithotomy position. After exploring the abdominal cavity, the ascending and descending segments of the large intestine are mobilized by incising along the lateral peritoneal reflections with careful sweeping of the mesentery off the retroperitoneum. The transmural nature of Crohn's disease can cause retroperitoneal inflammation and mesenteric shortening; therefore, care must be taken to not include the ureters or duodenum within the mobilized tissue. Once again, as with segmental resection, the entire lymphovascular drainage basin need not be resected unless a complicating carcinoma is suspected. With division of the blood vessels to the ascending colon, the integrity of the ileocolic artery is maintained to ensure adequate perfusion of the terminal ileum. Similarly, the terminal branches of the inferior mesenteric artery (superior rectal arteries) are left intact. The ileoproctostomy is created 15 to 16 cm from the anal verge using a circular stapling device or 000 polyglycolic acid suture. The hand-sewn anastomosis is formed by approximating the posterior walls with vertical-mattress su-

tures and an interrupted, single-layer closure of the anterior seromuscular layers. The completed anastomosis is then leak-tested using half-strength povidone-iodine instilled through the anus and proctoscopic air insufflation with the anastomosis submerged in saline.

Rarely, a patient will present with pancolonic Crohn's disease with significant upper rectal involvement. An ileoproctostomy is technically feasible but, as the anastomosis lies only 6 to 8 cm above the anal verge, function may be excessively impaired secondary to compromised compliance. In this instance, an ileal J-pouch is configured with 10-cm limbs and anastomosed to the disease-spared midrectum after total colectomy and proximal proctectomy. Although the recurrence rate is undoubtedly greater than that associated with total proctocolectomy and ileostomy, the patient may enjoy several years without a stoma.

Proctitis

In the rare patient with isolated proctitis secondary to Crohn's disease, Ritchie and Lockhart-Mummery[39] suggested disease resection with end colostomy. However, the colostomy should be constructed as an ileostomy with precise siting and spigot configuration, anticipating the high-volume, liquid effluent of Crohn's disease. Moreover, proctectomy alone should be avoided if the proximal or distal colon is segmentally involved as pancolonic disease will eventually develop. Therefore, unless significant small bowel has been resected or older age necessitates sparing of the large intestine's absorbing surface, proctocolectomy with end ileostomy is preferred over proctectomy and colostomy.

In the absence of malignancy or dysplasia, the rectum is mobilized so as to avoid damage to the lateral pelvic side-wall structures, including the autonomic innervation of the bladder and reproductive organs. The superior rectal vessels are identified at the level of the sacral promontory carefully sweeping the presacral sympathetic nerves posteriorly; following ligation and division of the vessels, the areolar space between the fascia propria of the mesorectum and the presacral fascia is entered. Sharp dissection continues distally in this plane dividing the rectosacral ligament as the levator hiatus is approached. Laterally, the reflections of the parietal peritoneum are incised to the depths of the genitorectal cul-de-sac, remaining close to the rectal wall. The anterior peritoneal reflection is incised dorsal to Denonvilliers' fascia, thereby protecting the seminal vesicles and prostate or vagina. The dissection cones down onto the muscularis propria of the rectum at the superior aspect of the lateral stalks. Distal to this point, the lateral and anterior mobilization continues on the rectal wall; inadvertent wandering out to the pelvic sidewalls risks needless injury to the nervi erigentes. The neurovascular structures of the fatty lateral stalks are divided using electrocautery to maintain hemostasis and reduce the potential for a postoperative pelvic abscess. Multiple times during the course of the lateral dissection, a large clamp is passed perpendicularly through the stalks creating "pseudo-pedicles" of tissue. By spreading the jaws of the clamp, the vessels within the tissue are compressed by traction. Electrocauterization, coupled with this technique, ensures better hemostatic division of the lateral stalks. Any bleeding that cannot be controlled with cauterization is stopped with suture ligation.

Once the levator ani muscles are reached circumferentially, the abdominal portion of the procedure is complete.

Following transabdominal mobilization of the rectum, an intersphincteric (endoanal) anorectal excision is performed. Perianal sutures efface the anal canal and expose the intersphincteric groove. Using electrocautery, a circumferential incision is made just outside the anoderm entering the intersphincteric plane. The dissection is carried cephalad to the level of the levators, meeting the previous point of transabdominal mobilization. The specimen, including internal sphincter, is then delivered from the operative field. Utilizing this technique, Leicester et al.[41] reported only a 4% incidence of permanent ejaculation difficulty without any instances of parasympathetic dysfunction.

Primary closure of the perineal wound is performed because it is associated with improved healing compared to healing by secondary intention. In all cases, the levators and puborectalis are closed, abscesses are drained with mushroom catheters, and fistulae are unroofed and curetted. If perineal sepsis is absent, the external sphincter and perianal skin are also approximated; otherwise, the remaining wound is packed with gauze.

Prior to abdominal wound closure, an attempt is made to fill the pelvic dead space. The pelvic parietal peritoneum is left open and the small bowel adequately mobilized so that it might migrate into the pelvis. A pedicle of omentum based on the left gastroepiploic vessel can be created and secured at the level of the levator hiatus. A transabdominally placed suction drain is positioned in the depths of the pelvis to prevent the collection of serosanguinous fluid, an ideal culture medium for bacteria. The purpose of these maneuvers is to avoid the unfortunate complication of an unhealed perineal wound with recalcitrant sinus. However, despite careful operative technique and attention to the above-mentioned details, some wounds will not readily heal. The majority of these wounds do not require early reoperative therapy as many of them will gradually heal over the ensuing 6 to 12 months. Instead, local wound care is recommended. Gauze packing and use of a WaterPik on a daily basis provides gentle tissue debridement that can complement more formal curettage in the office setting.

Proctocolitis

Total proctocolectomy with end ileostomy is indicated in those Crohn's colitics whose proctitis, sphincter dysfunction, or perianal sepsis is too severe for rectal preservation and ileoproctostomy.

The colon and rectum are excised as earlier described. Instead of primary proctectomy, Sher et al.[41] at Mount Sinai Hospital advocate a low Hartmann's closure of the rectum to allow regression of the anoperineal disease, thereby allowing subsequent perineal proctectomy to be performed in less inflamed tissues. Of 25 patients treated by a low Hartmann's pouch, 10 continued to demonstrate anoperineal sepsis that required intersphincteric perineal proctectomy. Despite this staged approach, 3 of the 10 proctectomy patients continued to suffer from an unhealed perineal wound.

Winslet et al.[42] reported on the use of ileostomy without resection for large intestinal Crohn's disease. Of 44 patients, 70% sustained disease remission with a reduction in steroid requirements and improvement in well being. Unfortunately,

16 patients needed subsequent proctocolectomy and only 4 (9%) had intestinal continuity successfully restored after an average follow-up of 99 months. Clearly, diversion alone is usually reserved only for those patients who refuse or would not tolerate proctocolectomy.

Anal/Perianal

The perianal abnormalities associated with Crohn's disease include edematous skin tags or hemorrhoids, cyanotic discoloration, fissures or ulceration, abscesses, fistulae, and anorectal stricture. Patients with colonic disease are more likely to have perianal manifestations than those with ileocolic or small bowel disease patterns. The perianal abnormalities can manifest themselves at any time in the disease course, but the intestinal symptoms usually antedate the perianal findings. Although the perianal disease component can be completely asymptomatic in some fortunate individuals, in others it can be the major source of disability.

The evidence of anal and perianal Crohn's disease is usually obvious upon inspection accompanied by digital examination, anoscopy, and rigid proctoscopy; however, individuals without a history of Crohn's disease can present a diagnostic challenge. Although biopsy is sometimes necessary, a multiplicity of abnormalities (e.g., laterally located fissures, cavitating anal canal ulceration, anorectal ring stenosis) are suggestive of Crohn's disease. If the patient is too uncomfortable for an adequate evaluation, a well-conducted examination under anesthesia is mandated. Computed tomography (CT) scanning, endoluminal ultrasonography, and magnetic resonance imaging have been suggested by some; however, their routine use adds little practical information to the above evaluation. Using the same modalities recommended for large intestinal disease, perianal manifestations of Crohn's disease necessitate thorough evaluation of the remaining alimentary tract.

The appropriate treatment of anal Crohn's disease is individualized to the specific patient with adherence to certain management principles. As there is no cure for Crohn's disease, the primary treatment goals are amelioration of the symptoms and prevention of future complications. However, the realization of these goals is not to be at the expense of harmful systemic side effects, impaired fecal continence, or increased risk of complications necessitating proctectomy. In general, a conservative medical, as well as operative, approach is adopted. A more aggressive attitude will often result in outcomes that are worse than the disease itself.

In part, evaluation of the entire intestinal tract prior to treatment of perianal Crohn's disease is based on the controversial notion that proximal disease control will improve more distal disease. Wolff[43] and Heuman et al.[44] noted persistence or recurrence of adult perianal disease when the proximal disease component was inadequately controlled after resection. Similarly, Hellers et al.[45] reported spontaneous healing of perianal fistula in 20 of 43 pediatric patients (47%) following resection of proximal disease. Orkin and Telander[46] offered a contrary opinion as they found improved perianal symptoms in only 5 of 17 children following enterectomy. Beyond the adolescent patient, other reports support a lack of improvement in perianal manifestations treated solely by resection of more proximal Crohn's disease.[47,48] Therefore, the proximal disease component of a patient with perianal Crohn's disease merits treatment only if the intestinal disease is independently symptomatic or obviously interrelated to the perianal component.

Skin Tags

Skin tags are a common occurrence in Crohn's disease and appear as large, painless growths that originate from the perianal skin. Contrarily, internal hemorrhoids are relatively rare and can cause discomfort as bulky, engorged tissue protrudes from its origin proximal to the dentate line. In either case, the lesion is usually secondary to loose, frequent stools as opposed to a primary manifestation of perianal disease. Consequently, treatment is typically nonoperative with therapy directed against the inciting diarrhea. Warm sitz baths and control of the causative bowel dysfunction are typically successful. Surgical treatment, whether conservative or aggressive, is associated with prohibitive morbidity. Excision of simple skin tags is often complicated by chronic, nonhealing ulcers. Moreover, excisional hemorrhoidectomy often has disastrous results as supported by the results of Jeffrey et al.[49] Of 21 individuals treated for hemorrhoids, 12 prior to the diagnosis of Crohn's disease and 9 after, postoperative complications occurred in 7 and 3 patients, respectively. Most disturbing is that, of the 10 patients with complications, 6 ultimately required proctectomy. Crohn's patients with symptomatic skin tags or hemorrhoids are best treated by local measures unless serious concerns (e.g., hemorrhage, suspected malignancy) supervene.

Fissures

Although typically considered a painless, eccentrically located lesion, the fissures of Crohn's disease can be very disabling and expansive. Some of the larger fissures actually appear as cavitating ulcers surrounded by undermined margins that encircle the anus and erode the sphincter mechanism. As with most perianal manifestations of Crohn's disease, nonoperative therapy in the form of topical agents, correction of diarrhea, and, possibly, oral corticosteroids may provide adequate symptom control. If a Crohn's fissure-in-ano becomes painful, a component of underlying sepsis should be suspected and a careful, yet thorough, examination is warranted. A patient with an uncomplicated fissure that does not improve by the previously mentioned measures may benefit from a lateral internal sphincterotomy, particularly if the rectum is spared of disease and manometry indicates an increased anal canal resting pressure. Fortunately, Crohn's fissures typically display a self-limiting course with only 10 of 53 patients (19%) in one series still afflicted after 10 years of follow-up.[47]

Symptoms secondary to the larger, virulent ulcers can often be controlled with oral azathioprine or intralesional injection of methylprednisolone; most of these patients, however, will eventually require proctectomy because of unrelenting pain, sepsis, or fecal incontinence.

Perianal Abscesses

Many of the perianal abscesses that occur in the Crohn's population are of a cryptoglandular origin whereas others represent complications of pre-existing fissures or fistulae. Most commonly, the abscess, regardless of its etiology, will manifest itself as a painful, indurated area with or without fluctuance. As discussed earlier, any suspected abscess of the Crohn's perianum mandates careful inspection. The principles applied to the treatment of perianal abscesses in the general population, also apply to the Crohn's patient. Unless perineal sepsis complicates the presentation, simple incision and drainage of the abscess will adequately relieve the acute symptoms and allow resolution of the inflammation. After anesthetizing the involved area, a stab incision is made into the medial aspect of the overlying skin, penetrating into the abscess itself. A mushroom-tipped catheter is then passed to the apex of the cavity and trimmed 2 to 3 cm beyond the skin level to allow egress of pus over the ensuing days. Further inspection for a potential fistula-in-ano is rarely performed in the acute setting; instead, a thorough search is reserved for a recurrent abscess. In addition, enteral antibiotics are needed only in patients with accompanying cellulitis, diabetes mellitus, immunosuppression, prosthetic implants, or valvular heart disease.

Anal Fistulae

The diagnosis and management of anal fistulae represents one of the most challenging dilemmas in the treatment of Crohn's disease. As in most components of this disease, therapy is directed at alleviating symptoms while avoiding untoward side effects. By no means does this imply that treatment should be delayed or withheld; rather, conservative medical and operative treatments should be initiated in a timely manner. At the extreme, aggressive surgical procedures are practical in only the occasional patient.

The treatment of this often difficult perianal manifestation is based on the individual patient's presentation considering the fistula's location and complexity, the presence or absence of concomitant proctitis, and the severity of accompanying anal canal disease. In addition, the physician should be cognizant of the known potential, albeit small, for malignant degeneration of the chronic fistula tract and caution the patient accordingly.

Most low-lying, simple fistulae without concomitant proctitis can be appropriately managed by fistulotomy. Many institutions have reported good success with fistulotomy for the Crohn's disease patient with normal continence and an intersphincteric or low transsphincteric fistula-in-ano. Fry et al.[50] reported complete healing in all 13 Crohn's disease patients within 4 months of undergoing intersphincteric fistulotomy. Levien et al.[51] reported excellent results in 18 of 21 patients following an intersphincteric or low transsphincteric fistulotomy. Fuhrman and Larach[52] as well as Sohn et al.[53] reported similar results when fistulotomy was combined with the postoperative use of metronidazole and sulfasalazine, respectively. Despite careful patient selection, an occasional fistulotomy will fail to heal and result in a chronic, relatively asymptomatic ulcer. Further operative treatment should then be avoided and previously mentioned medical management employed. If an overly generous sphincterotomy results in fecal incontinence, an overlapping sphincteroplasty with temporary diversion has been successful in select patients.[54]

If fecal continence would be compromised by partial sphincter division, a noncutting seton or rectal mucosal advancement flap is indicated for low-lying, simple fistulae without significant proctitis. Noncutting setons adequately satisfy the goals of therapy by reducing perianal drainage and pain without worsening fecal continence or risking proctectomy. The soft, nonreactive nature of Silastic vessel loops makes them an ideal seton material for long-term fistula management. The seton is passed through the curetted fistula tract and then loosely tied upon itself, encircling the perianal tissue. The seton establishes drainage of the fistula and minimizes the risk for future abscesses arising from the fistula tract. The seton rarely causes discomfort and does not interfere with adequate hygiene.

The rectal mucosal advancement flap is a versatile procedure that does not jeopardize continence or risk proctectomy. If rectal inflammation is limited and no cavitating ulceration or anal stenosis is present, the advancement flap may be used. The procedure is performed under regional or general anesthesia following mechanical and antibiotic bowel preparation. The patient is positioned with the internal opening of the fistula dependent; using effacing sutures or a self-retaining retractor, the anal canal is everted. The fistula tracts are carefully identified and curetted clean of granulation tissue. Normal saline with or without epinephrine is then injected into the submucosal plane to help identify the level of dissection. A 120° to 180° curvilinear incision is made in the rectal mucosa to include the internal opening in its most distal aspect. Taking care to maintain meticulous hemostasis, the mucosa of the flap is then elevated with a small portion of the underlying internal sphincter. After the flap has been widely mobilized, the sphincteric portion of the fistula tract is debrided and sutured closed; the mucosal site of the fistula is excised. The flap is then drawn distally over the now-closed muscular opening and secured without tension to the distal mucosal margin, which typically lies caudad to the dentate line. The external fistula sinuses are drained with mushroom-tipped catheters until the flap has healed and the tracts have collapsed. Temporary fecal diversion is not usually necessary unless the patient is undergoing a repeat advancement flap procedure or an excessive amount of fibrosis was encountered during flap mobilization. Fry et al.[50] reported successful closure in all three patients who underwent mucosal advancement flap repair of their simple Crohn's fistulae. Makowiec et al.[55] performed 36 advancement flaps in 32 patients with Crohn's disease. Their overall success rate of 60% at 20 months was improved if the rectum was spared of disease and the fistula was not anovaginal in nature.

In the event that the above situation is complicated by anal canal ulceration or stricturing, a rectal sleeve advancement with temporary ileostomy can be performed in select patients. This operation is a more extensive version of the rectal mucosal advancement flap whereby the full thickness of the rectum is circumferentially mobilized after excision of the ulcerated or strictured area. A formal proctoanal anastomosis is then performed in combination with diverting loop ileostomy. Although the mobilization can be done transanally in the majority of cases, the patient must be cautioned that transabdominal mobilization is sometimes necessary.

If proctitis complicates a low-lying, simple fistula, medical therapy is usually employed with or without a noncutting seton, thereby avoiding fistulotomy. Contrary to this opinion, Williams et al.[56] occasionally perform fistulotomies in this setting with 9 of 12 study patients demonstrating healed fistulae within 3 months of surgery.

In a patient with a high, complex fistula and no evidence of Crohn's proctitis, a rectal mucosal advancement flap is performed. One-third of complex fistulae treated in this fashion at the Cleveland Clinic completely healed.[57] If the anal canal is diseased, a rectal sleeve advancement may be attempted.

The presence of proctitis with a high, complex fistula prevents the successful use of an advancement flap and relegates the Crohn's disease patient to medical therapy in combination with seton drainage, temporary fecal diversion, or proctectomy. White et al.[58] reported a series of 10 patients with complex fistulae and proctitis treated by noncutting seton; excellent palliation was noted after 4 months to 7 years of follow-up. Despite severe proctitis in 6, none had required proctectomy. Once again, the experience of Williams et al.[56] was also encouraging with only 3 of 16 patients (19%) ultimately losing their rectum after seton management of a high, complex fistula.

Unfortunately, temporary ileostomy does not influence the long-term outcome of anal or perianal Crohn's disease. van Dongen and Lubbers[59] reported that only 22% of individuals treated by defunctioning ileostomy for fistulous perianal disease had restoration of intestinal continuity. At the Cleveland Clinic, only 5 of 15 patients underwent reversal of an ileostomy created solely to control perianal Crohn's disease; the remainder were subjected to proctocolectomy (unpublished data). The majority of patients who underwent closure required a secondary procedure (e.g., rectal mucosal advancement flap) while diverted.

Therefore, a loop ileostomy for severe perianal disease may acclimate the patient to life with a stoma and, in some instances, provide control of perianal sepsis or proctitis prior to mucosal advancement flap or proctocolectomy. However, the creation of a loop ileostomy as a planned definitive procedure is rarely indicated.

Endoanal proctectomy is necessary in approximately 5% of Crohn's disease patients solely to control their anal or perianal disease. Keighley and Allan[60] found that high, complex fistulae and deep ulcerations are among the disease characteristics likely to mandate proctectomy with permanent ostomy. The same proctectomy-associated complications mentioned earlier, particularly the unhealed perineal wound, can occur in this clinical situation.

Anovaginal Fistulae

Anovaginal fistulae typically originate from an anterior ulcer eroding into the vagina. However, the fistula may arise from a posterior cryptoglandular opening that has tracked to the vagina in a horseshoe fashion. The same examination outlined for a perianal fistula is used for a suspected anovaginal fistula. Despite this, anovaginal fistulae may be sometimes difficult to identify. Occasionally, a hypaque enema or infusion of methylene blue into the rectum with a tampon inserted in the vagina may be necessary to demonstrate the fistula. More commonly, careful examination under anesthesia with vaginoscopy and rectal insufflation while the vagina is filled with saline will identify the fistula tract.

As with all Crohn's disease perianal fistulae, several factors influence the appropriate therapeutic choice. Initial treatment is directed at control of the sepsis with catheter drainage, possibly in combination with placement of a noncutting seton or oral antibiotics. If the rectum is free or relatively spared of involvement, either a rectal mucosal advancement flap or a rectal sleeve advancement is performed depending on the state of the anal canal. Although some surgeons advocate an episioproctomy repair of an anovaginal fistula when rectal and anal disease are absent, we prefer the advancement flap as no sphincter division is necessary. In Crohn's patients with anovaginal fistulae, Crim et al.[57] reported 10 of 14 (71%) transanal advancement flaps ultimately healed after an average follow-up of 15 months. Fry and Kodner[61] reported an 80% healing rate in 10 women treated by this technique. Significant rectal or anal disease relegates the patient to nonoperative treatment or proctectomy.

Alternatively, Hesterberg et al.[62] reported the use of an anocutaneous flap to close anovaginal fistulae accompanied by proctitis. With 18 months of follow-up, only 3 of 10 fistulae have recurred.

Anourethral Fistulae

Although rare, an anourethral fistula can be treated in the same manner as a rectovaginal fistula. These fistulae can be successfully closed utilizing a mucosal advancement flap.[63]

COMPLICATION-SPECIFIC MANAGEMENT

Abscess

The majority of abdominal abscesses arise from transmural ulcers or fissures in segments of diseased bowel that are adherent to surrounding structures. As previously mentioned, inflammatory adhesions seal off the penetrating fistula and form the confines of the resultant abscess cavity. Riberio[64] reported on 129 intra-abdominal abscesses arising in Crohn's disease; 109 (84%) were intraperitoneal and 20 (16%) were retroperitoneal. Nearly half of the abscesses were associated with a synchronous fistula. Although an abdominal abscess is suspected when a patient presents with a painful, localized mass that is associated with tenderness, fever, and leukocytosis, spontaneous internal drainage or corticosteroids can mask these symptoms and signs. Of 653 patients with Crohn's disease, 110 were suspected of having an abscess or inflammatory mass after physical examination.[65] An abscess was confirmed at laparotomy in one-half of the subjects. Another 39 of the 653 patients were also found to have an abscess that was not suspected preoperatively. Therefore, almost 40% of abscesses were not detected by physical examination alone prior to operative intervention.

Enteroparietal

An enteroparietal abscess is ideally treated by initial external drainage using CT-guided techniques or surgical incision. As expected, the majority of patients will develop an enterocutaneous fistula over the ensuing weeks.[66] However, after a 6-week period the abscess cavity has usually collapsed; the intestinal source of the abscess can then be resected and a primary, nondiverted anastomosis safely created.

Interloop

Interloop abscesses are typically small in size and undiagnosed preoperatively. Alternatively, these subtle collections are usually discovered intraoperatively when matted segments of intestine are being separated. If the associated cavity and inflammation can be excised, the presence of an unsuspected interloop abscess should not alter the planned operative procedure.

Intramesenteric

Abscesses within the mesentery of the small bowel, colon, or rectum can present a challenging problem. An intramesenteric abscess generally originates from a penetrating ulcer located along the mesenteric margin of the bowel wall. In the case of midgut penetration, the abscess can develop between the mesenteric leaves and extend as far as the origin of the superior mesenteric vessels. With extensive abscesses, resection of the diseased segment and the associated mesentery can risk ischemia of nondiseased intestine, secondary contamination of the peritoneal cavity, and acute or delayed hemorrhage from the fragile vascular pedicles of the mesentery. An alternative and safer method of treatment is to confirm the presence of the cavity by needle aspiration, compress the mesenteric leaves toward the bowel wall, and attempt to establish retrograde drainage of the abscess into the bowel lumen. Bilateral exclusion of the diseased bowel is created by forming mucus fistulae with segments of intestine immediately proximal and distal to the involved area; bowel continuity is restored by enteroenterostomy of the uninvolved intestine. The excluded segment can be safely resected 6 months later. If retrograde drainage is impossible because of a multiloculated abscess, the individual abscesses are emptied by needle aspiration and external drainage catheters. Proximal diversion or an exclusion bypass is created with plans for resection and anastomosis to occur 6 months later.

Ideally, intramesenteric abscesses are treated by resection and primary anastomosis if no mitigating factors (e.g., undrained sepsis, peritoneal contamination, unprepared bowel, malnutrition) are present. However, large or complex abscesses are best managed by external drainage and proximal diversion with definitive resection and anastomosis delayed for 6 months. Of note, these abscesses associated with the hindgut can occasionally drain spontaneously through the perineum creating a complicated extrasphincteric fistula.

Fistula

The fistulae of Crohn's disease may be internal or external and relate to abscess formation. Penetrating ulceration of the diseased bowel may produce a contained bowel perforation and abscess, although the septic component may be occult or minimal. Fistulae develop when the abscess necessitates into an adjacent viscus or through a cutaneous wound. Not infrequently, ileoenteric, ileotransverse, or ileosigmoid fistulae will be observed. However, all hollow organs of the abdominal cavity, including such rarities as the common bile duct, ureters, seminal vesicles, and fallopian tubes, have been documented as components of intestinal fistulae in Crohn's disease.

Enteroenteric Fistula

Enteroenteric fistulae are the most common type of internal fistula in Crohn's disease. Greenstein[67] found internal fistulae occurred in 33% of 1,480 patients with Crohn's disease whereas external fistulae afflicted only 15%. Isolated enteroenteric fistulae usually cause few symptoms unless obstructive or septic sequelae complicate the clinical presentation. Broe et al.[68] showed that of 24 patients with internal fistulae initially managed by nonoperative methods, 10 required surgery within 1 year and an additional 8 patients within 9 years, mostly due to intractable disease. Azathioprine has been reported to promote healing of fistulae but appears to be of more benefit with anal fistulae than small bowel fistulae.[4]

In common with all internal fistulae due to Crohn's disease, the principles of surgical management include resection of the fistula source, freshening of the defect in the secondarily involved bowel loop by wedge excision, and suture closure of the latter defect. Primary bowel anastomosis can usually be safely performed after the ileal resection is completed. Although this is the procedure of choice for most enteroenteric fistulae, certain clinical situations may pose special considerations. If a phlegmonous reaction involving the sigmoid colon is part of an ileosigmoid fistula, suture closure of the sigmoid defect may be vulnerable to breakdown. Rather, a limited sigmoid resection with anastomosis should be performed. Of 27 ileosigmoid fistulae treated in this manner, no anastomotic dehiscences occurred.[69] However, this is a controversial issue as many surgeons attest to the safety of simple wedge excision, even in the presence of phlegmonous changes.

One of the most difficult management problems faced in Crohn's disease surgery is the treatment of an ileocoloduodenal fistula. This fistula typically arises from an ileocolic anastomotic recurrence overlying the duodenum and head of the pancreas. Apart from the technical difficulties of dissecting the recurrent disease from the pancreas and duodenum, closure of the duodenal defect is problematic. In this instance, a loop of proximal jejunum is brought up to the involved duodenum for a side-to-side duodenojejunostomy. The ileocolic recurrence is then resected and a neoileocolic anastomosis created.

Other varieties of these fistulae to the duodenum and stomach include ileoduodenal, ileogastric, and cologastric types. In each case, the appropriate procedure is resection of the diseased ileal or colonic segment with closure of the duodenal or gastric defect. For cologastric fistulae, the extent of colonic resection depends on the extent of disease; in most cases an extended colectomy with ileosigmoid or ileorectal anastomosis is performed.

Enterocutaneous

Enterocutaneous fistulae occur in the early postoperative period or at a late stage because of anastomotic dehiscence or recurrent disease, respectively. Rarely, a late fistula may result from residual sepsis associated with a previously contained anastomotic leak. With an early postoperative fistula, the fecal stream should be externally diverted proximal to the leak; this may be coupled with resection of the fistula and bowel anastomosis if peritoneal reaction is minimal. For later appearing septic fistulae (more than 10 postoperative days), re-entry into the peritoneal cavity can be dangerous because of dense adhesions and the risk of multiple enterotomies. In this instance, intravenous hyperalimentation and sepsis management usually provide an acceptable outcome.

Late enterocutaneous fistulae due to recurrent disease will usually require resection and anastomosis, when feasible. Very low output fistulae may be managed by nonoperative techniques in patients whose operative risk is significant. In such instances, azathioprine and cyclosporine have been valuable in augmenting fistula closure.

Enterovesical Fistula

Most patients with enterovesical fistulae manifest intestinal symptoms, although pneumaturia, dysuria, and urinary frequency are common. Cystography, cystoscopy, and barium enema are the preferred investigative tools. CT scanning may add to the diagnostic rate, although with all available studies, a correct diagnosis is usually achieved in only about 50% of cases. Although surgery is appropriate management in the vast majority of cases, there is usually no urgency. Patients can frequently be managed with urinary antimicrobial drugs with little or no risk of pyelonephritis.[70] At operation, the diseased bowel is pinched off the bladder and resected with the bladder defect then curetted. The defect is usually oversewn if reperitonealization is possible, although catheter drainage of the bladder for 7 to 10 days makes this largely unnecessary. Cystography is performed prior to catheter removal to confirm bladder integrity. In 61 such fistulae treated this way at the Cleveland Clinic, recurrence was rare.[71] Additionally, enterovesical fistulae are commonly associated with other varieties of internal and external fistulae.[72]

Enterovaginal Fistula

Enterovaginal fistulae may arise from Crohn's disease in the ileum, colon, or rectum. Commonly a previous hysterectomy has been performed when such fistulae arise from intraperitoneal intestine. The principles of management are identical to other intra-abdominal fistulae, namely detachment of the diseased intestine from the secondarily affected organ with resection of the diseased bowel. With enterovaginal fistulae, the vaginal defect may be trimmed and closed with polyglycolic acid sutures. If the bowel anastomosis is in proximity to the vaginal stump, an omental pedicle or muscle flap should be interposed between the anastomosis and vagina. Temporary fecal diversion is usually not required.

Malignancy and Dysplasia

Greenstein et al.[73] found the observed-to-expected ratio of small bowel adenocarcinoma to be 114:5 in patients with regional enteritis. Published literature reviews[14,74] accumulated 65 cases of small bowel cancer complicating pre-existing Crohn's disease. The average age at the time of cancer diagnosis was 48 years and one-third of affected patients were under the age of 40 years. The majority of the malignancies were reported in diseased terminal ileum; approximately 30% of the cancers were located in segments of bypassed jejunum or ileum. Greenstein et al.[75] studied 132 patients with bypassed segments of small bowel Crohn's disease and found 7 (5.3%) adenocarcinomas.

The incidence of large bowel adenocarcinoma complicating Crohn's disease is even greater. These adenocarcinomas usually demonstrate a worse histologic differentiation but their site distribution and propensity for regional or distant metastases are similar to colonic tumors in patients without Crohn's disease.

In Birmingham, England, the Cancer Epidemiology Research Unit reported a fourfold increase in the incidence of large bowel adenocarcinoma with extensive colonic Crohn's disease compared to a nondiseased cohort.[76] The likelihood of malignancy was directly related to duration and extent of disease involvement. Weedon et al.[77] examined this same association and reported that Crohn's disease patients under the age of 22 years when diagnosed with colitis experienced 20 times the incidence of colorectal cancer, especially affecting the right colon, contrasted to a demographically matched control population.

Greenstein et al.[78] substantiated these findings with a report of 579 patients with Crohn's disease followed for an average of 16 years. In addition, they reported that the cancers can develop in areas of bowel either microscopically or macroscopically affected by Crohn's disease. Similar to the small bowel, surgically excluded large bowel segments were at particular risk for malignancy. Many other series[79–82] observed adenocarcinomas arising in a section of bypassed colon or rectum.

Most recently, epidemiology studies from Europe have reported conflicting results regarding the association of large bowel Crohn's disease and adenocarcinoma. Ekbom et al.[83] studied a cohort of 1,655 patients with Crohn's disease in the Uppsala health care region, Sweden. They noted a 2.5 overall risk of colorectal cancer that was unaffected by duration of follow-up. The relative risk was 1.0 for patients with terminal ileum disease, 3.2 for terminal ileum and segmental colon involvement, and 5.6 for Crohn's disease isolated to the colon. More specifically, patients diagnosed with Crohn's disease before age 30 years with any component of colonic disease had a relative risk of 20.9. Contrarily, Munkholm et al.[84] did not find an increased risk in large bowel cancer among 373 Danish patients with Crohn's disease. Persson et al.[85] performed a population-based study of 1,251 patients with Crohn's disease diagnosed in Stockholm from 1955 to 1984 and followed until 1989. They found a greater incidence of small bowel carcinoma but no increase in the occurrence of colorectal cancer.

Like adenocarcinoma, lymphoma of the small intestine and colon is disease linked and has been reported in at least 13 patients with Crohn's disease.[86] In the majority of instances, the tumor originated in a segment of active inflammation.

The operative treatment of a malignancy arising in the midst of a diseased Crohn's segment obviously necessitates resection with inclusion of the associated lymphovascular pedicle. In the case of small bowel adenocarcinoma, however, care must be taken not to compromise the vascular supply to the remaining intestine while still providing at least 10-cm resection margins.

Operative treatment of colorectal tumors complicating Crohn's colitis requires adherence to basic oncologic techniques with high ligation of the involved mesenteric vessels. Additionally, consideration is given to resection beyond the directly involved colon as synchronous lesions have been described in one-third of patients.[78] In young patients with long-standing large bowel disease of an extensive nature or in those in whom future surveillance would be difficult, a subtotal colectomy with ileoproctostomy is the procedure of choice for a complicating colonic carcinoma.

The increased incidence of colorectal malignancy in Crohn's colitis has caused some authors to query as to whether an endo-scopic surveillance program should be instituted. However, the well-established colitis-dysplasia-carcinoma sequence of ulcerative colitis may not be as applicable in Crohn's disease.[87]

In support of this possible sequence, a strong correlation between dysplasia and adenocarcinoma in Crohn's colitis has been suggested by many authors. Richards et al.[88] found high-grade dysplasia in all five of their specimens resected for carcinoma complicating large bowel Crohn's disease. Petras et al.[89] of the Cleveland Clinic discovered dysplasia in five of six patients with colonic cancer and Crohn's disease; although the dysplastic mucosa was typically located in close proximity to the cancer, four patients demonstrated additional dysplasia remote from the tumor site. Similarly, Simpson et al.[90] reported on four patients with colonic Crohn's disease and colorectal carcinoma; two of the excised colons showed dysplasia remote from the index tumor. Finally, Hamilton[79] reported a series of nine patients with resectable colorectal cancer complicating their Crohn's colitis; all of the individuals harbored high-grade dysplasia near the tumor and six had dysplasia distant from the index lesion. The findings of these independent reports would suggest a causal relationship between dysplasia and carcinoma. However, the evolution of dysplasia from colitis is more ambiguous. Korelitz et al.[91] prospectively evaluated 356 patients with intestinal Crohn's disease for evidence of rectal dysplasia and synchronous or metachronous colorectal cancer. Over a 10-year period, rectal dysplasia was found in 18 patients. Of these 18 patients, two (11%) subsequently developed large bowel cancer. Lofberg et al.[92] used colonoscopic biopsy to monitor 24 patients with long-standing Crohn's colitis. Although none of the patients showed evidence of dysplasia, three displayed DNA aneuploidy with the subsequent discovery of an ascending colon cancer in one.

In summary, mucosal dysplasia is often observed when a malignancy is present, both in remote and adjacent mucosa. Given the difficult task of diagnosing colorectal cancer associated with long-standing Crohn's colitis and the relationship between dysplasia and carcinoma in this setting, the finding of dysplasia on colonoscopic biopsy or brushing, particularly in a worrisome area, warrants colonic resection. Moreover, albeit controversial, a colonoscopic surveillance program should be adopted in Crohn's patients at particularly high risk for the development of a colorectal malignancy.

Stricture

The incidence of Crohn's colonic stricture ranges from 5% to 17%.[93] Although luminal narrowing in Crohn's colitis is usually benign, carcinoma can arise in long-standing strictures, presumably secondary to chronic inflammation. Generally, strictures secondary to Crohn's colitis can be managed nonoperatively if they are not causing obstructive symptoms. However, in cases of high-grade obstruction, particularly with worsening symptoms, medical therapy is rarely successful and resection is usually required.

Any stricture occurring with Crohn's colitis should be endoscopically assessed for malignant degeneration. Yamazaki et al.[93] reported on 132 individuals with Crohn's disease complicated by colonic stricture; nine patients (6.8%) harbored a malignancy in the strictured segment. Although the benign strictures tended to be of longer length than the malignant variety, the clinical symptoms were no different. If colonoscopic biopsies or cytologic brushings from suspect areas identify a malignant focus, resection is indicated.

Anastomoses are commonly complicated by recurrent stricturing. Over a 20-year follow-up period, Trnka et al.[94] found a 69% symptomatic restricturing rate in 40 patients undergoing resection for Crohn's ileocolitis. Historically, these segments of stricture required resection and permanent ileostomy or neo-anastomosis. More recently, strictureplasty has been reported for strictures involving ileocolic and ileorectal anastomoses.[95] After an average of 2 years of follow-up, none of the 22 patients experienced clinical or operative recurrence at the site of anastomotic strictureplasty.

In a nonoperative approach, although still aggressive, endoscopic dilatation of the narrowed anastomotic lumen has been reported. Blomberg et al.[96] reported on 27 Crohn's patients in whom a balloon catheter was endoscopically positioned and controlled dilatation performed. Prior to the procedure, the strictures ranged from 0.5 to 3 cm in length and had diameters of 5 to 8 mm. In all cases, the lumens were successfully expanded to a diameter of at least 12 mm; complications occurred in three patients with two cases of hemorrhage requiring transfusion and one bowel perforation. After an average follow-up of 15 months, 67% of the patients were free of symptoms. Although more than one dilatation session was typically required, all of the patients preferred this form of treatment to repeat laparotomy. Breysem et al.[97] attempted to similarly dilate anastomotic strictures in 17 patients. They were successful in all but one instance and no patient experienced complications. One-half of the group remained asymptomatic an average of 25 months later. Hydrostatic dilatation was noted to be most successful in those patients whose stricture was fibrotic, relatively short (less than 8 cm), and without active disease involvement. As the experience and duration of follow-up with this new nonoperative therapy grow, its usefulness will become more defined.

Toxic Colitis and Megacolon

Toxic colitis is a potentially fatal complication of Crohn's colitis, especially if accompanied by megacolon. Although several attempts have been made to accurately define toxic colitis, an objective classification is useful whereby a "flare-up" of colitis and at least two of the following criteria must be present: hypoalbuminemia (less than 3.0 g/dL), leukocytosis (greater than 10.5×10^9 cells/L), tachycardia (greater than 100 beats/min), temperature elevation (greater than 38.6°C). Use of this relatively objective definition has assisted in the diagnosis and care of these colitics whose severe condition may be masked by high doses of steroids and immunosuppressants.

Initial treatment is directed at reversing physiologic deficits with intravenous hydration, correction of electrolyte imbalances, and blood product transfusions. Medical therapy is started using high doses of intravenous corticosteroids and, occasionally, bowel rest with nasogastric decompression. Broad-spectrum antibiotics directed against gut flora are prescribed to minimize the risk of sepsis from transmural inflammation or microperforation. Lichtiger et al.[98] described the use of cyclosporine as an adjunct treatment in severe ulcerative colitis refractory to conventional therapy. Although colectomy was avoided in 81% of the 32 patients, the routine use of high-dose

immunosuppressants for toxic Crohn's colitis is unproved and controversial. Anticholinergics, antidiarrheals, and narcotics are avoided as they may aggravate impaired colonic motility or conceal ominous symptoms. Toxic colitis is a life-threatening condition that warrants aggressive medical therapy accompanied by early surgical consultation, even if an operation does not appear imminent, to minimize the morbidity and mortality of these often youthful patients.

Increasing colonic dilation, free perforation, massive hemorrhage, peritonitis, and septic shock are indications for emergent operation after the patient has been adequately resuscitated. Otherwise, hyperalimentation is begun and the patient is closely observed with serial examinations and abdominal roentgenograms. Any worsening of the clinical course over the ensuing 24 to 72 hours mandates urgent laparotomy. Furthermore, if the patient improves minimally after 5 to 7 days of conventional therapy, the colitis is considered refractory and surgery is advised as the probability of obtaining a remission is low.

The principal operative choices in toxic colitis complicating Crohn's disease include subtotal colectomy with end ileostomy and rectosigmoid mucous fistula, total proctocolectomy with end ileostomy, and loop ileostomy with decompressive blow-hole colostomy. In the past decade, of the 50 Crohn's disease patients presenting to the Cleveland Clinic with toxic colitis, 38 individuals were treated with colectomy and ileostomy, 4 underwent proctocolectomy, and 8 patients were sick enough to require loop ileostomy with decompressive blow-hole colostomy (unpublished data). Seven of the 8 undergoing this latter procedure had accompanying toxic megacolon. Overall, only 4 operative mortalities (8%) occurred in these Crohn's colitics, all of which had toxic megacolon.

Subtotal colectomy with end ileostomy and rectosigmoid mucous fistula is the most widely practiced operation for toxic colitis. Upon entering the abdomen, the dilated colon is decompressed to minimize the risk of iatrogenic perforation. A large-bore needle is inserted through a taenia coli into the bowel lumen with intermittent suctioning of the luminal gases performed. Following decompression, the colon is mobilized and its mesentery divided as previously described. The most difficult aspect of the procedure is managing the distal bowel stump; the friable nature of the severely inflamed colon wall risks dehiscence of any stump closure. In order to reduce operative morbidity, our usual practice is to divide the individual sigmoid vessels, instead of the vascular trunk, to facilitate delivery of the distal limb to the anterior abdominal wall. The sigmoid colon is then divided and closed with sutures or staples so that it might lie without tension in the subcutaneous fat of the lower midline wound. Prior to closure of the incision, the seromuscular layers of the now-closed bowel are circumferentially sutured to the surrounding fascia so as to exclude the rectosigmoid stump from the peritoneal cavity. If the closure dehisces during the postoperative period, a mucous fistula develops, whereas if the divided bowel is left intraperitoneal, a pelvic abscess would likely result. In those instances when the bowel wall is too friable to hold sutures or staples, a mucous fistula is created primarily. Rarely, instead of creating the fistula, the rectosigmoid stump must be exteriorized and wrapped in gauze to prevent retraction with a mucous fistula safely fashioned 7 to 10 days later.

After subtotal colectomy and end ileostomy, the patient typically demonstrates rapid improvement and eventually returns to good health despite the diseased rectum left behind. If the previously discussed criteria (i.e., degree of inflammation, rectal compliance, sphincter function, perianal disease) are favorable, intestinal continuity may be restored by ileoproctostomy 6 months later. Otherwise, the diseased rectum, if not too bothersome, may be left in place. Regarding the fate of the retained rectum, the individual is counseled about the risk of malignancy and annual surveillance is recommended.[80] However, in those individuals where the rectum remains diverted, ongoing inflammation with stricturing can make adequate inspection impossible. If recurrent small bowel disease necessitates laparotomy, proctectomy is concomitantly performed. Conversely, in an otherwise asymptomatic patient, completion proctectomy is suggested for cancer prophylaxis if rectal scarring or patient compliance does not permit appropriate surveillance.

Proctocolectomy with end ileostomy is rarely performed in the severely ill toxic colitic because of the excessive mortality (9% to 30%) and morbidity rates.[99–101] Proctectomy increases the complexity of the procedure and risks bleeding as well as autonomic nerve damage. In rare instances, such as rectal perforation, profuse colorectal hemorrhage, or in the less severely ill patient who would not be a candidate for future ileorectal anastomosis, proctocolectomy may have a role. The surgeon must be cautioned, however, that the macroscopic and microscopic differentiation of ulcerative colitis from Crohn's proctocolitis is especially difficult in the fulminant case. Primary proctocolectomy would nullify the future option of a pelvic pouch procedure in the ulcerative colitic.

With improved medical recognition and more sophisticated management of toxic colitis, the need for loop ileostomy combined with decompression blow-hole colostomy has all but disappeared. Developed and championed by Turnbull, this procedure markedly reduced the mortality associated with toxic megacolon in the 1960s.[15] The operation is valuable in extremely ill patients or those in whom colectomy would be particularly hazardous (e.g., contained perforation, high-lying splenic flexure, pregnancy). Contraindications to the procedure are associated colonic hemorrhage, intra-abdominal abdominal abscess, free perforation, or the colon that can be readily excised.

The decision to create an ileostomy and blow-hole colostomy is typically made preoperatively based on criteria mentioned above. Consequently, a relatively small infraumbilical midline incision is made for abdominal exploration. If no reason for a major laparotomy is detected, a segment of terminal ileum is selected and delivered through a transrectus incision in the right lower quadrant for the creation of a loop ileostomy. The location of the dilated transverse colon is marked on the epigastric midline and the lower abdominal wound closed. A separate vertical incision is then made over the colon measuring 4 to 6 cm in length. The incision is carried down into the peritoneal cavity with the seromuscular layer of the dilated colon sutured to the linea alba so as to quarantine the wound and a segment of colonic serosa from the remaining peritoneal cavity. The colon is then deflated with a large-bore needle and opened transversely. The mucosa is gently pulled to the skin margins, or subcutaneous fat if relatively immobile, and the blow-hole colostomy created. The loop ileostomy is then matured in a routine everting fashion.

The ileostomy and blow-hole colostomy is a temporizing operation, as is the previously mentioned subtotal colectomy, with a definitive procedure usually performed 6 months later.

Perforation

Free perforation of the small bowel usually occurs at or just proximal to a strictured site. The treatment alternatives include simple suture closure, resection with anastomosis, and resection with proximal ileostomy; the latter is the preferred choice. Greenstein et al.[102] reported a 41% and 4% mortality rate with simple suture and resection, respectively.

Management of large bowel perforation depends on the clinical scenario. If the perforation occurs with toxic colitis or megacolon, the colon and site of perforation must be resected, even if this mandates resection of a portion of rectum. If iatrogenic perforation occurs during colonoscopy for symptomatic disease, the diseased segment and site of perforation should be resected; an anastomosis with or without proximal diversion may be considered based on principles discussed earlier. If iatrogenic perforation occurs during colonoscopy for surveillance of disease, the site of perforation should be treated by suture closure or resected, with the latter procedure preferred.

Hemorrhage

Hemorrhage is an infrequent complication of Crohn's disease and may complicate both small bowel and colonic patterns of the disease. More commonly, entities unrelated to Crohn's disease involvement may lead to intestinal bleeding. Peptic ulcer disease is known to accompany Crohn's disease in as many as 15% of patients. In addition, aspirin-containing compounds and nonsteroidal anti-inflammatory drugs, which are frequently used by patients with Crohn's disease, may induce upper intestinal irritation, ulceration, and hemorrhage. Consequently, gastric aspiration and esphagogastroduodenoscopy are required to exclude sources of hemorrhage indirectly associated with Crohn's disease.

If the bleeding originates from a diseased segment within the small bowel, surgery has been notoriously difficult due to inexact methods of identifying the bleeding site. In older series, angiography was not frequently used; subsequently, rebleeding rates and mortalities were high.[103] Should massive hemorrhage occur from an ulcerated area within a portion of small intestine affected by extensive Crohn's disease, choosing the appropriate segment to resect may be extraordinarily difficult and ineffective. On the other hand, some authors[10] have reported a more favorable experience with wide resection.

Expertise with mesenteric angiography has greatly enhanced our ability to identify the small bowel bleeding site. Moreover, this diagnostic tool can become therapeutic once the site is identified. Selective angiographic infusion of vasopressin will often provide definitive control of the hemorrhage. Of 139 patients treated by strictureplasty (3.8 strictureplasties per patient), 13 (9.3%) bled in the early postoperative period from small bowel strictureplasty sites.[104] Although none of the patients required laparotomy, selective mesenteric infusion of vasopressin was necessary in two patients with identifiable bleeding.

In the preoperative patient in whom hemorrhage cannot be controlled with vasopressin, the mesenteric catheter is left in place so that intraoperative angiography can be done.[105] At surgery, metallic clips are placed at 25-cm intervals along the mesenteric margin of the bowel and intra-arterial contrast material injected. This enables accurate identification of the bleeding site with appropriately limited bowel resection.

Even if angiography is not available, laparotomy and resection with or without anastomosis is required if the patient's hemodynamic state cannot be sustained, when bleeding persists after 4 to 6 units of blood have been transfused, or if another indication for surgery exists.

Hemorrhage in Crohn's colitis is equally rare. Similar to small bowel bleeding, mesenteric angiography is currently the diagnostic procedure of choice for major colonic hemorrhage. But, because the colonoscope is being used with increasing frequency as a primary investigative tool for many forms of colonic hemorrhage, its use in colonic bleeding secondary to Crohn's disease must be considered. However, colonoscopy should be used discriminantly for bleeding Crohn's colitis because such hemorrhage in Crohn's disease is usually a manifestation of fulminant colitis. In this case, colectomy with ileostomy is advised regardless of the endoscopy that might risk perforation.

Unhealed Perineal Wound

Unhealed perineal wounds are defined as those in which the healing process has completely arrested 6 to 12 months following proctectomy. If a symptomatic perineal sinus persists after this time interval, intervention is warranted. Initial investigative studies should include a sinogram and small bowel follow-through roentgenograms to exclude the possibility of an enteroperineal fistula, especially with patients who require several pads each day to collect the sinus drainage. If a pelvic abscess is suspected, a CT scan is indicated. Adequate inspection of the area is often difficult in the office setting; therefore, examination of the perineum under anesthesia is usually necessary. At that time, biopsies of the sinus tract are obtained and reviewed for the presence of granulomas indicative of local Crohn's involvement. During this initial examination, the wound can be debrided of necrotic tissue and epithelium that impede proper healing.

A conservative operative approach to this difficult problem is surprisingly successful if the surgeon and, more important, the patient are diligent and fastidious in their care of the wound. Multiple visits to the operating suite for curettage of the fibrotic cavity walls coupled with daily home wound care utilizing a WaterPik will often promote healing, or at least size reduction, of the cavity. When the configuration and condition of the sinus are conducive, skin grafting has been quite successful.

However, some instances of a persistent perineal sinus mandate a more aggressive approach. In these cases, treatment is directed at obliteration of the thick-walled cavity, which is incapable of collapse. In the past, coccygectomy and distal sacrectomy permitted adequate mobilization of the perineal soft tissue into the pelvic space by eliminating the posterior bony boundary. However, this extensive procedure fell into disfavor as muscle and musculocutaneous flaps were described.[106] These vascular-based grafts have afforded the benefits of a single-stage procedure with a relatively high success rate and low morbidity. Only those local muscles whose use will not produce functional

impairment are utilized. Accordingly, the gracilis, gluteus maximus (inferior or superior half), gluteal thigh, and rectus abdominis muscle flaps are recommended for perineal reconstruction after thorough wound debridement. The particular flap of choice depends on muscle availability, wound size, and necessary skin coverage with muscle availability determined by the patient's position during the procedure, the status of the individual muscle's vascular pedicle, and the operative wound approach.

An enteroperineal fistula can exist with an existing perineal sinus or result from aggressive curettage of a nonfistulous sinus; injury to a loop of small bowel within the pelvis may create a fistula. Management of enteroperineal fistulae consists of laparotomy, mobilization of small bowel loops out of the pelvis, resection of the fistula source, and anastomosis. The sinus component, although detached from the enteric source, will commonly persist and may necessitate later treatment.

Diverticulitis

Although Crohn's disease typically begins in early adulthood, a bimodal distribution in the age of onset has been reported in a large number of epidemiologic studies; these older patients demonstrate a propensity for distal colonic involvement. As expected, diverticular disease is as common among elderly patients with Crohn's colitis as it is in the general elderly population. Therefore, a diagnostic dilemma occasionally ensues that may potentially lead to delays in diagnosis with misguided therapy. Clinically, the differentiation between these two entities is of great importance. The failure to recognize that presumed diverticulitis is actually Crohn's disease, or diverticulitis superimposed on pre-existing Crohn's disease, often leads to a suboptimal surgical outcome.[107]

Crohn's colitics and patients with diverticulitis may present with similar symptoms and signs of abdominal pain, constipation, fever, palpable mass, or fistulae. However, whereas Crohn's disease is usually indolent in its presentation, diverticulitis is typically acute. Additionally, rectal bleeding occurs in the majority of Crohn's colitics but rarely with diverticulitis. Physical examination with proctosigmoidoscopy may show perianal disease or evidence of proctitis suggestive of Crohn's disease. Radiologic studies may assist in the diagnostic process; although intramural defects and fistulae are common to both diseases, ulceration within the rectum or distant from the disease site are suggestive of Crohn's disease. Furthermore, longitudinal sinus tracts along the mesenteric aspect of the bowel, particularly greater than 10 cm in length, are more typical in Crohn's disease than diverticulitis.[108]

Berman et al.[109] at the Lahey Clinic reported on older patients with histologically proven diverticulitis and unsuspected Crohn's colitis. In their 25 patients, the concurrence of these two disease entities resulted in failure of diversionary treatment to improve the distal colonic disease (76%), multiple operations (68%), and frequent mortality secondary to pelvic sepsis (16%). Similarly, elderly patients with unrecognized Crohn's disease undergoing resection for presumed, yet absent, diverticulitis experience a high rate of complications including anastomotic dehiscence, sepsis, fistulization, and reoperation.[110] Obviously, if a patient fails to readily recover following a segmental resection for diverticulitis, the diagnosis of Crohn's disease should be entertained.

When operating for presumed diverticulitis, and Crohn's disease is actually encountered, the principles discussed earlier regarding segmental Crohn's colitis should be recalled with resection margins dictated by the disease distribution. Conversely, if diverticulitis is found superimposed on underlying Crohn's disease, the diverticulitis should also be appropriately addressed. In diverticulitis with Crohn's disease uncomplicated by abscess or free perforation, the bowel should be divided proximally where muscular hypertrophy and significant mucosal changes are no longer present and distally at the confluence of the tenia coli demarcating the proximal rectum; primary anastomosis may be considered. If an abscess is present and can be incorporated into the resected specimen without spillage, the same guidelines prevail; otherwise, as in the case of free perforation, only the directly involved segment needs resection with the creation of a colostomy and, if possible, a mucous fistula. If a primary anastomosis is constructed, the imperatives detailed earlier are critical. Temporary diversion should be carefully considered, particularly if the patient demonstrates moderate proctitis, malnutrition, or the need for high doses of steroids.

Ileal Reservoir

Deutsch et al.[111] from the University of Toronto published their experience on five patients found to have histologic evidence of Crohn's disease after the creation of a pelvic reservoir. With nearly 3 years of surveillance, two of the patients have lost their ileal pouches due to severe perianal disease whereas the other three patients remain asymptomatic. Grobler et al.[112] found complications, pouch excision, and persistent proximal ileostomy were more common in 20 patients with possible Crohn's disease compared to 61 patients with ulcerative colitis. Medich et al.[113] at the Cleveland Clinic were able to stratify their 59 patients treated by ileal pouch-anal anastomosis in whom the postoperative pathologic diagnosis was reported as Crohn's proctocolitis. They found a previous history of perianal disease or subtotal colectomy for toxicity was associated with a significant likelihood for pouch loss.

Therefore, total proctocolectomy with the creation of an ileal pouch and pouch-anal anastomosis is contraindicated in a patient with a preoperative diagnosis of Crohn's disease, regardless of the disease distribution. In addition, if a patient with ulcerative or indeterminate colitis has a history of perianal abscess, fistula-in-ano, or anal canal stenosis, Crohn's disease must be suspected and the patient cautioned against an ileal pelvic reservoir. Intraoperatively, the pouch procedure should be abandoned at the surgeon's discretion when signs of small bowel Crohn's disease are present or if the open specimen displays the macroscopic appearance of Crohn's colitis with skip lesions or "bear claw" ulcerations. When the postoperative pathologic review indicates unsuspected Crohn's disease after the creation of a pelvic reservoir for alleged ulcerative or indeterminate colitis, the pouch does not necessarily require excision; instead, the patient is counseled about the possible implications of this diagnosis. In this instance, the diverting loop ileostomy that was created at the time of the initial operation is closed after the customary 3-month interval assuming a preoperative contrast enema indicates no leaks from the ileal pouch and the patient has not demonstrated any extracolonic signs of Crohn's disease. If pouch excision is eventually necessary for

pouch involvement or perianal disease, loss of the 25 to 30 cm of terminal ileum used to construct the reservoir should have little impact on intestinal function. Absorption after excision of the ileal pouch for intestinal disease, however, will be influenced by the distribution and extent of the small bowel involvement.

For reasons similar to ileal pelvic reservoir, most surgeons do not advise constructing a continent ileostomy for patients afflicted with Crohn's proctocolitis necessitating operative treatment. Occasionally, a patient will be diagnosed with ulcerative colitis and then, after total proctocolectomy and the creation of a continent ileostomy, manifest symptoms or signs of Crohn's disease. Initial management of the disease is similar to any patient with symptomatic small bowel Crohn's disease (e.g., antibiotics, 5-aminosalicylic compounds, and/or steroids). If the continent ileostomy is involved, topical therapy can be delivered directly into the reservoir through the stoma. In the event that the ileal reservoir is diseased, excision with conversion to a conventional end ileostomy is recommended. However, if the Crohn's disease is limited to small bowel remote from the reservoir, therapy is directed toward the diseased segment and the continent ileostomy is undisturbed. Of 16 patients at the Cleveland Clinic with a continent ileostomy who were subsequently found to have Crohn's disease, 4 individuals developed fistulae and 8 eventually lost their reservoir secondary to symptomatic disease.[114] Barnett[115] had a comparable experience in 15 Crohn's disease patients, as 3 of the ostomates underwent pouch excision shortly after its construction. Kock et al.[116] and Dozois et al.[117] have reported similarly disappointing outcomes. Most recently, Handelsman et al.[118] published their results with 100 consecutive continent ileostomies. All 8 of the patients with indeterminate or Crohn's colitis suffered complications whereas only 17 of the 87 ulcerative colitics had difficulties.

Despite these findings, Bloom et al.[119] have advocated the creation of a continent ileostomy in select patients with Crohn's disease. Operating only on those individuals who had been off systemic steroids and free of symptoms for a minimum of 5 years, they described good results in seven Crohn's disease patients with a continent ileostomy after 4 to 50 months of follow-up. With a longer postoperative interval, this success may lessen. Clearly, the continent ileostomy should be considered in few patients with known Crohn's disease and then only after preoperative counseling regarding potential disease recurrence.

RECURRENCE

The single most frustrating issue in the management of a patient afflicted by Crohn's disease is the incurable nature of the disorder. Although up to 90% of individuals with Crohn's disease will ultimately fail appropriate medical therapy and need operative treatment, the majority of this latter group will experience a recurrence of their disease. The risk of reoperation is greatest in the first 5 postoperative years with 40% to 70% of patients requiring at least one additional procedure by 15 years.[120–122] Despite universal acknowledgment of this characteristic disease recurrence, controversy exists. The confusion originates, in part, from the accepted definition of "recurrence." Depending on the study cited, "recurrence" may be defined as endoscopic, clinical, or reoperation recurrence. Regardless, the type of operative procedure and length of follow-up significantly influence reported recurrence rates. For example, bypass of the disease segment is known to have a significantly higher recurrence rate compared to resection; therefore, inclusion of these patients will distort the reported operative outcome.

Albeit controversial, an increased risk for recurrence has been suggested to be directly influenced by the site and pattern of disease, early age of disease onset, and short duration of disease prior to resection. The risk for recurrent disease requiring an operation appears to be least for colonic Crohn's disease and greatest for patients with ileocolic involvement.[120] On the other hand, symptomatic recurrence has been reported as highest in the large intestine group undergoing segmental resection and least in the patients with a small bowel disease pattern.[122] This apparent disparity may be explained by Koch et al.[123] who found ileal disease tends to recur proximal to an anastomosis and colonic disease distal to the same, independent of initial disease distribution.

Resection With Ileocolostomy

After a decade of follow-up, small bowel disease and ileocolic disease have reoperation rates of 29% and 44%, respectively.[124] With comparable surveillance, Scammell et al.[125] found a 35% recurrence rate after small bowel resection. As elaborated earlier, resection margins and type of procedure may artificially skew the observed recurrence rates, particularly for small bowel involvement.

Resection With Colocolostomy or Coloproctostomy

Segmental colonic disease treated by limited resection with colocolonic or colorectal anastomosis for Crohn's disease of the large bowel has been described by a number of institutions over the past 3 decades (Table 33-3). Although the majority of patients will experience symptomatic recurrence, over 75% will maintain intestinal continuity for more than a decade after their initial resection with anastomosis. Despite the symptomatic recurrence rate, it is important to recall that segmental colonic resection delays the need for permanent ileostomy and partially conserves a portion of the the large intestine's functional absorbing surface.

Table 33-3. Operative Recurrence After Segmental Resection and Anastomosis

Authors	No. Patients	Recurrence (%)	Follow-Up (Years)
Howel Jones et al. (1966)[129]	18	22	1–10
de Dombal et al. (1971)[120]	42	37	15
Sanfey et al. (1984)[130]	13	8	7
Stern et al. (1984)[131]	5	20	5
Longo et al. (1988)[132]	18	62	5
Allan et al. (1989)[133]	36	66	15

Table 33-4. Operative Recurrence After Colectomy and Anastomosis

Authors	No. Patients	Recurrence (%)	Follow-Up (Years)
Flint et al. (1977)[134]	37	41	6
Buchman et al. (1981)[135]	105	30	8
Ambrose et al. (1984)[136]	63	48	10
Goligher et al. (1988)[137]	47	49	15
Allan et al. (1989)[133]	63	53	15
Longo et al. (1992)[126]	131	65	10

Resection With Ileoproctostomy

Crohn's colitis with relative rectal sparing can be adequately treated by colectomy with ileoproctostomy as described earlier. Longo et al.[126] reviewed the Cleveland Clinic's experience utilizing this technique. The procedure was safely performed in 131 patients over a 26-year period. After an average 10 years of follow-up, 65% of patients maintained intestinal continuity with a functioning ileoproctostomy. Chevalier et al.[127] similarly reported the cumulative proportion of patients with a functioning ileoproctostomy to be 77% and 63% at 5 and 10 years, respectively. The success of this operation is independent of patient age and duration of symptoms, but inversely linked, in part, to the presence of concomitant small bowel disease at the time of anastomosis. Many other authors have reported similar favorable findings (Table 33-4).

Colostomy for Proctitis

In appropriately selected patients, the operative recurrence rate following colostomy for isolated rectal disease is comparable to that of ileostomy for proctocolitis (Table 33-5).

Ileostomy for Proctocolitis

One of the most common components of Crohn's disease that manifests itself following proctocolectomy is recurrence of disease in the ileostomy or remaining small bowel. Scammell et al.[128] reported a 19% and 24% cumulative reoperative rate for recurrence at 5 and 10 years, respectively. The majority (89%) of recurrences occurred within 25 cm of the stoma. Although the rates vary, these values largely agree with the experience of others.[37]

Table 33-5. Operative Recurrence After Proctectomy and Colostomy

Author	No. Patients	Recurrence (%)	Follow-Up (Years)
Ritchie et al. (1973)[39]	24	11	10
Stern et al. (1984)[131]	7	0	5

REFERENCES

1. Mekhijian HS, Sweitz DM, Watts HD et al (1979) National cooperative Crohn's disease study: factors determining recurrence of Crohn's disease after surgery. Gastroenterology 77: 907–913

2. Farmer RG, Hawk WA, Turnbull RB Jr (1976) Indications for surgery in Crohn's disease: analysis of 500 cases. Gastroenterology 71:245–250

3. Korelitz BI, Present DH (1985) Favorable affect of 6-mercaptopurine in fistulae of Crohn's disease. Dig Dis Sci 30:58–64

4. O'Brien JJ, Bayless TM, Bayless JA (1991) Use of azathioprine or 6-mercaptopurine in the treatment of Crohn's disease. Gastroenterology 101:39–46

5. Michelassi F, Testa G, Pomidor WJ et al (1993) Adenocarcinoma complicating Crohn's disease. Dis Colon Rectum 36: 654–661

6. Homer DR, Grand RJ, Colodny AH (1977) Growth, course and prognosis after surgery for Crohn's disease in children and adolescents. Pediatrics 59:717–725

7. Abscal J, Diaz-Rojas F, Jorge J et al (1982) Free perforation of the small bowel in Crohn's disease. World J Surg 6:216–220

8. Bundred NJ, Dixon JM, Lumsden AB et al (1985) Free perforation in Crohn's colitis: a ten-year review. Dis Colon Rectum 28:35–37

9. Softley A, Camp SE, Bouchier IAD et al (1988) Perforation of the intestine in inflammatory bowel disease. An OMGE survey. Scand J Gastroenterol, 23,(suppl. 144):24–26

10. Homan WP, Tang CK, Thorbjarnason B (1976) Acute massive hemorrhage from intestinal Crohn's disease. Arch Surg 111:901–905

11. Driscoll RH, Rosenberg IH (1978) Total parenteral nutrition in inflammatory bowel disease. Med Clin North Am 62: 185–201

12. Lashner BA, Evans AA, Hanauer SB (1989) Preoperative total parenteral nutrition for bowel resection in Crohn's disease Dig Dis Sci 34:741–746

13. Homan WP, Dineen P (1978) Comparison of the results of resection, bypass and bypass with exclusion for ileocecal Crohn's disease. Ann Surg 187:530–538

14. Faintunch J, Levin B, Kirsner JB (1985) Inflammatory bowel disease and their relationship to malignancy. Crit Rev Oncol Hematol 2:323

15. Turnbull RJ, Jr, Hawk WA, Weakley FL (1971) Surgical treatment of toxic megacolon—ileostomy and colostomy to prepare patients for colectomy. Am J Surg 122:325–331

16. Alexander-Williams J, Fielding JF, Cooke WT (1972) A comparison of results of excision and bypass for ileal Crohn's disease. Gut 13:973–974

17. Berman L, Krause U (1977) Crohn's disease: A long-term study of the clinical course. Scand J Gastroenterol 12:937

18. Karesen R, Serch-Hansen A, Thorensen BO, Hertzberg J (1981) Crohn's disease: long-term results of surgical management. Scand J Gastroenterol 16:57

19. Lindhager T, Ekelund G, Leandeer L et al (1983) Crohn's disease in a defined population; course and results of surgical treatment. I. Small bowel disease. Acta Chir Scand 149: 407–413

20. Papaioannau N, Piris J, Lee ECG, Kettlewell MGW (1979) The relationship between histological inflammation in the cut ends after resection of Crohn's disease and recurrence. Gut 20:A916

21. Pennington L, Hamilton SR, Bayless TM, Cameron JL (1980) Surgical management of Crohn's disease. Influence of disease at margin of resection. Ann Surg 192:311–318

22. Chardavayne R, Flint GW, Pollack S, Wise L (1986) Factors affecting recurrence following resection for Crohn's disease. Dis Colon Rectum 29:495–502

23. Speranza V, Zimi M, Leardi S, DelPap M (1986) Recurrence of Crohn's disease: Are there any risk factors? J Clin Gastroenterol 8:640–646

24. Adolff M, Armaud JP, Ollier JC (1987) Does the histological appearance at the margin of resection affect the postoperative recurrence rate in Crohn's disease? Am Surg 53:543–546

25. Heuman R, Boeryd B, Bolin T, Sjodahl R (1983) The influence of disease at the margin of resection on the outcome of Crohn's disease. Br J Surg 70:519–521

26. Hamilton SR, Reese J, Pennington L et al (1985) The role of resection margin frozen section in the surgical management of Crohn's disease. Surg Gynecol Obstet 160:57–62

27. Kotanagi H, Kramer K, Fazio VW, Petras RE (1991) Do microscopic abnormalities at resection margins correlate with increased anastomotic recurrence in Crohn's disease? Retrospective analysis of 100 cases. Dis Colon Rectum 34: 909–916

27a. Fazio VW, Marchetti F, Church JM et al (1996) Effect of resection margins on the recurrence of Crohn's disease in the small bowel. A randomized controlled trial. Ann Surg 224: 563–573

28. Scott NA, Sue-Ling HM, Hughes LE (1995) Anastomotic configuration does not affect recurrence of Crohn's disease after ileocolonic resection. Int J Colorectal Dis 10:67–69

29. Katariya RN, Sood S, Rao PG et al (1977) Strictureplasty for tubercular strictures of the gastrointestinal tract. Br J Surg 64:496–498

30. Lee ECG, Papaioannou N (1982) Minimal surgery for chronic obstruction in patients with extensive or universal Crohn's disease. Ann R Coll Surg Engl 64:229–233

31. Ozuner G, Fazio VW, Lavery IC et al (1996) How safe is strictureplasty in the management of Crohn's disease? Am J Surg 171:57–60

32. Tjandra JJ, Fazio VW (1992) Techniques of Strictureplasty, WB Saunders, Philadelphia

33. Post S, Herfarth C, Schumacher H et al (1995) Experience with ileostomy and colostomy in Crohn's disease. Br J Surg 82:1629–1633

34. Nugent FW, Roy MA (1989) Duodenal Crohn's disease: an analysis of 89 cases. Am J Gastroenterol 84:249–254

35. Danzi JT, Farmer RG, Sullivan BH Jr et al (1976) Endoscopic features of gastroduodenal Crohn's disease. Gastroenterology 70:9–13

36. Block GE (1980) Surgical management of Crohn's colitis. N Engl J Med 302:1068–1070

37. Goligher JC (1985) The long-term results of excisional surgery for primary and recurrent Crohn's disease of the large bowel. Dis Colon Rectum 28:51–55

38. Keighley MRB, Buchmann P, Lee JR (1982) Assessment of

anorectal function in selection of patients for ileo-rectal anastomosis in Crohn's colitis. Gut 23:102–107

39. Ritchie JK, Lockhart-Mummery HE (1973) Non-restorative surgery in the treatment of Crohn's disease of the large bowel. Gut 14:263–269

40. Leicaster RJ, Ritchie JK, Wadsworth J et al (1984) Sexual function and perineal wound healing after intersphincteric excision of the rectum for inflammatory bowel disease. Dis Colon Rectum 27:244–248

41. Sher ME, Bauer JJ, Gorfine S, Gelernt I (1992) Low Hartmann's procedure for severe anorectal Crohn's disease. Dis Colon Rectum 35:975–980

42. Winslet MC, Andrews H, Allan RN, Keighley MR (1993) Fecal diversion in the management of Crohn's disease of the colon. Dis Colon Rectum 36:757–762

43. Wolff BG (1986) Crohn's disease: the role of surgical treatment. Mayo Clin Proc 61:292–295

44. Heuman R, Bolin T, Sjodahl R, Tagesson C (1981) The incidence and course of perianal complications and arthralgia after intestinal resection with restoration of continuity for Crohn's disease. Br J Surg 68:528–560

45. Hellers G, Bergstrand O, Ewerth S, Holmstrom B (1980) Occurrence and outcome after primary treatment of anal fistulae in Crohn's disease. Gut 21:525–527

46. Orkin BA, Telander RL (1985) The effect of intra-abdominal resection or fecal diversion on perianal Crohn's disease in pediatric Crohn's disease. J Pediatr Surg 20:343–347

47. Buchmann P, Keighley MRB, Allan RN et al (1980) Natural history of perianal Crohn's disease. Ten year follow-up: a plea for conservation. Am J Surg 140:642–644

48. Marks CG, Richie JK, Lockhart-Mummery HE (1981) Anal fistulas in Crohn's disease. Br J Surg 68:525–527

49. Jeffery PJ, Ritchie JK, Parks AG (1977) Treatment of hemorrhoids in patients with inflammatory bowel disease. Lancet 1:1084–1085

50. Fry RD, Shemesh EI, Kodner IJ, Timmcke A (1989) Techniques and results in the management of anal and perianal Crohn's disease. Surg Gynecol Obstet 168:42–48

51. Levien DH, Surrell J, Mazier WP (1989) Surgical treatment of anorectal fistulas in Crohn's disease. Surg Gynecol Obstet 169:133–136

52. Fuhrman GM, Larach SW (1989) Experience with perirectal fistulas in patients with Crohn's disease. Dis Colon Rectum 32:847–848

53. Sohn N, Korelitz BI, Weinstein MA (1980) Anorectal Crohn's disease: definitive surgery for fistulas and recurrent abscesses. Am J Surg 139:394–397

54. Scott A, Hawley PR, Phillips RK (1989) Results of external sphincter repair in Crohn's disease. Br J Surg 76:959–960

55. Makowiec F, Jehle EC, Becker HD, Starlinger M (1995) Clinical course after transanal advancement flap repair of perianal fistula in patients with Crohn's disease. Br J Surg 82:603–606

56. Williams JG, Rothenberger DA, Nemer FD, Goldberg SM (1991) Fistula-in-ano in Crohn's disease. Dis Colon Rectum 34:378–384

57. Crim RW, Fazio VW, Lavery IC (1990) Rectal advancement flap repair in Crohn's patients—factors predictive of failure. Dis Colon Rectum 33:P3

58. White RA, Eisenstat TE, Rubin RJ, Salvati EP (1990) Seton management of complex anorectal fistulas in patients with Crohn's disease. Dis Colon Rectum 33:587–589

59. van Dongen LM, Lubbers EJC (1986) Perianal fistulas in patients with Crohn's disease. Arch Surg 121:1187–1190

60. Keighley MRB, Allan RN (1986) Current status and influence of operation on perianal Crohn's disease. Int J Colorectal Dis 1:104–107

61. Fry RD, Kodner IJ (1989) Management of anal and perineal Crohn's disease. Infect Surg 209–219

62. Hesterberg R, Schmidt WU, Muller F, Roher HD (1993) Treatment of anovaginal fistulas with an anocutaneous flap in patients with Crohn's disease. Int J Colorectal Dis 8:51–54

63. Fazio VW, Jones IT, Jagelman DG, Weakley FL (1987) Rectourethral fistulae in Crohn's disease. Surg Gynecol Obstet 164:148–150

64. Ribeiro HB (1991) Intra-abdominal abscess in regional enteritis. Ann Surg 213:32

65. Michelassi F, Finco C (1995) Indications for surgery in inflammatory bowel disease: The surgical perspective. pp. 771–783. In Kirsner JB, Shorter RG (eds): Inflammatory bowel disease. Williams & Wilkins, Baltimore

66. Nagler SM, Poticha SM (1979) Intra-abdominal abscess in regional enteritis. Am J Surg 137:350–354

67. Greenstein AJ (1987) The surgery of Crohn's disease. Surg Clin North Am 67:573–596

68. Broe PJ, Bayless TM, Cameron JL (1982) Crohn's disease: are enteroenteral fistulas an indication for surgery? Surgery 91:249

69. Fazio VW, Wilk PJ, Turnbull RB Jr, Jagelman DG (1977) Ileosigmoidal fistula complicating Crohn's disease. Dis Colon Rectum 20:381–386

70. Glass RE, Ritchie JK, Lennard-Jones J et al (1985) Internal fistulas in Crohn's disease. Dis Colon Rectum 28:557–561

71. McNamara MJ, Fazio VW, Lavery IC et al (1990) Surgical treatment of enterovesical fistulas in Crohn's disease. Dis Colon Rectum 33:271–276

72. Schraut WM, Chapman C, Abraham VS (1988) Operative treatment of Crohn's ileocolitis complicated by ileosigmoid and ileovesical fistulae. Ann Surg 207:48–51

73. Greenstein AJ, Sachar DB, Smith H et al (1981) A comparison of cancer risk in Crohn's disease and ulcerative colitis. Cancer 48:2742–2745

74. Hawker PC, Gyde SN, Thompson H, Allan RN (1982) Adenocarcinoma of the small intestine complicating Crohn's disease. Gut 23:188–193

75. Greenstein AJ, Sachar DB, Pucillo A et al (1978) Cancer in Crohn's disease after diversionary surgery. Am J Surg 135:86–90

76. Gyde SN, Prior P, McCartney JC et al (1980) Malignancy in Crohn's disease. Gut 21:1024–1029

77. Weedon DD, Shorter RG, Ilstrup DM et al (1973) Crohn's disease and cancer. N Engl J Med 289:1099–1103

78. Greenstein AJ, Sachar DB, Smith H et al (1980) Patterns of neoplasia in Crohn's disease and ulcerative colitis. Cancer 46:403–407

79. Hamilton SR (1985) Colorectal carcinoma in patients with Crohn's disease. Gastroenterology 89:398–407

80. Lavery IC, Jagelman DG (1982) Cancer in the excluded rectum following surgery for inflammatory bowel disease. Dis Colon Rectum 25:522–524

81. Shorter RG (1983) Risk of intestinal cancer in Crohn's disease. Dis Colon Rectum 26:686–689

82. Victor DW Jr, Thompson H, Allan RN, Alexander-Williams J (1982) Cancer complicating defunctioned Crohn's disease. Clin Oncol 8:163–165

83. Ekbom A, Helmick C, Zack M, Admami HO (1990) Increased risk of large bowel cancer in Crohn's disease with colonic involvement. Lancet 336:357–359

84. Munkholm P, Langholz E, Davidsen M, Binder V (1993) Intestinal cancer risk and mortality in patients with Crohn's disease. Gastroenterology 105:1716–1723

85. Persson P-G, Karlen P, Bernell O (1994) Crohn's disease and cancer: a population-based cohort study. Gastroenterology 107:1675–1679

86. Glick SN, Teplick SK, Goodman LR et al (1984) Development of lymphoma in patients with Crohn's disease. Radiology 153:337–339

87. Lofberg R, Brostrom O, Karlen P et al (1990) Colonoscopic surveillance in longstanding total ulcerative colitis—a fifteen year follow-up study. Gastroenterology 99:1021–1031

88. Richards ME, Rickert RR, Nance FC (1989) Crohn's disease-associated carcinoma: a poorly recognized complication of inflammatory bowel disease. Ann Surg 209:764–773

89. Petras RE, Mir-Madjilessi SH, Farmer RG (1987) Crohn's disease and intestinal carcinoma. Gastroenterology 93:1307–1314

90. Simpson S, Traube J, Ridell RH (1981) The histologic appearance of dysplasia (precancerous change) in Crohn's disease of the small and large intestine. Gastroenterology 81:492–501

91. Korelitz BI, Lauwers GY, Sommers SC (1990) Rectal mucosal dysplasia in Crohn's disease. Gut 31:1382–1386

92. Lofberg R, Brostrom O, Karlen P et al (1991) Carcinoma and DNA aneuploidy in Crohn's colitis—a histological and flow cytometric study. Gut 32:900–904

93. Yamazaki Y, Ribeiro MB, Sachar DB et al (1991) Malignant strictures in Crohn's disease. Am J Gastroenterol 86:882–885

94. Trnka YM, Glotzer DJ, Kasdon EJ et al (1982) The long-term outcome of restorative operation in Crohn's disease. Influence of location, prognostic factors, and surgical guidelines. Ann Surg 196:345–355

95. Tjandra JJ, Fazio VW (1993) Strictureplasty for ileocolic anastomotic strictures in Crohn's disease. Dis Colon Rectum 36:1099–1103

96. Blomberg B, Rolny P, Jarnerot G (1991) Endoscopic treatment of anastomotic strictures in Crohn's disease. Endoscopy 23:195–198

97. Breysem Y, Janssens JF, Coremans G et al (1992) Endoscopic balloon dilation of colonic and ileocolonic Crohn's strictures: long-term results. Gastrointest Endosc 38:142–147

98. Lichtiger S, Present DH, Kornbluth A et al (1994) Cyclosporine in severe ulcerative colitis refractory to steroid therapy. N Engl J Med 330:1841–1845

99. Scott HW, Sawyers JL, Gobbel WG Jr et al (1974) Surgical management of toxic dilatation of the colon in ulcerative colitis. Ann Surg 179:647–656

100. Binder SC, Miller HH, Deterling RA Jr (1975) Emergency and urgent operations for ulcerative colitis; the procedure of choice. Arch Surg 110:284–289

101. Koudahl G, Kristensen M (1975) Toxic megacolon in ulcerative colitis. Scand J Gastroenter 10:471–421

102. Greenstein AJ, Sachar DB, Mann D et al (1987) Spontaneous free perforation and perforated abscess in 30 patients with Crohn's disease. Ann Surg 205:72–76

103. Sparberg M, Kirsner J (1966) Recurrent hemorrhage in regional enteritis. Report of 3 cases. Am J Dig Dis 2:652–657

104. Ozuner G, Fazio VW (1995) Management of gastrointestinal hemorrhage after strictureplasty for Crohn's disease. Dis Colon Rectum 38:297–300

105. Fazio VW, Zelas P, Weakley FL (1980) Intraoperative angiography and the localization of bleeding from the small intestine. Surg Gynecol Obstet 151:637–640

106. Mann CV, Springall R (1986) Use of a muscle graft for unhealed perineal sinus. Br J Surg 73:1000–1007

107. Hoffman WA, Rosenberg MA (1972) Granulomatous colitis in the elderly. Am J Gastroenterol 58:508–512

108. Marshak RH, Lindner AE, Pochaczevsky R et al (1976) Longitudinal sinus tracts in granulomatous colitis and diverticulitis. Semin Roentgenol 11:101

109. Berman IR, Corman ML, Coller JA et al (1979) Late onset Crohn's disease in patients with colonic diverticulitis. Dis Colon Rectum 22:524

110. Schmidt GT, Lennard-Jones JE, Morson BC et al (1968) Crohn's disease of the colon and its distinction from diverticulitis. Gut 9:7

111. Deutsch AA, McLeod RS, Cullen J, Cohen Z (1991) Results of the pelvic-pouch procedure in patients with Crohn's disease. Dis Colon Rectum 34:475–477

112. Grobler SP, Hosie KB, Affie E et al (1993) Outcome of restorative proctocolectomy when the diagnosis is suggestive of Crohn's disease. Gut 34:1384–1388

113. Medich DS, Ziv Y, Oakley JR, Strong SA (1994) Determinants of failed ileal pouch-anal anastomosis for unsuspected Crohn's disease. Dis Colon Rectum 37:P2–P3

114. Fazio VW, Church JM (1988) Complications and function of the continent ileostomy at the Cleveland Clinic. World J Surg 12:148–154

115. Barnett WO (1989) Current experiences with the continent intestinal reservoir. Surg Gynecol Obstet 168:1–5

116. Kock NG, Myrvold HE, Nilsson LO (1980) Progress report on the continent ileostomy. World J Surg 4:143–148

117. Dozois RR, Kelly KA, Beart RW (1980) Improved results with the continent ileostomy. Ann Surg 193:319–324

118. Handelsman JC, Gottlieb LM, Hamilton SR (1993) Crohn's disease as a contraindication to Kock pouch (continent ileostomy). Dis Colon Rectum 36:840–843

119. Bloom RJ, Larsen CP, Watt R, Oberhelman HA Jr (1986) A reappraisal of the Kock continent ileostomy in patients with Crohn's disease. Surg Gynecol Obstet 162:105–108

120. de Dombal FT, Burton I, Goligher JC (1971) Recurrence of Crohn's disease after primary excisional surgery. Gut 12:519–527

121. Farmer RG, Hawk WA, Turnbull RB (1975) Clinical patterns

in Crohn's disease: a statistical study of 615 cases. Gastroenterology 68:627–635

122. Himal HS, Belliveau P (1981) Prognosis after surgical treatment for granulomatous enteritis and colitis. Am J Surg 142: 347–349

123. Koch TR, Cave DR, Ford H, Kirsner JB (1981) Crohn's ileitis and ileocolitis. A study of the anatomical distribution of recurrence. Dig Dis Sci 26:528–531

124. Lock MR, Farmer RG, Fazio VW et al (1981) Recurrence and reoperation for Crohn's disease: the role of disease location in prognosis. N Engl J Med 304:1586–1588

125. Scammell BE, Ambrose NS, Alexander-Williams J et al (1985) Recurrent small bowel Crohn's disease is more frequent after sub-total colectomy and ileorectal anastomosis than panproctocolectomy. Dis Colon Rectum 28:770–771

126. Longo WE, Oakley JR, Lavery IC et al (1992) Outcome of ileorectal anastomosis for Crohn's colitis. Dis Colon Rectum 35:1066–1071

127. Chevalier JM, Jones DJ, Ratelle R et al (1994) Colectomy and ileorectal anastomosis in patients with Crohn's disease. Br J Surg 81:1379–1381

128. Scammell BE, Andrews H, Allan RN et al (1987) Results of proctocolectomy for Crohn's disease. Br J Surg 74:671–674

129. Howel Jones J, Lennard-Jones JE, Lockhart-Mummery HE (1966) Experience in the treatment of Crohn's disease of the large intestine. Gut 7:448–452

130. Sanfey H, Bayless TM, Corman JL (1984) Crohn's disease of the colon. Is there a role for limited resection? Am J Surg 147:38–42

131. Stern HS, Goldberg SM, Rothenberger MD et al (1984) Segmental versus total colectomy for large bowel Crohn's disease. World J Surg 8:118–122

132. Longo WE, Ballantyne GH, Cahow E (1988) Treatment of Crohn's colitis. Segmental or total colectomy? Arch Surg 123:588–590

133. Allan A, Andrews MB, Hilton CJ et al (1989) Segmental colonic resection is an appropriate operation for short skip lesions due to Crohn's disease in the colon. World J Surg 13: 611–616

134. Flint G, Strauss R, Platt N, Wise L (1977) Ileorectal anastomosis in patients with Crohn's disease of the colon. Gut 18: 236–239

135. Buchmann P, Weterman IT, Keighley MR et al (1981) The prognosis of ileorectal anastomosis in Crohn's disease. Br J Surg 68:7–10

136. Ambrose NS, Keighley MRB, Alexander-Williams J, Allan RN (1984) Clinical impact of colectomy and ileo-rectal anastomosis in the management of Crohn's disease. Gut 25: 223–227

137. Goligher JC (1988) Surgical treatment of Crohn's disease affecting mainly or entirely the large bowel. World J Surg 12:186–190

34

INFECTIVE DISEASES

Michael J. G. Farthing

Intestinal infections are the most common disorders of the gastrointestinal tract worldwide. Prevalence is highest in the developing world where water quality and sewage disposal are often inadequate, but during the past 10 to 20 years there has been a progressive increase in infectious diarrheas in the United Kingdom and other European countries and in North America.[1] This relates in part to an increase in foodborne bacterial and viral enteropathogens and also to the increase in foreign travel, such that 300 million people leave their country of domicile each year, 30 million of whom travel to the developing world.[2] At least 30% of these individuals can expect to suffer an episode of infective diarrhea. The importance of opportunistic infection in the gastrointestinal tract has been highlighted by the continued spread of the human immunodeficiency virus (HIV) epidemic and the increasing use of anticancer drugs.

Many infections of the gastrointestinal tract are short-lived and generally not confused with nonspecific inflammatory bowel disease or other organic disorders of the gastrointestinal tract. However, other infections, particularly those due to invasive enteropathogens that cause ileocolitis, may mimic ulcerative colitis or Crohn's disease and thus it is essential to distinguish rapidly between these conditions because inappropriate use of corticosteroids or delay in administering an antibiotic is highly undesirable. In the past, misdiagnosis of amebiasis has occurred with inappropriate use of corticosteroids or colectomy, on some occasions leading to litigation. Intestinal tuberculosis continues to increase in the United Kingdom and in other Western countries and in its most common form, ileocecal tuberculosis, it may easily be confused with Crohn's disease.[3] Some self-limiting infectious colitides will resolve despite administration of corticosteroid and salicylate drugs, but it would be wrong to commit such an individual to maintenance therapy when future problems would not be anticipated. An accurate prognosis clearly demands precision in diagnosis.

Thus, although 20 to 30 years ago diarrheal disease in the southern hemisphere was largely infective and inflammatory bowel disease and colon cancer relatively rare, the distinction is now less clear with intestinal infections becoming more common in industrialized societies and nonspecific inflammatory bowel disease being increasingly recognized in many developing countries. Thus, it is now essential to confidently exclude intestinal infection in all patients presenting with diarrhea, including patients with known inflammatory bowel disease who are in relapse. Intestinal tuberculosis should always be considered in obstructive ileocecal disease particularly, in Asian immigrants, and infectious proctitis is now increasingly recognized.

EPIDEMIOLOGY OF INTESTINAL INFECTION

Reservoirs

The relative prevalence of the different intestinal infections depends on geographic location. However, infections such as amebiasis and giardiasis, which are usually regarded as tropical infections, are now well established in Europe and North America, although prevalence is substantially lower than in many regions of the developing world. The reservoirs of human gastrointestinal infection are predominantly other humans and in some instances animals. Infection such as shigellosis and amebiasis are restricted exclusively to humans, whereas *Salmonella enteritidis* and *Campylobacter jejuni* are found in 70% to 80% of factory-reared chickens in the United Kingdom, and appear to be the main vehicle for the dramatic increase in reporting of these infections.[4] The protozoan *Cryptosporidium parvum* is common in cattle and readily transmitted to healthy farm workers. There is increasing evidence to suggest that *Giardia lamblia* is carried by a variety of wild and domestic animals and that the same strains may be the source of human infection. Human reservoirs include not only individuals with symptomatic infection but also asymptomatic healthy carriers, examples of the latter being *E. histolytica*, *G. lamblia*, and *Salmonella* spp.

Transmission

Spread of intestinal infection is usually always by the fecal-oral route. This may occur through a vehicle such as water or food, or by direct person-to-person contact. Water may become

Table 34-1. Microbial Pathogens Responsible for Food Poisoning

Organism	Source	Incubation Period (h)	Symptoms	Recovery
Bacteria that colonize the gut				
Salmonella sp.	Eggs, poultry	12–48	Diarrhea, blood, pain, vomiting, fever	2–14 days
Campylobacter jejuni	Milk, poultry	48–168	As above	7–21 days
Vibrio parahaemolyticus	Seafood	2–48	As above (blood less common)	2–10 days
Yersinia enterocolitica	Milk, pork	2–144	Diarrhea, fever, pain	2–30 days
Clostridium perfringens	Spores in food, especially meat	8–22	Diarrhea, pain	1–3 days
Preformed toxins				
Staphylococcus aureus	Transmitted to food by humans	2–6	Nausea, vomiting, pain (diarrhea)	Few hours
Bacillus cereus	Spores in food, reheated rice	1–2	As above	Few hours
Clostridium botulinum	Spores in home-bottled or home-canned food	18–36	Transient, diarrhea paralysis	10–14 days

contaminated either directly by human contact or indirectly through inadequate separation of water supplies and sewage systems. Giardiasis and cryptosporidiosis have entered domestic water supplies and caused major outbreaks, in some instances affecting many thousands of individuals. The cysts of both organisms are able to survive in municipal water supplies despite adequate chlorination. Swimming pools have also been described as a source of these infections. Recently outbreaks of dysentery have been described in swimmers in freshwater lakes in Oregon. The organisms responsible were *Shigella* spp. and enterohemorrhagic *Escherichia coli* 0157:H7, which produces an illness indistinguishable from ulcerative colitis.

Chicken carcasses are commonly contaminated with *Salmonella* sp. and *Campylobacter* sp. but the organisms will be destroyed by adequate cooking. However, some bacteria may survive on the hands of a food preparer and then be transferred to uncooked salads, fruit, or vegetables by direct contact. *Salmonella* spp. infect not only the intestinal tract of chickens but also the genital tract, thus allowing the organisms to be included in chicken eggs. Providing eggs are stored at 4°C and then adequately cooked this does not usually cause a problem, although outbreaks are well recognized to occur in foods in which eggs are used raw or only partially cooked. A variety of other bacteria and bacterial toxins are responsible for food poisoning (Table 34-1).

Person-to-person transmission occurs commonly between infants and young children in daycare centers, schools, and other residential institutions. Infections such as giardiasis and shigellosis, which require relatively few organisms to transmit the disease, are among the most common. Many enteropathogens can be transmitted during sexual contact, and this has been described most clearly in homosexual men in whom many of the common enteropathogens are found more commonly than in a heterosexual population, irrespective of whether they are infected with HIV or have diarrhea.

High-Risk Groups

Although no individual is excluded from acquiring intestinal infection, a number of groups within the general population have been identified as being at increased risk.

Infants and Young Children

Infective diarrhea is most common in infants and young children with an estimated worldwide incidence of 1 billion attacks of acute diarrhea per year. Despite improvements in public health infrastructures and case management, more than 3 million preschool children die each year of intestinal infections. In most industrialized countries, and in many countries in the developing world, rotavirus is responsible for 30% to 60% of acute diarrhea episodes, followed closely in the developing world by enterotoxigenic *E. coli*. Young children are particularly at risk of the complications of shigellosis such as convulsions and the hemolytic-uremic syndrome. At least 50% of deaths in the developing world are now attributable to persistent diarrhea, which is a condition of diverse etiology whose pathogenesis is poorly understood.

Travelers

A traveler is exposed to a wide variety of enteropathogens (Table 34-2) that will closely reflect the geographic region visited. The spectrum of illness varies from self-limiting *watery diarrhea* due to enterotoxigenic *E. coli*, to the more severe *dysenteries* caused by *Shigella* spp. and *E. histolytica* and *persistent diarrhea* due to infection with *G. lamblia* and *Strongyloides stercoralis*.[5] War veterans from Southeast Asia, such as the British troops who worked on the Burma railroad and the American war veterans from Vietnam, are at risk of carrying *S. stercoralis*. Infection can exist without producing symptoms, although some individuals do present with chronic diarrhea and malabsorption. However, even in the asymptomatic host, exposure in later life to immunosuppressive drugs or the development of an immunsuppressive disease may lead to escalation of the infection, leading to systemic strongyloidiasis, which has an extremely high mortality. Travelers are also exposed to other helminths but infection is uncommon. However, acute schistosomiasis is being increasingly recognized in visitors to Africa, particularly those who swim in Lake Victoria and other East and Central African lakes and rivers.[6]

Immunodeficiency

Common variable immunodeficiency has been known to predispose to certain small intestinal parasitic infections such as giardiasis and isosporiasis for several decades. However, with the emergence of HIV infection, the range of bacteria, viruses, and parasites that are able to produce intestinal disease has expanded rapidly[7] (Table 34-3). The most clinically important infections are those due to the intracellular protozoa (*C. parvum, Microsporidia, Cyclospora cayatenensis*), which are predominantly small bowel enteropathogens, but all can infect the colon, *Mycobacterium avium*-complex, and the other invasive dysenteric enteropathogens including cytomegalovirus.[8] Although *E. histolytica* is commonly isolated in homosexual men, it is almost invariably one of the avirulent strains.

Anticancer chemotherapy often produces diarrhea in its own right but is commonly associated with intestinal infections, particularly *Clostridium difficile* infection. This probably relates to a combination of immunocompromise and the frequent use of broad-spectrum antibiotics.

Antimicrobial Chemotherapy

Antibiotic-associated diarrhea and pseudomembranous colitis are common in hospitalized patients. They are most commonly seen in patients receiving prolonged courses of broad-spectrum antibiotics and have their most devastating effects in the elderly.

Table 34-2. Prevalence of Microbial Enteropathogens in Travelers' Diarrhea

Enteropathogens	Reported Isolation Rates (%)	Estimated Prevalence (%)
Bacteria		
ETEC	20–75	40[a]
Salmonella spp.	0–16	3
Shigella spp.	0–30	8
Campylobacter jejuni	1–11	5[a]
Aeromonas and Plesiomonas spp.	1–57	5
Vibrio parahaemolyticus	1–16	1[b]
EIEC	5–7	2
Protozoa		
Giardia lamblia	0–9	2
Entamoeba histolytica	0–9	<1
Cryptosporidium parvum	1–10	1[b]
Microsporidia, Cyclospora	?	?
Helminths		<1
Viruses		
Rotavirus Norwalk virus family	0–36	10
Multiple pathogens	9–22	20
No pathogens isolated	15–55	20

Abbreviations: ETEC, enterotoxigenic *Escherichia coli*; EIEC, enteroinvasive *Escherichia coli*.
[a] Seasonal variation.
[b] Marked regional variation.

Table 34-3. Prevalence of Gastrointestinal Infections in Patients With HIV Infection and Diarrhea in Europe and North America

Pathogen	Prevalence (%)
Viruses	
Cytomegalovirus	7–46
Herpes simplex virus	4–18
Bacteria	
Salmonella spp.	5–25
Shigella spp.	1–5
Campylobacter spp.	9–11
Mycobacterium avium-complex	5–12
Chlamydia trachomatis	11
Vibrio parahaemolyticus	4
Clostridium difficile	7
Protozoa	
Cryptosporidium parvum	15–16
Microsporidium spp.	
Cyclospora cayetanensis	?
Isospora belli	2
Giardia lamblia	4–15
Entamoeba histolytica	11–25

C. difficile infection accounts for 60% to 70% of antibiotic-associated diarrhea but it is highly likely that other unidentified anaerobes also contribute to the syndrome.

Gastric Hypoacidity

The importance of the gastric acid barrier has been recognized for many decades. Achlorhydric individuals with pernicious anemia or following gastric surgery have been considered to be at increased risk, but there is now increasing evidence that long-term pharmacologic inhibition of gastric secretion with H_2-receptor antagonists or proton pump inhibitors results in increased risk of intestinal infection, particularly with bacterial infections such as *Salmonella* spp.[9] Individuals who are traveling to locations where intestinal infection is more common might consider modifying the time of administration of the drug so that the maximal acid inhibition occurs at night, a time when exposure to enteropathogens would be minimal.

CLINICAL PATTERNS OF INTESTINAL INFECTION

Intestinal infections can present as a variety of clinical patterns, each of which can masquerade as nonspecific inflammatory bowel disease. The most common presentations are those of (1) diarrhea with blood (dysentery), (2) persistent diarrhea with or without the clinical features of intestinal malabsorption, (3) subacute intestinal obstruction, and (4) proctitis and perianal disease.

Diarrhea With Blood

The presence of frank blood in the stool generally indicates the presence of a destructive process in the mucosa or deeper layers of the wall of the intestine.[10] A variety of infective agents can

Enteropathogens Causing Bloody Diarrhea

Bacteria

Shigella spp.

Salmonella spp.

Enteroinvasive *E. coli* (EIEC)

Enterohemorrhagic *E. coli* (EHEC)

Campylobacter jejuni

Yersinia enterocolitica

Mycobacterium tuberculosis

Protozoa

Entamoeba histolytica

Balantidium coli

Viruses

Cytomegalovirus (immunocompromised)

Helminths

Schistosoma spp.

Trichuris trichiura

be responsible for dysentery, which may be indistinguishable from nonspecific inflammatory bowel disease.[11] These invasive infections are generally associated with marked lower abdominal cramping pain, which is often the most debilitating symptom for the sufferer. Fever may also be a prominent feature during the initial phase of the illness, together with profound prostration. Tenesmus may also occur and in young children, shigellosis may result in excessive straining and rectal prolapse. Toxic megacolon can complicate any severe invasive infection of the colon.[12] Although bacterial dysenteric infections often begin with a brief episode of short-lived watery diarrhea, stool volume subsequently decreases and dehydration is usually much less profound than with the enterotoxin-mediated acute diarrheas. The onset of symptoms is usually moderately abrupt with the bacterial dysenteries, but *E. histolytica* may present as an indolent illness with apparent relapses and remissions over the course of weeks or months. Although infection with *Salmonella* spp., *Shigella* spp., and *C. jejuni* are usually self-limiting illnesses, they tend to persist longer than the watery diarrheas, with symptoms lasting for 2 to 3 weeks or even longer. Infection due to enterohemorrhagic *E. coli* 0157:H7, which may also present with a relatively protracted course of bloody diarrhea, is increasingly confused with ulcerative colitis. The macroscopic appearances at endoscopy can be identical to ulcerative colitis and the histologic appearances of the mucosa, once the infection is established, will not reliably distinguish the two conditions. It is therefore essential to take a full dietary history during the 2 to 3 days prior to the onset of symptoms, because EHEC 0157:H7 is most commonly transmitted through beef or beef products, particularly hamburgers. Infection often occurs in outbreaks and thus other individuals eating similar food or food from the same restaurant may also have been infected.

Aeromonas and *Plesomonas* spp. are relatively uncommon organisms but have been reported to produce an illness indistin-

guishable from ulcerative colitis. They are found in the industrialized countries but may also be imported by travelers. Diagnosis depends on fecal culture but the organisms are relatively slow growing and thus positive cultures may not be apparent for several days.

Cytomegalovirus can cause devastating bloody diarrhea with fever, severe abdominal pain, and marked weight loss in the immunocompromised.[7] Patients with HIV infection generally already have a diagnosis of AIDS and so this does not usually pose a major diagnostic problem.

Helminth infection of the colon, sufficient to produce bloody diarrhea, is usually only found in geographic regions where these infections are highly prevalent, and in the case of schistosomiasis, only in locations where the infection can complete its life cycle due to its absolute dependence on specific varieties of freshwater snail, the intermediate host. However, acute schistosomiasis (Katayama fever) is being increasingly recognized in travelers to endemic areas, particularly East Africa, and if untreated can progress to produce colorectal inflammation (*S. mansoni* and *S. haematobium*).[6] Advanced colonic schistosomiasis, particularly as seen in Egyptian farmers, can produce a severe colitis with extensive polypoid change, often associated with anemia and protein-losing enteropathy.

Persistent Diarrhea and Intestinal Malabsorption

Diarrhea that lasts longer than 2 weeks is considered to be persistent. Many enteropathogens can produce persistent diarrhea, the most profound effects being in immunocompromised individuals and those with severe undernutrition. In adults the most common enteropathogen is the protozoan *G. lamblia*, which causes an illness associated with anorexia, abdominal bloating, and if it persists for 4 to 6 weeks generally causes substantial weight loss.[13,14] Long-standing infections may result in overt steatorrhea. The intracellular protozoa (*C. parvum*, *Microsporidia*, *Cyclospora*) can produce persistent diarrhea in both the immunocompetent and immunocompromised, and like *Giardia* produce villous shortening in the small intestine.[8,15]

S. stercoralis infection may also cause chronic diarrhea and malabsorption, although this is more common in the hyperinfection syndrome. In children, enteropathogenic *E. coli* is an important organism to consider as a cause of persistent diarrhea. Amebic colitis can also produce a low-grade, fluctuating persistent diarrhea without obvious macroscopic blood loss. Tropical sprue should be considered in individuals returning from abroad, particularly the Indian subcontinent and Southeast Asia.

Subacute Intestinal Obstruction

Some chronic infections, such as intestinal tuberculosis and schistosomiasis, cause stricturing in the small and large intestine and can give rise to obstructive symptoms.[3,16] This may or may not be associated with diarrhea. Other associated features include fever, malaise, and weight loss and in ileocecal tuberculosis, there may be an associated tender mass in the right iliac fossa. Colonic strictures do not necessarily produce overt obstructive symptoms with pain but merely cause irregularity of bowel function. Occasionally, very heavy infections with the

Causes of Persistent Diarrhea

Protozoa

Giardiasis

Amebiasis

Cryptosporidiosis

Microsporidiosis

Isosporiasis

Balantidium coli

Cyclospora cayetanensis

Bacteria

Salmonella spp. infection[a]

Campylobacter spp. infection[a]

Intestinal tuberculosis/*Mycobacterium avium*-complex

Trophyrema Whippelii (Whipple's bacillus)

Helminths

Strongyloides

Colonic schistosomiasis

Miscellaneous

Inflammatory bowel disease

Tropical sprue

Postinfectious irritable bowel

---

[a] Mostly acute illness but may be prolonged.

roundworm *Ascaris lumbricoides* can cause small intestinal obstruction as a result of an entangled mass of worms.

Proctitis and Perianal Disease

It is now well established that *Chlamydia trachomatis*, *Neisseria gonorrhoeae*, and herpes simplex virus (HSV) produce inflammatory disease in the rectum. The appearances of *C. trachomatis* proctitis are indistinguishable from those of nonspecific proctitis, but HSV produces typical vesicles in the rectum with periodic proctitic symptoms. The lymphogranuloma venereum strain of chlamydia results in chronic inflammatory changes in the rectum that can progress to stricturing similar to that seen in anorectal Crohn's disease. Rectal tuberculosis may produce discrete ulceration in the rectum with fistulation. One study from India indicated that *M. tuberculosis* was detected in 15% of anal fistulae.[17] Infectious causes of proctitis are shown in the accompanying box.

DIAGNOSIS OF INTESTINAL INFECTION

Distinguishing intestinal infection from nonspecific inflammatory bowel disease is essential for management. This is of particular relevance for the severely ill patient when delay in starting appropriate treatment may significantly alter the clinical out-

come. Similarly, inappropriate use of corticosteroids may lead to rapid deterioration of amebic colitis and may result in unnecessary surgery. Confident exclusion of infection is rarely achieved in less than 24 to 48 hours and although imprecise, clinical assessment may be a useful guide to management during the early phase of the illness.

Clinical Assessment

It should be stated at the outset that clinical assessment cannot be used to reliably ascertain the specific etiology of an intestinal infection or confidently distinguish infection from nonspecific inflammatory bowel disease. However, there are certain aspects of the history and examination that may give direction to the diagnostic process.

In the history, special emphasis should be placed on the speed of onset of symptoms, the presence and severity of abdominal pain, and the occurrence of fever. Rapid onset, severe lower cramping abdominal pain, and the presence of fever would favor colonic infection rather than nonspecific inflammatory bowel disease. The possible geographic origins of an infection should be sought, remembering that travel to tropical or subtropical regions is not necessary for the acquisition of intestinal infection. Inquiries should be made about other risk factors, such as immunodeficiency, food recently ingested, and close contacts with other potential carriers or sufferers. Patients with established nonspecific inflammatory bowel disease are also at risk of superadded infection, and an apparent relapse in such an individual, whether they have traveled abroad or not, could be due to infection. In addition, patients may present with a first attack of nonspecific inflammatory bowel disease following foreign travel.[18]

General physical examination rarely distinguishes between infection and nonspecific inflammatory bowel disease unless there are obvious perianal stigmata of Crohn's disease, the cutaneous signs of typhoid (rose patch), HIV infection (Kaposi's sarcoma, hairy leukoplakia, or oropharyngeal candidiasis), or extraintestinal manifestations of inflammatory bowel disease such as erythema nodosum, aphthous ulceration, pyoderma gangrenosum, and arthralgia. Joint symptoms, however, may accompany intestinal infections, particularly those due to *Yersinia* and *Campylobacter*, when they can form part of a Reiter's syn-

Microbial Agents Causing Proctitis

Neisseria gonorrhoeae

Chlamydia trachomatis (LGV)

Chlamydia trachomatis (non-LGV)

Treponema pallidum

Herpes simplex virus

Abbreviation: LGV, lymphogranuloma venereum.

drome. The Guillain-Barré syndrome is now well recognized to be associated with *Campylobacter* infection.

Intestinal Imaging

Endoscopic examination of the rectum is an important step in the diagnostic process to confirm or exclude proctocolitis. It is important to emphasize at this stage, however, that a normal rectum at rigid sigmoidoscopy does not exclude proximal infective or nonspecific inflammatory bowel disease. If the rectum is normal and proximal disease is suspected clinically then it would be entirely reasonable to examine the proximal colon with a flexible colonoscope and to take multiple mucosal biopsies, particularly if stool microscopy and culture is negative. Even when the rectum is macroscopically involved it is often not possible to make a specific diagnosis. Bacterial dysentery can produce appearances in the rectum identical to ulcerative colitis. There are a number of "specific" abnormalities that may be apparent on proctoscopy that may provide a clear lead toward diagnosis. The presence of discrete ulceration occurs in a variety of conditions, but histologic examination of biopsy material and microscopy and culture of slough from ulcer bases would be required to make a specific microbiologic diagnosis. The presence of pseudomembrane strongly suggests *C. difficile* infection although this also occurs in intestinal ischemia. Patchy ulceration and stricturing occurs in Crohn's disease but may also be found in tuberculosis and lymphogranuloma venereum. Sexually transmitted diseases of the rectum do have some relatively specific features, although chlamydia proctitis is clinically indistinguishable from nonspecific proctitis.

Barium contrast examinations of the small and large intestine have a limited place in the diagnosis of intestinal infection. However, the cone-shaped cecum is typical of amebic colitis (Fig. 34-1) and granulomatous masses in the colon (amebomata)

Diseases Producing "Specific" Abnormalities in the Rectum

Deep ulcers

Crohn's disease

Amebiasis

Tuberculosis

Syphilis

Pseudomembrane

Clostridium difficile infection

Vesicles

Herpes simplex virus infection

Beads of pus

Gonorrhea

---

may resemble carcinoma. Ileocecal involvement in tuberculosis may resemble Crohn's disease (Fig. 34-2). Colonic strictures may also occur in tuberculosis (Fig. 34-3) but endoscopy and biopsy are required to differentiate specific and nonspecific inflammatory bowel disease. Occasionally, a barium follow-through examination or enteroclysis may reveal ileal abnormalities such as superficial ulceration in yersiniosis. Again the presence of ileal ulcers does not provide a specific diagnosis, and

---

Infections and Inflammatory Conditions of the Colon in Which the Rectum May Be Spared

Infections

Amebiasis

Pseudomembranous colitis

Yersiniosis

Campylobacter jejuni

Tuberculosis

Cryptosporidiosis

Salmonellosis

Shigellosis

Inflammatory Conditions

Crohn's disease

Ulcerative colitis

Microscopic colitis

Collagenous colitis

Behçet's disease

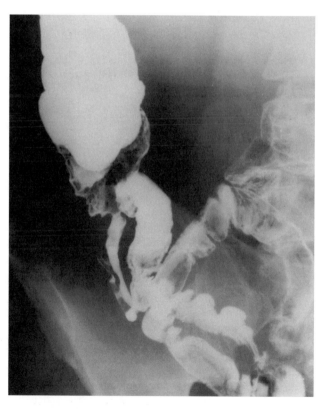

Figure 34-1. Double-contrast barium enema examination showing the typical cone-shaped cecum in amebic colitis.

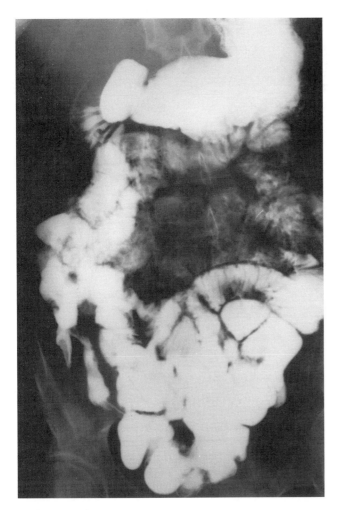

Figure 34-2. Barium follow-through examination showing ileocecal tuberculosis closely resembling Crohn's disease.

further microbiologic or serologic tests would be required to make a definitive diagnosis.

Laboratory Investigations

It is generally not possible to make a specific microbiologic diagnosis of intestinal infection without the use of laboratory tests. Many intestinal infections are self-limiting and the majority of cases of acute diarrhea resolve without a specific diagnosis having been made. For self-limiting illnesses for which specific therapy is not required, there is no compelling reason to obtain a precise diagnosis. However, for diarrhea and other associated abdominal symptoms that persist for more than 14 days, a specific diagnosis should be sought. Most bacterial infections of the intestinal tract and many parasitic infections can be diagnosed by conventional stool microbiologic tests. At least three fecal specimens collected on separate days should be submitted to light microscopy and microbiologic culture ensuring that this includes the conditions for isolation of *C. jejuni* and *Yersinia enterocolitica*. Microscopy of a direct saline wet mount of feces may reveal the typical, highly motile *C. jejuni* on direct dark-field or phase-contrast microscopy or the erythrophagic

trophozoites of *E. histolytica* (fresh fecal specimen). Cysts of *E. histolytica* may also be present, but the presence of cysts alone is inadequate to confirm the diagnosis of invasive amebic colitis. Concentration techniques may be required to isolate cysts of *G. lamblia*, but in florid cases trophozoites may be present in the stool or in duodenal aspirates. The oocysts of *Cryptosporidium parvum* and *Microsporidium* spp. can also be identified by direct microscopy using a modified acid-fast stain. Spores of the newly identified intracellular protozoan *C. cayetanensis* can also be detected in fecal specimens by an experienced observer by use of a trichrome stain.

Stool culture is required to isolate *Salmonella* spp., *Shigella* spp., *C. jejuni*, *Y. enterocolitica*, and *Aeromonas* and *Plesiomonas* spp. The identification of the various types of pathogenic *E. coli* is usually not performed in routine laboratories although it is now possible to use molecular genetic–based technologies, incorporating specific DNA probes for virulence factors that characterize the major *E. coli* variants. *Mycobacterium tuberculosis* is rarely cultured from feces but may be isolated from colonic or ileal biopsy specimens. In patients where there is diffuse abdominal tuberculosis, the organism may also be isolated from ascitic fluid, lymph node aspirates, or peritoneal biopsy specimens.

Rectal swabs taken at proctoscopy are required to isolate *N. gonorrhoeae* by culture, but chlamydia usually requires the use of a tissue culture cell line for its identification. *E. histolytica* trophozoites may be identified in material removed from rectal ulcers.

Serology

Serologic tests for the diagnosis of intestinal infection have overall been of limited value. There are, however, some notable exceptions. Serology is of value in patients with invasive amebic colitis in whom 85% to 95% have anti-*E. histolytica* IgG antibodies in serum. This test should always be performed in patients suspected of amebiasis although a negative test does not exclude amebiasis. Similar positivity rates are found in patients with amebic liver abscess. Serology can also be of value in the diagnosis of yersiniosis when a rise in titer can usually be demonstrated within 10 to 14 days after presentation. However, in the majority of cases the infection is self-limiting and generally resolves by 2 to 3 weeks. Thus, the role of serology in acute infection is questionable, particularly as false-positive tests do occur because of cross-reactivity of some *Y. enterocolitica* antigens with other gram-negative bacteria.

Serology has become much less important in the diagnosis of typhoid and paratyphoid because the organisms can generally be cultured from blood or bone marrow aspirates. Enzyme-linked immunosorbent assay (ELISA) tests are now available for strongyloidiasis and schistosomiasis and are now regarded as the most appropriate screening tests for these infections.[19]

A variety of attempts have been made to develop a serologic test for giardiasis. Anti-*Giardia* IgG antibodies are unhelpful as titers remain elevated for months or even years after acute infection, particularly in endemic areas. However, a specific anti-*Giardia* IgM response can be detected in acute infection and has been shown to have diagnostic value both in the industrialized and developing world. This test, however, is not widely available in routine diagnostic laboratories.[20]

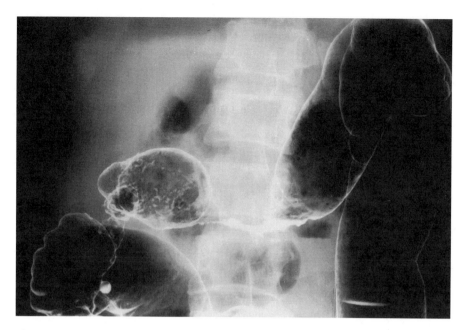

Figure 34-3. Double-contrast barium enema examination showing colonic strictures due to tuberculosis.

Bacterial Toxins

Many of the enteropathogens responsible for infective diarrhea synthesize a variety of entero- and cytotoxins that produce the secretory diarrhea related to enterotoxigenic *E. coli* and cholera infections and the epithelial damage associated with invasive microorganisms such as *C. jejuni, E.histolytica, Shigella* spp., and *Salmonella* spp. However, the only toxin that is routinely searched for in clinical practice is that of *C. difficile.* This toxin may be detected either by its cytopathic effects on cells in tissue culture or immunologic methods such as ELISA or latex agglutination. Although the organism may be isolated on culture, the presence of toxin confirms the organism's etiologic importance in diarrheal illness. Approximately 3% of healthy adults excrete *C. difficile* but in the absence of toxin. However, up to 80% of healthy neonates excrete both organism and toxin without any ill effects on the host.

Fecal Antigen Detection

An alternative approach to culture and microscopic identification of enteropathogens is to use immunologic techniques to detect pathogen-specific antigen.[19] There are often difficulties in producing ELISAs that work reliably on fecal extracts, although this method has been widely used for the detection of rotavirus. Fecal ELISAs have also been reported for the detection of *G. lamblia*, although the sensitivity and specificity of these assays may not be sufficiently good as yet for management to be made solely on their results. There are, however, a number of commercially available fecal antigen ELISAs for giardiasis. Other assays are under development for other organisms that are not routinely cultured such as *E. histolytica.*

Molecular Genetic Approaches to Diagnosis

A variety of DNA probes have been developed that appear to be useful in the identification of fecal enteropathogens.[21] DNA probes are selected from known gene sequences of highly spe-cific virulence factors, such as from the genes encoding for enterotoxins, invasion antigens, or other species-specific antigens. Use of amplification techniques such as the polymerase chain reaction can markedly increase the sensitivity of this approach. Ultimately, it might be anticipated that probes will be available for the full spectrum of enteropathogens, allowing fecal specimens to be screened rapidly for all common organisms. In some instances culture will still be required to establish drug sensitivity.

Histopathologic Examination of Mucosal Biopsies

Biopsy specimens should be taken from the rectum at proctosigmoidoscopy irrespective of whether the rectum appears macroscopically normal. When clinically indicated, colonoscopy should be performed and biopsies taken from the distal ileum and throughout the colon. Enteropathogens can sometimes be detected in mucosal biopsies such as the trophozoites of *E. histolytica* at the margins of ulcers, ova of schistosomes that can often be speciated on the basis of egg morphology, and other parasites including *C. parvum.* The only reliable method for confirming a diagnosis of cytomegalovirus infection is on the basis of the typical owl's eye inclusion bodies usually present in the submucosa. Bacterial infection cannot usually be accurately diagnosed on the basis of mucosal histopathology although the presence of caseating granulomata would be diagnostic of tuberculosis.

With the exception of the above examples where histopathology can provide a specific diagnosis, most histopathologists admit great difficulty in distinguishing infective colitis confidently from early nonspecific inflammatory bowel disease. Distorted crypt architecture and chronic inflammatory cell infiltrates favor a diagnosis of nonspecific inflammatory bowel disease, although these appearances may also be present in up to 30% of acute self-limited colitis.[22] Interpretation is further limited by 25% interobserver variation between histopathologists. Isolated basal giant cells, epithelial surface erosions, and epithelial granulomata are probably the most reliable histopathologic features of early inflammatory bowel disease. Some investigators, however, have been able to use histologic examination as a highly discriminatory test in distinguishing acute self-limited colitis from ulcerative colitis, infection being suggested by the presence of marked edema, preservation of crypt architecture, neutrophil infiltration in the lamina propria, and the migration of neutrophils through the crypt epithelium.[23] In practice, most histopathologists remain cautious in the interpretation of biopsies from acute colitis of any cause unless a specific pathogen can be identified in the tissue. An additional difficulty is that the appearances will change with time although differentiation may be possible within the first few days of infection; the two conditions appear to merge histopathologically as the illness progresses.

TREATMENT

The vast majority of acute intestinal infections will resolve without specific antimicrobial chemotherapy. However, there are situations when it is appropriate to use antibiotics both for enteropathogens producing dysentery (Table 34-4) and persistent diarrhea (Table 34-5).[5,24–26] Standard supportive management such as restoration of fluid and electrolyte balance, correction of acidosis,[27,28] and relief of obstructive symptoms should be initiated while awaiting a precise microbiologic diagnosis and the initiation of specific antimicrobial chemotherapy.

Treatment of Dysentery

An approach to the overall management of dysentery is outlined in Figure 34-4. Invasive amebic colitis should be treated with oral metronidazole or another nitroimidazole derivative for 10 days. This should be followed by a second agent such as diloxanide furoate to clear intraluminal encysted forms of the parasite. The majority of other forms of dysentery, providing they are of mild or moderate severity, are usually self-limiting and require no specific treatment. Shigella dysentery has proved difficult to treat because of widespread resistance to standard drugs such as ampicillin and trimethoprim-sulfamethoxazole. Because of the severe complications that can follow *S. dysenteriae* type I infection, antibiotics are usually given and resistant strains have been treated with nalidixic acid. More recently, the 4-fluoroquinolone drugs have been used and shown to be an excellent alternative. They are contraindicated in infants and young children because of their potential adverse effects on developing cartilage. *Salmonella enteritidis* gastroenteritis usually resolves spontaneously but ciprofloxacin reduces the duration of diarrhea. *C. jejuni* infection is usually self-limiting and its course is not influenced by erythromycin, which has been the treatment of choice for a number of years. Disseminated *Y. enterocolitica* infection requires antibiotics such as tetracycline, trimethoprim-sulfamethoxazole, aminoglycosides, chloramphenicol, or a third-generation cephalosporin. Uncomplicated

Table 34-4. Antimicrobial Chemotherapy for Dysentery

	First Line	Second Line
Bacteria		
Shigella spp.	Ampicillin, trimethoprim-sulfamethoxazole, fluoroquinolone	[a]Cephalosporin, nalidixic acid
Salmonella spp.	[b]Fluoroquinolone	
EIEC	? as *Shigella* spp.	
EHEC	?	
Campylobacter jejuni	Erythromycin, tetracycline, cephalosporin	Fluoroquinolone
Yersinia enterocolitica	Fluoroquinolone	Aztreonam, imipenem
Clostridium difficile	Metronidazole	Vancomycin
Mycobacterium tuberculosis	Quadruple therapy:	
	Rifampicin — 10 months	
	Isoniazid — 10 months	
	Pyrazinamide — 2 months	
	Ethambutol — 2 months	
Protozoa		
Entamoeba histolytica	Metronidazole/tinidazole plus diloxanide furoate	Paromomycin
Balantidium coli	Tetracycline	Metronidazole, paromomycin
Helminths		
Schistosoma spp.	Praziquantel	
Trichuris trichiura	Albendazole, mebendazole	Oxantel-pyrantel
Virus		
Cytomegalovirus	Ganciclovir	Foscarnet

Abbreviations: EIEC, enteroinvasive *E. coli*; EHEC, enterohemorrhagic *E. coli*.
[a] Third generation.
[b] Usually only for bacteremia.

Table 34-5. Antimicrobial Therapy for Persistent Diarrhea

	First Line		Second Line
Bacteria			
Salmonella/Shigella spp.	See Table 34-4		
Campylobacter jejuni	See Table 34-4		
Mycobacterium tuberculosis	See Table 34-4		
Tropheryma Whippelii	Penicillin plus streptomycin	14 days	
	TMP-SMZ	1 yr	
Protozoa			
Giardia lamblia	Metronidazole/tindazole		Albendazole
Entamoeba histolytica	See Table 34-4		
Cryptosporidium parvum	? Paromomcyin		
Isospora belli	TMP-SMX		
Microsporidia	Albendazole		
Cyclospora cayetanensis	TMP-SMX		
Helminths			
Strongyloides stercoralis	Thiabendazole		Albendazole, ivermectin
Schistosoma spp.	Praziquantel		
Miscellaneous			
Tropical sprue	Tetracycline		
	Folic acid		

Abbreviation: TMP-SMX, trimethoprim-sulfamethoxazole.

Figure 34-4. A systematic approach to the diagnosis and treatment of bloody diarrhea. IBD, inflammatory bowel disease; Eh, *Entamoeba histolytica*. *Consider appropriate antimicrobial therapy (see Table 34-4).

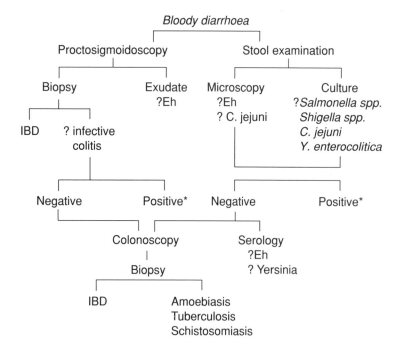

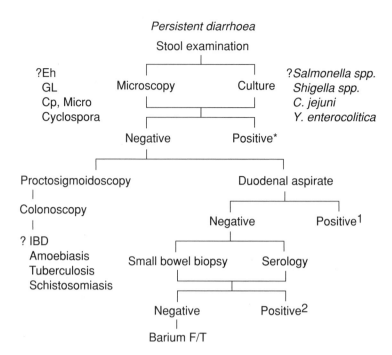

Figure 34-5. A systematic approach to the diagnosis and treatment of persistent diarrhea. IBD, inflammatory bowel disease; Eh, *Entamoeba histolytica*; GL, *Giardia lamblia*; Cp, *Cryptosporidium parvum*. *Consider appropriate antimicrobial therapy (see Table 34-5). [1] *?Giardia* or *Strongyloides stercoralis.* [2] *?Giardia* or *Strongyloides stercoralis.* ?enteropathy such as tropical sprue.

enteritis or mesenteric adenitis due to *Y. enterocolitica* do not usually require antibiotic therapy.

Treatment of Persistent Diarrhea

An approach to the overall management of persistent diarrhea is shown in Figure 34-5. Many of the classic bacterial enteropathogens such as *Salmonella* spp. and *Shigella* spp. can cause persistent diarrhea over a number of weeks, in which case it is appropriate to treat symptomatic individuals with antimicrobial chemotherapy. However, the more common infective causes of persistent diarrhea are due to the protozoa, namely *G. lamblia* and the intracellular protozoa (*C. parvum*, *Microsporidium* spp., and *Cyclospora*). Giardiasis in adults is treated with metronidazole 2 g as a single dose on 3 successive days or tinidazole 2 g as a single dose on 1 day. Treatment failures occur, possibly due to drug resistance. Alternative drugs include albendazole,

which has recently been shown to be highly effective in giardiasis and relatively free from adverse effects; mepacrine; and furazolidone. *C. parvum* does not respond to any known antimicrobial agent but microsporidiosis often responds well to albendazole, particularly the newly recognized variety, *Septata intestinalis*, which can often be eradicated. The more established variety, *Enterocytozoon bieneusi* may respond symptomatically in the shortterm, but infection almost invariably recurs. In immunocompetent individuals *C. cayetanensis* can be cleared with trimethoprim-sulfamethoxazole.

Strongyloidiasis is treated with thiabendazole. In severe infections, particularly in the hyperinfection syndrome in immunocompromised individuals, broad-spectrum antibiotics should be given with thiabendazole in an attempt to prevent septicemia and septic shock. Tropical sprue is treated with tetracycline for at least 10 to 14 days, although prolonged treatment is required for some individuals. It is also conventional to give folic acid and replace any other micro- or macronutrient deficiencies.

REFERENCES

1. Farthing MJG, Keusch GT (1989) Global impact of intestinal infection. pp. 3–12. In Farthing MJG, Keutsch GT (eds): Enteric Infection: Mechanisms, Manifestations and Management. Chapman & Hall, London

2. Farthing MJG, Du Pont HL, Guandalini S et al (1992) Treatment and prevention of travellers' diarrhoea. Gastroenterol Int 5:162–175

3. Farthing MJG (1992) Mycobacterial disease of the gut. pp. 174–189. In Phillips R, Northover J (eds): Modern Coloproctology. Edward Arnold, London

4. Rampling A (1993) *Salmonella enteritidis* five years on. Lancet; 342:317–318

5. Farthing MJG (1991) Prevention and treatment of travellers' diarrhoea. Aliment Pharmacol Ther 5:15–30

6. Chapman PJC, Wilkinson PR, Davidson RN (1988) Acute schistosomiasis (Katayama fever) among British air crew. Br Med J 297:1101

7. McCowan I, Weller I (1990) AIDS and the gut. pp. 133–156. In Pounder RE (ed): Recent Advances in Gastroenterology. Churchill Livingstone, London

8. Farthing MJG, Kelly MP, Veitch AM (1996) Recently recognised microbial enteropathies and HIV-infection. J Antimicrob Chemother 37(Suppl B):61–70

9. Neal KR, Brij SO, Slack RCB et al (1994) Recent treatment with H_2 antagonists and antibiotics and gastric surgery as risk factors for *Salmonella* infection. BMJ 308:176

10. Farthing MJG, Walker-Smith JA (1990) Infective diarrhoea. pp. 1513–1529. In The Metabolic and Molecular Basis of Acquired Disease. Bailliere Tindall, London

11. Farthing MJG (1987) Gut infections. pp. 127–141. In Dawson AM, Besser GM (eds): Recent Advances in Medicine 20. Churchill Livingstone, London

12. Snowden JA, Young MJ, McKendrick MW (1994) Dilatation of the colon complicating acute self-limited colitis. Q J Med 87:55–62

13. Farthing MJG (1989) Host-parasite interactions in human giardiasis. Q J Med 70:191–204

14. Farthing MJG (1994) Giardiasis as a disease. pp. 15–37. In *Giardia:* From Molecules to Disease and Beyond. CAB International, Cambridge, England

15. Ravdin JI, Weikel CS, Guerrant RP (1988) Protozoal enteropathies: cryptosporidiosis, giardiasis and amoebiasis. Bailliere's Clin Trop Med Commun Dis 3:504–536

16. Farthing MJG, Butcher PD (1989) Mycobacterium tuberculosis and paratuberculosis. pp. 3–12. In Farthing MJG, Keusch GT (eds): Enteric Infection: Mechanisms, Manifestations and Management. Chapman & Hall, London

17. Shukla HS, Gupta SC, Singh G, Singh PA (1988). Tubercular fistula in ano. Br J Surg 75:38–39

18. Harries AD, Myers B, Cook GC (1985) Inflammatory bowel disease: a common cause of blood diarrhoea in visitors to the tropics. BMJ 291:1686–1687

19. Pritchard DI, Tighe PJ, Billett EE (1995) Intestinal helminths—new approaches to diagnosis. pp.247–265. In Enteric Infection 2: Intestinal Helminths. Chapman & Hall, London

20. Farthing MJG, Goka AKJ, Butcher PD et al (1987) Serodiagnosis of giardiasis. Serodiagn Immunother 1:233–238

21. Char S, Farthing MJG (1990) DNA probes for diagnosis of gut infection. Gut 32:1–3

22. Allison MC, Hamilton-Dutoit SJ, Shillon AP, Pounder RE (1987) The value of rectal biopsy in distinguishing self-limited colitis from inflammatory bowel disease. Q J Med 65:985–995

23. Nostrant TT, Kumar NB, Appelman HD (1987) Histopathology differentiates acute self-limited colitis from ulcerative colitis. Gastroenterology 92:318–323

24. Keusch GT (1988) Antimicrobial therapy for enteric infections and typhoid fever: state of the art. Rev Infect Dis 10:S199–205

25. Sack RB (1986) Antimicrobial prophylaxis of travellers' diarrhoea. Rev Infect Dis, 8, (suppl. 2):160–166

26. Kelly MP, Farthing MJG (1997) Infections of the gastrointestinal tract. pp. 708–720. In O'Grady, Lambert, Finch, Greenwood (eds): Antibiotic & Chemotherapy. 7th Ed.

27. Hirschhorn N (1980) The treatment of acute diarrhea in children. An historical and physiological perspective. Am J Clin Nutr 33:63

28. Farthing MJG (1988) History and rationale of oral rehydration and recent developments in formulating and optimal solutions. In Advances in Oral Rehydration Seminar. Drugs, 36, (suppl. 4): 80–90

35

CONSTIPATION

Michael A. Kamm

Constipation is a symptom, most commonly regarded as infrequent or difficult defecation. For the purposes of standardization of clinical and epidemiologic studies this has been more precisely defined as a bowel frequency of less than twice per week, or the need to strain at defecation more than 25% of the time, based on normal data derived from the non–health-care-seeking population.[1] However, for patients the term may also mean that the stool is hard or incompletely evacuated, or may encompass a range of functional symptoms including bloating and pain.

EPIDEMIOLOGY

The prevalence of constipation is similar in most Western countries. In one study of British factory workers less than 1% had fewer than two stools per week, although 16% took laxatives.[2] Those with infrequent bowel actions were all women. The perception of normality plays a large part in determining health-care-seeking behavior, as reflected in the fact that less than a quarter of those who took laxatives considered themselves constipated.

Straining at stool is more common. Approximately 10% to 20% of British, American, and Australian populations often strain at stool.[2–4]

In childhood, constipation is more common in males. In adults with a normal diameter colon, constipation is much more common in women, and more common with increasing age. In one study it affected 3% of young adults compared with 8% of the middle-aged and 20% of elderly subjects.[3] In adults with an idiopathic megacolon the proportion of males and females affected is similar.

PATHOPHYSIOLOGY

Many different pathophysiologic processes may result in constipation. For example, the pathogenic mechanism producing constipation in children is unlikely to be the same as that in women of reproductive age or patients with a megacolon. Attempts to subdivide patients into distinct clinical syndromes allow different pathophysiologic processes to be identified.

Factors that affect the function of the large bowel and stool formation include (1) colonic factors such as abnormalities of enteric muscle, intrinsic nerves, absorption, and luminal contents. The colon may be the site of primary abnormalities, such as in Hirschsprung's disease, or affected as part of some other systemic condition such as myxedema; (2) extrinsic nerve supply which can be affected in the pelvis, spinal cord, or brain; (3) circulating hormones, gastrointestinal and nongastrointestinal; and (4) pelvic floor abnormalities. The effects of changes in dietary intake, drugs, and bile acids will be via one of these control mechanisms. Mechanical obstruction always needs to be excluded.

Motility Disturbance

Normal colonic activity is characterized by irregular segmenting activity that is not coordinated between different colonic segments, and is largely responsible for colonic mixing. Several times per day high-pressure peristaltic waves (mass movements) traverse a large part of length of the colon and transport colonic contents. Some of these mass movements progress distally and are associated with defecation.

Early distal colonic studies demonstrated an increase in segmenting activity in constipated patients. Recent studies involving the whole colon have shown a reduction in the frequency and duration of mass movements in severely constipated women with a normal diameter colon. In one study of 14 such patients and 18 healthy volunteers, the mean number of mass movements observed over a 24-hour period was 6.1 in the healthy subjects, but only 2.6 in the constipated patients.[5] Four of the patients had no recorded mass movements in 24 hours.

Fiber

The fiber content of the diet is thought to have a major influence on colonic function. Fiber can be regarded as mixed cell-wall material, nonstarch polysaccharide, or whole vegetable food with the cell walls intact. This group of carbohydrates contains a diverse group of substances that vary in their physical properties and possibly in their effect on the colon.

Dietary fiber intake is one of the determinants of bowel function. The mean transit time is shorter, and the frequency of defecation and wet weight of feces is greater, in adults with a higher fiber intake.[6]

Dietary fiber may act by several different mechanisms. Some types of fiber may draw water into the colonic lumen, whereas others may indirectly increase the fecal bacterial mass. Fermentation of fiber produces short chain fatty acids that may stimulate colonic activity. Fermentation may also allow for the release of adsorbed bile acids, which also stimulate the colon. The irritating effect of insoluble particles may also act to increase motility; larger particles of the same fiber type have a greater effect on transit time.

A deficiency of fiber in the diet is not the cause of constipation in patients with the irritable bowel syndrome or severe idiopathic constipation in whom fiber intake is normal. The administration of fiber will benefit patients with mild constipation and shorten the gut transit time, but will not help patients with more severe constipation.

Genetic Factors

Genetic causes are poorly defined in patients with idiopathic constipation and a normal size intestine. One study of fingerprint patterns, which are a genetic marker, in constipated patients suggested the influence of a genetic factor in patients with the onset of constipation before the age of 10.[7]

In a small minority of adults with chronic idiopathic intestinal pseudo-obstruction, due to a visceral myopathy or neuropathy, there is a clearly inherited basis, either autosomal dominant or recessive.

Sex Hormones

Sex hormones may have some influence on gut transit. Men have a faster transit time than women, and a greater proportion of adult women than men are constipated. Relaxation of gastrointestinal smooth muscle by progesterone may be the reason for the increased incidence of constipation during pregnancy, although changes in other hormones such as motilin may also be important.

Patients with severe idiopathic constipation and a colon of normal diameter are almost exclusively women, usually of reproductive age. Although these women do have a consistent reduction in adrenal and ovarian steroid hormones, this appears to be secondary to changes in the steroid hormone enterohepatic circulation and is unlikely to account for the motility disturbance.[8]

Psychological Factors

Psychological factors are an important determinant of bowel function. Personality profiles have been shown to correlate with stool weight in healthy subjects, and individuals with higher self-esteem and more extroverted personalities produce heavier more frequent stools.[9] Normal healthy subjects can suppress defecation and thereby slow colonic transit voluntarily, providing direct evidence of cerebral control over colonic function.[10]

Young women with severe constipation have a higher incidence of psychosexual problems, adverse early life events, and personality difficulties than asymptomatic healthy women.[11–14] In a group of patients having surgery for severe constipation, there was a higher depression score on psychometric testing compared with a control group with other surgical conditions.[15] Furthermore, patients who did not benefit from surgery had significantly higher anxiety and depression scores than those who did well.[15] Another study compared two groups of severely constipated women including those with a measured slow intestinal transit time and those with a normal transit time. Those with a normal transit time demonstrated the most psychopathology on psychometric testing whereas those with slow transit resembled healthy controls.[16]

There are several possible mechanisms by which gastrointestinal function might be affected by psychological factors:

1. Efferent autonomic pathways exert an effect on colonic motility and this may be affected by stress. Recent studies have demonstrated the importance of central neurotransmitters such as corticotropin-releasing factor in determining the colonic motor response to stress.[17]
2. Neurotransmitters that are common to both the enteric nervous system and the brain may be abnormal.
3. Psychological problems may disturb the regulation of hormones that affect colonic motility.

Alternatively, the persistent symptoms of severe constipation and abdominal pain may lead to depression and other neurotic symptoms.

Abnormalities of Extrinsic Innervation

Although the enteric nervous system demonstrates a large degree of physiologic independence from the central nervous system, injury to its extrinsic innervation at any level may result in constipation. The integrity of the extrinsic autonomic supply to the large intestine appears to be necessary for normal function.

The constipation observed in patients with spinal cord lesions is likely to be related to an absent sacral parasympathetic supply to the large bowel. Animal studies have shown that lesions of the spinal cord affect colonic transit[18] and patients with complete lesions of the thoracic spinal cord show decreased colonic compliance and an abnormal rectosigmoid motility response to a meal.[19]

Certain surgical procedures may result in damage to the extrinsic innervation of the bowel leading to constipation. Pelvic surgery that affects the sacral nerves has been shown to cause intractable constipation.[20] Hysterectomy produces constipation in a small proportion of patients although the exact mechanism is not clear. The effect may be via extrinsic nerve damage, or via altered local pelvic reflexes.[21] Alternatively the problem may be behavioral, as evidenced by the reversibility achieved by biofeedback treatment in some patients. Constipation can follow difficult childbirth rarely, also presumably due to pelvic nerve damage or disturbance of pelvic floor coordination.

Patients undergoing abdominal rectal mobilization and fixation (rectopexy) for rectal prolapse often have an abnormal bowel habit preoperatively, but as many as half who were not constipated before surgery become so after the operation. Division of the lateral rectal ligaments, which may carry some of the autonomic innervation to the distal bowel, leads to a higher incidence of this complication.[22]

Constipation developing after sacral trauma is believed to be due to damage to the parasympathetic innervation to the left colon.

Abnormalities of the Enteric Nervous System

The enteric nervous system is capable of coordinating patterns of colonic motility, while the brain and spinal cord modify this activity. Processes that directly affect the intramural plexuses of the bowel may result in constipation.

Aganglionosis of the distal bowel occurs as a congenital defect in Hirschsprung's disease. Although the intrinsic nerves are absent, extrinsic innervation by adrenergic and cholinergic nerves is still present.

In patients with severe idiopathic constipation there is both morphologic and functional evidence for an abnormality of the intrinsic colonic innervation. In an in vivo study in which internal anal sphincter relaxation was induced by electrical stimulation of the rectal wall, a larger current was required to produce maximal sphincter relaxation in constipated patients compared with healthy controls.[23]

Silver staining of the myenteric plexus in these patients reveals a decrease in the number and morphologic abnormalities of argyrophilic neurons.[24] However, oral laxatives have been shown to induce changes in the myenteric plexus in animal experiments. It is therefore not clear whether these changes are primary or secondary to these drugs.

Enteric neurotransmitters are responsible for the regulation of colonic motility. In two studies the concentration of vasoactive intestinal peptide (VIP) in the descending[25] and sigmoid colon[26] of patients with idiopathic constipation was found to be reduced. Decreased levels of this inhibitory neurotransmitter may relate to the decrease in propulsive mass movements seen in this condition. Levels of serotonin have also been found to be raised in the circular muscle and mucosa of the sigmoid colon in patients with severe idiopathic constipation[27]; this increase in serotonin may correlate with the manometrically observed increase in nonpropulsive segmenting activity found in this condition.

A study of mucosal biopsies from severely constipated subjects found a decreased concentration of substance P[28] but this was not found in a study of resected colons from constipated patients.[25] One study, using immunohistochemistry, found an increase in the number of nerve fibers immunoreactive to CGRP but no difference in the number of VIP staining fibers.[29]

The extrinsic cholinergic nerves provide an important motor innervation to the bowel, but there may be an abnormality that also involves intrinsic cholinergic nerves. In vitro studies of the taenia coli from constipated patients have shown reduced activity of cholinergic nerves in response to electrical field stimulation.[30] Clinical evidence for a subclinical disturbance of autonomic function comes from a study of impaired sweating in response to acetylcholine in women with severe constipation.[31]

An abnormality of endogenous central, circulating, or local gut opiates or enkephalins may affect gastrointestinal motility. Opioid and enkephalins receptors are found in the brain and throughout the gastrointestinal tract in endocrine cells,[32] extrinsic nerves,[33] and the myenteric plexus.[25] In a study of healthy volunteers, morphine was shown to decrease the frequency of bowel movements and decrease proximal colonic transit. Naloxone, an opioid antagonist, accelerated transit in the transverse and rectosigmoid colon without affecting bowel movements.[34] Evidence for a colonic wall abnormality involving opioid receptors comes from in vitro sucrose gap studies that show reduced activity of enkephalin receptors in colon from constipated patients.[35] However, constipated patients treated with naloxone or nalmefene, a well-absorbed opioid antagonist, show no improvement in transit time.

Circulating Gastrointestinal Hormones

The plasma levels of the peptides β-endorphin, neurotensin, somatostatin, substance P, and motilin were assessed in constipated patients. Apart from reduced levels of motilin there was no difference from controls.[36] The measured plasma levels may, however, be normal despite marked abnormalities of the myenteric plexus.

Some regulatory circulating gastrointestinal peptides are thought to modify colonic motor activity. Preston et al.[37] demonstrated a smaller than normal rise in serum gastrin and pancreatic polypeptide in severely constipated subjects following an oral water stimulus. Motilin also rises less than normal in these subjects postprandially.[36,37]

Different results were obtained by van der Sijp et al.[38] in response to a standard meal. They showed normal basal and postprandial blood levels of insulin, glucagon-like-peptide-1, gastric inhibitory polypeptide, motilin, neurotensin, and peptide tyrosine tyrosine (PYY) in patients with severe constipation. However, plasma levels of somatostatin, an inhibitory hormone, were markedly elevated and showed a diminished response to a meal.

Chronic Intestinal Pseudo-Obstruction

In patients with chronic idiopathic intestinal pseudo-obstruction careful examination of the gut wall using special stains and electron microscopy will usually reveal an abnormality of either the nerve plexuses (visceral neuropathy) or one or both of the muscle coats (visceral myopathy).[39]

A similar clinical, radiologic and motility disorder can be seen with other chronic abnormalities of the nerve plexuses or muscle coats. Progressive systemic sclerosis produces fibrous tissue replacement of one or both of the muscle coats, rendering propulsion ineffective. Inflammation of the nerve plexuses is seen in Chagas disease, and as a nonmetastatic effect in some tumors, especially small cell tumors of the lung.

Pelvic Floor Abnormalities

When patients with idiopathic constipation are asked to strain, they often inappropriately contract, rather than relax, the pelvic floor and anal striated muscles.[40] When testing rectal evacuation these patients, unlike healthy subjects, are unable to expel a balloon from the rectum,[41] expel a solid sphere, or evacuate even liquid barium or saline.[42–44] This phenomenon has been termed anismus, spastic pelvic floor syndrome, pelvic floor asynchronism, pelvic floor incoordination, and paradoxical puborectalis contraction. When these muscles contract on straining the anal canal pressure rises inappropriately. The pressure rise can be demonstrated using a manometric probe in the anal canal, and inappropriate contraction can be demonstrated by electromyography of the anal striated muscles.

The phenomenon of pelvic floor incoordination is more complex than was originally appreciated. Many patients with a variety of defecation disorders, such as solitary ulcer syndrome, idiopathic perineal pain,[45] and even fecal incontinence[46] demonstrate the same phenomenon, and it may also be observed in normal subjects in the anorectal laboratory. When other striated muscles, such as the external oblique and gluteus maximus, are monitored during straining they may also contract inappropriately.[47] The latter observation led Mathers et al. to conclude that pelvic floor incoordination is part of a dystonic phenomenon and not of direct relevance to the pathophysiology of the constipation.

It is likely that many of these patients do have pelvic floor incoordination that does involve more than just the sphincter muscles but that may well contribute to their constipation. When asked to squeeze their anal muscles many patients are unable to coordinate or recognize what they should be doing. There appears to be a loss of recognition about how to coordinate the full range of pelvic muscle maneuvers.[48] This incoordination may occur secondary to colonic inertia, in a vain attempt to empty the bowel. Alternatively it may be inappropriately learned defecatory behavior. Many of these patients have experienced sexual abuse early in life[49]; lack of awareness of pelvic coordination may relate to a subconscious desire by the patients to dissociate themselves from their own pelvis and genitalia.

Constipation sometimes follows pelvic surgery such as a hysterectomy. This has previously been attributed to pelvic nerve damage, but may relate to temporary interference with pelvic structures. Alternatively temporary constipation after pelvic surgery may become entrenched in a new abnormal pattern of behavior. There may even be grief associated with hysterectomy, which leads to subconscious abnormal behavior.

Different measurement techniques of pelvic floor contraction often give conflicting results. Miller et al.[50] studied 24 patients with constipation, 13 with measured slow transit and 11 with normal transit. Videoproctography and external sphincter electromyography were performed simultaneously. Electromyographic paradoxic contraction did not consistently correlate with the ability to evacuate the rectum on proctography or with symptoms of ''obstructed defecation.''

Similar observation were reported by Wald et al.[51] who evaluated 36 patients with chronic constipation by evacuation proctography and anorectal manometry. Twenty patients also had a colonic transit study, 10 having normal and 10 having delayed transit. Poor rectal emptying on proctography did not correlate with a paradoxic rise in anal pressure on straining. When manometry was abnormal only one-third of patients had an abnormal proctogram. Conversely when manometry was normal the proctogram was also normal in 88% of patients.

Intrarectal pressure and external sphincter electromyography can be performed simultaneously during evacuation proctogra-

phy[52] but this has provided less additional useful information than might have been expected.

Measurements of pelvic floor activity and incoordination in the laboratory have been criticized on the basis that the patient is straining in an unnatural way, without emptying the bowel, and in a left lateral position while being observed. This may be true, although non constipated subjects observed under the same circumstances usually do relax their pelvic floor normally. Ambulatory studies of the anorectum, using solid-state strain gauge transducers and fine wire electromyography of the external anal sphincter, have been undertaken in patients with constipation and pelvic floor contraction diagnosed in the laboratory. These studies have shown that when attempting to defecate on the toilet at home many of these patients do apparently relax their pelvic floor.

Paradoxic pelvic floor contraction is just one component of a complex functional and sometimes anatomic disorder. It can coexist with slow colonic transit, or with anatomic abnormalities such as a large rectocele defined as greater than 2 cm on a lateral radiograph.[53] Constipation can persist after correction of slow transit by colectomy, surgical rectocele repair, or biofeedback to correct abnormal pelvic floor dynamics. This suggests that in many patients there is also a large bowel or sphincter neuromuscular abnormality that still defies adequate characterization. This disturbance may have its origins in the bowel, the extrinsic nerve supply, or even cerebral centers of control.

Recently the behavioral treatment of patients with pelvic floor incoordination, biofeedback, has led to decreased straining, increased bowel frequency, and improved colonic transit in patients with disordered defecation.[48,54] This would appear to justify the testing for pelvic floor incoordination in these patients.

Internal Anal Sphincter

Although it has been postulated that the internal anal sphincter may be abnormal in some patients with constipation there is little evidence to support this. The resting anal pressure and rectosphincteric reflex are normal in patients with constipation.

There has only been one condition described in which the internal anal sphincter is definitely the cause of constipation. This is a hereditary myopathy affecting the internal anal sphincter, which causes both proctalgia fugax and difficulty with rectal evacuation. There is gross thickening and dysfunction of the internal sphincter. Light and electron microscopy have shown abnormal polyglucosan inclusion bodies, and the condition responds to an internal anal sphincter strip myectomy.[55]

Noncolonic Abnormalities in Constipated Patients

Even in patients with a disorder that appears to be confined to the colon there is often an abnormality of the upper gastrointestinal tract, and sometimes other systems. Nausea is common in women with severe constipation[56] and these same patients have demonstrable abnormalities of esophageal motility, gastric emptying, and small bowel motility.[38,57,58]

Women with severe constipation also have an increased incidence of urogynecologic symptoms. Some studies have suggested an abnormality in the spinal control of pelvic function.[59,60]

ETIOLOGY AND CLINICAL PRESENTATIONS

Constipation of Unknown Cause

Asymptomatic But Low Bowel Frequency

Many asymptomatic individuals, mainly women, who have a low bowel frequency can be considered part of the normal range. Most are at the "slow" end of the physiologic spectrum, although in a few others factors that may play a part include inadequate intake of fluids or dietary fiber, sex hormone environment, mental state, or personality. A patient who has always had infrequent bowel actions and is otherwise asymptomatic does not require investigation or treatment.

Irritable Bowel Syndrome

Patients who experience constipation alternating with diarrhea, which is accompanied by bloating and abdominal pain, are regarded as having the "irritable bowel syndrome" in the absence of identifiable gut pathology. Other symptoms in these patients include excessive straining at stool, unsatisfied defecation, passage of mucus, and numerous nongastrointestinal symptoms such as general malaise, backache, and urinary symptoms. If measured, the intestinal transit time is usually normal. The constipation is usually easily treated by an increase in dietary fiber or simple symptomatic measures, although the patient's diet is not necessarily low in fiber content. The abdominal pain and bloating are often more resistant to treatment than the constipation in these patients.

Anorectal Problems

Some patients with a "functional" anorectal problem, such as solitary rectal ulcer, rectal prolapse, or anterior mucosal prolapse, may have constipation as their primary problem. In one prospective study one-half of all patients with rectal prolapse complained of difficulty with rectal evacuation.[22]

Constipation is likely to be a part of the disordered anorectal neuromuscular function, but is often over shadowed by other more prominent symptoms. The underlying motility disturbance should not be ignored, as it may be worsened by treatment of the pelvic floor disorder. For example, abdominal rectopexy for complete rectal prolapse can worsen existing or precipitate new constipation.

The main symptom for some patients with a normal bowel frequency and normal measured transit time is difficulty with rectal evacuation. Commonly applied terms for this problem include anismus, outlet obstruction, anorectal dyssynergia, and pelvic floor incoordination, because of the observation that many such patients have poor anal sphincter relaxation during defecation straining. These patients, who are most commonly female and often middle-aged, can spend several hours a day on the toilet. Many insert a finger into the rectum, to initiate or aid evacuation, or into the vagina to help rectal emptying. In some the onset is gradual with no obvious precipitating cause, whereas in others the condition follows, or is worsened by, hysterectomy, abdominal rectopexy, or other pelvic or anorectal surgery. Examination is usually normal. A study of the rate of evacuation may show slow incomplete rectal emptying.[61] Proctography may also show incomplete emptying or failure of anal relaxation, whereas in some there is evidence of a large "rectocele," that is, bulging of the anterior rectal wall. The relationship of this radiologic or anatomic change to symptoms is not clear. The same radiologic "abnormalities" can be seen in asymptomatic individuals, and women without a rectocele may complain of the same symptoms. Furthermore, correction of the anatomic abnormality does not always lead to resolution of symptoms.

Posthysterectomy constipation has been attributed to pelvic nerve damage. Transit studies in these patients have demonstrated left colonic delay and in vitro studies of resected left colon have shown postdenervation changes. However, in some patients the constipation appears to be reversible with biofeedback retraining techniques, suggesting that delayed colonic transit may result from a loss of normal coordination after pelvic surgery.

The Elderly

Constipation is common in the elderly. In one study 42% of all acute geriatric patients admitted to hospital had fecal impaction.[62] The pathogenesis of this problem is likely to be multifactorial, and includes depression or confusion, immobility, weakness, lack of physical activity, and drugs, many with anticholinergic or other constipating side effects.

Fecal impaction in the elderly affects both sexes in similar proportion. Patients demonstrate impaired rectal and anal sensory function. Rectal expulsion and sphincter relaxation appear to be relatively normal. The disturbance of sensory function may be a primary problem, or related to medications or previous laxative nerve damage.

Pregnancy

Constipation is common in pregnancy, as are other disturbances of gastrointestinal motility, and is thought to relate to the hormonal changes such as increased progesterone and decreased motilin.

Severe Idiopathic Constipation

Young adults with a grossly decreased bowel frequency and a colon of normal diameter are almost exclusively women.[24,43,56,58,63] Some of these patients have been constipated since birth, whereas in others the onset is in adolescence or young adulthood.[57] Whether each of these groups has the same etiology is not known, although they appear clinically identical. In most of these patients there is no obvious precipitating cause for their symptoms.[56] They complain of infrequent bowel actions, sometimes only every 2 to 4 weeks, difficulty with rectal evacuation, and abdominal pain and bloating. They do not give a history of soiling, and usually have an empty rectum on examination.[44] They have a high incidence of previous gynecologic surgery, appendicectomy, and laparotomy; this probably relates to previous misdiagnosis of their lower abdominal pain, as their reproductive organs appear to be normal.[64]

These patients are usually resistant to increased dietary fiber and large doses of oral laxatives.[56]

Idiopathic Megarectum or Megacolon

Patients with severe constipation may be subdivided on the basis of rectal and colonic diameter, as assessed by contrast studies,[65] into those with a normal diameter bowel and those with an idiopathically dilated rectum (with or without dilated

Table 35-1. Causes of Constipation

Idiopathic
  Dietary abnormality
  Pregnancy
  Old age
  Irritable bowel syndrome
  Severe idiopathic constipation ("slow-transit") in women
Structural disease of the colon, rectum, or anus
  Colonic or rectal stricture
    Tumor
    Inflammation
    Chronic infection
    Ischemia
    Diverticular disease
  Distal ulcerative colitis
  Colonic neuromuscular abnormality
    Hirschsprung's disease (congenital aganglionosis)
    Chagas disease
    Intestinal pseudo-obstruction
    Idiopathic megarectum ± megacolon
    Segmental megacolon
    Myotonic dystrophy
    Systemic sclerosis
    Dermatomyositis
    Ganglioneuromatosis
      Primary
      Von Recklinghausen's disease
      Multiple endocrine neoplasia type 2B
  Anal lesion
    Tumor
    Infection
    Anal fissure
    Ectopic anus
    Internal anal sphincter myopathy
Abnormality outside the colon
  Neurologic
    Central nervous system disorders
    Damage to the spinal cord or sacral outflow
    Autonomic neuropathy—primary, paraneoplastic
  Psychological
    Anorexia nervosa
    Depression
  Metabolic disorders
    Hypothyroidism
    Glucagonoma
    Hypercalcemia
    Diabetic autonomic neuropathy
    Porphyria
    Amyloidosis
    Uremia
    Hypokalemia
    Lead poisoning
  Drug-induced

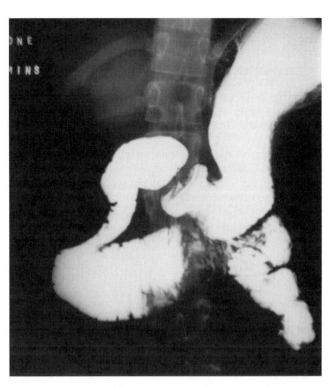

Figure 35-1. Barium follow-through examination of the stomach and small intestine of a 27-year-old woman with abdominal pain due to chronic idiopathic intestinal pseudoobstruction (CIIP) related to an inflammatory visceral neuropathy (see Figure 35-2). The third part duodenum is dilated. The duodenum is one of the most characteristic sites to pick up small bowel dilatation in patients with CIIP.

colon). Those with an idiopathically dilated rectum or rectum and colon appear to form part of a characteristic clinical group. Both sexes are affected equally. Those with onset of symptoms in childhood often have fecal soiling secondary to their impaction, a clinical feature that distinguishes them from patients with Hirschsprung's disease who very rarely soil. Other patients have onset of symptoms in adulthood; it is not known whether they acquire a megacolon or if it only becomes symptomatic later in life.

Secondary Causes of Constipation

Constipation may be related to a local colonic or anorectal cause, or may be secondary to some metabolic disorder, systemic illness, or neurologic lesion (Table 35-1).

Gastrointestinal Myopathy or Neuropathy

Patients with an abnormality of the muscle coats or the nerve plexuses in the gut may present with constipation. The best defined is Hirschsprung's disease, a congenital condition characterized by absent neurons within the bowel wall. The abnormal bowel extends for a variable proximal length from the anorectal junction, with proximal dilated normal bowel leading into the relatively narrow aganglionic segment. The affected segment ranges from very short to involving the whole colon. The most common presentation is during infancy, but occasionally patients may present for the first time even into old age, although the symptoms have been present since birth. This condition is described in more detail in Chapter 43.

The intramural nerve plexuses may be damaged in Chagas disease, caused by infection with *Trypanosoma cruzi*. Inflammation around the nerve ganglia and neuron degeneration leads to bowel dilatation and constipation.

Patients with chronic intestinal pseudo-obstruction may have prominent colonic disease with colonic dilatation and constipation.[54] The underlying disorder is one that affects either the gastrointestinal smooth muscle (i.e., a visceral myopathy), or one that affects the nerve plexuses (i.e., a visceral neuropathy) (Figs. 35-1 and 35-2). Those patients with a visceral myopathy often have just one of the two gut wall muscle coats affected. Most adult patients with this disorder are sporadic but a small minority have an inherited condition, which may be autosomal recessive or autosomal dominant. When the condition is inherited, different family members with a pathologically similar condition can have different severity of symptoms and degree of disability. Upper gastrointestinal symptoms are common, as the condition commonly affects the entire gastrointestinal tract. Some of these inherited syndromes have associated nongastrointestinal abnormalities.

A recently described myopathy of the internal anal sphincter can cause constipation, in particular difficulty with rectal evacuation, in association with proctalgia fugax. The internal anal sphincter in these patients is thickened and shows abnormalities of function and morphology.[55]

Extrinsic Neurologic Lesions

A neurologic lesion at different levels from the cerebrum to the extrinsic pelvic nerves can cause constipation. Patients with a cerebrovascular accident, including those who have had a subarachnoid hemorrhage, experience constipation in the early period after their stroke but this resolves with time. Some patients with Parkinson's disease have constipation that fluctuates with their general motor function. Either anterior or posterior pontine lesions may be associated with delayed colonic transit.

Constipation is common in patients with multiple sclerosis, occurring in 43% of affected individuals in one study.[66] It is more common in patients with moderate or severe disability, and correlates strongly with the duration of disease and the presence of genitourinary symptoms. Abnormalities of rectal compliance and absence of the normal postprandial colonic motor and myoelectrical response have been demonstrated in patients with advanced multiple sclerosis, suggesting a disturbance of the autonomic outflow to the gut.[67]

Constipation is common after spinal cord lesions.[68] The constipation may occur soon after the injury or even years later. It is thought to occur as a result of decreased extrinsic autonomic supply to the gut. Colonic compliance is markedly decreased, and there is a failure of postprandial increase in colonic motility.

In some patients constipation immediately follows either pelvic surgery or presumed trauma to the sacral outflow.[57] This can follow abdominal rectopexy, hysterectomy, or other pelvic surgery. The symptoms are of slow colonic transit with abdominal pain and bloating indistinguishable from those young women with idiopathic constipation, or of normal bowel fre-

Figure 35-2. Haematoxylin and Eosin stained section of a full-thickness small bowel biopsy from the patient shown in Figure 35-1. The longitudinal and circular muscle are seen on either side of the myenteric plexus, which is infiltrated by a large number of chronic inflammatory cells. The pseudo-obstruction in this case is caused by an inflammatory plexitis, which was later demonstrated to be due to Epstein-Barr virus infection.

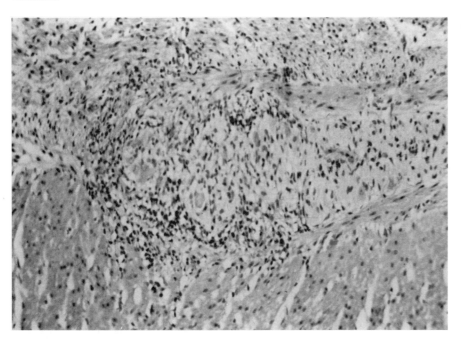

quency and colonic transit time but marked difficulty with rectal evacuation causing prolonged straining at stool. In one study, all patients who related the onset of their constipation to a previous hysterectomy had absent sacral reflexes and impaired urodynamics, suggesting extensive pelvic nerve trauma.[60]

Some patients experience profound constipation after sacral trauma, due to car accidents, spinal surgery, or even a simple fall onto the sacrum.[20,69] The presumed mechanism is damage to the sacral parasympathetic supply to the left colon, and occasionally this is accompanied by damage to the somatic voluntary muscles innervated by sacral motor roots. A similar syndrome of left colonic inertia may be produced by deliberate division of the nervi erigentes.[71] Pathologic examination of the resected colon in such cases demonstrates similar abnormalities of argyrophilic neurones in the myenteric plexus to those seen in severe idiopathic constipation.[24,69–71]

Metabolic Causes

Patients with hypothyroidism may present with constipation. In most cases this is related to the effect of thyroid hormone deficiency on the colonic muscle or neural control, without a change in colonic dimensions, but severe myxedema can be associated with infiltration of the colon and subsequent megacolon.[72]

Abnormalities of calcium and potassium metabolism probably affect the bowel by interference with intramural neural conduction, or a direct effect on smooth muscle. The transit abnormality is reversible.

The autonomic neuropathy seen in some patients with diabetes mellitus may result in constipation. These patients often give a history of several years of alternating diarrhea and constipation, followed by intractable unresponsive constipation. Diabetics with severe constipation have an absent gastrocolonic response to feeding. The colonic response to neostigmine is normal, suggesting that cholinergic postganglionic neurons are intact and that the colonic smooth muscle is capable of a normal motor response. Histologic abnormalities involving the myenteric plexus and parasympathetic nerve fibers have been described in the upper gastrointestinal tract of diabetic patients.[73]

ASSESSMENT AND INVESTIGATIONS

A careful history and precise definition of the patient's main complaints are essential. Some estimate of the amount and type of dietary intake is important. A drug history is important with particular attention to drugs that may have constipation as a side effect, and to laxatives. The age of onset of symptoms may give an important clue to the diagnosis. Constipation from birth in the absence of perianal soiling suggests congenital aganglionosis. Soiling from early childhood suggests a congenital megarectum or anorectal malformation. Symptoms developing in adolescence or as young adult suggest a motility disorder. Neoplasm should be excluded in a middle-aged or elderly patient developing new symptoms.

Examination

During the physical examination consider general causes such as hypothyroidism. Abdominal palpation may reveal fecal retention in those with a dilated or impacted bowel. Urinary reten-

tion may be present in those with a neurologic lesion. Digital examination of the lower rectum will show if there is fecal impaction or a rectal or pelvic tumor. If pain is present a fissure, abscess, or hemorrhoids should be excluded. Sigmoidoscopy is helpful in excluding a tumor or proctitis, and in confirming melanosis coli. The rectal size can also be appreciated. Reproduction of pain using air insufflation may suggest the irritable bowel syndrome.

Most young patients with mild long-standing symptoms do not require investigation. Those with severe symptoms of any age, or constipation of recent onset, require further investigation.

Radiologic Studies

In patients with a megarectum or megacolon a plain abdominal radiograph will often demonstrate the colonic dimension as well as fecal retention. In patients without megacolon a double-contrast barium enema after bowel preparation will exclude a primary colonic cause such as diverticular stricture or carcinoma. In patients with a megarectum or megacolon, including those with fecal impaction, a contrast study without preparation using a water-soluble contrast medium will provide a more useful picture of colonic size and morphology (Fig. 35-3). Bowel preparation in patients with megarectum or megacolon may reduce the bowel to normal size, giving a misleading impression about the extent of bowel dilatation. A further advantage is that unlike barium, a water-soluble contrast medium does not solidify. The maximum normal rectal diameter in a lateral radiograph at the pelvic brim is 6.5 cm; a diameter greater than this suggests that the rectum is enlarged.[65]

A contrast study may also show a distal narrow segment with proximal dilatation, suggestive of Hirschsprung's disease.

Bowel Transit Studies

In patients with severe constipation it is useful to determine whether the intestinal transit time is normal.

Radiopaque Markers

The most convenient way to measure transit is by the ingestion of radiopaque markers and a subsequent plain abdominal radiograph to determine the proportion of retained markers. Retention of more than 20% of markers 96 hours after ingestion reflects slow transit[74] (Fig. 35-4). The test should be conducted while the patient is on an adequate dietary fiber intake, and laxatives should be discontinued before the study. Severe constipation will usually be reflected by the retention of an excessive number of markers, although patients can have similar symptoms of abdominal pain, bloating, and difficult defecation, but demonstrate a normal intestinal transit time. Similarly, patients can have a normal bowel frequency but still have symptoms of difficult defecation and a slow measured intestinal transit time.

Radiographs can be taken at other times and the number of retained markers compared with a normal range.[75] The sensitivity of the test to detect an abnormal result can be further refined by ingesting three different sets of radiologically distinguishable markers on three successive days and taking a radiograph

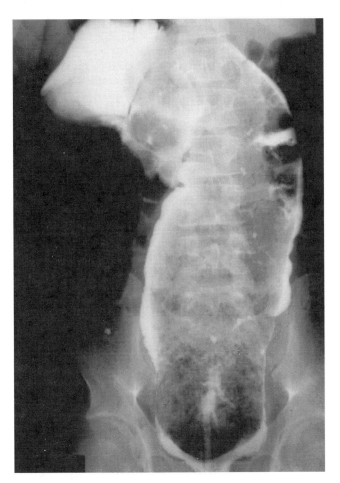

Figure 35-3. Water soluble unprepared contrast study of the large bowel in an 18-year-old boy with constipation and facal soiling since early childhood. The rectum and sigmoid are dilated and are typical of idiopathic megarectum. Note that the dilatation extends down to the pelvic floor, making Hirschsprung's disease unlikely. Other films showed the dilatation to involve only the rectum and sigmoid; the proximal colon was of normal diameter. He was managed with disimpaction and long-term maintenance with an osmotic laxative.

at 120 hours. These techniques can also be used to study the site of delay within the colon.[76]

Radioisotope Studies

More recently radioisotopes have been used to determine regional delay. They allow frequent imaging, thereby providing an accurate assessment of the site of colonic delay. The radioisotopes can be incorporated into a meal that provides information about gastric and small bowel, as well as colonic, transit.[38,77,78] Radioisotopes are more accurate at determining the site of colonic delay. For practical purposes, however, radiopaque markers are a satisfactory means of determining whether transit is normal, and the use of radioisotopes can be reserved for patients in whom surgery is contemplated and more information is required.

The usefulness of determining the site of regional delay in

choosing a particular medical or surgical treatment has not yet been proven.

Colonic Motility Studies

Although colonic motility studies are useful in a research context to characterize the motility disturbance, they have not been shown to provide information to influence management.

Studies of Defecation and Anorectal Physiology

Studies of rectal evacuation and anorectal physiology provide limited information and influence management in certain well-defined situations only.

Patients with severe constipation may fail to relax the pelvic floor on defecation straining. This can be demonstrated as a failure of relaxation of strained sphincter muscle, accompanied by a failure of the anal canal pressure to fall.[40] In a model of rectal evacuation, patients may be unable to expel a balloon

Figure 35-4. Abdominal radiograph 120 hours after ingestion of radio-opaque markers in a 32-year-old woman with severe idiopathic constipation. An excessive number of markers is retained, indicating slow intestinal transit. The sensitivity of the test can be increased by the ingestion of 3 sets of markers on successive days.

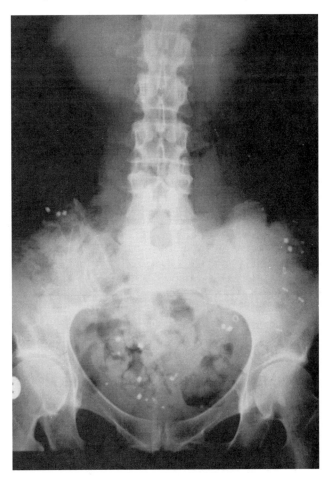

from the rectum.[41] An anal pressure or electromyographic tracing of external sphincter contraction during straining can serve as a useful signal for patients undergoing biofeedback treatment for constipation.

Evacuation proctography may demonstrate a reduced or absent ability to empty the rectum. Although this is often part of a picture of failure of pelvic floor relaxation, such a finding on its own is unhelpful in influencing management and has been shown to be unhelpful in predicting the outcome after colectomy for severe constipation.[79]

In older women whose main complaint is difficulty with rectal evacuation, proctography may also show a large rectocele or rectoanal intussusception. The radiologic signs are not specific, however, and therefore of questionable clinical significance. For example, the finding of a large rectoele correlates poorly with symptoms, since it may be seen in normal individuals without a defecatory disturbance.[80]

In patients with a dilated distal large bowel the rectoanal inhibitory reflex should be tested to distinguish idiopathic megarectum from Hirschsprung's disease. Balloon distension in the rectum causes a fall in anal pressure. This reflex, caused by a descending inhibitory neural pathway within the wall of the bowel, is absent in Hirschsprung's disease, owing to the absence of distal myenteric plexus. Some patients with idiopathic megarectum may give false-negative results owing to difficulty in distending an already dilated rectum.

Rectal Biopsy

Patients with a megarectum or megacolon and an absent rectoanal reflex should have a full-thickness rectal biopsy performed under anesthesia. This should be taken from the low rectum, but not within 2 cm of the dentate line, which can under normal circumstances have an absence of ganglia. Aganglionosis is diagnostic of Hirschsprung's disease. Staining for acetylcholinesterase demonstrates increased tissue levels in the affected aganglionic segment due to hypertrophied extrinsic nerves. This stain needs to be performed on fresh unfixed tissue. Other conditions occasionally identifiable on biopsy include systemic sclerosis and amyloidosis. Hypo- and hyperganglionosis are regarded by some clinicians to be disease entities. They are, however, largely qualitative diagnoses, based on apparent abnormalities in morphology or number of myenteric neurons. The correlation of such histologic changes with a definable clinical picture is disputed.

MEDICAL TREATMENT OF CONSTIPATION

Most patients with constipation can be managed symptomatically without investigations. This is especially true if the constipation is mild, there are no severe associated symptoms, and the condition is long-standing without recent changes.

The first step in treatment is a dietary assessment, with addition of fiber to the diet if this is deficient. Bringing the fiber intake up to 30 g/day will relieve mild constipation in many cases. Unprocessed bran, composed of large particles, can be added to breakfast cereal and is the most effective fiber supplement. Particle size as well as the type of fiber appears to be important. For patients who cannot tolerate the addition of bran to the diet, commercial fiber preparations, such as ispaghula or

sterculia, are often effective. Although the addition of fiber to the diet helps the constipation, it will cause increased wind and bloating and usually does not relieve abdominal discomfort.

If laxatives are to be used, they should be employed on a temporary basis if possible or if used long term they should be taken as infrequently as necessary. An osmotic laxative such as magnesium sulfate, or lactulose, is a satisfactory first choice. They are gentler in their action than many of the stimulant laxatives and avoid the theoretical problem of nerve plexus damage. If a stronger laxative is required, bisacodyl by mouth is often satisfactory. Senna may cause bowel nerve plexus damage but is an effective stimulant.

In the elderly who are otherwise well and not fecally impacted but who require a laxative, a senna-fiber combination appears to be more effective than lactulose.[81]

Suppositories or enemas are a good alternative to oral laxatives. Glycerine suppositories are gentle in their action, whereas bisacodyl suppositories are stronger, but leave some patients with cramps after defecation. Enemas are available as microenemas (sodium citrate) or larger phosphate enemas of 100 ml. Even in patients with severe constipation in whom oral laxatives are ineffective, rectal preparations are often helpful.

For the most severely constipated patients, stronger medication may be required intermittently. Oral stimulants include sodium picosulfate, or even electrolyte solutions such as are used for colonoscopy or radiograph preparation. These should be given with caution in patients who are extremely constipated or in those in whom bowel obstruction is a possibility Strong enemas include the use of a stimulant in water of a larger volume for example, bisacodyl rectal solution or oxyphenisatin. For the most intractable constipation a warmed enema consisting of 200 ml of one part treacle to two parts milk, is usually effective.

Patients with fecal impaction must be disimpacted prior to starting laxatives. Occasionally this can be done with sedation only, but often a general anesthetic is required. A plain abdominal radiograph is useful to confirm that the bowel has been adequately emptied.

Patients with an idiopathic megarectum or megacolon should also be disimpacted initially. They can then usually prevent further impaction by keeping the stool semiliquid, using magnesium sulfate or lactulose each day. This is usually necessary for life.

Biofeedback

Biofeedback conditioning for constipation was originally employed in the belief that abnormal pelvic floor contraction is a learned phenomenon that causes constipation. Bleijenberg and Kuijpers[82] used an intensive in-patient regimen to treat 10 patients with both delayed colonic transit and abnormal pelvic floor activity. Seven of these patients had a normal defecation frequency and feeling of urgency after treatment. Similar results were reported by Weber et al.[83] at the same time.

Biofeedback treatment involves teaching the patient how to relax the pelvic floor appropriately during defecation straining. The biofeedback component consists of the patient viewing a pressure trace derived from a pressure catheter in the anal canal, or an electromyographic trace derived from electrodes placed on the perianal skin or a plug electrode. Alternatively a balloon may be inserted into the rectum and the patient asked to expel it using abdominal muscles while simultaneously relaxing the anal sphincter.

Although biofeedback treatment was initially proposed for patients thought to have pelvic floor incoordination alone, it has also been shown to be effective in patients with documented slow colonic transit combined with pelvic floor dysfunction. It is possible that the treatment is useful in restoring bowel frequency and colonic transit time to normal, even if pelvic floor relaxation is initially normal.

The mechanism by which biofeedback treatment helps patients is currently unknown, although it is likely to be complex and to differ in different types of patients. In some, correction of the pelvic floor abnormality may be the most important element of the treatment. In these patients pelvic floor contraction may not only inhibit rectal evacuation but may promote retrograde peristalsis in the rectum and left colon. In others the behavioral therapy may disinhibit the cerebral control of colonic motility. In others discontinuing laxatives and relearning a routine for defecation, under supervision, may allow normal bowel function to re-express itself.

Biofeedback combined with relaxation training or other psychotherapeutic techniques may provide a greater success rate than biofeedback alone.[84] This behavioral treatment is dependent on a satisfactory relationship between the therapist and the patient. In addition to relearning pelvic floor relaxation, patients also learn about appropriate use of the thoracic and abdominal

muscles during straining. Many patients spontaneously talk about major personal concerns, including sexual problems, during biofeedback treatment. Although psychological therapy may well form a part of the treatment, patients may find the physical therapy of biofeedback more acceptable than initial psychotherapy.[19]

A large number of specialist centers have now reported their results using biofeedback treatment to treat intractable constipation. In most series approximately 50% to 80% of patients are symptomatically improved. The benefit appears to be sustained long term.[86] Although apparently effective in many patients, there are few controlled studies of the effectiveness of this technique against placebo. Studies are also required to show whether this treatment results in improved patient quality of life.

Botulinum A Toxin

Botulinum A toxin has been used in the treatment of disorders of the ocular muscles such as blepharospasm and strabismus and in torticollis. It is a neurotoxin produced by *Clostridium botulinum*, which causes irreversible neuromuscular blockade and a flaccid paralysis. Patients with inappropriate puborectalis contraction have been treated with injections into the muscle.[86] Although successful in decreasing voluntary anal contraction pressure, the amount of straining, and abdominal pain, it does not improve patients bowel frequency.

REFERENCES

1. Drossman DA, Sandler RS, McKee DC, Lovitz AJ (1982) Bowel patterns among subjects not seeking health care. Use of a questionnaire to identify a population with bowel dysfunction. Gastroenterology 83:529–534
2. Connell AM, Hilton C, Irvine G et al (1965) Variation of bowel habit in two population samples. BMJ 2:1095–1099
3. Thompson WG, Heaton KW (1980) Functional bowel disorders in apparently healthy people. Gastroenterology 79:283–288
4. Dent OF, Goulston KJ, Kubrzycki J, Chapuis PH (1986) Bowel symptoms in an apparently well population. Dis Colon Rectum 29:243–247
5. Bassotti G, Gaburri M, Imbimbo BP et al (1988) Colonic mass movements in idiopathic chronic constipation. Gut 29:1173–1179
6. Davies GJ, Crowder M, Reid B, Dickerson JWT (1986) Bowel function measurements of individuals with different eating patterns. Gut 27:164–169
7. Gottlieb SH, Schuster MM (1986) Dermatoglyphic (fingerprint) evidence for a congenital syndrome of early onset constipation and abdominal pain. Gastroenterology 91:428–432
8. Kamm MA, Farthing MJG, Lennard-Jones JE et al (1991) Steroid hormone abnormalities in women with severe idiopathic constipation. Gut 32:80–84
9. Tucker DM, Sandstead HH, Logan GM Jr et al (1981) Dietary fiber and personality factors as determinants of stool output. Gastroenterology 81:879–883
10. Klauser AG, Voderholzer WA, Heinrich CA et al (1990) Behavioral modification of colonic function: can constipation be learned? Dig Dis Sci 35:1271–1275
11. Preston DM, Pfeffer J, Lennard-Jones JE (1984) Psychiatric assessment of patients with severe constipation. Gut 25:A582–583
12. Brook A (1991) Bowel distress and emotional conflict. J R Soc Med 84:39–42
13. Devroede G (1994) A clinical perspective of psychological factors in constipation. pp. 101–116. In Kamm MA, Lennard-Jones JE (eds): Constipation. Wrightson Biomedical Publishing, Petersfield, UK
14. Denis P (1994), Biofeedback for constipation. pp. 340–353. In Kamm MA, Lennard-Jones JE (ed): Constipation. Wrightson Biomedical Publishing, Petersfield, UK
15. Fisher SE, Breckan K, Andrews HA, Keighley MRB (1989) Psychiatric screening for patients with faecal incontinence or chronic constipation referred for surgical treatment. Br J Surg 76:352–355
16. Wald A, Hinds JP, Caruana BJ (1989) Psychological and physiological characteristics of patients with severe idiopathic constipation. Gastroenterology 97:932–937
17. Gue M, Junien JL, Bueno L (1991) Conditioned emotional response in rats enhances colonic motility through the central release of corticotropin-releasing factor. Gastroenterology 100:964–970
18. Meshkinpour H, Harmon D, Thompson R, Yu J (1985) Effects of thoracic spinal transection on the colonic motor activity of rats. Paraplegia 25:272–276
19. Glick ME, Haldeman S, Meshkinpour H (1986) The neurovisceral and electrodiagnostic evaluation of patients with thoracic spinal cord injury. Paraplegia 24:129–137
20. Gunterberg B, Kewenter J, Peterson I, Stener B (1976) Anorec-

tal function after major resections of the sacrum with bilateral or unilateral sacrifice of sacral nerves. Br J Surg 63:546–554

21. Smith AN, Varma JS, Binnie NR, Papachrysostomou M (1990) Disordered colorectal motility in intractable constipation following hysterectomy. Br J Surg 77:1361–1366

22. Speakman CTM, Madden MV, Nicholls RJ, Kamm MA (1991) Lateral ligament division during rectopexy causes constipation but prevents recurrence: results of a prospective randomised study. Br J Surg 78:1431–1433

23. Kamm MA, Lennard-Jones JE, Nicholls RJ (1989) Evaluation of the intrinsic innervation of the internal anal sphincter using electrical stimulation. Gut 30:935–938

24. Krishnamurthy S, Schuffler MD, Rohrmann CA, Pope CE II (1985) Severe idiopathic constipation is associated with a distinctive abnormality of the colonic myenteric plexus. Gastroenterology 88:26–34

25. Koch TR, Carney JA, Go L, Go VLW (1988) Idiopathic chronic constipation is associated with decreased colonic vasoactive intestinal peptide. Gastroenterology 94:300–310

26. Milner P, Crowe R, Kamm MA et al (1990) Vasoactive intestinal polypeptide levels in the sigmoid colon are reduced in idiopathic constipation and increased in diverticular disease. Gastroenterology 99:666–675

27. Lincoln J, Crowe R, Kamm MA et al (1990) Levels of serotonin and 5-hydroxyindoleacetic acid are increased in the sigmoid colon in severe idiopathic constipation. Gastroenterology 98:1219–1225

28. Goldin E, Karmeli F, Selinger Z, Rachmilewitz D (1989) Colonic substance P levels are increased in ulcerative colitis and decreased in chronic severe constipation. Dig Dis Sci 34:754–757

29. Dolk A, Broden G, Holmstrom B et al (1990) Slow transit chronic constipation. An immunohistochemical study of neuropeptide-containing nerves in resected specimens from the large bowel. Int J Colorectal Dis 5:181–187

30. Burleigh DE (1988) Evidence for a functional cholinergic deficit in human colonic tissue resected for constipation. J Pharm Pharmacol 40:55–57

31. Altomare D, Pilot MA, Scott M et al (1992) Detection of subclinical autonomic neuropathy in constipated patients using a sweat test. Gut 33:1539–1543

32. Polak JM, Bloom SR, Sullivan SN (1977) Enkephalin-like immunoreactivity in the human gastrointestinal tract. Lancet 1:972–974

33. Lundberg JM, Hokelt T, Nilsson G et al (1978) Peptide neurons in the vagus splanchnic and somatic nerves. Acta Physiol Scand 104:499–502

34. Kaufman PN, Krevsky B, Malmud LS et al (1988) Role of opiate receptors in the regulation of colonic transit. Gastroenterology 94:1351–1356

35. Hoyle CHV, Kamm MA, Lennard-Jones JE, Burnstock G (1989) Reduced activity of enkephalins in the colon of patients with idiopathic constipation. Gut 30:A706

36. Sjolund K, Ekman R, Akre F, Lindner P (1986) Motilin in chronic idiopathic constipation. Scand J Gastroenterol 21:914–918

37. Preston DM, Adrian TE, Christofides ND et al (1985) Positive correlation between symptoms and circulating motilin, pancreatic polypeptide and gastrin concentrations in functional bowel disorders. Gut 26:1059–1064

38. van der Sijp, Kamm MA, Nightingale J et al (1993) Abnormal circulating somatostatin levels in patients with severe idiopathic constipation, abstracted. Gastroenterology 104:A593

39. Krishnamurthy S, Schuffler MD (1987) Pathology of neuromuscular disorders of the small intestine and colon. Gastroenterology 93:610–639

40. Preston DM, Lennard-Jones JE (1985) Anismus in chronic constipation. Dig Dis Sci 30:413–418

41. Barnes PRH, Lennard-Jones JE (1985) Balloon expulsion from the rectum in constipation of different types. Gut 26:1049–1052

42. Turnbull GK, Lennard-Jones JE, Bartram CI (1986) Failure of rectal expulsion as a cause of constipation: why fibre and laxatives sometimes fail. Lancet 1:767–769

43. Read NW, Timms JM, Barfield LJ et al (1986) Impairment of defaecation in young women with severe constipation. Gastroenterology 90:53–60

44. Waldron D, Bowes KL, Kingma YJ, Cote KR (1988) Colonic and anorectal motility in young women with severe idiopathic constipation. Gastroenterology 95:1388–1394

45. Jones PN, Lubowski DZ, Swash M, Henry MM (1987) Is paradoxical contraction of the puborectalis muscle of functional importance? Dis Colon Rectum 30:667–670

46. Johansson C, Nilsson BY, Mellgren A et al (1992) Paradoxical sphincter reaction and associated colorectal disorders. Int J Colorectal Dis 7:89–94

47. Mathers SE, Kempster PA, Swash M, Lees AJ (1988) Constipation and paradoxical puborectalis contraction in anismus and Parkinson's disease: a dystonic phenomenon? J Neurol Neurosurg Psychiatr 51:1503–1507

48. Koutsomanis D, Lennard-Jones JE, Kamm MA (1994) Prospective study of biofeedback treatment for patients with slow and normal transit constipation. Eur J Gastroenterol Hepatol 6:131–137

49. Drossman DA, Leserman J, Nachman G et al (1990) Sexual and physical abuse in women with functional or organic gastrointestinal disorders. Ann Intern Med 113:828–833

50. Miller R, Duthie GS, Bartolo DCC et al (1991) Anismus in patients with normal and slow transit constipation. Br J Surg 78:690–692

51. Wald A, Caruana BJ, Freimans MG et al (1990) Contributions of evacuation proctography and anorectal manometry to evaluation of adults with constipation and defecatory difficulty. Dig Dis Sci 35:481–487

52. Womack NR, Williams NS, Holmfield JHM et al (1985) New method for the dynamic assessment of anorectal function in constipation. Br J Surg 72:994–998

53. Siproudhis L, Ropert A, Lucas J et al (1992) Defecatory disorders, anorectal and pelvic floor dysfunction: a polygamy? Int J Colorectal Dis 7:102–107

54. Kamm MA (1994) Chronic intestinal pseudo-obstruction in adults. pp. 259–269. In Kamm MA, Lennard-Jones JE (eds): Constipation. Wrightson Biomedical Publishing, Petersfield, UK

55. Kamm MA, Hoyle CVH, Burleigh D et al (1991) Hereditary internal anal sphincter myopathy causing proctalgia fugax and constipation. A newly identified condition. Gastroenterology 100:805–810

56. Preston DM, Lennard-Jones JE (1986) Severe chronic consti-

pation of young women: "idiopathic slow transit constipation". Gut 27:41–48

57. Watier A, Devroede G, Duranceau A et al (1983) Constipation with colonic inertia. A manifestation of systemic disease? Dig Dis Sci 28:1025–1033

58. Reynolds JC, Ouyang A, Lee CA et al (1987) Chronic severe constipation. Prospective motility studies in 25 consecutive patients. Gastroenterology 92:414–420

59. Kerrigan DD, Lucas MG, Sun WM et al (1988) Manometric and electrophysiological investigation of anorectal and urethrovesical function in constipated females. Gastroenterology 94:A223

60. Varma JS, Smith AN (1988) Neurophysiology dysfunction in young women with intractable constipation. Gut 29:963–968

61. Kamm MA, Bartram CI, Lennard-Jones JE (1989) Rectodynamics-quantifying rectal evacuation. Int J Colorectal Dis 4: 161–163

62. Read NW, Abouzekry L, Read MG et al (1985) Anorectal function in elderly patients with faecal impaction. Gastroenterology 89:959–966

63. Shouler P, Keighley MRB (1986) Changes in colorectal function in severe idiopathic constipation. Gastroenterology 90: 414–420

64. Kamm MA, McLean A, Farthing MJG, Lennard-Jones JE (1989) Ultrasonography demonstrates no abnormality of pelvic structures in women with severe idiopathic constipation. Gut 30:1241–1243

65. Preston DM, Lennard-Jones JE, Thomas BM (1985) Towards a radiological definition of idiopathic megacolon. Gastrointest Radiol 10:167–169

66. Hinds JP, Eidelman BH, Wald A (1990) Prevalence of bowel dysfunction in multiple sclerosis. A population survey. Gastroenterology 98:1538–1542

67. Glick ME, Meshkinpour H, Haldeman S et al (1982) Colonic dysfunction in multiple sclerosis. Gastroenterology 83: 1002–1007

68. Glickman S, Kamm MA (1996) Bowel dysfunction in spinal cord injury patients. Lancet (in press)

69. Devroede G, Arhan P, Duguay C et al (1979) Traumatic constipation. Gastroenterology 77:1258–1267

70. Devroede G, Lamarche J (1974) Functional importance of extrinsic parasympathetic innervation to the distal colon and rectum in man. Gastroenterology 66:273–280

71. Preston DM, Butler MG, Smith B, Lennard-Jones JE (1983) Neuropathology of slow transit constipation. Gut 24:A997

72. Burrell M, Cronan J, Megna D, Toffler R (1980) Myxedema megacolon. Gastrointest Radiol 5:181–186

73. Smith B (1974) Neuropathology of the esophagus in diabetes mellitus. J Neurol Neurosurg Psychiatr 37:1151–1154

74. Hinton JM, Lennard-Jones JE, Young AC (1969) A new method for studying gut transit times using radio-opaque markers. Gut 10:842–847

75. Evans RC, Kamm MA, Hinton JM, Lennard-Jones JE (1992) The normal range and a simple diagram for recording whole gut transit time. Int J Colorectal Dis 7:15–17

76. Metcalf AM, Phillips SF, Zinsmeister AR et al (1987) Simplified assessment of segmental colonic transit. Gastroenterology 92:40–47

77. van der Sijp JRM, Kamm MA, Nightingale JMD et al (1993) Disturbed gastric and small bowel transit in severe idiopathic constipation. Dig Dis Sci 38:837–844

78. van der Sijp JRM, Kamm MA, Nightingale JMD et al (1993) Radioisotope determination of regional colonic transit in severe constipation. Gut 34:402–408

79. van der Sijp JRM, Kamm MA, Lennard-Jones JE (1992) Age of onset and rectal emptying: predicting outcome of colectomy for severe idiopathic constipation. Int J Colorectal Dis 7:35–37

80. Shorvon PJ, McHugh S, Diamant NE et al (1989) Defecography in normal volunteers: results and implications. Gut 30: 1737–1749

81. Passmore AP, Wilson-Davies K, Stoker C, Scott ME (1993) Chronic constipation in long stay elderly patients: a comparison of lactulose and a senna-fibre combination. BMJ 307: 769–771

82. Bleijenberg G, Kuijpers HC (1987) Treatment of spastic pelvic floor syndrome with biofeedback. Dis Colon Rectum 30: 108–111

83. Weber J, Ducrotte P, Touchais JY et al (1987) Biofeedback training for constipation in adults and children. Dis Colon Rectum 30:844–846

84. Turnbull GK, Ritvo PG (1992) Anal sphincter biofeedback relaxation treatment for women with intractable constipation symptoms. Dis Colon Rectum 35:530–536

85. Kamm MA (1993) Motility and functional diseases of the large intestine. Curr Opin Gastroenterol 9:11–18

86. Koutsomanis D, Lennard-Jones JE, Roy AJ, Kamm MA (1995) Controlled randomised trial of biofeedback versus muscle training alone for intractable constipation. Gut 37:95–99

87. Hallan RI, Williams NS, Melling J et al (1988) Treatment of anismus in intractable constipation with Botulinum A toxin. Lancet 2:714–716

36

SURGERY FOR CONSTIPATION

Peter M. Sagar
John H. Pemberton

It has been suggested that one in five healthy, middle-aged people has symptoms compatible with functional constipation and one in 10 experience outlet delay,[1] although larger epidemiologic studies estimate the prevalence of constipation at 1.2% to 4%.[2,3] Nevertheless, cathartics and laxatives are prescribed for up to 3 million patients in the United States each year and many patients, often young women, will experience distressing symptoms for days or even weeks before they gain relief from a successful bowel movement. For these patients in particular, surgical treatment can significantly improve their quality of life. Patient selection is of critical importance because an inappropriate decision to remove the colon may have disastrous, lifelong consequences.

HISTORIC PERSPECTIVE

Symptomatic constipation is a problem that dates back to ancient times when the Chinese used wooden rollers to massage the abdomen to evacuate stool.[4] Although constipation has been blamed for many illnesses since these times, Sir William Arbuthnot Lane was the first to report (in 1908) the use of colectomy with ileorectostomy as a treatment of colonic inertia.[5] He also advocated the procedure as a treatment for a variety of diseases such as thyrotoxicosis, arthritis, and tuberculosis, although most cases were patients with idiopathic megacolon. His results with ileorectostomy were superior to segmental resection, which had a high incidence of recurrent symptoms. Surgeons were reluctant to remove normal colon and the operation fell into disrepute. Even today, surgical treatment of constipation remains controversial, especially as many reported studies are incomplete or contradictory. Surgery for chronic constipation has been performed infrequently. One team performed 27 colectomies for chronic constipation during a 30-year period when they performed about 2,500 colectomies for colorectal cancer.[6]

PHYSIOLOGIC BASIS OF SURGICAL TREATMENT

In the absence of organic, anatomic, and extracolonic causes, constipation is the result of either colonic dysmotility or disordered defecation.

Normal Colonic Motility

Three types of colonic motility occur: retrograde movement, segmental nonpropulsive movement, and mass movement. Retrograde movements originate in the transverse colon, move to the cecum, and allow greater exposure of the colonic content to the mucosa for reabsorption of salt and water.[7-9] Segmental nonpropulsive movements are caused by localized, simultaneous contractions of colonic muscle, which isolates short segments and thereby pushes colonic content in either an oral or aboral direction.[10] Mass movements occur three or four times each day particularly in the transverse and descending colon.[11-13]

Studies using radiolabeled solids and liquids infused into the cecum have shown that liquids move ahead of solids in the ascending colon but are stored equally in the transverse colon. Whereas the descending colon acts mainly as a conduit, the sigmoid stores colonic content extensively.[14,15]

Colonic Dysmotility

Colonic dysmotility can occur with normal transit and be associated with abdominal pain, bloating, frequent, loose stools with the onset of pain; and incomplete evacuation—irritable bowel syndrome[16]—or it may occur with slow transit. This latter group has a radiographically normal colon and yet transit of radiopaque markers or a radioisotope-labeled meal along the colon is markedly prolonged.[17] Patients will show one of three patterns of transit: normal, rectosigmoid delay, or colonic inertia. The cause of delayed transit is unknown. Abnormalities of the myenteric plexus, impaired rectal sensation (and hence awareness of the need to defecate), laxative abuse, and decreased stool volumes have all been suggested. Defective cholinergic innervation has also been postulated. Constipated patients show little or no colonic motor activity in response to an injection of edrophonium.[18] In vitro preparations of the circular muscle layer from the sigmoid colon of patients with idiopathic chronic constipation show slower or longer nonadrenergic, non-cholinergic inhibitory neuromuscular transmission and are less likely to discharge trains of action potentials when the smooth muscle is depolarized compared with controls.[19]

Mechanism of Normal Defecation

The sigmoid colon is the main fecal storage organ. When the sigmoid is full, muscular contractions empty stool into the rectum. Conscious awareness of a full rectum is brought about by receptors in the rectal wall, pelvic floor, and upper anal canal. Rectal filling is recognized at a volume of about 50 ml. If the rectum continues to fill, the subject experiences an urge to defecate. This urge is probably mediated by stretch receptors in the pelvic floor, as placing a small balloon in the rectum and tugging against puborectalis will reproduce this sensation.[20] As the rectum distends, puborectalis is stretched. Distension of the rectum leads to relaxation of the internal anal sphincter and sampling of the contents. The external sphincter contracts. If the subject wishes to defecate, then intra-abdominal pressure is made to rise by contraction of the diaphragm, abdominal muscles, and the Valsalva maneuver. Puborectalis relaxes and allows the anorectal angle to become less acute.[21,22] Defecation is easier if the subject adopts the squatting position because this increases the anorectal angle more than can be achieved by flexion of the hips to 90° alone. Inhibition of pelvic floor activity allows descent of the pelvic floor by about 2 cm, which further straightens out this angle.[23] As the rectum empties, there is inhibition of the anal sphincter and anal pressure falls. If, however, the subject chooses not to defecate, contraction of the external sphincter allows the internal sphincter to recover and the rectal contents are propelled away from the anal canal by forceful contraction of puborectalis and the other pelvic floor muscles.

Obstructed Defecation

Obstructed defecation secondary to pelvic floor dysfunction occurs when the pelvic floor is immobile and fails to relax when the patient strains to defecate. The pelvic floor fails to descend and thus the anorectal angle fails to straighten. The normal response to defecation straining is silencing of electrical activity and therefore relaxation of sphincter muscles. In patients with obstructed defecation, puborectalis may actually increase its rate of firing and compound the obstruction at the outlet of the pelvic floor. Such patients are unable to initiate defecation, evacuate incompletely, and have to resort to digital evacuation. Three criteria are required to define obstructed defecation: demonstration of puborectalis electromyographic (EMG) recruitment greater than 50%, evidence of an adequate level of intrarectal pressure (greater than 50 cm H_2O on straining), and presence of defective evacuation.[24] EMG findings alone can be misleading and need to be related to radiologic evidence of incomplete evacuation.[25] Patients with obstructed defecation

fail to expel a rectal balloon and defecography shows persistence of the acute anorectal angle on straining and failure to open the anal canal.[26] In addition, there is impaired and delayed expulsion of artificial stool and prolonged transit along the rectosigmoid colon compared with patients with a mobile perineum.[27] EMG recordings of puborectalis show a paradoxic rise in activity when the patient performs a Valsalva maneuver. Such constipated patients with disordered evacuation may be distinguished from constipated patients with normal pelvic floor function by the simple clinical observation of failure of the perineum to descend more than 1 cm on straining.[27]

EVALUATION AND PHYSIOLOGIC ASSESSMENT

The symptom of constipation is variously described and largely depends on the patient's idea of normality. It refers to difficult, infrequent, or incomplete evacuation. Psychological factors play an important role. Some patients ascribe undue importance to a daily bowel action and become very concerned if they miss their daily movement. Conversely, some subjects repeatedly ignore the call to stool because of a busy lifestyle. Normal frequency of bowel action is between three times per day and three times per week.[28] Consistency and form of stool correlates well with time since previous bowel action. Slow intestinal transit is associated with hard pellet-like stools, whereas loose stools occur with rapid transit.[29] Small pellet-like stools are more difficult to evacuate than soft bulky ones.[30]

Assessment and Investigations

The indications for operation are poorly defined. Joint management between physician and surgeon is essential and should reduce the chance of major, unrecognized psychological problems being missed. Patients suitable for surgical intervention must be selected with great care. Thorough investigation will identify only a small proportion (10%) of all patients with constipation as being suitable candidates for surgery.

It is necessary to distinguish patients with colonic inertia from those with anorectal outlet dysfunction. A thorough history and careful examination are required. What does the patient mean by "constipation" and is the patient actually constipated? Frequency, consistency, and degree of straining should be determined. A sensation of persistent rectal fullness, rectal pain, the need to self-digitate or apply pressure to the posterior vaginal wall, and support of the perineum during defecation may be present. Excessive straining, self-digitation, failure of enemas, and abnormal balloon expulsion are indicative of outlet dysfunction. A sense of incomplete rectal evacuation is more typical of the irritable bowel syndrome. Dietary history, psychosocial factors, previous abuse of laxatives, or use of constipating drugs are all important. Gastrointestinal and metabolic causes of constipation should be ruled out with the usual tests. All patients must undergo a barium enema. Melanosis coli indicative of use of anthroquinone laxatives may be seen on flexible sigmoidoscopy.

The majority of patients with constipation will respond to increased daily fiber (greater than 25 g) and water.[31] Noncompliance is the usual reason for failure. Bowel training regimens have been described that involve discontinuation of laxatives, use of glycerin suppositories and enemas, and encouraging unrushed defecation as opposed to 45 seconds of straining on the toilet; 30 to 60 ml of milk of magnesia at night is also beneficial.

Patients who fail to respond to these measures are classified as having intractable constipation and warrant further evaluation. The key to selection of patients who will benefit from surgery is objective physiologic investigation:

Colonic Transit Studies

Colonic motor function may be tested by a number of methods of which the simplest is the ingestion of radiopaque markers. The markers are followed along the gastrointestinal tract with daily abdominal radiographs.[32] It is easy, inexpensive, reproducible, and repeatable. If a patient ingests 20 markers on day 0, then an abdominal radiograph on day 5 should show clearance of 80% of the markers from the colon. An alternative method requires ingestion of 20 distinctive radiopaque markers on each of the first 3 days and an abdominal radiograph taken on day 4.[33] This technique also gives information on segmental transit. Patients with transit times greater than 72 hours are classified as having slow transit constipation.

Scintigraphic methods to determine panintestinal transit are available that provide more reliable measures of segmental colonic transit and expose the patients to less radiation.[34] This technique quantifies gastric emptying and small bowel transit times as well as colonic transit times all within 24 hours. These techniques require repeat gamma scans and are not widely available. Segmental transit studies have been recommended by some authors as a means of limiting the extent of segmental colonic resection[35] but there are no convincing reports to suggest that these patients fare better than patients after total colectomy and ileorectostomy. Indeed, most authors have failed to find a significant degree of slowing in one segment compared with another and would advise against any resection less than total colectomy and ileorectostomy.[36]

Colonic Myoelectrical and Motor Function

Colonic myoelectrical activity is recorded by ring electrodes mounted on a polyvinyl tube while manometric recordings are made with point sensors.[37] Long duration bursts of spikelike activity have propulsive function but the propulsive function of the vast majority of colonic electrical activity and low amplitude manometric activity is unclear. Intraluminal measurements of colonic activity remain a research tool.

Anal Manometry

Anal manometry is not usually helpful with severe constipation. Very high resting anal pressures would suggest the presence of an anal fissure. Absence of the rectoanal inhibitory reflex raises the possibility of adult Hirschsprung's disease and the patients should then undergo a full-thickness rectal biopsy to confirm the absence of ganglion cells.

Defecating Proctogram

Defecating proctography in the constipated patient may demonstrate a rectocele, nonrelaxing puborectalis, or occult intussusception. Unfortunately, defecography will reveal similar abnor-malities in up to 50% of normal subjects.[38] Nevertheless, significant anatomic abnormalities may be identified and, although some will respond to increased dietary fiber, others will require surgical correction. For example, a severe internal intussusception with complete outlet obstruction secondary to funnel-shaped plugging at the anal canal or a large rectocele that fills preferentially at defecation rather than the barium being expelled through the anal canal are both readily amenable to surgical repair.

Inability to evacuate contrast during defecating proctography may be due to the unnatural, embarrassing nature of the test but if patients genuinely have difficulty evacuating the liquid barium then they may also have difficulty with evacuation of semiformed stool after colectomy.

Balloon Expulsion

Balloon expulsion evaluates the defecatory process and relaxation of puborectalis. A catheter with a balloon is placed in the rectum. The balloon is inflated to 50 ml. The patient is then asked to expel the balloon either while sitting on the toilet or in the left lateral position with the catheter suspended over a pulley. Weights are attached to the catheter (up to 200 g) until the balloon is expelled.[27] Failure to expel the balloon indicates outlet dysfunction and poor outcome after colectomy.[39] Fourteen of 25 patients who underwent a preoperative balloon expulsion test were unable to expel a 50-ml water-filled balloon. This group was much more likely to experience postoperative pain and require prolonged treatment with laxatives than patients who were able to expel the balloon.

Percentage Evacuation of Stool

Efficiency of defecation may be measured by calculating the percentage of artificial radiolabeled stool evacuated from the rectum.[40] Normal subjects will evacuate 60% ± 6% of stool in 10 seconds but this is significantly reduced in patients with obstructed defecation. This test can also be used to measure perineal descent and the anorectal angle at rest, squeezing, and straining. The anorectal angle fails to increase significantly at straining in patients with pelvic floor dysfunction.

Electromyography

The normal response to straining at defecation is silencing of electrical activity and relaxation of sphincter muscles. In patients with obstructed defecation, puborectalis may actually increase its rate of firing and compound the obstruction at the outlet of the pelvic floor. Three criteria help to define obstructed defecation: demonstration of puborectalis EMG recruitment greater than 50%, evidence of an adequate level of intrarectal pressure (greater than 50 cm H_2O on straining), and presence of defective evacuation.[24] EMG recordings of puborectalis show a paradoxic rise in activity when the patient performs a Valsalva maneuver. EMG findings alone, however, can be misleading and need to be related to radiologic evidence of incomplete evacuation.[25]

Table 36-1.   Tests of Anorectal Function for the Patient With Constipation

Test	Measures	Indication
Anal manometry	Increased RAP	Fissure-in-ano
	Increased MSP	Puborectalis spasm
	Absent rectoanal inhibitory reflex	Hirschsprung's disease
Radiopaque marker studies	Intestinal transit	Colonic inertia
Scintigraphic studies	Colonic transit	Colonic inertia
Defecating proctography	Dynamic movements of pelvic floor	Occult intussusception
Balloon expulsion	Ability to evacuate rectum	Obstructed defecation
% evacuation of stool	Efficiency of defecation	Obstructed defecation

Abbreviations: RAP, resting anal pressure; MSP, mean sphincter pressure.

Rectal Sensation

If megarectum is suspected, sensory perception of the rectum can be assessed by measurement of the first sensation volume and maximum tolerated volume as a balloon is inflated within the rectum. Patients with megarectum have greatly increased volumes due to chronic dilatation.

Studies with rectoanal manovolumetry during graded isobaric rectal distension have found that the pressure of distension needed to elicit a sensation of rectal filling and an urge to defecate may be abnormally high in a subgroup of patients who would otherwise be suitable for colectomy and ileorectostomy. Patients with blunted rectal sensation tend not to improve after colectomy.[41]

Classification of Constipation

On the basis of these functional studies, patients can be classified as having the following:

1. Slow transit constipation: colon transit significantly delayed, pelvic floor function normal.
2. Pelvic floor dysfunction: colon transit normal, pelvic floor function abnormal.
3. Slow transit constipation and pelvic floor dysfunction: colon transit significantly delayed, pelvic floor function abnormal.
4. Irritable bowel syndrome: colon transit normal, pelvic floor function normal. Patients with irritable bowel syndrome respond poorly to surgery.

The tests of central importance are colon transit studies to identify slow transit constipation and balloon expulsion to identify pelvic floor dysfunction.

Indications for anorectal tests in constipated patients are summarized in Table 36-1. An algorithm for the investigation of the constipated patient is shown in Figure 36-1.

TREATMENT

Surgical Treatment of Slow Transit Colon

The treatment of colonic inertia, assuming the failure of an aggressive prolonged trial of laxatives and fiber, is total colectomy with ileorectal anastomosis. Patients need to be told that the procedure is designed to treat the symptom of constipation and that other symptoms that the patient associates with constipation may not necessarily be relieved by achieving regular defecation.[42] Colectomy is carried out with conservative mesenteric dissection to the level of the sacral promontory with an anastomosis between the terminal ileum and upper rectum. The presacral space is entered with careful preservation of the sympathetic nerves.

Ileorectostomy is more successful than ileosigmoidostomy.[36] If any part of the sigmoid is left in place, constipation may recur whereas an anastomosis at a lower level may result in an unacceptably high frequency of bowel movements and sometimes fecal incontinence. As with segmental resection or partial colectomy,[43] removal of the colon but with preservation of the cecum and ileocecal valve has been shown to be associated with poor results. If the cecal reservoir is maintained, dilatation followed and constipation recurred.[44] In patients in whom a thorough physiologic evaluation has been undertaken,[34] with demonstration of convincing evidence of colonic inertia and no evidence of outlet obstruction, prompt and sustained relief of constipation can be expected.[36] Patients who continue to be constipated after ileorectostomy are likely to have abnormal pelvic floor function.[36]

Reported Series

The results of surgery for constipation vary considerably even in the recent literature, partly because the mechanisms of constipation are often not fully evaluated and heterogeneous groups of patients are operated upon. The outcome is then, not surprisingly, highly variable.

In a series from the Mayo Clinic of 277 patients who had undergone thorough evaluation as described above, 36 were found to have slow transit constipation with or without pelvic floor dysfunction. Colectomy and ileorectostomy were carried out in 34 and ileosigmoidostomy in 2 patients. There was no mortality. Return of bowel function was observed at 6 ± 4 days (mean ± 1SD). Recurrent constipation was only observed in one patient, who had undergone an ileosigmoidostomy, who later underwent successful conversion to ileorectostomy. Only 10% of patients had liquid stools 2 months after operation and eventually all patients described solid stools at a frequency of 2.0 ± 1.5 bowel movements a day without the need for antidiarrheal medication.[36] Although 14 of the 36 patients in this study had been shown to have pelvic floor dysfunction as well as slow transit constipation and would have been at risk of failure of ileorectostomy, each underwent pelvic floor retraining prior

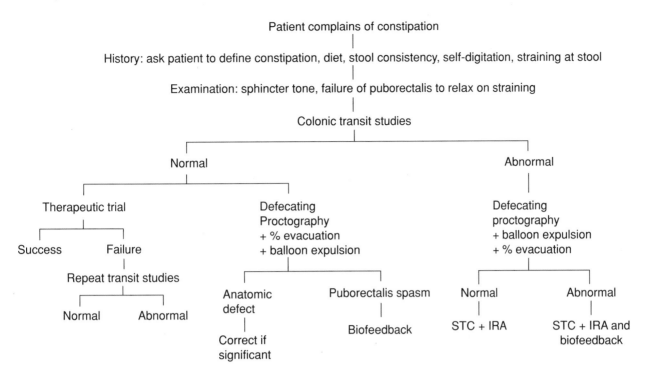

Figure 36-1. Investigation of idiopathic constipation. IRA, iliorectal anastomosis; STC, subtotal colectomy.

to surgery and were able to defecate spontaneously at completion of the program.

A similar physiologically based report of 163 patients who underwent assessment found only 16 patients to be suitable for total colectomy and ileorectostomy.[42] No mortality or significant postoperative morbidity was observed and the constipation was successfully treated in all patients with a frequency of bowel action of 3.5 per day (range 1 to 6 per day) at 15 months. Three patients required continued use of antidiarrheal medication.

A retrospective review of 52 patients found 79% of patients to be satisfied with their outcome with a frequency of bowel actions of 2.8 per day. Enemas were required by 20% of patients, however, probably because most of the patients had undergone ileodistal sigmoidostomy.[45] The incidence of postoperative complications in this series was unusually high but were largely technical and avoidable.

A series of 44 female patients from St. Mark's Hospital with a mean preoperative bowel frequency of one per month found that total colectomy with ileorectostomy resulted in normal bowel frequency in 50% and more than three stools per day in a further 39%. Constipation was reported in 11% of patients.[46] Disappointingly, further operations were required in 39% of patients although only 3 patients required reoperation for constipation.

Finally, the surgeon may encounter an occasional patient with severe idiopathic constipation in whom all medical treatment has failed, an ileorectostomy has not resolved the problem, and the patient refuses a stoma. The patient may be desperate for a solution and in such cases ileal pouch-anal anastomosis has been performed with satisfactory results.[47] Interestingly, one of two patients in the first report of the use of ileal pouch-anal

anastomosis for treatment-resistant constipation required self-catheterization despite having a J-pouch. A series of 13 patients who underwent ileal pouch-anal anastomosis for constipation included 8 patients who had previously undergone ileorectostomy. Postoperative morbidity was high but 85% of these patients gained symptomatic improvement and improved quality of life.[48]

The results of colectomy and ileorectostomy for idiopathic constipation are shown in Table 36-2.

Surgical Treatment of Outlet Obstruction

One would expect division of the posterior fibers of puborectalis to be beneficial in patients in whom the muscle paradoxically contracted at the time of defecation but this does not appear to be so. Attempts at surgical correction of obstructed defecation with partial division of puborectalis either in the posterior plane[49] or laterally[50] have been disappointing. Division of the inner fibers of puborectalis on either side of the midline produced symptomatic improvement in only 1 of 7 patients,[49] whereas lateral division of the muscle produced improvement in only 3 of 15 patients at the cost of minor incontinence.[50] Finally, posterior division also produced poor results (2 of 9 patients improved) with fecal incontinence developing in 5 patients.[51]

Anorectal myectomy has been used successfully for children with short segment Hirschsprung's disease.[52] A 2-cm wide strip of the internal sphincter and rectal circular muscle are excised from the anal canal and lower third of the rectum. Although the results in children were encouraging, results in patients over the age of 10 years have proved unsatisfactory with long-term follow-up.[53] At a mean period of follow-up of 2.5 years only

Table 36-2. Results of Surgery for Slow Transit Constipation With Patient Selection Based on Objective Physiologic Assessment

Author	Patients Studied	Patients Suitable for Surgery	Patients Operated On	Morbidity	Success Rate
Pemberton et al. (1991)[36]	277	43	38	11% SBO	100%
Wexner et al. (1991)[42]	163	16	16	0%	94%
Redmond et al. (1995)[62]	37	21 CI	37	ns	90% CI
		16 GID			13% GID
Mehendra et al. (1994)[63]	19	12	9	33%	88%
Sunderland et al. (1992)[64]	228	21	18	ns	88%

Abbreviations: SBO, small bowel obstruction; CI, colonic inertia; GID, generalized intestinal dysmotility.

17% of 63 patients could defecate spontaneously and 10% experienced minor fecal incontinence. There have been a few reports of the successful use of anal dilatation in children with fecal seepage or soiling complicating chronic constipation in the presence of high anal sphincter pressures[54] but there are no convincing data to support its use in adults.

Injection of *Clostridium botulinum* type A neurotoxin directly into puborectalis can produce excellent clinical results in some but may render others incontinent.[55] The results of surgery for anorectal outlet dysfunction are so unimpressive and the risks of incontinence unacceptably high that anorectal operations appear to have no role at the present time.

Biofeedback and relaxation training have been more successful[56] and, importantly, free of morbidity. Biofeedback can be used to train patients to relax their pelvic floor muscles during straining and to correlate relaxation and pushing to achieve defecation.[36] It is a relearning process in which the nonrelaxing activity of the pelvic floor is gradually suppressed. Biofeedback is also used in the treatment of fecal incontinence. There are, however, major differences in the use of biofeedback for fecal incontinence and constipation. The incontinent patient with intact neural pathways is able to appreciate a sensation of muscular contractile activity whereas the constipated patient has no similar sensation of muscular relaxation. In addition, sphincter squeeze is easily measured with manometry whereas manometry does not easily reflect relaxation. Nevertheless, biofeedback has been shown to reduce obstructive symptoms with an increase in the frequency of bowel actions, a more obtuse anorectal angle at the time of defecation, and more dynamic pelvic floor movements when the anal sphincter is contracted.[57] Quality of higher control of bowel function is improved. If pelvic floor dysfunction coexists with colonic inertia, then colectomy and ileorectal anastomosis may be carried out after pelvic floor retraining.[36]

Descending Perineum Syndrome

Constipation may also be seen in patients with "descending perineum syndrome." Such patients strain endlessly at stool but the rectum empties incompletely. The perineum is seen to bulge well below the plane of the ischial tuberosities. This abnormal perineal descent is probably secondary to injury to the sacral nerves from either childbirth or chronic straining at stool. Incomplete evacuation leads to more straining, more traction on the nerves, and progressive denervation of the external anal sphincter and puborectalis. In time, this scenario leads to fecal incontinence and thereby compounds the patient's misery. Surgery cannot correct this problem, which is best treated with biofeedback.

Rectal Intussusception

Occult rectal intussusception, and complete rectal prolapse, produce symptoms of obstructed defecation and incomplete evacuation. Again, repeated straining is counterproductive and increases the size of the prolapse. An occult intussusception will be apparent on defecography whereas rectal prolapse will be evident clinically. The latter responds well to surgical correction but the results of surgical treatment of the former are mixed at best.

Rectocele

A rectocele, the herniation of the anterior rectal wall into the lumen of the vagina, is often seen in a patient with constipation but the two are not necessarily related. It may be seen in healthy subjects particularly when childbirth has led to separation of the levator ani muscles but can also be a contributory factor in difficult evacuation. For a rectocele to cause outlet obstruction, two factors should be present: digital vaginal pressure to facilitate defecation and retained stool with a rectocele on defecography.[58] Symptoms of urinary incontinence are often present.[59] The anatomic lesion is due to a weakness in the circular muscle fibers of the lower rectal wall. Endoanal correction of a rectocele in these patients will alleviate symptoms of obstructive defecation.

Stoma

Many surgeons are surprised when a patient eventually requests a stoma because of constipation but it underlines the unhappiness that constipation can cause. A stoma may be a good option as it may be reversed but many patients have difficulty accepting a stoma perhaps because of the high incidence of psychological problems in this group of patients. Again, careful selection of patients is essential. A colostomy allows the possibility of colonic irrigation but a number of authors have reported unsatisfactory results because of persisting colonic inertia proximal to the site of the ostomy or a disorder of panintestinal motility. The best results appear to be in patients in whom a stoma is constructed as a primary procedure rather than after failed ileorectostomy.[60]

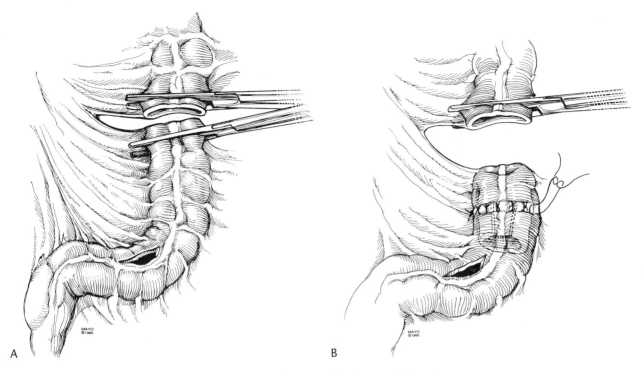

Figure 36-2. **(A & B)** Construction of a continent colonic conduit. (By permission of Mayo Foundation.)

A variation on the theme of a stoma is the recently described operation of a continent colonic conduit.[61] The sigmoid colon can be used as a continent conduit by transection at its midpoint, creation of a 3-cm longitudinal incision in the anterior wall of the distal colon 15 cm from the divided end, and intussuscepting a 5-cm segment of colon commencing 5 cm from the transected end to create a valve. The valve serves to prevent reflux of fecal material. The conduit is brought out onto the anterior abdominal wall and intestinal continuity is re-established by anastomosing the proximal sigmoid colon to the upper rectum (Fig. 36-2). Patients are taught to intubate and irrigate the conduit. The operation is successful in reducing the time the patient spends evacuating rectal contents and increases the number of bowel movements. The procedure is also reversible.

CONCLUSION

Many patients complain of constipation but only a small fraction will require surgical treatment. Careful physiologic evaluation is the cornerstone of management with the use of colon transit studies to identify slow transit constipation and the balloon expulsion test to identify outlet obstruction perhaps being the most useful. Colonic inertia responds to total colectomy with ileorectostomy whereas pelvic floor dysfunction is best managed with biofeedback.

REFERENCES

1. Talley NJ, Weaver AL, Zinsmeister AR, Melton LJ (1993) Prevalence of gastrointestinal symptoms in the elderly. A population-based study. Gastroenterology 105:781–790

2. Johanson JF, Sonnenberg A (1990) The prevalence of hemorrhoids and chronic constipation. An epidemiological study. Gastroenterology 98:380–386

3. Sonnenberg A, Koch TR (1989) Epidemiology of constipation in the United States Dis Colon Rectum 32:1–8

4. Schouten WR, Gordon PH (1992) Constipation. p. 908. In Gordon PH, Nivatvongs S (eds): Principles and Practice of Surgery for the Colon, Rectum and Anus. Quality Medical Publishing, St. Louis, Missouri

5. Lane WA (1908) The results of the operative treatment of chronic constipation. BMJ 126–130

6. Hughes ESR, McDermott FT, Johnson WR, Polglase AL (1981) Surgery for constipation. Aust NZ J Surg 51:144–148

7. Almy TP (1973) Constipation. In Sleisenger MH, Fordtran JS (eds): Gastrointestinal Disease. Philadelphia, WB Saunders

8. Thompson JC, Marx M (1984) Gastrointestinal hormones. Curr Probl Surg 21:6–24

9. Christofides ND, Ghatei MA, Bloom SR et al (1982) Decreased plasma motilin concentrations in pregnancy. BMJ 285: 1453–1454

10. Menardo G, Bausano G, Corazziari E et al (1987) Large-bowel transit in paraplegic patients. Dis Colon Rectum 30:924–928

11. Mahieu P, Pringot J, Bodart P (1984) Defecography. I. Description of a new procedure and results in normal patients. Gastrointest Radiol 247–251

12. Mahieu P, Pringot J, Bodart P (1984) Defecography. II. Contribution to the diagnosis of defecation disorders. Gastrointest Radiol 253–261

13. Barnes PRH, Lennard-Jones JE (1985) Balloon expulsion from

the rectum in constipation of different types. Gut 26: 1049–1052

14. Hammer J, Phillips SF (1993) Fluid loading of the human colon: effects on segmental transit and stool composition. Gastroenterology 105:988–998

15. Proano M, Camilleri M, Phillips SF et al (1990) Transit of solids through the human colon: regional quantification in the unprepared bowel. Am J Physiol 258:G856–862

16. Manning AP, Thompson WG, Heaton KW, Morris AF (1978) Towards positive diagnosis of the irritable bowel. BMJ 2: 653–654

17. van der Sijp JR, Kamm MA, Nightingale JM et al (1993) Radioisotope determination of regional colonic transit in severe constipation: comparison with radio opaque markers. Gut 34: 402–408

18. Bassotti G, Chiarioni G, Imbimbo BP et al (1993) Impaired colonic motor response to cholinergic stimulation in patients with severe chronic idiopathic (slow transit type) constipation. Dig Dis Sci 38:1040–1045

19. Hoyle CH, Kamm MA, Lennard-Jones JE, Burnstock G (1992) An *in vitro* electrophysiological study of the colon from patients with idiopathic chronic constipation Clin Auton Res 2: 327–333

20. Scarli AF, Kiesewetter WB (1970) Defecation and continence. Dis Colon Rectum 13:81–107

21. Womack NR, Williams NS, Holmfield JH et al (1985) New method for the dynamic assessment of anorectal function in constipation. Br J Surg 72:994–998

22. Barkel DC, Pemberton JH, Phillips SF et al (1986) Scintigraphic assessment of the anorectal angle in health and after operation. Surg Forum 37:183–186

23. Womack NR, Williams NS, Holmfield JH, Morrison JFB (1987) Anorectal function in the solitary rectal ulcer syndrome. Dis Colon Rectum 30:319–320

24. Roberts JP, Womack NR, Hallan RI et al (1992) Evidence from dynamic integrated proctography to redefine anismus. Br J Surg 79:1213–1215

25. Miller R, Duthie GS, Bartolo DC et al (1991) Anismus in patients with normal and slow transit constipation. Br J Surg 78:690–692

26. Nielson MB, Buron B, Christiansen J, Hegedus V (1993) Defecographic findings in patients with anal incontinence and constipation and their relation to rectal emptying. Dis Colon Rectum 36:806–809

27. Pezim ME, Pemberton JH, Levin KE et al (1993) Parameters of anorectal and colonic motility in health and in severe constipation. Dis Colon Rectum 36:484–491

28. Camilleri M, Thompson WG, Fleshman JW, Pemberton JH (1994) Clinical management of intractable constipation. Ann Intern Med 121:520–528

29. Heaton KW, Radvan J, Cripps H et al (1992) Defecation frequency and timing, and stool form in the general population: a prospective study. Gut 33:818–824

30. Bannister JJ, Davison P, Timms JM et al (1987) Effect of stool size and consistency on defecation. Gut 28:1246–1250

31. Cummings JH (1984) Constipation, dietary fibre and the control of large bowel function. Postgard Med J 60:811–819

32. Hinton JM, Lennard-Jones JE, Young AC (1969) A new method for studying gut transit times using radio-opaque markers. Gut 10:385–389

33. Metcalf AM, Phillips SF, Zinsmeister AR et al (1987) Simpli-

fied assessment of segmental colonic transit. Gastroenterology 92:40–47

34. Stivland TA, Vassallo M, Camilleri M et al (1990) Regional transit in the gut of patients with idiopathic constipation. Gastroenterology 98:A668

35. Schouten WR (1991) Severe longstanding constipation in adults, indications for surgical treatment. Scand J Gastroenterol 188:60–68

36. Pemberton JH, Rath DM, Ilstrup DM (1991) Evaluation and surgical treatment of severe chronic constipation. Ann Surg 214:403–413

37. Bueno L, Fioramonti J, Ruckebusch Y et al (1980) Evaluation of colonic myoelectrical activity in health and functional disorders. Gut 21:480–485

38. Goie R (1990) Anorectal function in patients with defaecation disorders and asymptomatic subjects. Radiology 174:121–123

39. van der Sijp JRM, Kamm MA, Evans RC, Lennard-Jones JE (1992) The results of stoma formation in severe idiopathic constipation. Eur J Gastroenterol Hepatol 4:137–140

40. O'Connell PR, Kelly KA, Brown ML (1986) Scintigraphic assessment of neorectal function. J Nucl Med 27:460–464

41. Akervall S, Fasth S, Nordgren S et al (1988) The functional results after colectomy and ileorectal anastomosis for severe constipation (Arbuthnot Lane's disease) as related to rectal sensory function. Int J Colorect Dis 3:96–101

42. Wexner SD, Daniel N, Jagelman DG (1991) Colectomy for constipation: physiologic investigation is the key to success. Dis Colon Rectum 34:851–856

43. McCready RA, Beart RW Jr (1979) The surgical treatment of incapacitating constipation associated with idiopathic megacolon. Mayo Clin Proc 54:779–783

44. Fasth S, Hedlund H, Svaninger T et al (1983) Functional results after subtotal colectomy and caecorectal anastomosis. Acta Chir Scand 149:623–627

45. Vasilevsky CA, Nemer FD, Balcos EG et al (1988) Is subtotal colectomy a viable option in the management of chronic constipation. Dis Colon Rectum 31:679–681

46. Kamm MA, Hawley PR, Lennard Jones JE (1988) Outcome of colectomy for severe idiopathic constipation. Gut 29:969–973

47. Nicholls RJ, Kamm MA (1988) Proctocolectomy with restorative ileo-anal reservoir for severe idiopathic constipation. A report of two cases. Dis Colon Rectum 31:968–969

48. Hosie KB, Kmiot WA, Keighley MRB (1990) Constipation: another indication for restorative proctocolectomy. Br J Surg 77:801–802

49. Keighley MRB, Shouler P (1984) Outlet syndrome: is there a surgical option? J R Soc Med 77:559–563

50. Kamm MA, Hawley PR, Lennard-Jones JE (1988) Lateral division of puborectalis in the management of severe constipation. Br J Surg 75:661–663

51. Barnes PRH, Hawley PR, Preston DM, Lennard-Jones JE (1985) Experience of posterior division of the puborectalis muscle in the management of chronic constipation. Br J Surg 72:475–477

52. Thomas CG, Bream CA, DeConninck P (1970) Posterior sphincterotomy and rectal myotomy in the management of Hirschsprung's disease. Ann Surg 171:796–809

53. Pinho M, Yoshioka K, Keighley MRB (1989) Long term results of anorectal myectomy for chronic constipation. Br J Surg 76:1163–1164

54. Loening-Baucke V (1984) Abnormal rectoanal function in children recovered from chronic constipation and encoparesis. Gastroenterology 87:1299–1304

55. Hallan RI, Williams NS, Melling J et al (1988) Treatment of anismus in intractable constipation with botulinum A toxin. Lancet 1:714–717

56. Wexner SD, Cheape JD, Jorge JMN et al (1992) Prospective assessment of biofeedback for the treatment of paradoxical puborectalis contraction. Dis Colon Rectum 35:145–150

57. Papachrysostomou M, Smith AN (1994) Effects of biofeedback on obstructive defecation—reconditioning of the defecation reflex? Gut 35:252–256

58. Sarles JC, Arnaud A, Selezneff I, Olivier S (1989) Endorectal repair of rectocele. Int J Colorect Dis 4:167–171

59. Siproudhis L, Dautreme S, Ropert A et al (1993) Dyschezia and rectocele—a marriage of convenience? Dis Colon Rectum 36:1030–1036

60. van der Sijp JRM, Kamm MA, Bartram CI, Lennard-Jones JE (1992) The value of age of onset and rectal emptying in predicting the outcome of colectomy for severe idiopathic constipation. Int J Colorect Dis 7:35–37

61. Williams NS, Hughes SF, Stuchfield B (1994) Continent colonic conduit for rectal evacuation in severe constipation. Lancet 343:1321–1324

62. Redmond JM, Smith GW, Barofsky I et al (1995) Physiological tests to predict long-term outcome of total abdominal colectomy for intractable constipation. Am J Gastroenterol 90: 748–753

63. Mahendrarajah K, Van der Schaff AA, Lovegrove FT et al (1994) Surgery for severe constipation: the use of radioisotope transit scan and barium evacuation proctography in patient selection. Aust NZ J Surg 64:183–186

64. Sunderland GT, Poon FW, Lauder J, Finlay IG (1992) Video-proctography in selecting patients with constipation for colectomy. Dis Colon Rectum 35:235–237

37

DIARRHEA AND IBS: A PRACTICAL APPROACH

Michael Camilleri

This chapter reviews the principles of the pathophysiology of "uncomplicated" diarrhea and irritable bowel syndrome (IBS) and proposes a practical, clinical appraisal of patients presenting with diarrhea. Specifically, a thorough clinical history with emphasis on positive identification of alarm symptoms, Manning's criteria for IBS and the salient features on physical and rectal examination are emphasized. In practice, chronic diarrhea is typically due to a handful of disorders, such as IBS, lactose intolerance, and inflammatory bowel disease. Therefore, investigations are geared to confirm the clinical diagnosis and should rarely involve more than a limited series of screening tests to exclude common and easily remediable disease, or to identify hematologic or biochemical abnormalities such as hypocalcemia, micro- or macrocytosis, hypoalbuminemia, or hypokalemia that mandate further assessment. Choice of treatment is determined by the diagnosis, and novel diagnostic and therapeutic approaches to the patient with IBS and diarrhea are discussed. "Complicated" diarrhea, that is, associated with hematologic or chemistry abnormalities to suggest malabsorption, and diarrhea associated with colonic mucosal lesions are not discussed in this chapter.

Chronic diarrhea is a relatively uncommon presentation in clinical practice; among patients seen in gastroenterology clinics, functional gastrointestinal disorders account for almost half of the patients evaluated, but the diarrhea-predominant form of (IBS) is probably the least common variant, as compared to constipation-predominant or IBS with alternating patterns of bowel movements. Chronic diarrhea may be the presenting symptom of a diverse group of disorders ranging from infectious to neoplastic diseases and, hence, a practical clinical strategy is necessary to efficiently, safely, and cost effectively manage these patients.

Traditionally, diarrhea is considered under three main pathophysiologic groups: osmotic, secretory, or motor. The typical approach involves measurement of stool osmolalities and electrolytes, and a 72-hour stool fat or measurement of stool volume during a 24-hour fast. Clearly, such an approach may be needed in a minority of patients, but the vast majority of patients require only a careful clinical appraisal, followed by a limited series of tests to confirm the clinical diagnosis.

BASIC PHYSIOLOGY OF FLUID ABSORPTION

Ingesta typically contribute 1 to 1.5 L of fluid to the intestines, but there is a total of about 7 L that reaches the proximal small intestine during the process of digestion and the interprandial periods each day. Salivary glands, gastric, hepatobiliary, and pancreatic secretions each contribute about 1 L of fluid per day.[1] Equilibration of osmolality and concentration gradients in the proximal small bowel draw the remaining 3 L toward the intestinal lumen. Corticosteroids and aldosterone exert a prolonged, modest controlling influence on salt and water absorption; gut hormones liberated locally after a meal limit the amount of absorption of salt and water at that time perhaps to maintain fluidity and facilitate digestion. More rapid short-term regulation of absorption is likely controlled by the enteric nervous system and paracrine cells.[2] Because only about 1.5 L enter the colon each day, and the stool weight is normally less than 200 g/day, it follows that the small bowel and colon are extremely effective in recovering the fluid load ingested or secreted during digestion. The main mechanisms for fluid and sodium absorption in the small intestine are solute drag and carrier-mediated coupled transport. These are reviewed elsewhere. Impairment of absorption (e.g., transport-carrier defect) or induction of secretion (e.g., hormonal diarrhea) may thus result in diarrhea if the capacitance, residence time, and reabsorptive capacities of the colon[3] are overwhelmed.

BASIC PHYSIOLOGY OF SMALL INTESTINAL AND COLONIC MOTILITY

The small bowel demonstrates cyclical motor activity, called the migrating motor complex (MMC), in the interdigestive period. The MMC consists of a phase I of quiescence, phase II

Categories of Common Disorders Resulting in Chronic Diarrhea

Functional: e.g., irritable bowel syndrome

Infectious: e.g., giardiasis

Inflammatory: e.g., chronic ulcerative colitis, Crohn's disease

Dietary intolerance: e.g., hypolactasia, sorbitol ingestion

Drug induced: e.g., laxatives, excessive use of magnesium-containing antacids

Malabsorption: e.g., celiac sprue, chronic pancreatitis

Neoplastic: e.g., colorectal cancer

Postsurgical: e.g., colectomy, ileal resection, cholecystectomy, or gastric surgery

of intermittent regular ("clustered") or irregular contractions, and phase III or the activity front of rhythmic contractions at a frequency characteristic for each segment of intestine, and showing an aboral frequency gradient that is highest in the proximal duodenum. This activity front may commence in the stomach or proximal duodenum and migrates through most of the small bowel, sometimes reaching the right colon. Small bowel transit time of solids and liquids is approximately equal, whereas ileal clearing of solid residue and liquids appears to be discriminated.[4] This is analogous to the process in the stomach, which retains solid particles until they are fully triturated while allowing fluids to empty more rapidly. Power or prolonged propagated contractions[5] that are typically identified in the terminal ileum but not elsewhere in the small intestine in health are considered important in clearing ileal content. Ileocolonic transit occurs in bolus movements,[6] but the motor mechanism responsible for these bolus transfers is unclear.[7] The ileocecal valve functions as a watershed between the ileum and colon, serving to prevent bacterial overgrowth in the small intestine by refluxed colonic content. Abnormal small bowel motility may thus result in diarrhea, either by accelerating transit as in a subgroup of patients with IBS,[8,9] or by virtue of the effects of bacterial overgrowth, which typically results from motor disorders that impair small bowel transit.

The colon's motility is less well understood. It appears that the ascending and transverse regions of the colon function as reservoirs; the descending colon functions as a conduit, and the rectum and sigmoid provide a further reservoir that facilitates final salvage of fluids within the colon, or stores stool until it is convenient to expel stool. Mass movements of colonic content are associated with high-amplitude propagated contractions (HAPCs), but these are relatively rare, on average five per day, and typically occur on awakening or within 1 hour of feeding. These HAPCs do not always result in mass movements, although they often precede the need to defecate. Bazzocchi et al.[10] showed that propagated colonic contractions are associated with development of functional diarrhea. Excessive postprandial colonic tone in carcinoid patients with diarrhea may reduce the colon's capacitance and contribute to the very rapid transit of residue through the reservoir sections of the colon.[11]

Maintenance of continence requires normal functioning of the anal sphincter mechanisms and maintenance of the rectoanal angle. Derangement of these functions may result in incontinence.

CLINICAL APPRAISAL

History

In the clinical history, identifying several specific positives or negatives is key to the overall appraisal of these patients. The key issues are listed in the form of questions in the accompanying box.

An increased frequency of bowel movements of normal consistency, "rabbity" or small caliber stools, abdominal discomfort prior to and relieved by having a bowel movement, bloating, mucus in the stool, and a sense of incomplete evacuation are quite characteristic and constitute the "Manning criteria" of IBS.[12] The syndrome should be positively sought with direct questioning to elicit this cluster of symptoms.

The presence of blood in the stool is an alarm feature[12] that should not be attributed to possible or known associated conditions such as hemorrhoids or colonic diverticulosis. Clinical features also facilitate identification of malabsorption, such as by the presence of foul-smelling, light-colored, floating stools, or undigested foods in the stool or objective findings such as anemia, edema, malnutrition, short stature, or clubbing. However, these objective abnormalities are unusual in the average patient presenting to a gastroenterologist with diarrhea.

Careful questioning is also necessary to differentiate diarrhea from incontinence, an often unvoiced symptom.[13] Stress incontinence for urine and stool is most indicative of external anal sphincter dysfunction and typically occurs during the daytime in middle-aged or elderly women. Multiparity[14] and unwanted anal penetration[15] are significant risk factors; external sphincter defects persist for several years after childbirth.[14] This weakness may also reflect a neurologic disorder such as a sacral root lesion or pudendal neuropathy. Questions about lower limb and urinary bladder function are key to identifying neurologic causes, and to intervening early enough to prevent potentially

Identifying Key Issues in the Clinical History

1. Is the consistency of the stool altered, or are stools of normal consistency passed more frequently?

2. Does the patient have diarrhea or incontinence? Is incontinence at daytime or nighttime?

3. Does the diarrhea alternate with constipation?

4. What is the diurnal frequency and periodicity of the symptom?

5. Does the patient pass blood per rectum with or without diarrhea?

6. Are there features suggestive of steatorrhea (oily, undigested food, difficult to flush)?

7. Are there other features (Manning's criteria) to positively diagnose irritable bowel syndrome?

catastrophic long-term incontinence. Soiling at night is more indicative of a lack of internal anal sphincter tone, which is a function of the muscle strength and its sympathetic neural input. Thus, nocturnal incontinence may be encountered in patients with systemic sclerosis or in disturbances of the sympathetic supply to the area, as in diabetes mellitus and other autonomic system degenerations. The history should also identify the duration and periodicity of diarrhea, aggravating dietary factors, relationship to medications, or a past medical history of a disorder that may cause diarrhea such as diabetes mellitus.

Physical Examination

The accompanying box summarizes the main features to be assessed during the physical examination. The presence of abdominal mass or tenderness should alert the clinician to the possibility of inflammatory bowel disease or a mass lesion. However, it is also common to find cecal or sigmoid tenderness in patients with IBS; right-sided constipation in functional disorders may be associated with an indentable cecal "mass" of stool. Hepatomegaly with nodularity may be the only finding in patients with carcinoid diarrhea, although flushing is also present in about 80% of patients.

Rectal examination is mandatory to assess the mucosa, wall defects (e.g., rectocele), or occult intussusception that may cause "overflow diarrhea" and to assess the anal continence mechanism. Resting anal sphincter tone reflects internal anal sphincter function, whereas the external sphincter contributes to about 85% of the anal squeeze pressures. Perianal excoriation or moisture and a patulous anus may be signs of sphincter weakness. Very rarely in adults, "diarrhea" results from "retention with overflow incontinence," but this is more common as incopresis in childhood or in the geriatric age group. "Retention" may be the result of internal mucosal prolapse, intussusception, or puborectalis spasm, which can also be suggested by the finding of a tender bar of muscle that fails to relax during the digital examination of the rectum. Excessive perineal descent or "ballooning" of the perineum during straining reflects a long history of excessive straining for constipation, ultimately resulting in stretch of the pudendal nerves and development of sphincter weakness and incontinence due to a pudendal neuropathy.

Initial Evaluation

To avoid unnecessary, costly, or potentially dangerous investigations in patients with suspected functional diarrhea, it is important to use relatively inexpensive "screening" tools and in-

terface therapeutic trials in the management process (Fig. 37-1). The first step is to carefully assess the patient's symptoms. Manning's criteria[12] can be used in a proactive, positive manner to raise the clinical suspicion of IBS.[16] The absence of rectal bleeding is helpful in excluding organic disease.[17] A limited series of initial investigations is necessary to exclude organic, structural, metabolic, or infectious diseases. These include hematology and chemistry tests; stool examination for occult blood, ova, and parasites; flexible sigmoidoscopy; and, in those over 40 years of age or with a first-degree relative with colon polyps or cancer, a barium enema.[18] The presence of abnormal hemoglobin, mean corpuscular volume (MCV), potassium, calcium, or albumin necessitates further investigation to exclude malabsorption or a secretory/hormonal diarrhea, usually by means of stool fat, small bowel aspirate and biopsy, and measurement of hormones in plasma (such as vasoactive intestinal polypeptide [VIP], gastrin, calcitonin) or urine (5HIAA). The finding of colitis or other mucosal lesions in the colon at flexible sigmoidoscopy or barium enema clearly requires further assessment and specific therapy. These "complicated" forms of diarrhea are not the major focus of this chapter and will not be considered further. We do not routinely obtain stool fat measurement in patients with diarrhea and normal screening tests because experience suggests the stool fat is rarely elevated in those patients, and because stool fats of up to 14 g/day may result from accelerated transit or an osmotic laxative[19] (i.e., the stool fat in the range of 7 to 14 g/day has a low specificity for malabsorption).

Some centers perform a colonic biopsy routinely at flexible sigmoidoscopy to detect microscopic or collagenous colitis in patients with unexplained diarrhea or melanosis coli in those with constipation. If the left side of the colon shows a macroscopically normal appearance, we do not routinely biopsy it because in two studies of patients with suspected IBS it was shown to not contribute any useful information other than the nonspecific effects of the phosphate enemas used to cleanse the lower colon.[20,21] A personality inventory may also be valuable in these initial evaluations. However, it is important to stress that if any of these initial tests is abnormal, further specific investigation or treatment is necessary, and the algorithm proposed in Figure 37-1 no longer applies.

Once organic, structural, or biochemical disorders are excluded, it is useful to actively reassure the patient of the negative results of these tests, and the importance of these normal findings. In patients with predominant diarrhea or pain-gas-bloat symptoms, a more detailed dietary history may identify factors that may be aggravating or, indeed, causing those symptoms, such as intolerance of lactose, fructose, or sorbitol.[22-25] Because there is such a high prevalence of lactose intolerance,[26] a lactose-hydrogen breath test[27] or lactose tolerance test should be performed because lactose-exclusion diets are not easy, and patients may ingest lactose unwittingly. If no specific dietary intolerance is identified, diarrhea should be treated symptomatically with antidiarrheal agents such as loperamide. Good evidence from controlled clinical trials suggests that loperamide will reduce the urgency and frequency of bowel movements in the subgroup of patients with diarrhea-predominant IBS[28] and, hence, these agents are the drugs of first choice. The tricyclic antidepressant, desipramine, 50 mg every 8 hours, significantly relieves diarrhea and associated pain[29]; these effects appear to

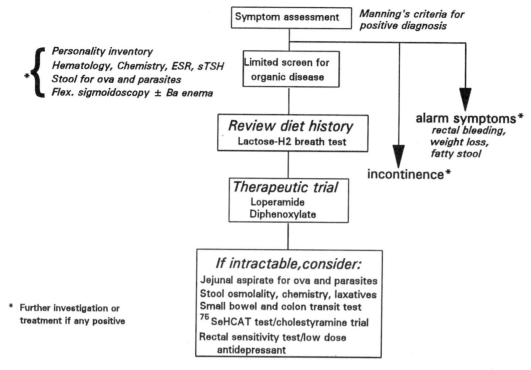

IRRITABLE BOWEL SYNDROME
Diarrhea-predominant

Symptom assessment

Manning's criteria for positive diagnosis

*
{
Personality inventory
Hematology, Chemistry, ESR, sTSH
Stool for ova and parasites
Flex. sigmoidoscopy ± Ba enema

Limited screen for organic disease

Review diet history
Lactose-H2 breath test

alarm symptoms*
rectal bleeding, weight loss, fatty stool

incontinence*

Therapeutic trial
Loperamide
Diphenoxylate

If intractable,consider:
Jejunal aspirate for ova and parasites
Stool osmolality, chemistry, laxatives
Small bowel and colon transit test
75 SeHCAT test/cholestyramine trial
Rectal sensitivity test/low dose antidepressant

* Further investigation or treatment if any positive

Figure 37-1. Algorithm for practical management of diarrhea in the irritable bowel syndrome.

be at least partly due to its anticholinergic actions. Calcium channel blockers, such as verapamil, 40 mg up to three times per day, or clonidine, 0.1 to 0.3 mg, may be used as a secondary treatment. Rarely, subcutaneous octreotide may be necessary; it is best to reserve this therapy as a last resort, because it is expensive and requires three subcutaneous injections daily. A depot preparation of a somatostatin analog is currently being investigated. We advise restriction of the cumulative dose of octreotide to less than 0.25 mg/day to avoid suppression of pancreatic exocrine function, which may result in fat malabsorption and worsening of the diarrhea.

INTRACTABLE DIARRHEA

In patients with persistent diarrhea (Fig. 37-1), we repeat the studies on stool and jejunal aspirates for ova and parasites, because these infestations are eminently treatable and these organisms may have been missed on examination of stool.[30] Stool osmolality, chemistry, and a screen for laxatives is helpful in identifying disaccharide or other malabsorption, and screening for surreptitious laxative abuse.[31,32] If these studies are negative, small bowel and colonic transit studies will assess the degree to which transit is accelerated (Fig. 37-2A). This provides the basis for further efforts to slow transit (for example, with higher doses of loperamide, up to 16 to 24 mg/day) in order to facilitate reabsorption of fluids and possibly osmotically active nutrients during their passage through the digestive tract.

At present, the generally available method for assessment of small bowel transit is the breath hydrogen tests[33] using a substrate such as lactulose or baked beans,[8] which are metabolized by colonic bacteria to produce hydrogen. A peak in breath hydrogen concentration indicates the arrival of the head of the substrate in the colon unless there is colonization of small bowel by colonic bacteria. Radiopaque marker methods[34–36] are used to identify delayed colonic transit in constipated patients by radiographs taken at defined intervals after the start of marker ingestion; however, this method has not been validated for the assessment of accelerated transit, and adaptation of this method by taking daily radiographs would expose the patients to considerable radiation. Importantly, there are no reported normal data for comparison with data from patients with accelerated transit.

A radioscintigraphic approach to measure colonic transit (Fig. 37-2) noninvasively has been developed at the Mayo Clinic.[37] By this method, radiolabeled 1-mm (average) resin pellets are delivered to the ascending colon by means of a delayed-release medication capsule. The latter is coated with the pH-sensitive polymer, methacrylate, and dissolves in the slightly alkaline pH in the ileum.[38] The isotope is delivered bound to the solid resin pellets in a single bolus and follows the normal transfer of solid residue from the terminal ileum to the colon.[6] Thus, detailed studies of ascending and transverse colon transit (Figs. 37-3 and 37-4) have been performed.[9,37] Using this method, it was shown that scans taken 4 and 24 hours after the capsule empties from the stomach (Fig. 37-2B)

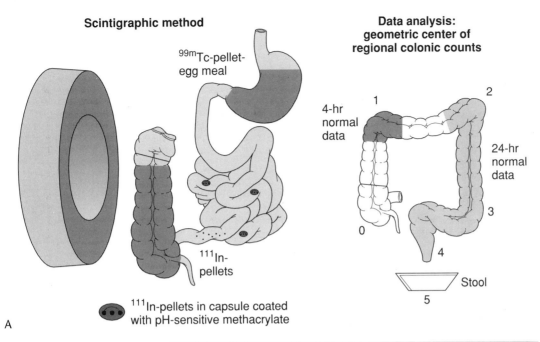

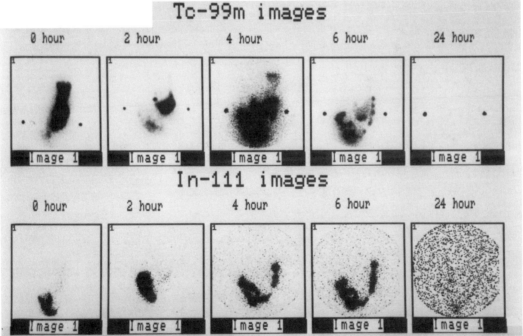

Figure 37-2. (**A**) Scintigraphic measurement of gastric, small bowel, and colonic transit. In this method, radiolabeled inert solid particles are incorporated in an egg meal to evaluate gastric and small bowel transit, and similar particles labeled with a different isotope are delivered to the colon in a delayed-release capsule coated with a pH-sensitive polymer. The geometric center refers to the weighted average of colonic counts, and shaded areas show normal data at 4 and 24 hours. (**B**) Sequential anterior scans of the abdomen showing ^{99m}Tc in images above and ^{111}In in images below at 0, 2, 4, 6, and 24 hours. Note the appearance of ^{99m}Tc and ^{111}In isotope in the sacculated left colon at 6 hours and the virtual disappearance of isotope from the abdominal field at 24 hours, suggesting rapid transit in this patient with diarrhea due to lactose intolerance.

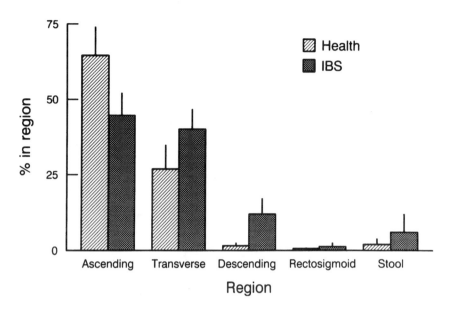

Figure 37-3. Proportion of radiolabel in different colonic regions at 36 hours in healthy and irritable bowel syndrome (IBS) groups. Note the small proportion of counts in the transverse and descending regions and the greater proportion in stool (*$P < .05$) in the IBS group. (From Vassallo et al.,[9] with permission.)

Figure 37-4. Representative examples of time-activity curves showing transit through different colonic regions in a control and patient with irritable bowel syndrome (IBS). Note the rapid regional emptying in the patient with IBS and diarrhea. (From Vassallo et al.,[9] with permission.)

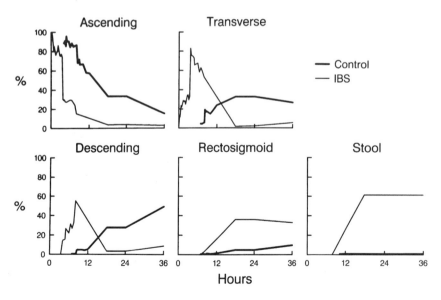

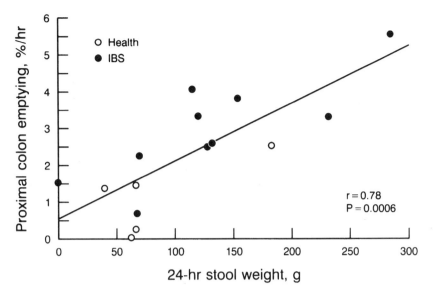

Figure 37-5. Correlation plot between fractional emptying rate of the proximal colon and 24-hour stool weight in healthy and irritable bowel syndrome (IBS) groups. (From Vassallo et al.,[9] with permission.)

provide data that allow discrimination of accelerated or delayed transit from normal transit.[39] The rate of emptying of the proximal colon correlates significantly with stool weight[9] (Fig. 37-5). At the same time, gastric and small bowel transit can be measured by incorporating a different isotope in a standard meal.[6] The prospective application of these methods to patients seen in a functional bowel clinic has proven the method to be clinically useful in screening for dysmotility syndromes and hence for choice of further diagnostic approaches or therapy.[40]

Another consideration in patients suffering intractable IBS with predominant diarrhea is the possibility of bile acid malabsorption secondary to idiopathic bile acid catharsis.[41] Because β-emitting isotopes are no longer permissible by many regulatory agencies, the standard C-14 cholylglycine breath test is no longer used to identify bile acid catharsis. The most widely applied method to demonstrate this phenomenon is the [75]selenium homocholic acid taurine ([75]SeHCAT) test,[42,43] which determines the proportion of radiolabeled bile acid retained in the body after 7 days. Retention is reduced below 10% after 7 days in patients with malabsorbed bile acids. In patients with functional diarrhea and proven bile acid catharsis,[44] cholestyramine treatment (up to 4 g, every 6 hours) is of proven benefit.[45] If this scintigraphic test is unavailable, a therapeutic trial with cholestyramine, 4 g every 6 hours, is reasonable, although it has been pointed out that such trials have up to 25% false-negative rates and an appreciable false-positive rate.[45] An alternative approach is to slow small bowel transit in order to facilitate absorption of bile acids. Data suggest that this approach is effective in stopping diarrhea[46,47] typically in patients with ileal resections of up to 50 cm and rates of [75]SeHCAT retention that are similar to those of patients with IBS and bile acid malabsorption.

If the transit profile is normal and there is no response to cholestyramine, it is likely that the "diarrhea" represents an increased frequency of bowel movements, typically of normal to slightly loose consistency. It is currently believed that this represents an increased sensitivity of the anorectum or pelvic colon[48] to the arrival of small volumes of stool, which results in a need to defecate associated with increased rectal contractility. As such, one of the best therapeutic approaches is to use low-dose antidepressants with anticholinergic effects to retard colonic transit somewhat and suppress visceral afferent function.[49]

CONCLUSION

Long-term studies of IBS show that these symptoms may disappear in time and that the survival of these long-suffering patients is unimpaired. Clearly, the practicing physician needs to find the right balance between, on the one hand, a careful, detailed appraisal of symptoms with a limited number of investigations to exclude organic disease and, on the other hand, the adoption of costly, laborious investigations to ensure that a rare cause of the patient's symptoms is not missed. Another practical dilemma arises between the choice of an empiric therapeutic trial to control symptoms or the pursuit of further studies to identify the pathophysiologic mechanism in the individual patient, in the hope that this may lead to better treatment. The latter approach is not cost effective unless restricted to patients with intractable symptoms. The current state of the medical art in IBS is still weighted toward positive symptomatic diagnosis. Intercalation of therapeutic and investigative approaches in the management of such patients can be achieved in practice. Novel methods are available to accurately and noninvasively assess motor function of the digestive tract. Malabsorption of bile acids or intolerance of nutrients are factors that "irritate" the digestive tract. Targeting therapy to the underlying mechanism causing diarrhea can be rewarding for the individual patient. A greater understanding of the mechanisms controlling motor and afferent functions in the digestive tract in health and IBS may allow the future development of new approaches to treatment as with serotonergic type 3 and 4 antagonists, the opioid agonists, and specific adrenergic agents. Meanwhile, the practicing physician must abide by the old dictum, ''primum non nocere,'' exclude organic disease efficiently and safely, and provide comforting, compassionate care while attempting symptomatic relief for this common, often distressing disorder.

REFERENCES

1. Phillips SF, Wingate DL (1979) Fluid and electrolyte fluxes in the gut, Review. Adv Intern Med 24:429–453
2. Turnberg LA (1984) Mechanisms of control of intestinal transport: a review. J R Soc Med 77:501–505
3. Debongnie JC, Phillips SF (1978) Capacity of the human colon to absorb fluid. Gastroenterology 74:698–703
4. Kerlin P, Phillips S (1983) Differential transit of liquids and solid residue through the human ileum. Am J Physiol 245: G38–43
5. Quigley EM, Phillips SF, Dent J, Taylor BM (1983) Myoelectric activity and intraluminal pressure of the canine ileocolonic sphincter. Gastroenterology 85:1054–1062
6. Camilleri M, Colemont LJ, Phillips SF et al (1989) Human gastric emptying and colonic filling of solids characterized by a new method. Am J Physiol 257:G284–G290
7. Hammer J, Camilleri M, Phillips SF et al (1993) Does the ileocolonic junction differentiate between solids and liquids? Gut 34:222–226
8. Cann PA, Read NW, Brown C et al (1983) Irritable bowel syndrome: relationship of disorders in the transit of a single solid meal to symptom patterns. Gut 24:405–411
9. Vassallo M, Camilleri M, Phillips SF et al (1992) Transit through the proximal colon influences stool weight in irritable bowel syndrome. Gastroenterology 102:102–108
10. Bazzocchi G, Ellis J, Villanueva-Meyer J et al (1991) Effect of eating on colonic motility and transit in patients with functional diarrhea. Simultaneous scintigraphic and manometric evaluations [see comments]. Gastroenterology 101:1298–1306
11. von der Ohe M, Camilleri M, Kvols LK, Thomforde GM (1993) Motor dysfunction of the small bowel colon in patients with the carcinoid syndrome and diarrhea. N Engl J Med 329: 1073–1078
12. Manning AP, Thompson WG, Heaton KW, Morris AF (1978) Towards positive diagnosis of the irritable bowel. BMJ 2: 653–654
13. Leigh RJ, Turnberg LA (1982) Faecal incontinence: the unvoiced symptom. Lancet 1:1349–1351
14. Sultan AH, Kamm MA, Hudson CN et al (1993) Anal-sphincter disruption during vaginal delivery. N Engl J Med 329: 1905–1911
15. Engel AF, Kamm MA, Bartram CI (1995) Unwanted anal penetration as a physical cause of faecal incontinence. Eur J Gastroenterol Hepatol 7:65–67
16. Thompson WG, Dotevall G, Drossman DA et al (1989) Irritable bowel syndrome: guidelines for the diagnosis. Gastroenterol Int 2:92–95
17. Kruis W, Thieme CH, Weinzierl M et al (1984) A diagnostic score for the irritable bowel syndrome: its value in the exclusion of organic disease. Gastroenterology 87:1–7
18. Camilleri M, Prather CM (1994) Axial forces during gastric emptying in health and models of disease. Dig Dis Sci 39: 14S–17S
19. Fine KD, Fordtran JS (1992) The effect of diarrhea on fecal fat excretion. Gastroenterology 102:1936–1939
20. MacIntosh DG, Thompson WG, Patel DG et al (1992) Is rectal biopsy necessary in irritable bowel syndrome? Am J Gastroenterol 87:1407–1409
21. Marshall JB, Singh R, Diaz-Arias AA (1995) Chronic, unexplained diarrhea: are biopsies necessary if colonoscopy is normal?. Am J Gastroenterol 90:372–376
22. Hyams JS (1983) Sorbitol intolerance: an unappreciated cause of functional gastrointestinal complaints. Gastroenterology 84: 30–33
23. McMichael HB, Webb J, Dawson AM (1965) Lactase deficiency in adults: a cause of functional diarrhoea. Lancet 2: 717–720
24. Newcomer AD, McGill DB (1983) Irritable bowel syndrome: role of lactase deficiency. Mayo Clinic Proc 59:339–341
25. Rumessen JJ, Gudmand-Hoyer E (1988) Functional bowel disease: malabsorption and abdominal distress after ingestion of fructose, sorbitol and fructose-sorbitol mixtures. Gastroenterology 95:694–700
26. Bayless TM, Rosensweig NS (1966) A racial difference in incidence of lactase deficiency: a survey of milk intolerance and lactase deficiency in healthy adult males. JAMA 197: 968–972
27. Bond JH, Levitt MD (1976) Quantitative measurement of lactose absorption. Gastroenterology 70:1058–1062
28. Cann PA, Read NW, Holdsworth CD, Barends D (1984) Role of loperamide and placebo in the management of irritable bowel syndrome (IBS). Dig Dis Sci 29:239–247
29. Greenbaum DS, Mayle JE, Vanegeren LE et al (1987) Effects of desipramine on irritable bowel syndrome compared with atropine and placebo. Dig Dis Sci 32:257–266
30. Kamath KR, Murugasu R (1974) A comparative study of four methods for detecting giardia lamblia in children with diarrheal disease and malabsorption. Gastroenterology 66:16–21
31. Morris AI, Turnberg LA (1979) Surreptitious laxative abuse. Gastroenterology 77:780–786
32. Phillips S, Donaldson L, Geisler K et al (1995) Stool composition in factitial diarrhea: a 6-year experience with stool analysis. Ann Intern Med 123:97–100
33. Bond JH, Levitt MD (1975) Investigation of small bowel transit time in normal subjects utilizing pulmonary hydrogen measurements. J Lab Clin Med 86:546–555
34. Arhan P, Devroede G, Jehannu B (1981) Segmental colonic transit time. Dis Colon Rectum 24:625–629
35. Hinton J, Lennard-Jones J, Young A (1969) A new method of studying gut transit times using radio-opaque markers. Gut 10: 842–847
36. Metcalf AM, Phillips SF, Zinsmeister AR et al (1987) Simplified assessment of segmental colonic transit. Gastroenterology 92:40–47
37. Proano M, Camilleri M, Phillips SF et al (1990) Transit of

solids through the human colon: regional quantification in the unprepared bowel. Am J Physiol 258:G856–G862

38. Fordtran JS, Locklear TW (1966) Ionic constituents and osmolarity of gastric and small intestinal fluids after eating. Am J Dig Dis 11:503–521

39. Camilleri M, Zinsmeister AR (1992) Towards a relatively inexpensive, noninvasive, accurate test for colonic motility disorders. Gastroenterology 103:36–42

40. Charles F, Camilleri M, Phillips SF et al (1995) Scintigraphy of the whole gut: clinical evaluation of transit disorders. Mayo Clin Proc 70:113–118

41. Thaysen EH, Pedersen L (1976) Idiopathic bile salt catharsis. Gut 17:965–970

42. Nyhlin H, Merrick MV, Eastwood MA, Brydon WG (1983) Evaluation of ileal function using 23-seleno-25-homotaurocholate, a Qgd-labelled conjugated bile acid. Gastroenterology 84:63–68

43. Sciarretta G, Fagioli G, Furno A et al (1987) [75]SeHCAT test in the detection of bile acid malabsorption in functional diarrhea and its correlation with small bowel transit. Gut 28:970–975

44. Hofmann AF (1967) The syndrome of ileal disease and the broken enterohepatic circulation: cholerrheic enteropathy. Gastroenterology 52:752–757

45. Merrick MV, Eastwood MA, Ford MJ (1985) Is bile acid malabsorption underdiagnosed? An evaluation of accuracy of diagnosis by measurement of SeHCAT retention. BMJ 290:665–668

46. Mainguet P, Fiasse R (1977) Double-blind placebo-controlled study of loperamide (Immodium) in chronic diarrhoea caused by ileocolic disease or resection. Gut 18:575–579

47. Olmos RV, den Hartog Jager F, Hoefnagel C, Taal B (1991) Effect of loperamide and delay of bowel motility on bile acid malabsorption caused by late radiation damage and ileal resection. Eur J Nucl Med 18:346–350

48. Ritchie J (1973) Pain from distension of the pelvic colon by inflating a balloon in the irritable bowel syndrome. Gut 14:125–132

50. Mayer EA, Gebhart GF (1994) Basic and clinical aspects of visceral hyperalgesia, review. Gastroenterology 107:271–293

38

DIVERTICULAR DISEASE

Philip H. Gordon

Diverticular disease is a ubiquitous condition in the Western world. Although many patients with diverticular disease may remain totally asymptomatic throughout life, symptoms can and do arise and complications when they do occur can be devastating and life threatening.

Diverticulosis is the presence of protrusions of the mucosa through the muscular wall. When there is superimposed inflammation, the term *diverticulitis* is used. Because many patients with this entity exhibit no evidence of inflammation, the encompassing term of *diverticular disease* is used to cover the entire spectrum of the clinical consequences of the presence of diverticula of the colon.

It is impossible to estimate the precise incidence of diverticular disease in the general population. Parks[1] estimated that 30% of the population over the age of 60 and perhaps 60% of the population over the age of 80 may be affected. Connell[2] estimated the probable risk of the aged population developing diverticular disease at nearly 50%. What is also evident is that the incidence steadily increases with age from about 5% in the fifth decade to about 50% in the ninth decade with a maximal incidence in the sixth, seventh, and eighth decades.[1] The incidence by sex varies from report to report but is probably comparable. Geographic location is important as it appears that diverticulosis is a disease of the Western world. Left-sided diverticula are predominant in the Western world. Right-sided diverticulosis is almost exclusively an Asian condition.[3]

ETIOLOGY AND PATHOGENESIS

It is generally agreed that colonic diverticula are acquired. They are considered pulsion diverticula that, under the influence of increased intraluminal pressure, represent mucosal herniations that protrude through points of the bowel wall rendered weakened by entry of blood vessels. Painter[4] hypothesized that it is a deficiency disease due to inadequate fiber brought about by the refining of carbohydrates.

The traditional belief is that diverticula develop as a result of elevated intraluminal pressures that arise due to segmentation of the colon. Segmentation of the colon is the mechanism by which the colon propels its contents or halts material moving through its lumen.[5] It involves the production of increased intraluminal pressures, which may exceed 90 mmHg. Figure 38-1 shows three longitudinal sections of colon, each containing three leads recording from different levels of the colon. In the top section the open lumen allows the colon's contents to move freely so that small movements of the colonic wall will result in no significant change of pressure. In the middle section the center segment is demarcated from its fellows by two contraction rings that narrow the lumen on each side of it. Further contraction of this segment will be resisted by its contents, which cannot flow freely into the neighboring bowel. A pressure change will be recorded by lead 2 but this pressure will not affect the adjacent segments. The bottom section shows the center segment contracted so that the lumen on each side of it is almost occluded. Further contraction of this segment would cause a very high pressure to develop. This would be recorded by lead 2 while lead 1 and lead 3, which lie in open bowel, would be unaffected. This center segment behaves like a "little bladder" whose outflow is obstructed and so generates very high pressures. These pressures cause the herniation of the mucosa.

Painter and Burkitt[6] further postulate that an unrefined diet containing adequate fiber may prevent diverticulosis for the following reasons: (1) the colon that copes with a large volume of feces is of a wide diameter, segments less efficiently, and is less prone to produce diverticula; (2) patients with a diet high in fiber have a shorter transit time. The colon absorbs water for less time and has to propel a less viscous fecal stream. Hence, the colon probably produces less pressure and is less apt to become trabeculated and to bear diverticula; (3) suppression of the call to stool favors drying of the feces and increasing generation of pressure. The swiftly passed soft stool subjects the sigmoid to less strain and does not favor the development of diverticula.

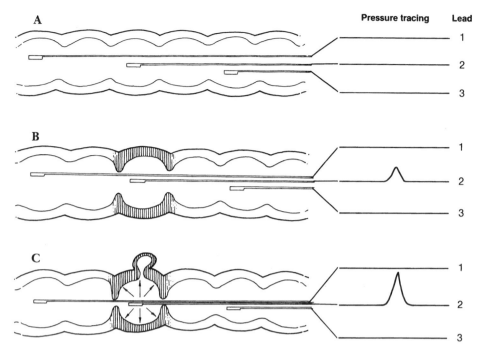

Figure 38-1. Segmentation causing high pressures and pulsation force responsible for diverticulosis.

In a departure from conventional teaching, Ryan[7] suggested that there are two kinds of diverticular disease: one is with the classic muscle abnormality, chiefly confined to the left colon and characterized by inflammation and perforative complications; the other is without muscle abnormality, but with diverticula throughout the colon in which bleeding is common, perhaps due to a connective tissue abnormality that, on the one hand, allows development of diverticula in the absence of abnormal intraluminal pressures, and on the other hand, provides inadequate support for vessels in the diverticular wall or for vascular malformations, which are therefore likely to bleed. His clinical evidence suggests both acute and chronic pain may be either inflammatory or associated with muscle spasm. He further proposed evidence that perforation may be due to abnormal intraluminal pressures rather than diverticular inflammation.

PATHOLOGY

The sigmoid colon in uncomplicated diverticular disease appears shortened and its wall thickened compared with normal. Characteristically, diverticula are of the pulsion type and were described by Whiteway and Morson[8] to occur in two rows between the mesenteric and antimesenteric taeniae. Occasionally protrusions may be situated in the antimesenteric intertaenial area. Myers et al.[8a] described four rows of diverticula, each related to a penetrating vasa recta.[8a]

The muscle abnormality is the most consistent and important feature in diverticular disease of the sigmoid colon.[3] When the colonic wall is sectioned, the interior aspect reveals round or slitlike openings that may at times be inconspicuous and detected only when fecal matter is in the orifice. Narrowing of the lumen may be due to these redundant folds but in part may be secondary to pericolic fibrosis.[3]

Microscopically, diverticula possess two coats: an inner mucosal and an outer serosal layer. An artery and vein as well as attenuated muscle may be seen close to the neck of the diverticulum.

In diverticular disease both muscle layers are greatly increased in thickness. Whiteway and Morson,[8] in their study of the thickened bowel, failed to reveal evidence of cellular hypertrophy or hyperplasia. Instead they attributed the thickening to the presence of elastic tissue specifically in the taeniae.[9] This progressive elastosis causes longitudinal foreshortening of the colon accentuating the semicircular corrugations of the shortened circular muscle.

About one-quarter to one-third of all specimens resected for diverticular disease fail to show evidence of inflammatory change.[3,10] When inflammation does occur, it is noted in the extramural pericolic tissues. The pericolitis may be due to micro- or macroperforation of a diverticulum.

NATURAL HISTORY

It is estimated that approximately 30% of patients with symptomatic diverticular disease of the colon will eventually require operative intervention.[1,11] Parks[1] summarized the following features of diverticular disease. There is no doubt the incidence increases with advancing years. There is an increased risk of hemorrhage in the elderly. The disease in young patients often pursues an aggressive course. There seemed to be a change in sex incidence with more recent reports recording a higher incidence in females. Progression of disease relative to number and size of diverticula does not occur in 70% of patients. It is doubtful that the frequency of attacks of diverticulitis is related to the number of diverticula present. The majority of patients with diverticula localized to the distal colon are not necessarily destined for the relentless progression of the disorder to involve additional segments subsequently. Progression is more often within the segment of bowel initially affected. Patients with extensive involvement are on the average no older, and may indeed be younger than those with localized disease. With regard to prognosis according to extent of disease, Parks noted severe complications to occur as commonly in patients with distal disease as in those with total colonic involvement. Indeed, following operation to eradicate distal disease, it was unusual for inflammatory complications to develop in the proximal bowel. However, where bleeding is concerned, hemorrhage was noted to occur more readily from the proximal bowel. He estimated that between 10% and 25% of patients with diverticular disease will develop an inflammatory complication. Such complications can cause major difficulties.

Relative to duration of symptoms, one-half of the patients with diverticular disease are in good health until approximately 1 month prior to presentation and three-quarters have symptoms for less than 1 year. Patients who present with serious complications may be asymptomatic until hours prior to admission. There is a poor correlation between symptoms and pathologic findings in that one-third of resected specimens fail to show evidence of inflammation. Nausea, vomiting, persistent urinary symptoms, and a palpable mass are associated with a high complication rate and worse prognosis. With respect to prognosis in inflammatory diverticular disease, many patients will have their initial attack respond to bowel rest and broad-spectrum antibiotics. Between one-third and two-thirds of patients will have recurrent attacks or continue to have symptoms. Approximately one-quarter of patients who resolve after conservative treatment will require further hospital admission for recurrent episodes of inflammation. More than 70% will continue to have intermittent symptoms and only 10% after a second hospital admission for diverticulitis will remain symptom free. Approximately one-half of the patients who require re-admission because of a second attack do so within 1 year of the first attack, and 90% are admitted within 5 years.

The outcome of recurrent attacks is different. Medical treatment of recurrent disease is less effective than the treatment of the presenting attack. The complication rate increases with subsequent attacks, being 23% for one attack and 58% for more than one attack. Although the addition of unprocessed bran to the diet of patients with diverticular disease will benefit approximately 80% of patients with respect to pain, it has not been shown that such a diet reduces the incidence of inflammatory attacks. It is estimated that 15% to 30% of patients that warrant hospital admission require operation. Follow-up studies reveal that 2% to 10% of these patients will have troublesome symptoms or a major recurrence, and up to 25% will have minor symptoms. Of the patients who have residual diverticula, more than 80% will be asymptomatic and only rarely will such a patient require further resection. Development of diverticula after resection of the affected segment does not often occur if there has been adequate resection of the distal bowel with the thickened muscle. The establishment of a colostomy, although a potentially helpful measure in the resolution of inflammation, in no way eliminates the possibility of an acute exacerbation of the disease. Closure of a colostomy without resection is associated with the inordinately high recrudescence rate in the order of 65% to 75% and is seldom justified. The immediate risk to

life for the elective operation is in the order of 2% to 3% and for the emergency situation 10% to 12%.

The association of hiatus hernia, cholelithiasis, and diverticular disease of the colon (Saint's triad) has been estimated to be 3% to 6%. It has been suggested the irritable bowel syndrome is related to diverticular disease of the colon and may, indeed, even be a prodromal phase of the disease, but reports have failed to demonstrate a clear association. Although seen in the same patient population, no causal relationship has been found between diverticular disease and carcinoma of the colon.

CLINICAL MANIFESTATIONS

Most often uncomplicated diverticular disease is asymptomatic. Some patients may experience an ill-defined left-sided abdominal discomfort. Associated symptoms of anorexia, flatulence, nausea, and alteration in bowel habits may occur. Patients may relate a history of passing "rabbit-ball" or narrow caliber stools or attacks of diarrhea. Rectal bleeding is uncommon in patients with uncomplicated diverticular disease.[12]

In patients with diverticulosis, no abnormal physical signs will be found on an abdominal examination. Similarly, digital rectal examination is unrevealing. A rigid sigmoidoscopic examination is also usually unrevealing because it is often not possible to examine beyond the rectosigmoid junction.

In the absence of specific symptoms and signs, the diagnosis is most often established by the use of a barium enema examination. The extent and severity of diverticulosis is also best obtained by barium enema. Diverticula may be distributed throughout the entire colon but it is the left colon, particularly the sigmoid, that is most often affected. A common radiologic finding is some degree of colonic spasm. In the chronic state, the lumen may become stenotic and the bowel will be more rigid.[13] Fistulae to adjacent viscera such as bladder may be seen. The use of the flexible sigmoidoscope may identify the presence of sigmoid diverticular disease. Colonoscopy has now proved to be a useful tool in differentiating diverticular disease from carcinoma. However, the endoscopist must be certain that he or she has traversed the area of narrowing in order to rule out a malignancy.

Kewenter et al.[12] found that minor rectal bleeding was uncommon in uncomplicated diverticular disease and patients with a history of rectal bleeding in whom a barium enema showed diverticular disease should be investigated as if the diverticula were not present.

The differential diagnosis includes carcinoma, irritable bowel syndrome, Crohn's disease, and ischemic colitis. Depending on the mode of presentation, other entities that may be included in the differential are ulcerative colitis, appendicitis, pelvic inflammatory disease, ureteral colic, small bowel obstruction, and endometriosis.

TREATMENT

Medical

Because of the demonstration of increased intraluminal pressures in patients with diverticular disease, a high-fiber diet has been recommended. A high-bulk diet reduces colonic pressure and removes the presumed underlying disorder in diverticular disease. Thompson and Patel[14] reviewed the results of seven placebo-controlled trials of bran and bulking agents in the treatment of diverticular disease. From these studies it was apparent that 20 to 30 g of bran is necessary to achieve a therapeutic effect. Coarse bran has been found to have a more significant effect on stool weight, speeds transit time, and reduces intraluminal pressure in the colon more than fine bran.[15] Because many patients find a high-fiber diet unpalatable, the addition of bulk-forming agents provides a suitable substitute. When analgesics become necessary, Demerol is probably the agent of choice because it decreases intraluminal pressure and is less likely to produce disorientation.[16] Morphine should not be used because it increases intracolonic pressure.[5] Based on the observed hypermotility of the sigmoid colon in many symptomatic patients with diverticular disease, the use of anticholinergic agents has been recommended. Their value has never been clearly documented.

Operative

Indications

At one time the indications for operation were reserved solely for the complications of the disease, namely perforation, the development of an abscess, fistula formation, obstruction, and massive hemorrhage. Based on the observation that operations for complicated diverticular disease carry a higher operative morbidity and mortality, some surgeons recommend a more aggressive attitude with regard to elective operations. Certain valid indications for elective resection have evolved.[17] Factors that enter the decision to recommend a resection include the patient's age, general health, life expectancy, severity of the episode(s), and the question of urinary tract involvement. Patients who suffer repeated attacks of diverticulitis (two or more) are candidates, but the absolute number is not the sole criterion. Consideration must be given to the severity of the attack (did it require hospitalization), the interval between attacks (e.g. every 9 months or 9 years), the association of urinary symptoms, and the bona fide nature of the attack (or simply transient left lower quadrant pain). Patients who harbor a persistent, tender mass are candidates. Patients who have persistence of symptoms attributed to colonic dysfunction associated with left lower quadrant discomfort might be considered for resection. However, caution must be exercised in recommending resection for this group of patients in that the surgeon should feel confident that these symptoms are attributable to the diverticular disease. A narrowed or marked deformity of the sigmoid on barium enema examination with the inability to exclude coexisting carcinoma is another valid criterion that is less frequently applicable today with the availability of colonoscopic assessment. Patients with persistent urinary symptoms suggestive of an impending colovesical fistula are also candidates. Elective resection has been advised following only one attack of diverticulitis, especially if the patient is less than 55 years of age or if there is radiologic evidence of a leak or obstruction.[18,19] However, one must be circumspect about advice for operation following only one episode of acute diverticulitis, even for the young patient.

Principles of Resection

For patients with a sound indication for operation, few surgeons would take issue with the concept of resection and primary anastomosis for uncomplicated diverticular disease. Preparation includes a general assessment of the patient's medical status as well as a mechanical and antibiotic bowel preparation.

The exact extent of the resection has varied from surgeon to surgeon. Ideally, the entire thickened contracted segment should be resected, not just the part involved in the inflammatory process. An anastomosis should not be performed in thickened bowel. It is also generally agreed that every diverticulum does not require resection. Follow-up of patients with previous resection have revealed that recurrent diverticulitis in diverticular proximal to the sigmoid is distinctly uncommon. A review by Benn et al.[20] of 501 patients who underwent elective resection for sigmoid diverticular disease has allowed the establishment of principles to determine the extent of resection. In the literature, overall recurrent diverticulitis develops in 7% of patients and 20% of these patients require reoperation. In this study symptoms and signs of recurrent diverticulitis developed in 10.4% of patients, 12.5% in whom the sigmoid colon had been used for the distal margin of anastomosis and 6.7% of those in whom the rectum had been used. Barium enema studies in 61 of these patients 5 to 9 years postresection revealed a progression of diverticula in 14.7%. They found the lowest incidence of recurrence when the descending colon was anastomosed to the upper rectum. Reoperation was required in 3.4% of patients in whom the sigmoid was used as the distal anastomotic site and in 2.2% of those in whom the rectum had been used. They therefore concluded that the entire distal sigmoid colon should be removed during resection for diverticular disease. From a purely technical point of view, if the descending colon is riddled with diverticula, common sense would dictate that the anastomosis be created through the distal transverse colon to avoid a difficult or hazardous anastomosis.

It is a sensible measure to obtain a preoperative intravenous pyelogram (IVP) to determine whether there is any obvious involvement of the ureter. Even with a normal IVP, it is wise to insert a left ureteral catheter prior to operation. It should be remembered that catheter placement does not eliminate intraoperative injury to the ureter but may prove helpful during the dissection.

Operative Options for the Elective Situation

The operation selected in the elective situation is almost invariably resection and primary anastomosis.[17] Upon entry of the abdomen, the sigmoid colon may be found adherent to a variety of viscera as well as the posterior and lateral walls. One of the first decisions the surgeon must make is whether or not the lesion is a carcinoma, a situation that would mandate a wider resection. The determination may be impossible, but when the surgeon is in doubt the disease is probably inflammatory in nature. Careful and often tedious dissection is necessary to separate attached viscera. In so doing, it is not uncommon to enter a pericolic abscess but this should not inhibit continued dissection. With adjacent viscera retracted, the sigmoid is then freed from the abdominal wall with special care taken to protect the left ureter. The inflammatory process rarely extends toward the rectum, and consequently a soft, pliable portion of proximal rectum can be prepared for the distal anastomosis. Proximally the anastomosis should be extended at least to the descending colon. Some surgeons recommend routine mobilization of the splenic flexure but this is not necessary in all cases. The technique for re-establishing intestinal continuity is according to the surgeon's preference. My preference is the use of the circular stapler to re-establishing intestinal continuity.

Some specific difficulties related to diverticular operations may be encountered. The colon is foreshortened and therefore the operator must be certain that there is no tension on the anastomosis. The mesentery is shortened and thickened and extra caution may be required in securing the blood supply. The appendices epiploica tend to be very fatty and these must be cleared in preparation for anastomosis. It must be remembered that diverticular enter the base of the fatty appendages and account must be made for this. In many patients who are undergoing resection for diverticular disease, the muscle wall is considerably thickened and it is unwise to create an anastomosis through this thickened wall. Should such thickening be identified at the level of transection, further excision is indicated. Occasionally the descending colon may contain such extensive diverticular disease that there is not a satisfactory portion through which an anastomosis can be performed. Under these circumstances, the surgeon should not hesitate to extend the resection proximally and anastomose the transverse colon to the upper rectum.

Myotomies, either longitudinal,[21] transverse,[22] or a combination of both,[23] have been advocated, but in general myotomy procedures have not caught on and there appears to be little enthusiasm for their use today.

Results

Breen et al.[10] reported that 94% of 82 patients operated on for diverticular disease were improved. Individuals from whom specimens with no histologic evidence of inflammatory changes were found were less likely to have favorable results. Preoperative factors that might predict the likelihood of a less successful outcome include the presence of bowel management problems for more than 1 year and abdominal pain not localized to the left lower quadrant. The results of elective resection and primary anastomosis for a selected series of patients are shown in Table 38-1.

COMPLICATIONS

The frequency with which complications occur in patients with diverticular disease is impossible to determine. To obtain a relative frequency of the various complications, the indications for operation were gleaned from the comprehensive report by Rodkey and Welch.[30] They include pericolic abscess (10.9%), perforation with local peritonitis or pelvic abscess (32.3%), generalized peritonitis (14.6%), obstruction (10.9%), bleeding (8.2%), fistula (9.7%), and pain (13.4%).

Acute Diverticulitis

Definition

When a segment of diverticula-bearing colon becomes acutely inflamed, the entity is referred to as *acute diverticulitis*. It is associated with fever, a leukocytosis, and sometimes a mass.

Incidence

It has been estimated that approximately 10% to 25% of patients with known diverticulosis will develop one or more bouts of diverticulitis.[1,2,31-33] Diverticulitis developed in about 15% of over 26,000 cases of diverticulosis seen at the Mayo Clinic.[34] Of those patients that require hospitalization, 10% to 20% require emergency operation,[35,36] and at operation generalized or fecal peritonitis is found in 20% to 60%.[37-39]

Clinical Features

Patients with acute diverticulitis usually present with steady left lower quadrant pain that may vary in intensity and may radiate to the suprapubic region, the back, or the left groin. It commonly persists for several days and then may disappear entirely. There may be an alteration in bowel habit with constipation or diarrhea. Should an element of obstruction be present, abdominal distension may develop. Occasionally, anorexia, nausea, and vomiting may supervene. Rectal bleeding is distinctly uncommon in the acute episode but slight bleeding may be noted. Should the inflammatory process involve the bladder, symptoms of dysuria, urgency, and frequency may develop. A low-grade fever is usually present.

Physical findings will depend on the severity of the inflammatory process. In milder cases, left lower quadrant tenderness

Table 38-1. Results of Elective Resection and Primary Anastomosis for Diverticular Disease

Author	No.	Operative Mortality (%)	Complication Rate (%)	1 Stage (%)	2 Stage (%)	3 Stage (%)
Smith et al., 1978[24]	38	0	34	95	—	—
Bokey et al., 1981[25]	47	4.3	21	64	36	—
Eisenstat et al., 1983[26]	135	2.2	—	100	—	—
Hackford et al., 1985[27]	86	1	18	—	—	—
Benn et al., 1986[20]	501	1.6	—	81	11	8
Levien et al., 1989[28]	46	0	60	89	7	—
Killingback, 1990[29]	146	1.4	—	75	12	12

and rebound can be demonstrated. A tender mass may be palpable. In more severe cases, abdominal distension may develop either secondary to an ileus or partial obstruction. Digital rectal examination reveals some tenderness in the pelvis or a mass might even be felt. Similarly, rigid sigmoidoscopy may be limited due to pain.

Diagnosis

In many cases, the clinical manifestations of the disease will allow the physician to arrive at the diagnosis with reasonable confidence. Associated constitutional disturbances may be present. The leukocyte count is not especially helpful. An abdominal series rarely offers any specific diagnostic information. The small bowel is involved in 7% of cases with manifestations including coloenteric fistula, small bowel obstruction, or inflammatory changes secondary to an associated mass.[40] A water-soluble contrast study may identify a perforation of a diverticulum. A spreading cellulitis and abscess adjacent to the diverticula produce roentgen alterations consisting of spasm, irritability, shortening, narrowing, rigidity, distension, and thickening of the folds.[13] Fiberoptic endoscopy yields little, if any, useful information and runs the risk of perforating an acutely inflamed bowel. It would therefore seem to be an unwise maneuver.

Parulekar[41] described sonographic findings of colonic diverticulitis. The wall of the inflamed bowel is hypoechoic and thickened. Abscesses and diverticula could be identified.

Hulnick and colleagues[42] performed computed tomography (CT) scans on 43 patients with diverticulitis. Their findings in decreasing order of frequency included inflammation of the pericolic fat (98%), diverticula (84%), thickening of the colonic wall (70%), a pericolic abscess (35%), peritonitis (16%), fistula (14%), colonic obstruction (12%), and intramural sinus tracks (9%). Secondary findings included a distant abscess (12%) and ureteral obstruction (7%). With the contrast enema, the extent of pericolic inflammation was underestimated in 41% of examinations. Labs et al.[43] also evaluated the role of CT in 42 patients with complications of diverticular disease. They found that CT correctly visualized acute complications in 21 of 22 patients and it excluded an abscess or fistula in all 20 patients with uncomplicated acute diverticulitis. Smith et al.,[44] in yet another study of the comparison of CT and contrast enema evaluation in diverticulitis, found both to be equally sensitive to an abnormality in approximately 90%. They concluded that contrast enema should be the primary mode of approach whereas CT was of value in follow-up when the diagnosis was still in doubt, when retrograde obstruction was present, or if management might be altered by additional information.

Medical Management

Patients who present with a mild case of diverticulitis may be treated on an outpatient basis. They are placed on clear liquids by mouth and a broad-spectrum antibiotic for a week or 10 days. As symptoms subside, solid food can be reintroduced into the diet.

For patients with a more severe inflammatory process, hospitalization is necessary. The mainstay of therapy is bowel rest, intravenous fluids, and broad-spectrum antibiotics including aerobic and anaerobic coverage as well as a penicillin for enterococcus coverage. Nasogastric suctioning may not be necessary unless there is evidence of obstruction or the patient develops nausea or vomiting. The use of morphine is contraindicated because of the well-documented increases in intraluminal pressure after its administration. The patient's symptoms should begin to subside within 48 hours and if resolution continues the patient investigated about 3 weeks later. If there is a failure of medical therapy, urgent operation may be required. If the patient presents with an acute abdomen with evidence of a spreading peritonitis, immediate operation would be mandatory. About one-third of patients admitted to the hospital with diverticulitis will require operation during the first admission.[30]

For the patient with an initial uncomplicated episode of diverticulitis, medical management is indicated because 70% of patients recovering from the attack will have no further recurrences.[45] In an extensive study by Parks[1] of 297 patients admitted to the hospital for medical treatment only and followed up for 2 to 16 years, 2% died of their diverticular disease, 4% were alive with severe symptoms of this condition, 26% were alive with mild symptoms of diverticulitis, and 40% were alive and entirely free of complaints referrable to the bowel. Of the original 297 patients, 25% had to re-enter the hospital for a second admission (half of them within 1 year), 4% for a third time, and 2% for a fourth time. Of the patients who were readmitted, 6.7% of the original 297 patients underwent operative treatment and 2% died.

Parks[1] reported that the complication rate increases with subsequent attacks with a 23% rate after one attack and 58% for more than one attack. In stark contrast, Haglund et al.[39] analyzed the short- and long-term outcome in 392 patients admitted to the hospital with an initial attack of acute diverticulitis. Emergency operation was required in 25% of patients after the first attack with an operative mortality of 20%. Of the 295 patients treated medically and followed 1 to 12 years, 25% developed recurrent attacks, almost one-half within 1 year after the first attack had subsided with a risk of an attack in the first year of about 10%. Once the initial attack had subsided, the yearly risk of suffering another attack was calculated to be about 3%. There were no perforations and medical treatment was uneventful in all. All perforations and the vast majority of other complications occurred in association with the initial attack. After the first attack the disease appeared to run a benign course and the risk of dying from unrelated diseases was greater than the risk of dying from acute diverticulitis or its complications. In view of their findings, they concluded that the increased risk of elective ''prophylactic'' sigmoid resection in early stages of diverticular disease or in patients who have recovered from acute diverticulitis can hardly be justified.

In a review by Larson et al.[45] of 99 patients treated medically for acute diverticulitis and followed for an average of 9.2 years, 73% had no further symptoms or hospital admissions once they recovered from their episode of acute diverticulitis. In light of these findings, it seems somewhat difficult to justify an operation after only one attack of diverticulitis.

Following complete resolution of an attack of acute diverticulitis, it has been customary to advise patients to partake in a high-fiber diet. Although the addition of unprocessed bran is helpful in control of the symptoms of pain, there is no evidence that it reduces the frequency of inflammatory attacks.

Operative Management

Operation is indicated for the patient who fails to respond to medical measures or for the patient who presents with generalized peritonitis. Failure of nonoperative therapy may declare itself within hours or may take 3 to 5 days. The decision to operate depends on the severity of peritoneal contamination judged by the degree and extent of tenderness and systemic disturbance. If signs are confined to the left lower quadrant, there is no urgency to operate. Urgent operation may be required in less than one-third of all emergency admissions with acute diverticulitis.[39]

When to resect after an acute episode of diverticulitis has resolved is controversial. There is no set time interval that must elapse before performing an elective resection. The inflammatory process usually resolves within a few weeks but may take longer if the initial process was extensive.

A number of operative options are available in the treatment of patients with complicated diverticular disease. The advantages and disadvantages of each option will be highlighted and together with available information provide reasons why certain trends in operative therapy have developed. The findings at laparotomy may influence the decision-making process. For example, Nagorney et al.[46] reported the operative mortality to be 9% for patients with spreading purulent peritonitis, 6% for those with diffuse purulent peritonitis, and 35% for those with fecal peritonitis. Nonetheless, certain trends have emerged.

Transverse Colostomy and Drainage (Three-Stage Procedure)

The traditional recommendation for patients who suffer from a perforated sigmoid diverticulitis with abscess formation has been a staged operation with an initial diversionary colostomy and drainage, a subsequent resection, and finally closure of the colostomy. Several disadvantages of the operation include the necessity to contend with a colostomy for some time and in some cases the stoma may be rendered permanent. Experience has shown that with this regimen the combined morbidity and mortality of the three stages is high and it is associated with long periods of hospitalization (Table 38-2). The presence of the perforated sigmoid colon and a column of stool in the left colon predictably permits a continuing focus of sepsis. How long to allow the inflammation to "cool off" is debatable. Recommendations have ranged from 6 weeks to 6 months.

In general, transverse colostomy and drainage is rarely, if ever, indicated, especially for patients with generalized peritonitis and overt perforation. A possible reasonable indication for this operation is in the elderly debilitated patient with intestinal obstruction due to diverticulitis or in the situation where the surgeon feels unable to mobilize the colon.

Exteriorization and Resection With Colostomy and Mucus Fistula (Mikulicz)

This operation entails the exteriorization of the perforated segment of bowel with the establishment of a proximal colostomy and mucus fistula side by side. Advantages of this procedure over simple diversion include the removal of the perforated segment of bowel from the peritoneal cavity, the establishment

Table 38-2. Results of Drainage and Proximal Colostomy for Perforated Diverticulitis

Authors	No.	Operative Mortality (%)
Alexander-Williams, 1976[47]	330	22
Greif et al., 1980[48] (ROL)	306	12[a]
	505	29[b]
Edelmann, 1981[37]	25	36
Sakai et al., 1981[49]	11	64
Wara et al., 1981[50]	50	26
Killingback, 1983[51]	59	12
Ryan, 1983[7]	23	30
Cullen et al., 1984[52]	25	58
Nagorney et al., 1985[46]	31	26
Lambert et al., 1986[53]	16	38
Finlay et al., 1987[54]	37	24

Abbreviation: ROL, review of the literature.
[a] Localized peritonitis.
[b] Generalized peritonitis.

of a sigmoid colostomy, which is easier to manage than a transverse colostomy, and it requires only two stages to effect intestinal continuity. It results in a single stoma but with difficulty in appliance placement.

The disadvantage of the operation is that with the foreshortened inflamed mesentery and distal extent of the disease there is seldom a distal length of bowel adequate to have the mucus fistula reach skin level.

In general this procedure is seldom applicable and appears to have no apparent advantage over resection with colostomy and mucus fistula.

Resection With Sigmoid Colostomy and Closure of Rectal Stump (Hartmann)

This operation entails the resection of the perforated segment of sigmoid colon along with closure of the rectal stump and the establishment of an end sigmoid colostomy (Fig. 38-2A). When technically feasible, most surgeons recommend that the distal bowel be brought out as a mucus fistula (Fig. 38-2B). In most circumstances the Hartmann operation is almost certainly the procedure of choice for patients suffering from a free perforation and generalized peritonitis. The advantages of this procedure are that the septic focus is removed by the primary operation, thus eliminating the continued source of contamination. The preventable mortality of this disease is due to immediate or delayed effects of sepsis. Disadvantages include the fact that the second stage of the operation requires a major abdominal procedure.

Upon opening the abdomen, the surgeon may easily be intimidated by the large phlegmonous mass. However, the acute inflammatory nature of the disease often permits blunt dissection to proceed without injury to adjacent structures, in particular, the small bowel and left ureter. The bowel distal to the inflammatory mass, usually at approximately the level of the sacral promontory, can be closed with a linear stapling device. The retrorectal space should not be dissected unless necessary for the drainage of an abscess. The bowel proximal to the inflamed

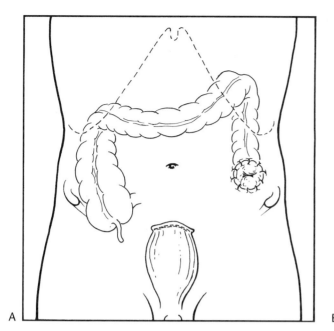
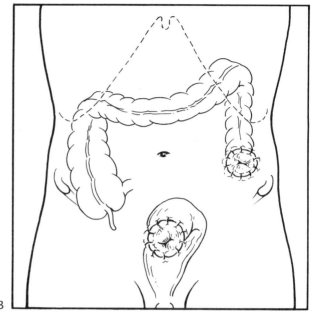

Figure 38-2. (**A**) Classic Hartmann's procedure. Resection of the perforated segment of sigmoid colon along with closure of the rectal stump and the establishment of an end sigmoid colostomy. (**B**) Sigmoid resection with the distal bowel brought out as a mucus fistula.

mass is then transected and an end sigmoid colostomy constructed. It is undesirable to mobilize the splenic flexure in the face of gross contamination.

One of the major criticisms of this procedure is the considerable difficulty encountered when intestinal continuity is to be re-established. Certain principles might best be considered when embarking upon this stage of therapy. First, timing of the second procedure is important. The more severe the initial contamination the longer will be the period required for resolution. In most cases 3 months is a reasonable convalescent period to allow for return to normalcy. Second, assessment must be made of the remaining colon for residual diverticular disease. Certainly any residual diverticular disease in the distal segment of bowel should be resected to allow the distal anastomosis to the proximal rectum. It is not essential to resect every diverticula-bearing portion of colon proximal to the anastomosis unless the disease is so extensive that there is not a satisfactory segment of colon in which to construct an anastomosis.

A number of intraoperative techniques have been described to assist the operation. The advent of the circular stapler with a trocar has dramatically facilitated the operation (Fig. 38-3). The colostomy is first mobilized and the edges freshened and a pursestring suture placed. The anvil is detached and inserted in the proximal bowel and the pursestring tied. If at the initial operation the distal bowel had been resected to the level of the proximal rectum, no further resection is required. The CEEA (US Surgical, Norwalk, CN) instrument with a piercing tip is applied to the central shaft and retracted in the cartridge. The instrument is then inserted through the anus and advanced to the apex of the rectum. The only part of the rectal stump that needs to be dissected is an area just large enough for the cartridge of the stapler. By simply turning the wing nut, the piercing tip and central shaft are protruded through the rectal stump,

and the anvil reunited with the central shaft. No pursestring is required on the distal bowel. The anvil is approximated to the cartridge and the instrument activated, thus creating the anastomosis. If a lesser distal resection is performed at the initial operation, removal of the distal sigmoid is indicated to allow anastomosis to the proximal rectum. Under these circumstances, the usual technique for establishing continuity with the circular stapler is utilized. The advent of laparoscopic techniques might obviate the need for a formal laparotomy to re-establish intestinal continuity.

Numerous reports on perforated diverticulitis have shown a decreased morbidity and mortality after primary resection of the disease segment compared to staged procedures. A tabulation of operative morbidity and mortality is provided in Table 38-3. The results of restoration of intestinal continuity are provided in Table 38-4.

In conclusion, the Hartmann procedure has evolved as the treatment of choice for patients with a purulent or fecal peritonitis. It is no longer the treatment of choice for a patient with an abscess, which should be treated primarily by percutaneous drainage. Should this be unsuccessful, the Hartmann procedure can then be considered.

Resection With Primary Anastomosis and Proximal Colostomy

Utilization of a resection and primary anastomosis with a proximal diverting transverse colostomy has the advantage that the diseased segment is resected and the anastomosis is created with no need to establish continuity in the area of the inflammatory process.

The disadvantage is that a further operation is required to close the colostomy, an operation that has its own attendant

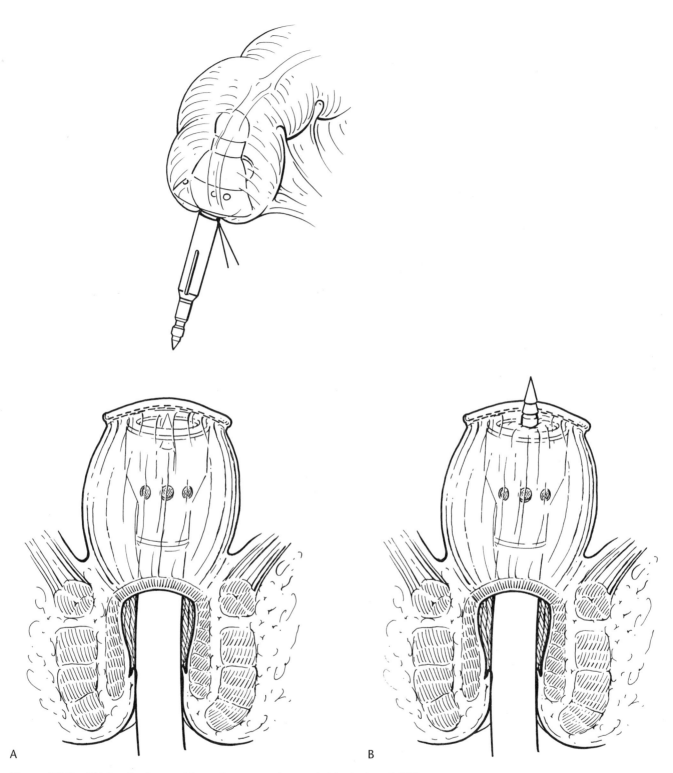

A   B

Figure 38-3. (**A**) Proximal pursestring suture secured around detached anvil. With trocar retracted into cartridge, CEEA stapler has been inserted into rectal stump. (**B**) Central shaft with contained trocar is extruded through rectal stump at its initial level of closure.

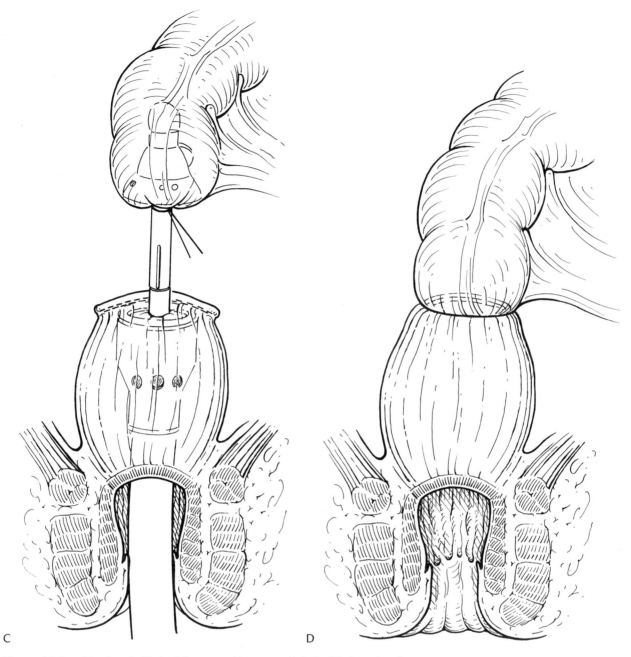

C   D

Figure 38-3.   *(Continued)* **(C)** Anvil is engaged into central shaft. **(D)** Completed
anastomosis.

complications. There is debate as to the timing of the closure
of the colostomy and recommendations have ranged from 6
weeks to 3 months. Prior to closure, the anastomosis should be
examined by sigmoidoscopy and barium enema to ensure healing has occurred. This operation is a viable option but is not
popular today.

Resection and Primary Anastomosis

A number of authors have adopted the operation of primary
resection and anastomosis without a protecting colostomy. Most
surgeons believe this is far too dangerous for general application. Anastomoses created following resection of inflamed unprepared bowel have been reported to suffer clinical leakage
rates as high as 17% to 30% and this complication proves fatal
in a substantial proportion of patients.[70] Mortality rates of 28%
to 50% have been reported after primary resection and immediate anastomosis.[69,70] Results of some series with obviously
highly selected patients and encouraging results are presented
in Table 38-5.

The introduction of on-table lavage has modified the thinking
of some surgeons. In selected cases, resection and primary anastomosis might be considered a suitable, safe operation.[70] Despite encouragement for greater use of this operation by some

Table 38-3. Results of the Hartmann Procedure for Perforated Diverticulitis

Authors	No.	Operative Mortality (%)	Complication Rate (%)
Greif et al., 1980[48] (ROL)	204[a]	2	—
	316[b]	12	—
Thiele, 1980[55]	12	0	—
Liebert et al., 1981[56]	18	0	33
Sakai et al., 1981[49]	15	20	20
Bakker et al., 1982[57]	19	37	74
Lubbers et al., 1982[58]	18	0	56
	170[c]	8	—
Eisenstat et al., 1983[26]	44	5	—
Killingback, 1983[51]	17	18	—
Bell et al., 1984[59]	78	3	35
Westen Underwood and Marks, 1984[60]	15	7	—
Auguste et al., 1985[61]	65	12	95
Hackford et al., 1985[27]	19	16	35
Krukowski et al., 1985[62]	14	14	—
Nogorney et al., 1985[46]	84	7	41
Lambert et al., 1986[53]	30	17	—
Mallonga et al., 1986[63]	38	5	13
Finlay et al., 1987[54]	38	21	—
Marien, 1987[64]	36	11	42
Haas et al., 1988[65]	76	3	—
Alanis et al., 1989[66]	26	15	23

Abbreviation: ROL, review of the literature.
[a] Localized peritonitis.
[b] Generalized peritonitis.
[c] Collected series.

Table 38-4. Results Following Restoration of Intestinal Continuity Following the Hartmann Procedure

Authors	No.	Operative Mortality (%)	Complication Rate (%)	Restored (%)
Bell, 1980[67]	70	3	33	—
Liebert et al., 1980[68]	25	4	20	—
Lubbers et al., 1982[58]	16	0	—	56
Eisenstat et al., 1983[26]	42	0	—	100
Irvin et al., 1984[69]	10	10	—	71
Hackford et al., 1985[27]	10	0	0	63
Krukowski et al., 1985[62]	12	0	—	86
Nagorney et al., 1985[46]	73	1	17	75
Lambert et al., 1986[53]	25	0	—	94
Mallonga et al., 1986[63]	30	0	3	83
Marien, 1987[64]	22	0	46	69
Haas et al., 1988[65]	32	—	—	42
Alanis et al., 1989[66]	14	—	—	64

Table 38-5. Results Following Resection and Primary Anastomosis for Acute or Perforated Diverticulitis

Authors	No.	Mortality Rate (%)	Complication Rate (%)
Eng et al., 1977[38]	50 (ROL)	10	—
Farkouh et al., 1982[71]	15	7	—
Ryan, 1983[7]	73 (ROL)	8	—
	12	0	—
Rodkey and Welch, 1984[30]	63[a]	0	—
	62[b]	5	—
	32[c]	3	—
Hackford et al., 1985[27]	86	1	18
Alanis et al., 1989[66]	29	3	50

Abbreviation: ROL, review of the literature.
[a] Localized perforation (pericolic abscess).
[b] Pelvic abscess.
[c] Obstruction.

surgeons, at the present time it would seem inappropriate to use it in patients with generalized peritonitis.

Percutaneous Drainage of Diverticular Abscesses

Ever-expanding technology has introduced a more palatable method of managing patients whose progression of their diverticulitis has resulted in a paracolic or pelvic abscess. In instances where the abscess is confined, it would seem that the most appropriate method of treatment is the CT- or ultrasound-guided percutaneous drainage under broad-spectrum antibiotic coverage.[72,73] Catheters are left to gravity until drainage ceases and there is resolution of pain and fever. Periodic flushing is performed to ensure patency. A repeat CT can be done at the time of catheter removal. Sinography may confirm closure of the fistula or collapse of the abscess cavity prior to catheter removal. In this way, patients can be discharged and after a period of about 4 to 6 weeks to allow resolution of the inflammatory process, the patient can return for an elective resection, thus converting a multiple to single-stage operation. The optimal time to wait before elective resection is not yet determined (10 to 28 days).

The only limitation to this procedure is the inability to find a safe access route such as occurs when an abscess is covered by bowel. Results of CT-guided percutaneous drainage of diverticular abscesses are listed in Table 38-6.

Table 38-6. Results of CT-Guided Percutaneous Drainage of Diverticular Abscesses

Authors	No.	Success[a]	Catheter-Related Complications
Mueller et al., 1987[74]	21	76%	0
Neff et al., 1987[75]	16	94%	0
Stabile et al., 1990[76]	19	74%	0

[a] Resolution of symptoms. Multistage operation not required.

Laparotomy and Incision and Drainage of Abscess

This treatment option, although once considered appropriate, is probably no longer a viable consideration. One exception to this conclusion occurs when the radiologist is unable to gain safe percutaneous access to the abscess. Under these circumstances an operative approach would be indicated. Most surgeons would perform a Hartmann procedure with drainage of the abscess but in exceptional circumstances drainage might be considered. Even then a complementary colostomy would probably be established.

Management in the Young Patient

Patients under 40 years of age comprise 2% to 5% of patients with diverticular disease.[19] In this age group there appears to be a preponderance of men.[77] It has often been suggested that diverticular disease in the young patient is associated with a more virulent course and is characterized by recurrent inflammatory episodes and a propensity for serious complications.[1,18,19,77,78] Hannan et al.[79] reported that 61% of patients under 45 years of age came to operation that was necessary for complications in 47% of patients after the first episode of diverticulitis. This is in contrast to the 20% to 30% of patients of all ages with diverticular disease expected to require operative intervention. Others support the aggressive management of patients with diverticulitis in patients younger than 40 years.[18,19,77,80]

Notwithstanding the urge to be more aggressive in determining indications for operation in the young patient, it must be remembered that Haglund et al.[39] found few serious complications in patients with subsequent attacks of diverticulitis. In light of their findings, caution should probably be exercised in recommending operation after only one attack of diverticulitis.

Chronic Diverticulitis

Chronic diverticulitis appears to be an ill-defined entity possibly characterized by a low-grade inflammation due to a local perforation in the past. Some patients show the muscle abnormality of left-sided diverticular disease with bowel symptoms. In some cases patients may have the irritable bowel syndrome. Indications for elective operation have already been described.

Perforation

Patients with perforated diverticulitis may have a variety of conditions ranging from a small abscess between the leaves of the mesocolon to a full-blown fecal peritonitis. Full credit for the introduction of some semblance of organization of the severity of the disease goes to Hughes et al.[81] These authors proposed a practical clinical classification based on operative findings to group patients according to severity of peritoneal contamination. They divided clinically acute diverticulitis into the following four main groups:

1. With local peritonitis
2. With local paracolic or pelvic abscess
3. With general peritonitis due to ruptured paracolic or pelvic abscess
4. With general peritonitis due to free perforation of the colon

Hinchey et al.,[82] in a classification almost identical to that of Hughes et al., divided their patients into four stages:

Stage I—pericolic or mesenteric abscess
Stage II—walled-off pelvic abscess
Stage III—generalized purulent peritonitis
Stage IV—generalized fecal peritonitis

The treatment recommended will depend on which one of these entities is present.

Localized (Pericolic, Intramesenteric) Abscess

A walled-off perforation or abscess is the most common complication of sigmoid diverticulitis. It may occur in the pericolic region or involve the mesentery. The clinical manifestations are confined to the left lower quadrant with varying degrees of pain and tenderness. Constitutional symptoms of tachycardia and leukocytosis are commensurate with the degree of inflammation.

Any contrast study should employ a water-soluble contrast medium. Dye may be seen tracking in the immediate pericolic region or toward the pelvis. Less commonly, the mass may increase in size to involve the abdominal wall, and on very rare occasions may even track toward the perineum via the ischioanal fossa. An abscess may be differentiated from a phlegmon with the use of ultrasound. CT scanning may indeed prove very valuable, both from a diagnostic and therapeutic point of view.

Initial management consists of broad-spectrum antibiotic therapy and bowel rest. If symptoms do not improve or worsen, the presence of an undrained abscess should be suspected. The development of the ability to percutaneously drain these abscesses under CT control has revolutionized the management of these patients. The tremendous advantage is that what was formerly treated as a two- or three-stage procedure can now be converted into a one-stage elective or at least semielective operation. Following the resolution of the acute inflammatory process, the patient can have a mechanical and antibiotic bowel preparation and proceed to an elective resection and primary anastomosis.

Pelvic Abscess

If a patient treated for acute diverticulitis fails to improve after 3 to 5 days of adequate medical therapy, a pericolic or pelvic abscess should be suspected. The signs and symptoms have already been described but ''protection'' by contiguous structures may initially mask the presence of a pelvic abscess. Rectal or vaginal examination may reveal a tender, bulging mass. Hypovolemia and gram-negative sepsis may occur. Once suspected, the diagnosis may be confirmed with an ultrasound or CT scan. The patient should be treated with intravenous fluids, broad-spectrum antibiotics, and CT- or ultrasound-directed percutaneous drainage.

Purulent Peritonitis

A purulent peritonitis may arise from a persistent leaking diverticulitis or the sudden rupture of a previous walled-off pericolic or pelvic abscess. This demands prompt operative treatment with the options outlined under the operative management of acute diverticulitis. The patient can no longer be considered too ill to withstand other than minimal emergency surgical procedures, but must be considered too ill to withstand other than primary resection. In perforation during acute diverticulitis, it is the disease and not the operation that causes death.

With respect to the general conduct of the operation, Fazio[83] has offered a number of guidelines for emergency operations on patients with generalized peritonitis secondary to perforated diverticulitis: (1) Resect the perforated segment; (2) do not do more than you have to do. Definitive operation is a more extensive procedure; (3) do not open up further avenues of sepsis by extensive peritoneal dissection, neither mobilization of the splenic flexure nor entry into the presacral space; (4) do not make a mucus fistula. The distal sigmoid can be stapled and delivered to the lower end of the abdominal wound. This will avoid a second appliance; (5) examine the open specimen before closure of the abdomen. If a malignancy is found, a wider resection can be entertained if the patient's general status is satisfactory. Following resection, copious irrigation with warm saline is helpful to dilute the bacterial inoculum. Opinion is divided whether an antibiotic irrigation is more efficacious. Opinion is also divided concerning the use of drains. The general peritoneal cavity cannot be drained but if an abscess cavity is present it might be appropriate to use suction catheters. At the time of definitive operation, the principles of the extent of operation are to be adopted as were described for elective procedures.

Fecal Peritonitis

The least common but potentially most devastating type of perforation is a free perforation in which the patient rapidly develops a generalized fecal peritonitis. It is associated with the greatest mortality.[46,70,82,84] The patient presents with a rather sudden onset of abdominal pain and distension. Examination may reveal a septic patient with constitutional signs of fever, tachycardia, and even hypotension in the advanced stage. Abdominal examination may reveal distension, tenderness, guarding, or rigidity. Leukocytosis of varying degrees will be present. An abdominal series will usually reveal free air.

These patients demand immediate treatment with replacement of fluids, restoration of blood volume, broad-spectrum antibiotics, and immediate operation. Emergency resection of the sigmoid colon is the best treatment for patients with generalized fecal peritonitis.[70] The general principles described in the previous section pertain.

Results

Operative mortality with respect to the type of operation is depicted in Tables 38-2 and 38-3. Factors identified with an increased risk of death include persistent sepsis, fecal peritonitis, preoperative hypotension, and prolonged duration of symptoms.

In an excellent review of the world literature, relative to emergency surgery for diverticular disease complicated by generalized and fecal peritonitis, Krukowski and Matheson[70] showed a clear advantage both in terms of immediate morbidity and mortality of primary resection over operations in which the colon was retained. The collective mortality relative to the various operation was as follows: drainage with or without suture (28.1%); colostomy with or without suture, with or without drainage (25.7%); exteriorization (13.1%); resection without anastomosis (12.2%); resection with anastomosis (9%); resection with anastomosis with colostomy (6.1%).

Silvis and Keeman[85] attempted to determine outcome relative to the stage of disease and type of operation performed. Patient mortality was low with either a staged resection (about 5%) or primary resection (no mortality recorded) for stage I. For stage II disease, mortality was also similar, about 8% and 5%, respectively. For stage III the operative mortality was about 17% for staged resection and 8% for primary resection. For stage IV, the operative mortality was 64% for staged resection and 28% for primary resection. The present trend is to preserve primary sigmoid resection and anastomosis for perforations in stages I and II and perform a Hartmann procedure for stages III and IV.

Fistula

Fistula formation is believed to evolve from a localized perforation to which an adjacent viscus becomes adherent. Ultimately the abscess or feces begin to drain through that viscus. Reports have varied from 5% to 33%, the larger percentages coming from referral centers.[86–88] The most common variety is the colovesical fistula, followed by colocutaneous, colovaginal, and coloenteric fistula.

The clinical manifestations depend on the type of fistula present. In the case of a colovesical fistula, the symptoms of cystitis (70% to 80%) namely dysuria, frequency, hematuria, lower abdominal pain (30% to 90%), pneumaturia (60%), and rarely fecaluria (40% to 70%) may be present.[89] Bowel symptoms may be absent in up to 36% of patients[90] and the presenting symptoms are those of a urinary tract infection. Very rarely the patient may pass urine from the rectum (10%). Systemic toxicity may be seen in 20% to 50% of patients and a mass is present in less than 30% of cases.

Ninety-five percent of colocutaneous fistulae develop following an operation whereas only 5% develop spontaneously.[91] The clinical manifestations of patients with small bowel fistula in addition to the obvious stool passing through the fistula include fever, a mass, obstruction, skin excoriation, rectal bleeding, or peritonitis. There is a high incidence of recent weight loss (40%) and hypoalbuminemia (47%). Factors leading to persistence of the fistulae included sepsis, distal obstruction, and the presence of Crohn's disease or carcinoma.

Patients with a colovaginal fistula may present with abdominal pain and a discharge of pus, stool, or flatus per vaginum. Vaginal examination will reveal an opening, usually at the apex of the vaginal vault (75%) or a mass may be detected on pelvic or abdominal examination. Many of these patients have previously undergone a hysterectomy.

The diagnosis of a colovesical fistula may be rather simple or difficult. The passage of stool per urethra is diagnostic but is uncommon. Unexplained recurrent urinary tract infections that fail to respond to appropriate antimicrobial therapy should alert the physician to the possible diagnosis. Pneumaturia that occurs at the end of voiding is strongly suggestive, but gas-producing organisms in the bladder might simulate the condition, particularly in patients with diabetes. The reliability of various investigative modalities has varied. An abdominal series may demonstrate an air fluid level in the bladder. A barium enema may demonstrate the communication in 5% to 80% of the cases but will show the diverticular disease. Cystoscopy may reveal a cystitis and the opening may be seen (46%).[89] Some abnormality was found in 92% of patients with bullous edema or localized cystitis.[89] An IVP may help in assessing renal function, in verifying the presence of two functioning kidneys, or other abnormalities. A series of dyes or charcoal have been ingested and if passed in the urine are diagnostic. Cystograms have demonstrated the fistula in up to 30% of cases. The Bourne test consisting of radiography of the centrifuged urine samples obtained immediately after a barium enema was positive in 9 of 10 patients, in 7 of whom it was the only positive evidence of an otherwise occult colovesical fistula.[92] CT scanning has detected the presence of a colovesical fistula. It may be useful in the assessment of the extent and degree of periocolonic inflammation, thus playing a role in the preoperative surgical planning as well as the diagnosis.

A barium enema will demonstrate the communication of a colovaginal fistula in about one-half the cases but if it is strongly suspected and unproven, a fistulogram can be used. Coloenteric fistulae can usually be demonstrated by barium enema. A hysterogram may demonstrate a colouterine fistula.

The general principle of treatment is to excise the offending organ. The operative management of patients with fistulae secondary to diverticular disease has dramatically changed over the years, but the trend is unquestionably toward a one-stage resection. In the case of a colovesical fistula, adherence along the bladder as well as the left ureter may be present. In the initial approach it is probably best to mobilize the colon proximal and distal to the fistula.[17] It may be possible to pinch the colon off the bladder by blunt dissection, but usually careful and often very tedious sharp dissection is necessary to remove the colon from the bladder. Caution must be exercised not to injure the left ureter. Often when the colon is freed from the bladder, an actual opening in the bladder is not seen. Should an opening be present, this can be closed in two layers. Despite the fact that there is induration in this portion of the bladder, there is no need for an excision of this portion of the bladder, as the induration will resolve after the colon has been excised. Interrupted absorbable sutures should be used. The diseased bowel is resected and usually a primary anastomosis is created. If suitable omentum is available, it may be placed with advantage between the bladder and bowel and tacked in place. At least 7 to 10 days of bladder drainage is required depending on the amount of bladder manipulation.

In the case of a colovaginal fistula when the colon is freed from the vaginal vault, there is no need for closure of the vagina. Similarly, a colouterine fistula requires no treatment of the uterine connection. Enteric openings clearly require closure or may even necessitate a small bowel resection.

In a series of patients in which a variety of internal fistulae (mostly colovesical) were operated on, Woods et al.[89] encountered a 3.5% operative mortality and a complication rate of 27%. In a series of patients with colocutaneous fistulae reported by Fazio et al.[91] 92 patients underwent operation, 80% having a one- or two-stage resection and anastomosis. There was one postoperative death and complications occurred in 48%.

Hemorrhage

Kubo et al.[93] reported diverticular hemorrhage in 3.9% of 1,124 cases, an incidence considerably lower than in Western countries (3% to 27%).[94–97] Concerning pathogenesis, in a review of collected cases from the literature Baer[98] found a pathologically proved ruptured vasa rectum within a diverticulum in 20 of 22 patients studied. The rupture can occur at the apex of the diverticulum or at the neck of the sac.

The characteristic presentation of patients with diverticular bleeding is one of otherwise healthy individuals who get the urge to move their bowels and suddenly pass a large amount of bright red or maroon-colored stool. Bleeding has been estimated to stop spontaneously in 70% of cases but 30% will continue to bleed and require emergency operative treatment.[96]

A number of algorithms have been suggested for the management of patients with massive lower gastrointestinal hemorrhage. In practice, the type of investigation and the order in which it is performed often depends on the preference of the surgeon, the availability of ancillary services, and the time of day which the patient is being assessed.

In the initial assessment the upper gastrointestinal tract should be ruled out as a bleeding source by gastric aspiration and possible gastroscopy. Sigmoidoscopy should be performed on all patients with lower gastrointestinal hemorrhage, despite the fact that it is usually not a fruitful examination. However, mucosal changes associated with neoplastic or inflammatory diseases may be seen.

For many years the barium enema was considered the initial examination to determine the source of bleeding. It has even been suggested that a barium enema may be therapeutic in stopping the bleeding.[99] However, as an initial study, the contrast will preclude the possibility of other investigations, and is therefore no longer favored. The demonstration of diverticula on a barium enema does not mean they are the source of the bleeding nor does it tell the examiner which diverticulum is the source if, in fact, it is.

When confronted with a patient with massive rectal bleeding, after sigmoidoscopy it is probably wise to perform a nuclear scan. Two radionuclide techniques have been described to detect active gastrointestinal bleeding. Technetium sulfur colloid scintigraphy uses a radiopharmaceutical that is rapidly cleared from the intravascular space ($T_{1/2}$ = 3 minutes in normal individuals).[100] The sensitivity is excellent but the disadvantage is that patients have to be actively bleeding during the few minutes in which the radiopharmaceutical is in the blood. An additional disadvantage of sulfur colloid is that this agent normally accumulates in the liver and spleen, which would make bleeding sites near these organs difficult to identify.

An alternative technique is the use of an intravascular tracer such as ^{99m}Tc-labelled red blood cells or albumin. For the bleeding site to be localized, 5 to 70 ml of blood are needed. The advantage of this technique is that the patient can be monitored for active gastrointestinal bleeding for as long as 24 hours after a single injection. Red blood cell scintigraphy can be used effectively to screen patients for arteriography, or if an operation is required, the surgeon can use the results to plan the operation. The disadvantage with the blood pool agent is that if imaging is not done precisely at the time of active bleeding (i.e., at the time of extravasation), the radioactive agent may propagate into the lumen because of peristalsis and during delayed imaging an erroneous localization may be made.

The use of colonoscopy in the setting of massive hemorrhage is debatable. Some authors have found the experience frustrating because of the amount of blood present and the failure to identify a source. Other authors have found the examination fruitful. Forde[101] has been able to identify a bleeding source in up to 80% of patients. In the face of massive bleeding, colonoscopy would seem to have limited application.

Selective angiography may prove helpful in identification of the bleeding source. If the radionuclide scan is negative, arteriography is probably not needed. If the study is positive, arteriography may not only confirm the finding but may prove therapeutic. The logical order of cannulation should be the superior mesenteric, inferior mesenteric, and finally the celiac if no source has yet been found. Angiographic abnormalities include extravasation of dye, or filling of a diverticulum. If a bleeding source is identified it may be controlled by the use of vasopressin infusion, but rebleeding may occur in 30% of patients after initial control with vasopressin. The treating physicians must be cognizant of the side effects of this agent, including decreased cardiac output, hypertension, and erythema. It also has an antidiuretic effect. Local problems related to the catheter insertion include embolism, bleeding around the puncture site, hematoma, and limitation of activity. Efficacy of this treatment has been reported in the 85% to 90% range.[102] Another therapeutic use of angiography is the employment of embolization of gel foam strips or autologous blood clot.[103–105] Patients, however, must be observed closely for potential necrosis of the bowel. For patients in whom angiography has failed to identify a bleeding site or in whom a site was identified but not controlled with vasopressin, barium enema might be considered in the next step as a therapeutic tool.

Despite the sometimes alarming nature of the bleeding, replacement of blood is usually followed by spontaneous cessation of bleeding. There is controversy as to how much blood should be administered prior to recommending an operation. After replacement of four units, the surgeon should be alerted to the possible necessity for operation. The elderly tolerate blood loss less well than young individuals and therefore early operative intervention is mandatory.

Concerning the appropriate operation, if a previous diagnostic investigation has revealed the source of the bleeding, the appropriate segmental resection should be performed. If no source has been identified, consideration can be given to intraoperative colonoscopy to identify a source. If there is still no evidence of a specific bleeding site, a total abdominal colectomy and ileorectal anastomosis should be performed. The rationale for the extended resection is based on the 30% rebleeding rate in cases having blind segmental resection.[96,106]

Bleeding of diverticular origin ceases spontaneously in 70% of cases but 30% of patients will continue to bleed and require emergency operation.[96] The frequency of delayed or recurrent bleeding is uncertain but estimated to be 10% to 25% of patients.[96,107] The frequency of recurrence of bleeding ranges from nil to 25%.[95] Within the first 24 hours it occurs in 20% of patients whereas late recurrence occurs in 12%.[96]

Obstruction

Obstruction secondary to diverticular disease is uncommon. It is usually a consequence of perforation or it may result from repeated episodes of inflammation with an acute on chronic presentation.[108] It may also result from a loop of small bowel becoming adherent to a diverticular mass. When obstruction supervenes, the usual symptoms of abdominal pain, distension, and constipation are present. Reliance is placed on confirmation of obstruction with plain films of the abdomen and water-soluble contrast enemas. Barium is withheld when any hint of peritoneal signs of leakage is present. The most specific finding is the deformed and spiculated inflamed diverticula. In a majority of patients there are radiologic findings of incomplete obstruction and possibly localized signs of sepsis.

Most patients with obstruction due to diverticular disease will respond to nonoperative management. Repeated bouts of obstruction or marked areas of narrowing require resection on an elective basis. Very rarely will a preliminary colostomy be required. In most circumstances in which the surgeon is forced to operate on a patient with obstruction secondary to diverticulitis, a resection (if technically feasible) is the treatment of choice. A Hartmann procedure would most commonly be employed.

RESULTS AND PROGNOSIS

Although diverticular disease as the cause of death is extremely low, it is recognized that the incidence of diverticular disease increases with age and the mortality rate from complications of diverticular disease increases with increasing age. Mendeloff[109] determined that diverticulitis as a cause of death ranked very low. For the population under age 64, it is 0.5 per 100,000. For ages 65 to 74, the rate was 6.2 for white females and males and 2.7 and 4.4, respectively, for nonwhite females and males.

RIGHT-SIDED DIVERTICULA

Right-sided diverticula may be seen in conjunction with universal diverticular disease or isolated to the right side only. Diverticula of the cecum and ascending colon occur at a younger age than diverticula of the left colon and are associated with an equal sex distribution. They are more common in Asians than in Caucasians and rarely occur in the West, where the incidence is 0.9% to 3.6%.[110] Right-sided diverticula are thought to be congenital and most are true diverticula (i.e., contain all layers of the intestine). Other authors believe most right-sided diverticula are false diverticula.[111]

The majority of patients with right-sided diverticula are asymptomatic and the diagnosis is made by radiologic investigation. Some patients may experience vague right-sided abdominal pain. The average age of patients with right-sided diverticula is 10 to 15 years less than that for patients with diverticula of the left colon.[112]

Right-sided diverticulitis mimics acute appendicitis but occurs at an average age of 40 years.[113] The patient will present with symptoms of pain, usually right lower quadrant but may be epigastric or right flank, pyrexia, nausea, or vomiting. Upon examination, there are varying degrees of tenderness, guarding, and rebound or a right lower quadrant mass. A leukocytosis is usually present. Plain films of the abdomen are generally not helpful. A nonspecific ileus or sentinel loop, a mass, or a fecalith may be seen but these are also in keeping with patients with appendicitis. CT scan may be useful in the early diagnosis of diverticulitis of the cecum and ascending colon.[114] It may show a thickened colonic wall, an extraluminal mass, haziness, and linear strands in the adjacent pericolic fat and thickened nearby fascial planes. The correct diagnosis is generally not made immediately; instead, as the patient is usually operated on for acute appendicitis and the diagnosis made at the time of laparotomy. Features that may help to distinguish the two diseases include the facts that (1) cecal diverticulitis tends to be more prolonged and less acute in presentation, (2) fever, anorexia, nausea, and vomiting occur less often, (3) a mass is more commonly present, and (4) patients tend to be older.[113] Patients may also present with bleeding of varying degrees.

Even at the time of laparotomy, the precise diagnosis may not be made because the inflammatory mass may be mistaken for carcinoma. In their review of the literature, Graham and Ballantyne[113] found that among 367 cases, the surgeon correctly identified cecal diverticulitis in 58% of instances and believed the diagnosis to be a neoplasm in 40% of instances. If there is a circumscribed area of inflammation and the diagnosis is certain as occurs in two-thirds of cases; diverticulectomy (local excision) is the preferred method of treatment.[110,111,113] If a large mass is present and there is a concern regarding the possibility of malignancy as occurs in the other one-third of cases, a right hemicolectomy is indicated.[110,113,115]

In the less acute case when the diagnosis of cecal diverticulitis is made before operation and where the patient may present with a mass, radiologic examination may suggest the correct diagnosis. Under these circumstances, nonoperative management with antibiotics and fluids may result in resolution of the symptoms.

Fischer and Farkas[116] compiled the treatment and operative mortality of 279 cases collected from the literature. Resectional therapy had an operative mortality of 1.7%. More recent reviews of the literature report a mortality of 1.4% to 2.5%.[110,113]

REFERENCES

1. Parks TG (1975) Natural history of diverticular disease of the colon. Clin Gastroenterol 4:53–69
2. Connell AM (1977) Pathogenesis of diverticular disease of the colon. Adv Intern Med 22:377–395
3. Morson BC (1975) Pathology of diverticular disease of the colon. Clin Gastroenterol 4:37–52
4. Painter NS (1982) Diverticular disease of the colon: the first of the Western diseases shown to be due to a deficiency of dietary fibre. South Afr Med J 61:1016–1020
5. Painter NS (1985) The cause of diverticular disease of the colon; its symptoms and its complications. J R Coll Surg Engl 30:118–122
6. Painter NS, Burkitt DP (1975) Diverticular disease of the colon. A 20th century problem. Clin Gastroenterol 4:3–21
7. Ryan P (1983) Changing concepts in diverticular disease. Dis Colon Rectum 26:12–18
8. Whiteway J, Morson BC (1985) Pathology of the ageing—diverticular disease. Clin Gastroenterol 14:829–846
8a. Myers MA, Volberg F, Katzen B (1973) The angioarchicture of colonic diverticula—significance in bleeding diverticulas. Radiology 108:249–262
9. Whiteway J, Morson BC (1985) Elastosis in diverticular disease of the sigmoid colon. Gut 26:158–166
10. Breen RE, Corman ML, Robertson WG et al (1986) Are we really operating on diverticulitis? Dis Colon Rectum 1986: 29:174–116
11. Ulin AW, Pearce AE, Weinstein SF (1981) Diverticular disease of the colon: surgical perspectives in the past decade. Dis Colon Rectum 24:276–281
12. Kewenter J, Hellzen-Ingemarsson A, Kewenter G et al (1985) Diverticular disease and minor rectal bleeding. S and J Gastroenterol 20:922–924
13. Marshak RH, Lindner AE, Maklansky D (1979) Diverticulosis and diverticulitis of the colon. Mt Sinai J Med 46:261–265
14. Thompson WG, Patel DG (1986) Clinical picture of diverticular disease of the colon. Clin Gastroenterol 1986:15:903–916

15. Smith AN, Drummond E, Eastwood MA (1981) The effect of course and fine Canadian Red Spring Wheat and French soft wheat bran on colonic motility in patients with diverticular disease. Am J Clin Nutr 34:2460–2463
16. Almy TP, Howell DA (1980) Diverticula of the colon. New Engl J Med 302:324–331
17. Gordon PH (1992) Diverticular disease of the colon. pp. 739–797. In: Gordon PH, Nivatvongs S (eds): Principles and Practice of Surgery for the Colon, Rectum, and Anus. Quality Medical Publishing, St. Louis, MI
18. Chodak GW, Rangel DM, Passaro E Jr (1981) Colonic diverticulitis in patients under age 40: need for earlier diagnosis. Am J Surg 141:699–702
19. Ouriel K, Schwartz SI (1983) Diverticular disease in the young patient. Surg Gynecol Obstet 156:1–5
20. Benn PL, Wolff BG, Ilstrup DM (1986) Level of anastomosis and recurrent colonic diverticulitis. Am J Surg 151:259–271
21. Reilly MCT (1979) The place of sigmoid myotomy in diverticular disease. Acta Chir Belg 78:387–390
22. Hodgson WJB, Schanzer H, Bakare S, et al (1979) Transverse caenia myotomy in localized acute diverticulitis. Am J Gastroenterol 71:61–67
23. Kettelwell MGW, Maloney GE (1977) Combined horizontal and longitudinal colomyotomy for diverticular disease; preliminary report. Dis Colon Rectum 20:26–28
24. Smith KR, Kovalcik PJ, Cross GH (1978) Diverticular disease of the colon. Surgical management at a military hospital. South Med J 71:1404–1405
25. Bokey EL, Chapuis PH, Phoils MT et al (1981) Elective resection for diverticular disease and carcinoma. Comparison of postoperative morbidity and mortality. Dis Colon Rectum 24:181–182
26. Eisenstat TE, Rubin RJ, Salvati EP (1983) Surgical management of diverticulitis. The role of the Hartmann procedure. Dis Colon Rectum 26:429–432
27. Hackford AW, Schoetz DJ Jr, Coller JA et al (1985) Surgical

management of complicated diverticulitis. Dis Colon Rectum 28:317–321

28. Levien DH, Mazier WP, Surrell JA et al (1989) Safe resection for diverticular disease of the colon. Dis Colon Rectum 32: 30–32

29. Killingback MJ (1990) Diverticulitis of the colon. pp. 222–231. In Fazio VW (ed): Current Therapy in Colon and Rectal Surgery. BC Decker Toronto

30. Rodkey GV, Welch CE (1984) Changing patterns in the surgical treatment of diverticular disease. Ann Surg 200:466–478

31. Boles RS, Jordan SM (1958) The clinical significance of diverticulosis. Gastroenterology 35:579–581

32. Horner JL (1958) Natural history of diverticulosis of the colon. J Dig Dis 3:343–350

33. Hackford AW, Veidenheimer MC (1985) Diverticular disease of the colon. Current concepts and management. Surg Clin North Am 65:347–363

34. Rankin FW, Brown PW (1930) Diverticulitis of the colon. Surg Gynecol Obstet 50:836–847

35. Kyle J, Davidson AI (1975) The changing pattern of hospital admissions for diverticular disease of the colon. Br J Surg 62:537–541

36. Parks TG, Connell AM (1970) The outcome of 455 patients adnitted for treatment of diverticular disease of the colon. Br J Surg 57:775–778

37. Edelmann G (1981) Surgical treatment of colonic diverticulitis: report of 205 cases. Int Surg 66:119–124

38. Eng K, Ranson JHC, Localio SA (1977) Resection of perforated segment: a significant advance in the treatment of diverticulitis with free perforation or abscess. Am J Surg 133: 67–72

39. Haglund U, Hellberg R, Johnsen C et al (1979) Complicated diverticular disease of the sigmoid colon. An analysis of short and long term outcome in 392 patients. Ann Chir Gynecol 68:41–46

40. Frager D, Wolf EL, Frager JD et al (1986) Small intestinal complications of diverticulitis of the sigmoid colon. JAMA 256:3258–3261

41. Parulekar SG (1985) Sonography of colonic diverticulitis. J Ultrasound Med 4:659–666

42. Hulnick DH, Megibow AJ, Balthazar EJ et al (1984) Computed tomography in the evaluation of diverticulitis. Radiol 152:491–495

43. Labs JD, Sarr MG, Fishman EK et al (1988) Complications of acute diverticulitis of the colon: improved early diagnosis with computerized tomography. Am J Surg 155:331–356

44. Smith HJ, Berk RN, Jones JO et al (1978) Unusual fistulae due to colonic diverticulitis. Gastrointest Radiol 2:387–392

45. Larson DM, Master SS, Spiro HM (1976) Medical and surgical therapy in diverticular disease. A comparative study. Gastroenterology 71:734–737

46. Nagorney DM, Adson MA, Pemberton JH (1985) Sigmoid diverticulitis with perforation and generalized peritonitis. Dis Colon Rectum 28:71–75

47. Alexander-Williams J (1976) Management of the acute complication of diverticular disease: the danger of colostomy. Dis Colon Rectum 19:289–292

48. Greif JM, Fried G, McSherry CK (1980) Surgical treatment of perforated diverticulitis of the sigmoid colon. Dis Colon Rectum 23:483–487

49. Sakai L, Daake J, Kaminski DL (1981) Acute perforations of sigmoid diverticula. Am J Surg 142:712–716

50. Wara P, Sorensen K, Berg V et al (1981) The outcome of staged management of complicated diverticular disease of the sigmoid colon. Acta Chir Scand 147:209–214

51. Killingback M (1983) Management of perforative diverticulitis. Surg Clin North Am 63:97–115

52. Cullen KW, Ferguson JC (1984) Diverticular disease as a surgical emergency. Br J Clin Pract 38:20–24

53. Lambert ME, Knox RA, Schofield PF et al (1986) Management of septic complications of diverticular disease. Br J Surg 73:576–579

54. Finlay IG, Carter DC (1987) A comparison of emergency resection and staged management in perforated diverticular disease. Dis Colon Rectum 30:929–933

55. Thiele D (1980) The management of perforated diverticulitis with diffuse peritonitis. Aust N Z J Surg 50:47–49

56. Liebert CW, de Weese EM (1981) Primary resection without anastomosis for perforation of acute diverticulitis. Surg Gynecol Obstet 152:30–32

57. Bakker FC, Hoitsma HFW, Otter GD (1982) The Hartmann procedure. Br J Surg 69:580–582

58. Lubbers EJC, de Boer HHM (1982) Inherent complications of Hartmann's operation. Surg Gynecol Obstet 155:717–721

59. Bell GA, Panton DNM (1984) Hartmann resection for perforated sigmoid diverticulitis. A retrospective study of the Vancouver General Hospital experience. Dis Colon Rectum 27: 253–256

60. Westen Underwood J, Marks CG (1984) The septic complications of sigmoid diverticular disease. Br J Surg 71:209–211

61. Auguste L, Borrero E, Wise L (1985) Surgical management of perforated diverticulitis. Arch Surg 120:450–452

62. Krukowski ZH, Koruth NM, Matheson NA (1985) Evolving practice in acute diverticulitis. Br J Surg 72:684–686

63. Mallonga ET, Brummelkamp WH, van Gulik TM et al (1986) The Hartmann procedure: its role in acute complicated diverticulitis. Neth J Surg 38:171–174

64. Marien B (1987) The Hartmann procedure. Can J Surg 30: 30–31

65. Haas PA, Haas GP (1988) A critical evaluation of the Hartmann's procedure. Ann Surg 54:380–385

66. Alanis A, Papanicolou GK, Tadros RR et al (1989) Primary resection and anastomosis for treatment of diverticulitis. Dis Colon Rectum 32:933–939

67. Bell GA (1980) Closure of colostomy following sigmoid colon resection for perforated diverticulitis. Surg Gynecol Obstet 50:85–90

68. Liebert CW, DeWeese BM (1980) Reconstructing colonic continuity after the Hartmann procedure. South Med J 73: 1576–1577

69. Irvin GL, Horsley JS, Caruana JA (1984) The morbidity and mortality of emergent operations for colorectal disease. Ann J Surg 189:598–603

70. Krukowski ZH, Matheson NA (1984) Emergency surgery for diverticular disease complicated by generalized and fecal peritoritis: a review. Br J Surg 71:921–927

71. Farkouh E, Hellou G, Allard M et al (1982) Resection and primary anastomosis for diverticulitis with perforation and peritonitis. Can J Surg 25:314–316

72. Gerzof SC, Johnson WC (1984) Radiologic aspects of diagno-

sis and treatment of abdominal abscesses. Surg Clin North Am 1984:64:53–66

73. Greco RS, Kamath C, Nosher JL (1982) Percutaneous drainage of peridiverticular abscess followed by primary sigmoidectomy. Dis Colon Rectum 25:53–55

74. Mueller PR, Saini S, Wittenburg J et al (1987) Sigmoid diverticular abscesses: percutaneous drainage as an adjunct to surgical resection in 24 cases. Radiology 164:331–335

75. Neff CC, van Sonnenberg E, Casola G et al (1987) Diverticular abscesses: percutaneous drainage. Radiology 163:15–18

76. Stabile BE, Puccio E, van Sonnenberg E et al (1990) Preoperative percutaneous drainage of diverticular abscesses. Am J Surg 159:99–105

77. Freischlag J, Bennion RS, Thompson JE (1986) Complications of diverticular disease of the colon in young people. Dis Colon Rectum 29:639–643

78. Kim U, Dreiling DA (1974) Problems in the diagnosis of diverticulitis in the young. Am J Gastroenterol 62:109–115

79. Hannan CE, Knightly JJ, Coffey RJ (1961) Diverticular disease of the colon in the younger age group. Dis Colon Rectum 4:419–423

80. Eusebio EB, Eisenberg MM (1973) Natural history of diverticular disease of the colon in the young patient. Am J Surg 125:308–311

81. Hughes ESR, Cuthbertson AM, Carden ABG (1963) The surgical management of acute diverticulitis. Med J Aust 1:780–782

82. Hinchey EJ, Schaal PGH, Richards GK (1978) Treatment of perforated disease of the colon. Adv Surg 12:86–109

83. Fazio VW (1989) Acute perforated diverticulitis. pp. 386–393. In Fischer JE (ed): Common problems in Gastointestinal Surgery. Year Book Medical Publishers, Chicago

84. Hollender LF, Meyer CH, Alexiou D et al (1981) Therapeutic principles in emergency colonic surgery. In Surg 66:307–310

85. Silvis R, Keeman JN (1988) Complicated diverticulitis in acute surgery. Neth J Surg 40:117–120

86. Hool GJ, Bokey EL, Pheils MT (1981) Diverticular coloenteric fistulae. Aust N Z J Surg 51:358–359

87. Corman ML (1984) Colon and Rectal Surgery. p. 505 Lippincott-Raven, Philadelphia

88. Colcock BP, Stahmann FD (1972) Fistulas complicating diverticular disease of the sigmoid colon. Ann Surg 175:838–846

89. Woods RJ, Lavery JC, Fazio VW et al (1988) Internal fistulas in diverticular disease. Dis Colon Rectum 31:591–596

90. Pheils MT (1972) Vesico-colic fistula due to diverticulitis. Aust N Z J Surg 41:237–240

91. Fazio VW, Church JM, Jagelman DG et al (1987) Colocutaneous fistulas complicating diverticulitis. Dis Colon Rectum 30:89–94

92. Amendola MA, Agha FP, Dent TL et al (1984) Detection of occult colovesical fistula by the Bourne Test. AJR 143:715–717

93. Kubo A, Kagaya T, Nakagawa H (1985) Studies on complications of diverticular disease of the colon. J J Med 24:39–43

94. Gennaro AR, Rosemond GP (1973) Colonic diverticula and hemorrhage. Dis Colon Rectum 16:409–415

95. Knutson OH, Wahlby L (1984) Colonic haemorrhage in diverticular disease—diagnosis and treatment. Acta Chir Scand 150:259–264

96. McGuire HH, Haynes BW (1972) Massive hemorrhage from diverticulosis of the colon: guidelines for therapy based on bleeding patterns observed in fifty cases. Ann Surg 175:847–855

97. Williams RA, Wilson SE (1980) Current management of massive lower gastrointestinal bleeding. Int Surg 2:157–163

98. Baer JW (1978) Pathogenesis of bleeding colonic diverticulosis: new concepts. CRC Crit Rev Diagn Imaging 11:1–20

99. Adams JT (1974) The barium enema as treatment for massive diverticular bleeding. Dis Colon Rectum 17:439–441

100. Markisz JA, Front D, Royal HD et al (1982) An evaluation of 99mT$_c$-labelled red blood cell scintigraphy for the detection and localization of gastrointestinal bleeding sites. Gastroenterology 83:394–398

101. Forde KA (1981) Colonoscopy in acute rectal bleeding. Gastrointest Endosc 27:219–220

102. Athanasoulis CA (1983) Angiography in the management of patients with gastrointestinal bleeding. Adv Surg 16:1–23

103. Goldberger LE, Bookstein JJ (1977) Transcatheter embolization for treatment of diverticular hemorrhage. Radiology 122:613–617

104. Matolo NM, Link DP (1979) Selective embolization for control of gastrointestinal hemorrhage. Am J Surg 138:840–844

105. Miller MD, Johnsrude IS, Jackson DC (1978) Improved technique for transcatheter embolization of arteries. Am J Roentgenol 130:183–184

106. Drapanas T, Pennington DG, Kappelman M et al (1973) Emergency subtotal colectomy: preferred approach to management of massive bleeding diverticular disease. Ann Surg 177:519–526

107. Lewis EE, Schnug GE (1972) Importance of angiography in the management of massive hemorrhage from colonic diverticula. Int J Surg 124:573–580

108. Jackson BR (1982) The diagnosis of colonic obstruction. Dis Colon Rectum 25:603–609

109. Mendeloff AI (1986) Thoughts on the epidemiology of diverticular disease. Clin Gastroenterol 15:855–877

110. Sardi A, Gokli A, Singer JA (1987) Diverticular disease of the cecum and ascending colon. A review of 881 cases. Am Surg 53:41–45

111. Tan EC, Tung KH, Tan L et al (1984) Diverticulitis of cecum and ascending colon in Singapore. J R Coll Surg Edinburgh 29:373–376

112. McFee AS, Sutton PG, Ramos R (1982) Diverticulitis of the right colon. Dis Colon Rectum 25:254–256

113. Graham SM, Ballantyne GH (1987) Cecal diverticulitis. Review of the American experience. Dis Colon Rectum 30:821–826

114. Crist DW, Fishman EK, Scatarige JC et al (1988) Acute diverticulitis of the cecum and ascending colon diagnosed by computed tomography. Surg Gynecol Obstet 166:99–102

115. Schuler JG, Bayley J (1983) Diverticulitis of the cecum. Surg Gynecol Obstet 156:743–748

116. Fischer MG, Farkas AM (1984) Diverticulitis of the cecum and ascending colon. Dis Colon Rectum 27:454–458

39

RECTAL PROLAPSE AND SOLITARY RECTAL ULCER SYNDROME

R. John Nicholls
Anjan Banerjee

Rectal prolapse and the solitary ulcer syndrome have many features in common. There is much evidence that the latter is associated with internal rectal prolapse. The term *rectal intussusception* is often used to define a group of patients with symptoms of difficulty in defecation and radiologic features of internal rectal prolapse on proctography. Many of these overlap with patients with the solitary rectal ulcer syndrome. An evacuation disorder as demonstrated by the inability to pass a water-filled rectal balloon is present in many patients in both groups. This clinical confusion is exacerbated by ignorance of the pathogenesis of evacuation disorders in general.

EXTERNAL RECTAL PROLAPSE

Incidence

There is an increased incidence of rectal prolapse in elderly women, with 50% of female patients being over the age of 70 years.[1] Rectal prolapse may be seen in nulliparous patients although the incidence of incontinence in the latter group of patients is considerably lower.[2] The female/male ratio is approximately 10:1. The age and sex ratios are shown in Figure 39-1. There is a great preponderance of elderly females in the older age group, but among younger patients the incidence is approximately equal. It is likely that prolapse at this age includes some patients with the solitary ulcer syndrome. Multiparous patients have a higher incidence of rectal prolapse with incontinence and have a lax pelvic floor as well as an intussusception and history of obstetric trauma or anal dilatation.[3] The pudendal nerve terminal nerve motor latency may be prolonged, giving a pattern similar to neuropathic fecal incontinence.[4] The majority of male patients are from tropical countries, particularly Egypt owing to an association with schistosomiasis and amebic dysentery.[5] Others include those affected by defecation disorders, for example, the solitary ulcer syndrome. Male patients with prolapse usually have normal continence and pelvic floor function.

Increased straining is likely to be an important causative feature both in these patients with behavioral difficulties and in others with an evacuation disorder. Prolapse has a high prevalence in a central European religious sect in which prolonged straining is part of ritual (Todd, unpublished observations). In senile patients prolapse may be a simple association between age itself and elderly and infirm patients in whom prolapse is common.[6]

Pathophysiology

In elderly patients there are two main factors present. These include a weak pelvic floor and an anatomically mobile rectum,[7–9] favoring intussusception[10] and sliding herniation.[11] Pelvic floor studies have shown weakness of internal and external sphincters with evidence of pudendal neuropathy.[4,12] The internal sphincter in patients with neurogenic incontinence is also abnormal with a reduced response to catecholamines, electrical field stimulation, and an abnormal electromyogram (EMG).[13] These changes may also be present in rectal prolapse. Studies on the rectal muscle itself are required. There is no evidence of abnormal hormone or neural transmitter distribution in the rectal wall.[14] Prolapse is a problem in some cauda equina lesions, and is also associated with generalized neurologic disorders, for example, demyelinating disease.

The peritoneal reflections of the rectum are also abnormal with a deep pouch of Douglas and, in many cases, a mobile mesorectum. These circumstances fit with the original concept of Moschowitz[11] of a sliding perineal hernia. More recently

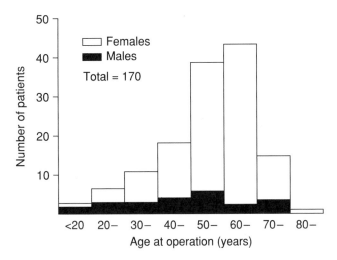

Figure 39-1. Age and sex distribution of rectal prolapse.

Broden and Snellman[10] using cineradiography suggested that an intussusception of the rectum from the rectosigmoid region was the main means by which prolapse originated. It is probable that both mechanisms occur in most patients but firm data on this point are lacking.[15,16]

Patients with rectal prolapse often have had a hysterectomy. It is not possible to state whether this is a causative factor or whether hysterectomy has been performed as a consequence of genital prolapse. The relationship of genital prolapse to rectal prolapse is itself not well known. Genital prolapse is associated with constipation[17] and defecation difficulty,[18] but there is as yet no long-term follow-up in such patients with regard to rectal prolapse. Sayer et al.[19] have described a group of patients in whom a generalized pelvic floor connective tissue weakness may predispose to uterine prolapse, cystocele, full-thickness prolapse of the rectum, as well as solitary rectal ulcer syndrome.

The relationship between rectal mucosal prolapse and complete rectal prolapse is, however, a little clearer.[20] Mucosal prolapse is a diagnosis made often by default. Some mucosal prolapse seen on proctoscopy during straining may well be a normal finding, yet this physical sign may be invoked as an explanation of symptoms, including perineal heaviness, difficulty in defecation, and the passage of blood and mucus. With this reservation, in a follow-up study of 94 patients with a diagnosis of mucosal prolapse followed over a 10-year period, only three (3%) ultimately developed complete rectal prolapse.[8]

In elderly patients we are left with the simplistic concept that a weak sphincteric mechanism is unable to retain a rectum with reduced intra-abdominal attachments. Neuropathy of the pelvic floor progresses with age, especially after 65 years[12] and also occurs after childbirth.[3,21] Interestingly, up to one-third of aged females with rectal prolapse are nulliparous.[22] Patients with spinal lesions do, however, have a high incidence of rectal prolapse. In patients without an obvious cause for neuropathy it might be that straining over many years due to long-standing constipation gradually weakens the pelvic floor. Until recently there has been little information on bowel function in patients with rectal prolapse.[23] Perhaps the first was a prospective study of 26 patients assessed before and after rectopexy. Of these, nine were constipated preoperatively.[24] Thus in some, but by no

means all patients, long-standing straining of stool and irritable bowel syndrome may be a factor although a direct relationship has not been shown. Younger patients with no history of incontinence and normal rectal emptying may have associated slow transit constipation.[25,26] Subtotal colectomy together with rectopexy may be beneficial in this group. Patients may have rectal prolapse and fecal incontinence coinciding with unpredictable episodes of diarrhea and colicky abdominal pain. They respond poorly to surgery because of the persisting hypermotile sigmoid colon.[27–29]

Clinical Features

Symptoms

Typical features include the prolapse itself, mucosanguinous discharge due to mucosal irritation and ulceration, and an erratic bowel habit of diarrhea or constipation with or without straining and incontinence. There may also be a feeling of incomplete evacuation after defecation. Incontinence of flatus, liquid, and solid stool occurs in over 50% of the older age group.[12] Patients with incontinence often have a weak internal anal sphincter as well as a conduction defect of the pudendal nerves resulting in weakness of the external sphincter.[30] The prolapse may bleed from trauma or as a result of venous congestion due to straining. It may secrete mucus that in turn may cause maceration of the perianal skin leading to pruritus. In some patients the rectum is irritable and contracts vigorously in response to rectal distension; these patients often have diarrhea.[20]

Signs

The diagnosis is made on inspection. The anal sphincter is usually patulous and perineal descent is apparent on straining. Usually the prolapse is obvious but in some cases it is not and may be missed unless the patient is asked to strain vigorously. If this does not succeed in demonstrating the lesion it may be necessary to examine the patient on the lavatory. In any patient complaining of fecal incontinence prolapse must be excluded. Proctography is occasionally helpful in showing a prolapse not seen by the clinician. There is often associated genital prolapse such as cystocele or rectocele but complete uterine prolapse is uncommon.

The rectovaginal septum may be atrophic and the perineal body deficient. Rectal examination may reveal loss of the normal anorectal angle due to a lax puborectalis. Occasionally a rectal prolapse may become incarcerated and gangrenous and require urgent perineal excision.[31–33]

Investigations

In elderly patients it may be argued that few investigations other than that of sigmoidoscopy are necessary. However, physiologic studies may help to predict the outcome of surgical treatment, particularly in younger patients.

Sigmoidoscopy may show proctitis, which may stop abruptly and resolves after surgical treatment of the prolapse. Histology is nonspecific; some patients may show features of the solitary rectal ulcer syndrome but recent work has demonstrated that this is associated with a particularly thick circular muscle wall and increase in rectal wall collagen content compared with rectal prolapse.[34] These features are not, however, evident on clinical examination.

Barium enema or colonoscopy may be useful if there is doubt about coexisting colorectal pathology.[35,36] These investigations may, however, be difficult to perform due to the lax anal sphincter preventing the retention of air or barium; occasionally a large bowel carcinoma may be found. Videoproctography may show an obtuse anorectal angle, a short anal canal, and excessive pelvic floor descent at rest or on straining. These findings may identify a group of patients who are likely to remain incontinent after rectopexy.[25]

Physiologic tests show reduced resting and squeeze anal pressures in most patients who have incontinence. The internal anal sphincter is impaired and is of predictive value in patients who are likely to remain incontinent after rectopexy.[37–39]

Tests of liquid continence show saline leak with much smaller volumes than in normal individuals and this is also predictive of a poor operative result.[30] The rectum may respond to intraluminal distension by abnormal motor motility suggesting irritability.[20] Rectal compliance is also reduced. The rectoanal inhibitory reflex and the anocutaneous reflex are often absent. With a patulous anus, it may be difficult to record changes of resting anal pressure owing to the difficulty of establishing physical contact with the anal balloon and the wall of the anal canal. Single-fiber EMG of the external sphincter and puborectalis is typical of nerve damage and attempted reinervation as evidenced by increased fiber density.[12] Pudendal nerve latency is prolonged, particularly in incontinent patients.

Colonic transit times show prolongation in constipated subjects with rectal prolapse and may indicate a subgroup of younger patients in whom subtotal colectomy should be considered in addition to rectopexy.[25,26]

Differential Diagnosis

Mucosal prolapse may be distinguished by careful examination being always anterior, never remaining prolapsed after straining, and being less often associated with a patulous anus. Bleeding, pain, constipation, perineal descent, and straining are often present. By contrast, complete prolapse reveals a ring of mucosa on straining, which then gives way to a complete eversion of the rectum. It often retracts spontaneously after cessation of straining but frequently remains visible until reduced manually.

Sphincter and pelvic floor deficiency may be associated with visible mucosa on inspection of the anus and may descend from 1 to 2 cm on straining. This is easily distinguished from a complete prolapse by anal examination when a sphincter defect will be readily seen when the patient is asked to contract the perineum.

It may be difficult to distinguish hemorrhoidal from rectal prolapse. This is largely a matter of degree. The former is limited to 2 or 3 cm and the hemorrhoidal swellings are clearly apparent with no palpable sulcus between the lateral aspect of the prolapse and the anal verge. Rectal prolapse is more extensive and where there is a degree of intussusception, a sulcus lateral to the prolapse is felt (Fig. 39-2).

A prolapsing adenoma should be easily distinguished from a rectal prolapse by its surface appearance and sigmoidoscopy. Some degree of reddening of the mucosa occurs with prolapse and this might be confused with proctitis. If there is real doubt, a biopsy should be performed. Solitary ulcer of the rectum may occur in association with an overt or internal rectal prolapse with a frequency ranging from less than 10% to 30% or more. The patient is often young and will give the typical history associated with the defecation disorder of this condition.

Treatment

In patients with an evacuation disorder associated with straining, abdominal symptoms of irritable bowel syndrome, and psychological disturbance, the initial treatment should be conservative. Such individuals are usually young and the aim should be to promote a strain-free regular evacuation through explanation with the help of laxatives and suppositories. In most cases, however, treatment of rectal prolapse is surgical. Surgery must be combined with the medical management of constipation in the hope of reducing the chance of recurrence. The operation aims to control the prolapse and also to restore continence while avoiding constipation and impaired evacuation. Selection of the correct operation should take into account the possible morbidity and mortality and also the patient's expectation of the likely functional result.

A variety of procedures is available. These may be classified into those that attempt to support the sphincter and pelvic floor and those that aim to reduce rectal mobility. The former include anal canal encircling devices and various forms of perineal repair. The latter include plication or excision of redundant rectum or rectal fixation. Techniques are available to achieve this either via a perineal or an abdominal approach, either open or laparoscopic.

Perineal Approach

Anal Encircling Devices

Thiersch[40] described a procedure in which a length of silver wire was inserted via the perineum to encircle the anus. Other materials including silastic, silicone implantable collars, or muscle have been described.[41–44] Although the operation is easy to perform and is well tolerated by the patient, it has almost completely disappeared from current practice owing to the poor results achieved. Complications include wire fracture, sepsis, and fecal impaction and there is a high recurrence rate.[45,46]

Delorme's Procedure

Delorme's procedure[47] is extremely well tolerated and can be carried out under local anesthetic if necessary. The mortality is very low.[48–52] In most cases, general anesthesia or regional anesthesia with sedation are easiest for the patient.

Either the lithotomy position with a steep Trendelenburg tilt or the prone jackknife position can be used and the bladder is catheterized. The bowel is prolapsed to its maximum extent by gentle traction on tissue forceps applied to the rectal wall and a 1:300,000 solution of adrenaline is infiltrated in the submucosal plane to raise the mucosa from the circular muscle and to induce some degree of vasospasm in the submucosal vessels. An incision in the mucosa is made 1 to 2 cm proximal to the dentate line (Fig. 39-3A) The submucosal plane is developed by scissor

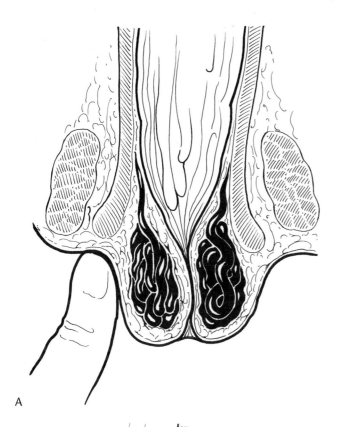

A

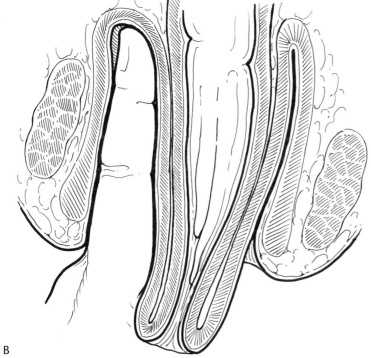

B

Figure 39-2. Differentiation of (**A**) hemorrhoidal from (**B**) complete intussuscepting rectal prolapse. In the former there is no sulcus between the prolapse and the edge of the anal canal.

or electrocautery dissection establishing hemostasis as the dissection progresses (Fig. 39-3B). This is then taken up beyond the apex for a distance equivalent to the length of the prolapse and the mucosa is then divided at that point (Fig. 39-3C). This more extensive dissection is often not included in the standard descriptions of the operation. Although there are no objective

data available, omission of this detail may be one reason for failure. Before division of the mucosa, it is wise to apply at least three stay sutures to the rectal wall and mucosa just proximal to the proposed point of division. This allows control of the rectal lumen, which can retract upward and out of site if it is not secured. The rectal muscular wall is thin and atrophic in many

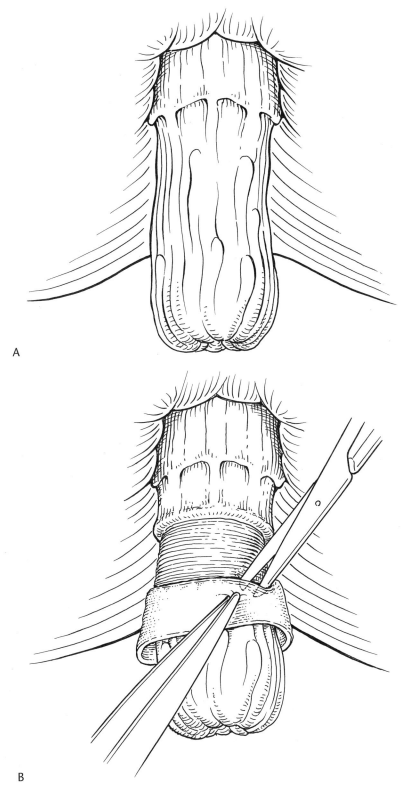

A

B

Figure 39-3. Delorme's operation. **(A & B)** *(Figure continues.)*

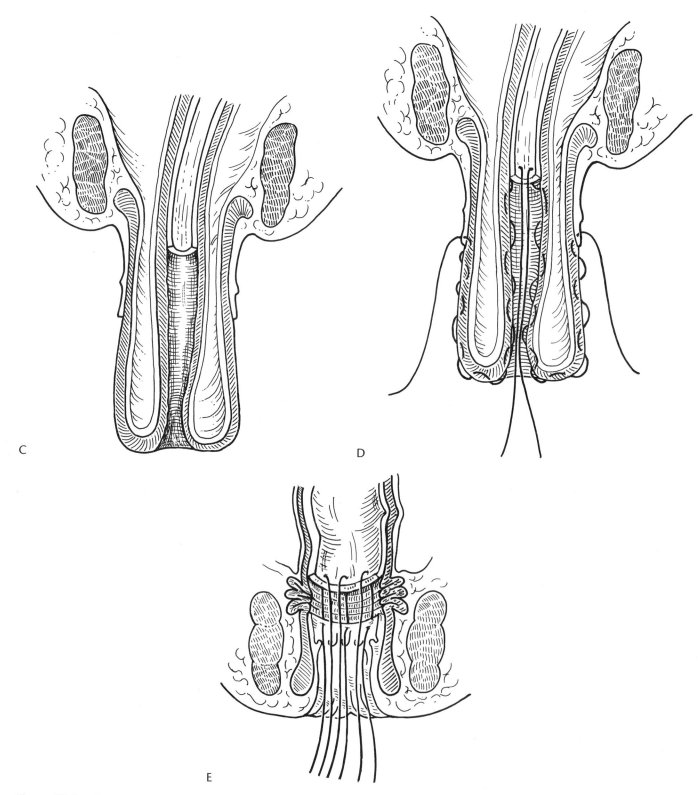

C

D

E

Figure 39-3. *(Continued)* **(C–E).** The mucosectomy is taken as far proximally as the length of the prolapse.

patients and is easy to breach. When it occurs, this is recognized by the appearance of extrarectal fat. In this event, the rectal wall should be repaired with interrupted sutures. The muscle cuff is then plicated by the insertion of a series (four to eight) of longitudinal sutures (Fig. 39-3D). A monofilament material slides more easily through the tissues. The sutures are tightened to achieve mucosal apposition. This creates a plication of redundant rectal muscular wall (Fig. 39-3E). It may be necessary to complete this by inserting further sutures using an endoanal technique. Postoperatively there is usually little pain unless the sutures have been placed too distally. A laxative should be prescribed and the patient mobilized.

Although the operation is well tolerated systemically, there may be early local complications including constipation, loss of anal sensation, incontinence, and secondary hemorrhage. Patients often have long-standing functional bowel disease and may have an erratic bowel habit for some time. Occasionally, a hematoma occurring within the plication may become infected; when suspected, careful examination with endoluminal drainage is necessary. Late complications include stricture formation and recurrence. Anal sensation recovers after several weeks and incontinence tends to improve spontaneously with time.

Results. Assessment of the long-term outcome for any procedure for rectal prolapse is complicated by two main factors. First, the life expectancy of many patients is short; second, accurate follow-up of the elderly, who are often confined to homes for the aged may be very difficult to achieve. Five-year recurrence rates sometimes quoted in the literature may be meaningless for these reasons.

With this caveat, reports of recurrence after Delorme's operation range from 7% to 17%[43–55] (Table 39-1). Thirty-two patients of mean age 70 years were followed for a mean of 24 months (4 months to 4 years). There were no operative deaths and 9 patients died of unrelated conditions. Thirteen of the patients had had 21 previous operations for prolapse. There were four (12.5%) recurrences, two in patients who had each had two previous procedures. Incontinence improved in 46%. No patient became constipated and 50% of those previously constipated improved postoperatively.[56,57]

Plusa et al.[58] reported clinical outcome and physiologic results in 19 women of mean age 77 years (range 57 to 94) before and after surgery. There was no significant defecation difficulty after Delorme's operation although there had been in several patients before. No change in anal sphincter pressures was observed but rectal capacitance and compliance both fell. The former might be interpreted as an improvement in rectal sensation. Thus the volume of first rectal sensation decreased from a median of 140 ml before surgery to 65 ml after, and the maximum tolerated rectal volume declined from a median of 249 ml to 120 ml. Rectal compliance was reduced from a median of 142.9 ml/kPa to 12.2 ml/kPa. Improved rectal sensation and lowered compliance appear, therefore, to be associated with a reduced incidence of defecatory problems after Delorme's procedure.[53,55,59,60]

Gant-Miwa Operation

A modified approach to the Delorme procedure is that of mucosal reduction and multiple rectal plication (Gant-Miwa plication). The rectal prolapse is delivered and a tag of mucosa is lifted off the muscle layers and ligated by suture. This is repeated so that 20 to 30 tags are created over the surface of the entire prolapse, which is then replaced. The tags disappear over a period of a few months and recurrence rates are usually less than 10%.

Rectosigmoidectomy

Rectosigmoidectomy was first described by Miles.[61] As a result of an early review of the outcome of the procedure from St. Mark's Hospital,[62] the procedure fell out of favor owing to the high rates of incontinence (46%) and recurrence (60%). Altemeier and colleagues[63] modified the technique to include a repair of the pelvic floor and reported improved results.

The principles of the operation used today[64,65] include excision of the prolapse, obliteration of the deep peritoneal pouch, and repair of the pelvic floor muscles. It has been recommended particularly for elderly patients deemed unfit for a major abdominal procedure.[63] The operation is associated with low morbidity and avoids dissection above the pelvic floor and the risks of nerve damage or presacral bleeding. It is the treatment of choice for gangrenous or incarcerated prolapse.

The main disadvantages include loss of the rectum with its reservoir capacity and the rare complication of ischemia, particularly if there has been a previous left colonic resection.

The operation may be performed in the lithotomy or prone jackknife positions under general or regional anesthesia. The prolapse is delivered and an incision is made anteriorly through the rectum just proximal to the dentate line (Fig. 39-4A). Two stay sutures are placed on the lateral aspect of the cut edge of the rectum to prevent it from slipping back into the anal canal and to act as markers. Once the anterior wall has been divided, the rectovaginal pouch will be exposed. The peritoneal coat should be opened transversely to reveal the sigmoid colon. This is then drawn down through the opened peritoneal pouch (Fig. 39-4B) and the vessels in the sigmoid mesentery are divided and ligated as the sigmoid colon is pulled progressively downward (Fig. 39-4C). At this point in the procedure the anterior fibers of the levator ani are identified and plicated. The proximal end of the sigmoid colon is then transected (Fig. 39-4D) and the rectal prolapse elevated upward to expose its posterior aspect. The rectal wall is then divided to expose the mesorectum and the posterior component of the puborectalis sling. The mesorectal vessels are divided between arterial clamps, and the

Table 39-1. Recurrence After Delorme's Procedure

	No.	Recurrence (%)
Uhlig and Sullivan, 1979[53]	44	3(7)
Christiansen and Kirkegard, 1981[54]	12	1(8)
Monson et al., 1986[55]	27	2(7)
Houry et al., 1987[51]	18	3(17)
Gundersen et al., 1985[50]	18	1(6)
Graf et al., 1992[49]	14	3(21)
Abulafi et al., 1990[48]	22	1(5)
Senapati et al., 1994[57]	32	4(12.5)
Lechaux et al., 1995[52]	85	11(13.5)

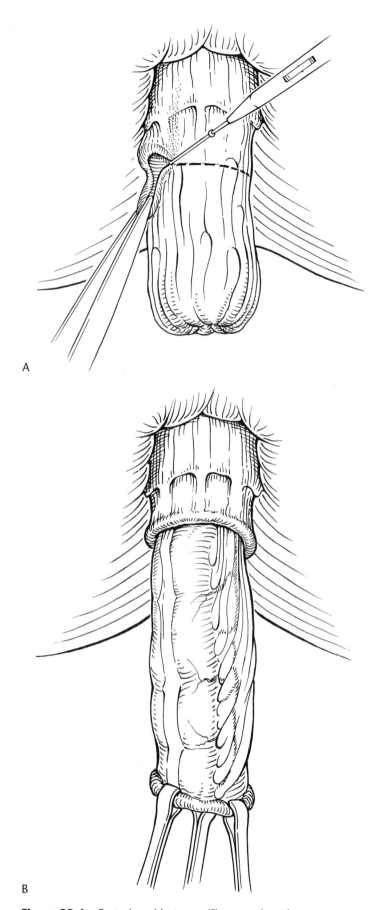

Figure 39-4. Rectosigmoidectomy. *(Figure continues.)*

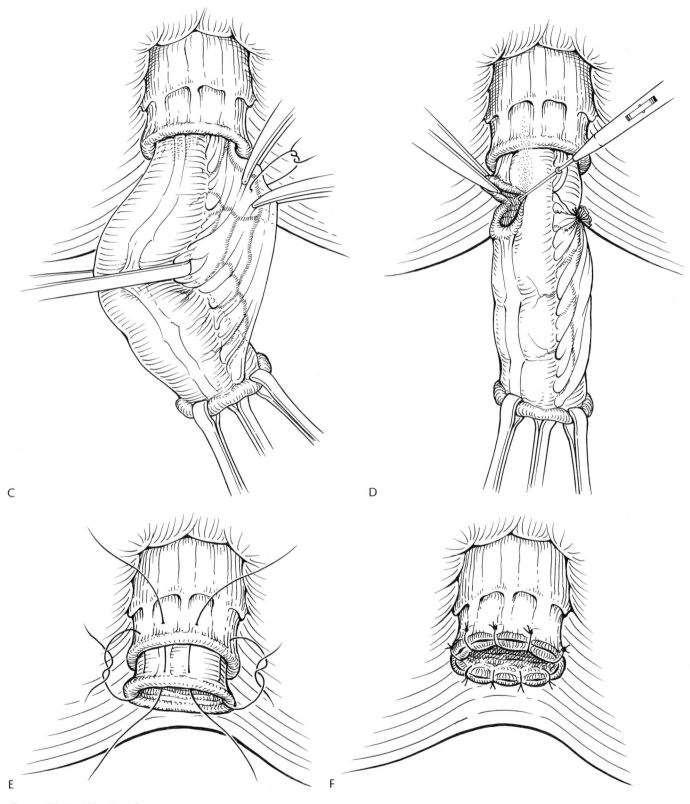

C

D

E

F

Figure 39-4.   *(Continued).*

Table 39-2. Recurrence After Rectosigmoidectomy

	No.	Recurrence (%)
Altemeier et al., 1971[63]	106	3(3)
Friedman et al., 1983[68]	27	13(48)
Gopal et al., 1984[191]	18	1(6)
Watts et al., 1985[192]	33	0(0)
Ramanujam and Venkatesh, 1988[31]	41	3(7.5)

entire rectal prolapse with the sigmoid colon is removed. The puborectalis muscle is repaired and the two divided ends of bowel may then be anastomosed with interrupted sutures[66,67] (Fig. 39-4E & F).

As with Delorme's operation, it is often difficult to determine the intermediate term results. There is considerable variation in reported recurrence rates. For example, Altemeier et al.[63] reported only three (3%) out of 106 patients compared with a much higher rate of 13 (48%) out of 27 patients operated on by Friedman et al.[68] Others have had excellent results (Table 39-2) but there are very few prospective studies comparing this method.

In a randomized trial comparing abdominal resection rectopexy ($n = 10$) with perineal rectosigmoidectomy ($n = 10$), both with pelvic floor repair, there were no recurrences of prolapse in the former group and one in the latter.[69] These authors examined function prospectively and found that continence to liquid and solid stool was achieved in nine patients with some soiling in two after resection rectopexy, and in eight with soiling in six following rectosigmoidectomy. The median (range) frequency of defecation was 1 (1 to 3) per day following resection rectopexy compared with 3 (1 to 6) per day after rectosigmoidectomy. There was an increase in the mean maximum resting pressure after resection rectopexy (19.3 cm H_2O) compared with a reduction following rectosigmoidectomy (-3.4 cm H_2O) ($P = .003$). Compliance was also greater after resection rectopexy than following rectosigmoidectomy. The study indicated that resection rectopexy gave better functional and physiologic results than rectosigmoidectomy although this result should be treated with caution given the small number of patients in the study.

A variety of different rectopexy techniques via the perineal approach have been described.[68,70,71] Although theoretically appealing these methods have high recurrence rates, even in combination with postanal levator repair.[72]

Abdominal Approach

The operation is based on the principles of rectal mobilization and fixation. The results suggest that abdominal rectopexy offers the patient the best prospect of cure with local recurrence rates lower than are achieved by perineal procedures. It is, however, an abdominal operation and can produce constipation associated with loss of rectal sensation. This is a difficult symptom to deal with. The extent of mobilization and whether the lateral ligaments should be divided have never been standardized. Various methods of fixation have been described.

Posterior Rectopexy

Some surgeons would argue that posterior rectopexy[73] remains the procedure of choice in most patients with full-thickness rectal prolapse owing to the low recurrence rates reported and the ease with which it is tolerated. Posterior fixation avoids the complications of stenosis and constipation, which are said to be more likely with anterior fixation procedures.[74–78]

The rectum is mobilized to the tip of the coccyx with or without division of the lateral ligaments. It is then fixed to the sacrum either by single sutures or by insertion of a synthetic mesh[73,79–82] (Fig. 39-5A). The type of foreign material used is perhaps the least important consideration and includes polyvinyl alcohol (Ivalon), polypropylene (Marlex), and polycarbon fluoride (Teflon). Polyvinyl alcohol sponge (Ivalon), which is widely used,[83–87] has several disadvantages. It holds sutures poorly, becomes soft when wet, and acts as a nidus of infection. Additionally, if reoperation is needed, the sponge may be encased in fibrous tissue.[88–91] which may rarely cause retroperitoneal fibrosis with ureteric obstruction. Polycarbon fluoride (Teflon) is rather soft but holds sutures well. Polypropylene is stiffer and is easy to handle. It is associated with a very low infection rate.[92] If sutures are used the rectum is mobilized to the pelvic floor and attached to the sacrum using a series of prolene, polydioxanone (PDS), or Ethibond sutures placed between the mesorectum and the periosteum of the sacrum.

A modification is to use a transabdominal plication technique by placing sutures through the rectal muscle in a method not dissimilar to the Delorme operation.[93] This approach is based on the theory that prolapse is due to intussusception of the rectum in its upper part.

Operative Technique. Bowel preparation is advised largely to prevent impaction in the postoperative period. General anesthesia is used with the patient placed in the Lloyd-Davies position. This permits access to the rectum and also allows a second assistant to stand between the abducted legs of the patient. The bladder is catheterized and antibiotics are administered. The abdomen is opened either through a midline or a Pfannenstiel incision, the peritoneum over the lateral aspect of the sigmoid is divided, and the sigmoid colon and rectum are mobilized. In so doing, the presacral nerves should be identified and safeguarded. The dissection is taken posteriorly to the tip of the coccyx between the presacral fascia and fascia propria of the rectum. There is no agreement about whether the lateral ligaments should be divided. A T-shaped strip of polypropylene mesh measuring 3.5 × 2.0 cm is cut. Several interrupted prolene sutures are placed between the mesh in the midline from pelvic floor to presacral fascia avoiding the presacral veins (Fig. 39-5B). The free margins of the mesh are then sutured to the lateral border of the rectum avoiding complete encirclement of the rectum and leaving at least a quarter of the circumference free anteriorly (Fig. 39-5C). pelvic peritoneum should be closed over the implant and the abdomen then sutured (Fig. 39-5D).

The main complications reported include intestinal obstruction, fecal impaction, infection of the mesh, and, rarely, ureteric obstruction due to retroperitoneal fibrosis.

Orr-Loygue Operation

Loygue et al.[94] have described a modification where, after mobilization, the rectum is fixed by nylon strips. These are sutured as far down as possible on each side of the rectum using a

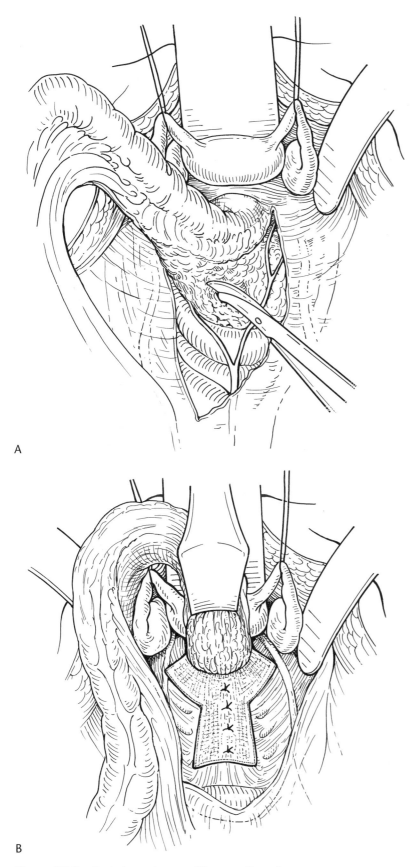

A

B

Figure 39-5.   Posterior rectopexy. *(Figure continues.)*

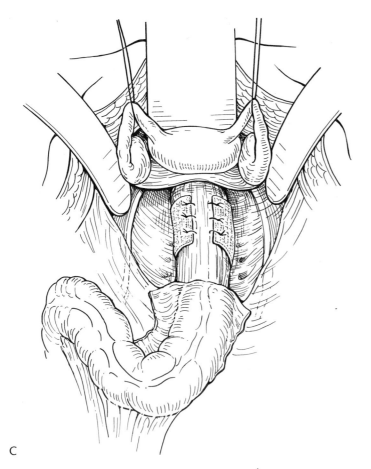

C

Figure 39-5. (Continued).

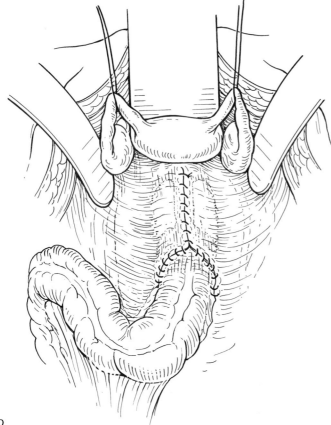

D

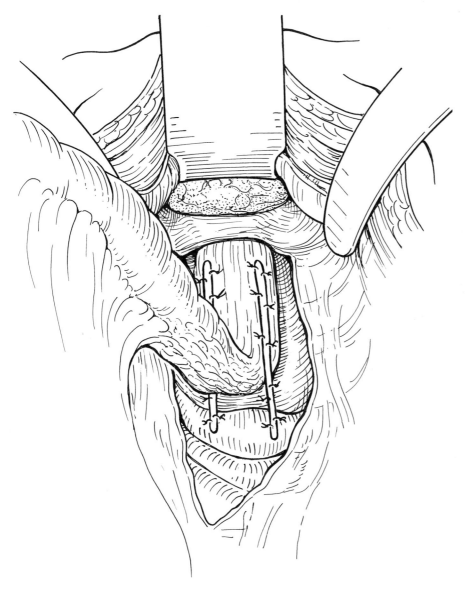

Figure 39-6. Orr-Loygue rectopexy.

double row of four or five nonresorbable stitches over a length of 5 cm. Gentle traction is then applied to the strips to pull up the anterior reflection of peritoneum to the level of the sacral promontory (Fig. 39-6). They are then sutured under moderate tension to the prevertebral fascia. The posterior peritoneum of the uterus is resected and the pouch of Douglas obliterated by suturing the cut edges of the peritoneum together.

Anterior Rectopexy

The principles underlying the Ripstein operation[95] include rectal mobilization and fixation of the rectum to the sacral promontory by a sling of material passed anteriorly around the bowel and fixed posteriorly to the sacrum.[96-100] The operation fixes the middle and upper rectum to the sacral curve, thereby preventing intussusception.

The operative technique is identical to posterior rectopexy as described above regarding mobilization of the rectum. A strip of the appropriate material is then hooked around the front of the rectum and sutured posteriorly[95,101,102] (Fig. 39-7) A triple suspension rectopexy has also been described.[103]

The major drawback of this operation is bowel dysfunction presumably due to angulation and fibrosis anteriorly. This may cause a constriction and stenosis. Constipation and fecal impaction occur in about 10% of patients.[90] Ulceration of the implant with perforation and extrusion rarely occurs.[95]

Lahaut's Operation

Lahaut's operation[104] involves a similar principle whereby the rectum is elevated and fixed by bringing the sigmoid colon through the posterior rectus sheath.[2]

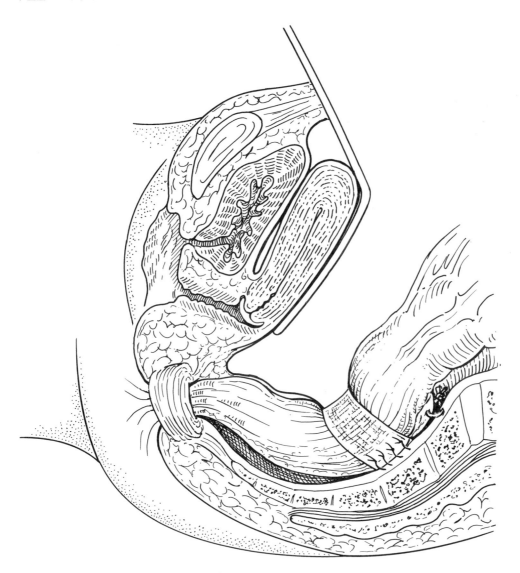

Figure 39-7. Anterior rectopexy.

Anterior Resection

Anterior resection was used in the past in some centers, notably the Mayo Clinic.[105] Good results concerning recurrence have been reported but the main disadvantage is the potentially serious complication of anastomotic dehiscence and the fear that some patients may develop incontinence. There is the possibility of morbidity from sepsis including anastomotic leakage, pelvic abscess, septicemia, and wound infection, which can occur in 20% of cases after low anterior resection. There is also the risk of late recurrence of about 10% at 10 years.[105] This approach has largely been abandoned owing to the lower morbidity of other methods. The operation largely practiced at Mayo in the last 20 years is anterior resection with rectopexy.[106]

Resection Rectopexy

In resection rectopexy a combination of resection and rectopexy is used.[106–108] The original rationale for this approach was to prevent early recurrence by exerting some upward traction on the rectum and improving evacuation. In patients who have

constipation preoperatively, resection with rectopexy is likely to result in superior functional results. The operative technique is identical to that of a standard high anterior resection, except a sutured rectopexy is performed to the presacral fascia usually prior to bowel resection[109,110] (Fig. 39-8).

Laparoscopic Rectopexy

The widespread success of laparoscopic cholecystectomy has led to the application of laparoscopic techniques to the large bowel including rectopexy.[111–114] With the catheterized patient in the Lloyd-Davies Trendelenberg position, four 10-to 12-mm ports are placed: two on the left side of the abdomen, one in the right iliac fossa, and one in the umbilical area. Standard insufflation is used and the plane lateral to the sigmoid colon is opened. Dissection is carried out posterior to the mesorectum and anterior to the presacral nerves with forward retraction on the rectosigmoid. Laparoscopic rectal mobilization and rectal fixation with sutures[115] or the use of Marlex mesh or a hernia stapler has been described.[116] Reports from trained laparoscopic

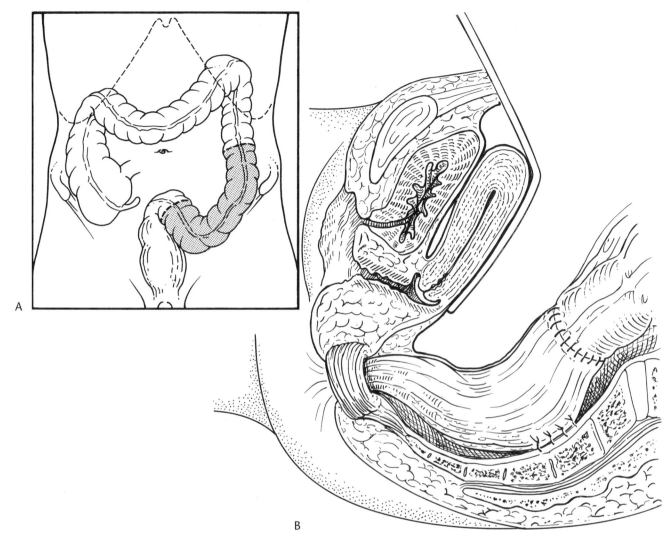

A

B

Figure 39-8. **(A & B)** Resection rectopexy.

surgeons show a low morbidity with a short hospital stay.[114] Complications (e.g., ureteric injury) have been encountered by others, indicating the need for thorough training in this technique.

Results

Recurrence. Recurrence rates reported in the literature are low (Table 39-3) with most below 10%. Most patients are aged and long-term follow-up is therefore not an important issue. Where it is, for example, in younger patients, recurrence is clearly a function of time. Thus, in a group of 26 patients under the age of 40 years having a posterior rectopexy with polyvinyl alcohol (Ivalon) insertion for external prolapse, recurrence was found in 5 (20%) at a median follow-up interval of 11 years.[77] This gradual increase with time should be taken into account when judging the relative effectiveness of procedures. In the absence of randomized controlled studies, the data available indicate that an abdominal approach is less likely to be followed by recurrence than is a perineal procedure.

Functional Outcome.

Incontinence. Short-term information on continence after rectopexy indicates that well over 50% of patients are improved to some extent.[1,26,101,110,117,118] Three mechanisms for this occurrence have been suggested.[117] These include a rise in resting anal pressure, improvement of rectal motility, and the abolition of high-pressure rectal waves leading to a reversal of the pressure gradient between the rectum and the anal canal. In a major prospective nonrandomized study comparing four techniques including suture rectopexy (10 cases), posterior rectopexy with polyvinyl implant (9 cases), anterior and posterior rectopexy with polypropyline (Marlex) implant (20 cases), and resection rectopexy (29 cases), Duthie and Bartolo[117] demonstrated an improvement of continence in all but the posterior rectopexy group. They showed that this could be associated with a rise in anal canal resting pressure, which occurred in patients having a sutured and resection rectopexy. It must be noted, however, that the rise was only of the order of 20 to 30 cm of water, supporting the possibility that other factors are important. It is probably significant that the improvement in

Table 39-3. Recurrence After Abdominal Rectopexy

	No.	Recurrence (%)
Posterior Rectopexy (Wells)		
Yoshioka et al., 1989[26]	135	2(1)
McCue et al., 1991[80]	53	2(4)
Boulos et al., 1984[97a]	25	5(20)
Kuijpers et al., 1988[193]	30	3(10)
Keighley et al., 1983[92]	100	0(0)
Penfold and Hawley, 1972[35]	101	3(3)
Posterior Rectopexy (Orr-Loygue)		
Loygue et al., 1984[1]	275	12(4)
Anterior Rectopexy (Ripstein)		
Ripstein, 1972[95]	500	0
Holmstrom et al., 1986[99]	97	4(4)
Launer et al., 1982[194]	54	7(13)
Anterior Rectopexy (Lehaut)		
Mortensen et al., 1984[2]	33	1(3)
Anterior Resection		
Schlinkert et al., 1985[105]	113	8(7)
Resection Rectopexy (Frykman-Goldberg)		
Watts et al., 1985[192]	138	2(1.4)
Madoff et al., 1992[110]	47	3(6)

[a] Mean follow-up 11 years.

continence was confined to the operation groups in which no implant of foreign material was made. Age and duration of follow-up were similar in all groups and the prolapse was controlled in all patients. Significantly improved continence was seen in all but the Ivalon group. There was no evidence of increasing postoperative constipation. Sphincter length and voluntary contraction were unaltered, but improved resting tone was seen in the resection and suture groups. This was not seen in the prosthetic groups. Improved continence correlated with recovery of resting pressure. Upper anal sensation was improved in all groups. Radiologic changes did not correlate with improved continence.[117,119]

In a study from the same unit, 22 patients with full-thickness rectal prolapse underwent ambulatory fine-wire EMG of the internal anal sphincter, external anal sphincter, and puborectalis, together with anorectal manometry, using a computerized system. Examinations were performed both before and 3 to 4 months after rectopexy. The median preoperative internal sphincter EMG frequency was 0.18 (0.05 to 0.31 interquartile range) Hz and the median preoperative resting anal pressure was 28 (15 to 64) cm H_2O. An improvement in the internal sphincter EMG frequency, and resting anal pressure, was recorded after surgery but these variables remained significantly lower than those found in normal controls. This suggests that repair of the prolapse allows the internal sphincter to recover by removing the cause of persistent rectoanal inhibition.[120]

A rise in resting anal canal pressure after rectopexy had been previously reported by Broden et al.[15] These authors reported a series of 15 patients of whom 10 had incontinence preoperatively. Only three were still incontinent after operation and in four cases a rise in resting pressure of 20 cm of water or more was correlated with this symptomatic improvement. In the re-

maining three cases it was not, however, indicating that other factors are likely to play a role. A rise of resting pressure in 26 patients undergoing rectopexy from 38 ± 26 SD to 49 ± 26 SD was reported by Madden et al.[118] Although undoubtedly useful, all these studies show only a modest increase to levels that only just approach normal values and seen in only a fraction of cases. Salvage procedures for patients whose incontinence does not respond to rectopexy may be worth considering. In one such report of postanal repair in 11 patients (nine women) with persistent fecal incontinence after rectopexy at a minimum follow-up of 5 years, one patient had required a colostomy and seven had improved continence, with all being continent to solid stool.[121]

Bowel Function. Rectopexy may induce constipation. This has been a clinical impression for many years and has recently been documented by a prospective study. In a series of 57 patients having a polyvinyl alcohol rectopexy, 19 were constipated before and 29 after. This increase was greater in patients who were incontinent preoperatively, rising from 18% to 46% compared with 48% to 55% in those who were continent. These changes were not sex related nor were they associated with hysterectomy.[74] In the first rigorous prospective study of function after rectopexy, Madden et al.[118] and Speakman et al.[24] from the same data base showed that although there was no significant change in bowel frequency there were alterations in the incidence of patients having to strain to defecate. Thus four of 11 patients who strained preoperatively were relieved of this symptom while straining was induced following the operation in five of 12 who did not strain before. Laxatives were required by 11 patients before and 19 after. Because the median bowel frequency was 21 motions per week before surgery and 17 afterward, the main determinant of constipation was straining. The study also indicated that rectal mucosal electrical sensitivity was reduced in some cases but this could not be related to function. There was evidence that constipation was more likely in patients who underwent a full rectal mobilization to the pelvic floor. A change in constipation occurred in 1 out of 12 patients having a limited dissection compared with 7 out of 14 in whom mobilization was extensive.[24] Twenty-one patients (91%) could expel a 50-ml balloon preoperatively and 18 could still do so postoperatively. This showed that rectal prolapse is occasionally associated with profoundly abnormal defecation. Although abdominal rectopexy improved continence, it may improve or worsen other bowel symptoms, including constipation.[118] It may be that denervation plays a part in causing dysfunction but mechanical factors including rigidity due to the implant angulation of the bowel above the implant may have an influence.[74]

Not all reports have shown constipation to occur after implant rectopexy; Duthie and Bartolo[117] found no difference in bowel frequency, straining, or incomplete emptying after various forms of rectopexy. Indeed there was an indication that function was improved in some cases. For example, these three variables before and after anteroposterior rectopexy in 20 patients were 3 (0.1 to 5) and 1.75 (1 to 5) per 24 hours; 13 (65%) and 11 (55%); and 13 (65%) and 8 (40%), respectively.

Rectal fixation combined with sigmoid resection, so-called resection rectopexy, appears to result in improved function when compared with standard mobilization with the insertion of an implant. The operation was originally described by Frykman and Goldberg[106] and long-term results have recently been reported.[110] In a review of the long-term functional results of colon resection and suture rectopexy for complete rectal prolapse in 47 patients followed for more than 3 years (mean 65 months), 33 patients underwent sigmoidectomy, 8 patients subtotal colectomy, and 4 patients sigmoidectomy, with subsequent subtotal colectomy. Three (6.3%) patients developed recurrent full-thickness prolapse, and four (8.5%) patients developed rectal mucosal prolapse. Twenty patients presented with constipation, 10 (50%) of whom improved after surgery. Constipation improved in seven (70%) patients who underwent subtotal colectomy. Twenty-one patients presented with incontinence, eight (38%) of whom improved. Continence worsened in six patients, and four patients developed significant diarrhea. These complications did not correlate with the extent of bowel resection. Three patients required a subsequent stoma. The authors concluded that colonic resection with rectopexy provides long-term control of rectal prolapse with an acceptable recurrence rate while being helpful to patients with associated preoperative constipation. Colonic resection of any magnitude does, however, risk chronic diarrhea with or without diminished continence although this is rare.[64,110]

In a prospective study a series of 39 patients followed up for a mean of 54 months after resection rectopexy were investigated.[122] Functional data were collected prospectively before the operation and at follow-up. These included clinical parameters, a constipation and incontinence score, anal manometry, proctography, and colonic transit studies. The postoperative complication rate was 7.1%, and mortality was 0%. No recurrence was seen. The prevalence of constipation improved from 43.6% to 25.6% ($P < .001$) and incontinence from 66.6% to 23.1% ($P < .001$). Anal resting pressure increased from 36.5 to 46.0 mmHg and squeeze pressure from 90.5 to 103.0 mmHg ($p < .001$). The anorectal angle changed little from 102° to 98°. The mean transit time decreased from 47.8 to 38.5 hours. These results indicate that rectopexy with sigmoid resection is a safe and effective procedure for rectal prolapse and leads to improved function of both bowel and sphincter.

Colorectal motility in 12 patients (10 females, aged 50.5 ± 5.2 years) complaining of severe constipation after Orr-Loygue rectopexy was compared with two control groups including 10 healthy volunteers and 12 patients with rectal prolapse. Before surgery, the rectopexy and prolapse groups were similar with respect to mean age, sex ratio, weekly stool frequency, other constipation symptoms, and anal incontinence. The former differed significantly from the latter in having a lower weekly stool frequency (2.5 ± 2.2 vs. 5.2 ± 3.7, $P < .01$) and a higher prevalence of abdominal pain. Colonic transit was 135.9 ± 38 hours and 51 ± 30.5 hours, respectively ($P < .01$).[82] These results indicate the possibility that the operation may induce changes in physiologic as well as clinical variables.

Although uncontrolled studies suggest that resection rectopexy results in a lower incidence of functional disturbance than conventional rectopexy, there are now firmer data to support this from a randomized controlled trial. Eighteen patients with full-thickness prolapse of the rectum were randomized to rectopexy alone (group 1) or with sigmoidectomy (group 2). Three months postoperatively, seven patients in group 1 and two in group 2 complained of severe constipation. Transit studies showed a significant increase in the number of markers at day 5 for those in group 1 (preoperative, 7.7 ± 2.6; postoperative, 14.6 ± 2.2) but no significant increase in group 2 (preoperative, 4.6 ± 2.2; postoperative 6.8 ± 2.3). No significant changes or differences between the groups were seen in the anorectal angle on proctography. Anorectal physiologic studies showed a significantly greater rectal compliance in group 1 compared with group 2 (group 1, 0.24 ± 0.02 mmHg/ml; group 2, 0.1 ± 0.02 mmHg/ml). The reason for these differences is unknown but it has been suggested that delayed transit may occur because the redundant loop of sigmoid colon causes hold-up of intestinal content and kinking at the junction between the sigmoid colon and the rectum.[103] Perhaps removal of some colon with poor motility may be a factor.

The main mechanisms of postoperative constipation can therefore be summarized as pre-existing slow colonic transit in some patients; the mechanical effects of surgery, which may include abnormal sigmoid configuration and perirectal fibrosis; and the possibility that rectal mobilization produces a partial denervation of the left colon thereby altering bowel function.[123–126]

Choice of Procedure

Given the many methods available, how should the individual surgeon decide on optimal management? To date, there are no good prospective randomized trials of a perineal versus an abdominal procedure including sufficient numbers of patients for adequate statistical analysis. With the simplicity and good results afforded by the Delorme procedure or rectosigmoidectomy, these operations are very suitable for frail elderly patients. Although the rate of recurrence may be greater than after abdominal rectopexy, the procedure can be repeated.

For a large prolapse, particularly in the younger patient, abdominal rectopexy offers a reasonably low chance of early recurrence with an excellent prospect of continence being restored. There is, however, evidence from studies reporting longer follow-up that recurrence gradually increases with time. Prospective data are now available showing that constipation can be induced by rectopexy, a complication that does not appear to follow perineal operations. This difficult problem can be minimized by combining rectal fixation with sigmoid resection without endangering improvement in continence. Despite the possibility of morbidity from the anastomosis, in the light of current knowledge it is reasonable to adopt this procedure as the treatment of choice where an abdominal operation is recommended. The uncertainty as to the best operation indicates the need for randomized comparative controlled trials.

SOLITARY RECTAL ULCER SYNDROME

Solitary ulcer of the rectum was described by Cruvehlier[127] in the 19th century, but it was not until the classic paper of Madigan and Morson[128] that it was identified as a clinical entity. The condition is rare with an estimated annual incidence of 1 per 100,000 population per year.[129] It can occur at almost any age from adolescence to over 50 years, but the greatest incidence is in the third decade of life. Most patients have symptoms for many months to years on average before the diagnosis is established. Solitary ulcer affects both sexes with a female/

male ratio of 3:1 reported in one series.[130] There is no known increased incidence of solitary ulcer running in families.

Clinical Features

Almost all patients complain of tenesmus, bleeding, and loss of mucus. About 50% have some degree of fecal incontinence and pain occurs in 20%. The diagnosis should be suspected on the history by the identification of the particular pattern of defecation abnormality. Although frequency of defecation itself may be normal, there may be a grossly abnormal bowel habit. Typically, the patient experiences many fruitless visits to the lavatory each day (e.g., 10 to 20 times), spending several minutes at each visit. Straining is nearly always present and is prompted by the feeling of a constant desire to defecate combined with a sensation of incomplete evacuation after defecation. Mucus is usually abundant but bleeding may not be. Solitary ulcer syndrome and villous adenoma are two conditions that produce abundant mucus. There may be a deep-seated pelvic ache, occasional anemia[131–133] and associations with irritable bowel syndrome and psychoneurosis.[134,135]

The essential features are seen on sigmoidoscopy. The rectum is seen to contain mucus within the lumen and there is mucosal reddening with or without ulceration. This is always located on one of the rectal valves, and on removing the window from the sigmoidoscope and asking the patient to strain, prolapse, of the lesion may be evident. In a series of 43 patients attending St. Mark's Hospital between 1974 and 1984, the lesion involved the anterior rectal wall in 39 (90%) (Nicholls, RJ, unpublished observations). Ulceration is not always present. It was found in about one-half of these patients but in 30% the mucosa was polypoid and in the remainder no more than an erythematous mucosal flush was seen.

Many patients have evident perineal descent with a rather lax resting tone. A polypoid lesion may simulate a carcinoma and histologic examination is essential.[136]

Histopathology

A typical solitary rectal ulcer varies between 1 and 5 cm^2, is shallow, and associated with a gray-white slough.[137] There may be considerable surrounding edema with an area of diffuse fibrosis. The ulcers may be round, oval, linear, serpiginous, or stellate. Histologically, there may be adjacent cysts or pseudopolyps with a surrounding area of inflammation.[138–140] They occur classically on the anterior wall of the anorectum opposite the puborectalis sling, 5 to 8 cm from the anal verge. The lesion is solitary in 50% to 90% of cases. Similar ulceration may occur elsewhere in the colon or on the apex of a stoma.

The lamina propria is replaced by collagen and there is fibromuscular replacement of the mucosa. There is intense fibrosis and a predominance of sialomucins. Muscle fibers are seen splaying into the lamina propria.[128,141–144] There is hypertrophy of the muscularis mucosae, crypt distortion, epithelial hyperplasia, and transitional mucosa (Fig. 39-9). Localized colitis cystic profunda is characterized by submucosal cysts.[145] The histology of solitary ulcer differs characteristically from that of full-thickness prolapse: the former has a markedly thickened circular muscle wall and abundance of collagen.[34] There are, however, marked similarities (including hypertrophy of the muscularis mucosae), which are also found in prolapsing hemorrhoids and mucosal prolapse.

Diagnosis

There is an extensive differential diagnosis but the typical history with the local endoscopic changes will exclude many other conditions. Microbiologic examination of the stool should be

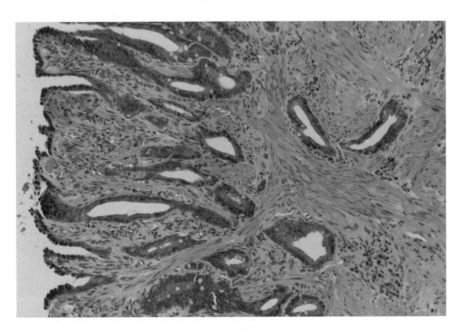

Figure 39-9. Histopathologic features of the solitary rectal ulcer syndrome. There is hypertrophy of the muscularis mucosae, crypt distortion, epithelial hyperplasia and fibroblast proliferation.

Differential Diagnosis of Solitary Rectal Ulcer

Inflammatory Bowel Disease

Crohn's disease

Ulcerative proctocolitis

Radiation proctocolitis

Infections

Actinomycosis

Amebiasis

Schistosomiasis

Others

Tumors

Carcinoma

Adenoma

Rare rectal tumors

Endometriosis

Stercoral Ulcer

requested. The diagnosis is confirmed by histopathologic examination of biopsy material. Almost any disease of the rectum can be mistaken for the solitary ulcer syndrome (see Box). On proctoscopy there is typically a considerable amount of mucus in the rectum; an extensive villous tumor is the only other condition that produces as much.

Etiopathology

Rectal Evacuation

The disease appears to be associated with a disorder of evacuation, the cause of which is unknown. With the introduction of defecating proctography, it had become appreciated that well over 50% of cases have evidence of internal rectal intussusception[146,147] (Fig. 39-10). It also appears that some cases with a primary diagnosis of rectal intussusceptiom can be shown to have a solitary ulcer.[148–151] To add to these considerations is the fact that the symptom complex found in both these conditions can occur without any evidence either of intussusception or rectal mucosal damage. For example, in the so-called descending perineum syndrome[152] or in patients with anterior mucosal prolapse,[3] many of the symptoms are common. With any pelvic floor disorder, it is often difficult to relate symptoms to physical signs. This makes the interpretation of proctographic evidence of internal prolapse or proctoscopic mucosal prolapse, or indeed of perineal descent, difficult when considering treatment.

Proctography itself may be difficult to interpret. Ihre and Seligson[153] have contributed to our understanding of intussusception and its relation to symptoms by cineproctography during straining. Proctographic features should, however, be interpreted with caution because radiologic abnormalities may occur in asymptomatic patients. Thus Shorvon et al.[154] have demon-

strated that up to 40% of normal individuals may show abnormalities on proctography including intussusception and rectocele. The picture is therefore confused. From a clinician's point of view, however, a diagnosis of internal intussusception or solitary rectal ulcer can only be made in the presence of symptoms.

It is possible to demonstrate a failure of evacuation using the balloon expulsion test in about 50% of patients with the solitary ulcer syndrome.[151] An overlap between this and rectal intussusception clearly occurs. Approximately 25% of patients diagnosed as having rectal intussusception have symptoms suggesting the presence of rectal ulceration,[150] such as mucus and bleeding. About 50% to 80%[146,147] of patients with the solitary ulcer syndrome have rectal intussusception on proctography and about 50% have a negative balloon expulsion test.[155,156] The significance of these interrelationships shown in Figure 39-11 is obscure.

Pelvic Floor Muscle Incoordination

Rutter and Riddell[157] have suggested that the sensation of urgency to defecate is due to an anterior mucosal prolapse that develops following many years of straining. Descent of the anterior mucosal prolapse may also be associated with reflex contraction of the pelvic floor (paradoxical puborectalis spasm) during straining (Fig. 39-12). There are some patients who have EMG evidence of hyperactivity of the puborectalis both at rest and during straining.[9] This paradoxical contraction of the puborectalis appears to be present in about 50% of cases.[158] One theory to explain solitary ulcer suggests that this paradoxical puborectalis muscle contraction results in trauma to the mucosal prolapse, thus rendering its tip ischemic. Ischemia results in fibromuscular obliteration of the lamina propria and the formation of the ulcer, which itself produces further urgency and worsening of mucosal damage.[159] Videoproctographic appear-

Figure 39-10. Proctography; internal intussusception.

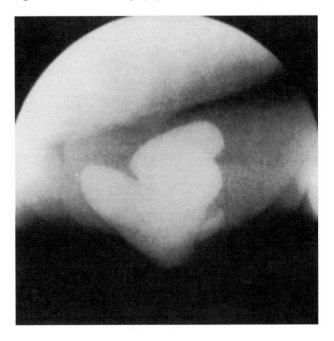

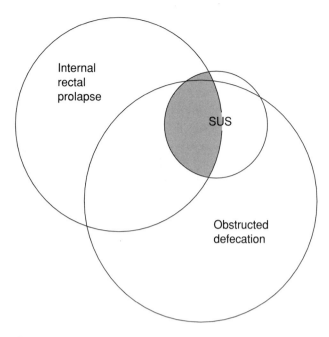

Figure 39-11. The interrelation of rectal intussusception, negative balloon expulsion, and the solitary rectal ulcer syndrome.

ances may in a minority of patients demonstrate a persistently closed anorectal angle during defecation despite perineal descent.[146,147] More commonly rectal invagination due to intra-anal intussusception, full-thickness prolapse, or anterior wall prolapse are seen.[160,161]

In a study using proctography with integrated measurements of external sphincter EMG and rectal pressure, Womack et al.[161] have reported raised intrarectal pressures during voiding. The significance of this is not known, but it may possibly have some traumatic effect on the rectal mucosa. Sun et al.[20] in a study of 11 patients with the solitary ulcer syndrome, observed higher rectal than anal pressures during straining, an observation that was found in patients with complete rectal and anterior mucosal prolapse, but not in normal controls. There was evidence of rectal contraction waves and a lower threshold of the desire to defecate on rectal distension. They concluded that the rectum is hypersensitive in the solitary ulcer syndrome.

Prolapse

The clinical association with rectal prolapse combined with the radiologic and histologic similarities suggest a common etiology. In a further attempt to explore this the physiologic features of patients with complete rectal prolapse and different degrees of solitary rectal ulcer syndrome were compared to determine

Figure 39-12. Electromyography of the external anal sphincter at rest and during straining.

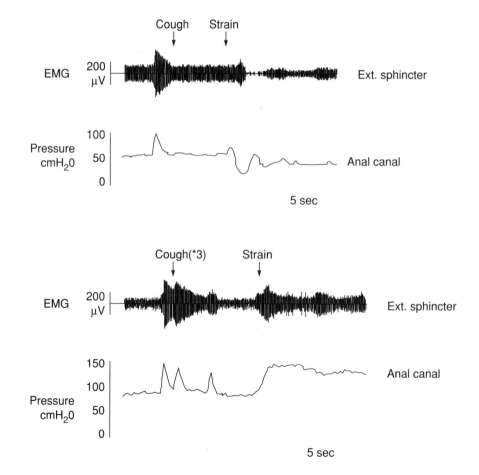

whether these conditions are likely to form part of the same disorder. Fifty-two patients with solitary rectal ulcer (median age 31 years, 40 females), and 15 complete rectal prolapse patients (median age 31, 12 females) were studied. Solitary rectal ulcer patients were divided into three groups, based on the extent of accompanying rectal prolapse (no prolapse, internal prolapse, or external prolapse). Solitary rectal ulcer patients without prolapse and with internal prolapse had significantly higher maximum anal resting ($P < .01$ for both groups) and squeeze pressures ($P < .05$ for both groups) than complete rectal prolapse patients. In contrast, solitary rectal ulcer patients with external prolapse were similar to those with complete rectal prolapse and had significantly decreased anal and rectal electrosensitivity when compared with healthy control subjects.[162] Solitary rectal ulcer patients therefore have a spectrum of clinical and physiologic features, suggesting that the condition may include various disease entities. It may also be that solitary rectal ulcer and complete rectal prolapse have different etiopathology. More work is required in this interesting condition.

The incidence of overt rectal prolapse ranges from 6% to 39%.[28,29] Indeed, in the report of Schweiger and Williams[163] 10 of the 12 cases reported had incomplete prolapse. Unlike patients with overt rectal prolapse, those with occult intussusception usually have no EMG or histologic evidence of pelvic floor neuropathy despite the presence of perineal descent.[164–166] In some patients increased external sphincter activity raises rectal pressure immediately adjacent to the intussuscepting rectum and this might be responsible for the ulcer. Alternatively, the intussusception initiates a desire to defecate even with an empty rectum, producing straining and resultant ischemic ulceration at the tip of the intussusception. Martin et al.[129] found that 34% of patients with solitary rectal ulcer syndrome had a complete prolapse, 25% had prolapse to the anal verge, 14% had occult prolapse, 11% had an anterior bulge, 7% had partial occult prolapse, and 9% were normal. Madigan and Morson[128] also described rectal prolapse in their cases.

Ischemia

Local ischemia at the apex of an intussusception or an anterior rectal prolapse may occur as described above. In a few patients, steal syndrome from the hemorrhoidal to the iliac vessels has been claimed to be responsible.[167] There are no objective data to support this, however. It may be that the local prolapsing process has an ischemic element but the histology is not typical of ischemia.[34]

Trauma

Rectal digitation is recorded in 50% to 70% of patients with solitary rectal ulcer syndrome and has been suggested as a cause of mucosal damage. These patients are unable to evacuate without digital assistance to remove feces directly from the rectum or indirectly by applying pressure on the posterior vault of the vagina.

This is, however, a consequence rather than the cause of the condition because anoreceptive homosexuals, chronically constipated paraplegics, and those with outlet obstruction do not develop solitary rectal ulcer syndrome despite experiencing some degree of trauma to the rectal mucosa.[29] Some patients

may produce self-inflicted injuries by traumatic insertion of objects whereas other associations include inflammatory bowel disease and insertion of suppositories. None of these conditions amounts to the solitary ulcer syndrome.

Treatment

Solitary ulcer syndrome is a physical manifestation of a functional disorder of unknown etiology. Medical management should be continued and surgery contemplated only in selected patients with severe symptoms in whom psychoneurosis is not a predominant feature.

Conservative

Treatment is difficult and should be conservative as far as is possible. The nature of the condition should be explained to the patient with appeals to avoid straining and to try and establish a regular strain-free bowel action.[168] This is very difficult in practice and medication with laxatives and suppositories is likely to fail. In a series of 190 patients, 95 were treated conservatively. Of this latter group 34% improved, 20% were worse, and 46% remained unchanged after 1 year of follow-up.[150] Tjandra et al.[169] reported improvement in 11 of 59 patients.

There is the further complicating factor of the patient's psyche and full attention should be given to this aspect. Local medication in the form of steroids or salicylic acid derivatives have been tried but there is no evidence that these are helpful.[170] Behavioral therapy such as biofeedback is currently being evaluated prospectively.

Surgery

A high proportion of solitary ulcers are resistant to therapy and seem to alter very little through a period of follow-up.[128,150] In patients who continue to have severe symptoms, surgery may be necessary. It appears to help only when there is an occult prolapse and then only about 70% in the medium term. An anal approach is possible only if there is a sliding prolapse at this level but otherwise an abdominal rectopexy will be required. However, the latter may result in constipation with apparent loss of rectal sensation and should therefore be advised with caution.

Where symptoms of irritable bowel disease or psychological disturbance predominate, it is unwise to offer surgery unless absolutely forced to do so by the severity of symptoms. Many treatments have been tried (Table 39-4) and with the exception

Table 39-4. The Results of Various Treatments in 43 Patients With the Solitary Ulcer Syndrome Seen at St. Mark's Hospital Between 1974 and 1984

	Treated	Improved
Rubber band ligation	4	1
Cryotherapy/diathermy	4	0
Local excision	8	1
Postanal repair	13	1
Posterior rectopexy	10	3
Colostomy	5	—
Anterior resection	5	0
Hartmann's operation	1	0
Total anorectal excision	2	2

of total rectal excision and rectopexy, the results are poor. There is some more recent information that mucosal excision (Delorme's operation) does help in selected cases. Patients who are so severely incapacitated by the condition that their life is completely taken over by the condition owing to the compulsion to visit the lavatory excessively may require surgery if medical treatment does not help.

In a retrospective study of 80 patients, it was found that 44% had polypoid lesions (the predominant finding in asymptomatic subjects), ulcerated lesions in 29% (always symptomatic), and edematous nonulcerated hyperemic mucosa in 29%. Management by bulk laxatives and bowel retraining led to symptom improvement in 19%. In 29%, symptoms persisted despite endoscopic healing of the lesion. Depending on the presence or absence of rectal prolapse, rectopexy or a conservative local procedure (such as local excision), respectively, appeared to be the optimal surgical treatment but surgery was needed in 34%. The polypoid variety tended to respond most favorably to treatment.[169]

Procedures No Longer Used

Local Excision

This is a difficult procedure and often results in a distorted, narrow rectum that may form a stricture. Symptoms usually persist or recur.[171]

Internal Sphincterectomy and Anorectal Myectomy

Excision of a strip of the sphincter and lower rectal smooth muscle has been tried but the functional disorder persists postoperatively,[172] as Yoshioka and Keighley[173] also found in applying this to a variety of defecation disorders.

Division of the Puborectalis

It may seem logical to treat by partial division of the innermost fibers of the puborectalis sling because paradoxical contraction of this muscle has been implicated in pathogenesis.[157,174,175] Some patients do appear to improve and none develop fecal incontinence. However, even in those with EMG evidence of abnormal pelvic floor contraction during straining, the majority are not cured.[158]

Anal Dilation

Almost all patients have marked perineal descent and evidence of a latent pudendal nerve lesion and hence this maneuver may cause incontinence and is therefore to be avoided.

Anterior Resection and Coloanal Sleeve Excision

This involves excision of the rectum to the dentate line and a low coloanal anastomosis. Very limited success has been reported although recurrence is likely.[176] In a small series of five patients, four failed within 2 years and required a colostomy (Sitzler et al., unpublished observations). This major procedure with potential serious morbidity cannot be recommended.

Procedures That May Be Helpful

Rectopexy

Rectopexy is a logical procedure in patients who have demonstrable evidence of prolapse. The results of posterior rectopexy have not been encouraging, but the Ripstein procedure is more logical given the anterior location of the ulcer.

Ihre and Seligson[153] reported a series of 90 patients of whom 40 had a Ripstein procedure. The series was expanded in a subsequent publication of 193 patients with internal rectal prolapse of whom 63 underwent a Ripstein rectopexy.[150] Among this latter group, the sensation of the constant desire to defecate was improved in 52%. Five of the patients had bleeding, suggesting the presence of the solitary ulcer syndrome. Of these bleeding was improved in four. Schweiger and Williams[163] reported 10 patients treated by Ripstein rectopexy with a follow up of 3 to 13 months. At that time no ulcer was present in 9 patients. All these cases, however, had an associated prolapse and the operation was not therefore really a test of rectopexy for the solitary ulcer syndrome without prolapse. In a series from Bristol where rectopexy was used for symptoms of obstructed defecation rather than in cases with rectal mucosal damage, only two patients of 17 had a good outcomes.[177] These cases did not have the solitary ulcer syndrome, however, since mucosal changes were absent. The results show that rectopexy should not be used for symptoms alone.

In an attempt to achieve anterior fixation, Nicholls and Simson[178] used a form of anteroposterior rectopexy mobilizing the rectum on all sides and placing a Marlex implant anteriorly as well as posteriorly. In an initial series of 12 patients followed for a mean of 17 months, there was a remarkable reduction in the number of visits to the toilet per 24 hours, from eight preoperatively to three postoperatively and the total time spent in the toilet per 24 hours decreased from 146 minutes preoperatively to 15 minutes postoperatively. The feeling of the constant desire to defecate and incomplete evacuation was eliminated in almost all patients. Bleeding and mucus discharge improved. Two patients, however, became severely constipated associated with a loss of rectal sensation. Both presented a difficult clinical problem.

A group of 23 patients underwent proctography before and after rectopexy. Prolapse was demonstrated in 19 of 23 patients before operation (internal in 12, external in 7) and in only 1 patient postoperatively. The rectal axis became more vertical at rest and on evacuation. The time taken to evacuate the contrast during the preoperative proctogram was related to outcome, being significantly longer in those with a poor result.[179] Thus, although rectopexy successfully corrects the prolapse in patients with solitary rectal ulcer syndrome this is not related to symptomatic outcome. Prolonged preoperative evacuation time is however, and may be a useful predictor of a poor result. Furthermore, surgery of this type should not be offered to patients who do not have evidence of prolapse of proctography.

Sitzler et al.[180] has reviewed a series of 66 patients who had surgical treatment for solitary ulcer more than 12 months previously. A rectopexy was carried out in 49. Of these, 19 (40%) required further procedures including stoma formation in 11 cases. The overall relief rate for symptoms was 51%, being slightly higher for anteroposterior (66%) than conventional posterior rectopexy (47%).

Excision of Mucosal Prolapse

Excision of the prolapsing mucosa can relieve the symptom of the persisting desire to defecate although it does not alter the fundamental underlying disorder of defecation. Where there is prolapse of the lower rectal mucosa it is usually possible to carry out an endoanal excision of the Delorme's type with ease. This procedure is not, however, appropriate in those patients in whom prolapse lies more proximal and should not be attempted. The results in a series of nine patients showed relief of the persisting desire to defecate in five (55%). There were four failures including two patients who developed a degree of fecal incontinence postoperatively, which was temporary in one (Sitzler, unpublished observations).

Stoma Formation

The formation of a stoma will relieve the defecatory symptoms and will be necessary in severe cases that do not respond to any other treatment. If carried out as a reversable maneuver preserving the rectum, patients may continue to complain of heaviness and pain in the perineum and discharge of mucus. Under these circumstances, the surgeon may need to remove the rectum. Creation of a stoma should be considered early in the postoperative course of patients who have had a failed rectopexy.

RECTOCELE

Rectocele is common in multiparous women. The symptoms include constipation in which classically the patient has incomplete evacuation that she may treat by digitating the posterior vaginal wall. Rectocele is associated with a weak pelvic floor and usually occurs in multiparous patients over 50 years of age.

Investigations are largely as outlined above under rectal prolapse and solitary rectal ulcer syndrome. EMG may show weak puborectalis function with increasing fiber density and prolonged pudendal nerve latencies. Proctography will confirm the diagnosis, showing an anterior rectal wall bulge during defecation; Sullivan et al.[17] maintain that a "rolling down" anterior rectal wall on proctoscopy is a prerequisite for suitability for surgical repair. Detailed assessment appears to show that rectocele is not associated with any physiologic change apart from a significant increase of pelvic floor descent.[181] The radiologic interpretation requires care because small rectoceles are a common finding in healthy individuals.[154] A rectocele projecting 2 cm or more from the contour of the rectal wall is significant if symptoms are present. A recent study found a prevalence of 27% in women presenting with disorders of defecation, but this depends on definition. Spence Jones et al.[18] studied the relationship between bowel symptoms and genital prolapse and showed a considerable overlap. Some degree of rectocele may be found in up to 80% of asymptomatic females, but only 16% of rectoceles larger than 2 cm are symptom free.[182] Other groups would place the lower limit of a clinically significant rectocele at 3 cm.[183] Yoshioka et al.[181] suggested that the size could be measured as the distance between the extended line of the ante-

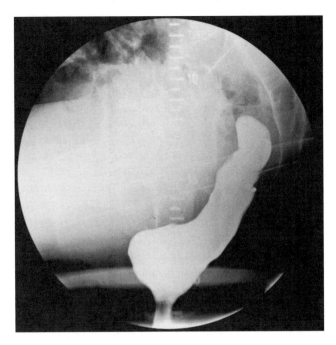

Figure 39-13.   Proctogram showing a clinically significant rectocele.

rior border of the anal canal and the tip of the rectocele. In an analysis of 2816 patients with defection disorders, 27% had rectocele and 19% had enterocele.[184] This latter report characterized rectoceles into three different sizes: small (less than 2 cm), medium (2 to 4 cm), and large (greater than 4 cm). In a study correlating defecography with magnetic resonance imaging (MRI), it was concluded that an anterior rectocele with a size of 2 cm or more on MRI corresponded well to symptomatic rectoceles seen on physical assessment and defecography and symptom improvement correlated well with rectocele size greater than 2 cm on defecography.[185] It would seem appropriate on the basis of these reports to consider 2 cm size of rectocele on defecography as clinically significant. (Fig. 39-13.)

Treatment

Treatment may be conservative but is indicated in selected symptomatic patients. Initial management should center on control of constipation because although there is an association, the latter symptom may not be wholly due to the outlet obstruction caused by the rectocele.[186]

Rubber Band Ligation

Rubber band ligation is a simple office procedure for the treatment of anterior mucosal prolapse and it has been suggested that it has a place in small rectocele.[187] However, no trials or long-term data are available on the efficacy of the technique and it could be argued that rectoceles smaller than 2 cm do not require intervention.

Endovaginal Repair

Prior to the mid 1960s endovaginal repair was the standard technique used by gynecologists. Briefly, the posterior vaginal mucosal wall is dissected and the underlying rectovaginal septum plicated with prolene sutures either transversely or longitudinally. The mucosa is then trimmed and closed. Although increasingly obsolete as a primary procedure, it may have a role in failed endorectal repair. In a retrospective review of 64 rectocele repairs (35 transanally and 29 transvaginal repairs), 80% had improvement postsurgery.[188] Persistent pain was more common after transvaginal repair but there was no difference in functional outcome between the two methods.

Endorectal Repair

Sullivan et al.[17] were the first to report good results using a peranal technique. Unfortunately no functional assessment is available in this or other reports but there is clearly a beneficial effect in many patients. The patient is placed in the prone jack-knife position and a transverse incision made in the anterior rectal mucosa about 8 cm from the anal verge. Adrenaline infiltration (1 in 300,000) will help in a bloodless dissection of the mucosa from underlying muscle. Interrupted 2/0 PDS sutures are placed to plicate the muscle, thus obliterating the rectocele. The mucosa is closed and the patient prescribed laxatives for 2 weeks. Good results have been reported with 80% improvement and no recurrence at 2 years of follow-up.[189]

Mesh Repair

Anterior levatorplasty with or without insertion of mesh is an option.[125] Although the perineal route is commonly used the procedure may be performed with a laparoscope transabdominally. Parker and Phillips described a technique for rectocele in which Marlex mesh is placed in the rectovaginal septum. Of four patients, three had normal defecation postoperatively and one was improved but still occasionally needed to use digital perineal pressure.[190] The original series has now been expanded with encouraging results (Phillips PKS, unpublished observations).

Analysis of Surgical Results

Following endorectal repair there is a significantly decreased urge to defecate on rectal distension and also a reduction in the size of rectocele on defecography. In a consecutive series of

Table 39-5. Comparative Outcomes of Various Surgical Series of Endorectal Repair of Rectocele

Series	Patients	Complications[a]	Good Result[b]	Follow-Up
Sullivan et al., 1968[17]	111	15%	80%	—
Schapayak, 1985[195]	355	6%	75%	—
Khubchandani, 1983[196]	59	7%	63%	—
Block, 1986[197]	60	7%	80%	1.5–4 years

[a] Fecal impaction, bleeding, wound breakdown, sinuses, rectovaginal fistula, stenosis, dysuria.
[b] Asymptomatic or considerable improvement.

76 patients anorectal function was improved in 70, with a reduction in rectal urge sensitivity being the most marked feature.[187] The outcome of several series of endorectal repair is shown in Table 39-5. It is perhaps appropriate after initial conservative measures, including rubber band ligation, to consider an endorectal technique. It is suggested that endorectal repair should be performed as the preferred procedure before vaginal correction owing to the persistence of anorectal symptoms after a vaginal repair alone and because of the risk of rectovaginal fistula in a combined vaginal and rectal repair. This can be a formal mucosal dissection, a muscle plication followed by mucosal closure, or a simple plication without lifting a mucosal flap. On analysis of the different series, a good symptomatic result has been reported in between 65% and 80% although long-term follow-up and detailed objective physiologic analysis is lacking. Complications appear generally to be minor and usually include hematoma formation or mucosal dehiscence.

Rectocele is associated with cystocele and uterine prolapse and these conditions should be deliberately looked for and treated as appropriate.

REFERENCES

1. Loygue J, Nordlinger B, Cunei O et al (1984) Rectopexy to the promontory for the treatment of rectal prolapse. Dis Colon Rectum 27:356–359
2. Mortensen NJMcC, Vellacott KD, Wilson MG (1984) Lahaut's operation for rectal prolapse. Ann R Coll Surg Engl 66:17–18
3. Andrews NJ, Jones DJ (1992) Rectal prolapse and associated conditions. BMJ 305:243–245
4. Henry MM, Parks AG, Swash M (1982) The pelvic floor musculature in the descending perineum syndrome. Br J Surg 69:470–472
5. Nwako F (1975) Rectal prolapse in Nigerian children. Int Surg 60:284–285
6. Mikulicz J (1889) Zur operativen Behandlung des Prolapsus Recti et Coli invaginati. Arch Klin Chir 38:74
7. Berman IR, Manning DH, Dudley Wright K (1985) Anatomic

8. Allen Mersh TG, Henry MM, Nicholls RJ (1987) Natural history of anterior mucosal prolapse. Br J Surg 74:679–682
9. Rutter KRP (1974) Electromyographic changes in certain pelvic floor abnormalities Proc R Soc Med 67:53–56
10. Broden B, Snellman B (1968) Procidentia of the rectum studied with cineradiography: a contribution to the discussion of causative mechanism. Dis Colon and Rectum 11:330–347
11. Moschowitz AV (1912) The pathogenesis, anatomy and care of prolapse of the rectum. Surg Gynecol Obstet 15:7–21
12. Neill ME, Parks AG, Swash M (1981) Physiological studies of the anal sphincter musculature in faecal incontinence and rectal prolapse. Br J Surg 68:531–536
13. Lubowski DZ, Nicholls RJ, Burleigh DE, Swash M (1988)

specificity in the diagnosis and treatment of internal rectal prolapse. Dis Colon Rectum 28:816–826

Internal anal sphincter in neurogenic faecal incontinence. Gastroenterology 95:997–1002

14. Dolk A, Broden G, Holmstrom B et al (1987) Endocrine cells in the human colorectal mucosa: immunocytochemical observations on patients with prolapse or internal procidentia of the rectum. Int J Colorectal Dis 2:77–81

15. Broden G, Dolk A, Holmstrom B (1988) Recovery of the internal sphincter following rectopexy: a possible explanation for continence improvement. Int J Colorectal Dis 3:23–28

16. Broden G, Dolk A, Holmstrom B (1988) Evacuation difficulties and other characteristics of rectal function associated with procidentia and the Ripstein operation. Dis Colon Rectum 31:283–286

17. Sullivan ES, Leaverton GH, Hardwick CE (1968) Transrectal perineal repair: an adjunct to improved function after anorectal surgery. Dis Colon Rectum 11:106–114

18. Spence Jones C, Kamm MA, Henry MM, Hudson CN (1994) Bowel dysfunction: a pathogenic factor in uterovaginal prolapse and urinary stress incontinence. Br J Obstet Gynecol 101:147–152

19. Sayer T, Dixon J, Hosker G, Warrell D (1990) A study of paraurethral connective tissue in women with stress incontinence of urine. Neurourol Urodynam 9:319–320

20. Sun WM, Read NW, Donnelly CT et al (1989) A common pathophysiology for full rectal prolapse, anterior mucosal prolapse and solitary rectal ulcer syndrome. Br J Surg 76:290–295

21. Snooks SJ, Swash M, Henry MM, Setchell ME (1986) Risk factors in childbirth causing damage to the pelvic floor innervation: a precursor of stress incontinence. Int J Colorectal Dis 1:20–24

22. Keighley MRB (1992) Rectal Prolapse. p. 316. In Henry MM, Swash M (eds): Coloproctology and the Pelvic Floor. 2nd Ed. Butterworth Heineman, Oxford

23. Kuijpers HC (1992) Treatment of complete rectal prolapse: to narrow, to wrap, to suspend, to fix, to encircle, to plicate or to resect? World J Surg 16:826–830

24. Speakman CTM, Madden MV, Nicholls RJ, Kamm MA (1991) Lateral ligament division during rectopexy causes constipation but prevents recurrence: results of a prospective randomised study. Br J Surg 78:1431–1433

25. Yoshioka K, Hyland G, Keighley MRB (1989) Anorectal function after abdominal rectopexy: parameters of predictive value in identifying return of continence. Br J Surg 76:64–68

26. Yoshioka K, Heyen F, Keighley MRB (1989) Functional results after posterior abdominal rectopexy for rectal prolapse. Dis Colon Rectum 32:835–838

27. Keighley MRB, Fielding JWL (1983) Management of faecal incontinence and results of surgical treatment. Br J Surg 70:463–468

28. Keighley MRB, Shouler PJ (1984) Abnormalities of colonic function in patients with rectal prolapse and faecal incontinence. Br J Surg 71:892–895

29. Keighley MRB, Shouler PJ (1984) Clinical and manometric features of the solitary rectal ulcer syndrome. Dis Colon Rectum 27:507–512

30. Metcalf AM, Loening-Baucke V (1988) Anorectal function and defecation dynamics in patients with rectal prolapse. Am J Surg 155:206–210

31. Ramanujam PS, Venkatesh KS (1988) Perineal excision of rectal prolapse with posterior levator ani repair in elderly high-risk patients. Dis Colon Rectum 31:704–706

32. Ramanujam PS, Venkatesh KS (1992) Management of acute incarcerated rectal prolapse. Dis Colon Rectum 35:1154–1156

33. Ramanujam PS, Venkatesh KS, Fietz MJ (1994) Perineal excision of rectal procidentia in elderly high-risk patients. A ten-year experience. Dis Colon Rectum 37:1027–1130

34. Kang YS, Kamm MA, Engel AF, Talbot IC (1996) Pathology of the rectal wall in solitary rectal ulcer syndrome and complete rectal prolapse. Gut 38:587–590

35. Banerjee AK, Jackson BT, Nicholls RJ (1986) Full thickness rectal prolapse associated with primary intraabdominal pathology. Postgrad Med J 62:303–304

36. Rashid Z, Basson MD (1996) Association of rectal prolapse with colorectal cancer. Surgery 119:51–55

37. Keighley MRB, Makuria T, Alexander-Williams J, Arabi Y (1980) Clinical and manometric evaluation of rectal prolapse and faecal incontinence. Br J Surg 67:54–56

38. Hiltunen KM, Matikainen M, Auvinen O, Hietanen P (1986) Clinical and manometric evaluation of anal sphincter function in patients with rectal prolapse. Am J Surg 151:489–492

39. Hiltunen KM, Matikainen M (1992) Improvement of continence after abdominal rectopexy for rectal prolapse. Int J Colorectal Dis 7:8–10

40. Thiersch (1891) quoted in Carrasco AB (1943) Contribution a l'etude du Prolapsus du Rectum. Masson, Paris

41. Hopkinson BR, Lightwood R (1966) Electrical treatment of anal incontinence. Lancet 1:297–298

42. Hopkinson BR, Hardman J (1973) Silicone rubber perianal suture for rectal prolapse. Proc R Soc Med 66:1095–1098

43. Jackman FR, Francis JN, Hopkinson BR (1980) Silicone rubber band treatment of rectal prolapse. Ann R Coll Surg Engl 62:385–387

44. Earnshaw J, Hopkinson BR (1987) Late results of silicone rubber perianal suture for rectal prolapse. Dis Colon Rectum 30:86–88

45. Vongsangnak V, Varma JS, Watters D, Smith AN (1985) Clinical manometric and surgical aspects of complete prolapse of the rectum. J R Coll Edinb 30:251–254

46. Vongsangnak V, Varma JS, Watters D, Smith AN (1985) Reappraisal of Thiersch's operation for complete rectal prolapse. JR Coll Edinb 30:185–187

47. Delorme R (1900) Sur le traitement des prolapsus de la muqueuse rectale ou rectocolique. Bull Soc Chir Paris 26:459

48. Abulafi AM, Sherman IW, Fiddian RV, Rothwell-Jackson RL (1990) Delorme's operation for rectal prolapse. Ann R Coll Surg Engl 72:382–385

49. Graf W, Ejerblad S, Krog M et al (1992) Delorme's operation for rectal prolapse in elderly or unfit patients. Eur J Surg 158:555–557

50. Gundersen AL, Cogbill TH, Landercasper J (1985) Reappraisal of Delorme's procedure for rectal prolapse. Dis Colon Rectum 28:721–724

51. Houry S, Lechaux JP, Huguier M, Moikhou JM (1987) Treatment of rectal prolapse by Delorme's operation. Int J Colorectal Dis 2:149–152

52. Lechaux JP, Lechaux D, Perez M (1995) Results of Delorme's procedure for rectal prolapse. Advantages of a modified technique. Dis Colon Rectum 38:301–307

53. Uhlig BE, Sullivan ES (1979) The modified Delorme operation: its place in surgical treatment for massive rectal prolapse. Dis Colon Rectum 22:513–521

54. Christiansen J, Krikegaard P (1981) Delorme's operation for complete rectal prolapse. Br J Surg 68:537–538

55. Monson JRT, Jones NAG, Vowden P, Brennan TG (1986). Delorme's operation: the first choice in complete rectal prolapse? Ann R Coll Surg Engl 68:143–145

56. Senapati A, Nicholls RJ, Thomson JPS, Phillips RKS (1992) Delorme's Operation—the St Mark's Experience. pp. 57–68. In Phillips RKS, Northover JMA (eds): Modern Coloproctology. Edward Arnold, London

57. Senapati A, Nicholls RJ, Thomson JP, Phillips RK (1994) Results of Delorme's procedure for rectal prolapse. Dis Colon Rectum 37:456–460

58. Plusa SM, Charig JA, Balaji V et al (1995) Physiological changes after Delorme's procedure for full-thickness rectal prolapse. Br J Surg 82:1475–1478

59. Oliver GC, Vachon D, Eisenstat TE et al (1994). Delorme's procedure for complete rectal prolapse in severely debilitated patients. An analysis of 41 cases. Dis Colon Rectum 37:461–467

60. Tobin SA, Scott IH (1994) Delorme operation for rectal prolapse. Br J Surg 81:1681–1684

61. Miles WE (1933) Rectosigmoidectomy as a method of treatment for procedentia recti. Proc R Soc Med 26:1445–1449

62. Goligher JC, Hughes ESR (1951) Sensibility of the rectum and colon: its role in the mechanism of anal continence. Lancet 1:543–548

63. Altemeier WA, Cuthbertson WR, Schowengerdt C, Hunt J (1971) Nineteen years experience with one stage perineal repair of rectal prolapse. Ann Surg 173:993–1001

64. Madoff RD, Watts JD, Rothenberger DA, Goldberg SM (1992) Rectal prolapse: Treatment. pp. 321–346. In Henry MM, Swash M (eds): Coloproctology and the Pelvic Floor. Butterworth Heinemann, Oxford

65. Williams JG, Rothenberger DA, Madoff RD, Goldberg SM (1992) Treatment of rectal prolapse in the elderly by perineal rectosigmoidectomy. Dis Colon Rectum 35:830–834

66. Finlay IG, Aitchison M (1991) Perianal excision of the rectum for prolapse in the elderly. Br J Surg 79:687–689

67. Johansen OB, Wexner SD, Daniel N et al (1993) Perineal rectosigmoidectomy in the elderly. Dis Colon Rectum 36:767–672

68. Friedman R, Muggia-Sulam J, Freund HR (1983) Experience with the one-stage perineal repair of rectal prolapse. Dis Colon Rectum 26:789–791

69. Deen KI, Grant E, Billingham C, Keighley MRI (1994) Abdominal resection rectopexy with pelvic floor repair versus perineal rectosigmoidectomy and pelvic floor repair for full-thickness rectal prolapse. Br J Surg 81:302–304

70. Wyatt AP (1981) Perineal rectopexy for rectal prolapse. Br J Surg 68:717–719

71. Graham W, Clegg JF, Taylor V (1984) Complete rectal prolapse repair by a simple technique. Ann R Coll Surg Engl 66:87–89

72. Prasad ML, Pearl RK, Abcarian H et al (1986) Perineal proctectomy, posterior rectopexy and postanal levator repair for the treatment of rectal prolapse. Dis Colon Rectum 29:547–552

73. Wells C (1959) New operation for rectal prolapse. Proc R Soc Med 52:602–604

74. Allen Mersh TG, Turner MJ, Mann CV (1990) Effect of abdominal Ivalon rectopexy on bowel habit and rectal wall. Dis Colon Rectum 33:550–553

75. Atkinson KG, Taylor DC (1984) Wells procedure for complete rectal prolapse: a ten year experience. Dis Colon Rectum 27:96–98

76. Blatchford GJ, Perry RE, Thorson AG, Christensen MA (1989) Rectopexy without resection for rectal prolapse. Am J Surg 158:576–576

77. Boulos PB, Stryker SJ, Nicholls RJ (1984) The long term results of polyvinyl alcohol (Ivalon) sponge for rectal prolapse in young patients. Br J Surg 71:213–214

78. Carter AE (1983) Rectosacral suture fixation for complete rectal prolapse in the elderly, the frail and the demented. Br J Surg 70:522–523

79. McCue JL, Thomson JPS (1990) Rectopaxy for internal rectal intussusception. Br J Surg 77:632–634

80. McCue JL, Thompson JPS (1991) Clinical and functional results of abdominal rectopexy for complete rectal prolapse. Br J Surg 78:921–923

81. Novell JR, Osborne MJ, Winslet MC, Lewis AA (1994) Prospective randomized trial of Ivalon sponge versus sutured rectopexy for full-thickness rectal prolapse. Br J Surg 81:904–906

82. Spiroudhis L, Ropert A, Gosselin A et al (1993) Constipation after rectopexy for rectal prolapse. Where is the obstruction? Dig Dis Sci 38:1801–1808

83. Naunton Morgan C, Porter NH, Kugman DJ (1972) Ivalon (polyvinyl alcohol) sponge in the repair of complete rectal prolapse. Br J Surg 59:846–848

84. Parks AG, Swash M, Urich H (1977) Sphincter denervation in anorectal incontinence and rectal prolapse. Gut 18:656–659

85. Penfold JCB, Hawley PR (1972) Experience of Ivalon sponge implant for complete rectal prolapse at St Mark's Hospital 1960–1970. Br J Surg 59:846–848

86. Porter NH (1962) Collective results of operation for rectal prolapse. Proc R Soc Med 55:1087–1091

87. Rogers J, Jeffrey PJ (1987) Post anal repair and intersphincteric Ivalon sponge rectopexy for the treatment of rectal prolapse. Br J Surg 74:384–386

88. Ross AH, Thomson JPS (1989) Management of infection after prosthetic abdominal rectopexy (Wells' procedure). Br J Surg 76:610–612

89. Sainio AP, Voutilainen PE, Husa AI (1991) Recovery of anal sphincter function following transabdominal repair or rectal prolapse: cause of improved continence? Dis Colon Rectum 34:816–821

90. Sainio AP, Halme LE, Husa AI (1991) Anal encirclement with polypropylene mesh for rectal prolapse and incontinence. Dis Colon Rectum 34:905–908

91. Winde G, Reers B, Nottberg H et al. Clinical and functional results of abdominal rectopexy with absorbable mesh-graft for treatment of complete rectal prolapse. Eur J Surg 159:301–305

92. Keighley MRB, Fielding JWL, Alexander-Williams J (1983) Results of Marlex mesh abdominal rectopexy for rectal prolapse in 100 consecutive patients. Br J Surg 67:54–56

93. Devadhar DSC (1965) A new concept of mechanism and treatment of rectal procidentia. Dis Colon Rectum 8:75–81

94. Loygue J, Huguier M, Malafosse M, Biotois H (1971) Complete prolapse of the rectum. A report on 140 cases treated by rectopexy. Br J Surg 58:847–848

95. Ripstein CB (1972) Procidentia: definitive corrective surgery. Dis Colon Rectum 15:334–336

96. Ahlbaack S, Broden B, Broden G et al (1979) Rectal anatomy following Ripstein's operation for prolapse studied by cineradiography. Dis Colon Rectum 22:333–339

97. Gordon PH, Hoexter B (1978) Complications of the Ripstein procedure. Dis Colon Rectum 21:277–280

98. Greene FL (1983) Repair of rectal prolapse using a puborectal sling procedure. Arch Surg 118:398–401

99. Holmstrom B, Broden G, Dolk A, Frenckner B (1986) Increased anal resting pressure following the Ripstein operation: a contribution to continence? Dis Colon Rectum 29:485–487

100. Kusminsky RE, Tiley EH, Boland JP (1992) Laparoscopic Ripstein procedure. Surg Laparosc Endosc 2:346–347

101. Roberts PL, Schoetz DJ, Coller JA, Veidenheimer MC (1988) Ripstein procedure Lahey Clinic experience 1963–1985. Arch Surg 123:554–557

102. Tjandra JJ, Fazio VW, Church JM et al (1993). Ripstein procedure is an effective treatment for rectal prolapse without constipation. Dis Colon Rectum 36:501–507

103. Soliman SM (1994) Triple suspension rectopexy for complete rectal prolapse. Ann R Coll Surg Engl 76:115–116

104. Lahaut J (1956) Cure radicale des grands prolapsus du Rectum. J Chirurgie 72:565–569

105. Schlinkert RT, Beart RW, Wolf BG, Pemberton JH (1985) Anterior resection for complete rectal prolapse. Dis Colon Rectum 28:409–412

106. Frykman HM, Goldberg SM (1969) The surgical treatment of rectal procidentia. Surg Gynecol Obstet 129:1225–1230

107. Luukkonen P, Mikkonen U, Jarvinen H (1992) Abdominal rectopexy with sigmoidectomy vs. rectopexy alone for rectal prolapse: a prospective, randomized study. Int J Colorectal Dis 7:219–222

108. McKee RF, Lauder JC, Poon FW et al (1992) A prospective randomized study of abdominal rectopexy with and without sigmoidectomy in rectal prolapse. Surg Gynecol Obstet 174:145–148

109. Sayfan J, Pinho M, Alexander Williams J, Keighley B (1990) Sutured posterior abdominal rectopexy with sigmoidectomy compared with Marlex rectopexy for rectal prolapse. Br J Surg 77:143–145

110. Madoff RD, Williams JG, Wong WD (1992) Long-term functional results of colon resection and rectopexy for overt rectal prolapse. Am J Gastroenterol 87:101–104

111. Baker R, Senagore AJ, Luchtefeld MA (1995) Laparoscopic-assisted vs. open resection. Rectopexy offers excellent results. Dis Colon Rectum 38:199–201

112. Cuesta MA, Borgstein PJ, de Jong D, Meijer S (1993) Laparoscopic rectopexy. Surg Laparosc Endosc 3:456–458

113. Cuschieri A, Shimi SM, Vander Velpen G et al (1994) Laparoscopic prosthesis fixation rectopexy for complete rectal prolapse. Br J Surg 81:138–139

114. Darzi A, Henry MM, Guillou PJ et al (1995) Stapled laparoscopic rectopexy for rectal prolapse. Surg Endosc 9:301–303

115. Graf W, Stefansson T, Arvidsson D, Pahlman L (1995) Laparoscopic suture rectopexy. Dis Colon Rectum 38:211–212

116. Kwok SP, Carey DP, Lau WY, Li AK (1994) Laparoscopic rectopexy. Dis Colon Rectum 37:947–948

117. Duthie GS, Bartolo DCC (1992) Abdominal rectopexy for rectal prolapse: a comparison of techniques. Br J Surg 79:107–113

118. Madden MV, Kamm MA, Nicholls RJ et al (1992) Abdominal rectopexy for complete prolapse: prospective study evaluating changes in symptoms and anorectal function. Dis Colon Rectum 35:48–55

119. Farouk R, Duthie GS, MacGregor AB, Bartolo DC (1994) Rectoanal inhibition and incontinence in patients with rectal prolapse. Br J Surg 81:743–746

120. Farouk R, Duthie GS, Bartolo DC, MacGregor AB (1992) Restoration of continence following rectopexy for rectal prolapse and recovery of the internal anal sphincter electromyogram. Br J Surg 79:439–440

121. Setti Carraro P, Nicholls RJ (1994) Postanal repair for faecal incontinence persisting after rectopexy. Br J Surg 81:305–307

122. Huber FT, Stein H, Siewert JR (1995) Functional results after treatment of rectal prolapse with rectopexy and sigmoid resection. World J Surg 19:138–143

123. Mann CV, Hoffman C (1988) Complete rectal prolapse: the anatomical and functional results of treatment by an extended abdominal rectopexy. Br J Surg 75:34–37

124. Mathai V, Seow-Choen F (1995) Anterior rectal mucosal prolapse: an easily treated cause of anorectal symptoms. Br J Surg 82:753–754

125. Miller R, Orrom WJ, Cornes H et al (1989) Anterior sphincter plication and levatorplasty in the treatment of faecal incontinence. Br J Surg 76:1058–1060

126. Spencer RJ (1984) Manometric studies in rectal prolapse. Dis Colon Rectum 27:523–525

127. Cruveilhier J (1830) Ulcere Chronique du Rectum. Ch. 25. Maladies du Rectum. Bailliere, Paris

128. Madigan MR, Morson BC (1969) solitary ulcer of the rectum. Gut 10:871–881

129. Martin CJ, Parks TG, Biggart JD (1981) Solitary rectal ulcer syndrom in Northern Ireland 1971–1980. Br J Surg 68:744–774

130. Madigan MR (1964) solitary ulcer of the rectum. Proc R Soc Med 57:403–404

131. Haskell B, Rovner H (1965) Solitary ulcer of the rectum. Dis Colon Rectum 8:333–336

132. Hershfield NB, Langevin JE, Kelly JK (1984) Endoscopic and histological features of the solitary rectal ulcer syndrome. Gastrointest Endosc 30:162–163

133. Hoffman MJ, Kodner IJ, Fry RD (1984) Internal intussusception of the rectum. Diagnosis and surgical management. Dis Colon Rectum 27:435–441

134. Meka R, Trinkl W, Sassaris M, Hunter F (1984) Colitis cystica profunda. Curr Concepts Gastroenterol 6:18–20

135. Lewis FW, Mahoney MP, Heffernan CK (1977) The solitary ulcer syndrome of the rectum: radiological features. Br J Radiol 50:227–228

136. Thomson G, Clark A, Handyside J, Gillespie G (1981) Solitary ulcer of the rectum—or is it? Br J Surg 68:21–24

137. Alborti-Florr JJ, Halters S Dunn GD (1985) Solitary rectal

ulcer as a cause of massive lower gastrointestinal bleeding. Gastrointest Endosc 31:53–54

138. Black HC, Gardner WA, Weidner MG (1972) Localised colitis cystica profunda, a benign lesion simulating malignancy Am Surg 38:237–239

139. Delaney H, Hitch WS (1974) Solitary rectal ulcer: a cause of life threatening haemorrhage. Surgery 76:830–832

140. Epstein SE, Ascari WQ, Ablow RC et al (1960) Colitis cystica profunda. Am J Clin Pathol 45:186–201

141. Boulay CED, Fairbrother J, Isaacson PG (1983) Mucosal prolapse syndrome: a unifying concept for solitary ulcer syndrome and related disorders. J Clin Pathol 36:1264–1268

142. Levine DS (1987) Solitary rectal ulcer syndrome and localised colitis cystica profunda, analogous syndromes caused by rectal prolapse. Gastroenterology 92:243–253

143. Howard RJ, Mannax SJ, Eusebio EB et al (1971) Colitis cystica profunda. Surgery 69:306–308

144. Martin JK, Culp CE, Welland LH (1984) Colitis cystica profunda. Dis Colon Rectum 27:153–156

145. Britto E, Borges AM, Swaroop VS et al (1987) Solitary rectal ulcer: 20 cases seen in an oncology centre. Dis Colon Rectum 30:381–386

146. Mahieu PHG (1986) Barium enema defaecography in the diagnosis and evaluation of the solitary rectal ulcer syndrome. Int J Colorectal Dis 1:85–90

147. Kuijpers HC, Schreve RH, Hoedemakers H ten cate (1986) Diagnosis of functional disorders of defaecation causing the solitary ulcer syndrome. Dis Colon Rectum 29:126–129

148. Kennedy DK, Hughes ESR, Masterton JP (1977) The natural history of benign ulcer of the rectum. Surg Gynecol Obstet 144:718–720

149. Kiff ES, Barnes PRH, Swash M (1984) Evidence of pudendal neuropathy in patients with perineal descent and chronic straining at stool. Gut 25:1279–1282

150. Johansson C, Ihre TM, Ahlback SO (1985) Disturbances in the defaecation mechanism with special reference to intussusception of the rectum (internal procidentia). Dis Colon Rectum 28:920–924

151. Mackle EJ, Mills JOM, Parks TG (1990) The investigation of anorectal dysfunction in the solitary rectal ulcer syndrome. Int J Colorectal Dis 5:21–24

152. Parks AG, Porter NH, Hardcastle JD (1966) The syndrome of the descending perineum. Proc R Soc Med 59:477–482

153. Ihre T, Seligson U (1978) Intussusception of the rectum—internal procidentia—treatment and results in 90 patients. Dis Colon Rectum 18:391–396

154. Shorvon PJ, McHugh S, Diamant NE et al (1989) Defecography in normal volunteers: results and implications. Gut 30:1737–1749

155. Feczko PJ, O'Connell DJ, Riddell PH, Frank PH (1980) Solitary rectal ulcer syndrome: radiological manifestations. Am J Roentgenol 35:499–506

156. Stuart M (1984) Proctitis cystica profunda: incidence, aetiology and treatment. Dis Colon Rectum 24:153–156

157. Rutter KP, Riddell RH (1975) Solitary ulcer syndrome of the rectum. Clin Gastroenterol 4:503–530

158. Snooks SJ, Nicholls RJ, Henry MM, Swash M (1985) Electrophysiological and manometric assessment of the pelvic floor in the solitary rectal ulcer syndrome. Br J Surg 72:131–133

159. Jones PN, Lubowski DZ, Henry MM, Swash M (1987) Is paradoxical contraction of puborectalis muscle of functional importance? Dis Colon Rectum 30:667–670

160. Womack NR, Williams NS, Holmfield JHM, Morrison JFB (1987) Anorectal function in the solitary rectal ulcer syndrome. Dis Colon Rectum 30:319–323

161. Womack NR, Williams NS, Holmfield JHM, Morrison JFB (1987) Pressure and prolapse—the cause of solitary rectal ulceration. Gut 28:1228–1233

162. Kang YS, Kamm MA, Nicholls RJ (1995) Solitary rectal ulcer and complete rectal prolapse: one condition or two? Int J Colorectal Dis 10:87–90

163. Schweiger M, Williams JA (1977) solitary ulcer syndrome of the rectum: its association with occult rectal prolapse. Lancet 1:170–171

164. Berman IR, Harris MS, Leggett JT (1987) Rectal reservoir reduction procedures for internal rectal prolapse. Dis Colon Rectum 30:765–771

165. Christiansen J, Zhu B-W, Rasmussen OO, Sorensen M (1992) Internal rectal intussusception: results of surgical repair. Dis Colon Rectum 35:1026–1029

166. Jalan KN, Brunt PW, Maclean N et al (1970) Benign solitary ulcer of the rectum: a report of 5 cases. Scand J Gastroenterol 5:143–147

167. White CM, Findlay JM, Price JJ (1980) The occult rectal prolapse syndrome. Br J Surg 67:528–530

168. Brant-Gradel V, Huibregtse K, Tytgat GNJ (1984) Treatment of solitary rectal ulcer syndrome with high fibre diet and abstention of straining at defaecation. Dig Dis Sci 29:1005–1008

169. Tjandra JJ, Fazio VW, Church JM et al (1992) Clinical conundrum of solitary rectal ulcer. Dis Colon Rectum 35:227–234

170. Zargar SA, Khuroo MS, Mahajan R (1991) Sucralfate retention enemas in solitary rectal ulcer. Dis Colon Rectum 34:455–457

171. Ford MJ, Anderson JR, Gilmour HM et al (1983) Clinical spectrum of solitary ulcer of the rectum. Gastroenterology 84:1533–1540

172. van Tets WF, Kuijpers JH (1995) Internal rectal intussusception—fact or fancy?. Dis Colon Rectum 38:1080–1083

173. Yoshioka K, Keighley MRB (1987) Anorectal myectomy for outlet obstruction. Br J Surg 74:373–376

174. Saul SH, Sollenberger LC (1985) Solitary rectal ulcer syndrome: its clinical and pathological underdiagnosis. Am J Surg Pathol 9:411–412

175. Pescatori M, Marta G, Mattana C et al (1985) Clinical picture and pelvic floor physiology in the solitary rectal ulcer syndrome. Dis Colon Rectum 28:862–867

176. Guy PJ, Ham M (1988) Colitis cystic profunda of the rectum treatment by mucosal sleeve resection and coloanal pull through. Br J Surg 75:289

177. Orrom WJ, Bartolo DC, Miller R et al (1991) Rectopexy is an ineffective treatment for obstructed defecation. Dis Colon Rectum 34:41–46

178. Nicholls RJ, Simson J (1986) Anteroposterior rectopexy in the treatment of solitary rectal ulcer syndrome without overt rectal prolapse. Br J Surg 73:222–224

179. Halligan S, Nicholls RJ, Bartram CI (1995) Proctographic changes after rectopexy for solitary rectal ulcer syndrome and preoperative predictive factors for a successful outcome. Br J Surg 82:314–317

180. Sitzler P, Kamm MA, Nicholls RJ (1996) Surgery for solitary ulcer syndrome. Int J Colorectal Dis 11:136

181. Yoshioka K, Matsui Y, Yamada O et al (1991) Physiologic and anatomic assessment of patients with rectocele. Dis Colon Rectum 34:704–708

182. Bartram CI, Turnbull GK, Lennard-Jones JE (1988) Evacuation proctography: an investigation of rectal expulsion in 20 subjects without defecatory disturbance. Gastrointest Radiol 13:72–80

183. Siproudhis L, Ropert A, Lucas J et al (1992) Defecatory disorders, anorectal and pelvic floor dysfunction: a polygamy? Radiologic and manometric studies in 41 patients. Int J Colorect Dis 7:102–107

184. Mellgren A, Bremmer S, Johansson C et al (1994) Defecography: results of investigations in 2816 patients. Dis Colon Rectum 37:1133–1141

185. Delamarre JBVM, Kruyt RH, Doornbos J et al (1994) Anterior rectocele: assessment with radiographic defecography, dynamic MRI and physical examination. Dis Colon Rectum 37:249–259

186. Karlbom U, Pahlman L, Nilsson S, Graf W (1995) Relationships between defecographic findings, rectal emptying and colonic transit time in constipated patients. Gut 36:907–912

187. Janssen LWM, van Dijke CF (1994) Selection criteria for anterior rectal wall repair in symptomatic rectocele and anterior rectal wall prolapse. Dis Colon Rectum 37:1100–1107

188. Arnold MW, Stewart WR, Aguilar PS (1990) Rectocele repair: four years experience. Dis Colon Rectum 33:684–687

189. Sarles JC, Arnaud A, Selezneff I, Oliver S (1989) Endorectal repair of rectocele. Int J Colorect Dis 4:167–171

190. Parker MC, Phillips PRKS (1993) Repair of rectocele using Marlex mesh. Ann R Coll Surg Engl 75:193–194

191. Gopal KA, Amshel AL, Shonberg IL et al (1984) Rectal prolapse in the elderly and debilitated patients: experience with the Altmeier procedure. Dis Colon Rectum 27:376–381

192. Watts JD, Rothenberger DA, Buls JG et al (1985) The management of procidentia: 30 years' experience. Dis Colon Rectum 28:96–102

193. Kuijpers HC, Moree H de (1988) Towards a selection of the most appropriate procedure in the treatment of complete rectal prolapse. Dis Colon Rectum 31:355–357

194. Launer DP, Fazio, Weakley FL et al (1982) The Ripstein procedure: a sixteen year experience. Dis Colon Rectum 25:41–45

195. Schapayak S (1985) Transrectal repair of rectocele—an extended armamentarium of colorectal surgeons: a report of 355 cases. Dis Colon Rectum 28:422–433

196. Khubchandani IT, Sheets JA, Stasik JJ, Hakki AR (1983) Endorectal repair of rectocoele. Dis Colon Rectum 26:792–796

197. Block IR (1986) Transrectal repair of rectocoele using obliterative suture. Dis Colon Rectum 29:707–711

40

INCONTINENCE

David A. Rothenberger
Kemal I. Deen

Anal incontinence is distressing and socially incapacitating. It is associated with reduced personal hygiene and frequently leads to social isolation and loss of self-esteem.[1–4] The condition is often taboo. Consequently, its true prevalence remains largely unknown. Studies have shown that individuals may not be forthcoming with symptoms of incontinence when questioned directly.[5] However, if questions are interspersed among an array of other questions on one's general health, a greater number of individuals admit to symptoms of anal incontinence.[6] The spectrum of symptoms ranges from occasional incontinence of gas to minor fecal soiling to frank leakage of feces. The pathophysiology underlying these manifestations is often multifactorial. This complexity partly explains the relatively slow progress achieved in fully understanding the nature of incontinence and in tailoring an effective treatment in the majority of patients.

In this chapter we discuss the prevalence, etiology, and pathophysiology of this condition with emphasis on recent clinical and basic scientific findings that have helped to better understand anal incontinence. Clinical and laboratory evaluations of the incontinent patient are described together with a variety of treatment modalities, including neoanal sphincters.

PREVALENCE OF FECAL INCONTINENCE

Based on questionnaire surveys, the prevalence of fecal incontinence in the general population has been reported to be as high as 7%.[7] A recent study using telephone interviews of 2,570 households comprising 6,959 individuals revealed anal incontinence in 2.2% of the general population.[8] Of those reporting incontinence, 36% were incontinent to solid stool, 54% to liquid feces, and 60% to flatus. Incontinence occurred more than once per week in 10%, restricted normal activities in 33%, required protective undergarments in 18%, and led to consultation with a physician in 36%. Independent risk factors for incontinence

included female gender, advancing age, poor general health, and physical limitations.

Thirty percent of the incontinent subjects were older than 65 years of age.[8] Incontinence is particularly common in elderly institutionalized individuals where constipation and overflow incontinence may also play a significant role. Thirty-nine percent of Wisconsin nursing home residents have fecal incontinence.[9]

Sixty-three percent of incontinent subjects in the study by Nelson et al.[8] were women. Vaginal delivery may result in anal sphincter damage and pelvic floor failure, resulting in lack of bowel control. A recent prospective study from the United Kingdom has indicated that between 4% and 6% of women who have vaginal deliveries will suffer from fecal incontinence.[10] Incontinence may also occur in men. The most common reported symptom in men is soiling without an underlying anorectal physiologic abnormality.[11]

In women, fecal incontinence often coexists with urinary incontinence and may signify pudendal nerve damage. Gee and Durdey[12] have indicated that the presence of stress incontinence of urine in women is a reliable clinical marker of pudendal nerve damage. Longer term follow-up is required to assess the incidence of fecal incontinence in these patients.

ETIOLOGY AND PATHOLOGY

Continence to gas and stool is the product of a complex interaction of central nervous system activity and that of the gastrointestinal tract, the pelvic floor, and the anal sphincter complex. Maintenance of continence is usually subconscious and involuntary, but voluntary control of the pelvic floor and anal sphincters becomes important if an individual has diarrhea or if the passage of bowel content is socially inconvenient. Continence may be altered either by generalized disorders (e.g., diabetes mellitus, which also affects other organ systems), or by local factors that damage the anal sphincter complex (e.g., obstetric trauma). This section reviews some of the disorders that may influence this physiologic pathway, which results in incontinence.

Cerebral and Psychological Factors

The function of the voluntary component of the anal sphincters and pelvic floor may be influenced by central nervous system activity.[13] In some individuals who experience fecal soiling and incontinence during sleep, combined synchronous electromyography and anal manometry have shown that the diminution of higher center electrical activity typical of sleep is associated with a corresponding reduction in the activity of the entire gut and the external anal sphincter.[14,15]

Cann et al.[16] reported a 25% incidence of incontinence in patients with irritable bowel syndrome chiefly due to intestinal overactivity. These patients were also found to have a weak anal sphincter, as evidenced by low anal squeeze pressures.

Psychological factors may play a role in incontinence and the resolution of symptoms with treatment. Incontinent patients who are lacking in motivation and are either anxious or depressed often have a poor result after treatment compared with well-motivated, psychologically stable individuals.[17] The unpredictable success of biofeedback therapy in patients with incontinence, often in those with a demonstrable neurophysiologic deficit of the anal sphincters, suggests that other unquantifiable factors may play a role in treatment.[18]

Hormonal factors may play a role. Kamm et al.[19] have shown that high estrogen levels may explain why some women may be more prone to have slow transit constipation. Hormonal imbalances may adversely affect bowel control in women with no obvious structural abnormality.[20] Obesity has been shown to reliably predict a poor result from surgery for fecal incontinence.[21]

Defects of Neurotransmission

Continence is threatened during periods of increased intra-abdominal pressure such as during coughing and sneezing. Reflex contractions of the external sphincter and the pelvic floor muscles, which are mediated at a spinal cord level and not the higher centers, prevent incontinence.[22] In patients with an upper motor neuron lesion, such as complete transection of the spinal cord, incontinence is rarely a problem unless there is soiling around a fecal bolus.[23] By contrast, in those with a lower motor neuron lesion (cauda equina, sacral spinal roots, pudendal nerve) the external sphincter and pelvic floor muscles are paralyzed. Continence is dependent solely on the internal anal sphincter, which may be insufficient to prevent involuntary defecation.[24,25]

Disorders of the Colon, Rectum, and Anus

Congenital Disorders

Anorectal malformations occur in approximately 1 in 5,000 live births.[26] These may range from imperforate anus to rectal agenesis. Incontinence may result from malposition of the anorectum and may persist despite surgical correction.

Inflammatory Disorders

Inflammatory disorders of the colon and rectum (e.g., ulcerative colitis, Crohn's colitis, or infectious colitis) cause rapid colonic transit and incontinence in patients with a weakened anal sphincter. Symptoms may range from frequency and urgency to frank incontinence. Anal fistulae, which may develop as a result of Crohn's disease or more commonly from cryptoglandular infection of the anal canal, may cause incontinence if the fistula tract bypasses the anal sphincter.[27]

Metabolic Disorders

Disorders such as diabetes mellitus may affect continence in a number of ways. Autonomic neuropathy may lead to deranged colorectal motility and transit, leading to diarrhea and incontinence. Pudendal neuropathy may be part of a generalized peripheral neuropathy associated with diabetes and other metabolic conditions, which leads to a weak anal sphincter.[28]

Neoplastic Disorders

Benign and malignant neoplasms of the anorectum may impair continence. A villous adenoma of the rectum may produce copious volumes of mucus resulting in soiling. By causing partial obstruction to the lumen, a rectal neoplasm may lead to overflow incontinence. A rectal or anal cancer can directly invade and damage the anal sphincter, or it can invade the rectovaginal septum, producing a fistula. Incontinence results from either situation.

Degenerative Disorders

Incontinence of feces is particularly distressing in the elderly and infirm. In geriatric patients, the combination of cerebral degeneration and impaired rectal sensation often causes incontinence, especially in the presence of a weak anal sphincter.[29,30]

Disorders of the Anal Sphincter and Pelvic Floor Musculature

The anal canal closure mechanism is complex. An acute anorectal angle is created by the forward pull of the slinglike puborectalis muscle, which has been thought by some to create a flap valve[31] and by others, a flutter valve[32] to maintain continence. It is now known that an obtuse anorectal angle is compatible with continence,[33,34] and the importance of the anorectal angle is unclear. By contrast, disruption of the external anal sphincter usually leads to episodes of urgency and urge incontinence.[35,36] If sphincter disruption is associated with denervation, as in some women after prolonged straining during labor or with chronic constipation, frank incontinence may result.[37] Defects of the internal anal sphincter may lead to incontinence independent of external anal sphincter damage.[38] Symptoms of internal sphincter damage are chiefly fecal soiling, particularly during sleep, when external anal sphincter activity is reduced. Although some authors have implied that the internal anal sphincter plays little or no role in continence, our own data assessing patients after lateral internal sphincterotomy for anal fissure prove otherwise. Approximately 38% of patients with an internal sphincter defect following sphincterotomy have reported alterations in continence.[39]

There is evidence that the hemorrhoidal cushions play a significant role in complete closure of the anal canal. Data from magnetic resonance images of the anal canal have shown that complete closure of the anal canal may only be achieved by the combined action of the anal sphincters with the anal cushions.[40] Hemorrhoidectomy can produce deficiencies of the anal cushions that may result in impairment of continence.

Obstetric Incontinence

The most common cause of sphincter disruption is obstetric injury.[35] Studies have shown that vaginal delivery but not cesarean section may result in disruption of the anal sphincter muscles, pudendal neuropathy, or both.[41] Disruption of the anal sphincters has been attributed to episiotomy, perineal laceration, and forceps extraction.[42,43] A prospective study of 150 women in whom the anal sphincters were imaged by anal ultrasound before and after vaginal delivery revealed anal sphincter disruption in 35%.[42] A proportion of these defects were occult. The same authors showed that women with external anal sphincter defects, presumably from previous obstetric trauma, were at a greater risk of incontinence from surgical procedures, such as lateral internal sphincterotomy.[44]

External Sphincter Defects

It appears that episiotomy may be directly related to the site of external anal sphincter disruption. In a study of women having posterolateral episiotomy in the United Kingdom, the site of anal sphincter disruption was in the anterolateral part of the sphincter complex.[45] In a similar study of women in the United States where a posterior midline episiotomy was routinely performed, the corresponding external sphincter defect was in the anterior midline.[46] Although a perineal laceration that extends to anal canal mucosa causes disruption of the anal sphincters, it is unlikely that episiotomy itself should directly damage the anal sphincter. It is possible that an episiotomy is performed such that the external sphincter muscle is cut without the obstetrician being aware of the extent of damage. An alternative explanation would be that rupture of the anal sphincters during vaginal delivery, irrespective of the cause, occurs in the line of least resistance: the site of episiotomy. The optimal site of episiotomy, therefore, remains unresolved.

Furthermore, it is unclear if episiotomy protects a woman from sustaining a third-degree tear. It has been estimated that up to 2% of all women having vaginal delivery will have a third-degree tear.[47] Of these, 85% will have an underlying anal sphincter defect compared with 33% without a tear. In a study of 8,553 women having vaginal delivery, Sultan et al.[47] found forceps-assisted delivery, primiparous delivery, occipitoposterior position, and birth weight greater than 4 kg to be risk factors associated with development of a third-degree tear.

Internal Sphincter Defects

Internal sphincter defects have been documented after obstetric injury. These defects may be isolated or more commonly associated with an external anal sphincter defect.[48] The majority of these defects are anterior, but some isolated posterior defects have also been recorded in women with no previous history of surgical intervention or anal sphincter damage.[38,49] It has been postulated that ischemia may play a role in posterior internal sphincter damage during periods of elevated intrapelvic pressure, as in the second stage of labor.

Disruption of the Perineal Body

Endosonographic studies of the anal sphincter in women with fecal incontinence have indicated that external sphincter defects are located chiefly at the level of the midpart of the anal canal, which corresponds to the superficial portion of the external sphincter.[45] A mid–anal canal sphincter defect may be found in association with an intact subcutaneous component of the external sphincter. Several theories may account for this appearance. First, it is possible that only a partial repair of the ruptured external anal sphincter was performed during primary repair of the episiotomy. This would have left a residual "tear drop" deformity of the anterior part of the sphincter.[50] It is also possible that rupture of the perineal body during traumatic childbirth may have resulted in damage to the superficial portion of the external sphincter, because contributory fibers from the external sphincter forming the perineal body arise chiefly from the superficial part, and not the subcutaneous part of the sphincter. The practical implication in sphincter repair after obstetric trauma is that it is essential to completely expose the entire length of the anal sphincter from the subcutaneous part to the level of the anterior levators to avoid missing an occult defect.

Rectovaginal Fistula with Incontinence

Rectovaginal fistula may coexist with anal sphincter damage in patients with obstetric trauma. It is thought to result from ischemic damage to the rectovaginal septum from pressure of the head of the fetus or from rupture of the perineal body during vaginal delivery (Fig. 40-1). It is essential to identify anterior anal sphincter disruption in these patients because repair of the fistula must be performed with concomitant anal sphincteroplasty to restore continence.[51,52]

Pudendal Neuropathy

The pudendal nerve (S-2,3,4) is a mixed nerve whose first branch, the inferior rectal nerve, traverses the fibro-osseous canal of Alcock in the side wall of the ischiopubic ramus to reach the external anal sphincter. Distal branches of the pudendal nerve include the superficial perineal nerve (sensory to genitalia, perineal region, and anal canal mucosa) and the deep perineal nerve, which supplies the transverse perineal muscles and sphincter urethra before continuing as the dorsal nerve of the penis or clitoris. Studies have shown that the external sphincter has a dual cross-over innervation.[24] In the majority of individuals, it has also been shown that the puborectalis muscle and the rest of the pelvic floor musculature is supplied directly by nerve roots from S3 and S4, not by the pudendal nerve.[24]

Electrophysiologic studies have suggested that the pudendal nerve may be damaged during the course of prolonged vaginal delivery, especially in the second stage. The result is a prolonged pudendal nerve latency (greater than 2.4 m sec).[53] This

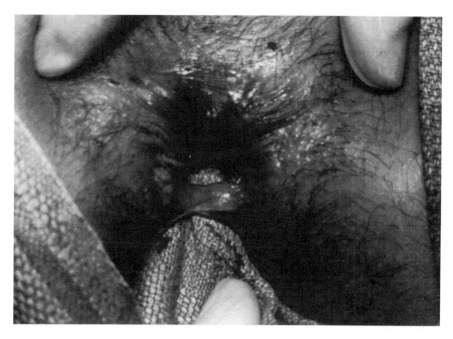

Figure 40-1. This woman had sustained a fourth degree tear during childbirth. The injury was recognized and repaired but did not heal successfully. The resulting defect in the anterior sphincter and the associated rectovaginal fistula are clearly demonstrated in this photograph. The patient is in the prone jackknife position just prior to a secondary repair.

injury has been shown to be reversible in 60% of women 3 months after vaginal delivery.[54] However, if pudendal neuropathy becomes established, studies have shown that nerve damage can be progressive.[55]

The injury to the pudendal nerve may be either unilateral or bilateral. The majority of women have unilateral damage and may not suffer from serious incontinence symptoms if the contralateral nerve trunk is intact and there is cross-over innervation.

It has been postulated that the nerve trunk undergoes demyelination consequent to stretching, although the exact site of nerve damage remains unclear. Some have postulated that edema and compression of the nerve during its intracanalicular course may be the chief cause of neuropraxia and permanent nerve injury.[54] If the latter were considered the only possibility, it would be difficult to explain how the puborectalis muscle, which derives its nerve supply from spinal nerve roots, becomes denervated. This would, therefore, seem to indicate that the site of nerve injury is proximal to the ischial spine and pudendal canal. However, studies of nerve conduction following spinal stimulation have shown apparently normal latencies of the nerve trunk proximal to the level of ischial spine.[56] Certainly the evidence is not unequivocal, and it is likely that a combination of stretch injury to the nerve trunk and compression injury within the pudendal canal coexist. Refinements in methodology, such as evoked potentials using magnetic electrodes and spinal nerve stimulation, may help resolve these uncertainties.

Autonomic Neuropathy

The internal anal sphincter receives an extrinsic sympathetic and parasympathetic as well as an intrinsic innervation in which the mediator substance has been shown to be nitric oxide.[57–59]

In vitro studies of strips of internal sphincter muscle have shown reduced sensitivity to noradrenaline under controlled conditions in patients with neuropathic fecal incontinence which suggests sympathetic denervation.[60] Based on these data, it has been suggested that the sympathetic nerves become stretched in a manner similar to that of the pudendal nerve during vaginal delivery.[60]

Diminished Anal Sensation

In a prospective study of women having vaginal delivery, Cornes et al.[61] have shown that there is a significant reduction in anal canal sensation after vaginal delivery, which may be transient. This may be due to pudendal nerve injury, rectal mucosal prolapse, or both. In the short term, there may be fecal soiling, but in the longer term, progressive mucosal prolapse may lead to impairment of evacuation and consequently constipation straining with further damage to the pudendal nerves.

Rectal Prolapse

Rectal prolapse is associated with incontinence in about 50% of patients.[62] It is essential to differentiate true incontinence of gas and stool from mucus leakage due to the prolapse itself, which may necessitate wearing of a pad. Several factors may be responsible for incontinence in these patients. Progressive and prolonged stretching of the external anal sphincter by the prolapse has been implicated in incontinence.[63] Studies have shown that some patients with prolapse also have gross perineal descent, which may result in pudendal neuropathy and consequently denervation of the anal sphincter.[64] Some patients with rectal prolapse, particularly women, have occult external sphincter defects, as demonstrated by anal ultrasound.[65] Furthermore, internal anal sphincter dysfunction may also lead to incontinence and soiling. Some have suggested that dilatation of the rectum by the prolapse itself causes reversible inhibition of the rectoanal inhibitory reflex.[66]

Aging

Fecal incontinence is particularly distressing in the elderly.[67,68] In geriatric patients, a combination of cerebral degeneration and impaired rectal sensation may lead to retention of feces with subsequent soiling, especially in the presence of a weak anal sphincter. Age-related degeneration of anal sphincter musculature is a well-known phenomenon. Several studies have shown a significant reduction in anal canal pressures in patients over the age of 60 years.[69,70] Swash et al.[71] have shown that with progressive age there is an increase in fibrosis in the anal sphincter. Laurbberg and Swash[72] have also shown an increase in pudendal nerve latency measurement in older patients with a corresponding increase in the fiber density of the external anal sphincter, confirming anal sphincter reinnervation. Internal anal sphincter tone is also reduced with increasing age chiefly due to diminished autonomic function. Furthermore, it has been documented that with increasing age there is an increase in fibrous tissue content in the internal sphincter, which alters its viscoelastic properties.[73] This explains the increasing thickness of the internal sphincter muscle in the elderly demonstrated by anal ultrasound.

Radiation

Radiation causes endarteritis, which results in diminished end organ nutrition and subsequently atrophy and fibrosis.[74] In large doses, radiation may induce necrosis. Anal incontinence after irradiation was recognized as a problem initially following treatment of women with cervical cancer using local irradiation. Similar techniques of local or endocavitary irradiation are now being employed in the treatment of anal and rectal cancers. Kollmorgen et al.[75] retrospectively assessed the long-term effect of postoperative chemoradiotherapy on bowel function in 41 patients who had undergone anterior resection for an Astler-Coller Stage B2 or C rectal cancer 2 to 5 years previously. Their postoperative anal function was compared with that of 59 patients who had undergone anterior resection for an Astler-Coller Stage A or B1 rectal cancer without any chemoradiotherapy. The group that had chemoradiotherapy had more bowel movements per day (median, 7 vs. 2), more clustering of bowel movements (42 vs. 3%), more nocturnal bowel movements (46 vs. 14%), more occasional or frequent episodes of incontinence (39% and 17 vs. 7 and 0%), more need to wear a pad (41 vs. 10%), more inability to defer defecation for more than 15 minutes (78 vs. 19%), more liquid stools, more use of antidiarrheal medications, more perianal skin irritation, more inability to distinguish stool from gas, and more need to repeat defecation within 30 minutes of a bowel movement.

Today, pelvic irradiation is often followed by sphincter-saving resection of the rectum. Whether preoperative adjuvant chemoradiation will have the same ill effects noted by Kollmorgen et al.[75] is open to study. The nature of anal sphincter damage and subsequent function require careful evaluation in these pa-

tients, as poor sphincter function and the risk of incontinence may preclude a sphincter-saving operation.

Trauma

Accidental trauma to the anal sphincter complex usually occurs after penetrating trauma, especially impalement injuries (Fig. 40-2). Manifestations may range from a subcutaneous hematoma in the region of the anal sphincters to a visible perianal laceration with complete anal sphincter disruption. Disruption of the anal sphincter is usually repaired as a primary procedure. A delayed repair may be necessary in the presence of gross contamination of the wound and other life-threatening injuries. Anal endosonography to map the anal sphincters after resolution of a perineal hematoma may be helpful, but misinterpretation of sphincter anatomy is possible because hematoma alone may cause a hypoechoic shadow.

In the male patient, impalement injury often causes concomitant rupture of the bulbar urethra, which may detract attention from proper assessment of the anal sphincters. Evaluation of a patient with perineal impalement injuries should include careful examination of the anal sphincter, urethra, and prostate. Occasionally, a degloving injury or crush injury of the pelvis and perineum from blunt trauma results in partial or total loss of the anal sphincter. Multiple surgical procedures to debride perineal wounds and care for other injuries may lead to iatrogenic anal sphincter damage and fecal incontinence. It is essential to fully understand the sphincter anatomy to avoid further injury to the sphincter complex.

Figure 40-2. This young woman was impaled on a boat dock during a water-skiing accident. Complete sphincter disruption resulted. Primary sphincter repair was done with restoration of near normal continence. The patient is in the prone jackknife position. (Photograph courtesy of Alan Times, M.D.)

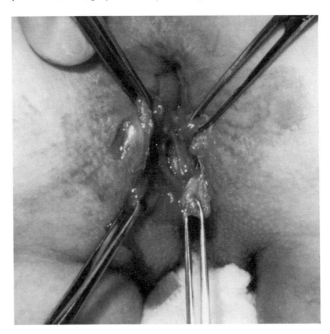

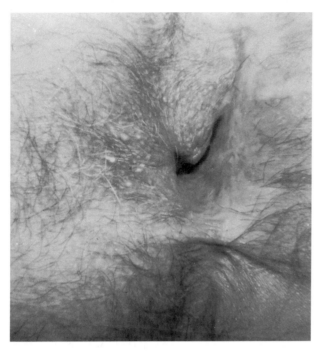

Figure 40-3.   Anal incontinence resulted from a posterolateral fistula operation. Sphincter repair was necessary to restore continence.

Iatrogenic injury can result in incontinence (Fig. 40-3. Table 40-1 lists operations that may result in partial or complete fecal incontinence.

EVALUATION OF INCONTINENCE

Clinical evaluation of the incontinent patient requires a careful history and examination that should determine the need for further evaluation by anorectal physiologic assessment and anal ultrasound. The ultimate goal is to determine the nature of incontinence (i.e., whether true or pseudo incontinence is present),

the degree of impairment, and finally the requirement for operative correction.

History

A clinical history is subjective, and patients may often be inconsistent in reporting symptoms chiefly because the meaning of terms such as soiling, leakage, frequency of stooling, and loss of control for feces varies. Hence, an objective assessment of incontinence is ideal. No perfect system exists, but our practice is to use a modified continence scale based on a continence score chart devised by Miller et al.[76] (Table 40-2). A patient with a score of 12 or greater is considered a potential candidate for operative correction. More recently we have used diaries that patients must maintain over a 7-day period in order to arrive at an incontinence score. Several authors have described a variety of incontinence scores based on similar questions.[77,78] Although none of these scales has proven to be unequivocally superior to the other, it is essential that assessment should incorporate an objective scale of evaluation to aid the surgeon in the choice of optimum treatment.

Physical Examination

General examination is performed to assess underlying systemic illnesses that may contribute to incontinence. The physical examination must include a neurologic assessment to exclude anal sphincter denervation.

Local examination involves inspection of the perineum and anal canal, including when possible a discreet inspection of the patient's underclothes. The presence of perianal soiling and the requirement for a protective pad is indicative of troublesome symptoms. On parting the buttocks, a patulous anus, indicative of loss of resting anal tone, may suggest internal anal sphincter injury or an occult rectal prolapse with neuropathy. The presence of scarring in the perianal area may suggest previous surgery or anal sphincter injury. Vaginal leakage of feces should alert the physician to the presence of an associated rectovaginal

Table 40-1.   Surgical Causes of Incontinence

Surgical Procedures	Mechanism of Sphincter Injury	Functional Deficit
Manual dilatation of anus	Damage to external and internal sphincters at multiple sites	Soiling to gross incontinence
Lateral internal sphincterotomy	Partial division of internal sphincter with intact external sphincter	Gas incontinence and soiling
	Partial division of internal sphincter with prior occult external sphincter injury	Urgency and incontinence
	Inadvertent division of external sphincter	Urgency and incontinence
Hemorrhoidectomy	Removal of anal cushions	Soiling and gas incontinence
	Internal sphincter damage	
Anal fistulectomy	Likelihood of damage to external sphincter	Urgency and incontinence
	Division of internal sphincter	Soiling and gas incontinence
Restorative ileoanal or coloanal procedures	Excision of proximal internal sphincter	Imperfect continence
	Dilatation of internal sphincter	
	Possibility of stapling injury to external sphincter	
Anal mucosal stripping	Damage to underlying internal sphincter	Soiling and nocturnal incontinence

Table 40-2. Incontinence Scoring System[a]

Frequency	Incontinence of Gas	Incontinence of Liquid	Incontinence of Solid	Significantly Alters Lifestyle
<1/month	1	4	7	10
>1/month but <1/week	2	5	8	11
>1/week	3	6	9	12

[a] The patient's "incontinence score" is determined by adding points from the above grid.
(From Miller et al.,[76] with permission.)

fistula. The perianal skin should be inspected for an external fistula-in-ano opening. The patient is then requested to squeeze the anal sphincter. During a voluntary squeeze one should observe complete and symmetric closure of the anal canal. Asymmetric closure of the anal sphincter ring indicates either unilateral sphincter injury or bilateral injury of unequal proportion. Perineal descent may be assessed by placing a finger on each of the ischial tuberosities while the patient strains. Gross perineal descent is indicated by descent below the level of the ischial tuberosities.

During palpation, the loss of touch sensation in the perianal area may suggest denervation injury, although extensive surgery and scarring may also be associated with sensory loss. The anal cutaneous or "wink" reflex may be assessed by observing anal sphincter contractility following stroking of the perianal skin. Loss of this reflex is suggestive of pudendal nerve injury.[79] Digital assessment of the anal canal is then performed to assess anal sphincter tone at rest and during maximum voluntary contraction. The anal sphincter is palpated along its entire length and circumference to detect a gap that is indicative of a sphincter defect. The absence of a palpable gap, however, does not exclude a sphincter defect because scar tissue may bridge a small defect. It is possible to assess the anorectal angle by curving the examining finger over the puborectalis sling at the posterior anorectal junction. By asking the patient to contract the sphincter, the examiner can assess the degree of pelvic floor mobility and "lift." Finally, bimanual assessment of the rectovaginal septum with a finger in the vagina and another in the anal canal may provide the examiner with an estimate of the thickness and integrity of this structure. Disruption of the anterior anal sphincter following obstetric injury usually involves the perineal body and the rectovaginal septum. By asking the patient to strain during the bimanual examination, the examiner may detect internal intussusception, rectocele, cystocele, or enterocele.

The anorectum is usually empty of stool. The presence of a fecal bolus during palpation of the rectal wall should alert the examiner to the possibility of overflow incontinence that is usually seen in elderly patients or in individuals with a megarectum. The underlying physiologic abnormality has been attributed to diminished sensation within the rectum and decreased response of the receptors within the pelvic floor to stretch stimuli.

Anoscopy and proctoscopy are then performed to assess the lumen and mucosa to exclude such conditions as proctitis or neoplasms. Most patients with incontinence will be observed to possess some degree of anorectal mucosal prolapse. Prolapse of the rectum, vagina, small bowel, or bladder may be detected by examining the perineum as the patient squats or strains.

In some patients it may be essential to evaluate the proximal colon with fiberoptic endoscopy and/or a barium enema. This decision should be based on features such as the presence of abdominal pain, the possibility of neoplasm, and the need to exclude proximal colitis.

Anorectal Physiology

Based on clinical findings, patients are referred for anorectal physiologic assessment for two main reasons. First, patients who are not considered subjects for operative repair may be assessed by physiologic studies to obtain baseline information that may direct nonoperative treatment or that may be helpful in serial follow-up. Secondly, for those who are candidates for surgery, anorectal physiology is useful to determine the extent of anal sphincter damage and to identify pudendal neuropathy and other related conditions, such as procidentia.

Several patterns of anal sphincter damage may be deduced from studies of anorectal physiology:

1. Anal sphincter disruption, which may be isolated to either the external sphincter or the internal sphincter, or may involve both muscles.
2. Nerve damage, which may be either unilateral or bilateral, complete or partial.
3. Combined anal sphincter disruption with prolonged pudendal nerve terminal motor latency.
4. Disorders of rectal or anal sensation, which may be isolated or found in association with any of the above injuries.
5. No detectable anorectal physiologic abnormality.

NONOPERATIVE MANAGEMENT

Nonoperative management should be offered to patients with minor incontinence such as occasional loss of control for gas and stool (i.e. incontinence score less than 12) (see Table 40-2). For those with no morphologic or physiologic abnormality, conservative treatment may be all that can be offered. Those patients with minor incontinence and underlying anorectal physiologic abnormalities or anatomic defects should also be treated initially with nonoperative means because success in relieving symptoms is often achieved.

Nonoperative management may consist of a bowel management program, biofeedback therapy, electrical stimulation, or a combination of these modalities. Treatment should be tailored to suit the individual.

Patient Education

Patient education and motivation are key factors in influencing the outcome of treatment. The direction and expertise of an interested clinician combined with consultation from a dietitian and a biofeedback therapist have been shown to be optimal.[80] Conservative management of fecal incontinence is time consuming, and much of this involves one-on-one sessions with the patient and technician or dietitian or both. To the patient, such nonoperative treatment may appear useless because the results are not dramatic. It is essential, therefore, that the physician discusses the disorder with the patient in a simple but meaningful way and outlines a plan of management from the outset. Realistic goals should be set that may require re-evaluation at frequent intervals. Ultimately, a well-motivated patient who understands the rationale for treatment is key to the likelihood of success. Patients should be warned against excessive straining at defecation, which is likely to further damage the pudendal nerves. Perianal hygiene should be attended to, chiefly to avoid pruritus. Absorbent cotton balls, adult diapers, and tampons should be used selectively. The goals are to improve the patient's ability to live with incontinence while slowly improving the patient's ability to maintain more normal continence.

Diet

Foods that induce loose stool and increase gastrointestinal transit (i.e., milk and milk products, prunes, and other fresh fruits) should be reduced or avoided. Foods that increase gas production (i.e., legumes) may need to be reduced or avoided. Fiber supplements are often helpful in improving stool bulk and sphincter control. However, excess fiber may be acted on by colonic microorganisms to cause gaseous distension and embarrassing passage of gas. Dietary advice may be enhanced by recruiting the help of a qualified dietitian.

Medication

Medications such as loperamide hydrochloride or diphenoxylate hydrochloride have been shown to increase internal anal sphincter response and are particularly useful in those with soiling.[81] In patients with loose stool, firming agents may also be helpful. Although prokinetic agents such as cisapride have been shown to be effective in the management of irritable bowel of upper gastrointestinal origin, these agents have not proven useful in colonic involvement by irritable bowel syndrome. A recent study demonstrated an increase in resting pressure by 10% or more in patients with spinal cord injury on cisapride.[82] Suppositories and enemas may also be used judiciously with variable frequency to ensure an empty rectum and thus reduce the stool load on the sphincter complex. In some patients where postevacuation soiling is a particular problem, the use of an irrigating water enema to cleanse the rectum is particularly helpful. Finally, diarrheal disorders must be fully investigated prior to appropriate therapy.

Biofeedback Therapy

Biofeedback therapy is becoming increasingly popular in the conservative management of fecal incontinence. During therapy, the patient is expected to learn to reproduce a normal sphincter contraction. The exact mechanism of success may not be clear in each individual. Data from this institution have shown that patients with prolonged pudendal nerve latencies have improved continence following a course of biofeedback therapy, although this was not mirrored by improvement in latency measurements.[18] It is possible that in some individuals regaining anal sphincter control is a learned response. In others, the feeling of attention and interaction with the biofeedback therapist may, in part, explain symptomatic benefit. Biofeedback therapy may be performed in several ways. Some prefer to initialize treatment with the patient in the hospital over a 10- to 14-day period with subsequent management performed on an outpatient basis.[83] Others perform treatment solely on an outpatient basis. At our institution, patients are managed by a biofeedback therapist in an office for approximately 3 to 6 months. The need for further treatment is based on response during this time.

The use of home trainers has added yet another dimension to therapy.[80] Patients are allowed home with portable equipment that enables them to monitor their performance during each session. At present, the equipment is expensive.

Anal sphincter response may be measured by anal manometry or electromyography, which can be measured with an intra-anal probe and longitudinally oriented electrodes.[84] Data are then displayed in graphic format that is easily understood by the patient. Most systems have either visual or auditory feedback. Although the greatest reported benefit of biofeedback for fecal incontinence has been around 60%, there is wide variation in results from different institutions. Recent data suggest that proper selection of patients, combined with the team approach (i.e., physician, therapist, and dietitian administering treatment over a minimum of 3 to 6 months) is likely to be most effective.[80]

Electrostimulation of the Pelvic Floor

Electrical stimulation of the anal sphincter and pelvic floor muscles has been employed by some using an intra-anal probe. The results of treatment, however, have been disappointing.[85]

OPERATIVE TREATMENT

Operative treatment is usually offered to patients with gross fecal incontinence who have an underlying correctable abnormality. Some of these patients with lesser degrees of incontinence who do not improve on conservative treatment may also be offered operative treatment. The outcome of operation depends on the extent of anal sphincter and associated neurologic injury. An isolated anal sphincter defect in a fit young individual offers the best prognosis for full recovery. In contrast, the presence of bilaterally prolonged pudendal nerve motor latencies is most likely to be associated with a poor result.

A number of operative approaches have been described in the literature. These range from simple overlapping external anal sphincter repair for a distal sphincter defect to repair of the entire pelvic floor for neuropathic fecal incontinence. In situations where these repairs have failed or in the presence of a nonfunctioning anal sphincter, which is commonly due to bilateral denervation, neoanal sphincter reconstruction may be an alternative. Finally, there is a group of patients who may require a stoma. Some authors have described creating either an appendicostomy or cecostomy through which an irrigating catheter may be introduced to empty the colon and rectum.[86] This technique has been particularly useful in children, and data from these studies have shown that it is acceptable and effective. An end colostomy may prove to be a better option, although it is often considered a last resort. Patients with a well-constructed, correctly located stoma usually have an excellent quality of life.

Timing of Repair: Primary Versus Secondary

Primary repair of the external anal sphincter is undertaken for most acute injuries to the sphincter. It is important to recognize the possibility of anal sphincter damage whenever there is a perineal tear associated with vaginal deliveries or pelvic-perineal injury after blunt or penetrating trauma.[43] The presence of extreme tissue edema or an expanding hematoma and the nature of the laceration may preclude primary repair of the sphincter. In such rare circumstances, it is advisable to repair the episiotomy or simply appose the skin edges and achieve tissue healing as a primary goal. If a patient is hemodynamically unstable, has multiple injuries, and extensive gross contamination of the perineal wounds, a diversion with distal washout and drainage is usually necessary. Repair of the sphincter is deferred until the patient is stabilized. Endoanal ultrasound can be used to map the extent of sphincter damage before performing a secondary repair as an elective procedure under optimal conditions when tissues are soft and pliable. This often requires waiting 3 or more months after the initial injury.

Primary Repair

Recognized acute sphincter injuries are usually best repaired immediately (Fig. 40-4). The muscle edges are freshened and repaired by direct apposition or by an overlapping technique using 2-0 polyglactin sutures in a horizontal mattress fashion without tension. Excessive lateral mobilization of sphincter muscle is usually unnecessary, but the entire length of the injury must be exposed to assure complete repair. The wounds are closed primarily, if possible, in the absence of gross contamination. Some authors use a closed suction drain. Usually, it is unnecessary to divert the fecal stream.

Secondary Repair

Secondary repair of the sphincter is often required in patients with obstetric injury. In most cases, a tear was recognized and repaired immediately after birthing, but the repair failed due to infection, ischemia, poor technique, or other causes. Sometimes no injury was noted and the woman presents months or years later with incontinence due to a sphincter injury. The remainder of the chapter deals mostly with methods of secondary repair.

Direct Sphincter Muscle Repair

Classically, direct sphincter repair has been used for incontinence secondary to a definite anatomic defect in the sphincter muscle. Less often, sphincteroplasty has been advocated for treatment of idiopathic fecal incontinence.[87,88] Although results

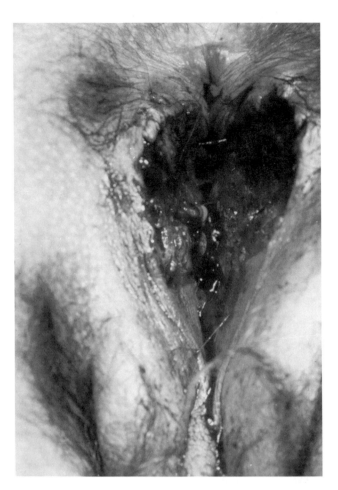

Figure 40-4. A severe, acute fourth degree tear secondary to birthing with complete disruption of the perineum is shown. Primary repair was performed with an excellent clinical result. The patient is in the prone jackknife position.

are not as good as for anatomic disruption, it appears that direct sphincter repair provides as good a result for idiopathic incontinence as any other operation.

The preferred direct surgical repair of incontinence secondary to a discrete sphincter injury is an overlapping sphincteroplasty of the affected muscle. If limited to an external sphincter injury, only the external sphincter muscle is overlapped. More often, a full-thickness injury is present. Repair requires overlap of both the external and internal sphincter muscles. Often the injury extends in a cephalad direction to disrupt not only the internal and external sphincter muscles, but also the levator ani muscles. In such cases, a full anterior repair is achieved by combining an overlapping sphincteroplasty with an anterior levatoroplasty.

Preliminaries

The patient undergoes an outpatient mechanical bowel preparation with either polyethylene glycol solution or a solution of sodium phosphate buffer. Intravenous prophylactic antibiotics are administered just prior to induction of anesthesia. A colostomy is not necessary in most cases. The operation is performed under general anesthesia, preferably with an epidural catheter inserted for postoperative pain control. A Foley catheter is placed in the bladder. The patient is positioned prone over a hip roll and the buttocks are taped apart. Proctoscopy is then performed to irrigate the rectum, and the perianal area, including the vagina, is prepared and draped. It is recommended that the surgeon performing the operation wear a fiberoptic headlight to provide adequate illumination of the operative field.

Incision and Anodermal Mobilization

A curved skin incision is made about 1.5 cm from the anal verge in the region of the sphincter defect and is extended as necessary in an arc of 200° to 240° to permit exposure of the retracted ends of the divided external sphincter muscle. Care must be taken to avoid injury to the inferior rectal nerves that enter the anal sphincter muscles from a posterolateral direction (Fig. 40-5).

The anoderm is elevated as a mucosal flap via an endoanal dissection. It is easiest to begin the dissection laterally and work medially to the area of scar and injury. A self-retaining retractor such as the Lone Star (Houston, Texas) is used to gently efface the anus and facilitate the endoanal dissection of the mucosa and submucosa from the underlying internal sphincter muscle. In the area of the injury, which is usually in the anterior midline, there is often only vaginal and anal mucosa with a small amount

Figure 40-5. An incision is made anterior to the anus through the middle of the perineum with the patient in the prone jackknife position. Extension beyond an arc of 240° risks injury to the underlying branches of the pudendal nerve.

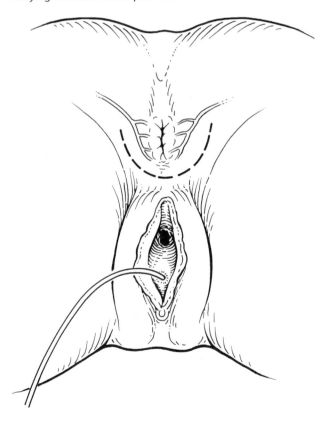

of intervening scar tissue. Placing a finger in the vagina can provide tactile sensation during this difficult dissection. The anodermal flap is mobilized in a cephalad direction to expose the entire length of the injury. Once normal planes of dissection cephalad to the injury are reached, the levator ani can be identified laterally to either side of the rectum.

Sphincter Mobilization

The external sphincter is mobilized from the scar and surrounding ischiorectal fat. The Lone Star retractor facilitates this procedure. It is again helpful to commence dissection laterally at a site remote from primary injury and to establish an appropriate plane of dissection lateral to all identifiable sphincter fibers. The dissection proceeds toward the site of sphincter injury. It is essential to identify the edges of the damaged sphincter muscle in order to achieve appropriate muscle overlap. Scar tissue is preserved. In addition to lateral mobilization of the anal sphincter, it is important to expose the entire length of the anal sphincter injury from the subcutaneous component distally to the level of the levator ani muscle proximally. This facilitates a full length repair of the sphincter. Deep exposure is facilitated by the use of narrow Deaver's retractors. In some cases of anterior anal sphincter injury where the defect is confined to a narrow band of scar tissue, one may encounter fusion between the fibers of the external sphincter muscle with those of the transverse perineal muscles at the level of the perineal body. It may then be necessary to divide these fusing fibers of the external sphincter in order to achieve complete mobilization necessary to perform an overlapping repair. Following complete mobilization and prior to sphincter reconstruction, the wound is irrigated and meticulous hemostasis is achieved. Venous bleeding in the posterior wall of the vagina may require suture ligation. If a concomitant rectovaginal fistula is present, direct repair of the vagina with 2-0 polyglactin sutures is now performed.

Anterior Levatoroplasty

When the injury extends proximally into the levator ani muscle, an anterior levatoroplasty is performed to plicate the anterior limbs of the muscle to the midline (Fig. 40-6). This may be achieved by using either 2-0 polyglactin or polypropylene sutures. If nonabsorbable sutures are used (e.g., polypropylene) it is essential to bury the suture knots deep to the muscle in order to avoid subsequent patient discomfort. Occasionally, it may not be possible to achieve side-to-side apposition of the levator ani, in which case construction of a lattice of sutures suffices. Anterior repair has been shown to increase the length of the anal sphincter high-pressure zone consistently. Prior to the advent of anal ultrasound, Miller et al.[87] reported excellent results from an anterior repair compared with patients who had postanal repair for neuropathic fecal incontinence. An improved result in patients undergoing anterior repair in this series was attributed to the finding of occult anterior anal sphincter defects in patients who may otherwise have had only a postanal repair.

Overlapping Sphincteroplasty

The sphincter reconstruction is completed by overlapping the mobilized edges of the external (and usually the internal) sphincter (Fig. 40-7). Four to eight horizontal mattress sutures

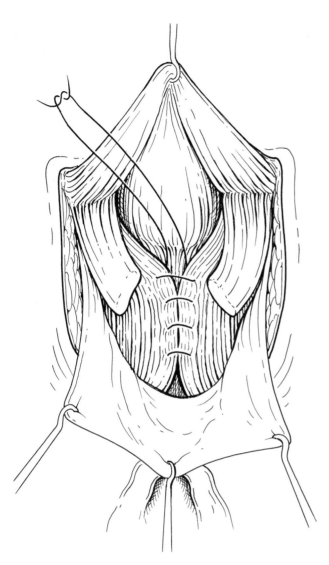

Figure 40-6. For injuries extending proximally into the levator ani muscle, an anterior levatoroplasty is performed by placing interrupted sutures to plicate the anterior limbs of the muscle to the midline.

of 2-0 polyglactin are placed and serially tied to achieve the desired degree of tightness. Sutures of 3-0 polyglactin are then placed as required between the principal anchoring sutures. Sutures must be ligated securely but not so tight as to result in ischemic muscle. Although there are reports of direct apposition repair achieving a similar outcome,[89] the overlapping technique is preferred because it uses the scar tissue, preserved at the severed ends of the muscle, to hold sutures and support repair and because the overlap provides a double thickness of muscle at the site of primary injury.

In some patients where anal sphincter injury is limited to gaps in the distal sphincter muscle in which the edges of healthy sphincter are linked by strands of remaining muscle tissue, it may not be necessary to divide the sphincter in the midline. In this situation, muscle is simply plicated and a sphincteroplasty performed to transpose functional muscle over nonfunctional fibrous scar tissue.

Wound Closure

After sphincter reconstruction the wound is irrigated and hemostasis achieved. One may plicate the vaginal wall with interrupted sutures of 3-0 polyglactin to provide added support to the rectovaginal septum. The wound is closed with interrupted vertical mattress sutures of 3-0 polyglycolic acid. The hemicircumferential incision is closed in a V-Y plasty to provide skin coverage over the thickened perineal body (Fig. 40-8). The anodermal flap is restored to its normal location with care taken to avoid mucosal ectropion. Small Penrose drains are placed laterally, extending to the cephalad portion of the dissection. An antibiotic ointment is applied to the suture line.

Postoperative Care

An epidural infusion is used to relieve pain as necessary, and a Foley catheter is left in the bladder until the epidural catheter is removed. Sitz baths are instituted as soon as the patient can ambulate. Patients are given a low-residue diet for the first 48 hours. A normal diet supplemented with bulk laxatives is commenced on postoperative day three. Fecal impaction, which may result in patient discomfort and destruction of the repair, is prevented by administering either a tap water or phosphate enema. Wounds must be checked at regular intervals for signs of infection or hematoma. Discharge from hospital is usually possible between the third and fifth postoperative days. Patients are instructed to continue with warm sitz baths and daily enemas if necessary, avoid straining and vigorous activities, and take analgesics as necessary for comfort. Patients are seen in the office or clinic approximately 3 to 4 weeks after discharge from the hospital.

Results of Direct Sphincter Repair

The reported outcome of anal sphincteroplasty from several centers varies from 60 to 90% for good to excellent results, depending in part on the etiology of the incontinence.[35,90–94] Direct sphincter repair achieves good to excellent results in 80 to 99% of patients whose incontinence is due to traumatic injury versus 60% of patients whose incontinence is idiopathic.[35,87,88,93] Researchers have attempted to analyze the value of anorectal physiologic tests and identify parameters that may predict a successful outcome following sphincteroplasty. Anal ultrasound has been shown to be valuable in preoperative and postoperative assessments of those patients who do not regain continence.[44] Ultrasound identifies breakdown of sphincter repair, which can help determine whether the patient should be subjected to a second procedure. Theoretically, repair of a denervated anal sphincter is unlikely to restore full continence. However, a recent review of 94 patients having overlapping sphincteroplasty at St. Mark's Hospital revealed pudendal neuropathy in 20%.[94] Analysis of this subset of patients showed an improvement in continence in 14 of 20 (70%) with pudendal neuropathy compared with 57 of 70 (77%) without neuropathy at a mean follow-up of 5 years. Thus, the presence of pudendal neuropathy does not appear to be a contraindication to anal sphincteroplasty.

Yoshioka and Keighley[91] and Fleshman et al.[92] have attempted to identify data on anal manometry that may predict

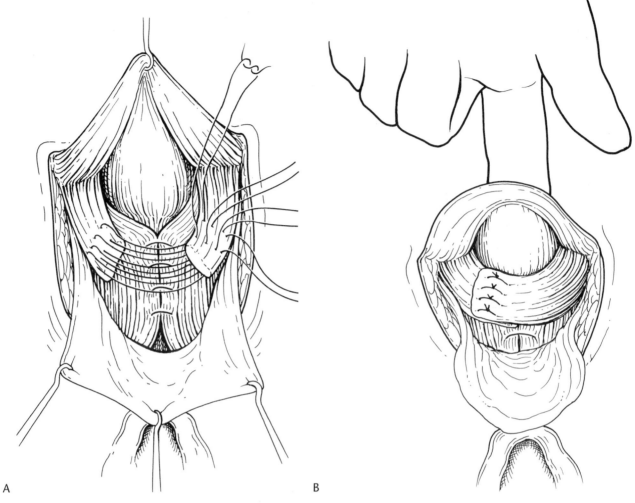

A   B

Figure 40-7. (**A**) Four to eight horizontal mattress sutures are placed through the edges of the mobilized external (and usually the internal) sphincter muscle. (**B**) The sutures are tied to achieve a snug but not overly tight overlapping sphincteroplasty.

a successful outcome in patients having sphincteroplasty. Both studies failed to identify such predictive data. However, Fleshman et al.[92] reported a significant increase in resting and squeeze pressures in patients who were continent after surgery, suggesting both anatomic and functional reconstruction of the sphincter. These authors, as well as others,[93] have indicated that improvement in the functional length of the sphincter corresponded to a successful outcome. This emphasizes the importance of a full-length sphincter reconstruction. A previous anal sphincter repair or the presence of a rectovaginal fistula in patients who require anal sphincteroplasty does not necessarily adversely affect the likelihood of a successful outcome.

Complications of Sphincter Repair

Documented complications after sphincter repair include urinary tract infection, hemorrhage and hematoma, infection of the repair site, and disruption of the repair. Both hematoma and infection at the site of repair may lead to sphincter disruption. Prophylactic antibiotics have helped reduce the incidence of

infection. Fecal diversion from the site of repair, unless grossly contaminated, appears to be of no benefit.

Role of Internal Anal Sphincter Plication

Several studies have reported the predictive value of resting anal pressure in the outcome of operation for fecal incontinence. In a study of anterior repair for fecal incontinence, Miller et al.[87] reported that patients who had a good clinical outcome were found to have an increase in their resting anal pressures. Their hypothesis was that plication of the internal anal sphincter during anterior sphincteroplasty may have contributed to this rise in resting pressure. Subsequently, Wexner et al.[93] performed a layered repair of the internal and external anal sphincters in an attempt to improve the clinical outcome in patients with fecal incontinence. These authors observed that the rise in resting anal pressure achieved in their study was significantly greater than that of other studies where internal sphincter plication was not undertaken. Based on these data, it was concluded that internal sphincter plication was helpful in anal sphincter repair for fecal incontinence.

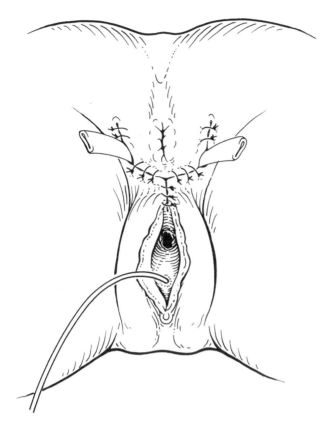

Figure 40-8. The hemicircumferential incision is closed in a V-Y plasty to provide skin coverage over the thickened perineal body. Small Penrose drains are placed laterally into the depths of the wound.

More recently, a randomized study was undertaken to evaluate the role of internal sphincteroplasty during pelvic floor repair.[95] Anal sphincter defects were mapped by anal endosonography. In patients with disruption of the internal sphincter, there was difficulty in achieving complete apposition of healthy edges of internal anal sphincter without undue tension at the site of repair and excessive lateral mobilization, which may have resulted in anal sphincter denervation. However, an attempt was made at longitudinal plication of the sphincter in which smooth muscle of the proximal anorectum was mobilized to fill the inferior deficiency in the sphincter. However, this procedure resulted in lowering of resting anal pressures and a reduced functional length of the anal canal. It is likely that autonomic denervation during this procedure may have resulted from the high intersphincteric dissection that was required to adequately mobilize the internal sphincter.

Others too have failed to achieve benefit from internal sphincter plication.[96] In conclusion, it is unlikely that separate plication of the internal anal sphincter will confer added benefit in patients with anal sphincter damage or neuropathic fecal incontinence.

Postanal Repair

The operation of postanal repair, described by Sir Alan Parks in 1975,[31] was based on the observation that patients with fecal incontinence had an obtuse anorectal angle. It was observed that in most continent individuals there is a double right angle between the anal canal and the distal rectum and midrectum. Parks theorized that re-creation of a more acute anorectal angle by plication of the posterior limbs of the puborectalis sling would improve continence by a flap valve effect. Early results of this operation were encouraging. However, long-term results have shown this to be a less than satisfactory treatment for incontinence, and its use has decreased significantly. Reasons for failure of this operation to regularly restore continence are multiple. Bartolo et al.[97] were unable to confirm the flap valve theory of incontinence and suggested that improvement after postanal repair is less related to the angle and more to improved muscular contractility.[87,88] This explains the observation that some individuals who are completely continent have an obtuse anorectal angle. Possible explanations for deterioration of continence following initial improvement after postanal repair may be the presence of missed occult anterior anal sphincter disruption, and/or the coexistence of denervation injury of the sphincter and pelvic floor.

Preoperative Preparation

Patients are given a full mechanical bowel preparation and prophylactic intravenous antibiotics are administered prior to induction of anesthesia. The procedure is performed under a general or regional anesthetic. The patient is positioned in the prone jackknife or lithotomy position, depending on the preference of the surgeon.

Operation

A curved incision is made midway between the posterior anal margin and the tip of the coccyx. Subcutaneous dissection is performed to the level of the intersphincteric groove posteriorly (Fig. 40-9A). Further dissection is performed in the avascular intersphincteric plane for about half the circumference. The external anal sphincter is mobilized posteriorly and retracted using malleable retractors. Intersphincteric dissection is then continued in a cephalad direction until the limbs of the puborectalis muscle are identified. The rectosacral fascia is then incised to expose the mesorectal fat (Fig. 40-9B). A deep retractor is placed to displace the anorectum anteriorly, thus exposing the limbs of the levator ani muscles. Between four and eight interrupted polypropylene sutures on a curved needle are then placed across both limbs of the ischiococcygeus, pubococcygeus, and puborectalis muscles (Fig. 40-9C). They are tied loosely to form a lattice across the pelvis at the cephalad aspect of the levator and to appose the most posterior limit of the puborectalis muscle (Fig. 40-9D). Parks suggested this would re-create an acute anorectal angle but that has not been shown to occur. The anal canal high pressure zone is lengthened. Finally, the external anal sphincter muscle is tightened posteriorly in an attempt to further narrow the anal canal. The incision is closed in the shape of a Y over suction drainage without fecal diversion.

Postoperative Care

Traditionally, pain relief was achieved with a combination of intramuscular analgesia followed by oral analgesics. More recently, epidural anesthesia and patient-controlled analgesic in-

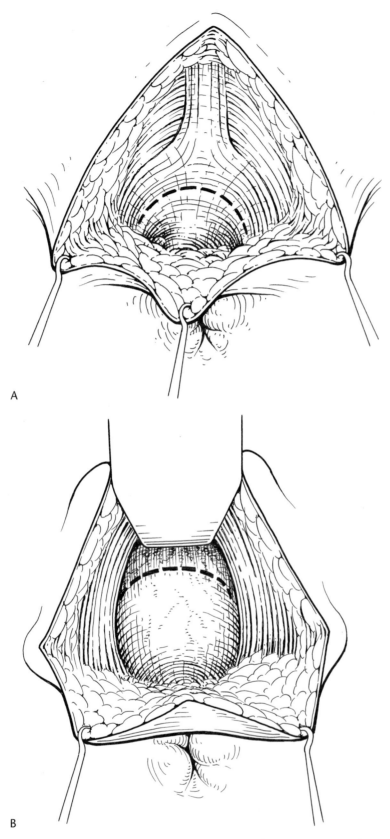

A

B

Figure 40-9. (**A**) The patient is in a prone jackknife position. A posterior curved incision is deepened to the intersphincteric groove posteriorly. (**B**) A retractor displaces the external sphincter posteriorly. The dissection is deepened in the avascular intersphincteric plane until the limbs of the puborectalis muscle are identified. The rectosacral fascia is then incised to expose the mesorectal fat. *(Figure continues.)*

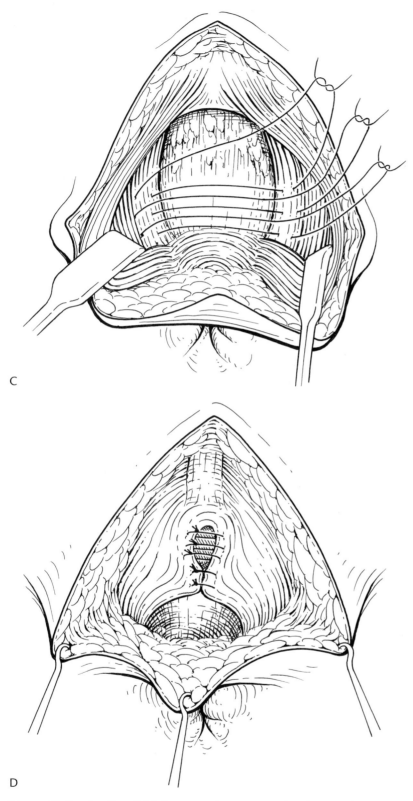

C

D

Figure 40-9. *(continued)* (**C**) Interrupted sutures are placed across the ischiococcygeus
and tied to form a lattice work across the pelvis at the cephalad aspect of the levator.
(**D**) A few additional plication sutures are placed across the pubococcygeus and
puborectalis muscles. The external sphincter muscle is also plicated.

fusions have been found to be more effective in providing immediate postoperative relief. A Foley bladder catheter is left for 2 to 3 days. The patient is started on a low-residue diet with a bulk laxative. If necessary, phosphate or tap water enemas may be used to cleanse the rectum and prevent fecal impaction. Patients are discharged after the first bowel movement, which is usually 2 to 3 days after operation.

Results of Postanal Repair

The reported results of this operation from various centers have been tabulated in Table 40-3. Although studies have shown improvement in up to 80% of patients in the short term, long-term evaluation has shown sustained improvement after postanal repair in only approximately 25%.

Total Pelvic Floor Repair

The operation of total pelvic floor repair incorporates an anterior repair with postanal repair for patients with neuropathic fecal incontinence.[98] The rationale for this operation was that most patients undergoing postanal repair had a concomitant anterior deficiency of the perineal body and anal sphincter complex as manifested by the presence of a rectocele. Furthermore, total pelvic floor failure was observed to be present in a proportion of patients with neuropathic fecal incontinence during video proctography. The purpose of this operation, therefore, was to achieve a circumferential buttress of the anorectum. In a small randomized trial of 36 patients in which anterior repair was compared with postanal repair and total pelvic floor repair, the greatest improvement in the short term was seen in those undergoing total pelvic floor repair.[45] The only physiologic parameter associated with improved outcome was an increase in the functional length of the anal canal. Longer term follow-up, however, has revealed deterioration in some patients. More recently, an attempt was made to identify parameters that could predict a satisfactory outcome in these patients. Unfortunately, no association between anal canal pressures or pudendal nerve latency and outcome was identified. Instead, obesity in patients was consistently found to be associated with a poor result.[21]

Neoanal Sphincter

A neoanal sphincter is indicated when the native anal sphincter is either lacking or is nonfunctional. In 1891 Thiersch described the use of an encircling wire to occlude the lumen of the anorectum. Labow[99] described the use of a Dacron-impregnated silastic sling for preservation of continence. Further studies have shown that these techniques are of little value chiefly due to the adynamic nature of the sphincter device. Others have used fascial slings around the anorectum to preserve continence.

Artificial Anal Sphincter

Recently, there has been a resurgence in interest in both non-biological and biological neoanal sphincters. The nonbiological neoanal sphincter is essentially a modified urologic sphincter, the successful use of which was first described by Christiansen and Lorentzen.[100] Subsequently, a pilot study was performed at the University of Minnesota in which the artificial anal sphincter (AMS-800, Minneapolis, Minnesota) was implanted in 10 patients.[101] This sphincter consists of an inflatable cuff of silicone rubber attached to a fluid-filled reservoir and pump via a valve mechanism. The pump and reservoir are implanted in a subcutaneous pocket at an easily accessible site and the cuff encircles the anorectum.

Technique

Two para-anal incisions are made and a circumanal tunnel is created through which the inflatable silastic cuff is inserted to surround the anal canal (Fig. 40-10). While the reservoir is inserted into a pocket created in the space of Retzius, the pump is implanted subcutaneously in the labium majus in women and within the scrotum in men. These are then connected to the cuff of the artificial sphincter via tubing placed in a subcutaneous tunnel. When activated, the cuff distends with fluid to occlude the anal canal and when deactivated, the cuff empties to allow defecation (Fig. 40-11).

Results

Ten patients having an artificial sphincter at the University of Minnesota have now been followed for 58 months (range, 30 to 76 months).[102] Three developed an infection of whom two required removal of the implant. Seven of 10 are completely continent, whereas one is occasionally incontinent of gas and liquid stool.

Skeletal Muscle Neosphincter

Several reports have described neoanal sphincters employing transposed striated muscle. Pickrell et al.[103] first described the successful use of a gracilis neoanal sphincter in children with anorectal agenesis. Subsequently, Cavina et al.[104] described a technique employing both gracilis muscles, which were wrapped around a perineal stoma following abdominal perineal excision of the rectum for cancer. Although a transposed striated

Table 40-3. Results of Postanal Repair

Author	Number	Continent to Solids and Liquid (%) (With or Without Gas Continence)
Parks (1975)[31]	75	83%
Keighley and Fielding (1983)[36]	89	63%
Henry and Simson (1985)[121]	129	56%
Habr-Gama et al. (1986)[122]	45	52%
Yoshioka et al. (1988)[34]	116	34%
Scheuer et al. (1989)[123]	39	15%
Athanasiadis et al. (1995)[124]	31	6%
Engel et al. (1994)[125]	38	21%
Jameson et al. (1994)[126]	36	28%
Setti Carraro et al. (1994)[127]	34	26%

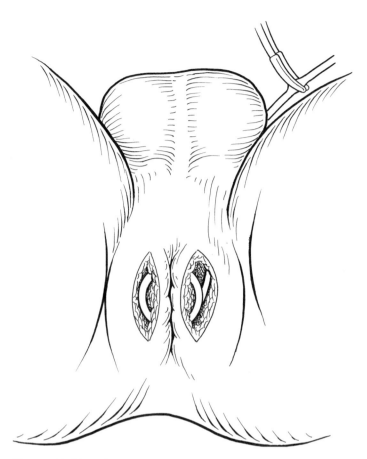

Figure 40-10. The inflatable silastic cuff has been wrapped around the anus within the circumanal tunnel and secured in position by a tab collar. Connecting tubing is then tunneled in the subcutaneous tissue to the site of the pressure-regulating balloon.

muscle neosphincter is capable of producing a voluntary contraction to occlude the anal canal, it is unable to preserve a closed lumen at all times. This is chiefly due to the lack of an inherent tone within this muscle, unlike the resting anal tone generated by the anal sphincter complex. Subsequently, Baeten et al.[105] reported on the feasibility of achieving total continence by means of an electrically stimulated gracilis neosphincter. In a larger series of patients Baeten et al.[106] and Williams et al.[62] employed low-frequency electrical stimulation of a gracilis neoanal sphincter to produce fused contractions and hence generate a resting anal pressure in the anal canal. Both authors reported that over 60% of patients were continent to solid and liquid stool. Furthermore, longer term follow-up in these patients has shown a sustained result from electrostimulation. Not all patients may require a stimulated neosphincter, however. In a long-term retrospective review of patients who had had a gracilis neosphincter without electrical stimulation, Foucheron et al.[107] reported an acceptable outcome in most patients. It is likely that these patients had reasonable internal sphincter function capable of preserving a closed anal canal. However, a proportion of patients in this series required electrical stimulation of their neosphincter to achieve satisfactory resting anal pressure and continence. The majority of series describe the use of a gracilis neoanal sphincter, but some authors have described successful continence with the aid of gluteus muscle transposition.[108]

Physiology of Electrostimulation

It is now known that striated muscle consists of a mixture of type 1 (slow twitch) and type 2 (fast twitch) muscle fibers arranged in a mosaic pattern. Based on physiologic, biochemical, and histologic parameters, type 1 fibers are slow twitch fatigue-resistant muscle fibers that derive their energy chiefly from aerobic metabolism. The diameter of these muscle fibers has been reported to be less than that of type 2 fibers. Furthermore, type 1 fibers possess a higher density of capillaries and mitochondria compared with type 2 fibers. In contrast, type 2 fibers are fast twitch, fatigue prone, large diameter muscle fibers that derive most of their energy from anaerobic metabolism. The external anal sphincter is composed of a greater proportion of type 1 fibers when compared with muscles such as the gracilis and the gluteus, hence the need for electrical stimulation. Salmons and Vrbova[109] were the first to demonstrate that low-frequency electrostimulation of striated muscle enabled conversion of type 2 to type 1 fibers in experiments on cats. Prior to use in humans, electrical stimulation was also employed in studies of thigh muscle neosphincters wrapped around stomas in dogs by several independent groups. Hallan et al.[110] demonstrated fiber-type conversion by electrostimulation in the sartorius muscle of dogs. Subsequently, Heine et al.[111] and Konsten et al.[112] demonstrated that the occlusive force developed in an

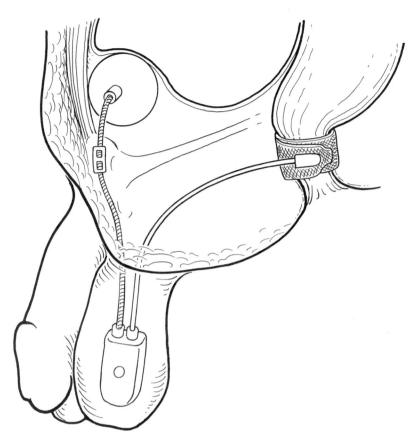

Figure 40-11. This drawing depicts the final placement of the inflatable silastic cuff, the pressure-regulating balloon, the control pump, and connecting tubing.

electrostimulated sartorius neosphincter was greater than that in nonstimulated neosphincters.

Most data on striated muscle electrostimulation have been derived from experimental stimulation of the latissimus dorsi, which has been used to provide ventricular assistance to failing cardiac muscle. For instance, it is not known whether electrical stimulation of a neosphincter should be preceded by a training period in which the amplitude and frequency of stimulation is progressively increased, thus enabling muscle to adapt to its new environment. Buie et al.[113] undertook a randomized study in dogs where a transposed neosphincter was continuously stimulated at low frequency from the outset and compared the result with an initial training period followed by continuous stimulation. Test groups were also compared with a nonstimulated control group. The data revealed greater fatigue resistance in electrically stimulated neosphincters compared with controls. However, there was no demonstrable difference in fatigue resistance in the group of neosphincters undergoing an initial training period versus those being continuously stimulated from the outset. These data suggest that an initial training period of electrostimulation of the neosphincter may be unnecessary.

Electrostimulated Gracioplasty: Technique

Preoperative Preparation. Preoperative stoma counseling is obtained if there is a likelihood of a diverting stoma. A full mechanical bowel preparation is performed and the patient is given intravenous broad-spectrum antibiotics just prior to surgery. The operation is performed under a general anesthetic with the patient placed supine with legs supported on Allen stirrups. Rectal lavage is performed to totally empty the rectum. The skin over the lower anterior abdominal wall, the perineum, and the entire lower limb is prepared. In the case of obese patients, it may be helpful to surface mark the course of the gracilis muscle preoperatively.

Incisions and Muscle Mobilization. The gracilis muscle may be exposed via three separate incisions in the lower limb. A 5- to 7-cm incision is first made in the upper thigh, followed by a 5-cm incision at the level of the midthigh and a 2-cm incision over the tibial tuberosity. Alternatively, one long medial thigh incision is used. The skin incision is deepened beyond the fascia lata to expose the muscles of the medial compartment of the thigh. The gracilis is a long cylindrical muscle that originates from the pubic bone proximally and attaches to the tibial tuberosity. It must be distinguished from the larger adductor longus muscle, which lies anterior to it. The fascia overlying the gracilis is incised and the muscle is encircled in its proximal portion. Further mobilization continues distally, taking care to ligate venous tributaries from this muscle at the level of the midthigh. Mobilization of the distal third of this muscle is performed via the thigh incision distally to the tibial tuberosity. At the level of the tibial tuberosity the tendon of the gracilis must be clearly distinguished from that of the sartorius and semitendinosus muscles by traction and countertraction on the muscle belly. Division of the gracilis tendon should be as far distal as possible to achieve maximum muscle length. The divided distal end of the muscle is delivered into the wound in the proximal thigh and upward mobilization continues by a combination of traction on the muscle belly and blunt fascial dissection. At this juncture it is essential to identify the anterior obturator neurovascular pedicle that must be preserved (Fig. 40-12). The neurovascular bundle usually enters the upper part of the muscle from an anterolateral direction. Hence, muscle dissection in the upper thigh may be performed with relative ease in the posteromedial region without risk of nerve damage. The nerve supply is then confirmed by means of a neurostimulator using the cathode as the stimulating electrode and the anode as the ground electrode. A voltage of between 1 and 2 volts is sufficient to produce visible muscle contraction.

Circumanal Wrap. The mobilized gracilis muscle is now prepared to be wrapped around the anal canal as a neosphincter (Fig. 40-13). During creation of the circumanal tunnel, damage to the posterior wall of the vagina should be avoided. The mobilized muscle is delivered to the circumanal incision and the thigh wounds are closed.

The goal of the muscle wrap should be to achieve 360° contact between the anal canal and muscle belly, not tendon. An epsilon configuration of muscle wrap has proven to be most

useful. The tension in the muscle wrap should be adjusted so that the anal canal feels snug around an examining fifth digit. Too tight a muscle wrap may cause anal canal ischemia and obstructed defecation. The tendon of the gracilis is anchored securely to the contralateral ischial tuberosity (Fig. 40-14). Occasionally, if there is insufficient length of muscle and tendon to reach the ischial tuberosity, the tendon may be anchored to the perianal skin. Hemostasis is achieved and the wounds are closed in layers, preferably over vacuum suction drains. This completes stage 1 of the procedure.

Stage 2 consists of implantation of the electrical stimulating device. The stimulating equipment consists of an implantable, fully programmable pulse generator attached to positive and negative terminal leads. The pulse generator is implanted in a subcutaneous abdominal wall pocket with the inscribed surface anterior. Our preference is to attach the stimulating electrodes around the proximal muscle belly at the point where the nerve to the gracilis muscle begins to divide. Others have described positioning these electrodes around the main nerve trunk. The electrodes are then tunneled subcutaneously to be attached to the implantable pulse generator (Fig. 40-15).

Stimulation Protocols. Although there are no fixed criteria for stimulation, we employ an initial training period of up to 8 weeks, during which time the pulse generator is switched on intermittently. A period of continuous stimulation then follows.

Figure 40-12. The gracilis muscle tendon has been divided distally at the tibial tuberosity and the muscle mobilized proximally to the level of the neurovascular pedicle, which enters the muscle from an anterolateral direction.

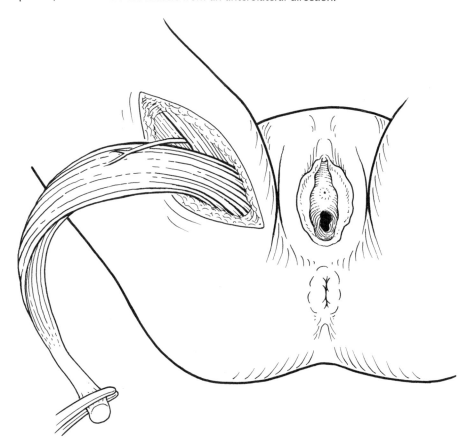

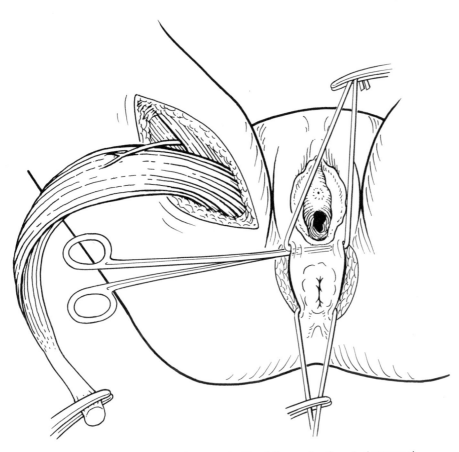

Figure 40-13.   An incision is made on each side of the anal orifice. A circumanal tunnel is created by gentle blunt dissection.

The stimulating voltage is usually around 2 volts with a pulse width of 210 msec and a frequency of up to 25 Hz, although this has to be adjusted so that fused contractions of the gracilis neosphincter are produced. Some have found that an increase in stimulation voltage was required through a period of 26 weeks after commencement of stimulation.[4] The longevity of the pulse generator set at these settings has been estimated to be 7 years.

Controversies.   *Vascular Delay.*   Williams et al.[62] have recommended that a period of vascular delay be employed during mobilization of the lower two-thirds of the gracilis muscle. It has been suggested that disconnection of the distal blood supply to this muscle is followed by a period during which collateral circulation becomes established. These authors have suggested that the use of vascular delay has improved muscle viability following a transposition. We do not routinely employ this technique of vascular delay, and have not encountered muscle ischemia or progressive muscle fibrosis consequent to ischemia.

Diverting Stoma.   We and others do not routinely employ fecal diversion during creation of a gracilis neoanal sphincter. However, the lack of fecal diversion precludes us from inserting the implantable pulse generator and stimulating electrodes at the same operation. Instead, this is performed 6 weeks later. By contrast, if the patient referred for a gracilis neoanal sphincter already has a stoma, then our policy has been to perform the

gracilis wrap and implant the stimulators at the same operation. A second operation is needed to take down the colostomy.

Postoperative Care.   Postoperative pain control is achieved either by an epidural or patient-controlled intravenous route. The patients are maintained on a low-residue diet and adequate fluid intake is ensured. The Foley catheter is left in the bladder until the patient is able to mobilize completely. The wounds are inspected daily. Mobilization and physical therapy to the donor thigh is commenced as soon as possible. Bulk laxatives are prescribed and the patient is discharged following a bowel movement. The operation of graciloplasty is associated with a complication rate that has been shown to be related to a learning curve.[114] Intraoperative complications include mobilization of the wrong muscle, damage to the proximal neurovascular pedicle, hematoma formation, and damage to the rectal and vaginal walls during creation of the subcutaneous neosphincter tunnel. Postoperative complications include infection and cellulitis of the thigh wound, fecal impaction and consequently obstructed defecation, perianal abscess formation, pressure necrosis of the anal canal, disruption of the distal tendinous attachment to the ischial tuberosity, muscle ischemia and chronic fibrosis, migration of implant, infection at the implant site, urinary tract infection, and deep vein thrombosis.

Results.   Early experience of graciloplasty in some series has been disappointing.[34] This has been chiefly due to infection.

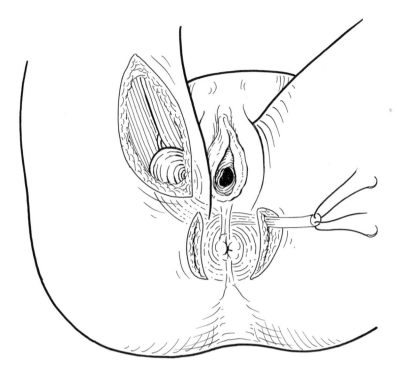

Figure 40-14. The gracilis muscle is wrapped around the anus and its tendon is sutured to the contralateral ischial spine. The ipsilateral leg is adducted to minimize tension on the muscle.

Figure 40-15. The perineal and thigh wounds are closed. The electrodes are attached to the muscle or nerve and led subcutaneously to an abdominal incision contralateral to the colostomy. The pulse generator is then inserted into a subcutaneous pocket on the abdominal wall.

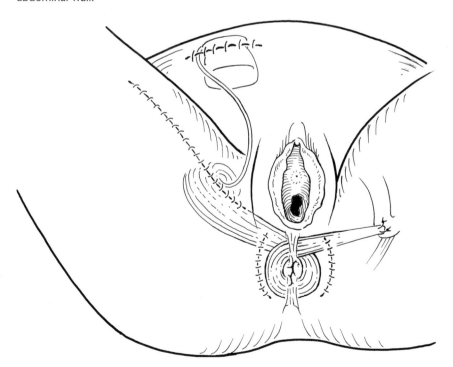

Table 40-4. Results of Gracilis Muscle Transposition

Author	Number	Electro-stimulated	Continent to Solid, Liquid, ± Gas (%)
Williams et al. (1991)[63]	20	Yes	60%
Baeten et al. (1995)[4]	52	Yes	73%
Leguit et al. (1985)[128]	10	No	90%
Yoshioka and Keighley (1981)[129]	6	No	0%
Christiansen et al. (1990)[130]	13	No	46%
Foucheron et al. (1994)[107]	22	No	55%
Cavina et al. (1991)[104]	47	Yes	65%
Madoff et al. (1994)[131]	9	Yes	78%
Gonzales et al. (1995)[114]	7	Yes	80%

However, subsequent studies of electrostimulated gracilis muscle transposition have shown a 75% continence rate in early and longer term follow-up studies.[4] Furthermore, patients having electrostimulated gracilis neosphincters have experienced a marked improvement in their quality of life. A comparative analysis of function after both stimulated and nonstimulated graciloplasty from various series is presented in Table 40-4.

Gluteus Maximus Transposition

The chief disadvantages of the gracilis muscle as a neosphincter are its occasional inadequate length, which prevents a circumferential wrap, and the presence of a thigh wound, which is often the site of cellulitis and discomfort in patients. Some authors have explored the possibility of the gluteus maximus muscle transposition as an alternative to gracilis neosphincters.[108,115] The gluteus maximus has been used in two different ways. First, some have employed partial gluteus maximus transposition with preservation of its proximal neurovascular bundle to support anal sphincteroplasty in which a large part of the native anal sphincter was found to be absent.[116] Others have used either a split unilateral transposition or bilateral gluteus maximus transpositions to achieve complete encirclement of the anal canal with some degree of success.

Stomas

Despite several recent developments in the treatment of fecal incontinence, some patients may ultimately require a stoma. Although longer term evaluation of patients with stomas has shown an increasing incidence of complications, such as parastomal herniation,[117] most patients with a stoma achieve a reasonable quality of life in the long term. In constructing a permanent stoma, it is ideal to incorporate the services of the enterostomal therapist who can improve patient motivation by proper preoperative patient counseling and help in rehabilitation of patients after operation. In general, an end sigmoid colostomy is the ideal stoma for patients with anal incontinence.

Appendicostomy

Some authors have described the use of the appendix to serve as a conduit for an irrigating catheter used to cleanse the entire colon and rectum.[86] This technique has been particularly useful in incontinent children. Although favorable results have been reported, it has not yet gained widespread popularity.

FUTURE PERSPECTIVES

Anal continence is primarily the result of a complex interaction of both muscular and sensory components of the anorectum. Much of the research in the past has focused on either restoring contractile function in the native anal sphincter or in recreating a neoanal sphincter. Research in current basic science may add considerably to improvement in sphincter function in the future. Johnson et al.[118] have explored the role of artificial electromagnetic sensors implanted in the anal canal that may restore anorectal sensation in some patients who may not receive adequate warning of impending evacuation or in those who have no warning at all. Artificial sensors may also be invaluable in automation of a neosphincter.

In a preliminary study, Shafik[119] has reported the value of submucosal injection of autologous fat or polytetrafluoroethylene in restoring the anal cushions, which aid complete anal canal closure. The technique appears to be simple and free of complications and is analogous to submucosal injection of collagen used by urologists for urinary incontinence. This may be of value in restoring continence in patients who become partially incontinent after internal sphincterotomy or hemorrhoidectomy.

Congilosi et al.[120] have reported successful restoration of anal tone and fiber typing similar to the native anal sphincter following cross innervation of the pudendal nerve to the innervation of transposed striated muscle. An intact pudendal nerve is a prerequisite for this technique, which would be of little value in neuropathic fecal incontinence. Although the technique may be of some use in patients having intestinal continuity restored after abdominoperineal excision for cancer, division of the main trunk of the pudendal nerve is likely to denervate the urethral sphincter complex and affect genital sensation. Instead, this technique may be refined by employing the inferior rectal nerves in cross innervation rather than the pudendal nerve trunk. Current research at our institution for neuropathic fecal incontinence is focusing on direct sphincter muscle stimulation with implanted electrodes and sacral nerve stimulation, which offer the advantage of being less invasive and provide a cosmetically better result compared with graciloplasty.

CONCLUSION

The cornerstone of treatment for fecal incontinence remains careful clinical history and physical examination supplemented by selective anorectal physiologic assessment. Patients should be well informed of the underlying abnormality and well motivated, as no treatment modality enables complete restoration of continence. In dealing with these patients, a multidisciplinary team approach appears to be most effective. Although researchers claim several surgical treatments improve the quality of life in these patients, longer term follow-up is necessary to determine ultimate prognosis. Currently, for end-stage neuropathic fecal incontinence there appears to be two major treatment modalities. The electrostimulated gracileoplasty may be effective in 75% of patients, but it is an expensive and still investigational technique. By contrast, the artificial anal sphincter is less invasive and may be less expensive. Further supportive studies, however, are required to justify its use. Future treatment and research in neuropathic fecal incontinence should focus on minimally invasive and cost-effective procedures that can be made available to the general population.

REFERENCES

1. Rothenberger DA (1989) Anal incontinence. pp.185–194. In Cameron (ed): Current Surgical Therapy. 3rd Ed. BC Becker, Toronto

2. Madoff RD, Williams JG, Caushaj PF (1992) Current concepts: fecal continence. N Engl J Med 326:1002–1007

3. Jorge JMN, Wexner SD (1993) Etiology and management of fecal incontinence. Dis Colon Rectum 36:77–97

4. Baeten CGMI, Geerdes BP, Adang EMM et al (1995) Anal dynamic graciloplasty in the treatment of intractable fecal incontinence. New Engl J Med 32:1600–1605

5. Enck P, Bielefeldt P, Rathmann W et al (1991) Epidemiology of faecal incontinence in selected patient groups. Int J Colorectal Dis 6:143–146

6. Denis P, Bercott E, Bizien C et al (1992) Prevalence of anal incontinence in adults. Gastroenterol Cliniq Biol 16(4):344–350

7. Talley NJ, O'Keefe EA, Zinsmeister AR, Melton JL (1992) Prevalence of gastrointestinal symptoms in the elderly: a population based study. Gastroenterology 102:895–901

8. Nelson R, Norton N, Cautley E, Furner S (1995) Community-based prevalence of anal incontinence. JAMA 274:559–561

9. Profile of Wisconsin Nursing Home Residents, 1992 (1994) Center for Health Statistics, Division of Health, Department of Health and Social Services, Madison, WI

10. Keighley MRB, Bick D, MacArthur C (1995) Prevalence and obstetric factors in childbirth-related fecal incontinence, abstracted. Dis Colon Rectum 38:14

11. Sentovich SM, Rivela LJ, Blatchford GJ et al (1995) Patterns of male fecal incontinence. Dis Colon Rectum 38:281–285

12. Gee AS, Durdey P (1995) Incontinence of urine is a marker of pudendal neuropathy in fecal incontinence, abstracted. Dis Colon Rectum 38:16

13. Sun WM, Read NW, Donnelly TC (1990) Anorectal function in incontinent patients with cerebral spinal disease. Gastroenterology 99:1372–1379

14. Miller R, Bartolo DCC, Cervero F, Mortensen NJ (1988) Anorectal sampling: a comparison of normal and incontinent patients. Br J Surg 75:44–47

15. Kumar D (1991) Sleep and the gut. Gastrointestinal mobility. pp.15–16. In Proceedings of the 12th BSG.SB International Workshop

16. Cann PA, Read NW, Holdsworth CD, Barends D (1984) The role of loperamide and placebo in the management of the irritable bowel syndrome (IBS). Dig Dis Sci 29:239–247

17. Fischer SE, Breckon K, Andrews HA, Keighley MRB (1989) Psychiatric screening for patients with fecal incontinence or chronic constipation referred for surgical treatment. Br J Surg 76:352–555

18. Jensen LL, Lowry AC (1993) Are pudendal nerve latencies a predictive factor in the success of biofeedback for fecal incontinence, abstracted. Dis Colon Rectum 36:30

19. Kamm MA, Farthing MJ, Lennard-Jones JE et al (1991) Steroid hormone abnormalities in women with severe idiopathic constipation. Gut 32:80–84

20. Kamm MA (1994) Obstetric damage and fecal incontinence. Lancet 344:730–733

21. Korsgen S, Deen KI, Vanden Akker O, Keighley MRB (1995) Outcome of total pelvic floor repair for neuropathic fecal incontinence: long-term follow up and predictive parameters, abstracted. Dis Colon Rectum 38:47

22. Taverner D, Smiddy FG (1959) An electromyographic study of the normal function of the external anal sphincter and pelvic diaphragm. Dis Colon Rectum 2:153–160

23. Melzack J, Porter NH (1964) Studies of the reflex activity of the external sphincter ani in spinal man. Paraplegia 1:277–296

24. Snooks SJ, Swash M (1986) The innervation of the muscles of continence. Ann R Coll Surg Engl 68:45–49

25. Womack NR, Morrison JFB, Williams NS (1986) The role of pelvic floor denervation in the etiology of idiopathic fecal incontinence. Br J Surg 73:404–407

26. Madoff RD (1991) Common etiologies of fecal incontinence. Presented at annual course, Principles of Colon and Rectal Surgery. University of Minnesota, Minneapolis

27. Belliveau P, Thompson JPS, Parks AG (1983) Fistula in ano: a manometric study. Dis Colon Rectum 26:152–154

28. Wald A, Tunuguntla AK (1984) Anorectal sensorimotor dysfunction in fecal incontinence and diabetes mellitus modification with biofeedback therapy. N Engl J Med 310:1281–1287

29. Barrett JA, Brockelhurst JC, Kiff ES et al (1989) Anal function in geriatric patients with fecal incontinence. Gut 30:1244–1251

30. Klosterhalfen B, Offner F, Topf N et al (1990) Sclerosis of the internal anal sphincter—a process of aging. Dis Colon Rectum 33:606–609

31. Parks AG (1975) Anorectal incontinence. Proc R Soc Med 68:681–690

32. Phillips SF, Edwards DAW (1965) Some aspects of anal continence and defaecation. Gut 6:396–405

33. Womack NR, Morrison JFB, Williams NS (1986) Prospective study of the effects of postanal repair in neurogenic fecal incontinence. Br J Surg 75:48–52

34. Yoshioka K, Hyland G, Keighley MRB (1988) Physiological changes after postanal repair and parameters predicting outcome. Br J Surg 75:1220–1224

35. Fang DT, Nivatvongs S, Herman FN et al (1984) Overlapping sphincteroplasty for acquired anal incontinence. Dis Colon Rectum 27:720–722

36. Keighley MRB, Fielding JWL (1983) Management of fecal incontinence and results of surgical treatment. Br J Surg 70:463–468

37. Snooks SJ, Barnes PRH, Swash M, Henry MM (1985) Dam-

age to the innervation of the pelvic floor musculature in chronic constipation. Gastroenterology 89:977–981

38. Burnett SJD, Spence-Jones C, Speakman CTM et al (1991) Unsuspected sphincter damage following childbirth revealed by anal endosonography. Br J Radiol 64:225–227

39. Garcia-Aguilar J, Belmonte C, Wong WD et al (1996) Open versus closed sphincterotomy for chronic anal fissure: long-term results. Dis Colon Rectum 39:440–443

40. Lestar B, Pennickx F, Rigauts H, Kerremans R (1992) The internal anal sphincter cannot close the anal canal completely. Int J Colorectal Dis 7:159–161

41. Snooks SJ, Swash M, Setchell M, Henry MM (1984) Injury to innervation of pelvic floor sphincter musculature in childbirth. Lancet 2:546–550

42. Sultan AH, Kamm MA, Hudson CN et al (1993) Anal sphincter disruption during vaginal delivery. N Engl J Med 329:1956–1957

43. Sorensen M, Tetzchner T, Rassmusen OO et al (1993) Sphincter rupture in childbirth. Br J Surg 80:392–394

44. Sultan AH, Kamm MA, Nicholls RJ, Bartram CI (1994) Prospective study of the extent of internal anal sphincter division during lateral sphincterotomy. Dis Colon Rectum 37:1031–1033

45. Deen KI, Oya M, Ortiz J, Keighley MRB (1993) Randomized trial comparing three forms of pelvic floor repair for neuropathic faecal incontinence. Br J Surg 80:794–798

46. Deen KI, Madoff RD, Finne CO et al (1995) Anal ultrasound and physiologic assessment in fecal incontinence: experience from a North American center, abstracted. Dis Colon Rectum 38:30

47. Sultan AH, Kamm MA, Bartram CI, Hudson CN (1994) Third degree obstetric anal sphincter tears: risk factors and outcome of primary repair. BMJ 308:887–891

48. Law PJ, Kamm MA, Bartram CI (1991) Anal endosonography in the investigation of faecal incontinence. Br J Surg 78:312–314

49. Deen KI, Kumar D, Williams JG et al (1993) The prevalence of anal sphincter defects in fecal incontinence: a prospective endosonic study. Gut 34:685–688

50. Motson RW (1985) Sphincter injuries: indications for and results of sphincter repair. Br J Surg suppl. 72:195–215

51. Mazier WP, Senagore AJ, Schiesel EC (1995) Operative repair of anovaginal and rectovaginal fistulas. Dis Colon Rectum 38:4–6

52. Khanduja KS, Padmanabhan P, Wise WE et al (1995) Reconstruction of rectovaginal fistula with sphincter disruption by combining advancement flap and sphincteroplasty, abstracted. Dis Colon Rectum 38:31

53. Kiff ES, Swash M (1984) Normal proximal and delayed distal conduction in the pudendal nerves of patients with idiopathic (neurogenic) faecal incontinence. J Neurol Neurosurg Psychiatr 47:820–823

54. Snooks SJ, Swash M, Henry MM, Setchell M (1986) Risk factors in childbirth causing damage to the pelvic floor innervation. Int J Colorectal Dis 1:20–24

55. Hill J, Mumtaz A, Kiff ES (1994) Pudendal neuropathy in patients with idiopathic faecal incontinence progresses with time. Br J Surg 81:1494–1495

56. Kiff ES, Swash M (1984) Slowed conduction in the pudendal nerves in idiopathic (neurogenic) faecal incontinence. Br J Surg 71:614–616

57. Lubowski DZ, Nicholls RJ, Swash M, Jordan MJ (1987) Neural control of internal anal sphincter function. Br J Surg 74:668–670

58. Carlstedt A, Nordgren S, Fasth S et al (1988) Sympathetic nervous influence on the internal anal sphincter and rectum in man. Int J Colorectal Dis 3:90–95

59. O'Kelly TJ, Brading A, Mortensen NJMc (1993) Nerve mediated relaxation of the human internal anal sphincter: the role of nitric oxide. Gut 34:689–693

60. Speakman CTM, Hoyle CHV, Kamm MA et al (1990) Adrenergic control of the internal anal sphincter is abnormal in patients with idiopathic faecal incontinence. Br J Surg 77:1342–1344

61. Cornes H, Bartolo DC, Stirrat GM (1991) Changes in anal canal sensation after childbirth. Br J Surg 78:74–77

62. Williams NS, Patel J, George BD et al (1991) Development of an electrically stimulated neoanal sphincter. Lancet 338:1166–1169

63. Williams JG, Wong WD, Jensen L et al (1991) Incontinence and rectal prolapse: a prospective manometric study. Dis Colon Rectum 34:209–216

64. Parks AG, Swash M, Urich H (1977) Sphincter denervation in anorectal incontinence and rectal prolapse. Gut 18:656–665

65. Deen KI, Grant EA, Billingham C, Keighley MRB (1994) Abdominal resection rectopexy with pelvic floor repair versus perineal rectosigmoidectomy and pelvic floor repair for full thickness rectal prolapse. Br J Surg 81:302–304

66. Farouk R, Duthie GS, Bartolo DCC, McGregor AB (1992) Restoration of continence following rectopexy for rectal prolapse and recovery of the internal anal sphincter electromyogram. Br J Surg 79:439–440

67. Leigh RJ, Turnberg LA (1982) Faecal incontinence: the unvoiced symptom. Lancet 1:1349–1351

68. Read NW, Cellik AF, Katsinelos P (1995) Constipation and incontinence in the elderly. J Clin Gastroenterol 20:61–70

69. Matheson DM, Keighley MRB (1981) Manometric evaluation of recal prolapse and fecal incontinence. Gut 22:126–129

70. McHugh SM, Diamant NE (1987) Effect of age, gender and parity on anal canal pressures. Dig Dis Sci 32:726–736

71. Swash M, Gray A, Lubowski DZ, Nicholls RJ (1988) Ultrastructural changes in internal anal sphincter in neurogenic fecal incontinence. Gut 29:1692–1698

72. Laurberg S, Swash M (1989) Effects of aging on the anal rectal sphincters and their innervation. Dis Colon Rectum 32:737–742

73. Jameson JS, Chia YW, Kamm MA et al (1994) Effect of age, sex and parity on anorectal function. Br J Surg 81:1689–1692

74. Mann WJ (1991) Surgical management of radiation enteropathy, review. Surg Clin North Am 71:977–990

75. Kollmorgen CF, Meagher AP, Wolff BG et al (1994) The long-term effect of adjuvant postoperative chemoradiotherapy for rectal carcinoma on bowel function. Ann Surg 220:676

76. Miller R, Bartolo DSS, Locke-Edmunds JC, Mortensen NJM (1988) Prospective study of conservative and operative treatment for fecal incontinence. Br J Surg 75:101–105

77. Browning GGP, Parks AG (1983) Postanal repair for neuro-

pathic faecal incontinence: correlation of clinical results and anal canal pressures. Br J Surg 70:101–104

78. Pescatori M, Anastasio G, Bottini C, Mentasti A (1992) New grading and scoring for anal incontinence: evaluation of 335 patients. Dis Colon Rectum 35:482–487

79. Varma JS, Smith AN, McInnes A (1986) Electrophysiological observations on the human pudendo-anal reflex. J Neurol Neurosurg Pyschiatr 49:1411–1416

80. Ferrara A, Lord SA, Larach SW et al (1995) Biofeedback with Home Trainer Program is effective for both incontinence and pelvic floor dysfunction, abstracted. Dis Colon Rectum 38:17

81. McKirdy H (1981) Effect of loperamide on human isolated internal anal sphincter. J Physiol 316:18

82. Longo WE, Vernava AM, Virgo KS, Johnson FE (1995) The effect of Cisapride on constipation in spinal cord injured patients: preliminary results of a pilot study, abstracted. Dis Colon Rectum 38:11

83. Grotz RL, Pemberton JH (1995) Anal incontinence. pp. 322–339. In Mazier WP, Levien DH, Luchtefeld M, Senagore AJ (eds): Surgery of the Colon, Rectum and Anus. WB Saunders, Philadelphia

84. Binnie NR, Kawimbe BM, Papachrysostomou M et al (1991) The importance of the orientation of the electrode plates in recording anal sphincter EMG by non-invasive anal plug electrodes. Int J Colorectal Dis 6:5–8

85. Scheuer M, Kuijpers HC, Bleijenberg C (1994) Effect of electrostimulation on sphincter function in neurogenic fecal continence. Dis Colon Rectum 37:590–593

86. Malone PS, Ransley PG, Kiely EM (1990) Preliminary report: the antegrade continence enema. Lancet 336:1217–1218

87. Miller R, Orrom WJ, Cornes H et al (1989) Anterior sphincter plication and levatorplasty in the treatment of faecal incontinence. Br J Surg 76:1058–1060

88. Orrom WJ, Miller R, Cornes H et al (1991) Comparison of anterior sphincteroplasty and post anal repair in the treatment of idiopathic fecal incontinence. Dis Colon Rectum 34:305–310

89. Arnaud A, Sarles JC, Sielezneff I et al (1991) Sphincter repair without overlapping for fecal incontinence. Dis Colon Rectum 34:744–747

90. Pezim ME, Spencer RJ, Stanhope CR et al (1987) Sphincter repair for fecal incontinence after obstetrical or iatrogenic injury. Dis Colon Rectum 30:521–525

91. Yoshioka K, Keighley MRB (1989) Sphincter repair for fecal incontinence. Dis Colon Rectum 32:39–42

92. Fleshman JW, Dreznik Z, Fry RD, Kodner IJ (1991) Anal sphincter repair for obstetric injury: manometric evaluation of functional results. Dis Colon Rectum 34:1061–1067

93. Wexner SD, Marchetti F, Jagelmann DG (1991) The role of sphincteroplasty for fecal incontinence re-evaluated: a prospective physiologic and functional review. Dis Colon Rectum 34:22–30

94. Londono-Schimmer EE, Garcia-Duperly R, Nicholls RJ et al (1994) Overlapping anal sphincter repair for fecal incontinence due to sphincter trauma: five-year follow-up functional results. Int J Colorectal Dis 9:110–113

95. Deen KI, Kumar D, Williams JG et al (1995) Randomized trial of internal anal sphincter plication with pelvic floor re-

96. Briel JW, Schouten WR, de Boer LM, Auwerda JJ (1995) Clinical outcome of anterior anal repair in patients with fecal incontinence, abstracted. Dis Colon Rectum 38:11

97. Bartolo DCC, Roe AM, Locke-Edmunds JC et al (1986) Flap valve theory of anorectal continence. Br J Surg 73:1012–1014

98. Pinho M, Ortiz J, Oya M et al (1992) Total pelvic floor repair for the treatment of neuropathic faecal incontinence. Am J Surg 163:340–343

99. Labow S, Rubin KJ, Hoexter B, Salvati EP (1980) Perineal repair of rectal procidentia with an elastic fabric sling. Dis Colon Rectum 23:467–469

100. Christiansen J, Lorentzen M (1987) Implantation of artificial sphincter for anal incontinence. Lancet August: 244–245

101. Wong WD, Rothenberger DA (1994) Artificial anal sphincter. pp.773–777. In Fielding LP, Goldberg SM (eds): Surgery of the Colon, Rectum, and Anus. 5th Ed. Butterworth-Heinemann, Oxford

102. Congilosi SM, Wong WD (1995) Anal incontinence. pp. 240–245. In Cameron JL (ed): Current Surgical Therapy. (5th Ed.) Mosby, St. Louis

103. Pickrell KL, Broadbent TR, Masters FW, Metzger JT (1952) Construction of a rectal sphincter and restoration of anal incontinence by transplanting gracilis muscle: a report of four cases in children. Ann Surg 135:853–863

104. Cavina E, Seccia M, Evangelista G et al (1991) Perineal colostomy and electrostimulated gracilis neosphincter after abdominal perineal resection of the colon and anorectum: a surgical experience and follow up study in 47 cases. Int J Colorectal Dis 6:63–64

105. Baeten CGMI, Spaans F, Fluks A (1988) An implanted neuromuscular stimulator for fecal continence following previously implanted gracilis muscle. Dis Colon Rectum 38:134–137

106. Baeten CGMI, Konsten J, Spaans F et al (1991) Dynamic graciloplasty for treatment of faecal incontinence. Lancet 338:1163–1165

107. Faucheron JL, Hannoun L, Thome C, Parc R (1994) Is fecal continence improved by nonstimulated gracilis muscle transposition? Dis Colon Rectum 37:979–983

108. Devesa JM, Vicente E, Enriquez JM (1992) Total fecal incontinence—a new method of gluteus maximus transposition—preliminary results and report of previous experience with similar procedures. Dis Colon Rectum 35:339–249

109. Salmons S, Vrbova G (1969) The influence of activity on some contractile characteristics of mammalian fast and slow muscles. J Physiol 210:535–549

110. Hallan RI, Williams NS, Hutton MRE et al (1990) Electrically stimulated sartorius neosphincter: canine model of activation and skeletal muscle transformation. Br J Surg 77:208–213

111. Heine JA, Rothenberger DA, Wong WD et al (1992) An electrostimulated skeletal muscle neosphincter in a canine model of fecal incontinence, abstracted. Dis Colon Rectum 35:8

112. Konsten J, Baeten CG, Havenith MG, Soeters PB (1994) Canine model for treatment of fecal incontinence using transposed and electrically stimulated sartorius muscle. Br J Surg 81:466–469

113. Buie WD, Johnson DR, Madoff RD et al (1993) Electrostimulated skeletal muscle neosphincter: effective chronic low fre-

quency stimulation on fatigue resistance, abstracted. Dis Colon Rectum 36:16

114. Gonzalez AP, Teoh TA, Wexner SD et al (1995) The stimulated gracilis neosphincter operation: initial experience, pitfalls and complications, abstracted. Dis Colon Rectum 38:19

115. Pearl RK, Prasad ML, Nelson RL et al (1991) Bilateral gluteus maximus transposition for anal incontinence. Dis Colon Rectum 34:478–481

116. Enriquez-Navascues JM, Devesa-Mugica JM (1994) Traumatic anal incontinence: role of unilateral gluteus maximus transposition supplementing and supporting direct anal sphincteroplasty. Dis Colon Rectum 37:766–769

117. Williams JG, Etherington R, Hayward MWJ, Hughes LE (1990) Paracolostomy hernia: a clinical and radiological study. Br J Surg 77:1355–1357

118. Johnson D, Buie WD, Paterson R et al (1993) Artificial anorectal sensation, abstracted. Dis Colon Rectum 37:44

119. Shafik A (1995) Perianal injection of autologous fat for treatment of sphincteric incontinence. Dis Colon Rectum 38: 583–587

120. Congilosi SM, Johnson DRE, Medot M et al (1995) Pudendal nerve innervation of a skeletal muscle neosphincter for fecal incontinence: a canine model, abstracted. Dis Colon Rectum 38:18

121. Henry MM, Simson JNL (1985) Results of postanal repair: a retrospective study. Br J Surg 72, suppl.:S17–19

122. Habr-Gamn A, Alves PA, DaSilva C et al (1986) Treatment of faecal incontinence by postanal repair. Colonoscopy 8: 244–246

123. Scheuer M, Kuijpers HC, Jacobs PP (1989) Postanal repair restores anatomy rather than function. Dis Colon Rectum 32: 960–963

124. Athanasiadis et al. (1995)

125. Engel AF, Kamm MA, Sultan AH, et al (1994) Anterior and sphincter repair in patients with obstetric trauma. Br J Surg 81:1231–1234

126. Jameson JS, Speakman CT, Darzi A et al (1994) Audit of postanal repair in the treatment of faecal incontinence. Dis Colon Rectum 37:369–372

127. Setti Carraro P, Kamm MA, Nicholls RJ (1994) Long term results of postanal repair for faecal incontinence. Br J Surg 81:140–144

128. Leguit R, van Baal JG, Brummelkauz WH (1985) Gracilis muscle transposition in the treatment of fecal incontinence: long term follow-up and evaluation. Dis Colon Rectum 28: 1–4

129. Yoshiok K, Keighley MRB (1989) Critical assessment of the quality of continence after postanal repair for faecal incontinence. Br J Surg 76:1054–1057

130. Christiansen J, Sevensen M, Rasmussen OO (1990) Gracilis muscle transposition for faecal incontinence. Br J Surg 77: 1039–1040

131. Madoff RD, Johnson DRE, Buie WD et al (1994) Initial North American experience with the electrically-stimulated skeletal muscle neosphincter. Podium presentation at American Society of Colon and Rectal Surgeons. 93rd Convention, May 8–13, 1994, Orlando, Florida

41

LOWER GASTROINTESTINAL BLEEDING

Adrian Francis Peng-Kheong Leong
Francis Seow-Choen

Acute lower gastrointestinal hemorrhage is relatively uncommon, accounting for approximately 1.5% of all surgical emergencies.[1] Bleeding is usually self-limiting rather than ongoing.[2] In 80% to 90% of cases the source of bleeding can be determined by conventional diagnostic endoscopy and radiology.[3] About 10% have severe and ongoing bleeding requiring hospitalization, resuscitation, urgent evaluation, and treatment.[4] Five percent bleed intermittently and chronically from an obscure source providing a diagnostic challenge.[3,5,6] Although an approach similar to that for upper gastrointestinal hemorrhage is desirable, internationally accepted protocols for the management of major lower gastrointestinal hemorrhage have yet to evolve.[7] The reasons for this include the diversity of causes for bleeding and the variable access to diagnostic services such as colonoscopy, angiography, and radionuclide scanning, especially in the emergency situation. Nevertheless, the role of different diagnostic modalities has become better defined and the selection of the appropriate investigation for the bleeding patient can be customized to local requirements.

The evolving nature of the management of lower gastrointestinal hemorrhage is reflected in the commonly held views of the likely cause of hemorrhage in the different decades of this century. In the early part of this century, colonic neoplasms were thought to be the main cause of most gastrointestinal hemorrhage. It was not until the 1950s that diverticular disease was recognized as an important cause of bleeding.[8] Blind segmental colectomy or subtotal colectomy would frequently be performed for bleeding patients with diverticular disease diagnosed on barium enema. Rebleeding rates following blind segmental colectomy varied between 35% and 40%.[9,10] In many of these cases, the presumption that diverticular disease was the cause of bleeding was evidently incorrect.

The advent of angiography in the 1960s markedly reduced the percentage of undiagnosed cases[11] and revealed the importance of vascular malformations in massive lower gastrointestinal hemorrhage. The introduction of therapeutic angiography was followed subsequently by diagnostic and therapeutic colonoscopy. Surgical procedures for undiagnosed acute lower gastrointestinal bleeding are now uncommon.[12]

CAUSES

Before subjecting patients with lower gastrointestinal hemorrhage to elaborate investigations, a bleeding diathesis should be excluded.[13,14] Platelet disorders, coagulopathies, and leukemias may present with active rectal bleeding. Drugs such as anticoagulants, nonsteroidal anti-inflammatory agents,[15] steroids, and enteric-coated potassium chloride can cause reversible lower gastrointestinal hemorrhage.

On the basis of a review of the available literature, Levinson et al.[16] estimated that moderate to severe lower gastrointestinal bleeding originated in 85% of cases from the colon, in 10% of cases from the upper gastrointestinal tract, and in 5% of the time from the small bowel. Massive bleeding from the upper gastrointestinal tract can result in the passage of fresh blood per rectum that may be indistinguishable from a lower gastrointestinal cause. Esophagogastric varices, peptic ulceration, and gastric erosions should be excluded as part of the investigation for acute lower gastrointestinal hemorrhage. Pancreatic carcinoma[17] and pseudocysts eroding into an artery[18,19] have been reported as causes of major gastrointestinal hemorrhage. In a patient with previous aortic surgery, an aortoenteric fistula needs to be considered as a cause of massive gastrointestinal bleeding.[20,21]

Anorectal conditions such as hemorrhoids and fissure are frequent causes of active, ongoing rectal hemorrhage.[22,23] Solitary rectal ulcer has also been known to cause massive lower gastrointestinal hemorrhage, generally in seriously ill patients.[24,25] Proctitis, particularly following radiotherapy,[26-28] diffuse hemangiomata,[29-31] and Dieulafoy-like lesions[32,33] have been reported to cause exsanguinating hemorrhage from the rectum. Dieulafoy lesions have been described in the colon[34–36] as well as the small bowel.[37,38] The lesion is characterized by a small mucosal defect with minimal inflammation and a large thick-walled artery at the base.[39] As a rule, an anorectal site for bleeding is more common in patients less than 50 years of age.[40]

Colonic causes are the most common source of lower gastrointestinal hemorrhage; of these, angiodysplasia and diverticular disease account for more than 60% of all cases of major hemorrhage in the older age group.[41] Bleeding occurs in between 3% and 5% of cases with colonic diverticula.[41–43] The site of bleeding is more likely to be from the proximal colon rather than from the sigmoid colon where diverticula predominate.[9,42,44–46] Hemorrhage from diverticular disease results from rupture of one of the branches of the vasa recta that enter the wall of the colon.[46] Cause of the rupture is uncertain and is generally believed to be a result of stercoral erosion (Fig. 41-1). Although colonic polyps and carcinoma are common causes of bleeding, they seldom cause massive blood loss. In a study by Noer et al.,[47] only 5% of 114 colonic neoplasms bled massively.

Colonic endometriosis is an unusual cause of lower gastrointestinal bleeding and is characterized by cyclical rectal hemorrhage with menstruation.[48,49] The sigmoid colon and rectum are the most commonly involved areas and preoperative diagnosis is often difficult as radiographic similarities with malignant lesions can cause diagnostic confusion.[50,51] A recent report describes successful diagnosis with endoscopy and biopsy.[52] Rarely, a colorectal ectopic pregnancy may also result in massive gastrointestinal hemorrhage.[53]

Extra-esophagogastric varices are uncommon but more than 70 cases of colonic varices have now been reported.[54,55] Although they are almost always secondary to portal hypertension, two patients from the same family have been described in whom colonic varices occurred without portal hypertension.[56] The most common location is in the rectosigmoid area.[57] Angiography and endoscopy are the primary means of diagnosis. On colonoscopy, they appear as serpinginous bluish collapsible structures.[54] Portosystemic shunt surgery has been used successfully for this condition.[54] Although rectal bleeding is common in ulcerative colitis, massive hemorrhage is rare.[58] Massive bleeding is slightly more common in Crohn's disease than in ulcerative colitis.[59,60] It may be the initial presentation in some patients with Crohn's disease.[61] Ischemic colitis may present with profuse bloody diarrhea[62] and it may be sometimes difficult to distinguish this clinically from idiopathic inflammatory bowel disease.

Other forms of colitis from infective causes such as *Campylobacter*,[63–66] *Escherichia coli*,[67] and tuberculosis[68] have been reported to present with lower gastrointestinal hemorrhage. Small bowel lesions that cause lower gastrointestinal hemorrhage include small bowel diverticula including Meckel's diverticulum, small bowel tumors, and diseases that also affect the colon such as radiation enteritis, angiodysplasia, hemangiomas, and Crohn's disease. Bleeding from jejunal diverticula is rare but has been reported as a source of massive gastrointestinal hemorrhage in more than 50 cases.[69] There is evidence that it is an acquired abnormality[70] resulting from a motility disorder of the jejunum.[71] Bleeding occasionally stops spontaneously but recurrent hemorrhage is the more common course. Segmental resection of the jejunum and primary anastomosis is required in the latter situation.

Unlike jejunal diverticulosis, Meckel's diverticulum is congenital. Bleeding occurs in childhood although it may occasionally present in adulthood. A bleeding Meckel's diverticulum invariably contains functioning heterotopic gastric mucosa,[72,73]

Figure 41-1. Bleeding diverticulum. A blood clot (arrow) is seen within the lumen of a diverticulum that has an outer layer of muscularis mucosa only. The diverticulum extends into the pericolic fat. (Courtesy of Dr. Jean Ho, Consultant Histopathologist.) (H&E ×20)

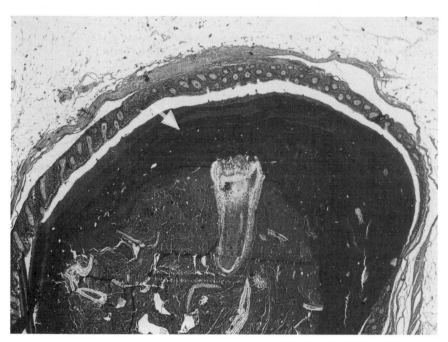

although bleeding has also been reported in a Meckel's diverticulum that had invaginated.[74] Technetium 99m pertechnetate that accumulates in the mucin-secreting cells of the heterotopic gastric mucosa may be used to detect Meckel's diverticulum,[75] although successful demonstration is rare.

Lower gastrointestinal bleeding can also occur from vasculitides including polyarteritis nodosa.[76-78] Henoch-Schöenlein purpura[79] and systemic lupus eythematosus[80] have all been reported to cause lower gastrointestinal hemorrhage due to ischemia and ulceration.

VASCULAR MALFORMATIONS OF THE COLON

The first report of a vascular lesion of the gastrointestinal tract was published in 1839.[81] In 1949, Gentry et al.[82] described vascular malformations as a distinct entity in a review of 283 cases from the world literature. Since that time, the advent of selective visceral angiography and colonoscopy has led to a large number of these vascular lesions being attributed as a cause for previously unexplained lower gastrointestinal hemorrhage.[11,83,84] The dramatic increase in the number of reports of vascular malformations in the last 20 years has been accompanied by confusion and controversy concerning nomenclature and classification.[59] The pathologic classification of vascular malformations shown in the accompanying box is useful and provides a framework based on biologic and histologic criteria rather than morphologic description.[85]

Angiodysplasia

Angioectasia or vascular ectasia or more commonly angiodysplasia (Fig. 41-2) are degenerative lesions associated with ageing. They should not be confused with congenital or neoplastic lesions in other age groups. Angiodysplasia occurs in the proximal part of the colon. The lesions may be single or multiple and are usually less than 5 mm in diameter.[86,87] They are thought to arise from the obstruction of tortuous submucosal veins as they pass through the muscularis propria of the colon. Repeated episodes of obstruction cause a gradual dilatation of the submucosal veins. Eventually, the venules and arteriolar-capillary units feeding these veins also dilate. Ultimately, the capillary rings

---

Classification of Vascular Malformations of the Gastrointestinal Tract

Type of Malformation

Degenerative
  Angiodysplasia
Hamartomatous
  Hemangioma
  Telangectasia
Neoplastic
  Hemangiosarcoma
  Kaposi's sarcoma
Connective tissue disorders
  Ehlers-Danlos

---

dilate, the precapillary sphincter becomes incompetent, and a small arteriovenous communication forms.[88] The latter is responsible for the "early-filling vein" that is seen on angiography. The predominance of these lesions in the right side of the colon is explained by Laplace's law. The largest initial luminal diameter and highest resting wall tension is in the cecum and ascending colon, giving rise to a greater degree of obstruction of submucosal veins in this area compared with that in other parts of the colon.

The prevalence of angiodysplasia varies in different reports. Boley et al.[86] found angiodysplasia in 25% of asymptomatic individuals above the age of 60 years. In a colonoscopic survey, Foutch et al.[89] reported a prevalence rate of 0.83% in 964 patients above the age of 50 years. In a prospective study, Hochter et al.[90] reported 59 patients with angiodysplasia out of 1938 who underwent total colonoscopy. Twenty percent of the patients with angiodysplasia had bleeding. The remainder were asymptomatic. The wide variation in the reported prevalence evidently arises from the differing criteria and method of diagnosis as well as the different study populations involved. The majority of subjects with angiodysplasia are above the age of 55 years and two-thirds are over the age of 70 years.[91,92]

Although "angiodysplasia" has been reported in the adolescent patient, these have not been accompanied by corroborating pathologic evidence.[93] Bleeding from angiodysplasia is usually subacute and recurrent but it is massive in 15% of patients. The nature of the stool may vary from bright red bleeding, maroon stools to melena, and occasionally such variation may occur in a single patient. Iron deficiency anemia and stools that test intermittently positive for occult blood may be the mode of presentation in 10% to 15% of patients.[94] About 50% of patients with angiodysplasia have cardiac disease and there appears to be an association with aortic stenosis[91,95-97] although the relationship to gastrointestinal hemorrhage[98-100] is controversial. In a critique of the literature on the association between angiodysplasia and aortic stenosis, Imperiale and Ransouhoff[101] found significant methodologic flaws in the controlled studies that supported the association.

Venous Ectasias

Phlebectasias or venous ectasias differ from angiodysplasia clinically and pathologically. These consist of dilated submucosal veins usually with a thin overlying mucosa. They have a normal endothelial lining and are non-neoplastic. Endoscopically, they appear as bluish-red nodules. In the lower gastrointestinal tract, they occur mainly in the rectum. Small bowel phlebectasias[102] have also been reported. Multiple phlebectasia is a rare cause of bleeding and is usually asymptomatic.

Hamartoma

Hemangiomas are hamartomatous lesions and are characterized by increased cell turnover of endothelium, mast cells, fibroblasts, and macrophages resulting in a proliferation of blood vessels.[103] They are rarely malignant. Pathologically, they are divided into capillary, cavernous, and mixed forms. Cutaneous cavernous hemangiomas of the blue bleb nevus syndrome[104,105] can also affect the gastrointestinal tract. The gastrointestinal

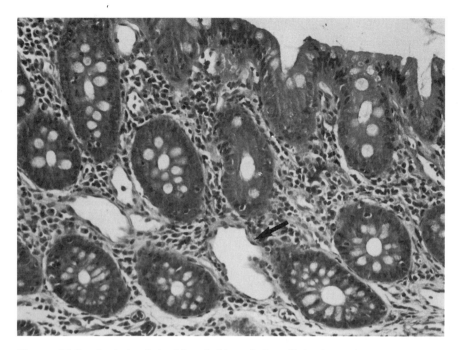

Figure 41-2. Angiodysplasia. Dilated, thin-walled capillaries (arrows) are present in the lamina propria between glands showing mild goblet cell depletion. There is no significant increase in the inflammatory cellular component of the lamina propria. (Picture courtesy of Dr. Jean Ho, Consultant Histopathologist.) (H&E ×20)

lesions manifest as intermittent rectal bleeding in childhood. Cavernous hemangioma of the gastrointestinal tract is an uncommon condition.[106] More than 200 cases have been reported in the world literature, of which half involve the rectum.[107] Recurrent bright red bleeding is the most prominent feature and is present in up to 90% of patients. Bleeding begins in adolescence and early adulthood.[108] Rectal examination may reveal a smooth compressible mass.[109] Endoscopic appearance is that of a bluish-red tumour.[110] Barium enema may show filling defects due to indentation of the bowel wall by the hemangioma. Multiple calcifications related to thrombosis within the tumor can be seen surrounding the bowel wall.[29,111,112] Computed tomography (CT) scan has been shown to reveal large vacuoles within a thickened mesentery.[29,113] Treatment for a bleeding colonic hemangioma is surgical resection.[114–116] If malignancy cannot be excluded segmental resection is the operation of choice. Local excision can be performed for benign tumors.[117] In the case of low rectal hemangiomas, abdominoperineal resection had been performed in the past,[118] although sphincter-saving procedures are possible in most cases. Resection with coloanal anastomosis[107,119] and rectal mucosectomy[120] have been used successfully for diffuse cavernous hemangiomas of the rectum. With the efficacious use of radiotherapy for hemangiomas at other sites, Chaimoff and Laurie[121] applied this technique for a low rectal hemangioma with complete remission.

Telangiectasia

Gastrointestinal telangiectasias tend to be diffuse, have a tendency to recur, and are associated with skin and mucous membrane lesions. They frequently occur as part of hereditary syndromes. These lesions differ from angiodysplasia in that the affected vessels are dilated through all layers of the bowel wall, not just the mucosa or submucosa as in angiodysplasia. Osler-Weber-Rendu syndrome or hereditary hemorrhagic telangiectasia[122,123] is inherited as an autosomal-dominant trait. It is characterized by discrete, red, small, superficial, punctate telangiectatic lesions on the skin or oronasopharyngeal mucous membrane. Epistaxis is the most common presenting symptom. Gastrointestinal bleeding occurs in about 15% of patients[6] and results from ulceration of telangiectatic lesions in the proximal small bowel and stomach. Turner's syndrome is also associated with gastrointestinal telangiectasis but bleeding occurs in less than 7% of patients.[124,125]

Connective Tissue Disorders

Connective tissue disorders such as Ehlers-Danlos syndrome may be associated with spontaneous arteriovenous malformations and can present with gastrointestinal hemorrhage.

DIAGNOSTIC ANGIOGRAPHY

Selective visceral angiography initially held the promise of demonstrating the site of bleeding[11,42,126] thereby avoiding blind extended colonic resections.[127] Using a modified Seldinger technique,[128] the superior and inferior mesenteric arteries and the celiac axis can be cannulated sequentially. Success rates of localization of bleeding in 69% to 87% of patients in an emergency setting have been reported.[11,126] Angiodysplasia demonstrates characteristic angiographic features such as a slowly emptying vein, vascular tuft, and early filling vein.[88]

Distinctions between bleeding from angiodysplasia and diverticular disease can be made with angiography resulting in appropriate treatment.[44,129,130]

Despite the success reported with the use of emergency angiography, the limitations are becoming apparent.[131] Poorer accuracy rates of between 40% and 60% have been reported even in experienced hands.[12,132,133] The efficacy of angiography is doubtful in centers that practice angiography infrequently.[134] Not surprisingly, angiography is seldom the primary investigation used for the diagnosis of lower gastrointestinal hemorrhage.[12]

The accuracy of diagnostic angiography depends on the presence of ongoing active hemorrhage. A bleeding rate of more than 0.5 to 1.0 ml/min[135,136] is required before angiography can demonstrate a source of hemorrhage. This makes the optimal timing for angiography difficult to judge. There are minute to minute variations in the rate of hemorrhage and this cannot be accurately determined by clinical assessment. The passage of a large amount of bloody stools may only represent an earlier episode of hemorrhage rather than active, ongoing bleeding. Further, only arterial or capillary bleeding can be detected by selective visceral angiography; venous bleeding is difficult to demonstrate.[44]

More recently, pharmacologic means have been used to precipitate or exacerbate bleeding in order to improve the diagnostic yield of angiography. Systemic heparinization, selective intra-arterial tolazoline vasodilatation, and thrombolytic agents such as streptokinase and urokinase have been used to prolong bleeding or induce recurrent bleeding.[3,137,138] Koval et al.[137] reported an increase of positive findings from 32% to 65% and a reduction of negative angiograms from 27% to 16% with the use of pharmacologic angiographic techniques. Major complications were rare in this small series. These methods may have a role in patients with continuing hemorrhage who have evaded previous expert attempts to localize the cause of bleeding.

Angiography has expanded its role in assisting localization of bleeding sites intraoperatively, particularly in the small bowel. Robertson and Gathright[139] have reported cannulation of segmental mesenteric vessel using a fine-bore needle and obtaining intraoperative angiograms of sequential segments. Fazio et al.[140] reported leaving the angiography catheter in-sites preoperatively and repeating the angiogram at surgery, marking the bowel with clips for easier localization. Methylene blue has been injected through an angiography catheter to stain the section of the bowel with an angiographically identified vascular malformation.[141,142] Lau et al.[141] have compared this with operative endoscopy and found the latter more precise, therefore allowing for a more limited resection.

THERAPEUTIC ANGIOGRAPHY

Localization of the bleeding point by selective angiographic catheterization can be followed by therapeutic maneuvers such as infusion of vasopressin or embolization. Vasopressin is a potent vasoconstrictor of smooth muscle especially of capillaries, arterioles, and venules. The efficacy of vasopressin in the treatment of gastrointestinal hemorrhage has been well reported.[42,137,138,143–147] Small intestinal hemorrhage is uncommon but has been reported to be controlled by selective intra-arterial vasopressin alone in 71% of patients.[145] Bleeding from

diverticular disease may be controlled by intra-arterial vasopressin in 80% to 90% of patients.[143–145] Massive lower gastrointestinal hemorrhage secondary to diverticular disease and arteriovenous malformations responded to intra-arterial vasopressin in 91% of patients in a large series.[42] There are side effects associated with the use of vasopressin, including hypertension, bradycardia, coronary vasoconstriction, bowel ischemia, peripheral vascular ischemia, and catheter-related thrombosis, plaque dislodgement, and sepsis with prolonged infusion.[148]

Initially, selective intra-arterial embolization was developed and used in patients in whom intra-arterial vasopressin therapy failed.[145,147,149–152] As experience with the use of this technique increased, embolization of bleeding sites with a variety of agents became the first choice for angiographic hemostasis.[148,149,153–157] Hemorrhage from small bowel causes may be better controlled by embolization than by vasopressin.[152] The major problems with performing embolization for colonic bleeding sites include ischemia and infarction leading to perforation. The rate of colonic infarction following embolization is approximately 15%.[152,155,157,158] There has been a report of colonic stricture formation following embolization in a patient who was bleeding from diverticular disease.[159]

In a recent series using a super-selectively placed catheter for delivering polyvinyl alcohol particles, no infarction occurred although two asymptomatic cases of mucosal ischemia were detected endoscopically.[160] Embolization at a super-selective site may cause less damage compared with vessel occlusion more proximally. The incidence of infarction may also be reduced by using the minimum of embolic particles to control the bleeding.[158] Therapeutic angiography may play a role in high-risk patients in whom surgery should be avoided or to allow surgery to be undertaken under elective conditions.

NUCLEAR MEDICINE TECHNIQUES

Two radioisotopic techniques have been found to be useful in the diagnosis of gastrointestinal bleeding. They include technetium(^{99m}Tc) sulfur colloid scintigraphy[161] and technetium-labeled red blood cell scintigraphy.[162] ^{99m}Tc sulfur colloid is rapidly cleared from the vascular space by the reticuloendothelial systems of the liver and spleen. It has the theoretical advantage of achieving better contrast between the background activity and the areas of extravasated radioisotope at the site of hemorrhage. Owing to the rapid clearance from the circulation, the patient must be actively bleeding at the time of the study for a positive result. In contrast, ^{99m}Tc-labeled red blood cells remain in the circulation longer and may produce a positive result on repeat scanning over 48 hours. It is useful in patients with intermittent bleeding and patients with bleeding but with low transfusion requirements.[163]

The disadvantage of ^{99m}Tc-labeled red blood cell scintigraphy is the necessity for repeated imaging and the inconvenience of the labeling procedure. Despite these limitations, most centers prefer ^{99m}Tc-labeled red cell scans over ^{99m}Tc sulfur colloid scans[164] given the intermittent nature of most lower gastrointestinal hemorrhage and the necessity for timing the latter during a period of hemorrhage.

The sensitivity of radioisotope scans appears to be greater than that of arteriography with many series reporting rates of over 90%.[165-168] Although the sensitivity of detecting hemorrhage appears high, there is concern about the radioisotope scan ability to localize bleeding sites accurately. Hunter and Pezim[169] studied patients who underwent ^{99m}Tc-labeled red cell scans for lower gastrointestinal hemorrhage and compared the result with the true site of bleeding determined by arteriography and surgery. The radioisotope scan was correct in the localization of a specific bleeding site in only 41% of patients. In 19 patients who underwent a surgical procedure directed by the radionuclide scan, 8 (42%) had incorrect procedures performed. Ryan et al.[170] reported in a recent review that ^{99m}Tc red blood cell scan localized the site of severe colonic bleeding in less than one-half of the patients whose site was confirmed by other means. Similarly, Bentley and Richardson[171] reported that ^{99m}Tc red blood cell tagged scans localized the site of bleeding in only 52% cases.

COLONOSCOPY

Colonoscopy has been used in the diagnosis of acute lower gastrointestinal hemorrhage for the past 25 years.[172] Initial experience established its use in patients with intermittent bleeding,[173,174] but its use in patients with massive bleeding was doubtful because of inadequate visualization of the entire colonic mucosa.[175,176]

Diagnostic success improved with the introduction of a pulsatile irrigation system[177] and the use of large-bore suction channels and fluoroscopic control.[178] More recently, the use of oral polyethylene glycol and sulfate purges has led to further enhancement of the yield of colonoscopy for diagnosis and therapy.[2,12,177,179-182] Fears that colonic lavage or irrigation would dislodge adherent clots and precipitate rebleeding are unfounded.[2,181] Jensen and Machiado[2] evaluated 80 consecutive patients with severe ongoing, lower gastrointestinal hemorrhage with colonoscopy after a saline or sulfate purge. They were able to identify lesions in all but 6% of patients. Similarly, whole gut irrigation is another approach to bowel preparation prior to emergency colonoscopy.[183] Treate and Forde[184] found that actual visualization of the bleeding vessel, the presence of fresh blood in a specific segment without blood proximal to it, and an adherent clot were all reliable signs of bleeding from a specific segment. There were no misleading diagnoses in patients with any of these three findings. The absence of these findings at the time of colonoscopy led to a 10% to 20% rate of inaccuracy.

The incidence of colonic angiomata causing severe bleeding appears to have increased after the use of oral purgative prior to colonoscopy.[2] Colonoscopy was the only modality to establish the diagnosis of angiodysplasia in 12% of patients and confirmed arteriography findings in a series reported by Max et al.[185] The use of colonoscopy in the management of angiodysplasia provides the opportunity for treatment with sclerotherapy, electrocoagulation, and laser therapy.[90,94,186-194] Steger et al.[195] warned that 22% of patients with known vascular lesions may be bleeding from other sites. The only way to be certain that the vascular lesion is the cause of bleeding is the observation of actual bleeding from the lesion. This warning has been echoed by Marx et al.[196]

The approach to bleeding diverticulosis has also been modified by colonoscopy. In a report of 100 consecutive patients,

17% had a diverticulum identified as the bleeding site on the basis of one of the following criteria: active bleeding from a single diverticulum, a nonbleeding visible vessel, and an adherent clot resistant to washing.[197] The same authors note that 73% of their patients with diverticulosis had a nondiverticular site of bleeding.[198] Patients with bleeding from a diverticulum may be treated by bipolar electrocoagulation[181] as well as the topical application of adrenaline solution.[199]

A "colonoscopy first" strategy in the management of patients with acute lower gastrointestinal hemorrhage has been advocated by several authors.[2,12,198,200] A definitive diagnostic rate of approximately 90%, the opportunity for therapy in up to 50% of patients, and a shorter hospital stay are cited as advantages.[12,198] This approach also enables the colonoscopic surgeon to be in direct control of the situation and lessens dependence on other services that may not be available in a bleeding emergency.

Provided that a reasonable degree of expertise is available in performing colonscopy, angiography, and nuclear medicine scanning, a useful algorithm for the management of acute lower gastrointestinal hemorrhage can be developed. (Fig. 41-3). First, bleeding diathesis should be excluded or identified. Although gastrointestinal hemorrhage in patients with a bleeding diathesis usually arises from a mucosal lesion,[201] it has been observed that the likelihood of diagnosing a remediable lesion decreases with a prolongation of prothrombin time.[13,14] An upper gastrointestinal cause of bleeding should then be identified with nasogastric aspiration or by esophagogastroduodenoscopy. Bleeding from an anorectal lesion must not be missed as these are easily identified by proctosigmoidoscopy.

MANAGEMENT OF BLEEDING

Assessment

Subsequently, management is dependent on the magnitude and progression of the bleeding. Patients with major ongoing bleeding should first be resuscitated before being subjected to diagnostic procedures. The investigation of choice in both patients with major, ongoing bleeding as well as minor, intermittent bleeding would be colonoscopy following an oral purge. The lesion should then be evaluated for the possible endoscopic therapy or definitive surgical treatment. Failure to identify a lesion will then necessitate the use of a second diagnostic modality. In patients with intermittent bleeding requiring fewer than two units of blood transfusion, radioisotope scanning should be the next investigation. In patients with a more rapid, ongoing hemorrhage, emergency angiography should be performed. If a bleeding site is identified, transcatheter therapy with intra-arterial vasopressin or embolization should be considered based on the physical state of the patient and the nature of the lesion. If no bleeding site is identified, consideration should be given to the use of pharmacoangiography with intravenous heparin, intra-arterial tolazoline, or urokinase.

Failure to identify a bleeding site by radioisotope scanning or angiography should lead to expectant management in patients who have elective conditions. If bleeding continues to be rapid and no bleeding site is identified by colonoscopy, radioisotope scanning, or angiography, emergency surgery is required. Intraoperative maneuvers such as antegrade irrigation with on-table

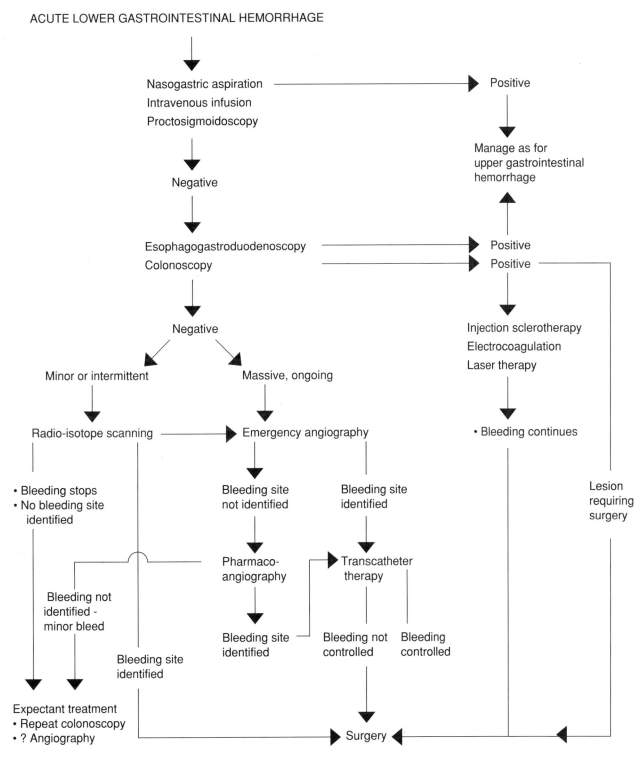

Figure 41-3. Management algorithm for acute lower gastrointestinal hemorrhage.

Table 41-1. Mortality and Rebleeding After Surgery for Lower Gastrointestinal Hemorrhage

Author	Blind Subtotal Colectomy			Directed Segmental Resection		
	No. of Patients	Mortality	Rebleed	No. of Patients	Mortality	Rebleed
Leitman et al., 1989[132]	5	2	0	23	3	1
Britt et al., 1983[203]	10	2	0	14	2	1
Browder et al., 1986[42]	18	4	4	17	0	0
Collachio et al., 1982[22]	12	4	1	46	10	5
Welch et al., 1978[91]	10	1	0	42	1	4

colonoscopy and enteroscopy should be used in order to achieve a precise, limited colorectal resection as opposed to blind extended total colectomy.

Surgical Treatment

If the bleeding point can be identified by angiography, radioisotope scanning, or colonoscopy, the appropriate therapy can be selected depending on the nature of the lesion and the clinical course. If surgery is required, a preoperatively identified bleeding point may lead to a directed,[22,42,44,91,132,202-204] as opposed to a blind segmental resection[9,10] or subtotal colectomy.[9,10,22,42,132,203]

The mortality and rebleeding rates from directed segmental resections have been compared with subtotal colectomy.[22,42,132,203,204] Mortality rates are significantly lower although rebleeding rates are approximately similar (Table 41-1).

Wright et al.[202] reported that 85% of patients with blood loss estimated at 1,500 ml or greater in the first 24 hours of hospitalization went on to surgery. In the patient who continues to bleed in whom the bleeding point has not been identified, intraoperative colonoscopy and enteroscopy has been advocated.[134,141,205-209] Preoperative preparation with enemas or routine methods is undertaken in patients in whom bleeding is inactive. For those with rapid, ongoing bleeding, on-table lavage is necessary.

The patient is placed in the Lloyd-Davies position and through a long midline incision, a laparotomy is performed. If an obvious source of bleeding is not present, an appendicostomy is performed and a Foley catheter inserted into the appendix stump. Normal saline is infused in the manner described for antegrade on-table lavage.[210] A large-bore proctoscope or suction tubing may be used in the anus to facilitate drainage and collection of the effluent. Once the colon is cleared, a colonoscope can be inserted through the anus and passed up through

the rectum and colon until the bleeding point is found. A large portion of the small intestine may also be visualized this way.

Excessive handling of the bowel is to be avoided as this may cause petechial hemorrhage giving rise to diagnostic confusion. If a lesion in the small bowel is suspected, a colonoscope may be passed orally. After the colonoscope is negotiated past the ligament of Trietz, the abdominal operators can assist the progress of the scope by manipulating the bowel over the tip of the instrument. Dimming the operating and room lights allows for better transillumination of the bowel wall. Dilated tortuous vessels, angioectatic blushing, ulcers, small tumors, and other lesions may be visualized.

Previously advocated methods such as multiple colotomies,[211,212] multiple applications of noncrushing clamps to observe segments for distension with blood,[213] and construction of a transverse colostomy to see if bleeding is from the right or left colon[214] are obsolete and probably have no place in modern surgical practice.

In the rare situation where the surgeon is operating on a patient with an unidentified bleeding site, the decision to perform a right, left, or subtotal colectomy has not been clearly addressed in the literature. Two studies[9,10] that attempted to answer this question were performed at a time when right-sided angiodysplasia was not widely recognized and many of the cases of massive lower gastrointestinal hemorrhage were ascribed rightly or wrongly to diverticular disease (Table 41-2). Milewski and Schofield[215] argued that a right hemicolectomy was the operation of choice when the bleeding site was not localized but "clues" to right-sided pathology were present. Such clues include nonbleeding lesions seen on angiography or colonoscopy, fresh blood on the right side at colonoscopy, and cecal thickening or abnormal serosal vessels at laparotomy. A subtotal colectomy is our operation of choice when the bleeding site cannot be localized after all preoperative and intraoperative investigations have been attempted. Extending surgery

Table 41-2. Mortality and Rebleeding After "Blind" Resections for Lower Gastrointestinal Hemorrhage

Author	Blind Segmental Resection			Blind Subtotal Colectomy		
	No. of Patients	Mortality	Rebleed	No. of Patients	Mortality	Rebleed
McGuire et al., 1972[9]	5	1	2	4	2	0
Drapnas et al., 1973[10]	23	7	8	35	4	0

from a right hemicolectomy to include the left colon does not take a great deal of additional time. The potential gain of a reduction in the rebleeding rate is worth the minimal increase in operative risk. However, the risk of diarrhea and incontinence in elderly patients should be borne in mind when considering subtotal colectomy.

REFERENCES

1. Stower MJ, Hardcastle JD, Bourke JB (1984) Surgical emergencies and manpower. Ann R Coll Surg Engl 66:117–119

2. Jensen DM, Machiado GA (1988) Diagnosis and treatment of severe haematochezia—the role of colonoscopy after purge. Gastroenterology 95:1569–1574

3. Rollins ES, Picus D, Hicks ME et al (1991) Angiography is useful in detecting the source of chronic gastrointestinal bleeding of obscure origin. AJR 156:385–388

4. Jensen DM (1995) Current management of severe lower gastrointestinal bleeding. Gastrointest Endosc 41:171–173

5. Spiller RC, Parkins RA (1983) Recurrent gastrointestinal bleeding of obscure origin: report on 17 cases and a guide to logical management. Br J Surg 70:489–493

6. Thompson JN, Salem RR, Hemingway AP et al (1987) Specialist investigation of obscure gastrointestinal bleeding. Gut 28:47–51

7. Berry AR, Campbell WB, Kettlewell MGW (1988) Management of major colonic hemorrhage. Br J Surg 75:637–640

8. Reinus JF, Brandt LJ (1994) Vascular ectasias and diverticulosis. Common causes of lower intestinal bleeding. Gastroenterol Clin North Am 23:1–20

9. McGuire HH, Haynes BW (1992) Massive hemorrhage from diverticular disease of the colon: guideline for therapy based on bleeding patterns in 50 cases. Am Surg 175:847–853

10. Drapnas T, Pennington DG, Kappeiman M et al (1973) Emergency subtotal colectomy. Preferred approach to management to massively bleeding diverticular disease. Ann Surg 177:519–525

11. Baum S, Nusbaum M, Blakemore WS, Finkelstein AK (1965) The operative radiography demonstration of intra-abdominal bleeding from undetermined sites by percutaneous selective celiac and superior mesenteric arteriography. Surgery 58:797–805

12. Richter JM, Christensen MR, Kaplan LM, Nishioka NS (1995) Effectiveness of current technology in the diagnosis and management of lower gastrointestinal hemorrhage. Gastrointest Endosc 41:93–98

13. Landefeld CS, Rosenblatt MW, Goldman L (1989) Bleeding in outpatients treated with wartarin: relation of prothrombin time and important remediable lesions. Am J Med 87:153–159

14. Wilcox OM, Truss CD (1988) Gastrointestinal bleeding in patients receiving long-term anticoagulant therapy. Am J Med 84:683–690

15. Schwartz HA (1981) Lower gastrointestinal side effects of non-steroidal anti-inflammatory drugs. J Rheumatol 8:952–954

16. Levinson SL, Powell DW, Callahan WT et al (1981) A current approach to rectal bleeding. J Clin Gastroenterol, suppl. 3:9–16

17. Lee P, Sutherland D, Feller ER (1994) Massive gastrointestinal bleeding as the initial manifestation of pancreatic carcinoma. Int J Pancreatol 15:223–227

18. Wu TK, Zaman SN, Gullick HD et al (1977) Spontaneous hemorrhage due to pseudocysts of the pancreas. Am J Surg 134:408–410

19. Lam AY, Bricker RS (1975) Pancreatic pseudocyst with hemorrhage into the gastrointestinal tract through the duct of Wirsung. Am J Surg 129:694–695

20. Wilson SE, Owens ML (1976) Aorto-colic fistula. A lethal cause of lower gastrointestinal bleeding: report of a case. Dis Colon Rectum 19:614–617

21. Reckless JPP, McColl J, Taylor GW (1972) Aorto-enteric fistula: an uncommon complication of abdominal aortic aneurysm. Br J Surg 59:458–460

22. Collachio TA, Forde KA, Patsos TJ, Nunez D (1982) Impact of modern diagnostic methods on the management of active rectal bleeding. Am J Surg 143:607–610

23. Lacey Smith J (1984) Approaches to the problem of lower gastrointestinal bleeding. Compr Ther 10:43–50

24. Delancey H, Hitch WS (1974) Solitary rectal ulcer: a cause of life-threatening hemorrhage. Surgery 76:830–832

25. Haycock CE, Suryanarayan G, Spiller CR et al (1983) Massive hemorrhage from benign solitary rectal ulcer of the rectum. Am J Gastroenterol 78:83–85

26. Seow-Choen F, Goh HS, Eu KW et al (1993) A simple and effective treatment for haemorrhagic radiation proctitis using formalin. Dis Colon Rectum 36:135–138

27. Viggiano TR, Zhigelbouis J, Ahlquist DA et al (1993) Endoscopic Nd:YAG laser coagulation of bleeding from radiation proctopathy. Gastrointest Endosc 39:513–517

28. Gilinsky NH, Burns DG, Barbezat GO et al (1983) The natural history of radiation-induced procto-sigmoiditis: an analysis of 88 patients. Q J Med 52:40–53

29. Bortz JH (1994) Diffuse cavernous haemangioma of the rectum and sigmoid. Abdom Imaging 19:18–20

30. Poggioli G, Marchetti F, Senei S et al (1993) Colo-anal anastomosis with colonic reservoir for cavernous haemangioma of the rectum. Hepatogastroenterology 40:279–281

31. Telander RL, Ahlquist D, Blaufum MC (1993) Rectal mucosectomy: a definitive approach to haemangiomas of the rectum. J Paediatr Surg 28:379–381

32. Abdulian JD, Santoro MJ, Chen YK, Collen MJ (1993) Dieulafoy-like lesion of the rectum presenting with exsanguinating haemorrhage: successful endoscopic sclerotherapy. Am J Gastroenterol 88:1939–1941

33. Franko E, Chardovoyne R, Wise L (1991) Massive rectal bleeding from a Dieulafoy's type ulcer in the rectum: a review of this unusual disease. Am J Gastroenterol 86:1545–1547

34. Barbier D, Luder P, Triller J et al (1985) Colonic haemorrhage from a solitary minute ulcer. Gastroenterology 88:1065–1068

35. Ma CK, Padda H, Pace EH et al (1989) Submucosal arterial malformation of the colon with massive haemorrhage. Report of a case. Dis Colon Rectum 32:149–152

36. Richards WO, Grove-Maloney D, Williams LF (1988) Haem-

orrhage from a Dieulafoy-type ulcer of the colon: a new cause of lower gastrointestinal bleeding. Am Surg 54:121–124

37. Matuchansky C, Babin P, Abadie JC et al (1978) Jejunal bleeding from a solitary large submucosal artery: report of two cases. Gastroenterology 75:110–113

38. Chen KTK (1985) Intestinal bleeding from a caliber-persistent submucosal artery in the ileum. J Clin Gastroenterol 7:289–291

39. Juler GL, Labitzke HG, Lamb R et al (1984) The pathogenesis of Dieulafoy's gastric erosion. Am J Gastroenterol 79:195–200

40. Makela JT, Kivinerui H, Laitenen S et al (1993) Diagnosis and treatment of acute lower gastrointestinal bleeding. Scand J Gastroenterol 28:1062–1066

41. Boley SJ, Di Biase A, Brandt LJ et al (1979) Lower intestinal bleeding in the elderly. Am J Surg 137:57–64

42. Browder W, Cerise EJ, Litwin MS (1986) Impact of emergency angiography in massive lower gastrointestinal bleeding. Ann Surg 204:530–536

43. Quinn WC (1961) Gross hemorrhage from presumed diverticulosis of the colon. Ann Surg 153:851–860

44. Casarella WJ, Karter IE, Seamen WB (1972) Right-sided colonic diverticula as a cause of acute rectal hemorrhage. N Engl J Med 296:450–453

45. Lewis EE, Schnug GE (1972) Importance of angiography in the management of massive hemorrhage from colonic diverticula. Am J Surg 124:573–580

46. Meyers MA, Alonso DR, Gray GF et al (1976) Pathogenesis of bleeding diverticulosis. Gastroenterology 71:577–583

47. Noer RJ, Hamilton JE, Williams DJ, Broughton DS (1962) Rectal hemorrhage:moderate and severe. Ann Surg 155:794–805

48. Leber RE, Hume HA (1966) Endometriosis requiring colonoscopy and resection: a case report and review of the literature. Am J Proctol 17:380–387

49. Levitt MD, Hodby J, VanMerwyk AJ, Glancy RJ (1989) Cyclical rectal bleeding in colorectal endometriosis. Aust NZ J Surg 59:941–943

50. Athmanathan N, Sehdev VK, Walsh TH (1990) Endometriosis of the sigmoid colon: a diagnostic problem. Br J Clin Pract 44:658–660

51. Eyers T, Morgan B, Bignold L (1978) Endometriosis of the sigmoid colon and rectum. Aust NZ J Surg 45:639–643

52. Bozdech JM (1992) Endoscopic diagnosis of colonic endometriosis. Gastrointest Endosc 38:568–570

53. Seow-Choen F, Goh HS (1993) Massive bleeding from an ectopic pregnancy. Ann Acad Med 21:818–820

54. Gudjonsson H, Zeiler D, Gamelli RL et al (1986) Colonic varices: report of an unusual case diagnosed by radionuclide scanning with review of the literature. Gastroenterology 91:1543–1547

55. Orozco N, Takahashi T, Mercado MA et al (1992) Colorectal variceal bleeding in patients with extrahepatic portal vein thrombosis and idiopathic portal hypertension. J Clin Gastroenterol 14:139–143

56. Beermann EM, Lagaay MB, VanNouhuys JM, Overbosch D (1988) Familial varices of the colon. Endoscopy 20:270–271

57. Boley SJ, Brandt LJ, Mitusudo SM (1984) Vascular lesions of the colon. Adv Intern Med 29:301–326

58. Robert JH, Sachar DB, Aufses AH Jr, Greenstein AJ (1990) Management of severe hemorrhage in ulcerative colitis. Am J Surg 159:550–555

59. Boley SJ, Brandt LJ, Frank MS (1981) Severe lower intestinal bleeding: diagnosis and treatment. Clin Gastroenterol 10:65–91

60. Ciccarelli O, Coley GM (1986) Massive rectal bleeding in Crohn's colitis. Conn Med J 50:301–303

61. Corona FE, Dyck WP (1973) Massive gastrointestinal hemorrhage as the sole manifestation of regional enteritis. Am J Dig Dis 18:1001–1004

62. Abel ME, Russell TR (1983) Ischaemic colitis: comparison of surgical and non-operative management. Dis Colon Rectum 26:113–115

63. Mee AS, Shield M, Burke M (1985) Campylobacter colitis—differentiation from acute inflammatory bowel disease. J R Soc Med 78:217–223

64. Stoll BJ, Glass LRI, Huq MI et al (1982) Obscure causes of lower gastrointestinal bleeding. BMJ 285:1185–1188

65. Blaser MJ, Parson RB, Lou-Wang (1980) Acute colitis caused by Campylobacter fetus ss. jejuni. Gastroenterology 78:448–453

66. Butzler JP, Skirrow MB (1979) Campylobacter colitis. Clin Gastroenterol 20:141–148

67. Pai H, Gordon RR, Sims H, Bryan LE (1984) Sporadic cases of haemorrhagic colitis associated with Escherichia coli 0157:H7. Ann Intern Med 101:738–742

68. Seow-Choen F, Chua CL, Kee SG, Ng BK (1989) Gastrointestinal tuberculosis presenting as massive melena. Asian J Surg 12:17–19

69. Miller LS, Barbarevech C, Friedman LS (1994) Less frequent causes of lower gastrointestinal bleeding. Gastroenterol Clin North Am 23:21–52

70. Wilcox RD, Shatney CH (1988) Massive bleeding from jejunal diverticula. South Med J 81:1386–1391

71. Krishnamurthy S, Kelly M, Rohrmann C et al (1983) Jejunal diverticulosis: a heterogenous disorder caused by a variety of abnormalities of the smooth muscle or myenteric plexus. Gastroenterology 85:538–547

72. Elsenberg D, Sherwood CE (1975) Bleeding Meckel's diverticulum diagnosed by arteriography and radio-isotope imaging. Dig Dis 20:573–576

73. Ghahremani GG (1986) Radiology of Meckel's diverticulum. Crit Dev Diagn Imaging 26:1–43

74. Wong TY, Enriquez RE, Modlin IM et al (1990) Recurrent hemorrhage from an invaginated Meckel's diverticulum in a 78 year old man. Am J Gastroenterol 85:195–198

75. Duzynski DO, Jewett TC, Allen JE (1971) Tc 99m pertechnetate scanning of the abdomen with particular reference to small bowel pathology. AJR 113:258–262

76. Cabal E, Holtz S (1971) Polyarteritis as a cause of intestinal hemorrhage. Gastroenterology 61:99–105

77. Harvey MH, Neoptoplemos JP, Fossard DP (1984) Abdominal polyarteritis nodosa—a possible surgical pitfall? Br J Clin Pract 38:282–283

78. Lopez LR, Schocket AL, Standford RE et al (1980) Gastrointestinal involvement in leucocytoclastic vasculitis and polyarteritis nodosa. J Rheumatol 7:677–684

79. Goldman LP, Lindenberger RL (1981) Henoch-Schoenlein purpura: gastrointestinal manifestations with endoscopic correlation. Am J Gastroenterol 75:357–360

80. Gore RM, Marn CS, Ujiki GT et al (1983) Ischaemic colitis associated with systemic lupus erythematosus. Dis Colon Rectum 26:449–451

81. Phillips B (1839) Letter to the editor. London M Gaz 1:514

82. Gentry RW, Dockety MB, Clagett OT (1949) Vascular malformations and vascular tumours of the gastrointestinal tract. Int Abstr Surg 88:281–323

83. Stewart WB, Gathright JB Jr, Ray JE (1979) Vascular ectasias of the colon. Surg Gynecol Obstet 148:670–674

84. Wolff KD, Grossman MB, Shinya H (1977) Angiodysplasia of the colon: diagnosis and treatment. Gastroenterology 72:329–333

85. Rees HC (1992) Vascular disease of the small and large intestine. pp. 1208–1209. In McGee James O'D, Isaacson PG, Wright NA (eds): Oxford Textbook of Pathology. Vol.2a. Oxford University Press, London

86. Boley SJ, Sammartano R, Adams A et al (1977) On the nature and etiology of vascular ectasias of the colon. Gastroenterology 72:650–660

87. Athanasoulis CA, Galdabini JJ, Waltman AC et al (1977–1978) Angiodysplasia of the colon: a cause of rectal bleeding. Cardiovasc Radiol 1:3–13

88. Boley SJ, Sprayregen S, Sammartano RJ et al (1974) The pathophysiologic basis for the angiographic signs of vascular ectasias of the colon. Radiology 125:615–621

89. Foutch PG, Rex DK, Lieberman DA (1995) Prevalence and natural history of colonic angiodysplasia among healthy asymptomatic people. Am J Gastroenterol 90:564–567

90. Hochter W, Weingart J, Kuhner W et al (1985) Angiodysplasia in the colon and rectum. Endoscopic morphology, localization and frequency. Endoscopy 17:182–185

91. Welch CE, Athanasoulis CA, Galdabini JJ (1978) Hemorrhage of the large bowel with special reference to angiodysplasias and diverticula disease. World J Surg 2:357–368

92. Boley SJ, Sammartano R, Brandt LJ, Sprayregen S (1979) Vascular ectasias of the colon. Surg Gynecol Obstet 149:353–358

93. Hemingway AP, Allison DJ (1982) Angiodysplasia and Meckel's diverticulum: a congenital association? BMJ 69:493–496

94. Boley SJ, Brandt LJ (1986) Vascular ectasias of the colon—1986. Dig Dis Sci suppl. 31:26S–42S

95. Ross EG, Rozenbaum JM (1971) Bleeding from the right colon associated with aortic stenosis. Am J Dig Dis 16:269–276

96. Greenstein RJ, McElhinney AJ, Reuben D, Greenstein AJ (1986) Colonic vascular ectasias and aortic stenosis: coincidence or causal relationship? Am J Surg 151:347–351

97. Weaver GA, Alpern HD, Davis JS et al (1979) Gastrointestinal angiodysplasia associated with aortic valve disease: part of a spectrum of angiodysplasia of the gut. Gastroenterology 77:1–11

98. Heyde EC (1988) Gastrointestinal bleeding in aortic stenosis. N Engl J Med 259:196–198

99. Love JW, Jahnke EJ, Zacharias D et al (1980) Calcific aortic stenosis and gastrointestinal bleeding. N Engl J Med 302:968

100. Shbeeb I, Prager E, Love J (1984) The aortic valve—colonic axis. Dis Colon Rectum 27:38–41

101. Imperiale TF, Ransohoff DF (1988) Aortic stenosis, idiopathic gastrointestinal bleeding and angiodysplasia: is there an association? A methodologic critique of the literature. Gastroenterology 950:1670–1676

102. Peoples J, Kartha R, Sharf S (1981) Multiple phlebectasia of the small intestine. Am Surg 47:313–376

103. Mulliken JB, Glowacki J (1982) Haemangiomas and vascular malformations of infants and children: a clarification based on endothelial characteristics. Plast Reconstr Surg 69:412–420

104. Oranje AP (1986) Blue rubber bleb nevus syndrome. Pediatr Dermatol 3:304–310

105. Golitz L (1980) Heritable cutaneous disorders that affect the gastrointestinal tract. Med Clin North Am 64:829–846

106. Ghahremani GG, Kangarloo H, Volberg F, Meyers MA (1976) Diffuse cavernous haemangioma of the colon in Klippel-Trenaunay syndrome. Radiology 118:673–678

107. Wang CH (1985) Sphincter-saving procedure for treatment of diffuse cavernous haemangioma of the rectum and the sigmoid colon. Dis Colon Rectum 28:604–607

108. Valette FN (1970) Cavernous haemangioma of the rectum. Dis Colon Rectum 13:344–345

109. Parker GW, Nurney JA, Kendyer WL (1960) Cavernous haemangioma of the rectum and rectosigmoid. Dis Colon Rectum 3:358–363

110. Skovgaard S, Sorensen FH (1976) Bleeding haemangioma of the colon diagnosed by colonoscopy. J Pediatr Surg 11:83–84

111. Bailey TJ, Barrick CW, Jenkinson EL (1956) Haemangioma of the colon. JAMA 160:658

112. Hollingsworth G (1951) Haemangiomatous lesions of the colon. Br J Radiol 24:220

113. Aylward CA, Orangio GR, Lucas GW, Fazio VW (1988) Diffuse cavernous haemangioma of the rectosigmoid: CT scan a new diagnostic modality and surgical treatment using sphincter saving procedures: a report of 3 cases. Dis Colon Rectum 31:797–802

114. Coppa GF, Localio SA (1984) Surgical management of diffuse cavernous haemangioma of the colon, rectum and anus. Surg Gynecol Obstet 159:17–22

115. Lyon DT, Mantia AG (1984) Large bowel haemangiomas. Dis Colon Rectum 27:404–414

116. Pontecorvo C, Lombardi C, Mottola L et al (1983) Haemangiomas of the large bowel: report of a case. Dis Colon Rectum 26:818–820

117. Head HD, Baker JQ, Muir RW (1973) Haemangioma of the colon. Am J Surg 126:691–694

118. Hellstrom J, Hultborn KA, Engelstedt L (1955) Diffuse haemangioma of the rectum. Acta Clin Scand 109:277–283

119. Poggioli G, Marchetti F, Seneri S et al (1993) Colo-anal anastomosis with colonic reservoir for cavernous haemangioma of the rectum. Hepatogastroenterology 40:279–281

120. Telander RL, Ahlquist D, Blaufuss MC (1993) Rectal mucosectomy: a definitive approach to extensive haemangioma of the rectum. J Pediatr Surg 28:379–381

121. Chaimoff C, Laurie H (1978) Haemangioma of the rectum. Clinical appearance and treatment. Dis Colon Rectum 21:295–296

122. Russell Smith C, Bartholomew LC, Cain JC (1963) Hereditary haemorrhagic telangiectasia and gastrointestinal hemorrhage. Gastroenterol 44:1–6

123. Jacobson G, Krause V (1970) Hereditary haemorrhagic telangiectasia localized to the gastrointestinal tract. Scand J Gastroenterol 5:283–288

124. Haddad H, Wilkins L (1959) Congenital anomalies associated with gonadal aplasia: review of 53 cases. Pediatrics 23: 885–902

125. Engel E, Forbes A (1965) Cytogenetic and clinical findings in 48 patients with congenitally defective or absent ovaries. Medicine 44:135–164

126. Allison DJ, Hemingway AP, Cunnigham DA (1982) Angiography in gastrointestinal bleeding. Lancet 11:30–33

127. Talman EA, Dixon DS, Gutirerrez FE (1979) Role of arteriography in rectal hemorrhage due to arteriovenous malformations and diverticulosis. Ann Surg 190:203–213

128. Seldinger SI (1953) Catheter replacement of needle in percutaneous arteriography: new technique. Acta Radiol 39: 368–376

129. Shapiro MJ (1994) The role of the radiologist in the management of gastrointestinal bleeding. Gastroenterol Clin North Am 23:123–181

130. Reinher E, Sonnenfeld T (1986) Angiodysplasia of the colon requiring emergency surgery. Acta Clin Scand Suppl 530: 61–62

131. Ng BL, Thompson JN, Adam A et al (1987) Selective visceral angiography in obscure postoperative gastrointestinal bleeding. Ann R Coll Surg Engl 69:237–240

132. Leitman IM, Paull DE, Shires GT (1989) Evaluation and management of massive lower gastrointestinal hemorrhage. Ann Surg 209:175–180

133. Uden P, Jiborn H, Jonsson K (1986) Influence of selective mesenteric angiography on the outcome of surgery for massive lower gastrointestinal hemorrhage: a 15 year experience. Dis Colon Rectum 29:561–566

134. Cussons PD, Berry AR (1989) Comparison of the value of emergency mesenteric angiography and intra-operative colonoscopy with antegrade colonic irrigation in massive rectal hemorrhage. J R Coll Surg Edin 34:91–93

135. Van der Vliet AH, Kalff V, Sacharias N, Kelly MJ (1985) The role of contrast angiography in gastrointestinal bleeding with the advent of technectium labelled red blood cell scans. Australs Radiol 29:29–45

136. Baum S (1982) Angiography of the gastrointestinal bleeder. Radiology 143:569–572

137. Koval G, Benner KG, Rosch J et al (1987) Aggressive angiographic diagnosis in acute lower gastrointestinal hemorrhage. Dig Dis Sci 32:248–253

138. Rösch J, Keller FS, Wawrukiewicz AS et al (1982) Pharmaco-angiography in the diagnosis of recurrent massive lower gastrointestinal bleeding. Radiology 145:615–619

139. Robertson HD, Gathright JB (1985) The technique of intraoperative segmental artery angiography to localize vascular ectasias. Dis Colon Rectum 28:274–278

140. Fazio VW, Zelas P, Weakly FL (1980) Intraoperative angiography and the localization of bleeding from the small intestine. Surg Gynecol Obstet 151:637–640

141. Lau WY, Wong SY, Ngan H et al (1988) Intraoperative localization of bleeding small intestinal lesions. Br J Surg 75: 249–251

142. Athanasoulis CA, Moncure AC, Greenfield AJ et al (1980) Intraoperative localization of small bowel bleeding sites with combined use of angiographic methods and methylene blue injection. Surgery 87:77–84

143. Baum S, Rösch J, Dotter CT et al (1973) Selective mesenteric arterial infusion in the management of massive diverticular hemorrhage. N Engl J Med 288:1269–1272

144. Athanasoulis CA, Baum S, Rosch J et al (1975) Mesenteric arterial infusions of vasopressin for hemorrhage from colonic diverticulosis. Am J Surg 129:212–216

145. Clark RA, Colley DP, Eggers FM (1981) Acute arterial gastrointestinal hemorrhage: efficacy of transcatheter control. AJR 136:1185–1189

146. Rösch J, Dotter CW, Rose RW (1971) Selective arterial infusions of vasoconstrictors in acute gastrointestinal bleeding. Radiology 99:27–36

147. Waltman AC (1980) Transcatheter embolization versus vasopressin infusion for the control of arteriocapillary gastrointestinal bleeding. Cardiovasc Intervent Radiol 3:289

148. Gomes AS, Lois JF, McCoy RD (1986) Angiographic treatment of gastrointestinal hemorrhage: comparison of vasopressin infusions and embolization. AJR 146:1031–1037

149. Rösch J, Dotter CT, Brown MJ (1972) Selective arterial embolization: a new method for acute gastrointestinal bleeding. Radiology 102:303–306

150. Bookstein JJ, Naderi MJ, Walter JF (1978) Transcatheter embolization for lower gastrointestinal bleeding. Radiology 127: 345–349

151. Goldberger LE, Bookstein JJ (1977) Transcatheter embolization for treatment of diverticular hemorrhage. Radiology 122: 613–617

152. Walker WJ, Goldin AR, Shaff MI, Allibore GW (1980) Per catheter control of hemorrhage from the superior and inferior mesenteric arteries. Clin Radiol 31:71–80

153. Encarnion CE, Kadir S, Beam CA, Payne CS (1992) Gastrointestinal bleeding: treatment with gastrointestinal arterial embolization. Radiology 183:505–508

154. Guy GE, Shetty PC, Sharma RP et al (1992) Acute lower gastrointestinal hemorrhage: treatment by superselective embolization with polyvinyl alcohol particles. 159:521–526

155. Lawler G, Bircher M, Spencer J et al (1985) Embolization in colonic bleeding. Br J Radiol 58:83–84

156. Palmaz JC, Walter JF, Cho KJ (1984) Therapeutic embolization of small bowel arteries. Radiology 152:377–382

157. Uflacker R (1987) Transcatheter embolization for treatment of acute lower gastrointestinal bleeding. Acta Radiol 28: 425–430

158. Rosenkrartz H, Bookstein JJ, Rosen RJ et al (1982) Post embolic colonic infarction. Radiology 142:47–51

159. Mitty HA, Efremidis S, Keller RJ (1979) Colonic stricture after transcatheter embolization for diverticular bleeding. AJR 133:519–521

160. Guy GE, Shetty PC, Sharma RP et al (1992) Treatment of acute lower gastrointestinal hemorrhage with superselective delivery of polyvinyl particles: further observations and outcomes in 19 patients. Radiology 185 RSNA:135

161. Alavi A (1982) Detection of gastrointestinal bleeding with 99m Tc-sulphur colloid. Semin Nucl Med 12:126–138

162. Pavel DG, Zimmer AM, Patterson VM (1977) In vivo labelling of red blood cells with 99m Tc: a new approach to blood pool visualization. J Nucl Med 18:305–308

163. Winzelberg GG, McKusick KA, Waltman AC, Greenfield AJ (1979) Evaluation of gastrointestinal bleeding by red blood cells labelled in vivo with technectium-99m. J Nucl Med 20: 1080–1086

164. Bunker SR, Lull RJ, Tanasecu DE et al (1984) Scintigraphy of gastrointestinal hemorrhage: superiority of 99mtc labelled red blood cells over 99m Tc sulphur colloid. AJR 143: 543–548

165. Alavi A, Ring EJ (1981) Localization of gastrointestinal bleeding: superiority of 99m Tc sulphur colloid compared with angiography. AJR 137:741–748

166. Lau WY, Fan ST, Wong SH et al (1987) Preoperative and intraoperative localization of gastrointestinal bleeding of obscure origin. Gut 28:869–877

167. Winzelberg GG, Froelich JW, McKusick KA, Staun HW (1981) Scintigraphic detection of gastrointestinal haemorrhage. Radiology 139:465–469

168. Olsen PR, Neilsen L, Dyrbye M, Hansen LK (1983) Colorectal bleeding localized with gamma camera. Acta Clin Scand 149:793–795

169. Hunter JM, Pezim ME (1990) Limited value of technectium 99m-labelled red cell scintigraphy in localization of lower gastrointestinal bleeding. Am J Surg 159:504–506

170. Ryan P, Styles CB, Chmiel R (1992) Identification of severe colon bleeding by technectium-labelled red cell scan. Dis Colon Rectum 35:219–222

171. Bentley DE, Richardson JD (1991) The role of tagged red blood cell imaging in the localization of gastrointestinal bleeding. Arch Surg 126:821–824

172. Deyhle P, Blum AL, Nuesch HJ, Jenny S (1974) Emergency colonoscopy in the management of acute peranal hemorrhage. Endoscopy 6:229–232

173. Knoepp LF Jr, McCulloch JH (1978) Colonoscopy in the diagnosis of unexplained rectal bleeding. Dis Colon Rectum 21:590–593

174. Tedesco FJ, Waye JD, Raskin JB et al (1978) Colonoscopic evaluation of rectal bleeding: a study of 304 patients. Ann Intern Med 89:907–909

175. Waye JD (1976) Colonoscopy in rectal bleeding. S Afr J Surg 14:143–149

176. Shinya H, Cwern M, Wolf G (1982) Colonoscopic diagnosis and the management of rectal bleeding. Surg Clin North Am 62:897–903

177. Forde KA (1981) Colonoscopy in acute rectal bleeding. Gastrointest Endosc 27:219–220

178. Veidenheimer MC, Corman ML, Coller JA (1978) Colonic hemorrhage. Surg Clin North Am 58:581–590

179. Caos A, Benner KG, Mauler J et al (1986) Colonoscopy after Golytely preparation in acute rectal bleeding. J Clin Gastroenterol 8:46–49

180. Vellacot KD (1986) Early endoscopy for acute lower gastrointestinal hemorrhage. Ann R Coll Surg 88:243–244

181. Savides T, Jensen DM, Machicado G, Hiribayashi K (1994) Colonoscopic haemostasis of recent diverticular hemorrhage associated with a visible vessel: a report of three cases. Gastrointest Endosc 40:70–73

182. Rossini FP, Ferrari A, Spandre M et al (1989) Emergency colonoscopy. World J Surg 13:190–192

183. Van Gompel A, Rutgeets P, Agg HO et al (1984) Vascular malformations of the colon. Coloproctology 5:247–253

184. Treate MR, Forde KA (1983) Colonoscopy, technectium scanning and angiography in acute rectal bleeding—an algorithm for their combined use. Surg Gastroenterol 2:135–138

185. Max MH, Richardson JD, Flint LM Jr et al (1981) Colonoscopic diagnosis of angiodysplasia of the gastrointestinal tract. Surg Gynecol Obstet 152:195–199

186. Schrock TR (1989) Colonoscopic diagnosis and treatment of lower gastrointestinal bleeding. Surg Clin North Am 69: 1309–1325

187. Hunter JG, Bowers JH, Burt RW et al (1984) Lasers in endoscopic gastrointestinal surgery. Am J Surg 148:736–741

188. Fruhmorgen P, Bodem F, Reidenbach HD (1976) Endoscopic laser coagulation of bleeding gastrointestinal lesions with report of the first therapeutic application in man. Gastrointest Endosc 23:73–76

189. Trudel JL, Fazio VW, Sivak MV (1988) Colonoscopic diagnosis and treatment of arteriovenous malformations in chronic lower gastrointestinal bleeding: clinical accuracy and efficacy. Dis Colon Rectum 31:197–210

190. Santos JCM Jr, Aprilli F, Guimaraes AS, Rocha JJR (1988) Angiodysplasia of the colon: endoscopic diagnosis and treatment. Br J Surg 75:256–258

191. Rutgeets P, Van Gompel F, Geboes K et al (1985) Long-term treatment of vascular malformations of the gastrointestinal tract by neodynium YAG laser photocoagulation. Gut 26: 586–593

192. Cello JP, Grendell JH (1986) Endoscopic treatment for gastrointestinal vascular ectasias. Ann Lutern Med 104:352–354

193. Gostout CJ, Bowyer BA, Ahlquist DS et al (1988) Mucosal vascular malformations of the gastrointestinal tract: clinical observations and results of endoscopic neodynium: yttrium-aluminium-garnet laser therapy. Mayo Clin Proc 63: 993–1003

194. Howard OM, Buchanan JD, Hunt RH (1982) Angiodysplasia of the colon. Experience of 26 cases. Lancet 2:16–19

195. Steger AC, Galland RB, Hemingway A et al (1987) Gastrointestinal hemorrhage from a second source in patients with colonic angiodysplasia. Br J Surg 74:726–727

196. Marx FW Jr, Gray RK, Duncan AM, Bakhtiar L (1977) Angiodysplasia as a source of intestinal bleeding. Am J Surg 134: 125–130

197. Jensen DM, Machicado GA (1994) Management of severe lower gastrointestinal bleeding. pp. 201–208. In Barkin JS, O'Phelan CA (eds): Advanced Therapeutic Endoscopy. 2nd Ed. Lippincott-Raven, Philadelphia

198. Jensen DM (1995) Management of severe lower gastrointestinal bleeding. Gastrointest Endosc 41:171–173

199. Mauldin JL (1985) Therapeutic use of colonoscopy in active diverticular bleeding. Gastrointest Endosc 31:290–291

200. Schuman BM (1984) When should colonoscopy be the first study for active lower intestinal hemorrhage? Gastrointest Endosc 30:372–374

201. Chu DZJ, Shivshanker K, Stroelein JR, Nelson RS (1983) Thrombocytopenia and gastrointestinal hemorrhage in the cancer patient: prevalence of unmasked lesions. Gastrointest Endosc 29:269–272

202. Wright HK, Pellicia O, Higgins EF et al (1980) Controlled, semi-elective, segmental resection for massive colonic hemorrhage. Am J Surg 139:535–538

203. Britt LG, Warren L, Moore OF (1983) Selective management of lower gastrointestinal bleeding. Am Surg 49:121–125

204. Smith GF, Ellyson JH, Parks SN et al (1984) Angiodysplasia of the colon: a review of 17 cases. Arch Surg 119:532–536

205. Scott HJ, Lane IF, Glynn MJ et al (1986) Colonic hemorrhage.

A technique for rapid intraoperative bowel preparation and colonoscopy. Br J Surg 73:390–391

206. Campbell WB, Rhodes M, Kettlewell MG (1985) Colonoscopy following intraoperative lavage in the management of severe colonic bleeding. Ann R Coll Surg Engl 67:290–292
207. Mendoza CB, Watne AL (1982) Value of intraoperative colonoscopy in vascular ectasia of the colon. Am Surg 48:153–156
208. Whelan RL, Buls JG, Goldberg SM et al (1989) Intraoperative endoscopy: University of Minnescta experience. Am Surg 55:281–286
209. Batch AJ, Pickard RG, DeLacey G (1981) Preoperative colonoscopy in massive rectal bleeding. Br J Surg 68:64–67
210. Radcliffe AG, Dudley HAF (1983) Intraoperative antegrade irrigation of the large intestine. Surg Gynecol Obstet 156:721–723
211. Stahlgren LH, Ferguson LK (1958) The surgical management of massive melena. Am J Surg 96:515–521
212. Beychock IA (1978) Precise diagnosis in severe hematochezia. Arch Surg 113:634–636
213. Maynard EP, Voorhees AB (1956) Arterial hemorrhage from a large bowel diverticulum. Gastroenterology 31:210–211
214. Hagihara PF, Sachatello CR, Mattingly SS et al (1982) Massive rectal bleeding of colonic origin: localization of the bleeding site. Surgery 92:589–597
215. Milewski PJ, Schofield PE (1989) Massive colonic hemorrhage—the case for right hemicolectomy. Ann Roy Coll Surg Engl 71:253–258

42

INTESTINAL ISCHEMIA

Hak-Su Goh

Disorders of the mesenteric circulation include acute mesenteric ischemia, chronic mesenteric ischemia, mesenteric venous thrombosis, and ischemic colitis. Management of these potentially lethal conditions is based on a clear understanding of the anatomy and pathophysiology of the mesenteric circulation. Recent advances in diagnostic modalities and treatment procedures, including the amelioration of ischemic injury at the cellular level, have given rise to new hope for improved outcome for these disorders.

MESENTERIC CIRCULATION

Like the blood supply of other parts of the body, the mesenteric circulation is subject to considerable anatomic variation, dating from embryonic development.[1] A good understanding of these variations is essential for the correct interpretation of mesenteric arteriograms and successful operative intervention.

The celiac and the superior mesenteric arteries supply the stomach and duodenum, the liver and biliary tract, the pancreas, the spleen, and the small and large intestine, the latter only up to the proximal two-thirds of the transverse colon. The inferior mesenteric artery supplies the splenic flexure, left colon, and rectum. Whereas the blood supply to all the abdominal gastrointestinal organs is referred to as the splanchnic circulation, the mesenteric circulation refers only to the intestinal portion, which receives about one-quarter of the cardiac output at rest.

The celiac axis arises at right angles from the anterior aspect of the abdominal aorta, opposite the junction of the T12 and L1 vertebrae. It is the largest of the three visceral arterial trunks. It gives rise to the left gastric artery and then branches into the common hepatic and splenic arteries. These two arteries send branches, the gastroduodenal and the dorsal pancreatic arteries, inferiorly to form the pancreaticoduodenal arcade, which is the main communicating site of the celiac and superior mesenteric arterial systems.

The superior mesenteric artery (SMA) comes off the aorta at a 20° to 30° angle, about 2 cm below the celiac axis. It is 1 cm in diameter at its origin, and runs in the small bowel mesentery, giving off right and left branches. The right branches include the inferior pancreaticoduodenal artery, which loops upward to communicate with the pancreaticoduodenal arcade, the middle colic artery, whose origin is the common site for an embolus to lodge, the right colic artery, and the ileocolic artery. Of these, the ileocolic is the most constant, as the right colic and the middle colic could be absent. The left branches, which number 15 to 20, are the jejunal and ileal branches.[2–5]

The inferior mesenteric artery is one-half the diameter of the SMA. It originates from the aorta just below the third part of the duodenum at the level of the L3 vertebra. It gives rise to the left colic artery, the sigmoidal branches, and the superior hemorrhoidal artery.

The ileocolic, right colic, and middle colic branches of the SMA and the left colic and superior hemorrhoidal branch of the inferior mesenteric artery fan out to anastomose with each other to form the marginal artery of Drummond.[6] The marginal artery is usually a continuous artery that runs parallel to the colon. There are two weak or watershed points; the Griffiths' point at the splenic flexure where branches of the middle colic and left colic meet, and the less important Sudek's point where the last sigmoid branch and the superior hemorrhoidal artery meet. These points, especially the one at the splenic flexure, are frequently the sites affected in segmental ischemic colitis.

It is generally accepted that colonic, as compared to small bowel, anastomoses are more hazardous because of poorer blood supply. Weight for weight, the colon has less blood flow than other parts of the gastrointestinal tract.[7] Active colonic peristalsis, which increases intraluminal pressure, also reduces blood supply.[8]

Collateral Circulation

The mesenteric circulation has a rich system of collateral communications, such that the intestines can remain viable when one, two, or even three of the main trunks are occluded. In chronic ischemia, usually two or more of the main trunks are occluded before symptoms of ischemia become apparent. The collateral communications are between (1) the celiac and superior mesenteric arteries, (2) the superior and inferior mesenteric arteries, (3) the inferior mesenteric and branches of the internal iliac arteries, and (4) the visceral and parietal branches of the aorta.

Although the pancreaticoduodenal arcade is the main collateral communication between the celiac and superior mesenteric arteries and it can perfuse adequately the liver and the stomach when the celiac axis is occluded, other types of communication sometimes exist. These include the branches of the middle colic and the dorsal pancreatic arteries, and the embryonic remnant anastomotic artery between the main celiac and superior mesenteric trunks.

The best known of the collateral communications is between the superior and inferior mesenteric arteries at the splenic flexure of the colon. Here, the anastomotic site of the marginal artery is known as Griffiths' point, which may be lacking in 5% of individuals.[9] In about 60% of individuals, an additional communication known as the arch of Riolan, or the meandering mesenteric artery, is present.[10,11] It arises from a branch of the left colic and a branch of the superior mesenteric arteries. In surgery for abdominal aortic aneurysm, ligation of the inferior mesenteric artery together with the meandering anastomotic artery can lead to disastrous ischemia of the left colon when the collaterals of the marginal artery are defective. This can be averted if the meandering anastomotic artery is preserved.

The inferior mesenteric and hypogastric collateral communications arise from the middle and inferior hemorrhoidal branches of the internal iliac arteries and the superior hemorrhoidal artery, which is the terminal branch of the inferior mesenteric artery. Being the narrowest of the visceral arterial trunks, the inferior mesenteric artery is most often occluded by atheroma. The low sigmoid and rectum are then maintained by collaterals from the hypogastric branches. In performing low anterior resections for rectal cancer, ligation of the inferior mesenteric artery and the lateral ligaments would compromise blood supply to the rectum. It is important to keep the rectal stump very short to avoid catastrophic anastomotic breakdown.

Other collateral communications, such as those between the splenic and left colic arteries, and those involving branches of the ileolumbar and the superior and inferior epigastric arteries, are less common, but are no less important because they sometimes maintain viability of the gastrointestinal tract in the presence of total occlusion of all three main visceral trunks.

Mesenteric Microcirculation

Although it is important to note that embolus, especially from thrombus originating in the heart, tends to lodge in the SMA because of its size and the angle of its origin relative to the aorta, and that arteriosclerotic occlusion tends to affect the inferior mesenteric artery because of its smaller caliber, it is ultimately the circulation to the mucosa and bowel wall that determines the clinical manifestations of mesenteric ischemia. The main arteries branch repeatedly to form arcades within the mesentery, more in the small than in the large bowel, ending with a marginal artery that lies close to the bowel wall. End arteries or vasa recta arise from this to penetrate the bowel wall and these

branch further. Arteries become arterioles when their diameter is about 25 μm. Arterioles contain smooth muscle that controls their internal caliber, so they act as resistance vessels. Arterioles later become capillaries, which are thin walled and function as exchange vessels. At the termini of the arterioles, precapillary sphincters are present, which act as gatekeepers to the blood flow through the capillaries. They are responsible for blood-shunting and control blood distribution to the capillary beds.

The capillaries drain into venules, which are thin-walled vessels with smooth muscle. These act as capacitance vessels, holding most of the blood in the mesenteric circulation. When needed, such as during exercise, the vessels contract to shift blood from this mesenteric reservoir to the general circulation.[12]

Regulation of Mesenteric Blood Flow

Mesenteric blood flow is tightly controlled by extrinsic and intrinsic factors acting on its vascular resistance. The predominant extrinsic control is through the sympathetic component of the autonomic nerves and through circulating neurohumoral substances, such as catecholamines, histamine, vasopressin, and angiotensin II.

Sympathetic discharge can greatly reduce mesenteric blood flow by increasing arteriolar resistance, by causing contraction of the precapillary sphincters to shunt blood from the capillary beds, as well as shifting blood from the mesenteric venous reservoirs by venous contraction. In acute ischemia, excessive and prolonged sympathetic activity may aggravate mucosal damage, even after the cause of the ischemia has been removed.

Mesenteric blood flow is also regulated by intrinsic factors, such as absorbed digested products, mucosal metabolites, and transmural mechanical pressure. All these factors make possible the fine adjustment of the blood flow to match intestinal activity. During digestion, absorption of chyme causes vascular dilatation, which increases blood flow, resulting in postprandial mucosal hyperemia. During intestinal contraction, increased transmural pressure causes vascular contraction, which reduces blood flow. With prolonged increase in transmural pressure, such as in intestinal obstruction, ischemic changes, including gangrene, can occur.[13]

One important feature of the mesenteric circulation is the countercurrent exchange mechanism in the mucosal villi, primarily evolved to enhance the absorption of nutrients. The vascular core of each villus consists of an arteriole and an accompanying venule with blood flowing in the opposite direction. In addition to the other gradients, an oxygen tension gradient is also set up between the two, which is greatest at the base of the villus. This gradient allows for some oxygen diffusion. It is exaggerated during episodes of ischemia and the increased diffusion of oxygen from the arteriole to the venule further deprives the tip of the villus of oxygen, which may lead to sloughing of the villus. This sloughing is an early event in intestinal ischemia, and helps account for the massive third space fluid loss found in this condition.[14,15]

Pathogenesis of Ischemia

Mesenteric ischemia causes both structural and metabolic changes.[16–19] In acute ischemia, microscopic changes in mucosal cells become evident after 10 minutes, and are extensive after 30 minutes. There is also increase in vascular permeability, causing increased capillary filtration and intestinal edema.[20] These changes are now thought to be mediated by oxygen radicals, such as the superoxide radical, hydrogen peroxide, and hydroxyl radicals, produced at the time of diminished perfusion and during reperfusion. Experimental models show that ischemia leads to accumulation of hypoxanthine from adenosine triphosphate (ATP) metabolism, and induction of the enzyme xanthine oxidase. Upon reperfusion, xanthine oxidase catalyses the conversion of hypoxanthine to superoxide radicals. These are reduced to produce reactive hydroxyl radicals that cause lipid peroxidation and damage to the lipid cellular membrane.[21]

During ischemia, neutrophils accumulate and they undergo degranulation during reperfusion and release numerous inflammatory substances, such as the interleukins, tumor necrosis factor, proteases, and oxygen free radicals. These substances cause injury not only to intestinal mucosa, but also to other organs such as the liver, heart, and lungs.[22,23]

Understanding the mechanism of ischemia-reperfusion injury could lead to novel treatments. Ideas such as the use of oxygen free radical scavengers (superoxide dismutase), enzyme inhibitors (allopurinol, lodoxamide), anti-inflammatory agents (diclofenac sodium), neutrophil extraction, and tumor necrosis factor monoclonal antibody, are all being investigated in the management of mesenteric ischemia.[24-28]

Diagnosis of Ischemia

Early diagnosis is the key to a successful outcome of mesenteric ischemia, because supportive measures, ameliorating agents, and timely surgery can be instituted early to limit the ravages of ischemia. Despite clinical awareness of the condition, diagnosis is often made late, particularly in the critically ill or unconscious patient.[29,30]

Severe leukocytosis and metabolic acidosis are not specific to mesenteric ischemia, and intramural or portal vein gas on plain abdominal radiographs are late signs. Even selective mesenteric angiography, which is still the "gold standard," can be difficult to interpret because ischemia can occur without vascular occlusion, while conversely, vascular occlusion does not necessarily mean ischemia.

Barium enema is traditionally used for the diagnosis of ischemic colitis, which has the characteristic features of thumb-printing and pseudotumor.[31] However, colonoscopy is now the investigation of choice, as it is readily available and can be performed at the patient's bedside. It is also one of the most reliable means of diagnosing ischemic colitis because of the characteristic appearance.[32,33] The small bowel can now be visualized with a 250-cm video enteroscope, a procedure that can be performed in about 90 minutes.[34] This may become an important additional test to the diagnosis of small bowel ischemia, but has yet to be evaluated.

Computed tomography (CT), because of its cross-sectional capabilities, provides a noninvasive means of assessing thickening and high attenuation of the bowel wall, as well as edema of the mesentery.[35-37] Although not specific, these features, when correlated with clinical and pathophysiologic findings, are highly sensitive for mesenteric ischemia. Magnetic resonance imaging (MRI) is more specific because it can recognize changes in water content of tissues. Ischemia is diagnosed by the thickening of the bowel wall and increase in signal activity on T_2-weighted images.[38-41]

Other novel but more experimental methods of diagnosing ischemia include the measurement of intraluminal pCO_2 by mass spectrometry, and excreted contrast medium in the urine with high-performance liquid chromatography (HPLC).[42,43] Intestinal ischemia leads to a rapid and sustained rise of intraluminal pCO_2, which can be correlated with severity of mucosal damage. Ischemia leads to increased mucosal permeability, which is measured by urinary recovery of iodixanol, an oral water-soluble contrast medium. The amount of urinary iodixanol is strongly correlated with the degree of ischemia and this test appears to be able to differentiate between arterial and venous ischemia.

Diagnostic laparoscopy is invasive, but has a role in cases where a full diagnostic laparotomy is contemplated.[44] Serosal color change in transmural ischemia is obvious through the laparoscope, but mucosal or muscular changes are not. The sensitivity of laparoscopy can be improved with fluorescein-assisted laparoscopy, which uses an argon laser instead of the normal light source.[45]

Operative assessment of intestinal viability can be difficult because mucosal damage is more extensive than would be indicated on the serosal surface. Although colonic resection is often not a problem, in resection of small bowel the surgeon is often caught between the need to avoid the short bowel syndrome by taking too much, and the risk of anastomotic breakdown from removing too little. The use of fluorescein under a modified Wood's lamp, as well as color Doppler, can help greatly in determining intestinal viability.[46,47] This may also be enhanced by the recent introduction of laser Doppler flowmetry.[48-50]

ACUTE MESENTERIC ISCHEMIA

Acute mesenteric ischemia is caused either by sudden occlusion of the SMA by an embolus or by thrombosis, or by sudden reduction of blood flow from low cardiac output. In its most severe manifestation, there is gangrene of the whole of the small bowel from the duodenojejunal junction down to the proximal two-thirds of the transverse colon. This is usually fatal. In less severe cases, the challenge is to diagnose the condition and re-establish blood flow before irreversible gangrene sets in.[51]

Pathogenesis

Most emboli originate in the heart, either from rheumatic heart disease, or atrial fibrillation. Some are derived from atheroma from the aorta or the proximal portion of the main vascular trunks. Embolus usually involves the SMA because of its caliber and the acute angle it makes with the aorta. Emboli usually lodge at the branching of the middle colic and jejunal arteries. The first jejunal branches are usually spared, preserving perfusion to the proximal jejunum. When the embolus lodges more distally, the ischemic segments will be correspondingly smaller or patchy.

Acute thrombosis of the SMA is nearly always due to a pre-existing atheromatous stenosis within the first centimeter of the beginning of the artery. A Finnish autopsy study on 120 patients showed that 67% of the subjects over the age of 80, but only 6% below the age of 40, had mesenteric artery stenosis.[52] Because the occlusion is at the origin of the SMA, ischemia often involves the whole of the small bowel from the duodeno jejunal junction down to the proximal two-thirds of the transverse colon.

Nonocclusive mesenteric ischemia is caused by a low-flow state of the mesenteric circulation as a result of cardiovascular insufficiency or severe vasoconstriction from drug ingestion. Ischemic injury occurs during the vasoconstriction period, as well as during reperfusion.[53]

Clinical Presentation

Acute mesenteric ischemia represents 1% to 2% of all gastrointestinal disease. Its incidence has increased over the last few decades because of the aging population, increased number of critical care patients, and major cardiovascular surgical procedures.[54,55]

The condition presents with sudden onset of abdominal pain. The pain is colicky in nature and is usually diffuse and periumbilical, but may sometimes be localized to a specific area, such as the epigastrium, right or left abdomen, or suprapubic region. As ischemia progresses and peritonitis sets in, the pain becomes more constant. It is associated with profuse sweating, vomiting, and diarrhea and the patient is greatly distressed.[56]

However, abdominal pain may be atypical or absent. In a review of 82 cases of SMA embolism, 23% of patients had atypical or no abdominal pain. This is particularly so in elderly patients, who may present with an acute confusional state instead of abdominal pain or tenderness.[57,58]

The abdomen is initially soft and nontender to palpation. Bowel sounds are active, but may become reduced and absent when ischemia becomes more severe. The presence of abdominal tenderness, guarding, and rebound heralds the onset of peritonitis. By this time, leukocytosis and metabolic acidosis become severe and serum enzymes, such as amylase, creatinine phosphokinase, lactate dehydrogenase, and glutamic-oxaloacetic transaminases are elevated.[59-64]

Despite recent advances in ultrasound, CT, and MRI scanning, arteriography remains the mainstay of diagnosis for acute mesenteric ischemia. Although flush abdominal aortography with anteroposterior and lateral projections may visualize the main vascular trunks adequately, selective SMA angiography, particularly with digital subtraction, defines the artery and its branches clearly. It is useful for differentiating the three forms of acute mesenteric ischemia. Mesenteric embolus tends to lodge at the origin of the middle colic artery. This will be found 3 to 8 cm from the origin of the SMA and has an inverted meniscus appearance. Collateral vessels are usually absent. In acute thrombosis, the occlusion is at the origin of the SMA and because of pre-existing atherosclerosis, collateral vessels are usually demonstrated. In nonocclusive mesenteric ischemia, which is the most common form, no vascular obstruction is found.[65-67]

Treatment

If clinical awareness is the axiom for diagnosis of acute mesenteric ischemia, aggressive intervention is the axiom for treatment of this potentially fatal condition.[68] Initial treatment includes adequate fluid replacement, electrolyte and acid-base correction, antibiotic administration, and pain relief. Nasogastric decompression is important to reduce intestinal luminal pressure, and heparin is given to prevent clot propagation distal to the site of occlusion. Oxygen is administered to maintain a high blood oxygen tension, but hyperbaric oxygen is probably not effective.[69]

The bladder is catheterized for urine output measurement. A central venous line, arterial line, and Swan-Ganz catheter are inserted for continuous monitoring of cardiac function and fluid and oxygen replacement.

Vasopressive and other drugs acting on the cardiovascular system, including digoxin, are used only when absolutely necessary to maintain blood pressure or correct cardiac arrhythmias, because they can cause mesenteric vasoconstriction and aggravate the ischemia.

Massive resection of the gut is often fatal. This can sometimes be averted by revascularization, which can be done percutaneously or intraoperatively. With the angiographic catheter in the SMA, acute embolus can be dissolved by infusion of streptokinase.[70,71] It is particularly useful in elderly or critically ill patients where the operative risk is high. Although percutaneous transluminal angioplasty is more commonly applied in chronic mesenteric occlusive ischemia, it has been successfully exploited in acute mesenteric occlusion.[72,73] In nonocclusive ischemia, arteriolar constriction can be relieved by continuous infusion of papaverine, a potent and rapidly acting vasodilator.

Surgery for mesenteric ischemia covers revascularization, intestinal resection, and second-look procedures. In acute embolus, the clot is extracted from the SMA through a transverse arteriotomy at the level of the middle colic artery. The artery is approached through the inferior aspect of the transverse mesocolon and dissected as it emerges from beneath the pancreas. Further embolectomy is performed with a small balloon-tipped catheter threaded first distally and then proximally to clear the artery of clots. It is done gently to avoid damage to the arterial wall and resultant hematoma formation. After embolectomy, heparinized saline is instilled into the artery.[74]

For acute thrombosis of the SMA, revascularization is done with a saphenous vein bypass directly from the aorta to the SMA, which is transected proximally. Synthetic grafts, such as polytetrafluoroethylene prostheses have also been used, and results are not found to differ from saphenous vein grafts. Long-term objective patency assessment has shown that graft patency is high, even when inserted for acute thrombus.[75,76]

After revascularization, nonviable bowel has to be resected. The difficulty is in determining the length of bowel that needs to be removed. It is important to examine the mucosal surface, because mucosal ischemia is always more extensive than what is apparent on the serosal surface. Many techniques have been introduced to assess intestinal viability at operation, including laser Doppler, tonometric measurement of intraluminal pH, and oximetry. The two most reliable and simplest aids are Wood's lamp fluorescence following intravenous fluorescein and hand-held continuous-wave Doppler.[77]

If viability is still in doubt, it is prudent to avoid fashioning anastomoses. Resected bowel ends are brought out as cutaneous stomas for easy assessment, and at the same time, the risk of anastomotic breakdown is averted.[78]

When primary anastomosis is unavoidable because of short bowel length, a decision must be made to perform a second-look operation 24 to 36 hours later. Once the decision is made, the second operation must be carried out, even when the patient appears to be getting better. This is to assess bowel viability and effectiveness of the resuscitative and revascularization measures. Laparoscopic second-look procedures have been described, but these require further evaluation before they can be recommended widely.[79,80]

Outcome

The mortality of acute mesenteric ischemia ranges from 50% to 100%. In general, patients treated conservatively do much worse than those who have undergone surgery, thus underlining the need for an aggressive approach to management. Patients who survive are generally younger and have less extensive ischemic bowel. In one report, 80% of acute mesenteric emboli, 60% of nonocclusive ischemia, and only 20% of acute thromboses survive with minimal sequelae of nutritional deficits. The cause of death is usually sepsis or multiorgan failure.[81–85] Rarely acute ischemia without transmural infarction leads to segmental strictures of the small bowel and may be mistaken for Crohn's disease.[86]

CHRONIC MESENTERIC ISCHEMIA

Chronic mesenteric ischemia has been variously referred to as ''mesenteric intermittent claudication'' or ''intestinal angina.'' Although atherosclerosis of the visceral arteries is not uncommon among the elderly, chronic mesenteric ischemia is not common, principally because of well-developed collateral communications.

By far the most common cause of chronic mesenteric ischemia is atherosclerosis. Other causes include systemic lupus erythematosus, thromboangiitis obliterans (Buerger's disease), and aneurysms of the aorta or the SMA.

Clinical Presentation

Patients with intestinal angima tend to be younger, in their 50s and 60s. Many have other manifestations of widespread vascular disease. Abdominal pain is the predominant feature. This is characteristically postprandial, appearing about 15 minutes after food intake, and lasting 2 to 3 hours. The pain invariably leads to a fear of eating and severe weight loss.[87]

Diagnosis

Selective angiography is the mainstay for defining arterial occlusions of the main visceral trunks. However, it was the diagnosis of chronic mesenteric ischemia that led to the development of major noninvasive investigative procedures. These include abdominal duplex ultrasonography, laser Doppler flow analysis, and cine-phase contrast MRI. The latter measures SMA blood flow 30 minutes after food, which increases significantly in normal subjects, but does not do so in patients with mesenteric ischemia.[88–90]

Treatment

The treatment of chronic mesenteric ischemia is operative. It is indicated when the characteristic triad of postprandial pain, fear of eating, and weight loss is present. If left untreated, super-

imposition of thrombosis on the SMA stenosis may lead to acute mesenteric ischemia, which carries a high mortality. Percutaneous transluminal angioplasty of the SMA is effective in relieving symptoms of chronic mesenteric ischemia. When compared with surgical bypass, angioplasty is comparable in relieving symptoms, but it may need to be repeated. It is especially suitable in patients with high operative risks.[91]

Operative revascularization could either be by endarterectomy or aortomesenteric artery bypass. Endarterectomy is difficult because of vascular access. Therefore the main surgical procedure is through aorto-SMA bypass with a saphenous vein graft. The long-term results are good because of high graft patency rates.[92–94]

MESENTERIC VENOUS THROMBOSIS

Mesenteric venous thrombosis is an uncommon cause of intestinal ischemia. It is still a lethal disease in the 1990s, although it carries a better prognosis than ischemia of the SMA. Delay in diagnosis constitutes significantly to this mortality. It is therefore important to have a high index of suspicion for this condition so that effective investigations and treatments can be instituted promptly.

Pathogenesis

In a review of 72 patients with mesenteric venous thrombosis from 1972 to 1993 by Rhee et al.,[95] 57 patients had secondary mesenteric venous thrombosis. Previous abdominal surgical procedure and hypercoagulable states were the most prevalent causes. Thrombotic disorder, such as antithrombin III, protein S and protein C deficiencies, polycythemia vera, and sickle cell disease have all been shown to cause mesenteric vein thrombosis.[96–98] Oral contraceptives use as a cause of mesenteric venous thrombosis is well established.[99–101] Less well-known causes are mesenteric phlebitis and venulitis, myointimal hyperplasia, and renal transplantation.[102–105]

Thrombosis usually involves small tributaries of the superior mesenteric vein, causing segmental bowel ischemia. Less frequently, the main venous trunk is thrombosed, causing more diffuse ischemia. The main pathologic features are edema, hyperemia, and submucosal hemorrhage. Because of venous blockage, back-pressure leads to thrombosis of capillaries, arterioles, and even the main arterial trunk. Typically, this progression is slow in contrast to that of acute arterial occlusion. In some instances, the venous thrombosis is chronic and intermittent, leading to segmental strictures of the small bowel, a condition akin to stricturing ischemic colitis.[106]

Clinical Presentation

Mesenteric vein thrombosis occurs in younger patients, between the ages of 30 and 60 years. It presents most commonly with abdominal pain (83%), anorexia (53%), nausea and vomiting (50%), and diarrhea (43%). The pain is nonspecific and poorly localized. In contrast to the rapid abdominal catastrophe of acute mesenteric arterial occlusion, the symptoms of mesenteric vein thrombosis are more indolent. Three-quarters of patients have symptoms longer than 48 hours, and even for as long as 2 weeks. The median time lapse between onset of abdominal pain and hospitalization is 8 days. Abdominal signs are also nonspecific, but abdominal distension and ascites are common. Bowel sounds are initially active, but become absent when peritonitis sets in. Typically, the patient's subjective distress is disproportionate to the objective findings.[95,107–109]

Diagnosis

The most common laboratory findings are leukocytosis and a mild metabolic acidosis with raised lactate dehydrogenase. Abdominal CT is the most useful diagnostic procedure, as most patients have severe edema of the bowel wall and mesentery. In some cases, the venous thrombus can be visualized as a low-density lesion after contrast enhancement.[110,111] Abdominal ultrasound can also detect the presence of thrombus as echoic material. Selective arteriography of the SMA shows spasm of the artery and venous thrombosis is implied when the capillary phase of the examination is more intense and prolonged. Enteroscopic appearances of the small bowel have also been documented for mesenteric vein thrombosis.[112]

Treatment

In the presence of peritonitis, the patient is resuscitated as for acute mesenteric ischemia, and prepared for emergency surgery. In the absence of peritonitis, mesenteric vein thrombosis is treated with intravenous heparin and evaluated twice weekly with abdominal CT and ultrasound scans, until recanalization of the mesenteric vein. The average time for recanalization is 17 days.[111]

Acute mesenteric thrombosis has also been reported to be successfully treated with transjugular intramesenteric urokinase infusion or infusion through a catheter in the SMA.[113]

Surgery is necessary if bowel necrosis is present. In contrast to arterial disease, gangrene is less extensive and resection is life-saving without the constant risk of producing short bowel syndrome. Nevertheless, the risk of anastomotic breakdown is high in the presence of edematous bowel, which therefore must be resected if anastomosis is contemplated.

Mesenteric venous thrombectomy is not often feasible because thrombosis usually involves the smaller tributaries, but if the main veins only are involved, thrombectomy may reduce the length of bowel that needs to be resected.

Recurrent thrombosis is common and therefore anticoagulation must be started early, and in cases with severe coagulopathy, continued indefinitely. Second-look operations may be necessary if clot propagation is anticipated.[114]

Outcome for mesenteric vein thrombosis is better than for arterial disease because the patients are younger, gangrene is more limited, and because venous thrombosis is amenable to anticoagulant therapy. Nevertheless, recurrent thrombosis occurs in up to 36% of patients, and 30-day mortality is 27%.[95]

ISCHEMIC COLITIS

Ischemic colitis refers to a spectrum of disease entities, ranging from fulminant gangrenous colitis to imperceptible, transient colitis, where the underlying pathology is an inadequate blood supply to the colon. The rate at which ischemia occurs, the extent of the ischemia, as well as the general condition of the patient, determine the clinical picture and the outcome of the disease.

The term "ischemic colitis" was first coined by Marston et al.[115] in 1966, but it was Boley et al.[116] in 1963 who first described five cases of the condition and established its vascular etiology. Three types of ischemic colitis were described: gangrenous, stricturing, and transient. The condition was thought to be rare, and the gangrenous form was considered the most common clinical manifestation. However, with the introduction and subsequent widespread use of colonoscopy, ischemic colitis is now known to be more frequent than previously thought, and transient colitis, which is easy to miss, is increasingly being diagnosed.[117]

Like ischemic heart disease and stroke, ischemic colitis tends to affect those over the age of 60. Similarly, generalized atheroma, diabetes mellitus, systemic vasculitis, and hypercoagulopathies are predisposing factors. However, the specific blood supply to the colon, its physiologic function of storage and disposal of solid body waste, and its unique proximity to overwhelming and harmful bacteria and toxins, give ischemic colitis its own characteristics.[118] With better appreciation of colonic blood supply and its relationship to function, as well as better understanding of the pathogenesis of ischemia, a new perspective on ischemic colitis has emerged.

Classification

Ischemic colitis is best classified under two main groups: gangrenous and nongangrenous. The latter can be further classified as chronic and transient colitis. Chronic colitis can lead to stricturing, depending on the extent of fibrosis. The distribution of various types of ischemic colitis is as follows: gangrenous 20%, chronic nonstricturing 20%, stricturing 10%, and transient 50%.[119]

Pathogenesis

Colonic ischemia may be due to many causes. Major vessel occlusion may occur as in the entrapment of the superior mesenteric vessels by pancreatic cancer or severe pancreatitis, or following ligation of inferior mesenteric vessels during abdominal aortic aneurysm repair. Ischemia is however, most commonly encountered in colonic surgery, following ligature of colonic arteries. Anastomotic breakdown is usually due to inadequate blood supply because pulsatile marginal arterial blood flow had not been maintained. This is most dramatically demonstrated when an end-colostomy becomes ischemic 1 to 2 days after fashioning.

Segmental colitis is usually due to more distal or small vessel

Classification of Ischemic Colitis	
Gangrenous	20%
Nongangrenous	
Chronic nonstricturing	20%
Chronic stricturing	10%
Transient	50%

Intestinal Ischemia: Etiologic Factors

Major Vascular Occlusion

Pancreatic cancer occluding superior mesenteric artery

Ligation of inferior mesenteric artery

Small Vessel Disease

Diabetes mellitus

Systemic lupus erythematosus

Slow Flow State

Hypovolemia

Septicemia

Cardiogenic shock

Colonic Obstruction

Tumor

Volvulus

Adhesions

Coagulopathies

Drugs

Idiopathic

occlusion. Small vessel disease could be due to diabetes mellitus or systemic vasculitis, such as systemic lupus erythematosus.[120,121]

Slow flow states, due to shock of any kind whether hypovolemic, septicemic, or cardiogenic, is a major cause of colonic ischemia. Often, it gives rise to the gangrenous form with its ensuing high mortality. Here the major vessels are all patent, but the blood flow is inadequate to meet the metabolic demands of the colon.

Colonic obstruction either from a tumor, volvulus, or adhesions as a cause of ischemia is frequently not appreciated.[122] Colonic blood flow proximal to the obstruction is compromised by distension of the colon. This has practical implications in surgery for obstruction. Care must be taken to resect all the ischemic bowel adequately to avoid anastomotic breakdown.

More often than not, a cause is not found and the ischemia is designated idiopathic. This merely reflects a failure to understand the complex control of colonic microvascular circulation versus its physiologic demands, rather than the absence of a cause.

Clinical Presentation

Gangrenous ischemic colitis is more frequently seen in elderly patients already hospitalized for critical conditions, such as cardiac insufficiency, septic shock, open heart surgery,[123] abdominal aortic aneurysm repair,[124] and colonic obstruction.[122] In younger patients, specific causes such as oral contraceptive use, collagen disease, or cocaine abuse can often be elicited.[125–128] The onset of gangrenous ischemic colitis is heralded by a sudden deterioration of the patient's condition with development of severe abdominal pain, progressive abdominal distension, and shock. The patient looks ill and anxious, with a grayish-blue hue of cutaneous and mucosal hypoperfusion and toxemia. The abdomen is initially tender with active bowel sounds that gradually disappear. This is followed by abdominal distension. Later, palpable tenderness and guarding may disappear altogether, when the patient becomes too ill to react. Rectal examination may or may not reveal altered blood from colonic bleeding.

Blood tests show leukocytosis, which is often very high, and severe acidosis. The well-described radiographic signs of gas in the bowel wall or the portal tracts are usually absent.[129] Instead, paucity of gas shadows in the bowels is a common finding on plain abdominal radiograph, presumably as a result of expulsion from the intense intestinal spasms occurring at the onset of ischemia.

Gangrenous colitis is frequently diagnosed late because it occurs in patients who are already critically ill or who have just undergone open heart surgery or aortic aneurysm repair. Yet it is essential to diagnose and treat ischemic colitis early if these very ill patients are to have any chance of survival. Confirmation of the diagnosis is not made by laboratory tests or other investigations but more usually at laparotomy or autopsy.

Nongangrenous ischemic colitis presents with colicky abdominal pain of sudden onset, associated with diarrhea and passage of altered blood per rectum. The pain is often localized to the lower abdomen and bleeding is not excessive. Nausea, vomiting, and anorexia may be present, suggesting the presence of ileus. Physical signs such as fever, localized tenderness, and altered blood mixed in with stool at rectal examination are either nonspecific or absent altogether. The pulse rate and blood pressure are usually normal. There is mild leukocytosis, and localized ileus may be seen on plain abdominal radiographs. There are no specific features on CT apart from thickening of the bowel wall in affected areas.[130]

Diagnosis

Diagnosis of nongangrenous ischemic colitis can be made by the presence of thumb-printing or pseudotumor on barium enema. This is the result of the lifting of edematous colonic mucosa by submucosal hemorrhage. These signs disappear when the mucosa sloughs.

Colonoscopy is preferred for diagnosing ischemic colitis. It is more sensitive in detecting mucosal abnormalities compared with barium enema, and biopsies can be taken. A wide range of colonoscopic features are seen, depending on the stage and severity of the condition. These include submucosal swelling without discernible mucosal abnormalities, mucosal edema, hyperemia, nodularity, friability, and ulceration as well as cauliflower mass lesions that can be mistaken for cancer. The mass lesions are associated with surrounding mucosal friability and ulceration. (Fig. 42-1)

Histologically, there is intense inflammatory reaction with sloughing of mucosa, submucosal hemorrhage, and edema. There is loss of goblet cells and degeneration of normal crypt architecture (Fig. 42-2 and 42-3). In transient ischemic colitis, the clinical picture resolves within a few days and the colonoscopic features disappear completely within 3 to 6 weeks.

In chronic ischemic colitis, the diarrhea and abdominal pain

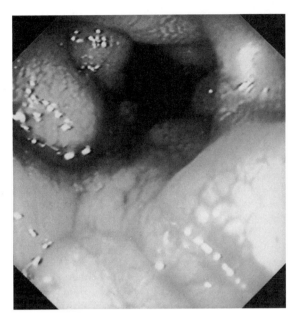

Figure 42-1. Transient ischemia with elevation and edema of mucosa.

persist with profuse mucus discharge, instead of bleeding to accompany the diarrhea. The endoscopic picture is that of a narrowed colonic lumen with a stiff bowel wall, and chronic ulceration with yellowish slough and granulation tissue (Fig. 42-4). Histologically, there is mucosal atrophy, granulation tissue with hemosiderin-laden macrophages, and fibrosis, that is most marked in stricturing ischemic colitis.

In patients with transmural infarction of the bowel wall, the endoscopic picture is that of green or black mucosa and submucosa (Fig. 42-5). In such patients, colonoscopy is best avoided because of the high risk of perforation.

Although colonoscopy is the investigation of choice in non-gangrenous ischemic colitis, it should be performed with care. Apart from the risk of perforation, distension of the bowel with air to pressures greater than 30 mmHg can reduce blood flow and aggravate the ischemia.[131,132] Insufflating carbon dioxide instead of air has been suggested to minimize this risk because carbon dioxide could cause vasodilatation and improve mucosal blood flow. However, in practice, gentle examination with constant suction during colonoscopy with air insufflation is safe.

Management

Management of ischemic colitis depends on its severity. Transient ischemic colitis is treated expectantly, with nasogastric tube suction to rest the bowel, intravenous fluid, and antibiotics.

Figure 42-2. Low power showing atrophic glands with goblet cell depletion. The glands gradually disappear toward the surface of the mucosa leaving empty spaces. (Courtesy of Dr. J. Ho) (H&E, ×40)

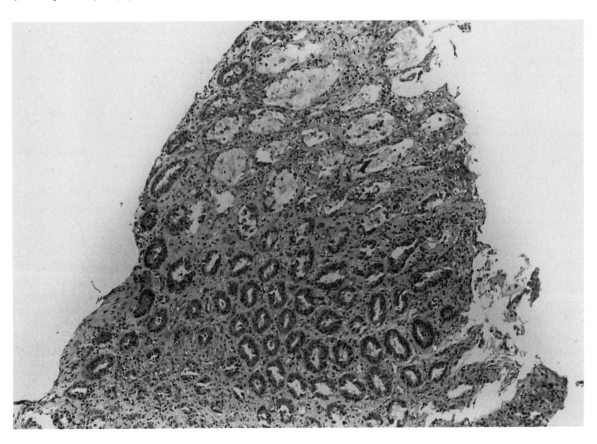

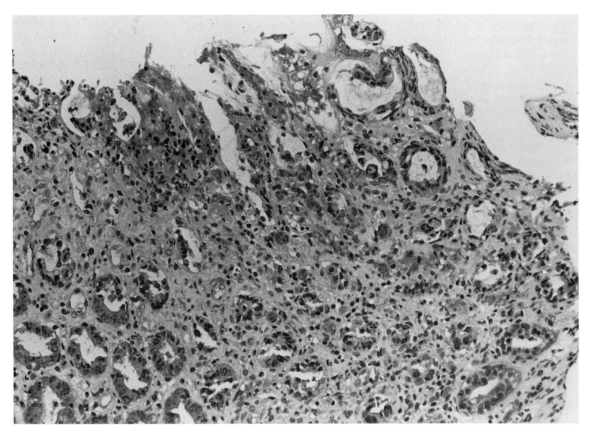

Figure 42-3. Higher magnification shows inflammatory cells in the lamina propria. (Courtesy of Dr. J. Ho) (H&E ×200)

Figure 42-4. Chronic ischemia with mucosal swelling, ulcerations, and sloughs.

Figure 42-5. Black mucosa of gangrenous ischemic colitis.

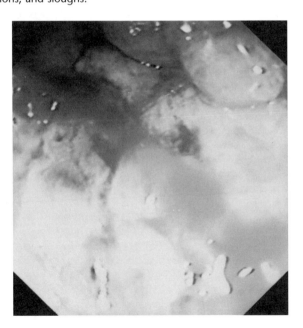

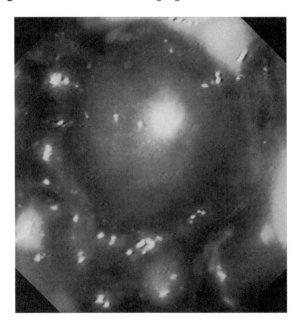

General measures are taken to ensure optimal blood oxygen saturation and perfusion. Drugs, including laxatives, that can aggravate bowel ischemia are withdrawn or avoided. Symptoms of abdominal pain and diarrhea should resolve quickly over 1 to 2 days. A repeat colonoscopy should be performed in 3 to 6 weeks, and the ischemic lesions should resolve completely.

Persistent symptoms over 10 days to 2 weeks indicate chronic colitis. This may lead to persistent fluid and protein loss, with ensuing debilitation and weight loss. Surgery is then indicated, even when stricture is not present. Care must be taken during surgery to ensure good blood supply and viability of bowel ends before any anastomosis. Ischemic stricture is also treated surgically.

If symptoms of ischemia persist and progress, especially to manifest signs of transmural infarction, such as fever, tachycardia, and peritonism, urgent surgery is indicated. As in gangrenous colitis, surgery is performed under antibiotic cover and adequate water and electrolyte replacement. In the presence of gangrene, there is a characteristic smell of dead bowel when the abdomen is opened. The extent of colonic resection is dependent on the extent of ischemia. Examination of the serosal surface may be misleading, as there may be extensive mucosal damage. It is therefore very important not only to look at the color of the serosa and pulsation of the marginal artery and vasa recta, but to establish the demarcation of the mucosa as well. Aids such as continuous-wave Doppler,[133] measurement of intramural pH,[5] or intravenous fluorescein[47] may be useful, but they cannot replace careful examination for the presence of a pink mucosa, healthy bleeding from the cut ends of the colon, and pulsatile blood flow from a cut marginal artery.

In cases with gangrenous colitis, it is prudent to avoid an anastomosis, because the underlying condition of the patient can cause further extension of the ischemia. The ends of the distal and proximal viable bowel are exteriorized whenever possible. When the rectum is involved, the distal end is closed and the proximal end exteriorized as in a Hartmann's procedure. Further resection may be necessary if the exteriorized portion becomes gangrenous. The extent of ischemia can be assessed by careful endoscopic examination through the colostomy.

The prognosis of ischemic colitis depends on the underlying condition of the patient. In general, gangrenous ischemic colitis requiring emergency resection carries a mortality of 50% to 100%. Ischemic colitis treated expectantly in the hospital has an overall mortality of 50%, as a proportion require surgery for progression of disease.[134–137]

REFERENCES

1. Ernst CB, (1995) Anatomy and collateral pathways of the mesenteric circulation. pp. 3–9. In Zuidema GD (ed): Shackelford's Surgery of the Alimentary Tract. 4th Ed. WB Saunders, Philadelphia
2. Michels NA, Siddarth P, Kornblith PL, Parke WW (1965) The variant blood supply to the descending colon, rectosigmoid, and rectum based on 400 dissections. Its importance in regional resections: a review of the literature. Dis Colon Rectum 8:251–278
3. Sonneland J, Anson B, Beaton L (1958) Surgical anatomy of the arterial supply of the colon from the superior mesenteric artery based upon a study of 600 specimens. Surg Gynecol Obstet 106:385–398
4. Steward JA, Rankin FW (1933) Blood supply of the large intestine: its surgical considerations. Arch Surg 26:843–891
5. Griffiths JD (1956) Surgical anatomy of the blood supply of the distal colon. Ann R Coll Surg Engl 19:241–256
6. Drummond H (1913) Some points relating to the surgical anatomy of the arterial supply of the large intestine. J R Soc Med 7:185–193
7. Kaminski DL, Herrmann VM (1986) Ischemic colitis. pp. 110–114. In Cameron J (ed): Current Surgical Therapy. 2nd Ed. BC Decker, Toronto
8. Kvietys PR, Granger DN (1982) Regulation of colonic blood flow. Fed Proc 41:2106–2110
9. Harnsberger JR, Longo WE, Vernava AM (1994) Vascular anatomy. Semin Colon Rectal Surg 5:2–13
10. Kornblith PL, Boley SJ, Whitehouse BS (1992) Anatomy of the splanchnic circulation. Surg Clin North Am 72:1–30
11. Moskowitz M, Zimmerman H, Felson B (1994) The meandering mesenteric artery of the colon. Am J Roentgenol 92:1088–1099
12. Jacobson LF, Noer RJ (1952) The vascular pattern of the intestinal villi in various laboratory animals and man. Anat Rec 114:85–101
13. O'Mara CS, Ernst CB (1995) Physiology of the mesenteric circulation. pp. 10–16. In Zuidema GD (ed): Shackelford's Surgery of the Alimentary Tract. 4th Ed. WB Saunders, Philadelphia
14. Hallback DA, Hulten L, Jodal M et al (1978) Evidence for the existence of a countercurrent exchange in the small intestine in man. Gastroenterology 74:683–690
15. Lundgren O (1974) The circulation of the small bowel mucosa. Gut 15:1005–1013
16. Price AB (1990) Ischaemic colitis. Curr Top Pathol 81:229–246
17. Brandt LJ, Boley SJ (1992) Colonic ischemia. Surg Clin North Am 72:203–229
18. Puglisi RN, Whalen TV, Doolin EJ (1995) Computer analyzed histology of ischemic injury to the gut. J Pediatr Surg 30:839–844
19. Weixiong H, Aneman A, Nilsson U, Lundgren O (1994) Quantification of tissue damage in the feline small intestine during ischaemia-reperfusion; the importance of free radicals. Acta Physiol Scand 150:241–250
20. Robinson JWL, Winistorfer B, Mirkovitch V (1980) Source of net water and electrolyte loss following intestinal ischemia. Res Exp Med 176:263–275
21. Schoenberg MH, Beger HG (1993) Reperfusion injury after intestinal ischemia. Crit Care Med 21:1376–1386
22. Simpson R, Alon R, Kobzik L et al (1993) Neutrophil and nonneutrophil-mediated injury in intestinal ischemia-reperfusion. Ann Surg 218:444–453
23. Yao YM, Sheng ZY, Yu Y et al (1995) The potential etiologic role of tumor necrosis factor in mediating multiple organ dysfunction in rats following intestinal ischemia-reperfusion injury. Resuscitation 29:157–168

24. Garcia JG, Cruz MD, Rollan CM et al (1995) Superoxide dismutase (SOD) and neutrophil infiltration in intestinal ischaemia-revascularization. Int Surg 80:95–97

25. Schmeling DJ, Caty MG, Oldham KT, Guice KS (1994) Cytoprotection by diclofenac sodium after intestinal ischemia-reperfusion injury. J Pediatr Surg 29:1044–1048

26. Sisley AC, Desai T, Harig JM, Gewertz BL (1994) Neutrophil depletion attenuates human intestinal reperfusion injury. J Surg Res 57:192–196

27. Sorkine P, Setton A, Halpern P et al (1995) Soluble tumor necrosis factor receptors reduce bowel ischemia-induced lung permeability and neutrophil sequestration. Crit Care Med 23: 1377–1381

28. Raul F, Galluser M, Schleiffer R et al (1995) Beneficial effects of ʟ-arginine on intestinal epithelial restitution after ischemic damage in rats. Digestion 56:400–405

29. Heys SD, Brittenden J, Crofts TJ (1993) Acute mesenteric ischaemia: the continuing difficulty in early diagnosis. Postgrad Med J 69:48–51

30. Dorudi S, Lamont PM (1992) Intestinal ischaemia in the unconscious intensive care unit patient. Ann R Coll Surg Engl 74:356–359

31. Wolf EL, Sprayregen S, Bakal CW (1992) Radiology in intestinal ischemia. Plain film, contrast, and other imaging studies. Surg Clin North Am 72:107–124

32. Seow-Choen F, Chua TL, Goh HS (1993) Ischaemic colitis and colorectal cancer: some problems and pitfalls. Int J Colorectal Dis 8:210–212

33. Brewster DC, Franklin DP, Cambria RP et al (1991) Intestinal ischemia complicating abdominal aortic surgery. Surgery 109:447–454

34. Dykman DD, Killian SE (1993) Initial experience with the Pentax VSB-P2900 enteroscope. Am J Gastroenterol 88: 570–573

35. Bartnicke BJ, Balfe DM (1994) CT appearance of intestinal ischemia and intramural hemorrhage. Radiol Clin North Am 32:845–860

36. Mirvis SE, Shanmuganathan K, Erb R (1994) Diffuse small-bowel ischemia in hypotensive adults after blunt trauma (shock bowel): CT findings and clinical significance. AJR Am J Roentgenol 163:1375–1379

37. Frager D, Baer JW, Medwid SW et al (1996) Detection of intestinal ischemia in patients with acute small-bowel obstruction due to adhesions or hernia: efficacy of CT. Am J Roentgenol 166:67–71

38. Temes RT, Kauten RJ, Schwartz MZ (1991) Nuclear magnetic resonance as a noninvasive method of diagnosing intestinal ischemia: technique and preliminary results. J Pediatr Surg 26:775–779

39. Park A, Towner RA, Langer JC (1993) Diagnosis of intestinal ischemia in the rat using magnetic resonance imaging. J Invest Surg 6:177–183

40. Park A, Towner RA, Langer JC (1994) Diagnosis of persistent intestinal ischemia in the rabbit using proton magnetic resonance imaging. J Invest Surg 7:485–492

41. Kaufman AJ, Tarr RW, Holburn GE et al (1988) Magnetic resonance imaging of ischemic bowel in rabbit model. Invest Radiol 23:93–97

42. Bass BL, Schweitzer EJ, Harmon JW, Kraimer J (1985) Intra-luminal pCO2: a reliable indicator of intestinal ischemia. J Surg Res 39:351–360

43. Andersen R, Stordahl A, Hoyseth H et al (1995) Increased intestinal permeability for the isosmolar contrast medium iodixanol during small-bowel ischaemia in rats. Scand J Gastroenterol 30:1082–1088

44. Duh QY (1993) Laparoscopic procedures for small bowel disease. Baillieres Clin Gastroenterol 7:833–850

45. Kam DM, Scheeres DE (1993) Fluorescein-assisted laparoscopy in the identification of arterial mesenteric ischemia. Surg Endosc 7:75–78

46. Horgan PG, Gorey TF (1992) Operative assessment of intestinal viability. Surg Clin North Am 72:143–155

47. Bergman RT, Gloviczki P, Welch TJ et al (1992) The role of intravenous fluorescein in the detection of colon ischemia during aortic reconstruction. Ann Vasc Surg 6:74–79

48. Johansson K, Ahn H, Lindhagen J (1986) Assessment of small-bowel ischemia by laser Doppler flowmetry. Some case reports. Scand J Gastroenterol 21:1147–1152

49. Johansson K (1988) Gastrointestinal application of laser Doppler flowmetry. An experimental and clinical study in cat and man. Acta Chir Scand Suppl 545:1–64

50. Johansson K, Ahn H, Lindhagen J (1989) Intraoperative assessment of blood flow and tissue viability in small-bowel ischemia by laser Doppler flowmetry. Acta Chir Scand 155: 341–346

51. Krausz MM, Manny J (1978) Acute superior mesenteric arterial occlusion: a plea for early diagnosis. Surgery 83:482–485

52. Jarvinen O, Laurikka J, Sisto T et al (1995) Atherosclerosis of the visceral arteries. Vasa 24:9–14

53. Lock G, Scholmerich J (1995) Non-occlusive mesenteric ischemia. Hepatogastroenterology 42:234–239

54. Schneider TA, Longo WE, Ure T, Vernava AM 3rd (1994) Mesenteric ischemia. Acute arterial syndromes. Dis Colon Rectum 37:1163–1174

55. Kaleya RN, Boley SJ (1992) Acute mesenteric ischemia: an aggressive diagnostic and therapeutic approach. 1991 Roussel Lecture. Can J Surg 35:613–623

56. Moore WM Jr, Hollier LH (1991) Mesenteric artery occlusive disease. Cardiol Clin 9:535–541

57. Finucane PM, Arunachalam T, O'Dowd J, Pathy MS (1989) Acute mesenteric infarction in elderly patients. J Am Geriatr Soc 37:355–358

58. Mishima Y (1988) Acute mesenteric ischemia. Jpn J Surg 18:615–619

59. Brooks DH, Carey LC (1973) Base deficit in superior mesenteric artery occlusion, an aid to early diagnosis. Ann Surg 177:352–356

60. Jamieson WG, Lozon A, Durand D, Wall W (1975) Changes in serum phosphate levels associated with intestinal infarction and necrosis. Surg Gynecol Obstet 140:19–21

61. Jamieson WG, Marchuk S, Ronsom J, Durand D (1982) The early diagnosis of massive intestinal ischemia. Br J Surg 69: S52–S53

62. Barnett SM, Davidson ED, Bradley EL (1976) Intestinal alkaline phosphatase and base deficit in mesenteric occlusion. J Surg Res 20:243–246

63. Lamor W, Woodard L, Statland BE (1978) Clinical implications of creatine kinase BB isoenzyme. N Engl J Med 299: 834–853

64. Graeber GM, Cafferty PJ, Reardon MJ et al (1981) Changes in the serum total creatine phosphakinase (CPK) and its isoenzymes caused by experimental ligation of the superior mesenteric artery. Ann Surg 193:499–505

65. Sachs SM, Morton JH, Schwartz SI (1982) Acute mesenteric ischemia. Surgery 92:646–653

66. Clark RA, Gallant TE (1984) Acute mesenteric ischemia: angiographic spectrum. Am J Roentgenol 142:555–562

67. Batellier J, Kieny R (1990) Superior mesenteric artery embolism: eighty-two cases. Ann Vasc Surg 4:112–116

68. Levy PJ, Krausz MM, Manny J (1990) Acute mesenteric ischemia: improved results—a retrospective analysis of ninety-two patients. Surgery 107:372–380

69. Dockendorf BL, Frazee RC, Peterson WG, Myers D (1993) Treatment of acute intestinal ischemia with hyperbaric oxygen. South Med J 86:518–520

70. Vujic I, Stanley J, Gobien RP (1984) Treatment of acute embolus of the superior mesenteric artery by topical infusion of streptokinase. Cardiovasc Intervent Radiol 7:94–96

71. McBride KD, Gaines PA (1994) Thrombolysis of a partially occluding superior mesenteric artery thromboembolus by infusion of streptokinase. Cardiovasc Intervent Radiol 17:164–166

72. VanDeinse WH, Zawacki JK, Phillips D (1986) Treatment of acute mesenteric ischemia by percutaneous transluminal angioplasty. Gastroenterology 91:475–478

73. Hallisey MJ, Deschaine J, Illescas FF et al (1995) Angioplasty for the treatment of visceral ischemia. J Vasc Interv Radiol 6:785–791

74. Lazaro T, Sierra L, Gesto R et al (1986) Embolization of the mesenteric arteries: surgical treatment in twenty-three consecutive cases. Ann Vasc Surg 1:311–315

75. McMillan WD, McCarthy WJ, Bresticker MR et al (1995) Mesenteric artery bypass: objective patency determination. J Vasc Surg 21:729–740

76. Johnston KW, Lindsay TF, Walker PM, Kalman PG (1995) Mesenteric arterial bypass grafts: early and late results and suggested surgical approach for chronic and acute mesenteric ischemia. Surgery 118:1–7

77. Ballard JL, Stone WM, Hallett JW et al (1993) A critical analysis of adjuvant techniques used to assess bowel viability in acute mesenteric ischemia. Am Surg 59:309–311

78. Stephenson BM, Thomas AJ, Shute K et al (1993) Acute intestinal ischaemia: options in surgical management. Ann R Coll Surg Engl 75:312–316

79. Nassar A (1994) 'Second-look' laparoscopy in the management of acute mesenteric ischemia. Br J Surg 81:1083

80. Chagla L, Kiff R (1994) 'Second look' laparoscopy in the management of acute mesenteric ischemia. Br J Surg 81:1083

81. Jrvinen O, Laurikka J, Salenius JP, Tarkka M (1994) Acute intestinal ischaemia. A review of 214 cases. Ann Chir Gynaecol 83:22–25

82. Tsai CJ, Kuo YC, Chen PC, Wu CS (1990) The spectrum of acute intestinal vascular failure: a collective review of 43 cases in Taiwan. Br J Clin Pract 44:603–608

83. Benjamin E, Oropello JM, Iberti TJ (1993) Acute mesenteric ischemia: pathophysiology, diagnosis, and treatment. Dis Mon 39:131–210

84. Allen KB, Salam AA, Lumsden AB (1992) Acute mesenteric ischemia after cardiopulmonary bypass. J Vasc Surg 16:391–395

85. Gennaro M, Ascer E, Matano R et al (1993) Acute mesenteric ischemia after cardiopulmonary bypass. Am J Surg 166:231–236

86. Feurle GE, Haag B (1991) Acute small bowel ischemia without transmural infarction. Z Gastroenterol 29:349–352

87. Cormier JM, Fichelle JM, Vennin J et al (1991) Atherosclerotic occlusive disease of the superior mesenteric artery: late results of reconstructive surgery. Ann Vasc Surg 5:510–518

88. Hallett JW Jr, James ME, Ahlquist DA et al (1990) Recent trends in the diagnosis and management of chronic intestinal ischemia. Ann Vasc Surg 4:126–132

89. Li KC, Whitney WS, McDonnell CH et al (1994) Chronic mesenteric ischemia: evaluation with phase-contrast cine MR imaging. Radiology 190:175–179

90. Li KC, Hopkins KL, Dalman RL, Song CK (1995) Simultaneous measurement of flow in the superior mesenteric vein and artery with cine phase-contrast MR imaging: value in diagnosis of chronic mesenteric ischemia. Work in progress. Radiology 194:327–330

91. Crotch Harvey MA, Gould DA, Green AT (1992) Case report: percutaneous transluminal angioplasty of the inferior mesenteric artery in the treatment of chronic mesenteric ichaemia. Clin Radiol 46:408–409

92. MacFarlane SD, Beebe HG (1989) Progress in chronic mesenteric arterial ischemia. J Cardiovasc Surg Torino 30:178–184

93. Calderon M, Reul GJ, Gregoric ID et al (1992) Long-term results of the surgical management of symptomatic chronic intestinal ischemia. J Cardiovasc Surg Torino 33:723–728

94. Johnston KW, Lindsay TF, Walker PM, Kalman PG (1995) Mesenteric arterial bypass grafts: early and late results and suggested surgical approach for chronic and acute mesenteric ischemia. Surgery 118:1–7

95. Rhee RY, Gloviczki P, Mendonca CT et al (1994) Mesenteric venous thrombosis: still a lethal disease in the 1990s. J Vasc Surg 20:688–697

96. Porter J, Vesely M, Jane S, Stebbing MA (1993) Mesenteric venous thrombosis with protein S deficiency. Am J Gastroenterol 88:2143

97. Montany PF, Finley PK Jr (1988) Mesenteric venous thrombosis. Am Surg 54:161–166 98. Wilson C, Walker ID, Davidson JF, Imrie CW (1987) Mesenteric venous thrombosis and antithrombin III deficiency. J Clin Pathol 40:906–908

99. Graubard ZG, Friedman M (1987) Mesenteric venous thrombosis associated with pregnancy and oral contraception. A case report. S Afr Med J 71:453

100. Nesbit RR Jr, Deweese JA (1977) Mesenteric venous thrombosis and oral contraceptives. South Med J 70:360–362

101. Milne PY, Thomas RJ (1976) Mesenteric venous thrombosis associated with oral contraceptives; a case report. Aust N Z J Surg 46:134–136

102. Corsi A, Ribaldi S, Coletti M, Bosman C (1995) Intramural mesenteric venulitis. A new cause of intestinal ischaemia. Virchows Arch 427:65–69

103. Genta RM, Haggitt RC (1991) Idiopathic myointimal hyperplasia of mesenteric veins. Gastroenterology 101:533–539

104. Flaherty MJ, Lie JT, Haggitt RC (1994) Mesenteric inflam-

matory veno-occlusive disease. A seldom recognized cause of intestinal ischemia. Am J Surg Pathol 18:779–784

105. Salaman JR, Mahmood K (1974) Recurrent mesenteric venous thrombosis complicating renal transplantation. Br J Urol 46:257–260

106. Eugene C, Valla D, Wesenfelder L et al (1995) Small intestinal stricture complicating superior mesenteric vein thrombosis. A study of three cases. Gut 37:292–295

107. Boley SJ, Kaleya RN, Brandt LJ (1992) Mesenteric venous thrombosis. Surg Clin North Am 72:183–201

108. Sack J, Aldrete JS (1982) Primary mesenteric venous thrombosis. Surg Gynecol Obstet 154:205–208

109. Carr N, Jamison MH (1981) Superior mesenteric venous thrombosis. Br J Surg 68:343–344

110. Kim JY, Ha HK, Byun JY et al (1993) Intestinal infarction secondary to mesenteric venous thrombosis: CT-pathologic correlation. J Comput Assist Tomogr 17:382–385

111. Rahmouni A, Mathieu D, Golli M et al (1992) Value of CT and sonography in the conservative management of acute splenoportal and superior mesenteric venous thrombosis. Gastrointest Radiol 17:135–140

112. Wade TP, Jewell WR, Andrus CH (1992) Mesenteric venous thrombosis. Modern management and endoscopic diagnosis. Surg Endosc 6:283–284

113. Rivitz SM, Geller SC, Hahn C, Waltman AC (1995) Treatment of acute mesenteric venous thrombosis with transjugular intramesenteric urokinase infusion. J Vasc Interv Radiol 6: 219–223

114. Levy PJ, Krausz MM, Manny J (1990) The role of second-look procedure in improving survival time for patients with mesenteric venous thrombosis. Surg Gynecol Obstet 170: 287–291

115. Marston A, Pheils MT, Thomas L, Morson BC (1996) Ischemic colitis. Gut 7:1–15

116. Boley SJ, Schwartz S, Lash J, Sternhill V (1963) Reversible vascular occlusion of the colon. Surg Gynecol Obstet 116: 53–60

117. Bower TC (1993) Ischemic colitis. Surg Clin North Am 73: 1037–1053

118. Taylor GE, Hebra A, McGowan KL et al (1995) Octreotide does not prevent bacterial translocation in an infant piglet model of intestinal ischemia-reperfusion. J Pediatr Surg 30: 967–969

119. Gandhi SK, Hanson MM, Vernava AM et al (1996) Ischemic colitis. Dis Colon Rectum 39:88–100

120. Ho MS, Teh LB, Goh HS (1987) Ischaemic colitis in systemic lupus erythematosus—report of a case and review of the literature. Ann Acad Med Singapore 16:501–503

121. Reissman P, Weiss EG, Teoh TA et al (1994) Gangrenous ischemic colitis of the rectum: a rare complication of systemic lupus erythematosus. Am J Gastroenterol 89:2234–2236

122. Seow-Choen F, Chua TL, Goh HS (1993) Ischaemic colitis and colorectal cancer: some problems and pitfalls. Int J Colorectal Dis 8:210–212

123. Visser T, Bove P, Barkel D et al (1995) Colorectal complications following cardiac surgery: six-year experience. Dis Colon Rectum 38:1210–1213

124. Maupin GE, Rimar SD, Villalba M (1989) Ischemic colitis following abdominal aortic reconstruction for ruptured aneurysm: a 10-year experience. Am Surg 55:378–380

125. Deana DG, Dean PJ (1995) Reversible ischaemic colitis in young women. Association with contraceptive use. Am J Surg Pathol 19:454–462

126. Matsumoto T, Iida M, Kimura Y et al (1994) Clinical features in young adult patients with ischaemic colitis. J Gastroenterol Hepatol 9:572–575

127. Gurbuz AK, Gurbuz B, Salas L et al (1994) Premarin-induced ischemic colitis. J Clin Gastroenterol 19:108–111

128. Brown DN, Rosenholtz MJ, Marshall JB (1994) Ischemic colitis related to cocaine abuse. Am J Gastroenterol 89: 1558–1561

129. Scholz FJ (1993) Ischemic bowel disease. Radiol Clin North Am 31:1197–1218

130. Philpotts LE, Heiken JP, Westcott MA, Gore RM (1994) Colitis: use of CT findings in differential diagnosis. Radiology 190:445–449

131. Brandt LJ, Boley SJ, Sammartano RJ (1986) Carbon dioxide and room air insufflation of the colon: effects on colonic blood flow and intraluminal pressure in the dog. Gastrointest Endosc 32:324–329

132. Wheeldon NM, Grundman MJ (1990) Ischaemic colitis as a complication of colonoscopy. BMJ 301:1080–1081

133. Ambrosett P, Robert J, Mathey P, Rohner A (1994) Left-sided colon and colorectal anastomoses: doppler ultrasound as an aid to assess bowel vascularization. A prospective evaluation of 200 consecutive elective cases. Int J Colorectal Dis 9:211–214

134. Fiddian-Green RG, Amelin PM, Herrmann JB et al (1986) Prediction of the development of sigmoid ischemia on the day of aortic operations. Arch Surg 121:654–660

135. Reeders JW, Tytgat GN, Rosenbusch G, Gramata S (1984) Ischemic Colitis. pp. 17–28, 145–151. Martinus Nijoff, The Hague

136. Parish KL, Chapman WC, Williams LF (1991) Ischemic colitis: an ever-changing spectrum? Am Surg 57:118–121

137. Guttormson NL, Bubrick MP (1989) Mortality from ischemic colitis. Dis Colon Rectum 32:469–472

43

CONGENITAL ANOMALIES

Robert L. Telander
William S. Brennom

HIRSCHSPRUNG'S DISEASE

In 1887 Hirschsprung[1] published his classic paper describing postmortem findings in infants with constipation and abdominal distension from birth. He described a distended colon with muscular hypertrophy proximal to a smaller rectum of more normal size. It was initially thought that the dilated distended proximal colon was the pathologic portion of the bowel, but in the 1930s investigators observed abnormal ganglion cells in the distended segment near the junction of the contracted distal segment. In 1938 Robertson and Kernohan[2,2a] and others including Zueler and Wilson in 1948 reported a group of children in whom the absence of ganglion cells was observed in the distal contracted segment and more normal appearing ganglion cells in the proximal distended segment.

In the 1940s, Swenson and Bill[3] as well as Ehrenpreis appreciated that children with aganglionic megacolon did well after a colostomy. These observations encouraged them to develop a surgical procedure removing the aganglionic distal rectum and sigmoid colon and bringing down the proximal colon with normal ganglion cells to the anus. Others working in this area (including Duhamel,[5] Soave,[6] and Boley[7]) also developed operative procedures that successfully corrected the problem. All of them surgically bypassed or removed the abnormal distal rectum (with an absence of ganglion cells), bringing proximal bowel with normal ganglion cells to the anal opening.

The incidence of Hirschsprung's disease is approximately 1 in 5,000 births. In patients with Hirschsprung's disease in whom the transition zone occurs in the typical location of the rectosigmoid, the male predominance is approximately 4:1. With a progressively longer segment of bowel involved with aganglionosis, there is a decreased male/female sex ratio. Of interest is the fact that in children with a transition zone in the small bowel the increased inherited risk approaches 30%. Other associated anomalies are few, and specific gene mapping has to date been unsuccessful.

Etiology

Hirschsprung's disease is characterized by the absence of ganglion cells in the rectum and rectosigmoid. Ganglion cells originate from the precursors found initially in the neural crest cells, which migrate cephalad to caudad in the intestine.[8] The cells ultimately reach the distal rectum by the end of the first trimester.[9] The migration can be seen in Auerbach's and Meissner's plexus at this stage of development. Later, neuroblasts appear in Henley's deep submucosal plexus and Meissner's superficial plexus. The neuroblasts mature to ganglion cells in both Auerbach's and Meissner's plexus. This maturation may not be complete at birth and is continued into the second year. Failure of this normal migration is thought to result in Hirschsprung's disease.

Other theories presented suggest immunologic destruction of neural elements. The presence of an immunologic response in the pathogenesis of Hirschsprung's disease has recently been studied again because of recent reports noting a marked elevation of MHC class II antigens involving the entire intestinal wall of aganglionic colon. Localization (in particular in the mucosa, lamina propria, and hypertrophic nerve trunks), was observed.[10] A recent study looked at the expression of intracellular adhesion molecule-1 (ICAM-1) and MHC class II antigens in patients undergoing bowel resection for Hirschsprung's disease. Strong expression of ICAM-1 and MHC class II antigens was found on the hypertrophic nerve trunks, both in the submucous and myenteric plexus of the aganglionic colon and on small ganglia in the myenteric and submucous plexus within the transition zone. In addition, there was no staining of ganglia or nerve cells in the ganglionic colon from the patients with Hirschsprung's disease.[11] Elevated class II antigen levels have also been demonstrated in patients with neuronal intestinal dysplasia.[12]

Pathophysiology

The aganglionic colon does not permit normal peristaltic waves to occur. Manometric studies have demonstrated a progressive wave of normal peristalsis in the normal colon proximal to the aganglionic segment. Progression of the normal peristaltic wave from the ganglionic segment to the aganglionic distal bowel is absent. The normal internal anal sphincter reflexly relaxes in response to rectal distension in normal individuals, but contracts after rectal distension in patients with Hirschsprung's disease. A functional obstruction thus occurs.

Clinical Findings

The infant may present with the appearance of complete colonic obstruction with or without overwhelming enterocolitis in the newborn. With the older infant or child, the presentation may vary. It may be much more subtle, with constipation, abdominal distension, and sometimes poor nutrition. Hirschsprung's disease was described by the late Dr. W. B. Keiswetter as the great masquerader because of the myriad of clinical pictures seen in children presenting with this problem.

Swenson emphasized that 94% of normal term neonates stooled in the first 24 hours, whereas 94% of neonates with Hirschsprung's disease do not stool in the same period.[13] This finding currently varies because of the numerous premature infants seen in neonatal intensive care units in the 1990s, but clearly it is highly unusual for infants not to pass meconium during the first 48 hours of life; such babies should be considered for diagnostic studies. Currently over one-half of all children diagnosed with Hirschsprung's disease are seen in the neonatal period with abdominal distension and obstructive symptoms, including bilious emesis. At times they may have diarrhea along with vomiting and sepsis, which are features of enterocolitis associated with the colonic obstruction.

Most children with idiopathic constipation have soiling because of the close proximity of the dilated rectum to the underclothing, whereas children with Hirschsprung's disease have a longer separation of the functional colon from the anus, and do not soil in this fashion. In addition, children with chronic constipation have little abdominal distension, although fecal material can be palpated on examination of the abdomen. Children with Hirschsprung's disease tend to have extreme abdominal distension because they are unable to pass the flatus in addition to the stool.

In the neonatal patient, physical examination should include a careful rectal examination to rule out anorectal anomalies and to establish the presence or absence of normal meconium. On introduction of the finger in the infant a stool may be produced, which may allow passage of a meconium plug thereby diminishing the possibility of the diagnosis of Hirschsprung's disease. A meconium plug may exist in an otherwise normal infant, but it may also be associated with Hirschsprung's disease. Because not all affected infants manifest the full clinical picture, some are prescribed feeds and the diagnosis does not become apparent until after the addition of cereals and strained foods and a more solid diet.

Diagnosis

The history of a child failing to pass stools within the first 24 to 48 hours, along with abdominal distension and bilious vomiting, is a strong predictor of possible Hirschsprung's disease and an indication for diagnostic studies.[14] The occurrence in older children of abdominal distension associated with chronic constipation as described also points toward the possibility of Hirschsprung's disease. Abdominal plain films are helpful by identifying intestinal obstruction in the distal colon rather than the small bowel, thus indicating the need for a barium enema examination.[14a]

The diagnosis is usually easily made on barium enema, which identifies the area of transition from the collapsed aganglionic distal bowel to the distended proximal ganglionic bowel. In problem cases, as in the newborn, a follow-up film taken 24 hours after the barium enema may demonstrate barium remaining in the colon at the transition zone, an appearance quite diagnostic of Hirschsprung's disease. Sometimes in the newborn the amount of dilation of the proximal bowel may be inadequate to show the characteristic change in size of the colon on the barium enema. When clinical suspicion still exists, it is necessary to proceed with a rectal biopsy. An important technical point is to avoid irrigation of the colon before the radiologic examination; such irrigation may remove the evidence of narrowed segment with proximal detection. The insertion of a balloon catheter into the rectum for the barium enema may dilate an otherwise narrow distal rectum, giving a false negative result.

Rectal biopsy is the definitive diagnostic technique for Hirschsprung's disease, showing the absence of ganglion cells and the presence of hypertrophied nonmyelinated nerve fibers in the mucosa. The pathologist may utilize a histochemical stain for excessive acetylcholinesterase present in the lamina propria.[15] A suction biopsy of the rectum is frequently used, and the technique is helpful in providing a small piece of mucosa and submucosa. Three biopsies 2 to 3 cm above the pectinate line should be taken. Some pathologists prefer a full-thickness rectal biopsy, which they claim demonstrates more certainly the absence of ganglion cells and the presence of hypertrophied nerves. Full-thickness rectal biopsy remains the standard against which other techniques are evaluated. Diagnostic difficulty may occur when the biopsy is performed too distally toward the pectinate line. It is essential therefore to perform the biopsy at least 2 cm above the pectinate line in a neonates and at least 3 cm in the older child. Performing a full-thickness rectal biopsy in the very young infant can be difficult owing to the small size of the anal canal. The Lonestar retractor, however, permits excellent visualization and greatly simplifies this procedure. With suction and full-thickness biopsies, permanent rather than frozen sections may be utilized. Multiple staining techniques, including hematoxylin and eosin and acetylcholinesterase should be used.[15]

The differential diagnosis includes the *left colon syndrome*, which is seen in children whose mothers are diabetic. Children with a meconium plug may occasionally have Hirschsprung's disease, but most do not and are greatly improved by contrast enema leading to the passage of a large meconium stool. The removal of a meconium plug is enhanced by utilizing a water-soluble hypertonic solution such as Gastrografin. A colostomy is avoided by this maneuver, which leads to rapid improvement.

In childhood, chronic constipation due to idiopathic megabowel may be confused with Hirschsprung's disease. The controversial question of short-segment Hirschsprung's disease arises when the patient fails to respond to the usual therapy for this condition. Short-segment Hirschsprung's disease can occasionally occur, and in this circumstance a rectal biopsy will identify the child who appears on contrast enema to have some of the features of Hirschsprung's disease but not the classic picture. Hirschsprung's disease is also characterized by absence of the recto-sphincteric inhibition reflex.

Treatment

In infancy, once the diagnosis has been established it is essential to perform a colostomy promptly to halt the disease process and to decrease the risk of enterocolitis. Sieber[16] emphasized the life-saving nature of a colostomy in the ill newborn child with abdominal distension. Many pediatric surgeons perform a definitive pull-through procedure in the newborn, while some prefer an initial colostomy and carry out the pull-through procedure after the child is at least 6 months old. In older children, lavage irrigation may be used to prepare the bowel for a definitive pull-through procedure.

The colostomy is made just proximal to the point of transition. Thus a sigmoid colostomy is the most frequent stoma performed when the surgeon decides on a two-stage treatment. Some surgeons continue to utilize the three-stage procedure, including an initial transverse colostomy in the newborn followed by a pull-through procedure several months later with subsequent closure of the stoma.[17,18] A protective colostomy after the pull-through procedure greatly reduces the possibility of anastomotic leakage and pelvic sepsis, which is the most common cause of serious morbidity and death.

Three procedures are currently in use for treating Hirschsprung's disease (Fig. 43-1A–E). All appear to be effective in relieving the constipation, although minimal differences exist in postoperative complications and functional results. The Swenson procedure (Fig. 43-1A) was the first of these to be described. The dissection is carried out close to the wall of the aganglionic rectum down to the anus, at which level it is divided. The proximal colon with normal ganglia is then anastomosed to the anal canal just above the pectinate line.

The Duhamel operation (Fig. 43-1B,C) was introduced with the intention of minimizing the pelvic dissection by confining this to the posterior aspect of the rectum. The proximal bowel with normal ganglion cells was then brought down behind the rectum to be anastomosed to the anal canal just above the pectinate line. Before doing so the rectum is transected, leaving a short stump, and the adjunct posterior rectal and anterior colonic walls are divided by linear stapling introduced per anum to create a common reservoir.

Soave[19] described the endorectal pull-through procedure which was modified by Boley[7] (Fig. 43-1D&E) and has become the most widely utilized technique.[20] Here the rectum is dissected and transected in its lower part. The mucosa is excised from the residual stump and the ganglionic colon is brought down through the rectal muscular sleeve to be anastomosed to the anal canal.

Authors' Preferred Approach

The diagnosis of Hirschsprung's's disease is made by rectal biopsy; in the acute situation a proximal colostomy is performed. Currently we are performing the definitive Soave pull through in early infancy with or without the protective colostomy. A Soave endorectal pull-through operation is carried out at 6 to 9 months of age. This has been modified by carrying out the rectal mucosectomy endoanally, minimizing the operative time. The transanal mucosectomy is done while the abdomen is being opened and the colostomy taken down.

The patient is placed in the lithotomy position, which is modified according to the age of the patient. In the infant, padded footplates are placed beneath the mattress, extending beyond the end of the table. A rectal tube is inserted and the rectum irrigated with saline followed by povidine-iodine solution (50 ml). A transverse lower abdominal incision is made to divide part of the right and all of the left rectus abdominis muscle. It then is curved superiorly to the left of the lower abdomen. This incision can be extended superiorly to expose the splenic flexure if needed.

The level of aganglionosis is established by biopsy if this has not previously been determined. The bowel is divided with a stapling device (GIA Auto sutures) just proximal to the transitional zone. Dissection is then carried out close to the wall of the rectum as in a classic Swenson procedure and is continued down to the level of the levators, where it encounters the mucosal dissection that has been already performed from below.

The transanal simultaneous mucosectomy is carried out utilizing the Lonestar retractor, which provides excellent exposure (Fig. 43-2A). In addition, electrocautery allows a rapid but meticulous dissection of the mucosal tube, starting at 1 cm above the pectinate line.

On completion of the submucosal and rectal dissection, a ring forceps is passed through the anal canal to withdraw the ganglionated rectum with the mucosal sleeve through the anus. The bowel is then divided to effect removal of the aganglionic bowel and mucosal sleeve. The ring forceps is again passed through the anus and short muscular cuff to grasp the ganglionated normal colon and deliver it to the perineum (Fig. 43-2B). A two-layer anastomosis is then made with Polyglactin (vicryl) sutures (30) and the abdomen closed either with or without a colostomy, depending on the surgeon's assessment of the procedure.

Complications

In the absence of a colostomy, an anastomotic leak can be serious. Its presence is suggested by fever, ileus, and abdominal pain. An emergency colostomy should be performed when a leak is confirmed. Appropriate radiologic contrast studies may be helpful in diagnosis. In the authors' hands, anastamotic leakage has not occurred owing to the practice of performing a proximal colostomy. If an anastomotic leak occurs, scarring with permanent damage to the sphincter and incontinence may result.

Regardless of the type of pull-through procedure, postoperative enterocolitis may develop, especially in children who presented with enterocolitis initially. This serious condition is manifested by sepsis, lethargy, and abdominal distension. Rectal examination is followed by forceful evacuation of a large amount of foul-smelling liquid stool. Therapy primarily consists of antibiotics combined with gentle rectal saline irrigations,

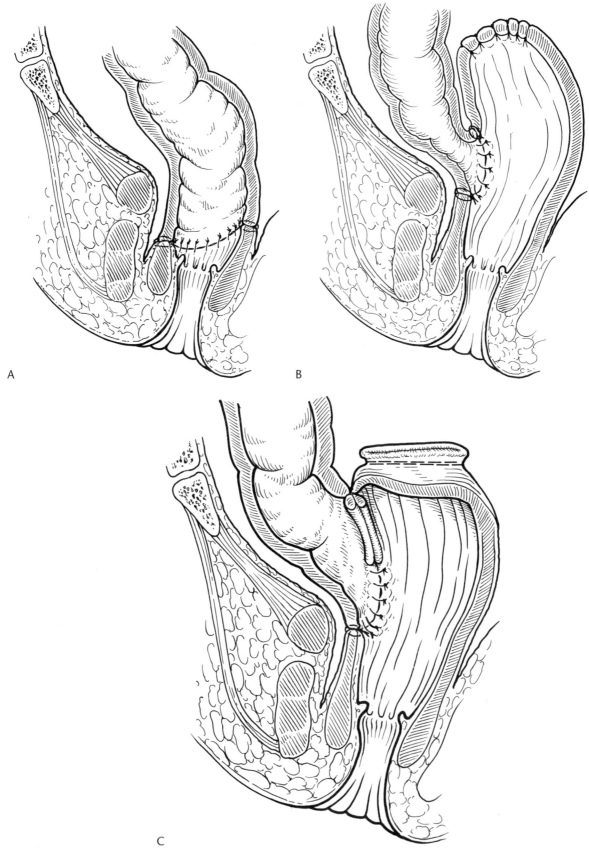

Figure 43-1. Diagrams of the three most common surgical procedures for Hirschsprung's disease. (**A**) In Swenson's procedure the bowel containing ganglion cells is anastomosed 1 to 2 cm above the pectinate line. (**B & C**) Duhamel's procedure; anastomosis between colon posteriorly to the remaining aganglionic rectum. Division of the spur between colon and rectum (**C**). (*Figure continues.*)

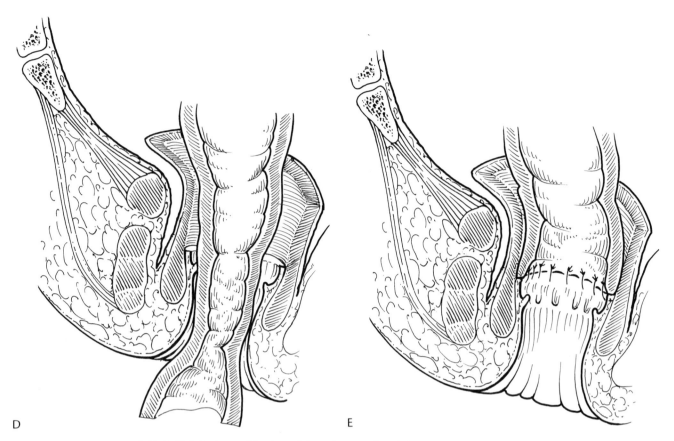

Figure 43-1. *(continued)* (**D & E**) Boley's modification of Soave's procedure brings innervated colon to 1 cm from the anal verge.

intravenous fluids, and electrolyte replacement. Such an episode may be life threatening and must be treated promptly and aggressively. Patients with enterocolitis may have palpable narrowing at the anastomosis, but usually they do not. A posterior sphincterotomy of the internal sphincter carried distally may provide relief, but no real evidence supports this notion. Subsequent management includes continued daily rectal irrigations at home by the mother, especially on any hint of abdominal distension. Some children experience recurrent attacks and may continue to be at risk as late as the teenage years, although the condition is primarily seen in the first 3 years of life and generally decreases later.

Anastomotic strictures and fecal incontinence can occur following a pull-through procedure. Long-term follow-up of patients in whom the transanal approach was used has demonstrated satisfactory clinical results with neither of these complications.

Total Aganglionosis

Patients with involvement of the entire colon extending even into the small bowel account for 5% to 10% of all children with Hirschsprung's disease and pose greater difficulty in management. Removal of the affected bowel with rectal mucosectomy and J-pouch reconstruction has produced excellent results in the authors' experience.

In the rare but severe cases of aganglionosis extending up into the jejunum, a much greater problem is presented. Myotomy of the aganglionic jejunum has been described, but long-term results are uncertain.[21] Parenteral nutrition is required in these children, and the associated incidence of central line sepsis and morbidity and mortality may become very high.

ANORECTAL MALFORMATIONS

Anorectal malformations affect approximately 1 in 5,000 live births, with a nearly equal distribution between males and females. The severity of the malformation depends on the timing of its development during fetal life. Embryonic differentiation of the hindgut and urinary system is due to a failure of descent of the urorectal septum. The separation of the urinary tract and the hindgut is determined by the level to which the urorectal septum descends. It is important to be aware of the numerous other anomalies often associated with anorectal malformations. Children born with an anorectal malformation should be evaluated for the other anomalies including esophageal atresia with tracheoesophageal fistula (10%) and cardiac (8%) and genitourinary (30%) anomalies. The VACTERL syndrome (*v*ertebral, *a*nal, *c*ardiac, *t*racheoesophageal, *r*enal,) and *l*imb anomalies) is more an association of anomalies than a syndrome.

Numerous classifications of anorectal malformations have been described. The first of these was developed by Gross,[22] and refinements were made by Stephens and Smith.[22] From a surgical point of view, the lesions can be classified according

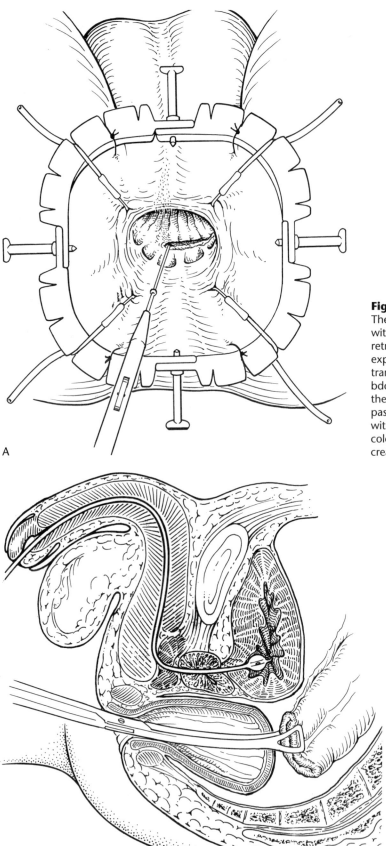

A

B

Figure 43-2.   Soave procedure. (**A**) The transanal dissection is performed with electrocautery with the Lonestar retractor in place to provide excellent exposure. (**B**) Upon completion of the transanal mucosal dissection and intra-bdominal dissection with removal of the aganglionic bowel, a forceps is then passed through the anal canal and withdraws the ganglionated normal colon. A two layer anastomosis is then created using absorbable suture.

Table 43-1. Classification of Anorectal Anomalies

	Level of Occlusion	Clinical Description
High	Above levator ani	Anorectal agenesis with[a] or without fistula
Intermediate	Within surrounding area of levator ani	Anorectal agenesis with[b] or without fistula
Low	Below levator ani, within anal canal	Anal stenosis with[c] or without fistula

[a] Female: rectovaginal; male: rectoprostatic or rectourethral.
[b] Female: rectovaginal or rectovestibular; male: rectobulbar or rectourethral.
[c] Female: anovestibular or anocutaneous; male: anocutaneous.

to the distal level of the occluded rectum. This may be high (supralevator), intermediate (partially translevator), or low (fully translevator). Most males with this malformation have a rectourethral fistula; the most common female equivalent is a rectovestibular fistula. A contrast study with the patient inverted demonstrating the rectal pouch provides adequate information to identify whether the end of the rectum is above, at, or below the pubococcygeal line. A rectum that ends above the pubococcygeal line is supralevator, or high. If it ends below the pubococcygeal line, but above the I point, or ischium, the defect is intermediate. A low defect (i.e., below the I point) will lend itself to surgical correction through the perineum shortly after birth, whereas the high anomalies are best treated by colostomy followed by reconstruction at 6 to 12 months of age. At that time a sacroperineal or abdominal sacroperineal pull-through procedure should be carried out. A high anomaly may be associated with a degree of sacrococcygeal agenesis.

Clinical Findings

Whereas the diagnosis of imperforate anus is obvious, the location of an associated fistula and its connection to the perineum vagina or urinary tract may be difficult. In the male, a small fistulous tract may develop along the median raphe of the perineum, extending as far as the scrotum. This finding usually denotes a low imperforate anus. Here further studies are required. Anal stenosis or an anal membrane are diagnosed by inspection. If the infant voids meconium per urethrum or has air in the bladder, a rectourethral fistula is certain. A voiding cystourethrogram may demonstrate a fistula that generally extends into the prostatic urethra, although it may be as high as the bladder. The presence of a dark-stained subcutaneous covering generally suggests a low malformation as well as a bucket-handled deformity in the anal area, often associated with anal stenosis. Frequent re-evaluations clinically over the first 12 to 24 hours may reveal a small dot of meconium appearing on the perineum, or in the female appearing from the vaginal opening or vestibule immediately posterior to the hymen.

Diagnostic Studies

Diagnostic studies are carried out to identify other anomalies and to determine the level of the blind rectal pouch as well as any associated fistula. A nasogastric tube should be passed

immediately to rule out esophageal atresia. Chest films are helpful in evaluating and identifying any possible cardiac intrathoracic and spinal or vertebral anomalies. An inverted lateral radiograph that includes the pelvis with a marker at the external sphincter may be helpful in identifying the level of the rectal pouch. Male infants with a low imperforate anus usually have a discernable fistula in the perineum along the midline; in females the opening may be in the perineum or vestibule. These infants generally pass meconium within the first 24 hours of life. In those infants with a higher malformation, a voiding cystourethrogram and contrast study will be helpful in identifying the associated fistula. All patients with a fistula communicating with the urinary tract have a high malformation requiring a colostomy.

Surgical Treatment

Peña has devised a flowchart for management, (Fig. 43-3A& B), based on clinical assessment, with radiology giving further information in about 20% of cases. The sagittal anorectoplasty described by Peña and DeVries[24] is currently the most popular technique.

Low Lesions

The management of low lesions includes simple measures including dilation of a stenosis present near the anal opening. Hegar dilators are suitable, beginning with a very small fine dilator and continuing up to at least a Hegar #10. This may be accomplished over several days and allows the child to maintain defecation. If dilations are maintained regularly, often no further therapy is required. In cases that do not respond, anoplasty is required. This is often necessary, especially if the anal opening is placed slightly anteriorly. In this circumstance the child is likely to respond well to a limited sagittal anorectoplasty. Similarly, in males with a long subcutaneous fistulous opening, it may be necessary to carry out a limited sagittal anorectoplasty or a simple unroofing of a membrane over the anal opening should that be the anatomic abnormality.

Intermediate and High Lesions

Infants with intermediate and high lesions can be diagnosed by radiology within the first 24 hours of life. At that time a suitable colostomy, usually a sigmoid colostomy, is carried out. Sagittal anorectoplasty via a posterior sacral approach is the preferred subsequent treatment of choice. This is usually carried out at 6 to 12 months of age.

Surgical Repair

Rectourethral fistulae are repaired via a posterior sacral approach, as described by Peña[25] (Fig. 43-4A–C) The patient is placed in the prone jackknife position with flexion of the hips. A special electrical stimulator designed by Peña is used throughout the operation to identify the delicate striated fibers of the pelvic floor and any sphincter musculature, sometimes including the superficial and subcutaneous external sphincter.

A sagittal incision is made beginning from the coccyx to the external sphincter or the anterior margin of the anus. A needle-

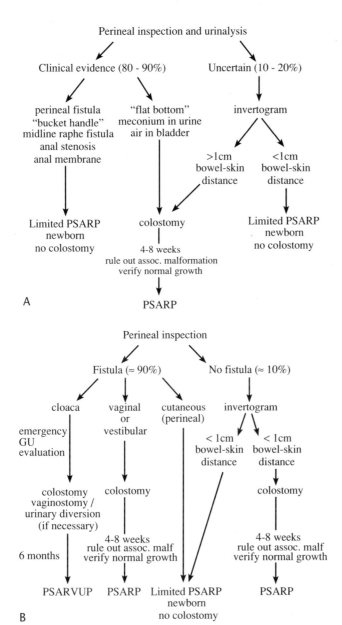

Figure 43-3. (**A**) Decision-making algorithm for the management of newborn male babies with anorectal malformation. PSARP, posterior sagittal anorectoplasty. (Courtesy of Alberto Peña). (**B**) Decision-making algorithm for the management of newborn female babies with anorectal malformation. PSARVUP, posterior sagittal anorectovaginourethroplasty; PSARP, posterior sagittal anorectoplasty.

tip cutting current is used for the incision and carried down in the midsagittal plane through the subcutaneous and superficial external sphincter muscle layers. This instrument is helpful in eliminating bleeding, which could obscure the fine muscle fibers that must be identified and divided, in the midline as far as is possible. The dissection is continued in the midline. Prolapsing fat indicates departure from this plane. Subsequently, the muscle fibers of the external sphincter and levators ani join and can be identified as forming the striated muscle complex. The dissection is continued to the levator ani if necessary. The

coccyx is split sagittally for exposure. On incising the levator ani, all layers of striated muscle are retracted laterally to expose the rectal pouch and its investing endopelvic fascia.

The dissection then continues around the rectum. Once this has been achieved, the rectal pouch is opened, and the fistula as it enters the urinary tract is identified (Fig. 43-4B). It is essential to carry out any dissection associated with the rectum directly on the rectum itself to avoid injury to the autonomic nerves and ganglia in the perirectal tissue. The fistula to the urethra can be seen and probed from within the bowel lumen. The rectal orifice of the fistula is circumcised and dissection continued to separate the fistula from the rectum and urethra (Fig. 43-4C). This is then closed, and the rectum is further mobilized superiorly until the seminal vesicles are visualized. If dilation of the rectum is present, the excessive rectal tissue is excised, but generally this is not necessary, and tapering of the rectum should not be carried out unless obvious distension is present.

The striated muscle complex of the levator and sphincter is subsequently mobilized to encircle the rectum (Fig. 43-4D). This is accomplished by placing the rectum itself in front of the reapproximated levator ani; the posterior edges of the striated muscle complex are then approximated and sutured to the edges of the distal rectum.

At 2 weeks, the anal opening is calibrated, and gentle gradual dilations are begun either with Hegar dilators beginning with #s 12 to 13, graduating to a # 14 to 15 dilator in the older child.

Surgical Repair in Females

Perineal Fistula

The diagnosis is made by inspection. If it is quite close to the center of the external sphincter, simple dilation with Hegar dilators may be adequate. If the fistula is positioned anteriorly, an anoplasty may be necessary. Generally a colostomy is not necessary unless the fistula lies far anteriorly adjacent to the vestibule.

Rectovestibular Fistula

A rectovestibular fistula is a much more difficult problem than it might seem. A colostomy is almost always required. A limited sagittal anorectoplasty is performed (Fig. 43-5). The orifice of the rectovestibular fistula is identified and fine stay sutures are placed circumferentially around the mucotaneous junction. The midline incision is then extended posteriorly, and the dissection is continued around the orifice to the wall of the rectum. The anterior rectal wall is in continuity with the vaginal wall, and the dissection is carefully carried out between these two structures. The dissection is extended superiorly to separate the rectum from the vagina. Unless this is complete, a risk of tension of the reconstruction exists after anastomosis with the skin. After the separation of the rectum from the vaginal wall, the repair is begun. The striated muscle complex is sutured about the rectum, approximating it anteriorly and posteriorly with fine sutures. The end of the rectum is carefully sutured to the skin and a Foley catheter is left in place for 3 to 5 days postoperatively. Antibiotics are given for 72 hours.

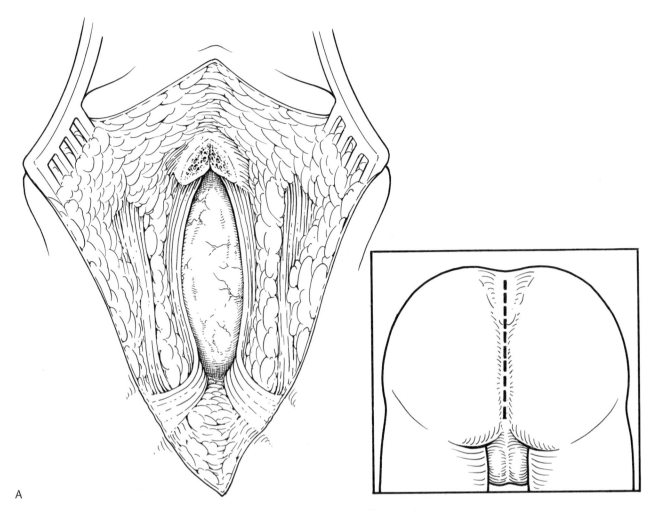

Figure 43-4. (**A**) Posterior sagittal incision. Separation of parasagittal fibers and exposure of the muscle complex. (*Figure continues.*)

Rectovaginal Fistula

Rectovaginal fistula is a much less common defect and requires a more extensive midline sagittal incision. This is because the higher the level of the rectovaginal fistula, the shorter the available rectum that must be mobilized. It is thus essential to carry out a much more extensive mobilization of the rectum in high rectovaginal fistula.

Postoperative Care

An examination under anesthesia is carried out 2 weeks later. The sutures are removed and calibration of the anal opening, usually to a Hegar dilator 10 to 12 is made. In some cases this can be carried out in the office. Daily dilation is then continued by the mother at home, gradually increasing the size of the dilator weekly. After approximately 2 to 3 months, when healing is complete and the anastomosis is soft and supple, the colostomy can be closed.

MALROTATION OF THE INTESTINE

Malrotation is usually due to failure of rotation or fixation of the midgut, or both. The earliest report of this abnormality was published in 1898 by Mall[26] and was later elaborated by em-

bryologic studies.[27] Normal rotation occurs between the 5th and 12th weeks of interuterine life, in which the fetal intestine undergoes the physiologic herniation and returns to the abdomen after undergoing a 270° rotation. The colon becomes fixed to the right posterior abdominal wall and the distal duodenum and proximal jejunum to the left of the origin of the superior mesenteric vessels at the ligament of Treitz. Under normal conditions this provides a broad base for the small intestinal mesentery from the ligament of Treitz to the cecum and prevents twisting of the entire midgut. All patients with malrotation display some degree of failure of rotation of the full 270° together with a narrowed base of the mesentery, which may allow the midgut to twist on itself. The surgical anatomy and approach standardized by Ladd[28] in 1936 with embryologic development, which was first described by Dott[29] in 1923. Failure of rotation or fixation of the midgut may include the proximal or duodenojejunal loop and/or the distal or colic loop.[30,31]

Clinical Manifestations

Malrotation leads to three clinical problems: acute or chronic midgut volvulus, chronic duodenal obstruction, and obstruction secondary to mesocolic hernia. Most patients with midgut vol-

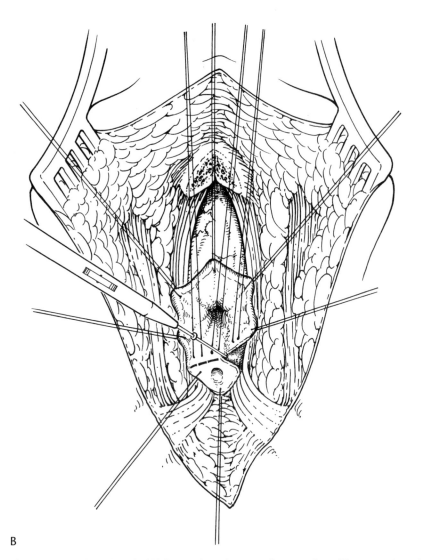

B

Figure 43-4 (*Continued*). (**B**) Separation of rectum from urethra. (*Figure continues.*)

vulus present with sudden bilious vomiting or bilious gastric aspirates within the first few months of life, although these symptoms may occur at any age. Physical examination may reveal abdominal distension and a palpable mass and abdominal tenderness. Infants with volvulus are usually full term, but the condition has been seen in stillborns and may present in premature infants, in whom it can be confused with necrotizing enterocolitis.[32]

If the volvulus of the midgut progresses, it may lead to strangulation of the bowel and gangrene of the entire midgut, resulting in a catastrophic loss of intestine. This disaster is associated with mortality of over 40%.[33]

Uncommonly, patients may present with chronic midgut volvulus and also recurrent abdominal pain from intermittent volvulus, which is often associated with lymphatic and venous obstruction. Chronic diarrhea or malabsorption and failure to thrive may also be present.[34,35]

Duodenal obstruction demands a search for acute midgut volvulus. Upper gastrointestinal contrast studies may reveal

duodenal atresia or partial obstruction from a high-grade duodenal stenosis or extrinsic compression by Ladd's bands passing from the colon to the right retroperitoneum. A mesocolic hernia occurs on the right side if the upper small bowel or duodenojejunal loop fails to rotate to the left of the superior mesenteric artery and remains trapped within the right mesocolon. It also may occur on the left, where a small bowel or duodenojejunal loop invaginates into the left mesocolon between the inferior mesenteric vein and the retroperitoneum. Such patients present with recurrent and intermittent signs of abdominal pain, vomiting, and obstruction[36] (Fig. 43-6).

Associated abnormalities in patients with malrotation include gastrochisis, omphalocele, and congenital diaphragmatic hernia with malrotation almost always present.[37] Malrotation has also been associated with duodenal atresia, small intestinal atresia, intussusception, esophageal atresia, prune belly syndrome, Hirschsprung's disease, pyloric stenosis, situs inversus, and heterotaxia.[38]

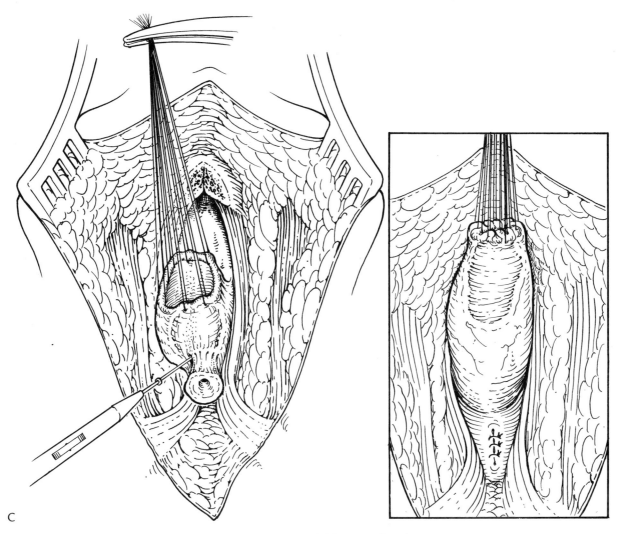

C

Figure 43-4 *(Continued)*. (**C**) Rectum is completely separated. (*Figure continues.*)

Diagnosis

In an infant with a clear clinical picture of midgut volvulus and plain films showing a dilated stomach with a nearly gasless abdomen, immediate exploration of the abdomen is preferable to further investigation.[39] Other patients with a less severe picture may present with a "double bubble" sign similar to that of duodenal atresia. In most cases, however, the diagnosis of midgut volvulus is made by upper gastrointestinal radiologic contrast study showing the characteristic corkscrew appearance of the duodenum or the pathognomonic "bird beak" narrowing of the duodenum. Recent research has shown that radiographic patterns are variable, but identification of these signs may strongly suggest malrotation and may lead to earlier surgical treatment.[40]

Surgical Treatment

Preoperative preparation includes a nasogastric tube decompression, fluid replacement, and antibiotic prophylaxis. The abdomen is explored through a transverse supraumbilical incision. If a midgut volvulus is present, the involved bowel should be delivered from the abdominal cavity and untwisted in a counterclockwise fashion. While the bowel is being examined for viability, attention should be paid to the exact position of the cecum and ligament of Treitz. In most cases in which no actual rotation is found, the entire midgut is suspended from a very narrow pedicle consisting of the superior mesenteric vessels flanked by the duodenojejunal segment on the right side and the ascending colon on the left. In other patients nonrotation of the colon may be found, with normal or incomplete rotation of the duodenojejunal loop. Rarely, reverse rotation is identified in which the duodenum passes anterior and cephalad and the colon inferior to the superior mesenteric vessels. A catheter inserted by the anesthetist from the mouth to the duodenum will rule out intrinsic obstruction at this site. "Ladd's" bands are rare, but when found can be divided to relieve compression on the duodenum. In cases without malrotation, the peritoneum on the anterior surface of the pedicle that encloses the neck of the midgut should be divided with scissors and further separation effected by blunt dissection. The duodenojejunal segment can then be placed over to the right retroperitoneum and the cecum to the left upper quadrant after an appendectomy. This

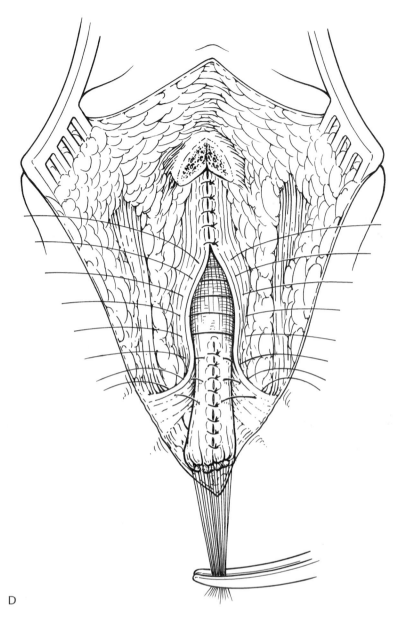

D

Figure 43-4 (*Continued*). (**D**) Rectum is passed in front of the levator muscle. Muscle complex sutures anchor the rectum. (*Figure continues.*)

maneuver has the effect of widening and restoring a broad base to the mesentery to prevent subsequent volvulus.[41]

Complications and Results

Morbidity and mortality of operations for midgut volvulus are directly related to the extent of gangrenous bowel and subsequent resection and the degree to which this will leave the patient with short bowel syndrome. When the bowel is of dubious viability after reduction, a second look operation 12 to 24 hours later will allow an assessment to determine the ultimate minimal length of bowel. It may also permit a decision of whether to withdraw further support for the patient. The most common cause of death in babies with short bowel syndrome is usually a complication of intravenous alimentation. Since older patients face the same risks of midgut volvulus as infants, the catastrophic loss of the midgut, and the subsequent short bowel syndrome, should be considered in all age groups.[33] As many as 8% of patients may experience recurrent volvulus postoperatively. Prophylactic fixation of the intestine has been recommended, but recurrence may occur despite this maneuver and for this reason is probably unhelpful.[42,43] In a review of over 400 cases, only two cases of recurrence were found.[44] In most patients with postoperative bowel obstruction, which may be partial or intermittent, the cause is probably secondary to adhesions. Unexplained symptoms of recurrent postoperative abdominal pain with or without vomiting, chronic constipation, or diarrhea have also been reported. Some of these patients may have an associated small intestinal motility disorder.[45–47]

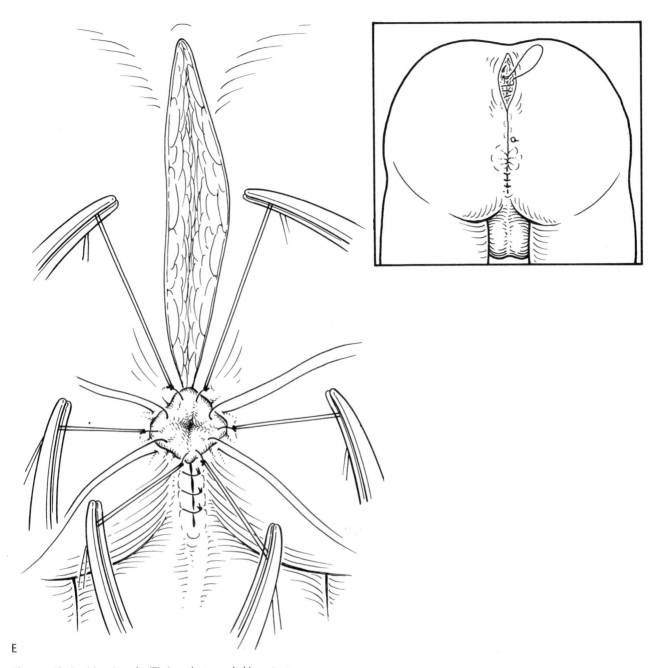

E

Figure 43-4 (*Continued*). (**E**) Anoplasty and skin suture.

TUMORS OF THE COLON AND RECTUM IN CHILDREN

Carcinoid Tumors

Carcinoid tumors, while rare, are nevertheless one of the more common neoplasms of the gastrointestinal tract occurring in childhood and early adulthood.[48] They are also referred to as argentaffin cell tumors[49] or Kultschitsky cell carcinoma,[50] being derived from APUD cells within the mucosa. The histopathogenesis of carcinoid tumors of the appendix differs from those in the small intestine.[51] Their relative incidence in the gastrointestinal tract also differs according to site: appendix

(50%), small bowel (28%), and rectum (17%).[52] This tumor has clearly been demonstrated to be malignant, but its specific natural history in children differs somewhat from that in the adult patient. To provide a comparison, a recent report from the Mayo Clinic described the institution's experience with carcinoid tumor of the appendix in all age groups.[48] This and our own analysis showed the disease to have a more benign course in children and young adults 20 years of age or younger.[53]

Clinical Presentation

The vast majority of children and young adults with carcinoid tumor of the appendix presented with signs and symptoms of an acute abdomen that led to an appendectomy. This is in con-

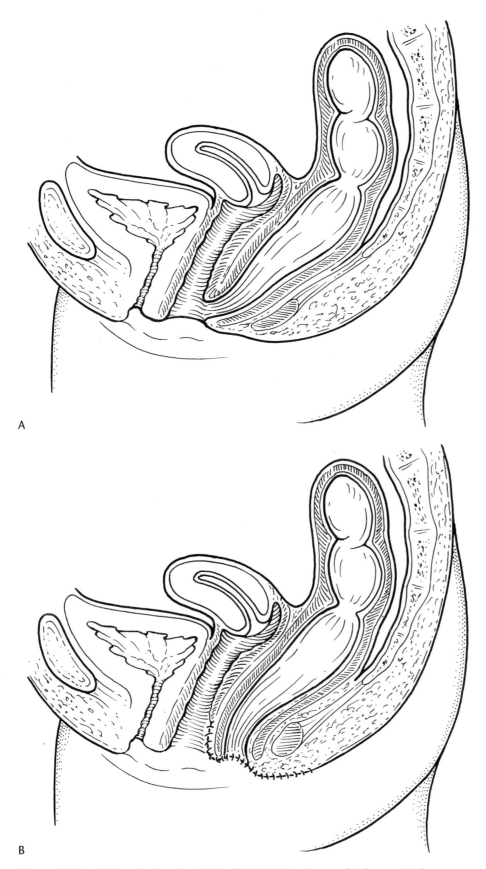

A

B

Figure 43-5. (**A**) Repair of rectovestibular fistula. Rectum is completely separated from vagina and perineal body is repaired. (**B**) Repair of vestibular fistula. Muscle complex sutures anchor the rectum. Normal intestinal rotation.

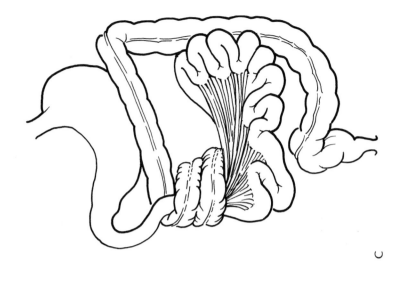

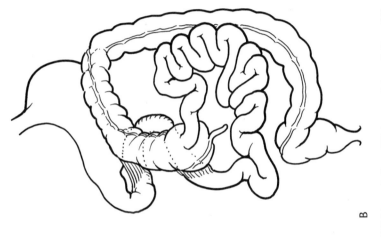

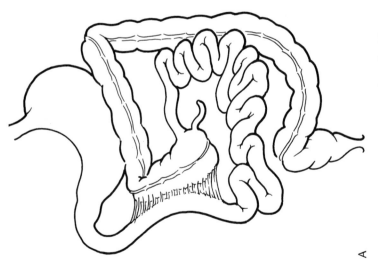

A

B

C

Figure 43-6. Pathologic narrowing of midgut mesentery. (**A**) Nonrotation. (**B**) Incomplete rotation. (**C**) Midgut volvulus.

808

trast to adult patients, in whom carcinoid tumors tended to be found during incidental appendectomy.

Histopathology

In our recent study of 23 children and young adults with carcinoid of the appendix, the tumor was located in the tip of the appendix in 12 and in the proximal appendix in 5. Analysis of invasiveness yielded some remarkable findings. Seven (30%) of the 23 tumors remained restricted to the appendiceal mucosa, 10 (43%) invaded to the serosa, and 6 (26%) had invaded the mesoappendix or appendiceal fat. Vascular invasion was not documented in any of the 18 tumors that were reviewed in detail. Invasion of lymphatics was present in all cases.

Surgical Therapy

The optimal management of these patients generally depends on tumor size and depth of invasion.[48,54–57] These tumors only rarely have evidence of metastatic diseases; over 95% of cases are nondisseminated. Thus the depth of invasion in this age group may not be as significant as it is in adults. In our series, 16 of the childhood tumors had penetrated to the serosa or beyond, and 6 of these had invaded to the mesoappendix or appendiceal fat, or both. No patient with invasion beyond the appendix was treated with anything more than simple appendectomy. Two of our 10 patients whose tumors invaded to the serosa underwent a right hemicolectomy and in both cases the tumor was 2 cm in greatest dimension. No metastatic tumor was encountered in either case. Another patient with a tumor 2.5 cm in diameter invading the serosa and mesoappendix was treated with a simple appendectomy only and was disease free at over 31 years of follow-up.

Current practice would suggest that patients with localized disease whose tumors exceed 2 cm in greatest dimension should be treated with right hemicolectomy. In our series of young patients with such tumors presenting to the Mayo Clinic, however, 12 were treated by simple appendectomy and only 1 had nodal metastastases, which developed 29 years later. This case was successfully salvaged by right hemicolectomy, with the patient alive and well 17 years later. Patients with tumors 2 cm or greater who ultimately died of their disease had metastases grossly evident at the time of diagnosis. Thus, 20 patients undergoing simple appendectomy were cured as well as the 3 undergoing right hemicolectomy. Based on these findings, carcinoid tumor of the appendix in children without metastasis at the time of diagnosis would appear to be a clinically more benign process than in adults, thus permitting a more conservative surgical approach. We could not document the need for second look surgery or right hemicolectomy except in certain carefully selected patients who are at risk of metastatic disease.

Adenocarcinoma of the Colon and Rectum

Whereas adenocarcinoma of the rectum and colon in children is exceedingly rare, it is nevertheless the most common cancer of the colon of childhood.[58] Diseases associated with adenocarcinoma in children often include familial adenomatous polyposis including Gardner's syndrome, Turcot's syndrome (a genetic disorder involving central nervous system tumors), and ulcerative colitis. It is of interest that most cases of adenocarcinoma of the rectum are not a complication of the above, but appear to be unrelated to them.[59] Devroede and colleagues[60] at the Mayo Clinic carried out a long-term follow-up of children with chronic ulcerative colitis. They evaluated the cancer risk and life expectancy of these children. Following the first 10 years of disease, the cancer risk was approximately 20% a decade thereafter.

Most of the children developing adenocarcinoma of the colon or rectum are over 10 years of age and tend to have a much more malignant course than in the adult patient. The poor prognosis is related at times to a delay in diagnosis, but also to an increased prevalence of mucinous or signet ring carcinoma, which is present in approximately half of the children developing this malignancy.[61,62]

Because of the predisposition of the colon to develop cancers in children with familial adenomatous polyposis or chronic ulcerative colitis, the sphincter-preserving operation associated with the endorectal pull-through procedure has been advocated at an early age, which has met with success.[63–66]

Treatment

The clinical findings of adenocarcinoma of the rectum in children are quite similar to those in adults. Because of the rarity of the lesion, children are generally evaluated and operated on for abdominal pain, possible appendicitis, intussusception, peritonitis, and so forth. They are most frequently noted to have melana with anemia, abdominal distension, and weight loss.[58,67] The choice of operation is no different than that in adults (see Ch. 23).

REFERENCES

1. Hirschsprung H (1887–88) Stuhlträgheit neugeborener in forge von dilatation und hypertrophic des colors. Jahrb Kuderh 27:1–7
2. Robertson E II, Kernohan JW (1938) The myenteric plexus in congenital megacolon. Proc Staff Meet Mayo Clin 13:123
2a. Whitehouse FR, Kernohan JW (1948) Myenteric plexus in congenital megacolon. Arch Int Med 82:75–111
3. Zueler WW, Wilson JL (1948) Functional intestinal obstruction on congenital neurogenic basis in infancy. Am J Dis Child 75:40–64
3a. Swenson O, Bill A II (1948) Resection of rectum and rectosigmoid with preservation of the sphincter for benign spastic lesions producing megacolon: an experimental study. Surgery 24:212
4. Ehrenpreis T (1946) Megacolon in the newborn: clinical and roentgenological study with special regard to the pathogenesis. Acta Chir Scand, suppl. 94:1–114
5. Duhamel B (1964) Recrorectal and transanal pull-through procedure for the treatment of Hirschsprung's disease. Dis Colon Rectum 7:455

6. Soave F (1964) Hirschsprung's disease: a new surgical technique. Arch Dis Child 39:116

7. Boley SJ (1964) New modification of the surgical treatment of Hirschsprung's disease. Surgery 56:1015

8. Okamoto E, Ueda T (1967) Embryogenesis of intramural ganglia of the gut and its relation to Hirschsprung's disease. J Pediatr Surg 2:437

9. Smith B (1968) Pre- and postnatal development of the ganglion cells of the rectum and its surgical implications. J Pediatr Surg 3:386

10. Hirobe S, Doody DP, Ryan DP et al (1992) Ectopic class II major histocompatibility antigens in Hirschsprung's disease and neuronal intestinal dysplasia. J Pediatr Surg 27:357–363

11. Kobayashi H, Hirakawa H, Puri P (1995) Overexpression of intercellular adhesion molecule-1 (ICAM-1) and MHC class II antigen on hypertrophic nerve trunks suggests an immunopathologic response in Hirschsprung's disease. J Pediatr Surg 30:1680–1683

12. Philippart AIN (1990) Hirschsprung's disease. pp. 358–371. Pediatric Surgery. 2nd Ed.

13. Sulaman M (1968) Anastomotic clamp for retro-rectal transanal pullthrough procedure in Hirschsprung's disease—a new modification of Duhamel's operation. Ann Chir Inf 9:63

14. Kosloske AM, Goldhorn JF (1984) Early diagnosis and treatment of Hirschsprung's disease in New Mexico. Surg Gynecol Obstet 158:233

14a. Saltzman DA, Telander MJ, Brennom WS et al (1996) Transanal mucosectomy: a modification of Soave's procedure for Hirschsprung's disease. J Ped Surg 31:1272–1275

15. Ehrenpreis T (1970) Hirschsprung's Disease. Year Book Medical Publishers, Chicago

16. Sieber WK (1978) Hirschsprung's disease. Curr Probl Surg

17. Nixon HH (1985) Hirschsprung's disease: progress in management and diagnostics. World J Surg 9:189

18. Sieber WK (1986) Hirschsrpung's disease. pp. 995–1022. In: Pediatric Surgery. 4th Ed. Vol. 2. Year Book Medical Publishers, Chicago

19. Soave F (1964) A new surgical technique for treatment of Hirschsprung's disease. Surgery 56:1007

20. Kleinhaus S, Boley SJ, Sheran M et al (1979) Hirschsprung's disease. A survey of the members of the surgical section of the American Academy of Pediatrics. J Pediatr Surg 14:588

21. Ziegler MM, Ross AJ, Bishop HC (1987) Total intestinal aganglionosis: a new technique for prolonged survival. J Pediatr Surg 22:82

22. Gross RE (1953) The surgery of Infancy and Childhood. WB Saunders, Philadelphia pp 349

23. Stephens FD (1984) Wingspread Conference on Anorectal Malformations, Racine, WI

24. Pena A, deVries P (1982) Posterior sagittal anorectoplasty. Important technical considerations and new applications. J Pediatr Surg 17:796–881

25. Pena A (1993) Imperforate anus and cloacal malformations. pp. 372–392. Pediatric Surgery. 2nd Ed.,

26. Mall FP (1988) Development of the human intestine and its position in the adult. Bull Johns Hopkins Hosp 997

27. Fraser JE, Robbins RH (1915) On the factors concerned in causing rotation of the intestine in man. J Anat Physiol 50:75

28. Ladd WE (1936) Surgical diseases of the alimentary tract in infants. N Engl J Med 215:704

29. Dott NM (1923) Anomalies of intestinal rotation: their embryology and surgical aspects, with report of five cases. Br J Surg 11:251

30. Bill AH Jr (1980) Malrotation and failures of fixation in the intestinal tract. pp. 346–355. In Holder TM, Ashcraft KW (eds): Pediatric Surgery, WB Saunders, Philadelphia

31. Snyder WH Jr, Chaffin L (1954) Embryology and pathology of the intestinal tract: presentation of 40 cases of malrotation. Ann Surg 140:368–380

32. Boulton JE, Ein BJ, Reilly, BT et al (1989). Necrotizing enterocolitis and volvulus in the premature neonate. J Pediatr Surg 24:901–905

33. Powell DM, Othersen HB, Smith CD (1989) Malrotation of the intestines in children: malrotation of the intestines in children: the effect of age on presentation and therapy. J Pediatr Surg 24:777–780

34. Howell CG, Vozza F, Shaw S et al (1982) Malrotation, malnutrition, and ischemic bowel disease. J Pediatr Surg 17:469–473

35. Firor HB, Steiger E (1983) Morbidity of rotational abnormalities of the gut beyond infancy. Cleve Clin Q 50:303–309

36. Callander (1993) pp. 320–330. In Holder TM, Ashcraft KW (eds): Pediatric Surgery, WB Saunders, Philadephia

37. Rescorla FJ, Shedd FJ, Grosfeld JL et al (1990) Anomalies of intestinal rotation in childhood. Analysis of 447 cases. Surgery 108:710

38. Smith EI (1986) Malrotation of the intestine. pp. 882–895. In Welch KJ, Randolph JG, Ravitch MM (eds): Pediatric Surgery. Yearbook Medical Publishers, Chicago

39. Kassner EJ, Kottmeier PK (1975) Absence and retention of small bowel gas in infants with midgut volvulus: mechanisms and significance. Pediatr Radiol 4:28–30

40. Schey WL, Donaldson JS, Sty JR (1993) Malrotation of bowel: variable patterns with different surgical considerations. J Pediatr Surg 28:96–101

41. Ladd WE (1936) Surgical diseases of the alimentary tract in infants. N Engl J Med 215:705–708

42. Bill AH, Grauman D (1966) Rationale and technique for stabilization of the mesentery in cases of nonrotation of the midgut. J Pediatr Surg 1:127–132

43. Stauffer UG, Hermann P (1980) Comparison of late results in patients with corrected intestinal malrotation with and without fixation of the mesentery. J Pediatr Surg 15:9–12

44. Andrassy RJ, Mahour GH (1981) Malrotation of the midgut in infants and children. Arch Surg 116:158–160

45. Brennom WS, Bill AH (1974) Prophylactic fixation of the intestine for midgut nonrotation. Surg Gynecol Obstet 138: 181–184

46. Spigland N, Brandt ML, Yazbeck S (1990) Malrotation presenting beyond the neonatal period. J Pediatr Surg 25: 1139–1142

47. Coombs RC, Buick RG, Gornall PG et al (1991) Intestinal malrotation: the role of small intestinal dysmotility in the cause of persistent symptoms. J Pediatr Surg 26:553–556

48. Moertel CG, Weiland LH, Nagorney DM et al (1987) The carcinoid tumor of the appendix: treatment and prognosis. N Engl J Med 317:1699–1701

49. Masson P (1928) Carcinoids (argentaffin cell tumors) and nerve hyperplasia of the appendicular mucosa. Am J Pathol 4: 181–212

50. Latham WP, Arnold HS, Ede S (1961) Kulschitsky cell carci-

noma (carcinoid) of the appendix with metastasis. Am J Surg 102:607–610

51. Lundqvist M, Wilander E (1987) A study of the histopathogenesis of carcinoid tumors of the small intestine and appendix. Cancer 60:201:206

52. Cheek RC, Wilson H (1970) Carcinoid tumors. Curr Probl Surg 4–31

53. Moertel CL, Weiland LH, Telander RL (1990) Carcinoid tumor of the appendix in the first two decades of life. J Pediatr Surg 25:1073–1075

54. Moertel CG, Dockerty MG, Judd ES (1968) Carcinoid tumors of the vermiform appendix. Cancer 21:270–278

55. Farringer JL, Tarasidis G (1964) Carcinoid tumors of the appendix. Arch Surg 88:354–356

56. Syracuse DC, Perzin KH, Price JB et al (1979) Carcinoid tumors—mesoappendiceal extension and nodal metastases. Ann Surg 190:58–63

57. Zakaria YM, Quam SHQ, Hajdu is (1975) Carcinoid tumors of the gastrointestinal tract. Cancer 35:588–591

58. Cain WS, Longino LA (1970) Carcinoma of the colon in children. J Pediatr Surg 5:527

59. Pratt CB, Rivera G, Shanks E et al (1977) Colorectal carcinoma in adolescents: implications regarding etiology. Cancer 40:2464

60. Devroede GJ, Taylor WF, Sauer WG et al (1971) Cancer risk and life expectancy of children with ulcerative colitis. N Engl J Med 285:17

61. Rao BN, Pratt CB, Fleming ID et al (1985) Colon carcinoma in children and adolescents: a review of 30 cases. Cancer 55:1322–1326

62. Symonds DA, Vickery AL Jr (1976) Mucinous carcinoma of the colon and rectum. Cancer 37:1891–1900

63. Telander RL, Spencer M, Perrault J et al (1990) Long-term follow-up of the illeoanal anastomosis in children and young adults. Surgery 108:717–725

64. Telander RL, Perrault J (1980) Total colectomy with rectal mucosectomy and ileoanal anastomosis for chronic ulcerative colitis in children and young adults. Mayo Clin Proc 55:420–424

65. Telander RL, Perrault J (1981) Colectomy with rectal mucosectomy and ileoanal anastomosis in young patients: its uses for ulcerative colitis and familial polyposis. Arch Surg 116:623–629

66. Telander RL, Dozois RR (1984) The endorectal ileoanal anastomosis. Probl Gen Surg 1:39–50

67. Goldthorn JG, Powars D, Hays DM (1983) Adenocarcinoma of the colon and rectum in the adolescent. Surgery 93:409

44

COLORECTAL INJURY

Michael P. Bannon

Injury to the colorectum threatens its victims with great risk of septic morbidity and mortality. Although new therapies based on evolving management principles avert many infectious complications, challenges persist. The challenges of penetrating injuries differ from those of blunt injuries. Penetrating colon wounds are readily recognized, and thousands have been reported. Nonetheless, the best operation for a given wound is not always clear, and surgeons continue to debate and refine options. Blunt colon injury, by contrast, often presents diagnostic dilemmas, occurs infrequently, and has generated only a sparse literature to guide therapy. Rectal injury often coexists with other severe and challenging pelvic injuries. Principles of colorectal trauma care thus remain dynamic; they are best understood within a general approach to critically injured patients. Colorectal injury per se can be treated only after the trauma victim has been evaluated and resuscitated, the indication for operation recognized, and hemostasis obtained. This chapter introduces these general issues and reviews the specific treatment of penetrating and blunt colorectal injuries.

INITIAL ASSESSMENT OF THE TRAUMA PATIENT

Initial assessment of all trauma patients must be organized and methodical. Evaluation follows the systematic approach of Advanced Trauma Life Support: primary survey, resuscitation, secondary survey, and definitive care.[1] All body systems are routinely evaluated in every patient; consideration of the specific trauma mechanism focuses indices of suspicion for particular injuries and directs special investigations. Upon the patient's emergency room arrival, the surgeon performs a primary survey to identify life-threatening injuries demanding immediate treatment. This rapid physical assessment follows the ABCDE guidelines: airway, breathing, circulation, neurologic disability, and exposure of the patient (Table 44-1). As deficiencies are recognized, they are treated prior to performing the next assessment step. Thus, primary survey and resuscitation are concurrent, not sequential activities. As the final step of primary sur-

vey, the trauma team completely disrobes the patient to allow thorough physical examination. The surgeon then documents all penetrating wounds and specifically searches for wounds potentially hidden between the buttocks, within the gluteal folds, or on the perineum.

Secondary survey combines scrupulous physical examination with judiciously chosen and expeditiously performed diagnostic studies. This phase identifies subtle injuries associated with minimal physiologic derangement and injuries that are not life threatening. Abdominal assessment is performed during the secondary survey; the goal is to identify the presence or absence of injury requiring celiotomy—not to diagnose specific organ injuries. Diagnostic peritoneal lavage (DPL) is the mainstay of abdominal evaluation for patients incurring penetrating trauma and hemodynamically unstable blunt trauma.[2] Hemodynamically stable patients incurring blunt injury may be evaluated with either DPL or abdominopelvic computed tomography (CT).[3] Two newer modalities of abdominal assessment, laparoscopy[4–6] and ultrasound,[7,8] hold much promise but at present lack universally accepted roles and indications.

DPL may be performed with either a percutaneous Seldinger (Fig. 44-1), semi-open Seldinger, or open cut-down technique.[9] Immediately upon placement, the lavage catheter should be aspirated; return of 10 ml gross blood dictates immediate celiotomy. Negative aspiration prompts lavage of the peritoneal cavity with 1 L of lactated Ringer's solution (10 ml/kg in children). A volume of at least 200 ml must return for analysis to yield accurate results. Lavage fluid with 100,000 red blood cells (RBC)/mm^3 or more (lower RBC counts are used in some penetrating trauma settings, as discussed below), 500 white blood cells (WBC)/mm^3 or more, 175 U amylase/100 ml or more, bacteria, bile, or vegetable matter prompts celiotomy.[10]

CT findings that prompt celiotomy include an appropriate grade of solid organ injury, pneumoperitoneum, or extravasation of gastrointestinal (GI) contrast. The latter two findings are rare. As discussed later, CT that reveals free intraperitoneal fluid without solid organ injury suggests hollow viscus or mes-

Table 44-1. Primary Survey and Resuscitation

Component	Assessment	Therapeutic Options
Airway	Quality of phonation	Chin lift/jaw thrust
	Air movement at mouth/nares	Placement of nasal/oral airway
	Presence/absence of obstructive sounds	Endotracheal intubation
Breathing	Comparison of bilateral breath sounds	Oxygen
	Use of accessory respiratory muscles	Tube thoracostomy
	Rate and depth of respirations	Mechanical ventilation
Circulation	Radial and femoral pulses	Intravenous access
	Capillary refill	Crystalloid infusion
	Skin color/temperature	Blood transfusion
Disability	Responsiveness (alert; responsive to verbal stimuli; responsive to painful stimuli; unresponsive)	Mechanical hyperventilation
		Mannitol
	Comparison of bilateral pupillary size/reactivity	
Exposure	Removal of all garments	Not applicable
	Observation/palpation of back	
	Search for penetrating wounds	

(Concept from American College of Surgeons.[1])

enteric injury and dictates further evaluation. In addition to the abdomen, secondary survey evaluates the head and neck, chest, extremities, and central nervous system in a detailed fashion. With this complete, the trauma team summates the patient's injuries, formulates a plan, and renders definitive care in the operating room, the surgical intensive care unit, or elsewhere as appropriate.

INDICATIONS FOR CELIOTOMY

In 1888, Senn[11] reported that ''rectal insufflation of hydrogen gas [was] an infallible test in the diagnosis of visceral injury of the gastrointestinal canal in penetrating wounds of the abdomen'' after completing an elaborate series of experiments. A lighted taper placed at the cutaneous wound ignited a blue flame when hydrogen gas escaped, thereby heralding gastrointestinal perforation. Not surprisingly, a "feeble explosive report" accompanied at least one such flame test.

The infallibility of Senn's method notwithstanding, diagnosis of colorectal injury is most often identified during celiotomy performed for general indications. Only rarely will a specific

---

Trauma Scenarios

Gunshot wounds
    Transperitoneal
    Tangential abdominal
    Transpelvic
Stab wounds
    Anterior abdominal
    Posterior abdominal
    Thoracoabdominal
Blunt mechanism
    Abdominal injury
    Closed pelvic fracture
    Open pelvic fracture

---

diagnosis of colorectal injury be made preoperatively. Thus, successful management of colorectal injury requires knowledge of the indications for trauma celiotomy; these depend on the clinical setting.[12] Clinical scenarios relevant to colorectal injury are listed in the accompanying box; an approach to each follows. Other approaches may be appropriate, but patient care is best served by consistency at a given trauma center.

Colon injury occurs in almost 42% of abdominal gunshot wound victims.[13] All patients with gunshot wounds having obvious transperitoneal traverse must undergo abdominal exploration; they harbor injuries requiring repair in 96% to 98% of cases.[14,15] Similarly, all hemodynamically unstable patients with abdominal or thoracoabdominal gunshot wounds must undergo immediate celiotomy. Occasionally, an abdominal gunshot wound will appear to track tangentially along an extraperitoneal course through the abdominal wall of a stable patient. Celiotomy is necessary for a tangential wound from a high-velocity military weapon because "blast effect" may injure intraperitoneal structures even if the missile course is extraperitoneal. However, a definitively tangential wound from a low-velocity civilian weapon may be managed nonoperatively because ''blast effect'' is unusual in civilian trauma.[16] The clinical problem is to confirm the extraperitoneal nature of an apparently tangential tract. DPL reliably differentiates transperitoneal from abdominal wall trajectories in patients with low-velocity tangential injuries. Lavage fluid with 10,000 RBC/mm^3 should prompt celiotomy.[17] Recently, laparoscopy has also been utilized to make this distinction.[18]

Celiotomy is indicated for abdominal stab wounds associated with shock, pneumoperitoneum, blood from the GI or genitourinary tracts, evisceration, and/or peritonitis. In the absence of these clinical indications, patients require an objective evaluation of the peritoneal cavity to avoid delayed diagnosis or missed injury.

Anterior abdominal stab wounds lie between the inguinal ligaments and the costal margins anterior to the midaxillary lines. Of these, two-thirds penetrate the peritoneum, and one-fourth cause injury requiring repair.[19] An anterior abdominal

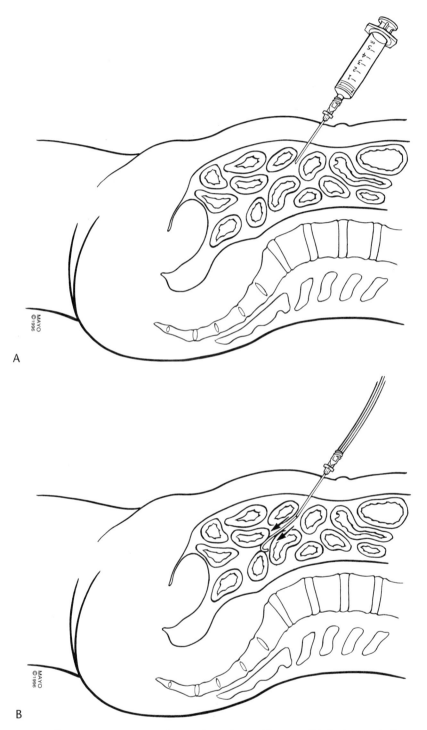

A

B

Figure 44-1. Percutaneous diagnostic peritoneal lavage. (**A**) During aspiration, a needle is placed through the infraumbilical midline, 45° from a coronal plane, toward the pelvis, and into the peritoneal cavity. (**B**) Needle is exchanged for guidewire. (*Figure continues.*)

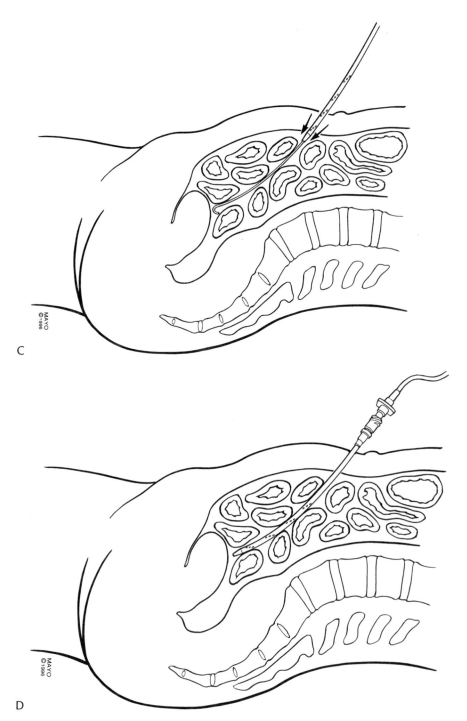

C

D

Figure 44-1. (*Continued*). (**C**) Guidewire is exchanged for lavage catheter. (**D**) One liter of warm saline is instilled into peritoneal cavity. Intravenous bag is then placed into dependent position to allow egress of fluid for analysis. (By permission of Mayo Foundation.)

stab wound without clinical indication for celiotomy should be extended and explored under local anesthesia to allow inspection of the fascia.[20] Those patients without fascial penetration are discharged. Those patients with wounds penetrating fascia are further evaluated with DPL. A lavage fluid RBC count of 100,000 cells/mm³indicates significant organ injury and dictates celiotomy.[20]

The thoracoabdomen lies deep to a circumferential band extending superiorly from the costal margin to the fourth intercostal space anteriorly and to the inferior tip of the scapula posteriorly. Celiotomy should be performed for thoracoabdominal gunshot wounds (Fig. 44-2). Objective evaluation of the peritoneal cavity in patients with stab wounds of the thoracoabdomen can be performed with DPL. Because thoracoabdominal stab

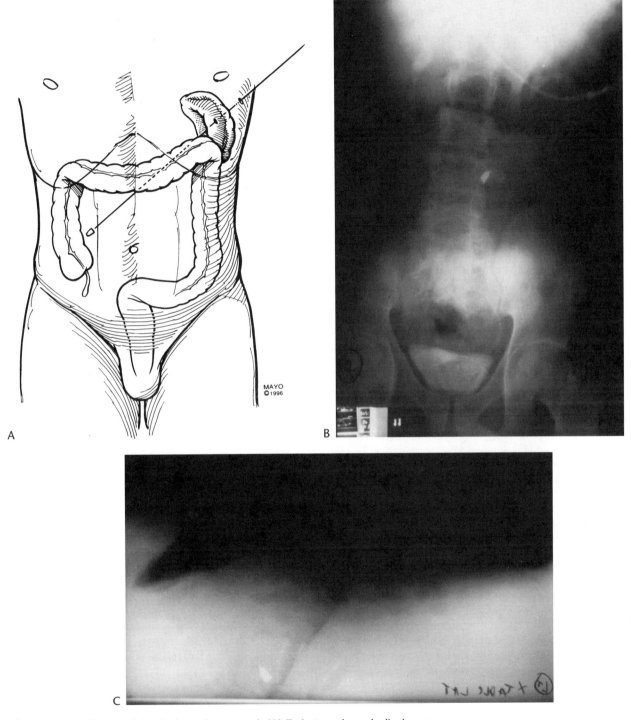

Figure 44-2. Thoracoabdominal gunshot wound. (**A**) Trajectory through diaphragm, spleen, and mesenteric aspect of transverse colon to infracolic compartment (**B** and **C**) Location of retained missile in lumbar spine. (*Figure continues.*)

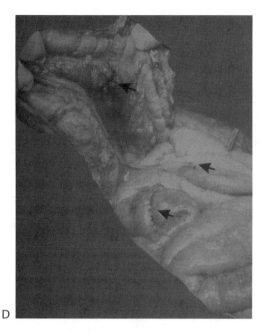

D

Figure 44-2. *(Continued)* **(D)** Primary suture closure of colonic and enteric injuries (arrows). (By permission of Mayo Foundation.)

wounds have the potential to penetrate the diaphragm, increased sensitivity is necessary, and the RBC count prompting celiotomy must be lower than that employed for anterior abdominal stab wounds. Although controversy abounds, a lavage RBC count of 10,000/mm³ is a reasonable criterion for celiotomy as it yields false negatives in only 1% and false positives in a modest 13%[21]. Initial experience suggests that laparoscopy can also reliably evaluate potential thoracoabdominal penetration.[5]

Stab wounds of the posterior abdomen lie between the iliac crests and the costal margin posterior to the midaxillary line; these have the potential to cause isolated retroperitoneal colon injury. However, only 2% of such wounds are associated with injury to retroperitoneal structures.[22] CT performed with intravenous, upper GI and lower GI contrast seems to screen reliably for injury in these cases.[23–25]

Transpelvic gunshot wounds cause colorectal injury in over 20% of patients; rectal injury per se occurs in over 7%.[26] Transpelvic injuries often arise from handgun wounds to the buttock inflicted as punishment by urban gangs. Buttock wounds in general are associated with rectal injury in 12 to 13% of patients.[27] Hypotensive patients require immediate celiotomy; associated vascular injuries are common. Hemodynamically stable patients may be managed without operation if workup is unrevealing.[26,28] DPL differentiates transperitoneal from extraperitoneal traverse. Proctoscopic examination is essential: with low-velocity missiles, rectal injury will appear as a subtle area of bloodied mucosal disruption; however, intraluminal blood may be the only sign of rectal injury. Fresh gross blood on digital examination must also lead one to diagnose rectal injury. Nonoperative evaluation of transpelvic gunshot wounds also includes cystography and a speculum exam of the cervix to examine the genitourinary outflow tracts. Displacement of the bladder on cystogram suggests a compressing hematoma from an iliac vascular injury.

Following blunt trauma, the abdomen may be evaluated with serial physical examinations if the patient is awake and alert, is free of intoxicants, has no abdominal pain or tenderness, and has no distracting pain from extra-abdominal injuries. Failure to meet these conditions necessitates an objective examination of the abdomen. Hypotensive patients should be evaluated with diagnostic peritoneal lavage; an RBC count of 100,000/mm³ necessitates celiotomy.[3,10] In the normotensive patient, CT is appropriate. CT provides both diagnosis and grade of solid organ injuries; appropriately severe grades prompt celiotomy. As discussed later, CT signs of colonic injury are most often nonspecific.

Blunt mechanisms may result in severe pelvic fractures associated with rectal laceration. On digital rectal examination, palpation of bony shards or retrieval of gross blood confirms diagnosis. Straddle injuries and hyperabduction injuries may cause open pelvic fractures with complex perineal lacerations.[29]

ANTIBIOTIC THERAPY

By definition all penetrating abdominal wounds are at least clean-contaminated, and transgression of colon or small bowel increases the wound class to contaminated. Colon injury significantly increases risk of postoperative infection.[30,31] Thus, patients with penetrating abdominal wounds should receive preoperative antibiotics. Because exogenous or endogenous contamination is present prior to antibiotic administration in all penetrating abdominal trauma patients, antibiotics are therapeutic rather than prophylactic.[32] Delay of antibiotic administration until the intraoperative or postoperative phases substantially increases infectious complications.[33,34]

Antibiotics chosen should be active against both aerobic and anaerobic organisms. The classic combination of an aminoglycoside and clindamycin provides such coverage but is no more efficacious than single-agent treatment with cefoxitin.[30] Aminoglycoside toxicity remains a concern. In general, single agents are as efficacious as multiple agents provided that anaerobic coverage is provided.[35] Recent studies have compared the efficacy of cefoxitin to cefotetan[31] and to ampicillin/sulbactam[36]; these studies revealed that ampicillin/sulbactam was superior to cefoxitin,[36] which was comparable to cefotetan.[31]

Prospective studies have shown that a 12-hour[37] or 24-hour[31] course of antibiotic treatment provides the same efficacy as longer courses. Even for patients with colon injury or severe multiple abdominal injuries, antibiotic therapy beyond 24 hours provides no added benefit.[31] Penetrating abdominal trauma patients should thus receive a 24-hour course of a single antibiotic active against aerobes and anaerobes including *Bacteroides fragilis*. The first dose should be given preoperatively. Antibiotics should be redosed intraoperatively if operative duration is long or blood loss significant. The dose chosen should account for the often increased volume of distribution present in trauma patients. These recommendations are also appropriate for blunt abdominal trauma patients undergoing celiotomy, although associated injuries, such as open fractures, may dictate specifics of antibiotic therapy in this setting.

TRAUMA CELIOTOMY

Trauma celiotomy mandates a generous midline incision. After rapid packing of the peritoneal quadrants to control hemoperitoneum, each quadrant is individually inspected for diagnosis and repair of hemorrhagic injuries. Running sutures, staples, or atraumatic clamps temporarily control contamination from leaking hollow viscus injuries until hemostasis is obtained. Missile and knife tracts must be defined in their anatomic entirety to avoid missed injury. Careful abdominal inspection and definitive repair of colorectal and enteric injuries follow. The small bowel is carefully examined in its entirety. Blood staining the retroperitoneum of the right or left paracolic gutters necessitates mobilization and inspection of the ascending and descending colon, respectively. Mesenteric hematomas encroaching on the mesenteric aspect of the small intestine or colon must be dissected free of serosa so that bowel injury can be identified and repaired or excluded with confidence.

Patients with abdominal hemorrhage require ongoing resuscitation during operation. Blood salvage with autotransfusion has emerged over the last 30 years as an expeditious means of restoring blood volume intraoperatively.[38] This technique minimizes reliance on banked blood and thus decreases risks of viral transmission and transfusion reaction. Originally developed for elective procedures, intraoperative autotransfusion is now employed during trauma celiotomy when bowel injury may potentially contaminate salvaged blood. Intraoperative autotransfusion has not increased infectious complications in patients with hollow viscus injury.[39,40] Only small numbers of patients receiving contaminated salvaged blood have been reported: 10 patients in the Ozmen study and 29 patients in the Horst study; thus, some caution is prudent. Nonetheless, these early encouraging results give the surgeon impetus to use intraoperative blood salvage and autotransfusion without reservation for exsanguinating hemorrhage combined with colon injury.

Following repair or hemostatic packing of hemorrhagic injuries, some patients remain unstable with persistent metabolic acidosis and hypotension. Nonsurgical bleeding from thrombocytopenia, dilution of coagulation factors, and/or disseminated intravascular coagulation may frustrate continued attempted dissection and manipulation of tissues. Hypothermia commonly accompanies trauma celiotomy, further impairs blood coagulation, and exacerbates the physiologic derangements of shock. Ongoing operation in the face of persistent hypotension, hypothermia, acidosis, and coagulopathy will prove fatal. In such circumstances, operation should be abbreviated and definitive management of bowel injury postponed.[41–45] GI perforations should be rapidly closed or resected with stapling devices, but restoration of GI continuity and creation of stomas should be deferred. Edema will often prevent primary fascial closure. The wound should be closed rapidly with towel clips, running cutaneous suture, or a prosthetic fascial patch. This abbreviated celiotomy allows timely retreat to the intensive care unit for rewarming, volume resuscitation, and correction of coagulopathy. After stabilization for 12 to 48 hours, the patient may be returned to the operating room for GI anastomosis and/or creation of intestinal stomas as appropriate.

MANAGEMENT OF COLON INJURY

Historic Trends

The primary issue surrounding the management of colon injury is colostomy. The current slow but steady trend away from colostomy toward primary repair follows the previous abrupt

abolition of primary repair by colostomy during the Second World War. How both changes represent progress for their respective times is best understood in a historical context. During the First World War, surgeons repaired most colon wounds primarily. In 1917, Cuthbert Wallace[46] described a 73% mortality for patients with isolated colon wounds treated with colostomy and a 50% mortality for those treated with primary repair. This difference in mortality certainly resulted from differences in injury severity and is overshadowed by the then dismal prognosis of colon injury managed by any means. Primary repair remained standard practice until the North African campaign of the Second World War. Ogilvie[47] reported a 59% mortality with colostomy and a 50% mortality with primary repair for colon wounds treated after the battles of Alem Halfa and Alamein. Complications of primary repair led Ogilvie to abandon this option in favor of mandatory colostomy. The Surgeon General soon dictated that all colon wounds be treated by colostomy, thus precipitously reversing the edict of primary repair advocated by military manuals prior to the war. Exteriorization of the injury as a stoma, resection with stoma, or repair with proximal diverting stoma thus became the only acceptable options. The mortality of colon injury fell dramatically to the range of 26% to 33% with late World War II experiences. This progress resulted in part from the practice of routine colostomy. However, other advances in resuscitation, blood banking, antimicrobial therapy, anesthesia, and postoperative care also contributed to improved outcomes. Problems unique to military wounds dictated mandatory colostomy; these included the extensive tissue destruction caused by high-velocity missiles and shrapnel, potential long durations from injury to operation, the variable experience of military surgeons, and potential delayed recognition of postoperative complications due to discontinuous care during evacuation. Despite the absence of these concerns with nonmilitary injuries, war-seasoned surgeons carried routine colostomy home to civilian practice after the war.

In 1951, however, Woodhall and Ochsner[48] challenged routine colostomy with their review of a civilian experience from Charity Hospital in New Orleans. In their words, ``. . . the wartime practice of exteriorization of colon wounds has been carried over into civilian practice too wholeheartedly for the patient's greatest good.'' Of 55 patients treated between 1944 and 1948, 22 were managed with primary suture of their colon wounds with a 9% mortality. Mortality for primary suture with proximal diversion and mortality for exteriorization were 60% and 23%, respectively. Retrospective in nature, these data did not suggest a better outcome with primary repair relative to colostomy for similar wounds, but they did suggest that some selected colon wounds could be treated adequately without colostomy. No other study could conclude differently for the next 40 years.

Despite Woodhall and Ochsner's plea, colostomy remained the primary treatment for colon injury during the next three decades. Mortality from colon injury continued to decline through the Korean conflict and was reported to be as low as 11.8% during the Vietnam era.[49] Suggestions that primary repair was appropriate for civilian injuries continued to appear.[50–52]

In 1979, Stone and Fabian[53] reported a randomized prospective trial of primary closure versus colostomy for colon injury. Given the prevailing conventional wisdom, which favored colostomy, the exclusion criteria were understandably broad; they included the following: the presence of preoperative shock, an intraperitoneal blood loss greater than 1L, injury to more than two intra-abdominal organ systems, significant peritoneal fecal soilage, initiation of operation more than 8 hours after injury, a colon wound so large as to necessitate resection, and major loss of abdominal wall or necessity for placement of abdominal wall mesh. These criteria excluded 48% of the patients seen during the study. Mortality was 1.5% and 1.4% in each of the groups randomized to primary closure (n = 67) and colostomy (n = 72), respectively, but it was 15% in the excluded patients (n = 129), reflecting the severe injuries of the latter. Comparison of the two randomized groups revealed that colostomy was associated with more frequent peritoneal sepsis (29% versus 15%), longer hospital stay (22 days versus 17 days), and higher cost. Also, patients randomized to colostomy experienced a 10% incidence of stoma-specific complications.

The Stone and Fabian[53] study is a landmark; it established clear advantages for primary repair relative to colostomy in *selected* patients. These patients were very highly selected, however. This paper also provided criteria for the obligatory performance of colostomy. Although these prudent criteria guided clinical practice, they were not derived from prospective data and were never tested clinically in a controlled fashion.

Stone and Fabian[53] heralded a trend toward primary repair. In 1986, Burch and others[54] from the Ben Taub General Hospital in Houston published a series of 727 patients with colon injury; 52.4% of these patients were treated with primary repair. Of those patients meeting the exclusion criteria of Stone and Fabian,[53] 42% were treated with primary repair. Mortality was 9.9%. The rate of fecal fistula was no different in those treated with colostomy (1.4%) versus primary repair (1.1%). However, the resection and colocolostomy subgroup (n = 9) experienced an 11.1% incidence of fecal fistula. This vast series demonstrated that experienced surgical judgement could identify patients appropriate for primary repair and that these patients comprised a slight majority. Later series revealed even higher percentages treated without colostomy.

In a 1989 paper, George et al.[55] further defined the group of patients appropriate for primary repair. In an unselected series of 83 patients, primary repair was performed without regard to severity of shock, extent of contamination, or associated injury; there were no suture line failures. Injuries requiring resection were treated with colostomy (n = 7) during the first half of the study, but primary anastomosis (n = 12) was performed during the latter half of the study, with one suture line failure (8.3%).

In 1991, Chappuis et al.[56] published the first randomized prospective trial of primary repair versus colostomy without exclusion criteria (n = 56 patients). No suture line failures occurred among the patients who underwent simple closure (n = 17) or anastomosis (n = 11). No mortality was reported. The incidence of intra-abdominal abscess in the primary repair/anastomosis group (10.1%) did not differ from that in the diversion group (14.2%); overall septic complications totalled 21.4 and 17.9% respectively. Although the number of patients studied was small, this study was the first to suggest that primary repair was safe in unselected patients.

Falcone et al.[57] prospectively randomized a small number of patients (n = 22) to primary repair versus colostomy. Patients in the former group had suture lines protected with an intracolonic bypass tube. Six patients incurred blunt trauma. Although many patients excluded from other series of primary repair were included, patients presenting more than 8 hours after injury and patients felt to be inappropriate by the operating surgeon were excluded. This latter exclusion criterion, randomization failures, a large proportion of blunt trauma, and the small population size limit the implications of this study. Nonetheless, no fecal fistulae were reported, and no differences were found between the two groups relative to duration of postoperative ileus, length of hospital stay, hospital charges, or incidences of septic and nonseptic complications.

Sasaki et al.[58] have corroborated Chappuis' findings in a slightly larger (n = 71) prospective randomized study also performed without selection criteria. No mortality and no fecal fistula were reported. In the primary repair group, 31 patients underwent simple closure, whereas 12 underwent resection and anastomosis. Intra-abdominal abscess occurred in 2.3% of those undergoing primary repair and 17.8% of those undergoing colostomy.

The studies reviewed above established that colostomy need not be *mandatory*. What remains at issue is which, if any, of the original Stone and Fabian[53] exclusion criteria remain valid for primary closure and which remain valid for primary anastomosis. The issue is hotly debated.[59,60] On one side of the debate are those that preach the abandonment of colostomy[60]; on the other are those that emphasize the statistical shortcomings of currently published trials.[59] The studies of Chappuis et al.[56] and Sasaki et al.[58] would seem to suggest that all exclusion criteria can be abandoned. However, the numbers of patients enrolled in these studies are small, and potential for type II statistical errors exists.[59] The numbers of patients undergoing resection and primary anastomosis (11 and 12, respectively) are especially troubling and comprise a seemingly trivial number of events from which to abandon logical (although not proven) surgical dicta.

Penetrating Colon Injury

A large collective experience with simple suture repair of colon injury reveals a low and acceptable incidence of leak and fecal fistula—less than 3% (Table 44-2). Even series with significant proportions of left colon injuries sutured primarily maintain this low incidence of leak (Table 44-2). Of more than 1,800 colon injuries reported in the 1990s, 63% have been repaired by suture closure (Tables 44-2 and 44-3). Prospective uncontrolled data suggest that leak after simple suture closure is not related to the presence of shock or severe contamination.[55] Definitive proof that simple suture repair can be performed in unselected patients without greater peritoneal infectious morbidity than colostomy would require a randomized series dramatically larger than the Chappuis and Sasaki studies combined.[59] The weight of current data makes randomization of all patients difficult, but randomization of patients with potentially high-risk colon wounds would be appropriate; these include patients with persistent shock and mild peritoneal inflammation. Currently, colon injuries not requiring resection should be sutured primarily unless these extenuating circumstances prevail. It should be emphasized that average time from admission to operation was 116 minutes in the Chappuis study and that the longest time

Table 44-2. Simple Primary Closure of Colon Injuries

Author	Year	No.	Primary Closure (% of series)[a]	Fecal Fistula No.[b]	%	Left Colon Closures No.	Left Colon Injuries (%)
Stone and Fabian[53]	1979	67	25.0[c]	1	1.5	NS	—
Thompson et al.[63]	1981	39	37.1	0	0	21	38.2
Karanfilian et al.[125]	1982	17	12.9	0	0	3	3.9
Adkins and Zirkle[126]	1984	27	48.2	0	0	NS[d]	—
Shannon and Moore[127]	1985	80	35.1	1	1.2	19	33.3
Burch et al.[54]	1986	328	49.3	3	0.9	77[e]	31.8
Dawes et al.[128]	1986	21	15.3	0	0	7	20.0
Nallathambi et al.[129]	1987	46	51.1	0	0	0[f]	—
George et al.[55]	1989	83	81.4	0	0	NS	—
Chappuis et al.[56]	1991	17	30.3[c]	0	0	NS[g]	—
Naraynsingh et al.[130]	1991	57	93.4	1	1.8	NS	—
Demetriades et al.[131,h]	1992	76	76.0	2	2.6	NS	—
Ivatury et al.[132]	1993	159	63.1	1[i]	0.6	NS	—
Schulz et al.[67]	1993	40	40.0	0	0	NS[j]	—
Sasaki et al.[58]	1995	31	43.7[c]	0	0	15	41.7[c]

Abbreviation: NS, not specified.
[a] See Table 44-4 for percentages treated with anastomosis.
[b] Tabulated as nil if report failed to document fecal fistula or suture line leak.
[c] Randomized series; percentage does not reflect selection bias.
[d] Of 29 left colon injuries, 17 repaired with simple closure or anastomosis.
[e] Excludes patients with multiple wounds.
[f] Report limited to right colon injuries.
[g] Of 25 left colon injuries, 12 repaired with simple closure or anastomosis.
[h] Series limited to gunshot wounds.
[i] Abscess with questionable radiographic evidence of fistula.
[j] Of 34 left colon injuries, 11 repaired with simple closure or anastomosis.

was 90 minutes in the Sasaki study. Although time to operation and degree of contamination were not exclusion criteria, severe peritoneal inflammation would not likely have developed in these time intervals, and thus the surgeon should continue to show the inflamed peritoneal cavity its due respect. Wounds in a segment of inflamed, friable bowel and wounds associated with frank peritonitis should not be closed primarily.

The experience with resection and primary anastomosis is small (Table 44-4), reflecting that patients are more stringently selected than for simple suture closure. Furthermore, the num-ber of patients reported with primary anastomosis does not allow analysis of risk factors in most series. Indications for primary anastomosis are thus less clear than indications for simple suture closure. It is disturbing that the largest experience (n = 43) was associated with a 14% incidence of anastomotic leak.[61] Furthermore, chronic disease or massive blood loss (or both) was associated with anastomotic leak in 42% of patients.[61] Thus, anastomosis should not currently be performed when these risk factors are present. Large multicenter studies are needed to define further the indications and contraindications

Table 44-3. Primary Repair of Colon Injuries[a]

Author	Year	Suture Closure (no.)	Primary Anastomosis (no.)	Total (no.)	Fecal Fistula No.	%	Primary Repair (% of series)
Nelken and Lewis[64]	1989	34	3	37	1	2.7	48.7
Levison et al.[133]	1990	98	8	106	1	0.9	44.3
Burch et al.[62]	1991	564	50	614	13[b]	2.2	61.0
Falcone et al.[57,c]	1992	NS	NS	11	0	0	50.0[d]
Taheri et al.[124]	1993	NS	NS	55	0	0	37.7

Abbreviation: NS, not specified.
[a] Series reporting morbidity for suture closure and primary anastomosis combined.
[b] Denominator = 593.
[c] Selected series of left colon anastomoses performed with intracolonic bypass tube.
[d] Randomized series; percentage does not reflect selection bias.

Table 44-4. Resection and Primary Anastomosis for Colon Injuries

Author	Year	Anastomoses, All Locations				Anastomoses, Left Colon			
		No.	% of Series[a]	Fecal Fistula No.[b]	%	No.	%[c]	Fecal Fistula No.[b]	%
Thompson et al.[63]	1981	11	10.5	0	0	3	5.4	0	0
Karanfilian et al.[125]	1982	9	6.8	3	33.3	2	2.6	2	100
Adkins et al.[126]	1984	9	16.1	0	0	NS	—	—	—
Shannon and Moore[127]	1985	30	13.2	0	0	6	10.5	0	0
Burch et al.[54]	1986	28	4.2	1	3.6	1	0.4	NS	—
Dawes et al.[128]	1986	13[d]	9.5	1	7.7	0	—	—	—
Nallathambi et al.[129]	1987	19	21.1	0	0	0[e]	—	—	—
George et al.[55]	1989	12	11.8	1	8.3	NS	—	1	—
Carpenter et al.[71]	1990	NA[f]	—	—	—	9	NA[f]	0	0
Chappuis et al.[56]	1991	11	19.6[g]	0	0	NS	—	—	—
Ivatury et al.[132]	1993	26	10.3	2	7.7	0	—	—	—
Schultz et al.[67]	1993	17	17.0	0	0	NS	—	—	—
Stewart et al.[61,h]	1994	43	13.6	6	13.9	15	NS	2	13.3
Sasaki et al.[58]	1995	12	16.9[g]	0	0	5	13.9[g]	0	0

Abbreviations: NS, not specified; NA, not applicable.
[a] See Table 44-2 for percentages treated with suture closure.
[b] Tabulated as nil if report failed to document anastomotic fistula or leak.
[c] Percent of all left colon injuries treated with resection and anastomosis.
[d] Includes two patients with wounds at multiple unspecified locations.
[e] Report limited to right colon injuries.
[f] Selected series of left colon anastomoses performed with intracolonic bypass tube.
[g] Randomized series; percentage does not reflect selection bias.
[h] Report limited to injuries requiring resection (n = 60); 316 injuries treated during study period.

for primary anastomosis after resection of destructive colon injuries.

In the absence of such studies, the surgeon must exercise judgment in the performance of primary anastomosis for trauma by honoring classic principles and turning to available retrospective data for guidance. Because trauma celiotomy may be attended by shock or pre-existing contamination (or both), classic anastomotic principles of particular relevance are those calling for good blood supply and good mechanical apposition of noninflamed tissue.

Consideration of three likely clinical situations helps to organize an approach to colonic anastomosis when the patient has been in shock. The first situation is shock, with the patient easily resuscitated prior to anastomosis; blood supply will be adequate, tissue derangements unlikely, and suture line healing should not be impaired. Anastomosis should be safe. The second situation is prolonged shock, with the patient resuscitated prior to anastomosis. Blood supply should be adequate, but colonic tissue may be edematous and/or harbor persistent metabolic abnormalities. Until randomized prospective data with good power suggest otherwise, I recommend colostomy in most of these instances. The third situation is ongoing shock. Shock present during anastomosis will compromise blood supply and likely impair healing. Current trauma principles dictate that anastomoses not be performed during shock irrespective of concerns for colonic healing. Shock that persists after surgical bleeding has been stopped obliges the surgeon to defer re-establishment of intestinal continuity and creation of stomas, to abbreviate and terminate celiotomy, and to move to the intensive care unit for hemodynamic resuscitation. Shock and volume resuscitation will render bowel edematous; at secondary celiotomy, the ends of such edematous colon are best exteriorized as stomas rather than anastomosed. Colonic perforations not requiring resection should be rapidly closed with stapling devices to control contamination in the hemodynamically unstable patient (Fig. 44-3); if inspection at secondary celiotomy reveals a staple line with questionable healing, it should be exteriorized as a colostomy.[62] I prefer to oversew staple lines with silk suture if the patient's condition permits.

All suture and staple lines must provide good mechanical apposition of noninflamed tissue in all circumstances. The aspect of this principle most relevant for trauma celiotomy is that tissue must be *noninflamed* for closure. Concerns regarding duration from injury to operation and degree of peritoneal contamination can be distilled into the need to respect this inviolable principle. As long as colonic tissue is of good quality, staple lines and suture lines should be safe. Bowel to be closed or anastomosed must be pliable, free of erythema and exudate, nonfriable, and hold suture well.

Much consideration has been given to differences between healing of unprepared right and left colon suture lines. A comparison of septic morbidity and healing in right and left colon injuries revealed no differences, but only three patients with left colon resection and anastomosis were included in this study.[63] Most primary anastomoses have been performed for right colon injuries, and no study reports a large number of primary anastomoses for left colon wounds; published experience is too small to define accurately the incidence of anasto-

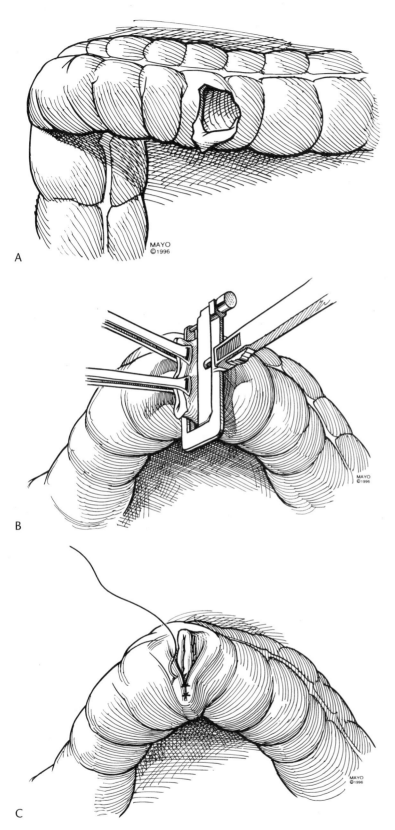

A

B

C

Figure 44-3.   Primary stapled closure of colonic injury. (**A**) Tangential injury to anterior wall, proximal transverse colon. (**B**) Margins of colonic wound controlled with Allis clamps. Stapling device ready to be fired. Tissue above staple line will be sharply debrided. (**C**) Staple line oversewn with seromuscular suture. (By permission of Mayo Foundation.)

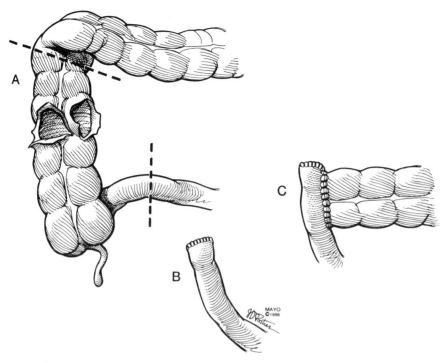

Figure 44-4.   (**A**) Destructive lesion of right colon. (**B**) Closure of distal ileum. (**C**) Side-to-end ileocolostomy. (By permission of Mayo Foundation.)

motic fistula associated with left colon wounds. Without this information, the surgeon must proceed carefully. Ileocolostomy and colocolostomy may indeed heal similarly after trauma, but as a practical matter clinical experience with the latter is particularly sparse, and caution must be exercised. Right colon resection with ileocolostomy is appropriate when the previously outlined principles are followed (Fig. 44-4); however, currently minimal precident exists for left colon resection with primary anastomosis (Table 44-4).

Contraindications to primary anastomosis based on the above principles are listed in the accompanying box.

Although it is important to know the incidence of fecal fistula associated with primary closures and primary anastomoses, other septic complications of colon injury are unrelated to suture lines. Although one can never eliminate the selection bias from

retrospective studies, the incidence of septic complication is greater for colostomy than primary repair even when injury severity is controlled.[64] Mildly to moderately severe injuries have been defined by a Penetrating Abdominal Trauma Index[65] less than 25, Injury Severity Score[66] less than 25, and Flint colon grade[34] less than 2; primary repair is clearly associated with fewer complications than colostomy for these injuries.[64] Comparison was difficult for severe injuries in this study because very few primary repairs were performed.[64] Overall, one can expect wound infection in 5 to 15% of patients,[54,55,64,67] abdominal abscess in 9 to 14%,[54,55,64] and multiple organ failure in 4%.[64] The mortality of patients with colon injury is about 10%[62]; however, recent studies excluding early death from hemorrhagic shock generally report mortality less than 3%.

Contraindications to Primary Colonic Anastomosis for Trauma

Absolute
    Massive blood loss
    Persistent shock
    Inflamed colonic tissue
    Blunt injury with gross fecal contamination
Relative
    Chronic disease
    Resuscitated, prolonged shock
    Prior abbreviated celiotomy
    Left colon location

Flint Colon Injury Grade

Grade 1
    Isolated colon injury, minimal contamination, no shock, minimal delay
Grade 2
    Through-and-through perforation, lacerations, moderate contamination
Grade 3
    Severe tissue loss, devascularization, heavy contamination

---

(From Flint et al.,[34] with permission.)

Proposed adjuncts to primary repair include exteriorization of the repair, intraoperative colonic lavage, and protective intracolonic bypass. With exteriorized repair a sutured colonic loop is brought through an abdominal wall stoma and protected with dressings so it may be directly observed for 5 to 10 days. If the colonic suture line remains healthy and intact, the loop is returned to the peritoneal cavity. If the suture line fails, the loop is converted to colostomy. Although good results have been reported,[68] so have frequent failures, and few surgeons continue to employ this technique.[69] Intraoperative prograde colonic lavage (bowel prep) could also potentially decrease septic complications by eliminating proximal fecal load. However, a prospective study of exteriorized and intraperitoneal repairs, each randomized to lavage versus no lavage, failed to show improvement in mortality or septic morbidity with this technique[70]; it currently has no established role. Finally, placement of an intraluminal latex tube to isolate the suture line from the fecal stream comprises a novel approach to anastomotic protection. Good results have been reported in small numbers of selected penetrating and blunt trauma patients undergoing left colon anastomosis (n = 9)[71] and either right or left colon suture closure or anastomosis (n = 11)[57]; no suture line leaks occurred. However, without data from a large randomized study, intracolonic bypass cannot be recommended.

Blunt Colon Injury

Blunt trauma to the large bowel is rare. Colon injury occurs in 0.5% of patients incurring blunt trauma.[72] Of those undergoing celiotomy, about 10% have colonic injury,[72] and 1.3% to 3.7% require major colonic operation.[72,73] Blunt injury occurs across a broad spectrum of severity (see box); the injuries of most concern are full-thickness laceration and devascularizing mesenteric tear. Because a great deal of blunt force must be dissipated to induce colonic injury, most patients are multiply injured and critically ill. Blunt intestinal injury occurs via two general pathophysiologic mechanisms: (1) an external anterior force may crush bowel against the vertebrae or pelvis posteriorly, or (2) deceleration may shear bowel and mesentery at points of fixation where retroperitoneal segments of colon become intraperitoneal on a mesentery.[74] A third purported mechanism—burst from increased intraluminal pressure—seems less likely. Injury by other mechanisms may occur in specific circumstances. Sigmoid perforation from pelvic fracture has been reported.[75] Rarely, pre-existing colonic abnormalities may predispose to blunt injury. For example, Crohn's disease has led to colon perforation after an otherwise trivial blow.[76] In addition, blunt colon transections have occurred at sites of undiagnosed malignancy,[72] and blunt trauma-associated hypotension has led to necrosis of previously irradiated rectosigmoid.[77]

Seat belts play an important role in the pathophysiology of blunt colon injury through the first general mechanism outlined above. Although they decrease fatalities from motor vehicle crashes,[78] seat belts increase incidence of colon, small bowel, and mesenteric injuries.[79–81] Colon and small bowel injuries are much more likely to occur in belted victims subjected to frontal impact than in unrestrained victims or victims of lateral impact.[82] However, fatal intra-abdominal solid organ injuries and other severe extra-abdominal injuries are more common in unbelted victims.[81] Seat-belt-associated injuries seem to be minimized by appropriate use of a shoulder harness. In a Finnish study of more than 3,500 motor vehicle crashes involving at least one fatality each, 9.5% of 42 seat-belted victims with predominantly abdominal injury suffered colonic contusion and another 9.5% suffered colonic rupture.[81]

The timely diagnosis of blunt colon perforation or devascularization presents one of the most difficult dilemmas in blunt trauma management.[83,84] This diagnosis is made preoperatively in only 5% of cases.[72] Delayed diagnosis certainly leads to unnecessary morbidity and mortality, yet delay may be difficult to avoid because early signs of blunt colon injury are nonspecific and often subtle. Severe deceleration, use of a lap belt,[79] anterior abdominal wall abrasion and ecchymosis in a characteristic "seat belt sign"[85] (Fig. 44-5), or presence of pelvic or lum-

Figure 44-5. "Seat-belt sign". Hypogastric contusion, ecchymosis, and abrasion. (By permission of Mayo Foundation.)

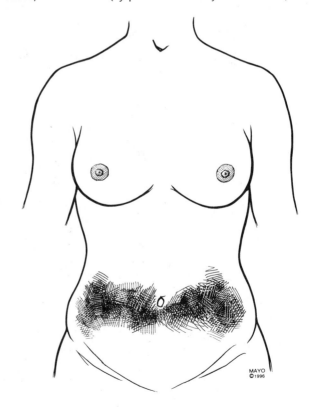

Table 44-5. Blunt Colon Injury

Indications for celiotomy (n = 286)	%
Diagnostic peritoneal tap or lavage	59.8
Initial physical findings	20.3
Computed tomography	9.1
Chest X-ray	3.5
Delayed findings or sepsis	7.3

(Data from Ross et al.[72])

bar spine[79,86] fracture should heighten suspicion for bowel injury. Although the vast majority of evaluable patients with bowel injuries (98%) demonstrate abdominal tenderness, physical examination will not confirm the diagnosis except by way of prompting celiotomy when peritonitis is present.[87] Further limiting its usefulness, abdominal examination is not reliable in patients with head injury, intoxication, or distracting extra-abdominal pain. Serum amylase does not differentiate those patients with bowel injury from those without.[87] Loss of psoas

shadow on plain abdominal radiograph suggests colon injury, but this finding is nonspecific, and plain abdominal radiographs are not routinely employed during blunt trauma evaluation. Recognition of blunt colon injury rests on performance of diagnostic peritoneal lavage (which leads to diagnosis at celiotomy), or CT (which may lead to celiotomy for other injuries or may suggest colon injury per se). Indications for celiotomy from a recent review of blunt colon injury are outlined in Table 44-5 DPL findings prompting celiotomy have been reviewed above; none are specific for the diagnosis of colon injury. However, one might expect DPL WBC count to be of particular relevance given the potential inflammation incited by colon injury. Unfortunately, DPL WBC count adds little to the sensitivity and specificity of DPL RBC count for diagnosis of colon injury.[88–90]

CT scans for trauma are performed after administration of intravenous and upper GI contrast material. CT findings of bowel injury include pneumoperitoneum, extraluminal GI contrast, free intraperitoneal fluid without solid organ injury (Fig. 44-6), thickened bowel wall, and streaks of high-density infiltration within low-density mesenteric fat.[91,92] Pneumoperitoneum and extraluminal contrast are absolute indications for celiotomy. The latter three findings are indirect signs of hollow viscus

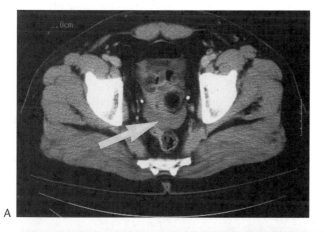

A

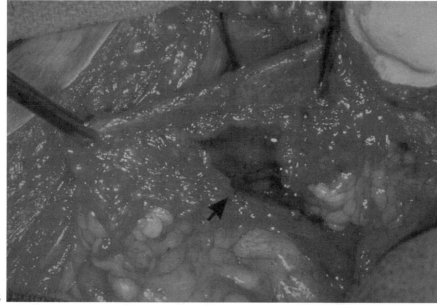

B

Figure 44-6. A 27-year-old man who had been involved in motor vehicle crash. (**A**) Computed tomography scan revealed free intraperitoneal and pelvic (arrow) fluid but no injury to solid organs. This prompted laparoscopy, which revealed persistent bleeding from sigmoid mesocolon. (**B**) Sigmoid colon with mesocolic defect. Mesenteric bleeding controlled. Colon is well vascularized. (By permission of Mayo Foundation.)

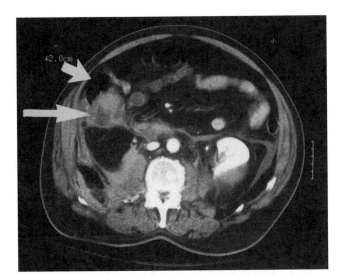

Figure 44-7. Computed tomography scan of 77-year-old man crushed by falling telephone pole reveals mesenteric hematoma (long arrow) displacing right colon (short arrow) anteriorly and laterally. Leukocytosis and abdominal tenderness prompted celiotomy 48 hours after injury. Ischemic right colon was resected with primary ileocolostomy. (By permission of Mayo Foundation.)

or mesenteric injury. Mesenteric hematomas may also be apparent (Fig. 44-7) Patients with CT scans demonstrating these findings must be observed closely. Emergence of peritoneal irritation, unexplained fever, or leukocytosis necessitates celiotomy in search of colon or small bowel perforation or devascularization. In place of serial examinations, the author has found diagnostic laparoscopy useful to confirm or exclude the presence of blunt hollow viscus injury suggested by indirect CT signs.

Blunt injuries are rather equitably distributed among the ascending, transverse, and sigmoid colon; descending colon lesions are relatively rare.[72,87,93-95] Approximately one-fourth of blunt colon injuries result in perforation or devascularization.[72]

Treatment of blunt colon trauma must be tailored to the specific injury present. Small stable mesenteric hematomas require no treatment. Ongoing bleeding from a mesenteric hematoma will often stop with simple application of manual pressure. Large or expanding mesenteric hematomas should be explored so that control of specific bleeding vessels can be obtained. If hemostasis results in devascularization of a colonic segment, resection is necessary. Seromuscular tears may be closed with interrupted seromuscular sutures of 3-0 silk or—if superficial—left untreated. Rarely, large deep seromuscular lacerations will require resection. Although small intramural hematomas may require no specific therapy, large intramural hematomas may be associated with obstruction, delayed perforation, or late stenosis; for this reason, large intramural hematomas should be resected.[96] A degloving injury of the colon has been described in which the serosa and muscularis are stripped from the remaining bowel wall, leaving a mucosal tube.[97] Because this lesion threatens the mechanical integrity of the bowel and is likely to be associated with compromised blood supply, it should be resected. Full-thickness lacerations may be treated by primary repair, resection and primary anastomosis, or colostomy. The latter two treatments are options for mesenteric injuries associated with devascularized and ischemic colon.

The issue of primary suture closure/primary anastomosis versus colostomy exists for blunt as well as penetrating trauma. However, because blunt colon injury is infrequent relative to penetrating injury, we have fewer data on which to base treatment recommendations. Most surgeons apply primary repair more conservatively for blunt than for penetrating trauma.[74] Early studies suggested that primary repair of blunt colon injury was associated with an increase in colon-specific mortality.[94] Blunt colon injury more often occurs in multiply injured patients, who will poorly tolerate the septic complications of colonic suture line breakdown. For these reasons, one's threshold for performing primary colon repair should be higher for blunt injury than for penetrating injury. Nonetheless, in some circumstances, blunt colon perforation may be safely treated with primary closure or primary anastomosis. A multicenter retrospective study of 286 patients with blunt colon injury suggested that gross fecal contamination should dictate colostomy as this finding predicted infectious and systemic complications in patients undergoing primary repair but not in patients undergoing diversion.[72] In this series, operative delay, shock, and timing of antibiotic administration did not affect morbidity; data regarding effects of prolonged shock were not available. Thus, gross fecal contamination, prolonged shock, and inflammation of the colonic wall at the site of potential suture lines should comprise contraindications to primary repair or anastomosis after blunt colon trauma.

Blunt trauma may be complicated by colonic obstruction months or years after injury. This results from an insidious cicatricial process incited by colonic hematoma or ischemia, or both. Resection is required.[98]

MANAGEMENT OF EXTRAPERITONEAL RECTAL INJURY

No distinctions need be made between the management of intraperitoneal rectal injuries and colon injuries. Extraperitoneal rectal injuries require special considerations, however. Penetrating rectal injury may be present in any patient with a wound of the abdomen, buttock(s), perineum, or proximal thigh(s). The innocuous appearance of gluteal stab wounds may belie significant underlying injury including rectal laceration.[99] Digital examination of the rectum is performed during the secondary survey of all trauma patients; the finding of gross blood suggests rectal injury.[100] Guaiac testing does not play a role since a negative result does not exclude injury, and missile trajectory or wound proximity will prompt proctoscopy without it.[101] All patients with wounds raising suspicion of rectal injury should undergo rigid proctoscopic examination. Proctoscopic visualization of a mucosal defect confirms the presence of injury; fresh intraluminal blood strongly suggests injury. If index of suspicion is high based on the trajectory of the wounding agent, rectal injury should be presumed and treated despite the absence of definitive proctoscopic findings. Hemodynamically unstable patients will require celiotomy without preoperative proctoscopic examination and may force definitive action on a presumptive diagnosis of rectal injury. Rarely, a rectal defect will be palpated. Little experience has been gained with fluoroscopic water-soluble contrast studies. They may be useful in select circumstances.

Both unequivocal and presumed rectal injuries require fecal

Diversion for Rectal Injuries

Loop colostomy

Colostomy and mucous fistula

Loop colostomy with closure distal limb

Colostomy with closure rectum (Hartmann-type procedure)

diversion. Although multiple options exist, loop sigmoid colostomy is generally favored for injuries without significant rectal destruction (Fig. 44-8). Care must be taken to construct the loop with an adequate common wall spur to ensure complete fecal diversion.[102,103] Destructive injuries necessitating resection should be diverted with a Hartmann-type procedure. Both loop and end colostomies should be matured immediately. It is essential to bring a 2-cm length of bowel onto the abdominal wall with good blood supply and without tension prior to maturation.

The presacral space should be drained for all extraperitoneal rectal injuries. Lack of presacral drainage has been associated with greater septic morbidity.[104] Transperineal drains have most commonly been recommended, although transperitoneal drains are acceptable if the rectum is mobilized from the presacral space in the process of repairing pelvic injuries. With a transperineal approach, a curvilinear incision is made between the coccyx and anus, the presacral space is entered by sharp division of Waldeyer's fascia, and then blunt dissection is continued to

Figure 44-8. Transverse loop colostomy with supporting bar beneath spur. (By permission of Mayo Foundation.)

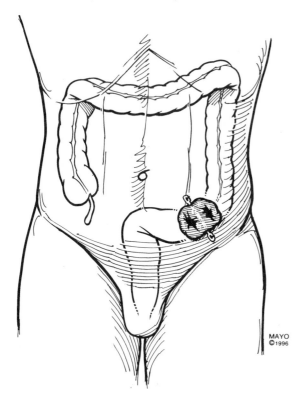

the level of the injury. Penrose drains placed through the resulting wound have generally been advocated. However, the author prefers placement of closed suction drains, which exit the perineum laterally with closure of the postanal incision (Fig. 44-9).

Whereas diversion and drainage of extraperitoneal rectal injuries are cornerstones of therapy, the roles of injury repair and distal rectal washout are controversial. The latter adjuncts appeared to limit mortality in a Vietnam experience but are of questionable benefit in civilian practice.[105]

Small, low-velocity extraperitoneal rectal injuries need not be repaired. Exposure of distal injuries may be difficult and may result in unnecessary opening of the presacral space. Closure of proximal injuries and injuries encountered during exposure of other pelvic lesions is reasonable to perform. Single-layer closure with interrupted 3-0 polydioxanone suture is preferred. Treatment of injuries involving significant loss of rectal wall by resection with end sigmoid colostomy (Hartmann-type procedure) rather than closure and diversion minimizes the risk of rectal fistula or sinus.

Distal rectal irrigation has some advocates among civilian trauma surgeons, but its purported benefit has not been well established and indeed has been seriously challenged. Nonetheless, it appears to be a safe practice and does not lead to extrusion of stool into the presacral space; to safeguard against this latter concern, the anus should be dilated before irrigation is initiated, and its patency should be maintained with an anorectal retractor during the procedure. Distal rectal irrigation is reasonable to perform at the discretion of the individual surgeon.

OPEN PELVIC FRACTURE

Most blunt injuries to the extraperitoneal rectum are associated with pelvic fracture.[106] A pelvic fracture is compound, or open when the fracture site directly communicates with a rectal, vaginal, or cutaneous laceration. Open pelvic fracture comprises one of the greatest challenges in blunt trauma management (Fig. 44-10). Perineal lacerations have been reported in nearly 50% of patients and rectal injuries in 22%.[107] Pelvic fracture fragments puncture the rectum, causing laceration. Diverting colostomy is essential for all patients.[108,109] Patients are threatened immediately by severe hemorrhage and later by perineal or pelvic sepsis. However, aggressive management to control hemorrhage and sepsis has lowered the 50% expected mortality to 15% in one report.[107] During prehospital transport, pneumatic antishock garments provide a degree of fracture hemostasis; definitive control of bleeding requires perineal packing, external bony fixation, and/or arteriographic embolization. Celiotomy with pelvic hematoma exploration or hypogastric artery ligation (or both) is fraught with hazard and not recommended. Once hemorrhage is controlled, prevention of sepsis takes priority. Severe perineal soft tissue injury (Fig. 44-10) occurs as a result of hyperabduction of the hips or direct "straddle" impact. These injuries require intensely aggressive wound management to prevent pelvic abscess, soft tissue infection, and/or osteomyelitis.

The components of this management are fecal diversion, irrigation of the defunctionalized rectum, and debridement of perineal wounds, followed by repeated daily debridements and irrigations. Fecal diversion should be performed at the initial

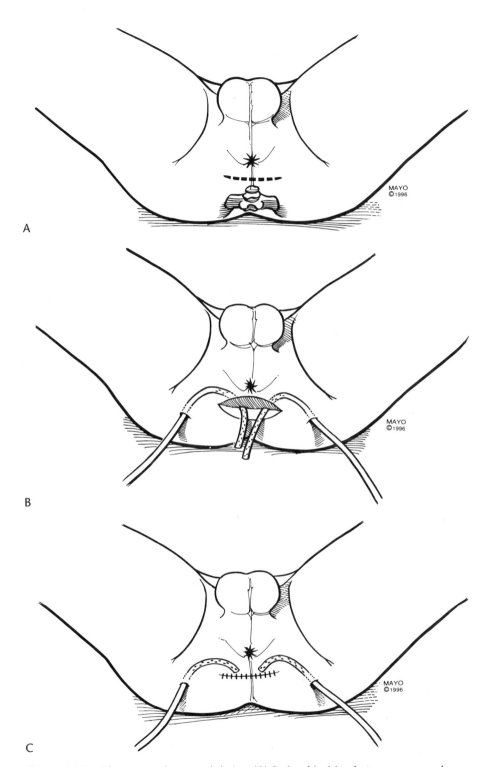

Figure 44-9. Placement of presacral drains. (**A**) Perineal incision between anus and coccyx. (**B**) Presacral space opened; drains exit perineum. (**C** & **D**) Drains advanced to level of rectal injury. *(Figure continues.)*

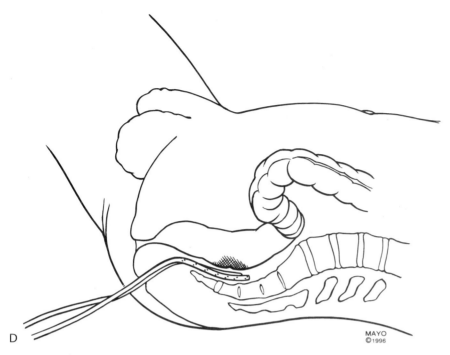

Figure 44-9. *(Continued)* (By permission of Mayo Foundation.)

trauma celiotomy immediately after life-threatening injuries have been addressed. Diverting loop colostomy or a colostomy with mucous fistula rather than a Hartmann-type procedure is recommended so that the distal limb may be irrigated to prevent uncontrolled perineal soilage. Infection of external fixator pin sites has not occurred despite proximity to stomas. Presacral drainage and closure of the laceration are desirable if safe to perform, but acute pelvic hematoma should not be disturbed.[74] The distal limb of the loop colostomy or the mucous fistula should be irrigated with warm saline and then Betadine solution until all residual stool has been removed. Perineal wounds are then debrided and packed with saline-moistened gauze. Dressings are changed three times daily in the intensive care unit, and the patient is returned to the operating room for repeated debridement and wound irrigation daily for the first 5 to 7 days after injury. This aggressive approach has dramatically minimized expected septic morbidity and mortality.[107,110]

Proctosigmoidoscopic examination should be performed at the initial procedure if possible. This will allow identification of rectal mucosal lacerations extending from the perineum so that they may be repaired. Assessment of the anal sphincter can be performed at the time of subsequent debridements; simple reapproximation can be performed at this time, but more complex repairs are best performed as interval procedures.

COLOSTOMY CLOSURE

Despite the ascendancy of primary repair, colostomy remains necessary for treatment of extraperitoneal rectal, severe colon, and extensive perineal injuries. Accordingly, colostomy closure is an essential of trauma care. Three aspects of colostomy closure deserve discussion: attendant morbidity, use of preclosure contrast studies, and timing.

As many as 30% of patients undergoing closure of trauma-related colostomy suffer a complication. Although reported morbidity is generally much lower, it remains significant (Table 44-6). The precise incidence of complications has been debated because purportedly excessive morbidity rates argue for primary repair. If colostomy is utilized only when necessary, the point becomes moot and the debate empty. Colostomy closure carries morbidity, but this is not so great as to influence the indications or contraindications for primary repair. When conditions at trauma celiotomy dictate colostomy, this should be performed without undue concern for closure-related complications. Unfounded fear of colostomy-closure morbidity should not overcome good judgment and drive the surgeon to perform inappropriate primary repair.

Adverse events that can frustrate colostomy closure include fecal fistula, stenosis, wound infection, small bowel obstruction, and general postoperative complications. Most, but not all[111] series have been free of mortality; in a compilation of nearly 1,500 trauma and nontrauma patients, mortality after colostomy closure was less than 1%.[112] Morbidity seems to be greater in those patients who suffer obstructive or septic complications following initial trauma celiotomy.[113] The type of stoma (end versus loop) should not influence morbidity.[114] Fecal fistula has been reported after closure of loop colostomy by suture of the anterior wall[115] and by resection and anastomosis.[116] Loop stomas can be safely sutured, but inflamed tissue and the mucocutaneous margin must be carefully debrided.

Concern for possible fistulae, sinuses, stenosis, or unsuspected nontraumatic pathology prompts barium examination of the large bowel prior to colostomy closure. The need for routine preclosure barium studies has been challenged,[117,118] since the vast majority are unrevealing.[119] Some caution is advisable, however. The number of reported patients studied with rectal injury has been small and thus the true incidence of positive

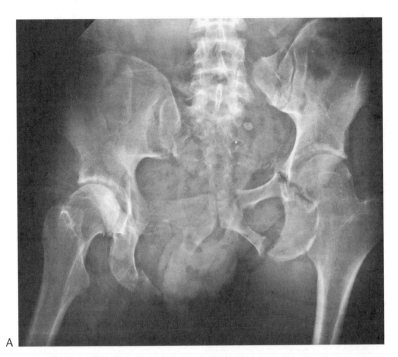

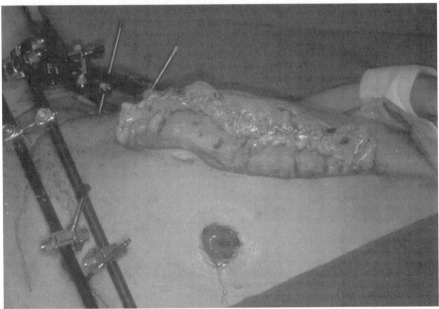

Figure 44-10. A 22-year-old man incurred open pelvic fracture with severe perineal injury in motorcycle crash. (**A**) Complex pelvic fracture: vertical displacement of left hemipelvis, fracture of pubic rami, diastasis of left sacroiliac joint, and fracture of left acetabulum. (**B**) External fixator and end-sigmoid colostomy. Bowel edema necessitated abdominal closure with Silastic "silo". *(Figure continues.)*

preclosure studies in this population is not well defined. Furthermore, anastomotic and septic complications following colostomy closure are morbid and costly; thus, even infrequent barium study findings that alter the operative plan so as to avert these complications may well justify most negative studies.[120] Until studies with larger numbers of patients allow rigorous cost-benefit analyses, continued routine contrast examination prior to colostomy closure is recommended. Patients with extra-

peritoneal rectal injuries should also undergo proctoscopy since some abnormalities in this region may be missed by barium examination alone.[121] Adequate anal sphincter function must be ensured with anorectal manometry in patients who have incurred central perineal lacerations lest colostomy closure result in fecal incontinence.[122]

The timing of colostomy closure is best based on the extent of postinjury abdominal sepsis, the severity of colonic and ex-

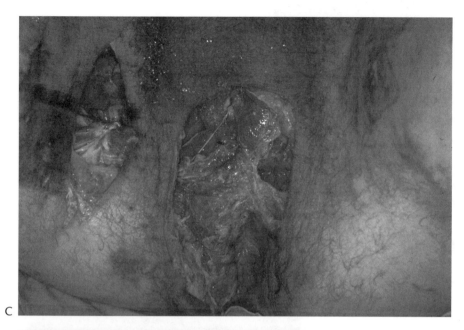

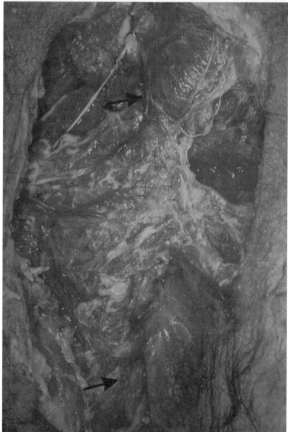

Figure 44-10. *(Continued)* (**C**) Perineal lacerations 4 days after injury. (**D**) Central perineum with anal sphincter mechanism exposed inferiorly and base of penis exposed superiorly (arrows). (By permission of Mayo Foundation.)

Table 44-6. Closure of Trauma-Related Colostomy (%; Selected Series)

Author	Year	No.	Penetrating Trauma	Type of Stoma End[a]	Type of Stoma Loop	Leak/ Fistula	Wound Infection	Total Morbidity	Mortality
Thal and Yeary[123]	1980	137	NS	32.8	67.2	1.5	5.1	10.2	0
Williams et al.[134]	1987	49	NS	NS	NS	2.0	2.0	6.1	0
Crass et al.[135]	1987	75	59	100.0	0	0	2.7	5.3	0
Livingston et al.[136]	1989	121	83	79.0	21.0	3.3	5.8	9.9	0
Pachter et al.[137]	1990	87	89	91	9.0	0	9.0	25.0	0
Taheri et al.[124]	1993	110	NS	71.6	28.4	0.9	3.6	18.2	0
Rehm et al.[138]	1993	25	68	NS	NS	0	0	8.0	0
Renz et al.[115,b]	1993	16	NS	12.5	87.5	12.5[c]	12.5[c]	18.8	0
Sola et al.[113]	1993	86	95	62.8	37.2	2.3	10.5	24.4	0

Abbreviation: NS, not specified.
[a] Includes Hartmann-type procedures.
[b] Same-admission colostomy closure for rectal trauma.
[c] Wound infections occurred in patients with fistula.

tracolonic injuries, and the patient's general condition including nutritional status. Intestinal continuity should be re-established only after the patient has healed all injuries, has attained preinjury body weight, and has begun to regain physical strength. Optimal timing thus varies from patient to patient. Thal & Yeary[123] found no correlation between timing of closure and morbidity. Thirty-two of their 137 patients had colostomy closure within 4 weeks of injury (including 13 patients who had closure during their initial hospitalization), with morbidity comparable to that for patients with later closures. More recently, Renz et al.[115] reported two anastomotic leaks in 16 patients with rectal injuries who underwent closure during their initial hospitalization, but most patients had no difficulties. Examining intervals from injury to closure of 0 to 3 months, 3 to 6 months, and greater than 6 months, Taheri and colleagues[124] found no differences in morbidity.[124] No randomized data are available,

and others have found greater morbidity and more technically demanding operations among patients undergoing closure within 6 weeks of injury.[116] In summary, some patients can undergo uncomplicated early or even same-admission re-establishment of intestinal continuity, but without guidelines from large studies, prudent judgment must be exercised. Takedown of colostomy can be performed safely for most patients between 2 and 3 months after injury. Following trauma celiotomy complicated by severe intra-abdominal sepsis, closure should be deferred for at least 6 months to allow intense inflammatory changes to resolve.

ACKNOWLEDGMENTS

The author offers his deepest gratitude to Ms. Karma Krumwiede for her dedicated and persevering assistance with manuscript preparation.

REFERENCES

1. American College of Surgeons (1993) Advanced Trauma Life Support Course for Physicians. 5th Edi. Student Manual. American College of Surgeons, Chicago, IL

2. Root HD, Hauser CW, McKinley CR et al (1965) Diagnostic peritoneal lavage. Surgery 57:633–637

3. Sorkey AJ, Farnell MB, Williams HJ Jr et al (1989) The complementary roles of diagnostic peritoneal lavage and computed tomography in the evaluation of blunt abdominal trauma. Surgery 106:794–801

4. Salvino CK, Esposito TJ, Marshall WJ et al (1993) The role of diagnostic laparoscopy in the management of trauma patients: a preliminary assessment. J Trauma 34:506–515

5. Ivatury RR, Simon RJ, Stahl WM (1993) A critical evaluation of laparoscopy in penetrating abdominal trauma. J Trauma 34:822–828

6. Simon RJ, Ivatury RR (1995) Current concepts in the use of cavitary endoscopy in the evaluation and treatment of blunt and penetrating truncal injuries. Surg Clin North Am 75: 157–174

7. Rozycki GS (1995) Abdominal ultrasonography in trauma. Surg Clin North Am 75:175–191

8. Rozycki GS, Ochsner MG, Schmidt JA et al (1995) A prospective study of surgeon-performed ultrasound as the primary adjuvant modality for injured patient assessment. J Trauma 39:492–500

9. Cué JI, Miller FB, Cryer HM III, et al (1990) A prospective, randomized comparison between open and closed peritoneal lavage techniques. J Trauma 30:880–883·

10. Trunkey DD, Hill AC, Schecter WP (1991) Abdominal trauma and indications for celiotomy. pp. 409–426. In Moore EE, Mattox KL, Feliciano DV (eds): Trauma. Appleton & Lange, Norwalk, CT

11. Senn N (1888) Rectal insufflation of hydrogen gas: an infallible test in the diagnosis of visceral injury of the gastro-intestinal canal in penetrating wounds of the abdomen. JAMA 1: 767–777, 807–811

12. Moore EE, Marx JA (1985) Penetrating abdominal wounds: rationale for exploratory laparotomy JAMA 253:2705–2708

13. Feliciano DV, Burch JM, Spjut-Patrinely V et al (1988) Abdominal gunshot wounds: an urban trauma center's experience with 300 consecutive patients. Ann Surg 208:362–370

14. Lowe RJ, Saletta JD, Read DR et al (1977) Should laparotomy be mandatory or selective in gunshot wounds of the abdomen? J Trauma 17:903–907

15. Moore EE, Moore JB, Van Duzer-Moore S, Thompson JS (1980) Mandatory laparotomy for gunshot wounds penetrating the abdomen. Am J Surg 140:847–851

16. Edwards J, Gaspard DJ (1974) Visceral injury due to extraperitoneal gunshot wounds. Arch Surg 108:865–866

17. Merlotti GJ, Marcet E, Sheaff CM et al (1985) Use of peritoneal lavage to evaluate abdominal penetration. J Trauma 25:228–231

18. Sosa JL, Sims D, Martin L, Zeppa R (1992) Laparoscopic evaluation of tangential abdominal gunshot wounds. Arch Surg 127:109–110

19. Thompson JS, Moore EE, Van Duzer-Moore S et al (1980) The evolution of abdominal stab wound management. J Trauma 20:478–484

20. Feliciano DV, Bitondo CG, Steed G et al (1984) Five hundred open taps or lavages in patients with abdominal stab wounds. Am J Surg 148:772–777

21. Merlotti GJ, Dillon BC, Lange DA et al (1988) Peritoneal lavage in penetrating thoraco-abdominal trauma. J Trauma 28:17–23

22. Phillips TF (1989) Editorial comment. J Trauma 29:1229–1230

23. Phillips T, Sclafani SJA, Goldstein A et al (1986) Use of the contrast-enhanced CT enema in the management of penetrating trauma to the flank and back. J Trauma 26:593–601

24. Hauser CJ, Huprich JE, Bosco P et al (1987) Triple-contrast computed tomography in the evaluation of penetrating posterior abdominal injuries. Arch Surg 122:1112–1115

25. Meyer DM, Thal ER, Weigelt JA, Redman HC (1989) The role of abdominal CT in the evaluation of stab wounds to the back. J Trauma 29:1226–1230

26. Duncan AO, Phillips TF, Scalea TM et al (1989) Management of transpelvic gunshot wounds. J Trauma 29:1335–1340

27. Fallon WF Jr, Reyna TM, Brunner RG et al (1988) Penetrating trauma to the buttock. South Med J 81:1236–1238

28. Malangoni MA, Miller FB, Cryer HM et al (1990) The management of penetrating pelvic trauma. Am Surg 56:61–65

29. Maull KI, Sachatello CR, Ernst CB (1977) The deep perineal laceration—an injury frequently associated with open pelvic fractures: a need for aggressive surgical management. J Trauma 17:685–696

30. Nichols RL, Smith JW, Klein DB et al (1984) Risk of infection after penetrating abdominal trauma. N Engl J Med 311:1065–1070

31. Fabian TC, Croce MA, Payne LW et al (1992) Duration of antibiotic therapy for penetrating abdominal trauma: a prospective trial. Surgery 112:788–795

32. Feliciano DV, Spjut-Patrinely V (1990) Pre-, intra-, and postoperative antibiotics. Surg Clin North Am 70:689–701

33. Fullen WD, Hunt J, Altemeier WA (1972) Prophylactic antibiotics in penetrating wounds of the abdomen. J Trauma 12:282–289

34. Flint LM, Vitale GC, Richardson JD, Polk HC Jr (1981) The injured colon: relationships of management to complications. Ann Surg 193:619–623

35. Hooker KD, DiPiro JT, Wynn JJ (1991) Aminoglycoside combinations versus beta-lactams alone for penetrating abdominal trauma: a meta-analysis. J Trauma 31:1155–1160

36. Weigelt JA, Easley SM, Thal ER et al (1993) Abdominal surgical wound infection is lowered with improved perioperative enterococcus and bacteroides therapy. J Trauma 34:579–585

37. Dellinger EP, Wertz MJ, Lennard ES, Oreskovich MR (1986) Efficacy of short-course antibiotic prophylaxis after penetrating intestinal injury, a prospective randomized trial. Arch Surg 121:23–30

38. Williamson KR, Taswell HF (1990) Indications for intraoperative blood salvage. J Clin Apheresis 5:100–103

39. Ozmen V, McSwain NE Jr, Nichols RL et al (1992) Autotransfusion of potentially culture-positive blood (CPB) in abdominal trauma: preliminary data from a prospective study. J Trauma 32:36–39

40. Horst HM, Dlugos S, Fath JJ et al (1992) Coagulopathy and intraoperative blood salvage (IBS). J Trauma 32:646–653

41. Carrillo C, Fogler RJ, Shaftan GW (1993) Delayed gastrointestinal reconstruction following massive abdominal trauma. J Trauma 34:233–235

42. Hirshberg A, Mattox KL (1995) Planned reoperation for severe trauma. Ann Surg 222:3–8

43. Brenneman FD, Rizoli SB, Boulanger BR (1994) Abbreviated laparotomy for damage control: a case report. Can J Surg 37:237–239

44. Morris JA Jr, Eddy VA, Blinman TA et al (1993) The staged celiotomy for trauma: issues in unpacking and reconstruction. Ann Surg 217:576–586

45. Burch JM, Ortiz VB, Richardson RJ et al (1992) Abbreviated laparotomy and planned reoperation for critically injured patients. Ann Surg 215:476–484

46. Wallace C (1917) A study of 1200 cases of gunshot wounds of the abdomen. Br J Surg 4:679–743

47. Ogilvie WH (1944) Abdominal wounds in the western desert. Surg Gynecol Obstet 78:225–238

48. Woodhall JP, Ochsner A (1951) The management of perforating injuries of the colon and rectum in civilian practice. Surgery 29:305–320

49. Ganchrow MI, Lavenson GS Jr, McNamara JJ (1970) Surgical management of traumatic injuries of the colon and rectum. Arch Surg 100:515–520

50. Pontius RG, Creech O Jr, DeBakey ME (1957) Management of large bowel injuries in civilian practice. Ann Surg 146:291–295

51. Beall AC Jr, Bricker DL, Alessi FJ et al (1971) Surgical considerations in the management of civilian colon injuries. Ann Surg 173:971–978

52. LoCicero J III, Tajima T, Drapanas T (1975) A half-century of experience in the management of colon injuries: changing concepts. J Trauma 15:575–579

53. Stone HH, Fabian TC (1979) Management of perforating colon trauma: randomization between primary closure and exteriorization. Ann Surg 190:430–436

54. Burch JM, Brock JC, Gevirtzman L et al (1986) The injured colon. Ann Surg 203:701–711

55. George SM Jr, Fabian TC, Voeller GR et al (1989) Primary repair of colon wounds: a prospective trial in nonselected patients. Ann Surg 209:728–734

56. Chappuis CW, Frey DJ, Dietzen CD et al (1991) Management

of penetrating colon injuries: a prospective randomized trial. Ann Surg 213:492–498

57. Falcone RE, Wanamaker SR, Santanello SA, Carey LC (1992) Colorectal trauma: primary repair or anastomosis with intracolonic bypass versus ostomy. Dis Colon Rectum 35:957–963

58. Sasaki LS, Allaben RD, Golwala R, Mittal VK (1995) Primary repair of colon injuries: a prospective randomized study. J Trauma 39:895–901

59. Ryan M, Dutta S, Masri L et al (1995) Fecal diversion for penetrating colon injuries—still the established treatment. Dis Colon Rectum 38:264–267

60. Nance FC (1995) A stake through the heart of colostomy. J Trauma 39:811–812

61. Stewart RM, Fabian TC, Croce MA et al (1994) Is resection with primary anastomosis following destructive colon wounds always safe? Am J Surg 168:316–319

62. Burch JM, Martin RR, Richardson RJ et al (1991) Evolution of the treatment of the injured colon in the 1980s. Arch Surg 126:979–984

63. Thompson JS, Moore EE, Moore JB (1981) Comparison of penetrating injuries of the right and left colon. Ann Surg 193:414–418

64. Nelken N, Lewis F (1989) The influence of injury severity on complication rates after primary closure or colostomy for penetrating colon trauma. Ann Surg 209:439–447

65. Moore EE, Dunn EL, Moore JB, Thompson JS (1981) Penetrating abdominal trauma index. J Trauma 21:439–445

66. Baker SP, O'Neill B, Haddon W Jr, Long WB (1974) The Injury Severity Score: a method for describing patients with multiple injuries and evaluating emergency care. J Trauma 14:187–196

67. Schultz SC, Magnant CM, Richman MF et al (1993) Identifying the low-risk patient with penetrating colonic injury for selective use of primary repair. Surg Gynecol Obstet 177:237–242

68. Ivatury RR, Nallathambi MN (1996) Colon. pp. 657–668. In: The Textbook of Penetrating Trauma. Williams & Wilkins, Philadelphia, PA

69. Huber PJ Jr, Thal ER (1990) Management of colon injuries. Surg Clin North Am 70:561–573

70. Baker LW, Thomson SR, Chadwick SJD (1990) Colon wound management and prograde colonic lavage in large bowel trauma. Br J Surg 77:872–876

71. Carpenter D, Bello J, Sokol TP et al (1990) The intracolonic bypass tube for left colon and rectal trauma: the avoidance of a colostomy. Am Surg 56:769–773

72. Ross SE, Cobean RA, Hoyt DB et al (1992) Blunt colonic injury—a multicenter review. J Trauma 33:379–384

73. Cox EF (1984) Blunt abdominal trauma, a 5-year analysis of 870 patients requiring celiotomy. Ann Surg 199:467–474

74. Harrison AW, Whelan P (1990) Bowel injury from blunt abdominal trauma. pp. 265–271 In: Management of Blunt Trauma. Williams & Wilkins, Baltimore, MD pp. 265–271

75. Shapiro MJ, Wolverson MK (1989) Perforation of the retroperitoneal sigmoid colon secondary to fracture-dislocation of the left sacroiliac joint: case report. J Trauma 29:694–696

76. Johnson GA, Baker J (1990) Colonic perforation following mild trauma in a patient with Crohn's disease. Am J Emerg Med 8:340–341

77. Norotsky MC, Shackford SR (1992) Rectosigmoid ischemia following blunt abdominal trauma in a patient treated with radiation therapy: case report. J Trauma 33:931–932

78. Bohlin NI (1966) A statistical analysis of 28,000 accident cases with emphasis on occupant restraint value. Proceedings of the Eleventh Stapp Car Crash Conference, New York Society of Automotive Engineers. SAE Trans 76:2981–2994

79. Appleby JP, Nagy AG (1989) Abdominal injuries associated with the use of seatbelts. Am J Surg 157:457–458

80. Denis R, Allard M, Atlas H, Farkouh E (1983) Changing trends with abdominal injury in seatbelt wearers. J Trauma 23:1007–1008

81. Arajärvi E, Santavirta S, Tolonen J (1987) Abdominal injuries sustained in severe traffic accidents by seatbelt wearers. J Trauma 27:393–397

82. Siegel JH, Mason-Gonzalez S, Dischinger P et al (1993) Safety belt restraints and compartment intrusions in frontal and lateral motor vehicle crashes: mechanisms of injuries, complications, and acute care costs. J Trauma 34:736–759

83. Stahl KD, Geiss AC, Bordan DL et al (1985) Blunt trauma and delayed colon injury. Curr Surg January-February: 4–9

84. Winton TL, Girotti MJ, Manley PN, Sterns EE (1985) Delayed intestinal perforation after nonpenetrating abdominal trauma. Can J Surg 28:437–439

85. Doersch KB, Dozier WE (1968) The seat belt syndrome: the seat belt sign, intestinal and mesenteric injuries. Am J Surg 116:831–833

86. Ritchie WP, Ersek RA, Bunch WL, Simmons RL (1970) Combined visceral and vertebral injuries from lap type seat belts. Surg Gynecol Obstet 131:431–435

87. Wisner DH, Chun Y, Blaisdell FW (1990) Blunt intestinal injury: keys to diagnosis and management. Archi Surg 125:1319–1323

88. D'Amelio LF, Rhodes M (1990) A reassessment of the peritoneal lavage leukocyte count in blunt abdominal trauma. J Trauma 30:1291–1293

89. Jacobs DG, Angus L, Rodriguez A, Militello PR (1990) Peritoneal lavage white count: a reassessment. J Trauma 30:607–612

90. Soyka JM, Martin M, Sloan EP et al (1990) Diagnostic peritoneal lavage: is an isolated WBC count $\geq$ 500/mm^3 predictive of intra-abdominal injury requiring celiotomy in blunt trauma patients? J Trauma 30:874–879

91. Donohue JH, Federle MP, Griffiths BG, Trunkey DD (1987) Computed tomography in the diagnosis of blunt intestinal and mesenteric injuries. J Trauma 27:11–17

92. Nghiem HV, Jeffrey RB Jr, Mindelzun RE (1995) CT of blunt trauma to the bowel and mesentery. Semi Ultrasound CT MRI 16:82–90

93. Howell HS, Bartizal JF, Freeark RJ (1976) Blunt trauma involving the colon and rectum. J Trauma 16:624–632

94. Strate RG, Grieco JG (1983) Blunt injury to the colon and rectum. J Trauma 23:384–388

95. Dauterive AH, Flancbaum L, Cox EF (1985) Blunt intestinal trauma: a modern-day review. Ann Surg 201:198–203

96. Nance FC, Crowder VH (1968) Intramural hematoma of the colon following blunt trauma to the abdomen. Am Surg 34:85–87

97. Ho YH, Pritchett CJ (1990) Blunt abdominal trauma causing a 'degloving injury' to the colon. Injury 21:119–120

98. Mays ET, Noer RJ (1966) Colonic stenosis after trauma. J Trauma 6:316–331

99. Feigenberg Z, Ben-Baruch D, Barak R, Zer M (1992) Penetrating stab wound of the gluteus—a potentially life-threatening injury: case reports. J Trauma 33:776–778

100. Ferraro FJ, Livingston DH, Odom J et al (1993) The role of sigmoidoscopy in the management of gunshot wounds to the buttocks. Am Surg 59:350–352

101. Levine H, Simon RJ, Smith TR et al (1992) Guaiac testing in the diagnosis of rectal trauma: what is its value? J Trauma 32:210–212

102. Wangensteen OH (1947) Complete fecal diversion achieved by a simple loop colostomy. Surg Gynecol Obstet 84:409–414

103. Rambeau JL, Wilk PJ, Turnbull RB, Fazio VW (1978) Total fecal diversion by the temporary skin-level loop transverse colostomy. Dis Colon Rectum 21:223–226

104. Burch JM, Feliciano DV, Mattox KL (1989) Colostomy and drainage for civilian rectal injuries: is that all? Ann Surg 209:600–611

105. Lavenson GS, Cohen A (1971) Management of rectal injuries. Am J Surg 122:226–230

106. McKenzie AD, Beall GA (1972) Nonpenetrating injuries of the colon and rectum. Surg Clin North Am 52:735–746

107. Sinnott R, Rhodes M, Brader A (1992) Open pelvic fractures: an injury for trauma centers. Am J Surg 163:283–287

108. Kusminsky RE, Shbeeb I, Makos G, Boland JP (1982) Blunt pelviperineal injuries: an expanded role for the diverting colostomy. Dis Colon Rectum 25:787–790

109. Fallon WF Jr (1992) The present role of colostomy in the management of trauma. Dis Colon Rectum 35:1094–1102

110. Kudsk KA, McQueen MA, Voeller GR et al (1990) Management of complex perineal soft-tissue injuries. J Trauma 30:1155–1160

111. Yajko RD, Norton LW, Bloemendal L, Eiseman B (1976) Morbidity of colostomy closure. Am J Surg 132:304–306

112. Parks SE, Hastings PR (1985) Complications of colostomy closure. Am J Surg 149:672–675

113. Sola JE, Bender JS, Buchman TG (1993) Morbidity and timing of colostomy closure in trauma patients. Injury 24:438–440

114. Mileski WJ, Rege RV, Joehl RJ, Nahrwold DL (1990) Rates of morbidity and mortality after closure of loop and end colostomy. Surg Gynecol Obstet 171:17–21

115. Renz BM, Feliciano DV, Sherman R (1993) Same admission colostomy closure (SACC)—a new approach to rectal wounds: a prospective study. Ann Surg 218:279–293

116. Machiedo GW, Casey KF, Blackwood JM (1980) Colostomy closure following trauma. Surg Gynecol Obstet 151:58–60

117. Atweh NA, Vieux EE, Ivatury R et al (1989) Indications for barium enema preceding colostomy closure in trauma patients. J Trauma 29:1641–1642

118. Sola JE, Buchman TG, Bender JS (1994) Limited role of barium enema examination preceding colostomy closure in trauma patients. J Trauma 36:245–247

119. Demetriades D, Pezikis A, Melissas J et al (1988) Factors influencing the morbidity of colostomy closure. Am J Surg 155:594–596

120. Lewis FR (1994) Editorial comment. J Trauma 36:247

121. Ledgerwood AM (1987) Discussion of Crass. J Trauma 27:1238–1239

122. Engel AF, Kamm MA, Hawley PR (1994) Civilian and war injuries of the perineum and anal sphincters. Br J Surg 81:1069–1073

123. Thal ER, Yeary EC (1980) Morbidity of colostomy closure following colon trauma. J Trauma 20:287–291

124. Taheri PA, Ferrara JJ, Johnson CE et al (1993) A convincing case for primary repair of penetrating colon injuries. Am J Surg 166:39–44

125. Karanfilian RG, Ghuman SS, Pathak VB et al (1982) Penetrating injuries to the colon. Am Surg 48:103–108

126. Adkins RB Jr, Zirkle PK, Waterhouse G (1984) Penetrating colon trauma. Trauma 24:491–499

127. Shannon FL, Moore EE (1985) Primary repair of the colon: when is it a safe alternative? Surgery 98:851–859

128. Dawes LG, Aprahamian C, Condon RE, Malangoni MA (1986) The risk of infection after colon injury. Surgery 100:796–803

129. Nallathambi MN, Ivatury RR, Shah PM et al (1987) Penetrating right colon trauma: the ever diminishing role for colostomy. Am Surg 53:209–214

130. Naraynsingh V, Ariyanayagam D, Pooran S (1991) Primary repair of colon injuries in a developing country. Br J Surg 78:319–320

131. Demetriades D, Charalambides D, Pantanowitz D (1992) Gunshot wounds of the colon: role of primary repair. Ann R Coll Surg Engl 74:381–384

132. Ivatury RR, Gaudino J, Nallathambi MN et al (1993) Definitive treatment of colon injuries: a prospective study. Am Surg 59:43–49

133. Levison MA, Thomas DD, Wiencek RG, Wilson RF (1990) Management of the injured colon: evolving practice at an urban trauma center. J Trauma 30:247–253

134. Williams RA, Csepanyi E, Hiatt J, Wilson SE (1987) Analysis of the morbidity, mortality, and cost of colostomy closure in traumatic compared with nontraumatic colorectal diseases. Dis Colon Rectum 30:164–167

135. Crass RA, Salbi F, Trunkey DD (1987) Colostomy closure after colon injury: a low-morbidity procedure. J Trauma 27:1237–1239

136. Livingston DH, Miller FB, Richardson JD (1989) Are the risks after colostomy closure exaggerated? Am J Surg 158:17–20

137. Pachter HL, Hoballah JJ, Corcoran TA, Hofstetter SR (1990) The morbidity and financial impact of colostomy closure in trauma patients. J Trauma 30:1510–1513

138. Rehm CG, Talucci RC, Ross SE (1993) Colostomy in trauma surgery: friend or foe? Injury 24:595–596

45

FOREIGN BODIES

Yanek S. Y. Chiu

In the 1970s and early 1980s, there was a proliferation of surgical literature on the subject of management of colorectal foreign bodies,[1-7] perhaps reflecting a change in social mores, a new sexual permissiveness, and some unusual behavior in the gay population such as anal "fist" fornication.[1-7] The last 5 years have seen some definite changes. The well-publicized epidemic of the acquired immunodeficiency syndrome has resulted in city and state ordinances banning gay bath houses. Patients positive for the human immunodeficiency virus are under a variety of treatment protocols and are by and large abstaining from anal sexual contact. Excellent educational outreach projects, particularly in major cities such as San Francisco, Los Angeles, and New York, have succeeded, to a certain extent, in teaching and warning young men and women of all races and nationalities of the dangers of sexual promiscuity. The combination of all these factors may have contributed to a decrease in the incidence of sexual trauma to the anus and rectum, at least in my experience in San Francisco.

However, patients with colorectal foreign bodies continue to be seen and treated in emergency rooms with regularity. They can be from all walks of life and of all ages. In male patients, the foreign body is usually self-administered. The surgical literature is replete with documentation of every imaginable object being retrieved from the rectum.[8] These individuals need not always be gay. In fact, some of them are married, with a stable family lifestyle. Quite often, objects are introduced into the rectum in the act of autoeroticism. In female patients, foreign bodies are usually inserted by male partners during sexual encounters and are usually vibrators and dildos of all sizes and varieties, with or without batteries (Fig. 45-1).

EMERGENCY ROOM PROTOCOL

Since patients with colorectal foreign bodies are seen primarily in emergency rooms and quite often at odd hours, several important steps must be followed to ensure patient safety and success in retrieving the foreign bodies with minimal invasive maneuvers.

Invariably, these patients have a high level of anxiety and embarrassment. It is important to assess them quickly regarding any alcohol or drug ingestion history, the type of foreign body, how long it has been lodged in the rectum, and how many times attempts have been made to retrieve the object. The longer the foreign body has been in place, the more chance that suction action has pushed it further upward secondary to rectal mucosal edema. The many unsuccessful attempts at retrieval, usually at home, will mean more edema, trauma to the rectum, and discomfort to the patient at initial presentation to the emergency room.

RADIOLOGIC EVALUATION

Biplane abdominal and pelvic films must be taken to assess the size, shape, and exact location of the object.[1,9,10] It will also show whether free air is present, which will confirm the clinical diagnosis of peritonitis. Sometimes more than one object may be lodged in the rectum. A simple anteroposterior projection will not be adequate. This is particularly important in dealing with objects that may have a sharp edge. It is imperative to know the direction the sharp edge is pointing.

SURGICAL INTERVENTION

If no peritoneal signs are present, if abdominal films show no free air, if the object is low enough to be retrieved transanally, and if the patient can be adequately sedated with intravenous Versed or Valium in combination with a narcotic such as Demerol or morphine, a careful attempt at removal of the object can be carried out in the emergency room with adequate equipment and nursing assistance. Local anesthesia of the anal sphincter can be achieved with 1% lidocaine or xylocaine very quickly. However, when in doubt, one should always consider performing this procedure in the operating room with an anesthesiologist, just in case a spinal or even a general anesthetic is necessary, particularly when the object is lodged quite high

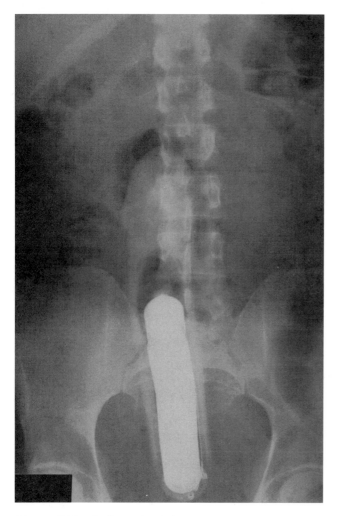

Figure 45-1. Radiograph of vibrator in rectum.

in the upper rectum or sigmoid colon and when peritoneal signs are equivocal. When the foreign body is made of glass (or worse still when the glass is broken), proper anesthesia is mandatory to avoid further trauma or injury to the rectum and sphincter.

It is rare that a lateral internal sphincterotomy will be needed after proper anesthesia. However, sometimes when a bulky object is being removed, this step should be undertaken to avoid laceration of the anal sphincter. A large operating proctoscope such as the Ferguson type is useful. If the object is low-lying, easily within reach of the index finger, anal retractors such as the Sawyer or even the Parks' self-retaining retractor will be very helpful. All foreign bodies must be retrieved under direct vision, using long grasping forceps or a sharp two-pronged tenaculum, frequently used in gynecologic surgery.[7] Since the advent of laparoscopic surgery, the ratcheted long grasping forceps used in cholecystectomy have become useful tools to hold on to the foreign bodies. If there is any evidence of rectal mucosal tear from the object itself or from the manipulation, intravenous antibiotics such as a broad-spectrum cephalosporin should be administered by the anesthesiologist before or during the procedure.

FOLEY CATHETER TECHNIQUE

If there is considerable edema in the rectum, thus causing an upward suction of the foreign body, inserting a few Foley catheters (20 to 22 Fr) alongside the object and pumping air into the rectum and lower sigmoid colon can break this negative suction.[10] The Foley catheter balloons can then be inflated with 30 to 50 ml of saline and gently pulled back to bring the object down to the rectum to be retrieved. I have rarely used this technique, because one has little control over the angle of the object as it is being pulled down by the Foley catheter. Nonetheless, it is a good way to break the negative suction pressure.

HOSPITAL ADMISSION AND FOLLOW-UP

It is a challenge if the foreign body is too proximal and beyond the reach of the rigid sigmoidoscope. If the object has no particularly sharp points and the patient has no evidence of peritoneal irritation, it is prudent to admit the patient for close observation, bed rest, and mild sedation for the next 12 to 24 hours. Usually within this period the object will descend into the rectum within reach to be retrieved.

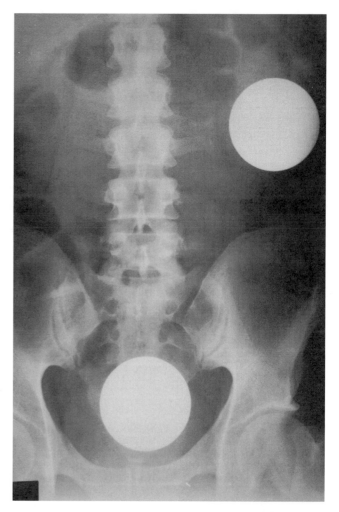

Figure 45-2. Radiograph showing two large metallic balls, one lodged in the rectum, the other in the splenic flexure.

If peritoneal signs exist, or if the object does not descend with patient observation after 24 hours, then urgent laparotomy will be needed. With the patient in the supine lithotomy position, a careful search for bowel ischemia, perforation, or mesenteric laceration should be carried out and if possible, the foreign body should be gently guided distally to come out of the anal canal to avoid contamination of the abdominal cavity. Should perforation occur, the object should still be brought out through the anal canal if at all possible. The colonic perforation can be repaired primarily and a diverting colostomy should be considered only if there is gross contamination.

After retrieval of the foreign body, regardless of the method, a rigid or flexible sigmoidoscopy should be performed to rule out any obvious laceration, hematoma or other traumatic injury to the rectum and lower colon.

EXTRAPERITONEAL SEPSIS FROM RECTAL TRAUMA

Although intraperitoneal colonic or rectal perforation is easy to detect, with free air under the diaphragm and obvious peritoneal

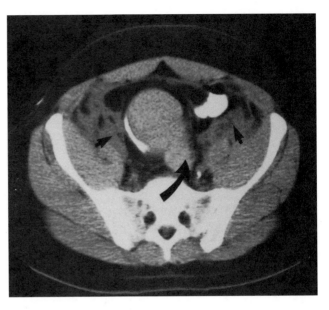

Figure 45-4. Computed tomography case shown in Figure 45-2 and 45-3 showing retrorectal inflammatory mass (large arrow) and abscess with air bubbles at psoas muscle level (small arrows).

signs on physical examination, extraperitoneal rectal perforation is rather difficult to diagnose. There is usually a delay of a few days before the pelvic and perineal sepsis becomes evident. The patient can suddenly become severely ill and septic shock with Fournier's gangrene has been reported.[3] If there is a high index of suspicion of extraperitoneal sepsis from rectal trauma, a combination of sigmoidoscopy (rigid or flexible), water-soluble contrast enema study such as Gastrografin, and computed tomography scan of the abdomen and pelvis will yield the correct clinical diagnosis. Appropriate treatment can then be carried out.[11] The unusual case of the metallic balls illustrates this point. Figure 45-2 is a plain abdominal film showing two large metallic balls, one lodged in the rectum and the other near the splenic flexure. Surprisingly, both balls were retrieved successfully transanally. However, after persistent fever and pelvic discomfort despite normal abdominal examination, Gastrografin enema (Fig. 45-3) indicated rectal perforation, confirmed on computed tomography. scan (Fig. 45-4), of the pelvis; the scan showed a retrorectal inflammatory mass (large arrow) as well as abscess formation with air bubbles at the psoas muscle level (small arrows).

SPHINCTER INJURY

Occasionally autoeroticism or sexual assault may result in sphincter injury. If the injury is fresh, the muscles can be repaired primarily. When the injury is of undetermined period and a chronic inflammatory reaction exists at the site of injury, it is usually best to treat conservatively. At the appropriate time, an elective sphincter repair or reconstruction can be undertaken to correct any incontinence.

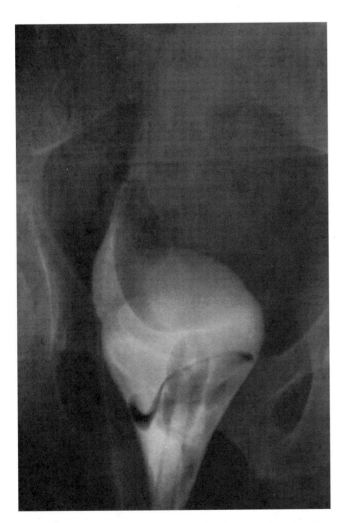

Figure 45-3. Gastrografin enema showing rectal perforation in the case shown in Figure 45-2.

REFERENCES

1. Abcarian H, Lowe R (1978) Colon and rectal trauma. Surg Clin North Am 58:519, 1978
2. Barone JE, Sone N, Nealon TF (1976) Perforations and foreign bodies of the rectum: report of 28 cases. Ann Surg 184:601–604
3. Barone JE, Yee J, Nealon TF (1983) Management of foreign bodies and trauma of the rectum. Surg Gynecol Obstet 156:453–457
4. Bercl G, Morgenstern L (1983) An operative proctoscope for foreign body extraction. Dis Colon Rectum 26:193–194
5. Crass RA, Trunbaugh RF, Kudsk KA, Trunkey DD (1981) Colorectal foreign bodies and perforations. Am J Surg 142:85–88
6. Eftaiha M, Hambrick E, Abcarian H (1977) Principles of management of colorectal foreign bodies. Arch Surg 112:691–695
7. Sohn N, Weinstein MA, Gonchar J (1977) Social injuries of the rectum. Am J Surg 134:611
8. Busch DB, Starling JR (1986) Rectal foreign bodies: case reports and a comprehensive review of the world's literature. Surgery 100:512–519
9. Abcarian H (1990) Rectal trauma. pp. 102–105. In Fazio VW (ed): Current Therapy in Colon and Rectal Surgery. BC Decker
10. Kingsley AN, Abcarian H (1985) Colorectal foreign bodies management update. Dis Colon Rectum 28:941–944
11. Fry RD (1994) Anorectal trauma and foreign bodies. Surg Clin North Am 74:1491–1505

46

IATROGENIC DISEASE

Philip. F. Schofield

In medicine in general the practitioner has to deal with a variety of diseases, both major and minor. All competent physicians will weigh potential good against potential harm. Unfortunately, in dealing with serious disease many effective treatments have a potential to produce side effects, and some of these side effects will produce significant harm. Most misadventures during treatment are unsought but inevitable consequences of the method of treatment; provided the patient is appropriately counseled, such complications of treatment will usually be accepted. However, patients have been increasingly inclined toward litigation: in the United States in the 1980s, litigation against doctors increased fivefold, an escalation that has continued into the 1990s.[1] The same process is beginning in the United Kingdom. My experience in medicolegal matters shows that many potential litigants have no claim in law; their attempt at litigation is based on some element of unsatisfactory outcome without manifest negligence on the part of the physician. On the other hand, in a number of cases management has been negligent. It is of interest to note that in the United States almost one-half the cases of litigation turn on diagnostic delay, with a slightly greater number based on medical or surgical error. Kern[2] reviewed litigation involving colon and rectal cases that came to court in the United States between 1971 and 1991. The most common cause for legal action was failure to establish the diagnosis at an appropriate time. The principal conditions involved were colorectal cancer and appendicitis and represented 43% of the total. Surgical iatrogenic injury was the next most common cause, with colorectal injury representing 25% of total cases and anal sphincter problems 10%. Medical complications (15%) and lack of informed consent (8%) made up the rest.

Within coloproctology in the United Kingdom most cases of negligence at the moment are due to medical or surgical error; few cases are due to delay. Since litigation is costly, adding 5% to the health budget in the United States, it is important that we have a good understanding of the potential pitfalls of investigation and treatment.[3] It is also of relevance that many cases of misfortune are not due to negligence. However, a better understanding may diminish the risks.

This chapter addresses injuries due to drugs, physical treatments, and investigations as well as some problems arising as a consequence of surgical operations.

INJURY DUE TO DRUGS

Laxatives

Although bulking agents such as bran are less likely to produce ill effects, they tend to produce flatulence and abdominal discomfort so that patients often prefer either osmotic or stimulant laxatives. These latter include senna, cascara, danthron derivatives, phenolphthalein, and bisacodyl. Stimulant and osmotic laxatives are in common use and are readily available. In the United States over 3 million people have laxatives prescribed, and many millions of dollars are paid for laxatives bought without prescription.[4] They have some capacity to produce harm.[5] Laxatives may produce mucosal injury in the colon; for example, castor oil has been shown to produce colitis in ponies.[6] Long-term use of anthraquinone is well known to produce pseudomelanosis coli, which has been considered benign for many years. Recently a colonoscopic study has suggested that pseudomelanosis coli caused by anthranoid laxative abuse increases the relative risk of colorectal cancer to 3.04.[7] It is important to recall that laxative abuse is a rare cause of an inexplicable diarrheal state.[8] Before colorectal surgery or colonoscopy the bowel is prepared, and purgation often plays an important part. Sodium picosulphate with magnesium citrate (Picolax), sennosides (X-prep), or castor oil and enemata are common methods of preparation. All these regimes produce some degree of dehydration with some sodium loss. This is of little clinical relevance in most patients, but it may be so in the elderly and frail.

Nasogastric bowel preparation was introduced 20 years ago.[9] Initially sodium chloride was used, but this caused salt and water retention and precipitated heart failure in elderly patients. A balanced electrolyte solution with an osmotic agent eliminated most of the metabolic problem. It has become common to take this combination by mouth for preparation using polyethylene glycol as the osmotic agent (Golytely; Klean-Prep). Mannitol was one of the best osmotic agents but has been abandoned because it did not eliminate the metabolic disturbance and was fermented in the colon by *Escherichia coli* with the production of methane, which may explode. In fact, occasional fatalities due to explosion were recorded.[10] Poor preparation may also be responsible for combustible gas in the colon.[11]

Antidiarrheals

The chief antidiarrhea drugs are opiate related and include codeine phosphate, diphenoxylate/atropine, and loperamide. They are effective in acute diarrhea and act through specific receptors in the colon that reduce colonic motility. Long-term use is associated with tolerance and addiction (dependency).

Antispasmodics

Antispasmodics are frequently prescribed for irritable bowel syndrome. Mebeverine hydrochloride and peppermint oil have uncertain therapeutic value but few side effects. The antimuscarinic preparations (e.g., propantheline bromide) have their effect on cholinergic receptors in the colon. Unfortunately they affect other cholinergic receptors and thus may precipitate acute retention of urine, glaucoma, and cardiac arrythmias as well as symptoms of dry mouth and blurred vision.

Drugs Used in Inflammatory Bowel Disease

Three principal types of agent are used in inflammatory bowel disease, namely, corticosteroids, aminosalicylates, and immunosuppressives.

Corticosteroids

Systemic corticosteroids have been used for many years and are known to be effective in suppressing acute attacks of colitis. They are best used in short courses, but there is a tendency among many physicians to continue with high to moderate doses of steroids for a longer period than is desirable. For this reason, it is important to note their effects. The adverse effects can be divided into those due to the mineralocorticoid element (causing salt and water retention with striae, acne, and hypertension) or the glucocorticoid effects of diabetes mellitus and osteoporosis, with its danger of vertebral collapse in the elderly.[12] Although the newer corticosteroids have less mineralocorticoid effect than the older ones, it is still present. It is important that other problems be recognized, in particular, mental disturbances with paranoia or depression, possibly leading to suicide; in children a significant risk of growth retardation exists. Corticosteroids may be given topically to the rectum as steroid enemas, suppositories, or foam. Some steroid is absorbed from the rectum, but this route is much less likely to produce side effects.

Aminosalicylates

Sulphasalazine (Salazopyrin) was the first effective therapy in ulcerative colitis.[13] The drug consisted of 5-amino-salicylic acid with sulphapyridine as a carrier molecule, allowing the salicy-

late to pass to the colon before being released. In a significant proportion of patients sulphasalazine is associated with side effects such as gastrointestinal disturbance or occasionally hematologic problems with marrow suppression or hemolytic anaemia. A further and more subtle effect is oligospermia, leading to infertility.[14] The side effects were due to the sulphonamide and occurred in slow acetylators.[15] These effects are reversible on cessation of the drug. Because of these problems, other methods of carriage of the 5-amino-salicylic acid were devised and are now commonly used. These are to link two molecules of 5-amino-salicylic acid together by a diazo bond (olsalazine) or, alternatively, to coat the 5-amino-salicylic acid with a resin (mesalazine/mesalamine). These drugs were shown to be as effective as sulphasalazine in controlling colitis but to have fewer side effects and no tendency to reduce sperm counts.

Immunosuppressives

Azathioprine/6-Mercaptopurine

The place of azathioprine is now established as a second-line agent in the treatment of inflammatory bowel disease. Its more consistent absorption makes it a more reliable drug than its metabolite 6-mercaptopurine. Although immunosuppresive drugs carry the risk of serious marrow suppression, this is very rare at the dose levels used in the treatment of inflammatory bowel disease. However, worries have been raised about the potential oncogenic effect of long-term use of an immunosuppressant. The worry was increased a decade ago when it was reported in a study of benign conditions (predominantly rheumatoid arthritis patients receiving long-term immunosuppression with azathioprine) that an apparent increase in neoplasia existed, especially lymphoma.[16] Evidence also shows excess lymphoma from long-surviving immunosuppressed patients in transplant programs. Sporadic reports exist of carcinomas developing in patients with inflammatory bowel disease treated with azathioprine; in a recent long-term study of patients with inflammatory bowel disease treated with azathioprine an excess of carcinomas was shown but no lymphomas among the patients. However, the excess did not reach statistical significance.[17] Whereas the suspicion of an oncogenic effect may persist, such an effect has not been demonstrated; if it exists at all, it must be very small.

Cyclosporin

Cyclosporin has been introduced very cautiously in inflammatory bowel disease because although it has little tendency to suppress the bone marrow a significant risk of complications exists, including renal damage and hypertension.[18] Since this is a much more recently introduced immunosuppressant in inflammatory bowel disease, relatively little is known about any long-term effects. Lymphoma has been reported in transplant patients treated with this drug.[19]

Antibiotics

Antibiotics are in common use by all medical practitioners, but all antibiotics may produce unwanted effects.

Allergy

It is possible to be allergic to any substance so that all antibiotics have the capacity to produce allergic reactions; some are more frequent causes than others. Penicillin still represents an appro-

<table>
</table>

Unwanted Effects of Antibiotics

Allergic reactions
Specific drug reactions
Antibiotic resistance
Antibiotic-induced diarrhea or colitis

priate model for the different types of drug allergy, which can range from the dramatic anaphylactic shock through skin reactions to serum sickness and allergic vasculitis. Most drug reactions are mediated by IgE, but the rare hemolytic anemias are mediated by IgG. In drug allergies, the time lapse between exposure and the first clinical symptom differs with the kind of syndrome so that anaphylactic shock or bronchospasm will occur within minutes and maculopapular rashes within hours, but other effects may take days or weeks to manifest. The so-called serum sickness syndrome is characterized by joint pains, lymphadenopathy, fever, and rash and is one of the late-developing allergic complications.[20]

Specific Drug Toxicity

The profile of drug toxicity complications differs with different antibiotics. In general, it can be said that whereas these may be seen with normal dosage of the antibiotic, they commonly occur due to overdosage, which allows the substance to reach toxic levels. For this reason, it is particularly important to be careful in prescribing antibiotics to patients with renal impairment. The toxic effects may be to the bone marrow, with depression producing either agranulocytosis or aplastic anemia; to the kidney, with decreasing renal function; to the liver, with cholestasis or even liver failure; or to the nervous system, especially the vestibuloauditory nerve.

Table 46-1 lists the common specific toxic reactions associated with the different antibiotic groups.

Resistance to Antibiotics

Bacteria may be resistant to the effects of antibiotics, either intrinsically or because they acquire resistance. The mechanisms of resistance are well understood in the penicillins and cephalosporins: the resistance is due to the degradation of the β-lactam by β-lactamase or the alterations of binding proteins.[21] Many enterococci are naturally resistant, but initially organisms such as *Staphylococcus aureus* were susceptible. However, an increasing number of enterococci and many staphylococci have now become resistant to the β-lactam antibiotics. In general, the influence of antibiotic administration on the development of antibiotic resistance depends on the kind of antibiotic and its frequency of use. Overuse of antibiotics aggravates the problem of drug resistance.

The development of newer antibiotics to deal with *S. aureus* has not fully kept pace with the problem, so we now have organisms resistant to methicillin. Methicillin-resistant *S. aureus* has become a major problem in many hospitals worldwide. The organisms tend to show multidrug resistance and easily produce problems throughout a hospital ward. For this reason many hospitals have had to close wards or departments temporarily in an attempt to eradicate the organism.

Alterations of Bacterial Flora

The use of antibiotics will cause differential death of bacteria in the normal resident population of the human body. The changes take place primarily in the upper respiratory tract, skin, and gastrointestinal tract. Foreign organisms may colonize these areas or antibiotic-resistant organisms may rapidly increase in number. This process may be totally asymptomatic, or it may lead to the replacement of the residual flora by *Candida albicans*, for example, or to superinfection.

Antibiotic-Associated Diarrhea and Colitis

Almost all the antibiotics may produce diarrhea. The frequency of this complication depends on the antibiotic and the specific indication for which the agent is being administered. The symp-

Table 46-1. Specific Antibiotic Reactions

Antibiotic Group	Toxic Reaction
Penicillins	Hypersensitivity reactions common but specific drug toxicity rare
	Rare hepatic or renal damage
Cephalosporins/carbopenems	Similar to the penicillins
Tetracyclines	Tooth discoloration in the growing fetus or child
	Fatty liver degeneration (rare)
Chloramphenicol	Gray syndrome in infants
	Marrow aplasia (allergic and rare)
Aminoglycosides (e.g., gentamicin, streptomycin)	Ototoxic (both vestibular and cochlear)
	Nephrotoxic
	Inhibition of neuromuscular transmission
Macrolides (e.g., erythromycin, and others)	Cholestatic jaundice
Lincomycin/clindamycin	*Clostridium difficile*-induced colitis
Metronidazole	Neuropathy
	Epileptiform seizures
Quinolones (e.g., ciprofloxacin)	Central nervous system disturbance including loss of dexterity
	Hemolysis in subjects with glycero-6-phosphate dehydrogenase deficiency
	Contraindicated in children because of possible arthropathy (animal experiment evidence)

toms can vary from a minor increase in frequency and looseness in the bowel action to gross diarrhea with toxemia.

These diarrheal states are due to alteration in the intestinal bacterial flora. In less severe cases, improvements have been produced through restoring the intestinal flora by taking lactobacillus,[22] and it has been suggested that *Saccharomyces boulardii* may be used to prevent the development of antibiotic-associated diarrhea.[23] Clinically, antibiotic-associated colitis should be considered in patients with severe disease within a month of completing a course of antibiotics.

In minor cases of diarrhea no objective physical signs are present; in more severe cases, the diarrhea has an increasing tendency to be associated with overgrowth of a particular organism. Recently, the most common organism causing severe diarrhea after antibiotics has been the toxigenic strain of *Clostridium difficile*, but other organisms such as *St. aureus* have also been implicated, producing diarrhea with severe and even fatal enterocolitis.

Diarrhea due to toxogenic *C. difficile* has become an increasing problem. We know that this organism can be associated with no symptoms, with mild diarrhea, with a nonspecific colitis, with pseudomembranous colitis, or with toxic megacolon. Two percent of the population are carriers,[24] 40% of newborn children have the toxigenic strain of *Cl. difficile* in their stools but undoubtedly have an effective defence mechanism as they are asymptomatic.[25] Less than one-third of patients with severe diarrhea but without demonstrable colitis are found to have *Cl. difficile*, but two-thirds of patients have the organism if there is endoscopic evidence of colitis and almost all have the organism if there is pseudomembranous colitis.[26,27] Figure 46-1 shows the typical changes of pseudomembranous colitis (PMC).

PMC was recognized as a pathologic entity before the discovery of antibiotics, but the disease has increased rapidly since their widespread use. Bartlett et al.[28] showed that the toxigenic strain of *C. difficile* was associated with PMC. Since that time

most but not all cases have been associated with antibiotic use. A few have been associated with cancer chemotherapy,[29] and some appear to have arisen without a precipitating cause.[30] The first antibiotics to be connected with PMC were the lincomycin/ clindamycin group, but it is now well established that virtually all antibiotics may be associated; cephalosporins and ampicillin/ amoxycillin seem to be the most common.[31] It is paradoxical that both vancomycin and metronidazole have been reported as causes of PMC, yet they are the two drugs used in the treatment of the condition.[32]

C. difficile produces two toxins, an enterotoxin (toxin A) and a cytotoxin (toxin B). The toxins are thought to be responsible for the effects of the disease. Although other tests have been advocated, the recognition of toxin B by an assay involving the cytotoxicity of HeLa cells in tissue culture is still the most reliable. The histology of the condition is quite typical and is well described by Price and Davies.[33]

Most patients settle after medical treatment with either metronidazole or vancomycin, but there is an approximately 15% relapse rate within a few days of completion of the treatment.[34] On rare occasions operation may be indicated in the fulminant case, in which medical treatment repeatedly fails and either toxic dilation or incipient perforation exists.[35] Under these circumstances, the best emergency operation may well be subtotal colectomy and ileostomy.[36]

Cancer Chemotherapy

It is important for all surgeons to have an understanding of cancer chemotherapy because the powerful drugs used produce significant side effects. These may simply affect patient management, but they may also be associated with oncologic gastrointestinal emergencies. Chemotherapeutic agents may be used singly but are commonly used in combination regimes of two, three, or four agents. Common complications occur in associa-

Figure 46-1. Operative specimen of pseudomembranous colitis. Note the typical white plaques.

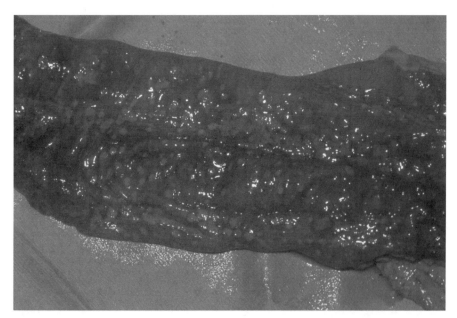

Table 46-2. Complications of Cancer Chemotherapy

Drug	Complication
Alkylating agents	Increase in acute leukemia
Cyclophosphamide	Infertility (not impotence)
Ifosfamide	Hemorrhagic cystitis
Cytotoxic antibiotics	Cardiotoxicity
	Pulmonary fibrosis
	Hemolytic uremic syndrome
Antimetabolites	Pneumonitis
5-Fluorouracil	Cerebellar syndrome (rare)
Mitotic inhibitors	
Vinca alkaloids	Peripheral amd autonomic
	neuropathy
Platinums	Nephrotoxic
	Ototoxic
	Peripheral neuropathy
	Epileptiform seizures

tion with many courses of chemotherapy, such as vomiting, alopecia, myelosuppression, mucositis, and effects on reproductive function. In addition, some drugs used have specific complications (Table 46-2).

Vomiting

Vomiting may either be acute at the time of the chemotherapy or delayed after 24 hours and can occasionally be anticipatory (i.e., before the chemotherapy). The severity of the symptom depends on the agent: for example, cisplatin, cyclophosphamide, and others produce a very high incidence of vomiting, whereas vincristine does not.

If a high likelihood of severe vomiting exists, then the patient is given appropriate treatment before and during chemotherapy. Lorazepam is useful in preventing anticipatory vomiting and is often coupled with dexamethasone. For the more severe case, management of acute vomiting underwent a revolution with the introduction of the serotonin antagonist ondansetron. This group of drugs is now often given with dexamethasone when severe vomiting is likely. The treatment of delayed vomiting is more difficult. Metoclopramide may be effective in high dosage but is likely to produce extrapyramidal side effects.

Effects on Reproductive Function

Virtually all cytotoxic drugs, especially alkylating agents, are teratogenic and should not be administered during pregnancy. Similarly, contraceptive advice should be given so that pregnancy may be avoided during a course of chemotherapy.

In the male, there is an effect on fertility, particularly by the alkylating agents. Since permanent sterility may occur, it is necessary to discuss this aspect with the patient and if desirable arrange for sperm storage.

Tumor Lysis Syndrome

On some occasions when the tumor responds rapidly to the chemotherapeutic agent, the breakdown of cells may produce a specific syndrome, tumor lysis syndrome. It is particularly likely to occur in the treatment of leukemia and non-Hodgkin's lymphoma, although it can occur with other tumors. The rapid breakdown of the tumor leads to hyperuricemia because of the massive accumulation of the breakdown products of the nucleic acids. In addition, hyperkalemia and hyperphosphatemia (associated with hypocalcemia) are present. If this process is untreated, there is a tendency for uric acid to be deposited in the renal tubules, leading to renal insufficiency and even renal failure. The hyperkalemia may lead to cardiac abnormalities and even cardiac arrest.

If it is possible, preventive measures should be taken when this syndrome is likely, such as pretreatment with intravenous hydration to prevent oliguria and allopurinol to decrease the formation of uric acid. Ideally the treatment should be started 24 hours before chemotherapy and continued for 7 to 10 days afterward. In the acute stage, an electrocardiogram is desirable to monitor any toxic effects of the high blood potassium so that this may be treated by glucose and insulin.

Intestinal Perforation in Chemotherapy

When chemotherapeutic agents are used to treat intra-abdominal tumors, in particular intra-abdominal lymphomas, the effective treatment may lead to perforation of the tumor. Peritonitis arising during or after chemotherapy is not always due to this cause because peptic ulcer disease may perforate or diverticulitis may be exacerbated. Ferrara et al.[37] studying patients undergoing chemotherapy for abdominal malignancy, found that two-thirds of the intestinal perforations occurred in organs not involved in tumor. My experience would indicate that in an oncologic institute, most perforations are through tumor tissue. At operation the area of perforation should be excised if this is possible, but primary anastomosis may often not be the best policy as healing may be compromised by the patient's poor nutritional state and sepsis.

Neutropenic Colitis

Neutropenic colitis has been described by various names, including typhlitis and the ileocecal syndrome as well as neutropenic enterocolitis. The initial descriptions were in children with acute leukemia or lymphoma undergoing chemotherapy, but it is now recognized that the condition may affect adults undergoing chemotherapy for hematologic malignancy or, more rarely, solid tumors.[38] The clinical picture is of a pyrexial illness with right-sided abdominal pain and tenderness, abdominal distension, and diarrhea. The signs and symptoms characteristically develop after neutropenia has lasted for a week or more. The condition must be differentiated from *C. difficile* colitis or other infective enteritis as well as appendicitis. The cause is uncertain.

It has been ascribed to low flow states or infection with *Clostridium septicum*. In severe cases, there is undoubtedly bacterial invasion of the mucosa of the right colon.[39] The condition varies in its severity and frequently settles with conservative treatment, gastrointestinal rest, broad-spectrum antibiotics, and intravenous fluids. These patients, however, do need to be closely monitored because surgical intervention should take place if the situation deteriorates. The appropriate operative treatment is right hemicolectomy with terminal ileostomy and mucous fistula.[40]

Gastrointestinal Hemorrhage

When a patient is undergoing cancer chemotherapy, bleeding may occur into the upper gastrointestinal tract, leading to hematemesis, or into the colon, with the passage of bright red blood per rectum. Intra-abdominal tumors themselves are rarely the source of hemorrhage, although occasionally there may be a bleed associated with regression of a tumor, especially a lymphoma. By far the most common cause of gastrointestinal hemorrhage either from the upper or lower gastrointestinal tract in patients undergoing chemotherapy is severe thrombocytopenia, although benign causes such as peptic ulcer may be responsible. The management is, in the main, supportive, with blood and platelet transfusion, although in many cases appropriate investigations by gastroscopy or colonoscopy to rule out a localized bleeding source are justified. Surgery in these cases should be approached with great reluctance as operation may not eliminate the problem: many of the disease processes involved are widespread and beyond the scope of surgery.

Diarrheal States

Although immunosuppression is well recognized in the acquired immunodeficiency syndrome (AIDS) and in patients after transplant, patients on long-term chemotherapy are also immunosuppressed to a degree and are subject to diarrheal problems. These are due to enterocolonic infections, in particular *Cl. difficile*, cryptosporidium, and cytomegalovirus as well as a higher incidence of the more usual gastrointestinal infections.

Anticoagulants

Heparin and low molecular weight heparin are currently in common use. When they are given at the time of surgery, it is unusual for these regimes to cause trouble, and any bleeding tendency is readily corrected. Oral anticoagulants, of which warfarin is the most usual, may cause complications in long-term use, and a significant number of people with cardiac, arterial, or venous problems are on warfarin long term. The initial dosage of warfarin is measured by the response of the prothrombin time as measured by the international normalized ratio (INR). A correct dosage can be achieved within a few days by observing the results of the dose of warfarin on the INR. However, when the patient is stabilized and goes into the community, intercurrent illness or other drugs may increase the INR so that the patient may develop bleeding. In the less severe states, hematuria or epistaxis may occur, which will often remit on withholding the warfarin. If, however, the INR is grossly elevated, then the patient should be given vitamin K by intravenous injection. If bleeding is catastrophic, then plasma hematinic factors may have to be transfused. Poor control of long-term anticoagulation may produce serious intra-abdominal problems with bleeding into the wall of the large or small bowel.[41] These patients present with signs of both peritoneal irritation and intestinal obstruction. They require intensive medical treatment and usually settle. However, the condition is unusual, so the clinican may not make the link with the anticoagulants. Under these

circumstances or when conservative treatment fails, operation is indicated.

Another site of surgical importance is retroperitoneal hematoma, which can present with a shock-like state and abdominal signs varying from distension to signs of peritoneal irritation.[42] Such patients require intensive medical treatment. The other serious problem that one should recognize is that warfarin is teratogenic; women at risk of pregnancy should be warned of this, particularly in the first trimester. If oral anticoagulants are given late in pregnancy, a risk exists of fetal hemorrhage and hemorrhage at delivery.

BLOOD TRANSFUSION RISKS AND TRANSMISSION

Transfusion

Immediate Reactions

The risk of a mismatched transfusion is low because of the grouping and cross-matching procedures. Careful checking that the identifying number as well as the name on the blood unit matches the number and name of the recipient is of prime importance, as mistakes are still occasionally made. A mismatched transfusion will result in hemolysis due to red cell incompatibility. If hemolysis occurs, the patient has rigors and loin pain, which may progress to renal failure. The transfusion must be stopped immediately and a high fluid intake maintained.

Allergic reactions due to foreign material in the blood may occur. These are usually confined to an irritant skin rash, but more severe reactions may occur. Treatment for the skin rash with intravenous hydrocortisone and antihistamine is usually effective.

Febrile reactions not associated with hemolysis are common. They appear to be associated with platelet or granulocyte antigens and can be reduced in frequency by white cell removal filters. This condition, which simulates a hemolytic reaction, is frightening but not serious and usually settles rapidly with the discontinuation of the responsible unit of blood.

Delayed Reactions: Infection

The most serious problem is transmitted infection, usually of a viral nature. All donated blood is screened for the known infective agents, such as syphilis, hepatitis B, hepatitis C, and the human immunodeficiency virus (HIV; 1 and 2).[43] Despite these measures the donor blood may contain an unknown transmissible agent, and some centers now add screening for cytomegalovirus and malaria antibodies.

The risks of infection depend on the product transferred. Whole blood and some plasma products cannot be pasteurized, so they carry more risks of transmitting virus than cell-free fractions such as cryoprecipitate. The risks of transfer are difficult to calculate and depend in part on the prevalence of the disease in the population.

The risks should not be underestimated as we recall the disaster of HIV infection in hemophiliacs. This appears to have been overcome by appropriate treatment of antihemophilic factor concentrates.[44] Whereas a good safety record exists for intramuscular injection of immunoglobulin, several cases of transmission of hepatitis C by intravenous immunoglobulin have been documented.[45]

Transmission of Infection Between Patients and Doctors

Surgeons run a risk when they operate on patients with hepatitis B or HIV infection. Although the commonest mode of transmission of both hepatitis B and AIDS is sexual, contact with infected blood at operation or at other times in patient care puts health care workers at particular risk. Fortunately, both HIV and hepatitis B are of low infectivity. However, it has been calculated that the chance of a surgeon contracting hepatitis B is 30% to 40% during a 40-year career.[46] The attack may be asymptomatic or may produce jaundice with illness of varying severity, but most individuals recover, with complete lifelong immunity. The risk of surgeons becoming chronic carriers is about 4%, and they will be HBs antigen positive but may not be infective unless their serum contains the e antigen (HBeAg). This situation precludes work as a surgeon; in the United Kingdom a surgeon was recently sentenced to 1 year in jail because he continued to work while knowing he was HBeAg positive. A vaccine is available for hepatitis B, and all health workers at risk are required to show evidence of satisfactory vaccination.

The risk of transmission of HIV to health care workers as a consequence of their work is small. Lifson and Castro[47] analyzed 49 health care workers with HIV infection. In 42 cases, factors other than occupational risk were identified. Needlestick injuries in workers caring for HIV patients are unlikely to cause HIV, with a rate of seroprevalence of 0.42%.[48] No cases of seroconversion except when contact is by blood have been recorded. In known cases of hepatitis B, AIDS, or HIV positivity, surgeons and staff should have full protection of eyes and body against contamination with body fluids or the occurrence of accidental injury while operating.

THERAPY CAUSING COLONIC DISEASE

Drug-Induced Intestinal Inflammation

It is important to recognize that many drugs may cause ulceration, stricture, perforation, or diffuse inflammation in both the small and large bowel.

Nonsteroidal Anti-inflammatory Drugs

It has been clearly demonstrated that nonsteroidal anti-inflammatory drugs (NSAIDs) not only injure the upper gastrointestinal tract but also affect the small bowel and colon. Bjarnason et al.[49] detailed the chronic changes in the small bowel: inflammation, bleeding, strictures, and perforation (Fig. 46-2). Although NSAID injury of the colon is unusual in any individual patient, many patients suffer from NSAID-induced colon injury because of the widespread use of these drugs. Tanner and Raghunath[50] estimated that patients taking NSAIDs had a five times greater risk of colonic inflammation than others and Gabriel et al.[51] estimated the risk as three fold. Gibson et al.[52] reviewed the literature and recognized four types of NSAID-associated disease (Table 46-3).

The NSAIDs most commonly involved were mefenamic acid, indomethacin, and diclofenac. Pucius et al.[53] described abnormalities of the right colon and ileum that simulated Crohn's disease but were due to NSAID use. Campbell and Steele[54] reported a statistically significant relationship between septic complications of diverticular disease and NSAID use. Bjarnason et al.[55] reviewed small and large bowel lesions and discussed the mechanism of injury, possibly loss of cytoprotection from prostaglandins in the colon through inhibition of cyclo-oxygenase production.

Figure 46-2. Operative specimen of ileum showing perforation due to nonsteroidal anti-inflammatory drugs.

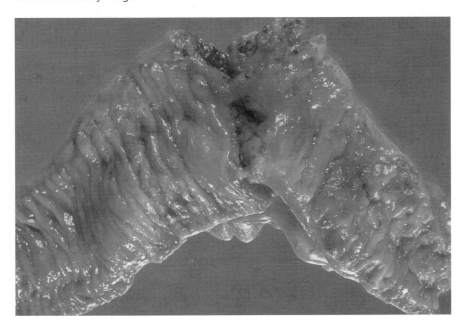

Table 46-3. Types of Nonsteroidal Anti-inflammatory Drug Colitis

Form of Colitis	Average Age at Onset (yr)	Duration Before Onset
De novo colitis	67	Months–years
Reactivation of quiescent colitis	42	1 week
Salicylate allergy	Any	minutes–hours
Suppository proctitis	60	—

Other Drugs

Many drugs have been reported to cause inflammatory responses in the large or small bowel. Potassium causes small bowel ulceration with stricture formation.[56] Irritant suppositories such as bisacodyl may cause proctitis.[57] Several drugs have been associated with enterocolitis or colitis including 5-fluorouracil,[58] methyldopa,[59] and gold compounds.[60] A specific histologic entity of large bowel strictures in children with cystic fibrosis receiving high-strength pancreatic enzyme supplements has been described and is termed fibrosing colonopathy.[61]

Drug-induced Colonic Ischemia

Most cases of colonic ischemia are not due to drugs, but occasional cases are. The cause of colonic ischemia is poor colonic perfusion due to either arterial or venous occlusion or a low flow state due to hypotension. Certain drugs, especially those containing ergot, and the contraceptive pill have been associated with colonic ischemia. It has been suggested that venous thrombosis may be the cause of ischemia in young women on oral contraceptives containing conjugated estrogen.[62] Symptomatically these patients present like other cases of ischemic colitis, although the cecum and right colon are the common site of injury.[63]

Long-term use of neuroleptics, especially phenothiazines, has been reported as a rare cause of necrosing enterocolitis due to vascular insufficiency secondary to colonic stasis.[64] Other causes of drug-induced ischemic colitis include vasopressin, digitalis overdosage, and diuretic abuse, which probably act by impairing tissue perfusion.[65] If colonic infarction has occurred, then speedy operation is indicated. However, most cases produce transient ischemic colitis that settles spontaneously and should be managed conservatively. Johnson and Berenson[66] report a case of transient right-sided ischemic colitis after self-administration of methamphetamine and note previous reports of ischemic colitis due to cocaine or similar substances used in drug abuse.

Sclerosing Peritonitis

A number of conditions may produce a chronic sclerosing peritonitis. Although historically tuberculosis was a common cause, in recent years iatrogenic injury has been more prominent. The drug Practolol, introduced in 1970, resulted in classic sclerosing peritonitis, which led to its withdrawal in 1976.[67] In this condition the whole of the large and small bowel was cocooned in a dense adhesive membrane and the patient presented with subacute obstruction. In the 1980s another cause was recognised associated with continuous ambulatory peritoneal dialysis in patients with renal failure. Evidence suggested that this was due to the chlorhexidine used to sterilize the catheters.[68]

Of historic interest only is a granulomatous peritoneal reaction produced by talc in glove powders. Its replacement by starch as a lubricant for gloves was found to lead to starch peritonitis.[69] In this condition the patient began to develop symptoms between 2 and 6 weeks after an apparently successful recovery from an abdominal operation. The symptoms were those of obstruction and possible ascites. At reoperation dense adhesions between loops of bowel were seen and histology showed birefrigent particles. Starch-free gloves were subsequently introduced.

Graft-Versus-Host Disease

Bone marrow transplantation for leukemia is a recognized therapy for some cases, but it may lead to graft-versus-host disease. Donor T cells may react against the patient's cells in liver, skin and intestine, causing jaundice, skin rash, and diarrhea.[70] There is ulceration within the colon, which is readily demonstrated at endoscopy or on barium enema. However, it is difficult to distinguish this condition from enteritis due to cytomegalovirus.[71] Therapy is extremely difficult, and operation appears to be unrewarding. The mortality of the acute condition is extremely high.

INJURY DUE TO PHYSICAL CAUSES

Diathermy Injury

Surgical diathermy is a technique that allows control of bleeding from small vessels by heat generated by passing an electric current through the tissues. In monopolar diathermy, a high current density is delivered to a localized area to produce coagulation, with the circuit being completed through a remotely situated large surface area indifferent plate. Bipolar diathermy involves the current passing between the two points of an insulated forceps. Monopolar diathermy is more frequently used but appears to carry more risks. The hazards are as follows:

Skin burn due to inadvertent contact with the skin, which can occur with either type

Inadvertent coagulation of pedicles; monopolar diathermy applied to the testis may cause cord damage, thrombosis, and testicular necrosis

Skin burns due to poor contact of the indifferent diathermy plate.

Adverse effects on cardiac pacemakers with arrythmia or death

Diathermy causing fire with inflammable skin preparation solutions; this is especially dangerous if solution collects in the groin or under the buttocks when the patient is in the lithotomy position

Explosions of flammable anesthetic gases (historic only) or intracolonic gases at endoscopy

During laparoscopic surgery, unintended diathermy injury may occur outside the view of the surgeon; the risk is high with a monopolar electrode, when the burn may occur due to a failure of insulation; it has also been postulated that energy may pass from a correctly insulated electrode to the cannula or irrigator and hence to any tissue in contact with it

Injuries are best avoided by using a bipolar electrode and avoiding high-voltage coagulation.[72]

INJURY INDUCED BY DIAGNOSTIC OR THERAPEUTIC RADIATION

Diagnostic Imaging

It is believed that some genetic mutations leading to malignant disease are due to background radiation. Thus any addition to the radiation for an individual must increase the risk of malignancy, albeit by a minute amount. However, it is apparent that radiographs should be used sparingly and not repeated too often. This is particularly relevant in chronic disease such as inflammatory bowel disease, in which imaging may be repeatably required over many years.

The average radiation dose of a chest x-ray is 0.02 mSv, that of a barium meal 5 mSv, and that of a barium enema or abdominal computed tomography (CT) 9 mSv. Since all radiation adds to the malignancy risk, it is better to employ imaging techniques not using ionizing radiation such as ultrasound or nuclear magnetic resonance imaging if appropriate. In the United Kingdom there is an estimated risk of between 100 and 250 additional deaths a year due to the cumulative effects of diagnostic radiology. However, the excess lifetime cancer risk for a basic barium enema is approximately 0.01 to 0.03%.[73] The excess risk to each individual is small and poses a risk that is acceptable in clinical practice provided radiation dosage is as low as possible. Most investigations using radionuclide scans are of relatively low radiation dosage.

Therapeutic Radiation

The purpose of therapeutic radiation is to produce a lethal effect on tumor cells while leaving surrounding normal tissue largely unaffected. This aim is difficult to achieve within the pelvis, which in effect is a small box with the urinary tract, genital tract, and large bowel all packed into a small volume. It is further complicated because the pelvic peritoneum descends between the genitourinary system and the bowel and within this pouch there may be small bowel or sigmoid colon. All these areas are at risk of receiving damaging irradiation as a byproduct of irradiating any tumor in the pelvis. The main tumors treated by radiation are carcinoma of the cervix uteri and carcinoma of the bladder, but in recent years radiotherapy has been increasingly used in the treatment of carcinoma of the prostate and rectum. Less commonly, pelvic radiotherapy is used for ovarian tumors.

Radiotherapy is delivered by either external beams from linear accelerators or telecobalt units. The desired radiotherapy field is mapped out, and the dose is calculated exactly. Doses were formerly expressed in rads, but they now seem to be expressed in either Grays or Siverts. The dose is fractionated into a number of treatments giving the desired amount of centiGrays

in each treatment. Fractionation allows normal tissue to recover and allows better tolerance to radiation. The biologic effect of a course of radiotherapy should be measured by the normal standard dose in which not only the total amount of radiation given is noted but also the length of time over which the course extends and the number of fractions. This is vitally important because a shorter course with the same total dose will have a greater biologic effect than the same dose given over a longer period. Thus 40 Gy over 3 weeks is a much more severe schedule than 40 Gy over 5 weeks.

Brachytherapy is defined as the placement of a radionuclide within or adjacent to a tumor to give a localized high dosage. This type of treatment is used in carcinoma of the cervix: intracavitary implants are placed, and then removed after a prescribed length of time. For many years radium was used for this intracavitary treatment, but in the last decade cesium has taken its place. The modern technique in carcinoma of the cervix involves remote afterloading, whereby preplaced "tubes" are filled with radionuclide by means of a mechanical device that allows the operator to remain remote from the radionuclide.

Carcinoma of the cervix is sometimes treated only by intracavitary methods, but usually it is treated by intracavitary plus external beam radiation from several sources. Carcinomas of the bladder, prostate, and other pelvic tumors are usually treated by external beam only. The effects of radiotherapy on the bowel or urinary tract after treatment for carcinoma of the cervix have been widely studied. They are conveniently classified into early, late, and remote effects. The major morbidity and mortality are due to the late effects.

Pathology

Early Effects

The early effects of radiotherapy in the normal rectum have been studied.[74] They include inflammatory changes with eosinophilic crypt abscesses, meganucleosis, and cell death. However, the cells at the base of the crypts survive, and repopulation occurs within 3 or 4 weeks. Symptoms of diarrhea often occur at the time and shortly after treatment but then remit. Occasionally, with pelvic or abdominal radiation, the reaction is acute, involving the small bowel with colic and diarrhea. The symptoms are sometimes quite alarming, but most cases settle quickly and surgery should only be considered if clear evidence of perforation exists, which happens on very rare occasions. Early symptoms in the urinary tract are minor frequency and dysuria, but because of inaccessibility the early histologic changes have not been well studied in the urinary tract.

Late Changes

The late changes appear to be due to vascular insufficiency.[75] Vessels of all sizes may be affected, but the brunt is borne by the medium-sized vessels in the bowel wall, which are occluded. This leads to ischemic ulceration with bleeding and possibly full-thickness loss of bowel wall with sepsis and subacute obstruction or rectovaginal or vesicovaginal fistula. These late manifestations occur between 6 and 24 months after treatment. Bleeding may appear earlier than the other problems and is more likely to undergo spontaneous resolution.

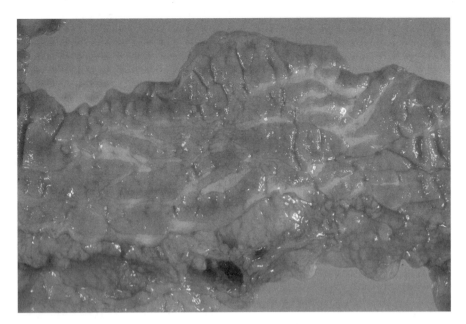

Figure 46-3. Radiation bowel disease. Mucosal aspect showing ulceration and mucosal edema.

The macroscopic changes may show thickening of the wall, ulceration, and cobblestoning of the mucosa (Fig. 46-3). Microscopically, in addition to the obvious vascular changes, submucosal edema and fibrosis are present throughout the wall, characterized by radiation fibroblasts (Fig. 46-4). Usually histologic evidence is present of mucosal ulceration and chronic infection.[76] In the urinary tract, the injury also appears to be caused by vascular damage, leading to fibrosis with bladder contraction and mucosal ulceration and telangiectasia. The lower ureters may also be involved and may become thickened and stenosed.

Several factors appear to be associated with an increased possibility of radiation damage to the gastrointestinal tract. These include previous pelvic surgery, diseases associated with vascular abnormality (e.g.,) diabetes mellitus, hypertension, and other arterial diseases),[77] and coincident chemotherapy.[78]

Remote Effects

Two or more years after radiotherapy, patients may present with fibrous strictures in either the small bowel or the colon. These can produce obstruction many years after radiotherapy. Other

Figure 46-4. Histology of radiation bowel disease. Note completely occluded blood vessel and surrounding fibrosis with plump fibroblasts. (H&E ×100.)

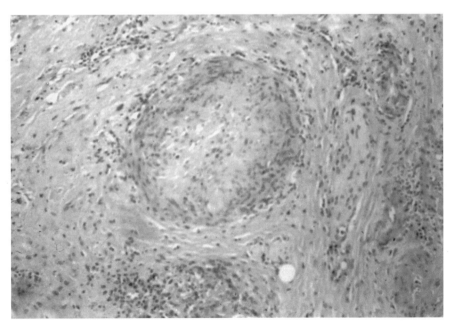

remote effects are metabolic problems from ileal disease, which may lead to vitamin B_{12} deficiency, bacterial overgrowth, or bile salt-induced diarrhea.

It is well recognized that an increased risk exists of malignant change some years after radiotherapy.[79] In my experience, there has been an excess of carcinoma of the rectum as a late complication of radiation to the cervix uteri,[79,80] which accords with the findings of others.[76]

It should be noted that previous pelvic radiotherapy may cause complications after aortic surgery. Rectal necrosis has been reported to occur after aortic bifurcation grafts in patients who had pelvic radiotherapy many years previously.[81]

Clinical Presentation

Radiation Bowel Disease

There are different presentations of radiation enteropathy, in which some symptoms may predominate. The mixure of presenting symptoms can be categorized as follows.

Rectal Bleeding

Rectal bleeding is the most common problem and comes from abnormally thin-walled vessels in the rectum. If mild, it may settle spontaneously, but if the patient requires repeated blood transfusions for anemia or has significant abdominal pain, then many of these patients require some form of surgery.[82]

Anal or Perineal Pain

Pain is usually due to anorectal ulceration; it is unusual after treatment of carcinoma of the cervix but appears to be more common after radiotherapy for carcinoma of the prostate. It occurs in the first few months after pelvic radiation and may produce quite severe and even intolerable pain so that the patients often have to be examined under anesthetic to establish the extent of the lesion. Ulceration may extend to deeper necrosis, leading to fistula formation; thus biopsy of an anterior rectal wall ulcer in females is contraindicated, as it may precipitate a fistula into the vagina. A proportion of these patients will settle, so local treatment may be appropriate; it is one of the few indications for which a defunctioning colostomy is justified in radiation injury. In some intractable cases, however, relief can only be achieved by excision of the anal canal and rectum with permanent colostomy.

Rectovaginal Fistula

The rectovaginal type is the commonest fistula and occurs at a mean of 15 months after treatment. It presents with incontinence and perineal excoriation. Examination under an anesthetic with biopsy is important to determine whether recurrent tumor is present.

Vesicovaginal Fistula

Vesicovaginal fistula usually occurs in association with severe bladder injury and also must be assessed and biopsied under anesthetic preparatory to treatment.

Chronic Perforation

Chronic perforation due to an ischemic necrosis is most commonly localized in the sigmoid colon, but it can occur in the ileum. The perforation is almost never free and presents as a localized abscess with relatively minor symptoms but significant abdominal pain and bowel upset. Such patients all require resectionable surgery.

Intestinal Obstruction

Intestinal obstruction tends to occur rather later than the other complications and is due to a fibrous stricture. The terminal ileum is more commonly affected than the colon. Typically attacks are recurrent and become gradually more severe. Radiation damage is a more usual cause of intestinal obstruction than recurrent tumor in patients who have had radiotherapy and present with small bowel obstruction.[83]

Radiation Urinary Tract Disease

Urinary tract problems (Table 46-4) may occur in isolation and are often seen in patients who have had gastrointestinal problems some months previously. It is difficult to distinguish between radiation injury and recurrent tumor. Even at operation the pathology may be uncertain. Thus it is necessary to have frozen section histopathology facilities available.

Cystitis/Hematuria. Significant radiation cystitis is said to occur in about 10% of patients who have had radiotherapy for carcinoma of the cervix. The symptoms vary from minor frequency, dysuria, and hematuria to severe pelvic pain and life-threatening hemorrhagic cystitis. Similarly, as the disease progresses, the bladder becomes contracted, with gross frequency and urgency due to reduced bladder capacity. Some of these patients also develop a vesicovaginal fistula. A stricture at the bladder neck or in the posterior urethra may develop following radiotherapy for carcinoma of the prostate.

Renal Symptoms. Progressive fibrosis of the lower ureter tends to cause a ureteric stricture with proximal dilation. Although this may be asymptomatic, it may produce renal pain and pyonephrosis. Renal outflow obstruction leading to diminished renal function is an important cause of morbidity that will require urologic intervention.

Management

Pilepich et al.[84] proposed a grading system for the severity of radiation injury after treatment of carcinoma of the prostate; this has a useful application for all radiation injury. The grading

Table 46-4. Radiation Urinary Tract Disease

Condition	Symptom
Radiation "cystitis"	Bladder contracture
Vesicovaginal fistula	Incontinence
Ureteric stenosis	Hydronephrosis

system is based on the requirement for treatment and its magnitude and the patient's performance status:

Grade I: minor symptoms that require no treatment

Grade II: symptoms that do not affect the performance status and can be managed by simple outpatient methods

Grade III: more severe symptoms altering performance status that may require admission for diagnostic procedures or minor surgery

Grade IV: Prolonged hospitalization with major surgical intervention

Grade V: fatal complications

Although occasional cases of rectal bleeding may be categorized as grade II and the telangiectatic areas in the rectum treated by laser as an outpatient, most patients who give concern are in grades III and IV. Smith and de Cosse[85] emphasized the importance of stabilizing and correcting anemia and metabolic defects before investigating the patient and constructing a treatment strategy.

Investigation

Clinical assessment is extremely important. A detailed symptomatic history is vital to decision taking. A diagnostic investigation has to be made because patients usually present many months or years after radiotherapy. Assessment should be directed toward the following factors:

The general state of the patient

Differentiation between recurrent tumor and radiotherapy injury

Localization of the radiotherapy injury

Differentiating between radiation disease and tumor recurrence can be very difficult. A chest x-ray to exclude pulmonary metastases is mandatory, as well as a CT scan of the liver to exclude metastatic disease. A tissue diagnosis is desirable, but it is frequently not possible to obtain material from biopsy before open surgery. To assess the extent of the disease a combination of endoscopy and imaging is useful, and flexible sigmoidoscopy or colonoscopy may demonstrate lesions in the sigmoid colon when there is rectal sparing, especially if a stricture exists at this level.

Contrast radiology of the colon will show degrees of distortion and narrowing, but the general experience has been that radiology tends to underestimate the severity of the radiation injury.[86] The most common abnormality is a stricture at the rectosigmoid junction or in the sigmoid colon itself. Small bowel contrast enema is the investigation of choice in the small intestine, but again this tends to underestimate the extent of injury. An intravenous urogram is indicated in cases with suspected ureteric stricture. Cystoscopy will show the changes within the bladder, and it is important that bladder capacity be measured. Contraction of the bladder can occur over a very few weeks, so repetition of this investigation will give a useful assessment of progression.

Medical Treatment

Medical management is largely symptomatic and supportive because no evidence has shown that any drug (including sulphasalazine, steroids, or antifibrinolytic agents) usefully influence the condition. Symptomatic treatment with dietary manipulation, stool softeners, and oral iron or transfusion for anemia may well help. Chronic small bowel disease with bacterial overgrowth may be improved with appropriate antibiotics, and deficiencies such as that of vitamin B_{12} may be corrected by injection.

Operative Treatment

Most severe problems, especially those in grade IV, will require surgery after appropriate preparation. Approximately 40% of patients present with signs of sepsis, intestinal obstruction, or rectovaginal fistula. Sufficient time for improvement of the general state before undertaking surgery is often possible.[80] Emergency surgery for complete obstruction or perforation is very rarely necessary. In cases with radiation enterocolitis, surgery will take the forms either of excision of abnormal bowel or bypass. At the present time, the consensus of surgical opinion leans toward excision as the best method of treatment if feasible.

The extent of radiation bowel disease has been mapped in pathologic specimens by vascular injection studies using dilute barium[87] (Figs. 46-5 and 46-6). It is conditioned by the technique of radidotherapy used. For example, in patients treated for carcinoma of the cervix with the intracavitary method alone, the lesion tends to be fairly localized, and a relatively short resection of the small or large bowel is adequate. Unfortunately, most patients have been treated by external beam radiotherapy in combination with intracavitary treatment; in this situation the lesion tends to be widespread and may be multiple.[88] For this reason, most radiation injuries require wide excision. In ileal disease it should be noted that it is unnecessary to remove much colon above the cecum, as the ascending and transverse colon are well away from the radiation field. The most common maximal injury in the ileum is 8 to 10 cm from the ileocecal valve but significant injury will be seen for at least 20 to 30 cm proximal to this. Thus, in patients who have had extensive radiotherapy it is rare for a resection of small bowel to be less than 40 cm.[87] Under these circumstances, primary anastomosis between the remaining ileum and the ascending colon is safe.[79] Similar considerations prevail in lesions of the rectosigmoid and rectum when, after combined intracavitary and external beam treatment, it is desirable to do a coloanal anastomosis after excision because the whole of the rectum is of doubtful viability.[88] More recently a colonic pouch has been used.

When a patient has been treated by external beam radiotherapy alone (as in carcinoma of the bladder or prostate), the situation is somewhat different. Although the radiation damage is more extensive compared with intracavitary irradiation, the colonic and rectal injury tends to be greater in bladder cases and less so in prostate cases. This may alter management, for it is usually possible to retain some rectum in bladder cases to permit a low colorectal anastomosis. In the prostate patient, however, it may well be that the anal sphincter and the pelvic floor are involved in the radiation process. When ulceration is very low and involves the anal canal, it is not unreasonable to temporize

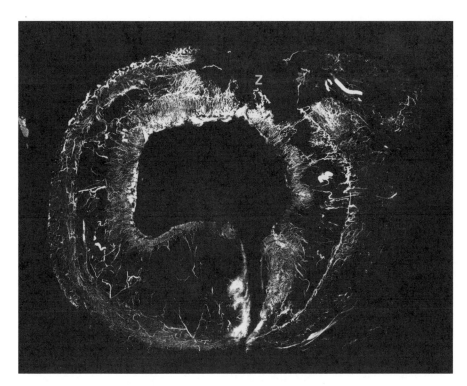

Figure 46-5. Microradiograph of fresh specimen of sigmoid colon after injection of blood vessels with dilute barium suspension (transverse section). Note small avascular area in muscularis propria labeled Z.

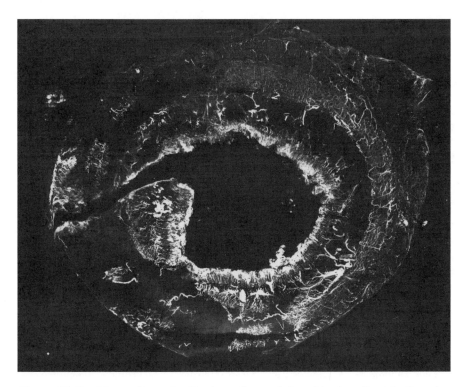

Figure 46-6. Microradiograph of fresh specimen of sigmoid colon after injection of blood vessels with dilute barium suspension (transverse section). Note extensive avascular changes involving almost half the circumference of the colon.

with a colostomy if surgery is necessary; in some instances the bowel will recover over a period of months. In patients with more extensive anorectal injuries, however, an abdominoperineal excision of the rectum has to be undertaken. In these cases serious thought should be given to combining this procedure with a repair of the perineum using a myocutaneous rectus abdominis flap or other plastic procedure.[89] Mobilization of the greater omentum and bringing it into the pelvis to add vascularized tissue has proved a useful adjunct to many procedures and is particularly relevant if the ureters have had to be widely dissected. It is, however, suitable for perineal reconstruction.

Local procedures for the repair of rectovaginal fistula have not been very successful in the experience of the author. It has been suggested that the interposition of well-vascularized tissue might increase the chance of healing. A fat pad from the labium major has been used, but the long-term results do not appear to be satisfactory as the fistula ultimately breaks down in most cases.[90] The gracilis muscle has been used for interposition, but the results have also been disappointing.[91] The policy I favor is to resect the damaged bowel whatever the level of the fistula and then carry out a coloanal anastomosis, possibly as a two-stage procedure with a covering colostomy. The procedure was initially described by Parks et al.[92] However, this left a large muscle sleeve, which may be undesirable as it can lead to cuff abscess. It is probably best to excise the rectum and sigmoid colon entirely and mobilize the left colon and splenic flexure. The colon can be anastomosed transanally with a series of full-thickness interrupted sutures. Bricker et al.[93] adopted a different approach using a method that does not require full mobilization of the rectum. They divided the sigmoid colon, opened up any stricture in the rectum, and then used the opened normal colon as a patch to eliminate the stricture and to exclude the fistula, which was separately divided. Bricker has devised several variations on this theme and has had good results.[94,95]

With regard to the urinary tract, severe bladder problems due to contraction may be dealt with by cystectomy and urinary diversion or by some reconstructive cystoplasty to increase bladder capacity. Ureteric problems may be dealt with by temporizing with cystoscopic dilation and stents or by excising the stricture and using an ileal interposition between the residual ureter and the bladder. The psoas hitch procedure is rarely possible in radiotherapy injury because the bladder is immobilized by fibrosis. If bladder and ureteric problems are being dealt with at the same time, lost ureteric length and bladder contraction can be handled by an ileocecocystoplasty. This operation should be approached with great circumspection, as the loss of the ileocecal region may lead to major worsening of any bowel problem because of the inevitable increase in bowel frequency.[96] Ureteric stents can be used as a long-term solution to ureteric obstruction. Replacement will be required at regular intervals, and this approach may relieve symptoms without recourse to major potentially dangerous surgery.

Progress After Surgery

Provided well-vascularized tissue is used, anastomotic failure is rare. Major complications are due to sepsis, and antibiotics are always indicated after such operations. Late morbidity and mortality in these patients are due to progressive radiation disease or recurrence of the tumor, the former being more likely than the latter. De Cosse et al.[77] reviewed 100 patients with radiation bowel disease and found that 55 subsequently developed urinary tract disease that was frequently severe. A few patients developed further progressive intestinal disease.

It has been suggested that patients who suffer from radiation bowel disease have a lesser tendency to recurrence of the tumor.[97] Harling and Balslev[98] looked at the life expectancy in patients after treatment for carcinoma of the uterine cervix. The 10-year survival rate was 52% in patients with bowel involvement compared with 58% of those without. Considering the problems that these patients have, this is a remarkable finding.

INJURIES DURING INVESTIGATION

Perforations of the rectum or colon have been recorded from many and various procedures, but endoscopy (especially colonoscopy) is now the most important. Perforations have been recorded after insertion of a rectal thermometer.[99] or administration of an enema for treatment,[100] or by the radiologist for diagnosis. They have been recorded after dilation of a rectal stricture, after colostomy irrigation,[101] or when inserting an intraperitoneal catheter for continuous ambulatory peritoneal dialysis.[102]

Rigid Sigmoidoscopy

With rigid sigmoidoscopy, perforation is rare and undoubtedly rarer than perforation complicating colonoscopy. The usual site is at the rectosigmoid junction due to forcible attempts to negotiate this area. Perforation has been reported to occur in 1 to 2 cases in 10,000 examinations (i.e., 0.01 to 0.02%).[103] Occasional significant rectal bleeding may occur after rectal biopsy, especially if the patient has a clotting disorder. It is obligatory to establish whether the patient is on medication likely to encourage bleeding before taking a biopsy.

Damage During Colonoscopy

Following the introduction of flexible colonoscopy, it soon became apparent that several (relatively rare) hazards can occur. Perforation and bleeding are the most common. Both are increased in frequency if biopsy or polypectomy has been undertaken.

Rare General Complications

Most endoscopies are carried out under intravenous sedation, and all sedative drugs depress cardiac and respiratory function. Rogers et al.[104] reported that during colonscopy there was an incidence for respiratory depression of 0.03%; for respiratory arrest of 0.02%; and for myocardial infarction of 0.01%. For this reason, all patients are monitored by pulse oxymetry during colonoscopy. Jonas et al.[105] described a distal proctocolitis due to glutaraldehyde used to disinfect colonoscopes. They noted that the condition was similar to pseudomembranous colitis, and subsequent animal experiments have indicated that glutaraldehyde was the cause.[106] Another rare complication of the procedure is bacteremia, which assumes significance in patients with a history of endocarditis, prosthetic cardiac valves, and possibly other implanted prostheses. The guidelines for antibiotic prophylaxis are set out by the American Society of Colon and Rectal Surgeons.[107]

Colonoscopic Perforation and Bleeding

Colonoscopic perforation and bleeding are worldwide problems and may lead to medicolegal action for negligence. Husson[99] of Le Sou Medical states that in France they handle 15 to 20 cases a year. The number of litigation cases in the United States is large, with the Physician Insurers Association of America logging 141 cases of endoscopic perforation in 1987.[108] Elfant et al.[109] stress the importance of informed consent, including both risks and benefits.

Perforation usually occurs because the tip of the instrument will not move onward due to an acute kink in the bowel or because the tip has passed into a diverticulum. The commonest site of injury is at the rectosigmoid junction or in the sigmoid colon. Pneumatic perforation may occur due to excessive amounts of air being insufflated.[110] An injury may occur during polypectomy by tenting the bowel wall into the snare or by applying excess current to the snare. This latter gives rise to the postpolypectomy coagulation syndrome, in which pyrexia with localized abdominal pain and tenderness occurs; these symptoms usually resolve spontaneously over 2 to 3 days but may progress to perforation at 6 to 12 hours.[111] Habr-Gama and Waye[112] pooled the information from several series of colonoscopy and concluded that after diagnostic colonoscopy the perforation rate was 0.17% and after polypectomy the significant bleeding rate was 1.4%. Bleeding may be immediate, but it can occur several days after the polypectomy when the slough separates.

Many series have recorded the incidence of perforation and bleeding associated with colonoscopy (0.1 to 3%). High rates are usually associated with polypectomy, in which the bleeding risk may rise to 5%.[113] The treatment of bleeding is initially conservative, with intravenous infusion and monitoring. If feasible, colonoscopy may be repeated and the area injected with adrenalin solution.[112] In patients in whom the bleeding is not controlled, laparotomy is indicated and hemostasis usually easily effected. Perforation may be noted by the colonoscopist during the procedure or it may only be diagnosed hours or even days after the procedure. If the perforation is noted at colonoscopy or if there are signs of a generalized or spreading peritonitis, immediate laparotomy is indicated. Perforation not associated with signs may be managed conservatively with antibiotics and intravenous fluids even in the presence of free gas on abdominal radiograph.[114] Similar conservative management can be employed in the postpolypectomy coagulation syndrome.

Barium Enema

The hazards of barium enema appear to be low, but if perforation occurs it carries a high mortality. Nelson et al.[103] reported that seven patients who sustained a barium perforation all died. Savia et al.[115] reported a mortality of 50% for intraperitoneal rupture during barium enema but less for extraperitoneal injury to the rectum. Why the mortality is so high is uncertain, but Sisel et al.[116] suggested that barium acted as an additive factor

in an already serious illness complicated by fecal peritonitis. Treatment includes peritoneal toilet, antibiotics, and colostomy.

COMPLICATIONS OF LAPAROSCOPY

In this decade there has been an explosion in the use of laparoscopy by abdominal surgeons. They have had to acquire new and different skills to bring laparoscopic operating into their range of techniques. This may have led some to venture beyond their expertise; too many accidents have been associated with the introduction of "key hole" surgery. Closed laparoscopy using a Veress needle for insufflation followed by blind insertion of the trocar to give access for the laparoscopic camera has been the usual initial mode of access to the peritoneal cavity. Alternatively, a short subumbilical incision to insert a Hassen's trocar and cannula has been advocated as a safer method.[117] Appropriate ports are then established for the necessary surgery.

Irrespective of any operation to be undertaken laparoscopically, certain hazards are intrinsic to the procedure. These include major vascular injury, hollow viscus perforation, thermal injury, complications of the pneumoperitoneum, and delayed complications.

Major Vascular Injury

In Germany, injury to the major retroperitoneal vessels was recorded at 3 to 10 in 10,000 laparoscopies.[118] In the United States a similar incidence was reported in a study of laparoscopic cholecystectomy.[119] The injury may be due to the trocar or the Veress needle.

Hollow Viscus Perforation

In the series of Deziel et al.[119] there was a 0.14% incidence of bowel injury. The injury was often not recognized but presented later as peritonitis, abscess, or fistula. Perforation of other organs from stomach to bladder have been reported.

Thermal Injury

Burns may occur with either monopolar diathermy or laser. The injury may not be observed at the time of operation.[72]

Complications of the Pneumoperitoneum

The absorption of carbon dioxide during a prolonged laparoscopic procedure may lead to hypercarbia, with potential cardiorespiratory problems. Gas embolus due to intravascular placement of the Veress needle occurs but is very rare. Tension pneumothorax is even rarer but has been reported.[120]

Delayed Complications

Delayed complications include hernia through the trocar site or, more rarely, through another port.[121] The other late complication of mounting concern is recurrence of tumor at a port site after laparoscopic colectomy for cancer. In a recent report, it was stated that more than 25 cases had appeared in the literature between 1993 and 1994.[122]

OPERATIVE ACCIDENTS

Abdominopelvic Operations

Sepsis

The bane of colorectal surgery used to be infection; although it still causes problems, they have been much less frequent since rational perioperative antibiotic policies have been added to careful surgical technique. A typical early study was by Washington et al.,[123] who showed a wound infection rate of 27% in the placebo group and 3% in the treatment group. The recognition of the importance of anaerobic organisms, especially *Bacteroides* species, in producing infection was key to evolving an effective antibiotic strategy.[124] Several randomized studies in the 1970s demonstrated conclusively that antibiotics acting at the time of surgery produced a dramatic fall in the infection rate. Krukowski et al.,[125] who stressed the importance of wound protection and surgical technique as well as the appropriate use of antibiotics, reported an infection rate of 1.8% in elective colorectal surgery.

A great number of antibiotic regimes have given good results; the basic principle is that they should be effective against a wide spectrum of anaerobic and aerobic organisms. When antibiotics are given for prophylaxis, some disagreement exists about the starting time and the number of doses. The combination of oral neomycin and erythromycin has had wide acceptance in the United States, but in the United Kingdom systemic antibiotics given immediately before operation as a single dose or continued for 24 hours is usual. Evidence shows that a single dose is effective if there is no contamination at the time of surgery.[126] Timing of the single dose to give an adequate blood level during operation is most important.[127]

The common combinations have been metronidazole with a cephalosprorin or aminoglycoside. There is no apparent advantage for second- or third-generation cephalosporins.[128] If contamination occurs during an operation, the risk of infection[129] is significantly increased, and antibiotics should be continued on a therapeutic basis.[130] Some believe that addition of a tetracycline lavage (1 g/L) reduces sepsis.[125] Most wound infections are relatively minor, but some may be serious and rarely fatal.

Synergistic Gangrene

Synergistic gangrene is a rapidly spreading necrosis of the skin and subcutaneous tissue that may be associated with gas and appears to spread in the subfascial planes. It occurs most often in the lower abdomen or perineum. The causative organisms are a mixture of anaerobic and aerobic bacteria. Treatment is urgent radical debridement and sytemic antibiotics.

Gas Gangrene

Gas gangrene is very rare; it is characterized by extreme toxemia associated with spreading necrotic infection and gas formation. Treatment is urgent debridement and massive doses of soluble penicillin.

Bacteremia/Septicemia

A risk still exists of intra-abdominal sepsis or septicemia after colonic surgery, which adds significant morbidity to an operation. There is no doubt that an asymptomatic bacteremia occurs at the time of many procedures involving the colon and rectum (Fig. 46-7). For this reason it is particularly important to have

Figure 46-7. Frequency of positive blood cultures in patients undergoing various operative procedures. Unpublished data accumulated before proplylactic antibiotics were used (personal series).

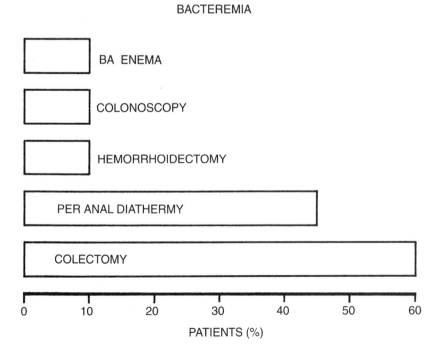

BACTEREMIA

adequate antibiotic cover even for minor procedures in patients who are at risk, such as those with heart or other prostheses or those who are immunosuppressed. Despite measures to reduce sepsis, it is still the chief cause of morbidity and mortality in colorectal surgery.

Splenic Injury

In many colorectal operations it is necessary to mobilize the splenic flexure. It is important to have adequate exposure and to divide the gastrocolic omentum and the peritoneum lateral to the descending colon alternatively until the two planes of dissection meet. Care is important because rough handling can produce a tear in the splenic capsule by traction. If this occurs, it must be recognized and dealt with appropriately. Tears in the splenic capsule can usually be dealt with effectively by the application of topical hemostatic agents. Parenchymatous injury is less common but can be repaired by splenorrhaphy.[131] If significant peritoneal contamination is present or if doubt exists about the efficacy of the splenorrhaphy, it is safer to accept the disadvantages and carry out a splenectomy.

Postsplenectomy Sepsis

Overwhelming sepsis in patients who had had a splenectomy was first described by King and Shumacker.[132] Although rare, it carries a high mortality. The risk is greatest within 3 years of splenectomy.[133] The loss of the spleen impairs the antibody response to infections caused by bacteria with a polysaccharide capsule (e.g., *Streptococus pneumoniae*, which is the commonest cause of overwhelming infection. Other organisms that are recognised to produce overwhelming infection are *Neisseria meningitidis*, *E. coli*, and *Haemophilus influenzae*. The risk appears to be greater in children than in adults but can be minimized by immunization against the common encapsulated bacteria.[134] The role of prophylactic antibiotics is less certain. They appear to lessen the risk in children but not in adults.[135] The advice in the United States and in the United Kingdom for prophylaxis is that asplenic patients should be given Pneumovax II, a 23-valent pneumococcal polysaccharide vaccine. In addition, in 1994 the Department of Health in the United Kingdom recommended immunization against *influenzae* type b and *N. meningitidis*.[136] It is further recommended that asplenic children under 16 should take penicillin V twice daily.

Urologic Complications

Ureteric Injury

During the course of a pelvic operation it is possible to injure either the bladder or the ureters. A ureteric injury may be apparent at the time, but it may not become manifest until some days after the operation.[137] Delayed presentation may occur because the injury was not noticed, or because the ureter has been rendered ischemic, leading to formation of a stricture or sloughing of the ureter, with fistula formation. This may be more likely following high-dose preoperative radiotherapy.

Prophylaxis. The ureters may be damaged deep in the pelvis when dividing either the lateral ligaments during rectal excision

or the uterine arteries at hysterectomy. The other site of injury is above the pelvis after the left ureter has been ligated or divided with the inferior mesenteric vessels. Graham and Goligher[138] reported a large series of rectal excisions with a 0.93% incidence of ureteric injury, and few more recent studies have improved on this figure.

Good surgical principles can prevent difficulties. It is important to start the dissection of the ureter above the field of operation and follow it down with minimal dissection to preserve the blood supply. Some believe that passing ureteric catheters before a difficult operation helps in identification. This does not prevent ureteric injury but it does aid immediate recognition.[139]

Treatment. When recognized, a divided ureter may occasionally be reanastomosed over a double J stent or reimplanted into the bladder with a psoas hitch. If it has been crushed, a J stent should be passed and left for several weeks. If the injury is not suspected at the time of operation, it may present as anuria if both ureters have been tied or urinary fistula if one ureter has been damaged. Treatment of the delayed complications should be carried out by a urologist.

Bladder Dysfunction

Bladder injury may occur during rectal excision for an adherent rectal carcinoma. An incidence of 2% is reported by Baumrucker and Shaw.[140]

The area at most risk is low down on the posterior bladder wall or trigone. It is desirable to open the fundus of the bladder in difficult dissections so that orientation becomes easier and an injury to the trigone is avoided. It is easy to close the fundus, but closing the trigone and bladder base are difficult because of the proximity of the distal ureter.

A major problem with the bladder after pelvic surgery is retention of urine. In older men this may be due to prostatic hypertrophy, but it may have been caused by injury to the motor parasympathetic nerves to the bladder detrusor muscle, leading to an atonic bladder. It may be clinically apparent which of these causes is the most likely, but urodynamic investigation will demonstrate the difference between obstruction and atonia. If the cause is prostatic hypertrophy, then a transurethral prostatectomy can be performed, if the cause is atonia, then a period of some weeks of catheterization will often allow the bladder to recover tone and permit adequate voiding.

Pelvic Nerve Injury

Nerve injury may affect the bladder or sexual function, with retention of urine or impotence. As noted above, there are causes other than nerve injury for urinary retention and the same applies to impotence. The accompanying box shows the causes of impotence.

Anatomy and Physiology

The bladder and genital tract are supplied by autonomic nerves that are in close relationship with the rectum and for this reason are at risk during rectal mobilization. The sympathetic nerves flow down in front of the aorta at the root of the mesentery and enter the pelvis in front of the promontory of the sacrum. They

Causes of Impotence/Ejaculatory Dysfunction

Vasculogenic causes
    Aortic disease
    Local arterial disease
Drugs
    Benzodiazepines
    Major tranquillizers
    Antidepressants
    Antipsychotics
    Digitalis
    Cimetidine
    Metoclopramide
    Antihypertensives
Neurologic causes
    Multiple sclerosis
    Diabetes mellitus
    Spinal injury
Operative neural damage
Endocrine causes
Psychological causes

can easily be seen as the presacral nerves dividing into two trunks, which pass to form the pelvic plexus on the side wall of the pelvis to be distributed to the pelvic organs by branches passing with the blood vessels or with the nervi erigentes. The parasympathetic supply is more difficult to see as it is situated deep in the pelvis. Contributions from S2, S3, and S4 form the nervi erigentes, which are distributed to the pelvic organs in the endopelvic fascia on the surface of the pelvic floor. The function of these nerves in the bladder and sexual organs is shown in Table 46-5.

Clinical Problems

Since the presacral nerves are situated well posterior or lateral to the rectum, it should not be difficult to avoid damage when operating for inflammatory bowel disease because the operation can keep close to the rectum. It may, however, be much more difficult to avoid injury in cases of malignant disease, when a more radical approach has to be taken. The nerves are in close relation to the lateral aspect of the rectum and mesorectum but can be nearly always seen and should be preserved in almost all cases. Damage to the parasympathetic nerves is more likely, as they lie close to the lateral aspect of the lateral ligaments posterolaterally to the bladder. They are at risk of damage by wide excision of the lateral ligaments. Although the nerves may

Table 46-5. Autonomic Nerve Function

Nerve System	Bladder	Sexual
Sympathetic	Sensation	Ejaculation
Parasympathetic	Contraction	Erection

be injured anterior to the rectum, this is extremely unusual owing to the presence of Denonvillier's fascia. Pelvic nerve injury is best avoided by identification and preservation of the sympathetic nerves early in the operation. Sharp dissection to mobilize the rectum in front of the presacral fascia and behind the prostate leads to a bloodless field. The lateral ligaments should be divided close to the rectum in inflammatory bowel disease. This technique should keep bladder and sexual dysfunction to a minimum. Unfortunately, a wide lateral excision in malignant disease is more likely to cause problems.[141] Modern series show that impotence is rare after rectal excision for inflammatory bowel disease with ileoanal pouch, but cases of retrograde ejaculation have been recorded.[142] However, impotence is reported in many patients after rectal excision for cancer.[143]

It is absolutely vital to discuss preoperatively the potential sexual and bladder complications with all males undergoing rectal surgery. Although the risk of impotence in patients undergoing operation for inflammatory bowel disease is low, such warnings are nevertheless vital because these patients are often young, and impotence will be a particularly severe disability.

Sexual problems in women after rectal surgery seem to be predominantly due to a local mechanical problem.[144] However, there is no doubt that some women have dyspareunia after rectal excision due to the vaginal vault falling back to the sacrum; this can be prevented or minimized by transposing the omentum or other tissue into the area in front of the sacrum. Dyspareunia has been reported in 7% to 28% of females after ileal pouch-anal anastomosis.[145]

Rectal Injury

Gynecologic Operations

Although the rectum may be damaged during any pelvic operation, the most common cause of inadvertent injury is gynecologic operations.[146] This is more likely to occur when endometriosis or tumor render the operation difficult. Provided the injury is not through diseased tissue, the defect can be closed; if the rectum is involved in a disease process, it is necessary to excise the affected area of the bowel. This is usually the rectosigmoid region, so primary anastomosis is possible in most cases.

Patients sometimes develop a fecal fistula or peritonitis in the postoperative period after hysterectomy due to an overlooked rectal injury or rectal necrosis occurring after diathermy coagulation. Treatment will depend on presentation, but urgent reoperation is required for patients with peritonitis. Low rectal injury may occasionally occur when the gynecologist is carrying out a posterior vaginal repair or a vaginal hysterectomy. Provided the injury is recognized, it may be readily repaired. If it is not repaired, a rectovaginal fistula into the mid- to low rectum will develop. Although small fistulae may heal, it is often necessary to carry out further surgery such as a rectal advancement flap for a low fistula or abdominal exploration and repair for a high fistula.[147]

Obstetric Trauma

Prolonged or obstructed labor, which is more frequently seen in third world countries, may produce pressure necrosis of the rectovaginal septum, causing a rectovaginal fistula in the midrectum. More frequently the pressure necrosis will lead to a vesicovaginal fistula.[148] Lawson,[149] who has great experience, uses a transvaginal approach to repair the high rectovaginal fistula in layers.

The usual obstetric fistula seen in the United Kingdom or North America is situated in the vagina but above the level of the anal sphincter into the rectum. It often arises as a complication of a failed repair of a third-or fourth-degree tear. Some will close spontaneously. Many, however, need to be repaired as a delayed procedure. It is important to recognize that many of these patients have a coexistent persisting sphincter injury that will need repair.[150]

Urologic Operations

Operations on the prostate or urethra are recognized as a possible cause of injury to the anterior rectum. An obvious injury should be treated by immediate repair. The injury may not be apparent at operation but may present in the postoperative period as sepsis progressing to a rectoprostatic fistula.[151]

A small fistula with flow from the bladder or urethra to the rectum may not require any treatment, but a large fistula with flow from the rectum to the bladder may produce serious illness with septicemia. In these patients surgery is obligatory. An initial defunctioning colostomy with broad-spectrum antibiotics is the safest preliminary step before definite treatment of the fistula. This can be achieved by a variety of approaches, including perineal with direct repair,[152] transanal with rectal advancement flap,[153] trans-sphincteric with direct transrectal repair,[154] or rectal excision with coloanal anastomosis.[92]

Vascular Surgery

Left-sided colonic infarction is well recognized as a complication of aortic surgery, especially emergency surgery for aneurism.[155] The incidence is reported to be 2% after emergency aneurism surgery but 0.7% after elective aortic surgery.[156] Colonic ischemia producing ischemic colitis after aortic surgery is much more common if patients are assessed postoperatively by endoscopy. Hagihara and Griffin[157] reported that 6% of patients after aortic surgery showed evidence of ischemic change in the sigmoid colon and a higher incidence after surgery for a ruptured aneurism. Previous pelvic radiotherapy increases the hazard of rectal necrosis after aortic surgery even if the radiotherapy was administered many years previously.[81]

Postoperative Complications

The frequency of anastomotic dehiscence, tumour recurrence, and stoma complications varies considerably among different surgeons. These topics are fully reviewed elsewhere in this book.

Anal Sphincter Injury

Injuries to the anal muscle complex may lead to incontinence. However, the term incontinence covers a wide area of disability, from minor occasional loss of gas to complete sensory or motor deficiency with total inability to control solid stool. Some patients are only incontinent if the stool becomes loose, some

> **Causes of Incontinence**
>
> Neurologic diseases
> Fecal impaction
> Rectal disease (urge incontinence)
> Idiopathic "neurogenic"
> Perineal descent/prolapse
> Sphincter injury
>   Surgical
>   Obstetric
>   Accident

have urgency resulting in incontinence, and some have minor contamination of the underclothes without true incontinence. This last is referred to as soiling to distinguish it from true incontinence. Although incontinence has many causes it is the anal sphincter injuries that are pertinent to this chapter.

The muscle complex that surrounds the terminal part of the large bowel consists of two concentric tubes. The inner tube terminates in an expansion of the circular smooth muscle of the gut, the internal sphincter, which is involuntary and has a dual autonomic innervation. It is responsible for most of the resting tone in the anal sphincter. The outer tube consists of the puborectalis-external sphincter complex, which is voluntary and supplied by the pudendal nerve (S2 to 4). The external sphincter displays tone at rest but can be contracted at will and so represents the incremental increase measured as squeeze pressure in physiologic studies. Injuries to either or both elements of the sphincter complex may lead to incontinence.

Surgical Sphincter Injury

Incontinence of a greater or lesser degree has been recorded after all types of anal canal operations.

Fistula-In-Ano

Operations for fistula-in-ano include laying open the fistula or excising it. These procedures involve some division of anal musculature in most patients. This becomes particularly hazardous if the fistula is high or if multiple operations have been performed for perineal sepsis. The subject of fistulae has been extensively reviewed by Seow-Choen and Nicholls,[158] who point out the dangers to continence in dividing substantial parts of the external sphincter even if the puborectalis is not damaged. Marks and Richie[159] showed that many patients had some degree of altered continence after successful fistula surgery but fecal incontinence was relatively rare. This has been confirmed by careful prospective study.[160] Loss of gas or occasional liquid appears to occur in approximately one-fourth of patients treated for a low anal fistula. Surgeons have become more conservative in treating fistulae, so more recent studies probably record a lower incidence of incontinence although soiling due to scar tissue is still a significant problem.[161]

Anal Dilation

Anal dilation had a vogue some time ago for the treatment of hemorrhoids.[162] It is still widely practiced for the treatment of fissure-in-ano. Many reports indicate that anal dilation leads to incontinence in some subjects, especially if they have a potentially weak sphincter complex before dilation.[163] Nielson et al.[164] reviewed patients after dilation for fissure and found minor incontinence in 13%. Speakman et al.[165] demonstrated internal sphincter injury in patients with incontinence after anal dilation by ultrasonography, which showed thinning with irregular disruption of the internal sphincter. Surgical repair has a poor prognosis, and dilation should be used with great caution or even not at all, particularly in females.

Other Anal Operations

Major incontinence is less common after other anal procedures. Bennett and Goligher[166] reported a 30% minor incontinence rate due to a "key hole" deformity after posterior sphincterotomy for anal fissure. Hoffman and Goligher[167] recorded a low but significant rate of incontinence after lateral internal anal sphincterotomy. In a series of 350 patients treated by lateral sphincterotomy, minor incontinence lasting more than 6 weeks was found in 6% of patients.[168] Hemorrhoidectomy has been reported as a rare cause of incontinence but a common cause of soiling.[169]

Obstetric Trauma

A report from Arizona indicated that 5% of all normal vaginal deliveries resulted in a major perineal tear involving the anal sphincter complex and that 10% of these women had wound disruption after primary repair.[170] Although occasional cases of incontinence may occur due to internal sphincter damage alone, almost all cases of incontinence follow either episiotomy or a tear involving the external sphincter. It appears that episiotomy does not give major protection against sphincter injury. Coats et al.[171] demonstrated that sphincter injury is more likely after midline than mediolateral episiotomy. Forceps delivery is another major factor associated with sphincter injury.[172]

The advent of anorectal ultrasound has revolutionized our understanding of fecal incontinence, especially of incontinence after childbirth. This modality has challenged the previous concept that most fecal incontinence is due to pudendal nerve neuropathy. It has become apparent that the vast majority of women with incontinence after childbirth have associated sphincter damage. Sultan et al.[173] studied pudendal nerve function prospectively in a series of women before and after delivery. There was some prolongation of nerve transit in 16% but this recovered rapidly in most. More significantly, these authors carried out anorectal ultrasound examination on 202 consecutive patients 6 weeks and 6 months after delivery.[174] Over one-third (35%) of primipara had sphincter damage, but new damage was seen in only in 4% of multipara. The changes observed at 6 weeks persisted at 6 months. Not all patients with sphincter abnormalities had incontinence, but all patients with incontinence had a sphincter abnormality.

An obstetric injury involving the anal sphincters is described as a third-degree tear. If the anal epithelium is also damaged, some describe this as a fourth-degree tear although the results of treatment are similar to third-degree tears.[175] If a third-or fourth-degree tear occurs, then incontinence is much more probable because immediate repair is often inadequate. Sorensen et al.[176] studied 38 women who had a third-degree tear repaired and found that 14 were incontinent 3 months after delivery. Another study of the effects of repaired third-degree tears in 34 women showed that 50% still had symptoms and 85% still had a demonstrable defect on ultrasonography.[175]

Treatment

The usual treatment of sphincter injury is direct surgical repair of the sphincter. It is important that bowel preparation be excellent and that prophylactic antibiotics be used at the time of surgery because sepsis is the biggest reason for imperfect results of operation. Most surgeons do not use a protective colostomy, but it may be of merit in obese patients or in patients with an associated fistula.

Parks and McPartlin[177] described a method where by most of the scar tissue was excised and the external sphincter repaired with overlap. Others preserve scar tissue for the overlap. Browning and Motson[178] reported the outcome in 97 patients, most of whom had problems after previous anal surgery. Complete continence was achieved in 78%, but the authors remarked that the few patients with a previous obstetric tear did less well.

Fang et al.[179] reported their results in a series with a preponderance of patients with old obstetric injuries and obtained complete continence in 55% after repair. In another study 9 of 35 patients still had incontinence after delayed sphincter repair for previous obstetric trauma.[150] Attempted repair of sphincter injury has had mixed results and may be difficult to categorize because the surgeon's view and the patient's view of the outcome may not coincide. In this respect Fleshman et al.[180] reported that surgeons felt they had a 94% success rate but 44% of patients admitted to some degree of incontinence when directly questioned.

If a substantial part of the external sphincter is lost, a muscle transfer may be used. Several muscles have been tried, but the results in general have been rather disappointing. Gluteus maximus transposition has been used by Devesa et al.[181] and Pearl et al.[182] who have had encouraging preliminary results with this procedure. Of great interest has been the use of gracilis as a sling around the anus.[183] The results were encouraging in only a few young patients. Williams et al.[184] and Baeten et al.[185] have refined the technique of gracilis transposition by employing an implanted nerve stimulator to convert the gracilis into a slow twitch muscle. The results indicate that around 60% of patients treated have acceptable continence. Long-term results of this procedure are not yet available.

REFERENCES

1. Pearse WH (1988) Professional liability: epidemiology and demography. Clin Obstet Gynecol 31:148–152

2. Kern KA (1993) Medical malpractice involving colon and rectal disease: a 20-year review of United States civil court litigation. Dis Colon Rectum 36:531–539

3. Halley MM (1989) Tort law impact on health care. p. 23. In Halley MM et al (eds): Medical Malpractice Solutions: Systems and Proposals for Injury Compensation. Charles C Thomas, Springfield, IL

4. Johanson JF, Sonnenberg A, Koch TR (1989) Clinical epidemiology of chronic constipation. J Clin Gastroenterol 11:525–536

5. Gattuso JM, Kamm MA (1994) Adverse effects of drugs in the management of constipation and diarrhea. Drug Safety 10:47–65

6. Johnson CM, Cullen JM, Roberts MC (1993) Morphologic characterization of castor oil-induced colitis in ponies. Vet Pathol 30:248–255

7. Siegers C-P, von Hertzberg-Lottin E, Otte M, Schneider B (1993) Anthranoid laxative abuse—a risk for colorectal cancer? Gut 34:1099–1101

8. Morris AI, Turnberg LA (1979) Surreptitious laxative abuse. Gastroenterology 77:780–786

9. Hewitt J, Reeve J, Rigby J, Cox AG (1973) Whole gut irrigation in preparation for large bowel surgery. Lancet 2:337–340

10. Zanoni CE, Gergamini C, Bertoncini M et al (1982) Whole gut lavage for surgery: a case of intra-operative colonic explosion after administration of mannitol. Dis Colon Rectum 25:580–581

11. Ambrose NS, Hohnson M, Burdon DW, Keighley MRB (1983) A physiological appraisal of polyethylene glycol and a balanced electrolyte solution as bowel preparation. Br J Surg 70:428–430

12. Compston JE 1995 Review article: osteoporosis, corticosteroids and inflammatory bowel disease. Aliment Pharmacol Ther 9:237–250

13. Svartz N (1942) Salazopyrin, a new sulfanilamide preparation. Acta Med Scand 110:577–598

14. Levi AJ, Fisher AM, Hughes L, Hendry WF (1979) Male infertility due to sulphasalazine. Lancet 2:276–278

15. Azad Khan AK, Howes DT, Piris J, Truelove SC (1980) Optimum of sulphasalazine for maintenance treatment in ulcerative colitis. Gut 21:232–240

16. Kinlen LJ (1985) Incidence of cancer in rheumatoid arthritis and other disorders after immunosuppressive treatment. Am J Med suppl. A 78:44–49

17. Connell WR, Kamm MA, Dickson M et al (1994) Long-term neoplasia risk after azathioprine treatment in inflammatory bowel disease. Lancet 343:1249–1252

18. Lennard-Jones JE (1990) Corticosteroids and immunosuppressive drugs. pp. 373–389. In Allan RN et al (eds): Inflammatory Bowel Disease. 2nd Ed. Churchill Livingstone, Edinburgh

19. Von Graffenried B (1989) Sandimmun (ciclosporin) in autoimmune disease: overview on early clinical experience. Am J Nephrol 9:51–56

20. Hoigne R, Neftel K, Cerny A et al (1992) Meyler's Side Effects of Drugs. 12th Ed. Elsevier Science Publishers, Amsterdam

21. Jacoby GA, Archer GL (1991) New mechanisms of bacterial resistance to antimicrobial agents. N Engl J Med 324:601

22. Gorbach SL, Chang TW, Goldin B (1987) Successful treatment of relapsing *Clostridium difficile* colitis with *Lactobacillus* GG. Lancet 2:1519

23. McFarland LV, Bernasconi P (1993) *Saccharomyces boulardii*: a review of an innovative biotherapeutic agent. Microbiol Ecol Health Dis 6:157–171

24. Aronsson B, Mollby R, Nord CE (1985) Antimicrobial agents and *Clostridium difficile* in acute enteric disease: epidemiological data from Sweden, 1980–1982. J Infect Dis 151:476

25. Viscidi R, Willey S, Bartlett JG (1981) Isolation rates and toxigenic potential of *Clostridium difficile* isolates from various populations. Gastroenterology 81:5

26. George WL, Rolfe RD, Finegold SM (1982) Clostridium difficile and its cytotoxin in feces of patients with antimicrobial associated diarrhea and miscellaneous conditions. J Clin Microbiol 15:1049–1053

27. Bartlett JG (1979) Antibiotic-associated colitis. Clin Gastroenterol 8:783

28. Bartlett JG, Chang TW, Gurwith M et al (1978) Antibiotic associated pseudomembranous colitis due to toxin producing clostridia. N Engl J Med 198:531–534

28. George WL, Rolfe RD, Finegold SM (1982) *Clostridium difficile* and its cytotoxin in feces of patients with antimicrobial associated diarrhea and miscellaneous conditions. J Clin Microbiol 15:1049–1053

29. Roda PI (1987) *Clostridium difficile* colitis induced by cytarabine. Am J Clin Oncol 10:451–452

30. Ellis ME, Watson BM, Milewski PJ, Jones G (1983) *Clostridium difficile* colitis unassociated with antibiotic therapy. Br J Surg 70:242–243

31. Committee on Safety of Medicines (1994) Antibiotic associated colitis. Curr Probl Pharmacovigilance 20:7–8

32. Bingley PJ, Harding GM (1987) *Clostridium difficile* colitis following treatment with metronidazole and vancomycin. Postgrad Med J 63:993–994

33. Price AB, Davies DR (1977) Pseudomembranous colitis. J Clin Pathol 30:1–12

34. Gebhard RL, Gerding DN (1988) *Clostridium difficile* disease. JAMA 259:3052

35. Trudel JL, Deschenes M, Mayrand S, Barkun AN (1995) Toxic megacolon complicating pseudomembranous enterocolitis. Dis Colon Rectum 38:1033–1038

36. Bradley SJ, Weaver DW, Maxwell MPT, Bouwman DL (1988) Surgical management of pseudomembranous colitis. Am Surg 54:329–332

37. Ferrara JJ, Martin EW, Carey LC (1982) Morbidity of emergency operations in patients with metastatic cancer receiving chemotherapy. Surgery 92:605

38. Keidan RD, Fanning J, Gatenby RA, Weese JL (1989) Recurrent typhilitis: a disease resulting from aggressive chemotherapy. Dis Colon Rectum 32:206–209

39. Koea JB, Shaw JHF (1989) Surgical management of neutropenic enterocolitis. Br J Surg 76:821–824

40. Vohra S, Prescott RJ, Banerjee SS et al (1992) Management of neutropenic colitis. Surg Oncol 1:11–15

41. Hafner CD, Granley JJ, Krause RJ et al (1962) Anticoagulant ileus. JAMA 182:947

42. Lowe GDO, McKillop JH, Prentice AG (1979) Fatal retroperitoneal haemorrhage complicating anticoagulant therapy. Postgrad Med J 55:18

43. Anonymous (1993) Managing patients with hepatitis C. Drug Ther Bull 31:61–62

44. Horowitz MS, Rooks C, Horowitz B, Hilgartner MW (1988) Virus safety of solvent/detergent-treated antihaemophilic factor concentrate. Lancet 2:186–189

45. Mollison PL (1993) Infectious agents transmitted by transfusion. pp. 724–725. In: Blood Transfusion in Clinical Medicine. 9th Ed. Blackwell Scientific Publications, Oxford

46. Lemmer JH, (1984) Hepatitis B as an occupational disease for surgeons. Surgery Gynecology and Obstetrics 159:91–100

47. Lifson A, Castro KG (1986) Health care workers with the acquired immunodeficiency syndrome. Second International Conference on AIDS, Paris.

48. Marcus R (1988) CDC Cooperative Needlestick Surveillance Group. Surveillance of the health care workers exposed to blood from patients infected with the human immunodeficiency virus (update). N Engl J Med 319:1118–1123

49. Bjarnason I, Zanelli G, Smith T et al (1987) Nonsteroidal antiinflammatory drug-induced intestinal inflammation in humans. Gastroenterology 93:480–489

50. Tanner AR, Raghunath AS (1988) Colonic inflammation and non-steroidal anti-inflammatory drug administration: an assessment of the frequency of the problem. Digestion 41:116–120

51. Gabriel SE, Jaakkimainen L, Bombardier C (1991) Risk for serious gastrointestinal complications related to use of nonsteroidal anti-inflammatory drug: a meta-analysis. Ann Inter Med 115:787–796

52. Gibson GR, Whiteacre EB, Ricotti CA (1992) Colitis induced by nonsteroidal anti-inflammatory drugs. Arch Intern Med 152:625–632

53. Pucius RJ, Charles AK, Adair HM (1993) Diaphragm-like strictures of the colon induced by non-steroidal anti-inflammatory drugs. Br J Surg 80:395–396

54. Campbell K, Steele RJC (1991) Nonsteroidal anti-inflammatory drugs and complicated diverticular disease: a case control study. Br J Surg 78:190–191

55. Bjarnason I, Hayllar J, Macpherson AJ, Russell AS (1993) Side effects of non-steroidal anti-inflammatory drugs on the small and large intestine in humans. Gastroenterology 104:1832–1847

56. Boley SJ, Schultz S, Kreiger H (1965) Evaluation of thiazides and potassium as a cause of small bowel ulcer. JAMA 192:763–768

57. Levy N, Gaspar E (1975) Rectal bleeding and indomethacin suppositories. Lancet 1:577

58. Floch MH, Hellman L (1965) The effect of 5-fluorouracil on rectal mucosa. Gastroenterology 48:430–437

59. Graham CF, Gallagher K, Jones JK (1981) Acute colitis with methyldopa. N Engl J Med 304:1044–1045

60. Jackson CW, Haboubi NY, Whorwell PJ, Schofield PF (1986) Gold-induced enterocolitis. Gut 27:452–456

61. Committee on Safety of Medicines (1995) Fibrosing colono-

pathy associated with pancreatic enzymes. Curr Probl Pharmacovigilance 21:11

62. Betancourt E, Farman J, Lawson JP (1968) Vascular occlusion of the colon and oral contraceptives. N Engl J Med 278:438–440

63. Clarke AW, Lloyd-Mostyn RH, Sadler MR de C (1972) "Ischaemic" colitis in young adults. BMJ 4:70–72

64. Faurel JP, Calmat A, Delast N (1981) Entercolites necrosantes après prise prolongée de neuroleptiques Med Chir Dig 10:9–13

65. Turnbull AR, Isaacson P (1977) Ischaemic colitis and drug abuse. BMJ 3:1000

66. Johnson TD, Berenson MM (1991) Methamphetamine-induced ischemic colitis. J Clin Gastroenterol 3:687–689

67. Brown P, Baddeley H, Read AE et al (1974) Sclerosing peritonitis, an unusual reaction to a beta-adrenergic-blocking drug. Lancet 2:1477–1481

68. Saklayen MG (1990) CAPD peritonitis: incidence, pathogens, diagnosis and management. Med Clin North Am 74:997–1010

69. Ellis H (1994) Pathological changes produced by surgical dusting powders. Ann R Coll Surg Engl 76:5–8

70. McGregor GI, Shepherd JD, Phillips GI (1988) Acute graft-versus-host disease of the intestine: a surgical perspective. Am J Surg 155:680–682

71. Jones B, Kramer SS, Saral R et al (1988) Gastrointestinal inflammation after bone marrow transplantation: graft-versus-host disease or opportunistic infection. Am J Radiol 150:277–282

72. McAnena OJ, Willson PD (1993) Diathermy in laparoscopic surgery. Br J Surg 80:1094–1096

73. National Radiation Protection Board (1986) A national Survey of Doses to patients Undergoing a Selection of Routine X-Ray Examinations in English Hospitals. NRPB-R200. HMSO London

74. Haboubi NY, Schofield PF, Rowland P (1988) The light and electron microscopic appearances of early and late phase radiation-induced proctitis. Am J Gastroenterol 3:1140–1144

75. Carr ND, Schofield PF, Hasleton PS (1985) Vascular changes in radiation bowel disease. Histopathology 9:517–534

76. Berthrong M (1986) Pathological changes secondary to radiation. World J Surg 10:155–170

77. De Cosse JJ, Rhodes RS, Wentz WB et al (1969) The natural history and management of radiation induced injury of the gastrointestinal tract. Ann Surg 170:369–384

78. Danjoux CE, Catton GE (1979) Delayed complications in colo-rectal carcinoma treated by combination radiotherapy and 5-fluorouracil. Eastern Cooperative Oncology Group (ECOG) Pilot Study. Int J Radiat Oncol Biol Phys 5:311–316

79. Sandler RS, Sandler DP (1983) Radiation induced cancers of the colon and rectum. Assessing the risk. Gastroenterology 84:51–57

79. Schofield PF, Carr ND, Holden D (1986) The pathogenesis and treatment of radiation bowel disease. J R Soc Med 79:30–32

80. Schofield PF, Lupton EW (1989) The Causation and Clinical Management of Pelvic Radiation Disease. Springer-Verlag, London.

81. Harling H, Balslev I, Larsen JF (1986) Necrosis of the rectum

complicating abdominal aortic reconstructions in previously irradiated patients. Br J Surg 73:711

82. Gilinsky NH, Burns DG, Barbezat GO (1983) The natural history of radiation induced proctosigmoiditis: analysis of 88 patients. Qu J Med 52:40–53

83. Walsh HPJ, Schofield PF (1984) Is laparotomy for small bowel obstruction justified in patients with previously treated malignancy? Br J Surg 71:933–935

84. Pilepich MV, Pajak T, George FW et al (1983) Preliminary report on phase III RTOG studies of extended-field irradiation in carcinoma of the prostate. Am J Clin Oncol 6:485–491

85. Smith DH, de Cosse JJ, (1986) Radiation damage to the small intestine. World J Surg 10:189–194

86. Johnson RJ, Carrington BM (1992) Pelvic radiation disease. Clin Radiol 45:4–12

87. Carr ND, Pullan BR, Hasleton PS, Schofield PF (1984) Microvascular studies in human radiation bowel disease. Gut 25:1448–1454

88. Carr ND, Holden D (1989) Experimental findings in radiation bowel disease. pp. 69–93. In Schofield PF, Lupton EW (eds): The Causation and Clinical Management of Pelvic Radiation Disease. Springer-Verlag, London

88. Cooke SAR, Wellsted MD (1986) The radiation-damaged rectum: resection with colonal anastomosis using the endoanal technique. World J Surg 10:220–227

89. Brough WA, Schofield PF (1991) The value of the rectus abdominis myocutaneous flap in the treatment of complex perineal fistula. Dis Colon Rectum 34:148–150

90. Aartsen EJ, Sindram IS (1988) Repair of the radiation induced rectovaginal fistulas without or with interposition of the bulbocavernosus muscle (Martius procedure). Eur J Surg Oncol 14:171–177

91. Graham JB (1965) Vaginal fistulas following radiotherapy. Surg Gynecol Obstet 120:1019

92. Parks AG, Allen CLO, Frank JD, McPartlin JF (1978) A method of treating post-irradition rectovaginal fistulas. Br J Surg 65:417–421

93. Bricker EM, Kraybill WG, Lopez MJ (1986) Functional results of postirradiation rectal reconstruction. World J Surg 10:249–258

94. Bricker EM, Johnston WD (1979) Repair of postirradiation recto-vaginal fistula and stricture. Surg Gynecol Obstet 148:499–506

95. Bricker EM, Johnston WD, Patwardham RV (1981) Repair of post irradiation damage to colo-rectum. A progress report. Ann Surg 193:555

96. Barnard RJ, Lupton EW (1989) Treatment of radiation urinary tract disease. pp. 123–139. In Schofield PF, Lupton EW (eds): The Causation and Clinical Management of Pelvic Radiation Disease. Springer-Verlag, London

97. Perez CA, Breau S, Bedwinek JM et al (1984) Radiation therapy alone in the treatment of carcinoma of the uterine cervix. II. Analysis of complications. Cancer 54:235–246

98. Harling H, Balslev I (1988) Long-term prognosis of patients with severe radiation enteritis. Am J Surg 155:517–519

99. Husson R (1994) Gastroenterologists in trouble. J Med Defence Union 1:4–5

100. Large PG, Mukheiber WJ (1956) Injuries to the rectum and anal canal by enema syringes. Lancet 2:596–599

101. Mazier WD, Dignon RD, Capehart RJ, Smith BG (1976) Ef-

fective colostomy irrigation. Surg Gynaecol Obstet 142:905–909

102. Rosenman JE, Allison DC, Smith DE (1984) Colonic perforation as a complication of peritoneovenous shunt: a case report. Surgery 100:619–622

103. Nelson RL, Abcarian H, Prasad ML (1982) Iatrogenic perforation of the colon and rectum. Dis Colon Rectum 25:305–308

104. Rogers BHG, Silvis SE, Nebel OT (1975) Complications of flexible fiberoptic colonoscopy and polypectomy. Gastrointest Endosc 22:73

105. Jonas G, Mahoney A, Murray J et al (1988) Chemical colitis due to endoscope cleaning solutions: a mimic of pseudomembranous colitis. Gastroenterology 95:1403

106. Durande L, Zulty JC, Israel E et al (1992) Investigation of an outbreak of bloody diarrhoea: association with endoscopy clean solution and demonstration of lesions in an animal model. Am J Med 92:476–480

107. American Society of Colon and Rectal Surgeons (1992) Practice parameters for antibiotic prophylaxis to prevent infective endocarditis or infected prosthesis during colon endoscopy. Dis Colon Rectum 35:277–285

108. Gerstenberger PD, Plumeri PA (1993) Malpractice claims in gastrointestinal endoscopy: analysis of an insurance industry data base. Gastrointest Endosc 39:132–138

109. Elfant AB, Korn C, Mendez L et al (1995) Recall of informed consent after endoscopic procedures. Dis Colon Rectum 38:1–3

110. Williams CB, Lane RH, Sakai Y, Hanwell AE (1973) Colonoscopy: an air-pressure hazard. Lancet 2:729

111. Waye JD (1981) The postpolypectomy cogulation syndrome. Gastrointest Endosc 27:184

112. Habr-Gama A, Waye JD (1989) Complications and hazards of gastrointestinal endoscopy. World J Surg 13:193–201

113. Waye JD, Lewis BS, Yessayan S (1992) Colonoscopy: a prospective report of complications. Lancet 15:347–351

114. Donckier V, Andre R (1993) Treatment of colon endoscopic perforations. Acta Chir Belg 93:60–62

115. Savia G, Volkmar P, Raoux M et al (1982) Les perforations recto-coliques au cours du lavement baryte. Lyon Chir 78:73–77

116. Sisel RJ, Donovan AJ, Yellin AE (1972) Experimental fecal peritonitis: influence of barium sulphate or water soluble radiographic contrast material on survival. Arch Surg 104:765–768

117. McMahon AJ, Baxter JN, O'Dwyer PJ (1993) Preventing complications of laparoscopy. Br J Surg 80:1593–1594

118. Riedell HH, Lehmann-Willenbrock E, Mecke H, Semm K (1989) The frequency distribution of various pelviscopic (laparoscopic) operations, including complication rates statistics of the Federal Republic of Germany in the years 1983–1985. Zentralbl Gynakol 111:78–81

119. Deziel MC, Millikan KW, Economou SG (1993) Complications of laparoscopic cholecystectomy: a national survey of 4292 hospitals and an analysis of 77604 cases. Am J Surg 165:9–14

120. Whiston RJ, Eggers KA, Morris RW, Stamatakis JD (1991) Tension pneumothorax during laparoscopic cholecystectomy. Br J Surg 78:1325

121. Boyce DE, Fligelstone LJ, Wheeler MH (1992) An unusual

complication of laparoscopic cholecystectomy. Ann R Coll Surg Engl 74:254–255

122. Jacquet P, Averbach AM, Stephens AD, Sugarbaker PH (1995) Cancer recurrence following laparoscopic colectomy: report of two patients treated with heated intraperitoneal chemotherapy. Dis Colon Rectum 38:1110–1114

123. Washington JA, Dearing WH, Judd ES, Elveback LR (1974) Effect of preoperation antibiotic regimen on development of infection after intestinal surgery. Ann Surg 180:567–572

124. Nichols RL, Condon RE, Gorbach SL, Nyhus LM (1972) Efficacy of preoperative antimicrobial preparation of the bowel. Ann Surg 176:227–232

125. Krukowski ZH, Stewart MPM, Alsayer HM, Matheson NA (1984) Infection after abdominal surgery: 5 years prospective study. BMJ 288:278–280

126. Rowe-Jones DC, Peel ALG, Kingston RD (1990) Single dose cefotaxime plus metronidazole versus three dose cefuroxime plus metronidazole as prophylaxis against wound infection in colorectal surgery. Multicentre prospective randomised study. BMJ 300:18–22

127. Classen DC, Evans RS, Pestotnik SL (1992) The timing of prophylactic administration of antibiotics and the risk of surgical-wound infection N Engl J Med 326:281–286

128. DiPiro JT, Bowden TA, Hooks VH (1984) Prophylactic parenteral cephalosporins in surgery. Are the newer agents better? JAMA 252:3277–3279

129. Allsop JR, Lee ECG (1978) Factors which influenced postoperative complications in patients with ulcerative colitis or Crohn's disease of the colon on corticosteroids. Gut 19:729–734

130. Tornqvist A, Forsgren A, Leandoer L, Ursing J (1987) Identification and antibiotic prophylaxis of high-risk patients in elective colorectal surgery. World J Surg 11:115–119

131. Langevin JM, Rothenberger DA, Goldberg SM (1984) Accidental splenic injury during surgical treatment of the colon and rectum. Surg Gynecol Obstet 154:139–143

132. King H, Shumacker HB (1952) Splenic studies: susceptibility to infection after splenectomy performed in infancy. Ann Surg 136:239–242

133. Chattopadhyay B (1989) Splenectomy, pneumococcal vaccination and antibiotic prophylaxis. Br J Hosp Med 41:172–174

134. Amman AJ, Addiego J, Wara DW et al (1977) Polyvalent pneumococcal polysaccharide immunisation of patients with sickle-cell anaemia and patients with splenectomy. N Engl J Med 297:897–900

135. Read RC, Finch RG (1994) Prophylaxis after splenectomy. J Antimicrob Chemother 33:4–6

136. MacInnes J, Waghorn DJ, Haworth E (1995) Management of asplenic patients in South Buckinghamshire: an audit of local practice. Communicable Dis Rep 5:R173–R177

137. Zinman LM, Libertino JA, Roth RA (1978) Management of operative ureteral injury. Urology 12:290–303

138. Graham JW, Goligher JC (1954) The management of accidental injuries and deliberate resections of the ureter during excision of the rectum. Br J Surg 42:151–160

139. Bothwell WN, Bleicher RA, Dent TL (1994) Propylactic ureteral catheterisation in colon surgery: a five-year review. Dis Colon Rectum 37:330–334

140. Baumrucker GO, Shaw JW (1953) Urological complications following abdomino-perineal resection of the rectum. Arch Surg 67:502–513

141. Santangelo ML, Romano G, Sassaroli C (1987) Sexual function after resection for rectal cancer. Am J Surg 154:502–504

142. Dozois RR (1985) Ileal "J" pouch-anal anastomosis. Br J Surg suppl. 72:S80

143. La Monica G, Audisio RA, Tamburini M et al (1985) Incidence of sexual dysfunction in male patients treated surgically for rectal malignancy. Dis Colon Rectum 28:937–940

144. Watts JMcK, de Dombal FT, Goligher JC (1966) Long-term complications and prognosis following major surgery for ucerative colitis. Br J Surg 53:1014–1022

145. Counihan TC, Roberts PL, Schoetz DJ (1994) Fertility and sexual and gynecologic function after ileal pouch-anal anastomosis. Dis Colon Rectum 37:1126–1129

146. Wiener I, Rojas P, Wolma FJ (1981) Traumatic colonic perforation. Am J Surg 142:717–720

147. Rothenberger DA, Goldberg SM (1983) The management of rectovaginal fistula. Surg Clin North Am 63:61–79

148. Kelly J (1992) Vesico-vaginal and recto-vaginal fistulae. J R Soci Med 85:257–258

149. Lawson J (1972) Rectovaginal fistulas following difficult labour. Proc R Soc Med 65:283–286

150. Khanduja KS, Yamashita HJ, Wise WE et al (1994) Delayed repair of obstetric injuries of the anorectum and vagina: a stratified surgical approach. Dis Colon Rectum 37:344–349

151. Kilpatrick FR, Mason AY (1969) Postoperative recto-prostatic fistula. Br J Urol 41:649–654

152. Goodwin WE, Turner RD, Winter CC (1958) Rectourinary fistula: principles of management and a technique of surgical closure. J Urolo 80:246–254

153. Parks AG, Motson RW (1983) Perianal repair of rectoprostatic fistula. Br J Surg 70:725–726

154. Jackson BT, Mason AY (1983) Rectoprostatic fistula. In: Eds. Todd IP and Fielding LP. Rob & Smith's Operative Surgery. 4th Ed. Butterworths, London

155. Smith RE, Szilagyi DE (1960) Ischemia of the colon as a complication in the surgery of the abdominal aorta. Arch Surg 80:806–821

156. Schroeder T, Christoffersen JK, Andersen J (1985) Surg Gynecol Obstet 160:299–303

157. Hagihara PF, Griffin WO (1979) Incidence of ischemic colitis following abdominal aortic rec onstruction. Surg Gynecol Obstet 149:571–573

158. Seow-Choen F, Nicholls RJ (1992) Anal fistula. Br J Surg 79:197–205

159. Marks CG, Ritchie JK (1977) Anal fistulas at St. Mark's Hospital. Br J Surg 64:84–91

160. Lunniss PJ, Kamm MA, Phillips RKS (1994) Factors affecting continence after surgery for anal fistula. Br J Surg 81:1382–1385

161. Shouler PJ, Grimley RP, Keighley MRB, Alexander-Williams J (1986) Fistula in ano is usually simple to manage surgically. Int J Color Dis 1:113–115

162. Lord PH (1969) A day case procedure for the cure of third degree haemorrhoids. Br J Surg 56:747–749

163. McDonald A, Smith A, Mcneill AD, Finlay IG (1992) Manual dilatation of the anus. Br J Surg 79:1381–1382

164. Nielsen MB, Rasmussen OO, Pedersen JF, Christansen J (1993) Risk of sphincter damage and anal incontinence after

anal dilatation for fissure-in-ano. An endosonograghic study. Dis Colon Rectum 36:677–680

165. Speakman CTM, Burnett SJD, Kamm MA, Bartram CI (1991) Sphincter damage following anal dilatation revealed by anal endosonography. Br J Surg 78:1429–1430

166. Bennett RC, Goligher JC (1962) Results of internal sphincterotomy for anal fissure. BMJ 2:1500–1503

167. Hoffman DC, Goligher JC (1970) Lateral subcutaneous internal sphincterotomy in the treatment of anal fissure. BMJ 3: 673–675

168. Lewis TH, Corman ML, Prager ED, Robertson WG (1988) Long-term results of open and closed sphincterotomy for anal fissure. Dis Colon Rectum 31:368–371

169. Felt-Bersma RJF, Janssen JJWM, Klinkenberg-Knol EC et al (1989) Soiling: anorectal function and results of treatment. Int J Color Dis 4:37–40

170. Venkatesh KS, Ramanujam PS, Larson DM, Haywood MA (1989) Anorectal complications of vaginal delivery. Dis Colon Rectum 32:1039–1041

171. Coats PM, Chan KK, Wilkins M, Beard RJ (1980) A comparison between midline and mediolateral episiotomies Br J Obstet Gynaecol 87:408–412

172. Sultan AH, Kamm MA, Bartran CI, Hudson CN (1993) Anal sphincter trauma during instrumental delivery. Int J Gynecol Obstet 43:263–270

173. Sultan AH, Kamm MA, Hudson CN (1994) Pudendal nerve damage during labour: prospective study before and after childbirth. Br J Obstet Gynaecol 101:22–28

174. Sultan AH, Kamm MA, Hudson CN, Bartram CI (1993) Anal sphincter disruption during vaginal delivery. N Engl J Med 329:1905–1911

175. Sultan AH, Kamm MA, Bartram CI, Hudson CN (1994) Third degree obstetric anal sphincter tears: risk factors and outcome of primary repair. BMJ 308:887–891

176. Sorensen M, Tetzschner T, Rasmussen OO et al (1993) Sphincter repair in childbirth. Br J Surg 80:392–394

177. Parks AG, McPartlin JF (1971) Late repair of injuries of the anal sphincter Proce R Soc Med 64:1187–1189

178. Browing GGP, Motson RW (1984) Anal sphincter injury. Management and results of Parks sphincter repair. Ann Surg 199:351–356

179. Fang DT, Nivatvongs S, Vermeulen FD et al (1984) Overlapping sphincteroplasty for acquired anal incontinence. Dis Colon Rectum 27:720–722

180. Fleshman JW, Peter WR, Shemesh EI, Fry RD, Kodner IJ (1991) Anal sphincter reconstruction: anterior overlapping muscle repair. Dis Colon Rectum 34:739–743

181. Devesa JM, Vincente E, Enriquey JM (1992) Total fecal incontinence—a new method of gluteus maximus transposition: preliminary results and report of previous experience with similar procedures. Dis Colon Rectum 35:339–349

182. Pearl RK, Prasad ML, Nelson RL (1991) Bilateral gluteus maximus transposition for anal incontinence. Dis Colon Rectum 34:478–481

183. Pickrell KL, Broadbent TR, Masters FW, Metzger JT (1952) Construction of a rectal sphincter and restoration of anal continence by transplanting the gracilis muscle. Ann Surg 135: 853–862

184. Williams NS, Patel J, George BD et al (1991) Development of an electrically stimulated neoanal sphincter. Lancet 338: 1166–1169

185. Baeten CGM, Konsten J, Spaans F et al (1991) Dynamic graccoloplasty for the treatment of faecal incontinence. Lancet 338:1163–1165

47

LAPAROSCOPIC SURGERY

Heidi Nelson

The success and widespread acceptance of laparoscopic cholecystectomy has encouraged the adaptation of laparoscopic techniques to increasingly complex abdominal procedures, including colectomy and proctectomy. In contrast to the rapid acceptance of laparoscopic cholecystectomy, laparoscopic colorectal procedures have been introduced at a slower, more controlled, pace. Such hesitation principally stems from the complexity of the techniques and the complexity and diversity of the colorectal diseases. It is well recognized that laparoscopic colectomy is challenging both to learn and to perform, for a number of reasons. Furthermore, whereas cholelithiasis is the principle indication for cholecystectomy, indications for colectomy range from benign inflammatory conditions (such as Crohn's disease and ulcerative colitis) to benign and malignant neoplastic conditions (such as polyps and cancers). Each condition presents special concerns and technical difficulties, such as the management of the phlegmon or fistula in Crohn's disease or the detection and management of a metastatic hepatic lesion in colon cancer. Indeed, whether laparoscopic procedures are indicated at all in malignancy is a matter of controversy. The goal of this chapter is to provide a status report on the application of laparoscopic techniques in colorectal surgery, commencing with indications, techniques, and feasibility, and closing with outcome analyses and controversies.

INDICATIONS

To date, laparoscopic techniques have been described for everything from simple colotomy and standard segmental resection to total abdominal colectomy and ileal pouch-anal anastomosis. Even though all of these procedures are technically feasible, at least one of them, total abdominal colectomy, does not offer sufficient patient-related benefits to warrant current application.[1] For this reason, diagnoses requiring total colectomy, such as ulcerative colitis, familial adenomatous polyposis, and colonic inertia, should be treated using standard open techniques. In the future, technical advances and increased experience may encourage surgeons to revisit this procedure. In the meantime, laparoscopic surgery may be indicated for diseases requiring segmental bowel resection, stoma formation, or proctectomy.

Current indications for laparoscopic segmental bowel resection include colon polyps, colon cancer, diverticular disease, volvulus, rectal prolapse, endometriosis, inflammatory bowel disease, and lipomas.[2-13] Laparoscopic intestinal stoma surgery may be indicated for purposes of fecal diversion, and laparoscopic proctectomy may be indicated for rectal cancer or more rarely for inflammatory bowel disease.[10,14-20] Although colon and rectal cancers have been resected using laparoscopic techniques, this application of laparoscopy remains highly controversial. The reader is referred to the discussion of controversies below.

CONTRAINDICATIONS

Although none are absolute, contraindications for systemic and primary bowel disease are described. Surgeons should be discouraged from performing laparoscopic bowel surgery on patients with severe systemic diseases such as cardiac failure with no margin for hemodynamic variability, liver failure with coagulopathy, and respiratory failure with no pulmonary reserve.[21,22] Regarding primary bowel disease, common sense should be applied. Potential benefits must be favorably balanced against surgical risks. For example, any large bulky lesion (such as an inflammatory phlegmon or tumor) that requires a generous incision for extraction will likely provide greater risk of harm than of postoperative recovery advantage. Similarly, the presence of dilated obstructed bowel will render abdominal entry and bowel manipulation risky and intra-abdominal visualization limited. Finally, although it is not a contraindication, I am biased against performing laparoscopic procedures in cases of unusual diagnoses or when the goals of surgery are not sharply defined because the efficacies of exploratory and resective laparoscopic techniques are not yet fully established. Obesity, previous surgery, and the risk of conversion do not contraindicate laparoscopic surgery. Having said that, patients with known dense adhesions or crisscrossing abdominal scars (or both) are often poor candidates for laparoscopic surgery.

PATIENT SELECTION

In addition to the indications and contraindications discussed above, a number of factors should be considered when selecting patients for laparoscopic bowel surgery. For those surgeons who are less experienced at laparoscopy, thin patients without previous surgery and with benign cecal disease are ideal candidates. Right colectomy, which is technically less challenging and has lower conversion rates, is probably the best procedure for initiates.[12] For technical reasons, transverse colon lesions that require full mobilization of both flexures are not ideally suited for laparoscopic resection. One final consideration is that of patient consent. Patients are only suitable if they are fully capable of understanding the potential risks and benefits of this new laparoscopic application, particularly in cases of malignancy.

PREOPERATIVE EVALUATION AND PREPARATION

Preoperative evaluations and preparations for laparoscopic surgery are generally the same as for open surgery. A few exceptions deserve discussion. First, since palpation is not possible with laparoscopy, precise preoperative colonic pathology localization is essential, especially since inadvertent resection of normal bowel has been described.[23] Colonoscopic localization is generally reliable when lesions are in close proximity to anatomic landmarks, such as the rectosigmoid junction and ileocecal valve. However, the area between the hepatic flexure and the distal sigmoid is a "no man's land"; confident localization in this area may be facilitated by taking a single abdominal radiograph during colonoscopy or performing a preoperative barium enema or intraoperative colonoscopy. A second exception involves the evaluation of parenchymal disease, such as liver metastases. Surface lesions may be visible, but intrahepatic metastases may be missed unless preoperative studies (computed tomography (CT) scan or hepatic ultrasound) are performed. Finally, for laparoscopic proctectomy, it is desirable to perform endorectal ultrasound, to ensure early stage disease.

Preoperative bowel preparation, with standard mechanical cleansing agents and antibiotics, is accomplished according to patient compliance, at home or in the hospital. Risk of deep venous thrombosis is minimized by the application of pressure stockings and sequential compression devices, and risk of injury to the stomach and bladder at surgery is minimized by nasogastric tube and urinary catheter decompression, respectively. Patients who are likely to need a temporary or permanent stoma are marked prior to surgery by a stoma therapist.

OPERATIVE TECHNIQUES

Although limited illustrations of laparoscopic techniques are warranted, the following is not a comprehensive surgical atlas. The technical descriptions illustrate key concepts for laparoscopic resection of the right colon, sigmoid colon, and rectum; as such, they can be adapted to virtually all colon and rectal procedures.

It must first be said that laparoscopic colectomy, although certainly feasible, is technically challenging. A number of factors contribute to the difficulty of learning and performing laparoscopic bowel resections, including the fact that it is necessary to shift exposures to allow dissection in multiple operative fields. The trick is to accomplish these exposures without creating reverse image fields for the surgeon and assistant. Additional impediments include the necessity for using the two-handed technique, ligating a large vascular pedicle, performing a bowel resection and anastomosis, and finally, removing a large specimen. Although a number of techniques have been described, only two basic approaches are used; intracorporeal laparoscopic colectomy[6] and laparoscopic-assisted colectomy (LAC).[24]

Intracorporeal colectomy accomplishes bowel resection using only laparoscopic techniques. All aspects of the operation are performed inside the abdomen, and the specimen is retrieved through large cannulas or per anus. Drawbacks to this approach include the fact that intracorporeal suturing is required, specimen retrieval is often difficult, and anastomotic leak rates are reported as high as 18%.[6] LAC is an alternate and more widely accepted technique; mobilization and vascular ligation are performed intracorporeally and using a small incision, resection and anastomosis are performed extracorporeally. LAC and protectomy, which have gained favor due to their relative simplicity and safety, are described below.

Equipment

It has generally been possible to perform laparoscopic colorectal procedures with only limited laparoscopic equipment. Basic reusable instruments include a 30-degree laparoscope, 5-mm graspers, curved or parrot scissors, and long (38-cm) babcocks. Typical disposables include 10/12-mm cannulas with 5-mm adaptors and stability threads, clip appliers, and linear vascular and bowel staplers. To economize, disposable instruments, although readily available, are only opened as needed. To facilitate ease and versatility of instrument repositioning, 10/12-mm cannulas with stability threads are used at all sites.

Right and Left Colectomy

Right and left colectomy are performed in essentially the same manner, only one is the reverse, or mirror image of the other. Because it is more commonly performed, the details of segmental right colectomy are described.[24]

The patient is positioned supine and secured to the table with ankle straps or a bean bag to prevent slippage during steep Trendelenburg positioning. The patient, operating personnel, and equipment are positioned as illustrated in Figure 47-1. A pneumoperitoneum of 10 to 12 mmHg is established using the Verres needle or open technique.[25,26] The first cannula is placed periumbilically; subsequent cannulas are placed in the left upper paramedian, left lower paramedian, and finally right midparamedian positions. Cannula positions often need to be adjusted individually to minimize cross-field interference in patients with short torsos and to maximize multiple field reach in patients with long torsos.

Once the abdominal cavity is explored, the camera is positioned in the left upper quadrant, the patient is placed left side

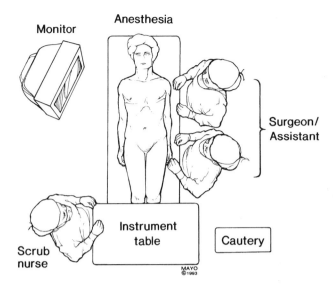

Figure 47-1. Operating room positions for right colectomy. The monitor and nurse are on the same side as the pathology, and the surgeon and assistant are on the side opposite. This minimizes reverse image problems. (From Elftmann et al.,[24] by permission of Mayo Foundation.)

down in steep Trendelenburg position, and dissection is commenced in the right lower quadrant (Fig. 47-2). Cecal dissection is started by dividing the lateral peritoneal attachments along the ileocecal junction. Entering the retroperitoneum at this point allows identification of the ureter caudad, and eventually the

duodenum cephalad. Even though it is possible to retract the bowel atraumatically, better retraction and less risk of bowel damage can be accomplished if the peritoneum adjacent to the bowel is grasped with a babcock.

In patients who have previously undergone appendectomy or gynecologic surgery, pelvic adhesions can be anticipated. Whereas a few filmy adhesions are readily managed, dense and extensive adhesions may require conversion. By assessing this promptly and converting early, frustration and complications may be avoided.

Next the hepatic flexure is exposed and dissected by reversing the Trendelenburg, surgeon, assistant, and camera positions. A large fatty omentum and adhesions from prior cholecystectomy are the greatest impediments to hepatic flexure mobilization.

Once the cecum, ileum, and hepatic flexure are fully mobilized, it is possible to perform mesenteric ligation either extracorporeally in a thin patient or intracorporeal (Fig. 47-3) in an obese patient. Intracorporeal ligation of the ileocolic vessel can be facilitated by grasping the ileocecal junction with a babcock and placing it on stretch. This maneuver usually displays the junction between the ileocolic and superior mesenteric vessels. Windows are developed on either side of the vessels, and then clips and loops or a linear vascular stapler are applied. Dividing the ileocolic vessel allows the bowel to be exteriorized for resection and anastomosis, even in obese individuals.

A small (less than 6-cm) incision is made either using the right paramedian (transverse, muscle splitting) or periumbilical (vertical, midline) port sites. If any difficulties are encountered, it is best to make the minimal access wound in the midline, so

Figure 47-2. Cecal dissection. As depicted in the inset, every attempt should be made to have the retracting instrument in the nondominant and the dissecting instrument in the dominant hand of the surgeon. (From Elftmann et al.,[24] by permission of Mayo Foundation.)

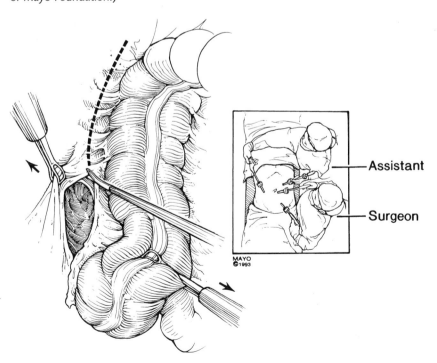

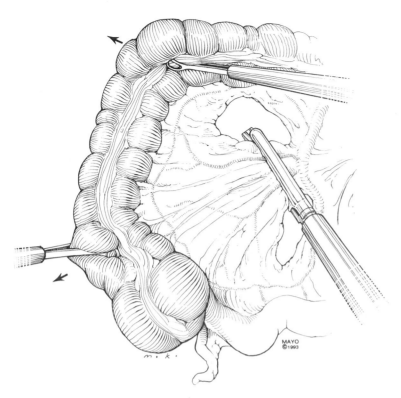

Figure 47-3. Intracorporeal vascular ligation. Vascular pedicle ligation can be performed using a 30-mm linear vascular stapler, readily introduced through 10/12-mm cannulas, or using clips and endoloops. (From Elftmann et al.,[24] by permission of Mayo Foundation.)

that conversion can be accomplished with one incision. For malignant disease, specimen isolation, using either a bowel bag or wound protector, is recommended. The bowel is exteriorized and the remaining vascular pedicles ligated, and standard resection and anastomosis are then performed (Fig. 47-4). After the bowel is returned to the abdominal cavity and the access wound closed, the pneumoperitoneum is re-established, operative fields and cannula sites are inspected for hemostasis, and all cannula site wounds are closed.

Sigmoid Resection

Except for the addition of a circular bowel stapler, equipment for laparoscopic resection of the sigmoid is the same as described for right colectomy. To facilitate abdominal and perineal exposure, the patient is placed in a legs-up position and the surgeon, two assistants, a nurse, and equipment are positioned as illustrated in Figure 47-5. Typical cannula placement includes periumbilical, left upper, and right lower paramedian positions and additional ports in the mid- and lower left paramedian positions as needed. Much of the sigmoid mobilization can be performed using three cannulas.

Using the same principles as those described for right colectomy, the patient is placed in steep Trendelenburg position with the right side down. As depicted in Figure 47-5, the surgeon works with a babcock and dissecting instrument, while the first assistant provides exposure with the laparoscope in the left upper quadrant. The second assistant helps to mobilize the sig-

moid and expose the ureter by gently retracting the peritoneum along the proximal bowel (Fig. 47-6) or along the lateral abdominal wall. When the sigmoid is densely adherent to the lateral abdominal wall due to inflammation or tumor, conversion should be considered early. Inability to identify the left ureter should prompt conversion. Once the presacral avascular plane is entered and the proximal rectum dissected, it is time to clear and divide the mesentery.

For malignancy, the superior hemorrhoidal and sigmoidal vessels are divided just below the take-off of the left colic (Fig. 47-7). For benign disease it is possible to divide the mesentery closer to the bowel, but this generally consumes more time and staplers. Next, the mesorectal tissue is cleared and the rectum prepared for transection (Fig. 47-7). Linear bowel staplers that can be introduced through 10/12-mm cannulas are now available. With the rectum divided, the reach of the descending colon to rectum can be assessed and if necessary the proximal colon can be further mobilized. The left gutter is generally easy to dissect; if required, the splenic flexure can be mobilized by repositioning the patient, head up and right side down.

The level of proximal transection is determined intracorporeally, making certain the proximal colon and rectum will anastomose comfortably without tension. It is now possible to exteriorize the proximal colon for removal of the specimen and placement of the detachable circular stapler anvil. A small (less than 6-cm) muscle-splitting transverse incision is made at the left midparamedian cannula site. The bowel is delivered and divided and the detachable anvil secured in the proximal colon.

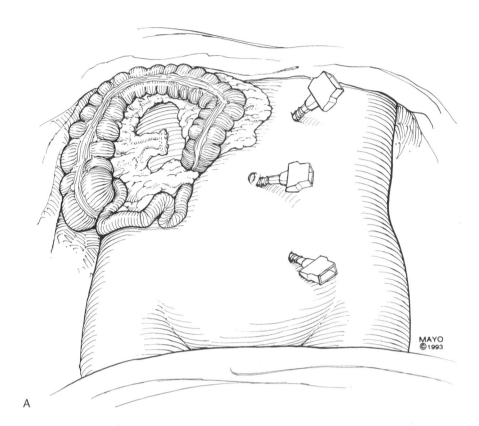

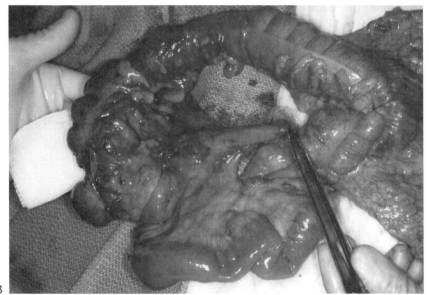

Figure 47-4. Bowel exteriorization. (**A**) A transverse right paramedian muscle splitting incision can be used for exteriorization, as depicted here, or the same effects can be accomplished with a small midline incision. Cannulas are left in place for one final laparoscopic inspection prior to completion. (**B**) Photograph. (From Elftmann et al.,[24] by permission of Mayo Foundation.)

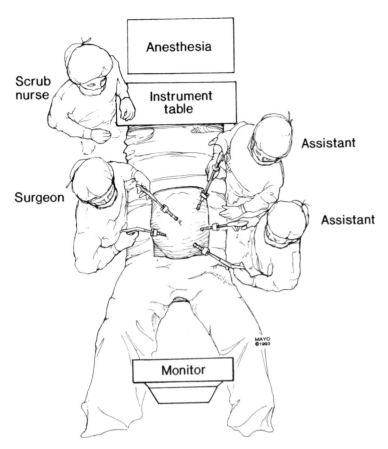

Figure 47-5. Operating room positions for sigmoid colectomy. Although a single monitor between the legs is generally sufficient, in some cases it may be more suitable to have two monitors, one on each side of the lower extremities. (From Elftmann et al.,[24] by permission of Mayo Foundation.)

The bowel with anvil is returned to the abdominal cavity and the wound closed and pneumoperitoneum re-established. The shaft of the stapler is gently introduced through the lubricated anus and advanced to the rectal staple line. Once the trocar pierces through the end of the rectum, the anvil is attached to the stapler shaft and the stapler closed and fired. Tissue rings are inspected for deficiencies and proctoscopy performed to test for leaks and hemostasis. Intra-abdominal inspection, cannula removal, and wound closure complete the procedure.

Abdominal Perineal Resection

The initial steps for rectal resection are nearly identical to those for sigmoid resection, with the exception that cannula placement varies slightly (Fig. 47-8). Even though cannula sites are slightly modified, the same personnel, equipment, and instrument positions are utilized. Sigmoid mobilization and vascular ligation are the same as described for sigmoid resection. However, instead of dividing the distal bowel, the proximal colon is divided at the junction of the descending and sigmoid colon. Next the rectum is dissected all the way to the levators (Fig. 47-9). The laparoscope generally provides clear exposure of the deep pelvis. To finish the procedure, the proximal colon is delivered through the previously marked transrectus stoma site,

which has been enlarged to accommodate the bowel. Perineal dissection is performed using standard techniques. Note that the pneumoperitoneum is not evacuated until the perineum and pelvis are contiguous; in this way the abdominal operator can facilitate perineal dissection.

POSTOPERATIVE CARE

Postoperative management following laparoscopic colorectal surgery differs little from corresponding open surgery, except for the faster pace of the recovery. Nasogastric and urinary catheters are removed early and oral intake instituted within 1 or 2 days after surgery and advanced as tolerated. Patients may be released from the hospital when they are capable of maintaining enteral nutrition. Since patients typically remain in the hospital for fewer postoperative days, stoma education and training should be started early and if necessary continued on an outpatient basis.

FEASIBILITY

The technical feasibility of any new procedure depends on whether it can be performed safely and efficiently. Current reports suggest that laparoscopic colorectal procedures can be

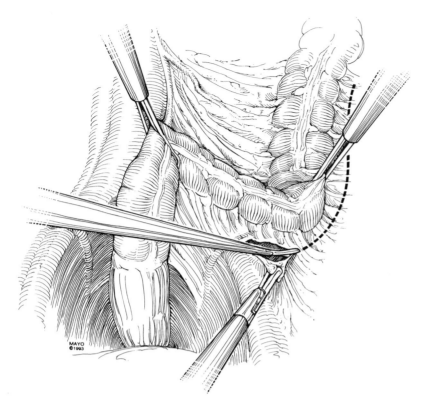

Figure 47-6. Sigmoid dissection. Mobilizing the sigmoid colon should allow confident visualization of the left ureter. (From Elftmann et al.,[24] by permission of Mayo Foundation.)

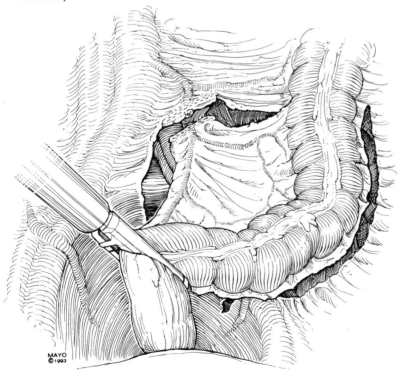

Figure 47-7. Intracorporeal rectal transection. After the proximal rectum is mobilized and the superior hemorrhoidal and sigmoidal vessels are ligated, the rectum can be divided using a linear bowel stapler. (From Elftmann et al.,[24] by permission of Mayo Foundation.)

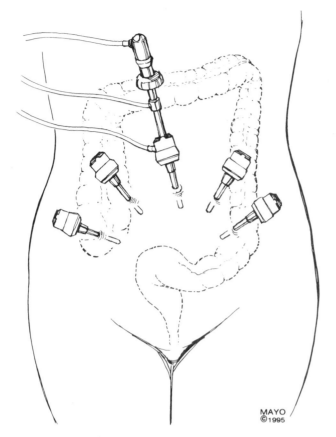

Figure 47-8. Cannula placement for abdominal perineal resection. To facilitate pelvic dissection of the rectum, cannula sites are modified slightly from those described for sigmoid resection. (From Thibault and Nelson,[71] by permission of Mayo Foundation.)

performed safely, with morbidity and mortality rates comparable to those of conventional coleotomy, and efficiently, with reasonable rates of conversion and operating times. The broader issue of feasibility (whether these procedures can be performed in all surgical practices) has not yet been thoroughly tested.

Safety

First and foremost, new procedures must be as safe as conventional procedures. To date, overall morbidity and mortality figures for laparoscopic colectomy, 14% and 0.6%, respectively, (Table 47-1) are comparable to those reported for conventional colectomy, 22 to 41% and 1.3 to 8%, respectively.[27,28] In a more direct comparison, Senagore and collegues[7] reported perioperative morbidity rates of 11%, 15%, and 17% for open, laparoscopic, and converted colectomies, respectively. In the largest series of 122 patients from the Mayo Clinic, no postoperative deaths occurred, but there were 13 (11%) complications, 7 intraoperative and 6 postoperative.[12] Intraoperative complications included two cases of small bowel perforation, and one case each of ureteral injury, bladder injury, hemorrhage, bowel rotation, and atrial fibrillation. Postoperative complications included four cases of prolonged ileus or obstruction, and one case each of urinary retention and recurrent prolapse. Neither

the rate nor the severity of laparoscopic colectomy complications appear to be different from conventional colectomy. This is in part true for laparoscopic abdominoperineal resection as well. Although a few laparoscopy-specific complications have been reported,[20] overall morbidity rates (23% for seven series totaling 35 patients) are comparable to those of conventional abdominoperineal resection.[6,18–20,29–31] In the same series of patients the mortality rate was 9%. This is higher than expected, and close scrutiny seems warranted.

Technical Efficiency

That laparoscopic bowel surgery can be performed safely raises a second feasibility issue, namely, that of technical efficiency. Can laparoscopic bowel surgery be performed in a timely fashion and with acceptable rates of conversion to open colectomy?

Operative Times

It can be anticipated, particularly early in the surgeon's experience, that laparoscopic bowel resections will require longer operative times than corresponding open resections. This has been well documented for LAC (Table 47-2). Although laparoscopic procedures always take longer than open procedures, converted procedures may be longer or shorter, depending on the surgeon's philosophy and practice of conversion. Those who convert early after rapid assessment of technical feasibility or after evidence of cause for conversion will likely experience less frustration and shorter times for converted cases. As alluded to above, operative times are experience dependent. A number of reports have graphically illustrated the learning curve for initiates in laparoscopic bowel surgery, with the typical plateau occurring somewhere between 10 and 20 cases.[5,10]

Conversion to Open Surgery

In the same manner as operative times are experience dependent, so are conversion rates, which are variably reported to be as low as 14% and as high as 48%.[3,5,7,12,32] Hoffman and colleagues[3] nicely illustrated the effects of experience with a decline in their conversion rate from 23% in the first half to 15% in the second half of their series of 80 patients. Reasons for converting to open surgery are diverse and include technical, complication, and disease-related indications.

A number of technical factors have provided cause for conversion, perhaps most often the finding of prohibitive adhesions or other factors causing poor visualization. Early in the Mayo Clinic experience, an attempt was made to identify risk factors for conversion. Even though adhesions were an often cited cause of conversion, history of a previous abdominal surgery was not predictive for conversion. Interestingly, the only factor that significantly predicted a high rate of conversion (75%) was weight exceeding 90 Kg.[12]

Since laparoscopic procedures are highly technical and rely on assistance from other operating room personnel, it may be necessary to convert for reasons of instrumentation or equipment failure. Having a consistent and well-trained team assisting with these procedures will help to reduce this risk. Another reported cause for conversion is prolonged operative time. One guideline that may help the initiate maintain enthusiasm for the

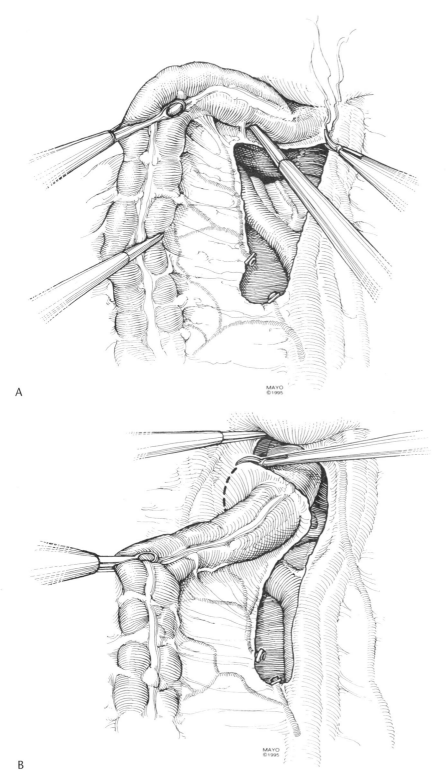

A

B

Figure 47-9.   Rectal dissection. (**A**) Use of the 30-degree laparoscope often facilitates exposure in a deep and narrow pelvis. (**B**) Cautery dissection follows the same planes as for open proctectomy. (From Thibault and Nelson,[71] by permission of Mayo Foundation.)

Table 47-1. Laparoscopic-Assisted Colectomy: Safety

| Author | No. of Patients | Complications | | Mortality (%) |
		No. of Patients	%	
Phillips et al., 1992[6]	51	4	8	2
Falk et al., 1993[10]	66	13	24	0
Peters and Bartels, 1993[5]	28	3	13	3.6
Dean et al., 1994[12]	122	13	11	0
Hoffman et al., 1994[3]	80	16	23	0
Totals	347	49	14	0.6

procedure is an early converting rule. The author typically has someone monitoring the clock and if progress in the bowel resection is not evident within 30 to 40 minutes, conversion is strongly considered.

If any time during the procedure a serious complication arises, converting to open surgery is advised. Many complications may be managed using laparoscopic techniques; therefore, it is up to the surgeon to distinguish between complications requiring conversion and those managed confidently without conversion. It is important to remember that conversion to open surgery should not be considered as a failure or complication, by surgeon or patient. If patients are properly counseled on the risks and reasons for conversion prior to surgery, most will accept the necessity for open surgery; that conversion is possible and safety a priority often provides reassurance.

Finally, a number of disease-related factors may influence the ability to complete the procedure using laparoscopic techniques. As described above, the purpose of the procedure may be defeated if the minimal access wound has to be enlarged, beyond 10 cm, to accommodate a large bulky inflammatory phlegmon or bulky tumor. Such disease processes may also render the procedure less feasible due to the obscuring of normal anatomy. If the left ureter can not be confidently identified when a large sigmoid lesion is being removed, conversion is appropriate. Variants in anatomy have also been reported as cause for conversion. Last but not least is the problem of laparoscopic tumor localization. As discussed above, it may be neces-

sary to supplement colonoscopic localization in some cases to avoid the embarassment of resecting normal bowel.

Proficiency and Applicability

A broader and more important issue of feasibility concerns whether laparoscopic bowel resection is feasible for all surgical practices. The time and expense required for proper training must not be underestimated.[33–35] In addition, laparoscopic bowel resection may not be appropriate in all cases; in fact, its purported merits have not been rigorously tested. Although only time will tell, most experts consider this technique viable and, furthermore, predict that it is destined to become part of colorectal surgical practices.[36]

CLINICAL RESULTS

Patient Benefits

It has been anticipated that patient-related advantages, as described for laparoscopic cholecystectomy, may be realized with laparoscopic bowel resection. This has generally been true. Reports on laparoscopic bowel resection describe more rapid return of bowel function and oral intake, and consequently reduced lengths of hospital stay (Table 47-3). That postoperative hospital stays can be reduced to 2 days shatters preconceptions that postoperative ileus is anastomosis dependent.[37] However, reasons for reduced length of postoperative ileus are not clear and may relate to reductions in postoperative pain, narcotic usage,[38] and operative bowel handling or to improvements in patient status and sense of well-being.[7] Experimental animal data demonstrating reductions in all phases of ileus, from gastric to colonic, with laparoscopic compared with open bowel resection strongly suggest physiologic rather than psychological bases for these clinical findings.[39]

Physiologic Measures of Outcome

Other physiologic measures that corroborate findings of more rapid return of bowel function include nitrogen balance studies and immune studies. In a comparative study of 10 open colecto-

Table 47-2. Laparoscopic-Assisted Colectomy (LAC): Operative Times (min)

| Author | No. of Patients | LAC | | Open |
		Completed	Converted	
Vayer et al., 1993[11]	38	196	—	167
Senagore et al., 1993[7]	38	174	204	126
Dean et al., 1994[12]	122	129	114	—
Hoffman et al., 1994[3]	80	221	244	183
Saba et al., 1995[51]	25	127	157	120
Tate et al., 1993[38]	11	205	—	123

Table 47-3. Laparoscopic Colectomy (LAC): Functional Outcomes and Length of Stay (days)

| Author | No. of Patients | Bowel Function[a] | | Hospital Stay | |
		LAC	Open	LAC	Open
Hoffman et al., 1994[3]	80	2[b]	4[b]	5.2	7.8
Peters and Bartels, 1993[5]	28	2.3	3.7	4.8	8.2
		2.3[b]	4.6[b]		
Senagore et al., 1993[7]	38	3	4.9	6	9.9
Saba et al., 1995[51]	25	1.1	3.9	3.6	8.1
		2.5[b]	5[b]		
Tate et al., 1993[38]	11	2.5	3.6	12.3	14.3
Falk et al., 1993[10]	66	—	—	5[c]	8

[a] Oral intake, unless otherwise specified.
[b] Flatus.
[c] Length of stay estimated from Figure 3 in the study by Falk et al., right and sigmoid combined.

mies and 9 LACS, Senagore and colleagues[40] found that urinary nitrogen losses were similar; however, significantly more LAC patients reached positive nitrogen balance on postoperative day 3.[40] Studies of interleukin-6, which rises in proportion to the degree of trauma, also support the hypothesis that surgical stress may be lessened with laparoscopic bowel resection.[41]

Whether these short-term advantages are paralleled by long-term advantages remains to be determined. One difference that could theoretically be significant is that of adhesion-related complications. In a prospective randomized trial, the occurrence of late adhesive formation, confirmed at second look laparoscopy, was significantly lower (10%) in patients who had undergone laparoscopic appendectomy compared with laparotomy and appendectomy (80%).[42] This reduction in adhesions may translate into reductions in the frequency of late obstructive ileus, which variably affects 5 to 15% of patients.[42,43] Current prospective trials will determine whether adhesion-related complications are reduced with laparoscopic large bowel resection.[44]

Finally, whether patients in poor health will fare better with minimal access colon and rectal surgery needs to be defined as it was for laparoscopic cholecystectomy. It has previously been noted that both morbidity and mortality rates are reduced in high-risk patients undergoing laparoscopic cholecystectomy.[45,46] Even though laparoscopic cholecystectomy has been advocated for use in elderly and high American Society of Anesthesiologists classification patients, this is not yet advised for LAC.

CONTROVERSIES

The resolution of two essential controversies is pivotal to the eventual success of laparoscopic colectomy. First and foremost to be resolved are concerns regarding cancer outcomes and second are concerns regarding cost effectiveness.

Cancer Issues

Most would agree that palliative laparoscopic bowel procedures are acceptable in patients with cancers beyond hope of surgical cure; however, such is not true for curable lesions. Debate regarding the appropriateness of laparoscopic bowel resection in curable cancer focuses on two essential issues. First, are laparoscopic and open bowel resections comparable cancer procedures? Second, does the technique of laparoscopy itself adversely influence patterns of recurrence?

Traditional goals of colectomy for cancer include examination for detection of metastatic disease; minimal tumor handling to prevent tumor dissemination; proximal vascular pedicle ligation for adequate lymphatic sampling; and wide bowel margins to prevent anastomotic recurrence. Staging information derives from both the macroscopic examination for intra-abdominal metastases and microscopic examination for lymphatic metastases. The challenge for laparoscopic surgery is to prove that accurate staging and adequate margins are provided.

Since laparoscopy does not afford opportunity for parenchymal hepatic evaluation, additional staging studies must supplement laparoscopic bowel resection. Two approaches are considered: first, the preoperative application of abdominal CT scans and second, the intraoperative use of ultrasound probes. CT of the abdomen, with a reported negative predictive value of 90%[47]

and a sensitivity of 100% compared with surgery,[48] should accurately supplement laparoscopic bowel resection. For those who do not routinely perform preoperative CT scans, the cost of this additional test must be considered in the cost-effectiveness equation. Although less experience is reported for laparoscopic ultrasonography (none in the setting of colorectal cancer), some enthusiasts have found success with these new devices. In a series of 43 patients with liver lesions destined for hepatic resection, the application of laparoscopic ultrasound increased the rate of resectability from 58% to 93%.[49]

The adequacy of lymph node sampling for staging purposes has been thoroughly addressed in both experimental and clinical studies. In a porcine model using mesenteric lymphangiography, no differences were noted in length of bowel resected, total number of nodes resected, number of labeled nodes resected, or number of unresected labeled nodes, when laparoscopic and open bowel resections were compared.[50] Clinical studies comparing lymph node harvests from open and laparoscopic approaches also demonstrate essentially no difference (Table 47-4).

Based on the results of lymphadenectomy specimens, it would be expected that extent of bowel margins would be similar in the two procedures and, in fact, they are. In keeping with the concept that laparoscopic resections should be identical to open ones, the extent of resection appears to be no different for laparoscopic versus open resection when the closest margins (5.8 cm versus 6.7 cm, respectively[3]) or lengths of bowel resections (15.7 cm versus 19.3 cm, respectively[51]) are evaluated. Whether extent of rectal resection with laparoscopic abdominoperineal resection is adequate awaits further study. One additional issue concerns resection of locally adherent (T4) cancers. In this author's opinion celiotomy with wide en bloc resection of adherent organs or structures is advised until such time as advanced laparoscopic techniques can ensure wide margins without risk of contamination.[52] Indeed, it is the issue of contamination, specifically wound contamination with laparoscopy, that has raised the greatest cause for alarm.

A number of reports announcing the occurrence of wound or trocar site tumors following laparoscopic bowel resection for malignancy have caused great concern. Although most laparoscopy-related wound recurrences are provided as anecdotal case reports,[53–59] a few reports do provide incidence figures. In the largest series of 208 patients undergoing bowel surgery for malignancy, registry data identified three cases of port or extraction

Table 47-4. Lymph Node Sampling for Laparoscopic Versus Open Colectomy

Author	No. of Lymph Nodes	
	Laparoscopic	Open
Peters and Bartels, 1993[5]	9.0	8.5
Falk et al., 1993[10]	14	9
Ota, 1995[69]	8.8	18.8
Hoffman et al., 1994[3]	8.0	6.1
Lacy et al., 1995[32]	12.7	12.8
Saba et al., 1995[51]	6	10
Fine et al., 1995[70]	8.7–10	10
Tate et al., 1993[38]	10	13

site recurrences for an overall incidence of 1.44%.[60] By contrast, the smallest series (14 cases for malignancy) reports the same number of recurrences (three), for an incidence of 21%.[61] Less extreme is the 3.5% incidence reported by Boulez and Herriot.[62] Critical of course is the comparison of these figures with those for comparable open colectomy.

The perception that wound recurrence does not occur with open surgery is not supported by the literature. The incidence of wound recurrence in fact depends on the time point examined (i.e., at first recurrence or at death with recurrence) and the rigor of the method of examination (clinical or autopsy). The incidence of wound recurrence using clinical methods of detection is reported to be between 0.6% and 2.5%.[63–65] When a series of patients subjected to second or symptomatic look laparotomy for colorectal cancer were examined for sites of recurrence, the incidence of wound implants was between 3.3% and 5.3%.[66,67] This same phenomenon was noted in a recent evaluation of 623 patients with recurrence in a series of 1,711 patients with curative colorectal cancer. Whereas the detection rate based on clinical examination alone was 1%, it was 3.4% in those undergoing laparotomy.[63] Finally, at the time of death, wound involvement based on autopsy findings is reported to be as high as 16.6%.[68]

It is evident from the reports noted above that in addition to great variability of reporting for wound involvement with laparoscopic colectomy, there is also great variability for open colectomy. The degree of variability suggests that not only is the risk of wound recurrence multifactorial, but so also is the risk of detection. This makes the comparison of studies very difficult and justifies the need for controlled trials.[44] If, in the meantime, the "clinical" incidence of wound recurrence for open versus laparoscopic surgery is considered, then the rate of wound involvement with laparoscopic surgery varies from comparable, at 1.4%,[60] to unreasonable, at 21%.[61] Although it would seem logical that such descrepant results must be due to either tumor or treatment-related factors, it is another matter to sort this out with current data. To resolve this issue, enthusiasts for the laparoscopic procedure are encouraged to participate in prospective trials.[69] In the United States, at least one large multi-institutional phase III trial is under way. With the intent of examining many factors (cancer outcomes, recurrence, and survival; safety, morbidity, and mortality; quality of life; and costs), 1,200 patients will be randomly assigned in this trial to undergo open colectomy versus LAC.[44]

COSTS

Anticipated cost savings, based on reductions in length of hospital stay, have not been universally realized for laparoscopic bowel resection as they have been for laparoscopic cholecystectomy. Results are mixed, with some reports describing higher and others describing lower costs associated with laparoscopic bowel surgery. Early on, total hospital costs were typically higher for laparoscopic colectomy, especially if converted and completed laparoscopic cases were analyzed together.[11] When examined independently, completed laparoscopic colectomies were cost competitive ($12,131) with open colectomies ($14,449), and converted cases were more expensive ($17,583).[7] Since cost reductions from expedited recovery are counterbalanced by increased costs generated in the operating room, high conversion rates offset overall potential gains.

Costs associated with laparoscopic colorectal surgery will likely soon become more competitive based on reductions in conversion rates and reductions in operating room costs. Operating room charges are typically higher for laparoscopic cases because of the additional time and equipment required for these cases.[3,51] With experience, operating times more closely approximate those of open bowel surgery. Further reductions are expected as better reusable equipment becomes available.

SUMMARY

Laparoscopic-assisted bowel resection, utilizing laparoscopic techniques for exploration, mobilization, and vascular pedicle ligation, together with extracorporeal techniques of resection and anastomosis, is feasible. Reports to date suggest that such resections can be accomplished safely and efficiently. It is apparent that both operative times and rates of conversion are experience dependent. Patient-related advantages, such as reductions in length of ileus and hospital stay are consistently reported, but do not yet translate into consistent cost savings. Although many colon and rectal diseases may be treated using laparoscopic techniques, considerable controversy still exists regarding the application of this technique to malignancy. Results from phase III trials will help to resolve this issue. Such results will be pivotal to the general acceptance of laparoscopic surgery for treatment of diseases of the colon and rectum.

REFERENCES

1. Wexner SD, Johansen OB, Nogueras JJ, Jagelman DG (1992) Laparoscopic total abdominal colectomy: a prospective trial. Dis Colon Rectum 35:651–655
2. Corbitt JD Jr (1992) Preliminary experience with laparoscopic-guided colectomy. Surg Laparosc Endosc 2:79–81
3. Hoffman GC, Baker JW, Fitchett CW, Vansant JH (1994) Laparoscopic-assisted colectomy: initial experience. Ann Surg 219:732–743
4. Milsom JW, Lavery IC, Church JM et al (1994) Use of laparoscopic techniques in colorectal surgery: preliminary study. Dis Colon Rectum 37:215–218
5. Peters WR, Bartels TL (1993) Minimally invasive colectomy: are the potential benefits realized? Dis Colon Rectum 36:751–756
6. Phillips EH, Franklin M, Carroll BJ et al (1992) Laparoscopic colectomy. Ann Surg 216:703–707
7. Senagore AJ, Luchtefeld MA, MacKeigan JM, Mazier WP (1993) Open colectomy versus laparoscopic colectomy: are there differences? Am Surg 59:549–554
8. Jacobs M, Verdeja JC, Goldstein HS (1991) Minimally invasive colon resection (laparoscopic colectomy). Surg Laparosc Endosc 1:144–150
9. Scoggin SD, Frazee RC, Synder SK et al (1993) Laparoscopic-assisted bowel surgery. Dis Colon Rectum 36:747–750

10. Falk PM, Beart RW Jr, Wexner SD et al (1993) Laparoscopic colectomy: a critical appraisal. Dis Colon Rectum 36:28–34

11. Vayer AJ Jr, Larach SW, Williamson PR et al (1993) Cost effectiveness of laparoscopic assisted colectomy, abstracted. Dis Colon Rectum 36:P34

12. Dean PA, Beart RW Jr, Nelson H et al (1994) Laparoscopic-assisted segmental colectomy: early Mayo Clinic experience. Mayo Clin Proc 69:834–840

13. Saclarides TJ, Ko ST, Airan M et al (1991) Laparoscopic removal of a large colonic lipoma: report of a case. Dis Colon Rectum 34:1027–1029

14. Kim LH, Chung KE, AuBuchon P (1992) Laparoscopic-assisted abdominoperineal resection with pull-through (sphincter saving). Surg Laparosc Endosc 2:237–240

15. Velez PM (1993) Laparoscopic colonic and rectal resection. Baillieres Clin Gastroenterol 7:867–878

16. Rehman SU (1993) Laparoscopic abdominoperineal resection of the rectum. Br J Surg 80:1080.

17. Sackier JM (1993) Laparoscopic abdominoperineal resection of the rectum (letter, comment). Br J Surg 80:1349.

18. Chindasub S, Charntaracharmnong C, Nimitvanit C et al (1994) Laparoscopic abdominoperineal resection. J Laparoendosc Surg 4:17–21

19. Geis WP, Kim C (1994) Improved efficiency in laparoscopic abdominoperineal resection: the Kim-Geis approach. Int Surg 79:226–227

20. Larach SW, Salomon MC, Williamson PR, Goldstein E (1993) Laparoscopic assisted abdominoperineal resection. Surg Laparosc Endosc 3:115–118

21. Evans RM, Hulbert JC, Reddy PK (1992) Complications of laparoscopy. Semin Urol 10:164–168

22. Safran DB, Orlando R III (1994) Physiologic effects of pneumoperitoneum. Am J Surg 167:281–285

23. Monson JRT, Darzi A, Carey PD, Guillou PJ (1992) Prospective evaluation of laparoscopic-assisted colectomy in an unselected group of patients. Lancet 340:831–833

24. Elftmann TD, Nelson H, Ota DM et al (1994) Laparoscopic-assisted segmental colectomy: surgical techniques. Mayo Clin Proc 69:825–833

25. Hasson HM (1978) Open laparoscopy vs. closed laparoscopy: a comparison of complication rates. Adv Planned Parenthood 13:41–50

26. Donohue JH, Grant CS, Farnell MB, van Heerden JA (1992) Laparoscopic cholecystectomy: operative technique. Mayo Clin Proc 67:441–448

27. Akwari OE, Kelly KA (1980) Anterior resection for adenocarcinoma of the distal large bowel. Am J Surg 139:88–94

28. Rouffet F, Hay JM, Vacher B et al (1994) Curative resection for left colonic carcinoma: hemicolectomy vs. segmental colectomy. A prospective, controlled, multicenter trial. The French Association for Surgical Research. Dis Colon Rectum 37:651–659

29. Dodson RW, Cullado MJ, Tangen LE, Bonello JC (1993) Laparoscopic-assisted abdominoperineal resection. Contemp Surg 42:42–44

30. Fuhrman GM, Ota DM (1994) Laparoscopic intestinal stomas. Dis Colon Rectum 37:444–449

31. Slim K, Pezet D, Stencl J Jr et al (1994) Prospective analysis of 40 initial laparoscopic colorectal resections: a plea for a randomized trial. J Laparoendosc Surg 4:241–245

32. Lacy AM, Garciá-Valdecasas JC, Delgado S et al (1995) Laparoscopic versus conventional surgery in colon cancer: preliminary results of a prospective and randomized trial. Surg Endosc 9:216

33. See WA, Cooper CS, Fisher RJ (1993) Predictors of laparoscopic complications after formal training in laparoscopic surgery. JAMA 170:2689–2692

34. Society of American Gastrointestinal Endoscopic Surgeons (1991) Granting of privileges for laparoscopic general surgery. Am J Surg 161:324–325

35. Soper NJ, Brunt LM, Kerbl K (1994) Laparoscopic general surgery. N Engl J Med 330:409–419

36. Beart RW Jr, Ballantyne G, Fleshman JW Jr et al (1994) Laparoscopic considerations in colon and rectal surgery. Perspect Colon Rectal Surg 7:245–263

37. Bardram L, Funch-Jensen P, Jensen P et al (1995) Recovery after laparoscopic colonic surgery with epidural analgesia, and early oral nutrition and mobilisation. Lancet 345:763–764

38. Tate JJT, Kwok S, Dawson JW et al (1993) Prospective comparison of laparoscopic and conventional anterior resection. Br J Surg 80:1396–1398

39. Davies W, Tu Q, Kollmorgen C et al (1995) Duration of postoperative ileus after laparoscopic and open segmental colectomy, abstracted. Gastroenterology 108:A1217

40. Senagore AJ, Kilbride MJ, Luchtefeld MA et al (1995) Superior nitrogen balance after laparoscopic-assisted colectomy. Ann Surg 221:171–175

41. Harmon G, Senagore A, Kilbride M et al (1993) Cortisol and IL-6 response attenuated following laparoscopic colectomy, abstracted. Surg Endosc 7:121

42. DeWilde RL (1991) Goodbye to late bowel obstruction after appendicectomy, abstracted. Lancet 338:1012

43. Dozois RR (1986) Restorative proctocolectomy and ileal reservoir. Mayo Clin Proc 61:283–286

44. Nelson H, Weeks JC, Wieand HS (1995) Proposed phase III trial comparing laparoscopic-assisted colectomy versus open colectomy for colon cancer. J Natl Cancer Insti Monogr 19:51–56

45. Massie MT, Massie LB, Marrangoni AG et al (1993) Advantages of laparoscopic cholecystectomy in the elderly and in patients with high ASA classifications. J Laparoendosc Surg 3:467–476

46. Feldman MG, Russell JC, Lynch JT, Mattie A (1994) Comparison of mortality rates for open and closed cholecystectomy in the elderly: Connecticut in statewide survey. J Laparoendosc Surg 4:165–172

47. Cance WG, Cohen AM, Enker WE, Sigurdson ER (1991) Predictive value of a negative computed tomographic scan in 100 patients with rectal carcinoma. Dis Colon Rectum 34:748–751

48. Fischer KS, Zamboni WA, Ross DS (1990) The efficacy of preoperative computed tomography in patients with colorectal carcinoma. The American Surgeon 56:339–342

49. John TG, Greig JD, Crosbie JL et al (1994) Superior staging of liver tumors with laparoscopy and laparoscopic ultrasound. Ann Surg 220:711–719

50. Cataldo PA, Hadick C, Resnikov P et al (1993) Laparoscopic vs. open colorectal resections for malignancy: assessment of lymphatic resection by mesenteric lymphangiography, abstracted. Dis Colon Rectum 36:33

51. Saba AK, Kerlakian GM, Kasper GC, Hearn AT (1995) Lapar-

oscopic assisted colectomies versus open colectomy. J Laparoendosc Surg 5:1–6

52. Orkin BA, Dozois RR, Beart RW Jr et al (1989) Extended resection for locally advanced primary adenocarcinoma of the rectum. Dis Colon Rectum 32:286–292

53. Alexander RJR, Jaques BC, Mitchell KG (1993) Laparoscopically assisted colectomy and wound recurrence. Lancet 341: 249–250

54. Walsh DCA, Wattchow DA, Wilson TG (1993) Subcutaneous metastases after laparoscopic resection of malignancy. Aust NZ J Surg 63:563–565

55. Fusco MA, Paluzzi MW (1993) Abdominal wall recurrence after laparoscopic-assisted colectomy for adenocarcinoma of the colon: report of a case. Dis Colon Rectum 36:858–861

56. Guillou PJ, Darzi A, Monson JRT (1993) Experience with laparoscopic colorectal surgery for malignant disease. Surg Oncol, suppl. 1, 2:43–49

57. O'Rourke N, Price PM, Kelly S, Sikora K (1993) Tumour inoculation during laparoscopy, letter; comment. Lancet 342: 368

58. Cirocco WC, Schwartzman A, Golub RW (1994) Abdominal wall recurrence after laparoscopic colectomy for colon cancer. Surgery 116:842–846

59. Nduka CC, Monson JRT, Menzies-Gow N, Darzi A (1994) Abdominal wall metastases following laparoscopy. Br J Surg 81:648–552

60. Ramos JM, Gupta S, Anthone GJ et al (1994) Laparoscopy and colon cancer: is the port site at risk? A preliminary report. Arch Surg 129:897–899

61. Berends FJ, Kazemier G, Bonjer HJ, Lange JF (1994) Subcutaneous metastases after laparoscopic colectomy, letter. Lancet 344:58

62. Boulez J, Herriot E (1994) Multicentric analysis of laparoscopic colorectal surgery in FDCL group: 274 cases. Br J Surg 81:527

63. Reilly WT, Nelson H, Schroeder G et al (1996) Wound recurrence following conventional treatment of colorectal cancer: a rare but perhaps underestimated problem. Dis Colon Rectum 39:200–207

64. Hughes ES, McDermott FT, Polglase AL, Johnson WR (1983) Tumor recurrence in the abdominal wall scar tissue after large-bowel cancer surgery. Dis Colon Rectum 26:571–572

65. Cass AW, Million RR, Pfaff WW (1976) Patterns of recurrence following surgery alone for adenocarcinoma of the colon and rectum. Cancer 37:2861–2865

66. Gunderson LL, Sosin H (1974) Areas of failure found at reoperation (second or symptomatic look) following "curative surgery" for adenocarcinoma of the rectum: clinicopathologic correlation and implications for adjuvant therapy. Cancer 34: 1278–1292

67. Gunderson LL, Sosin H, Sevitt S (1985) Extrapelvic colon—areas of failure in a reoperation series: implications for adjuvant therapy. Int J Radiat Oncol Biol Phys 11:731–741

68. Welch JP, Donaldson GA (1979) The clinical correlation of an autopsy study of recurrent colorectal cancer. Ann Surg 189: 496–502

69. Ota DM (1995) Laparoscopic colectomy for cancer: a favorable opinion. Ann Surg Oncol 2:3–5

70. Fine AP, Lanasa S, Gannon MP (1995) Laparoscopic colon surgery: report of a series. Am Surg 61:412–416

71. Thibault, Nelson (199X) Laparoscopic abdominoperineal resection for malignancy. In Cosgrove J (ed): Minimally Invasive Surgery: Principles and Outcomes. Harwood Academic Publishers

48

STOMAS

John M. MacKeigan

HISTORY

The earliest stomas were fecal fistulae resulting from war, trauma, or strangulated intestine.[1] Surgical intervention for the relief of obstruction was described in Aristotle's time (384–322 BC). Incisions were made to relieve the obstruction, but the results of the interventions were not described. In 1776 Pilore performed a cecostomy for an obstructing carcinoma, but the patient died on the 28th postoperative day from perforation of the rectal cancer. In the 1800s, colostomy was used more liberally, with frequent debate on the value of a lumbar colostomy to avoid transperitoneal contamination or inguinal stomas. Amussat reported on 29 patients with colostomy, 21 with imperforate anus. Twenty patients died, which he attributed to peritonitis. He considered the lumbar colostomy to be preferable in an effort to avoid the transperitoneal route.[2] In 1852, Hawkins reported on 44 patients noting no difference in results whether a transperitoneal or lumbar colostomy was utilized.[3]

Although von Mikulicz is credited with describing resection and exteriorization of the intestine, the techniques were suggested and described in 1798 by Schmalkalden.[4] In 1828 Dupuytren[5] described a clamp and a method of reanastomosing the two ends of the stoma. In 1903, von Mikulicz[6] described his method and ultimately reported on 16 patients on whom he used a two-stage procedure. Again, it was not von Mikulicz who did the first elective colon resection. It was performed at Guys Hospital in London in 1882 by Thomas Bryant[7] utilizing a double-barreled colostomy.

Resection with closure of the distal end of the colon (Hartmann procedure) may have first been performed by Martini in 1879. The method was further used in the late 1800s and continues as an appropriate management of resections deemed to require a colostomy.[8] Loop colostomy was first reported by Madyl in 1888 using a rigid rod passed beneath a loop colostomy to prevent retraction.[9] Since then, little has changed except the material and the increasing use of loop ileostomies (with or without a supporting rod).

Ileostomy

The first ileostomy accompanied a resection of a right colon cancer in 1879 by Baum[10] in Germany. The wider use of ileostomy grew out of the failure of cecostomy[11] and appendicostomy[12] with irrigation to improve ulcerative colitis. In 1912, Brown[13] (from St. Louis) described ileostomy after failure of cecotomy and irrigation for a number of disorders from colitis to cancer and obstruction. The unmatured stoma was drained by a catheter maintained in the stoma.[13] The stoma protruded 2 to 3 inches from the lower end of the incision. Brown[13] advocated this treatment for ulcerative colitis, and it gained in popularity as a treatment of last resort in the early half of this century.

The ileostomy created in this fashion caused serositis, scarring, and stenosis with dysfunction. Skin grafting of the stoma was tried as an alternative and to create a nipple for better skin control.[14] Brooke[15] is credited with suggesting direct maturing of the stoma to prevent serositis. At the same time, Crile[16] had suggested a similar method but with removal of the distal muscle and folding over of the mucosa. Turnbull and Crile[16] defined ileostomy dysfunction and its management with catheter drainage. Rupert Turnbull has to be credited with advancing the understanding and acceptance of stomas. He refined techniques, developed early stomal therapist education, and inspired surgeons to be aware of many aspects of management. With the use of karaya, plastic appliances, and stoma adhesive, the life of the stoma patient was advanced significantly.

Continent Stomas

Various methods were tried beginning in 1888 with Maydl to develop a sphincter for a colostomy.[9] Methods included muscle-splitting incisions, torsion of the stoma, plication of circular muscles of the colon, rectus muscle sphincters, and use of the ileocecal valve in the reversed position. Others used tunneling of the stoma through the abdominal wall with external pressure or developed a skin-grafted tube amenable to compression or folding.

In 1969, Nils Kock[17] developed an internal ileal reservoir drained periodically through the abdominal wall. Various methods have been developed to create a continent nipple and to minimize complications of leakage, obstruction and infection. The Kock pouch has a particular place for the ileostomy patient for whom the ileoanal pouch may not be appropriate or who has significant abdominal scarring or allergies, making appliances difficult to maintain in place.

PHYSIOLOGY

A distal colostomy may initially cause increased volume; it then adapts and approximates normal feces in amount and consistency. A proximal stoma has all the disadvantages of increased volume, with increased water and sodium loss.

With an ileostomy, the physiologic volume and solute changes are different from those of the normal ileum. The normal ileum presents 1,000 to 2,000 ml of fluid to the colon, which is then reabsorbed enough to provide 100 to 200 ml of fluid volume in normal feces. Early ileostomies discharge 1,000 to 1,800 ml of fluid a day but soon settle to 200 to 700 ml a day. Fasting may cause further reductions to 50 to 100 ml a day. Volume is increased with fiber and fruit content and inflammatory conditions such as Crohn's disease. A partial obstruction from ileal stenosis, serositis, or food bolus may cause an increased water output, which has been termed ileostomy dysfunction.

Although the colon probably plays some role in maintaining nutrition, with bacterial degradation of carbohydrates and proteins, its role in all but the chronically malnourished is probably small. Certainly, following proctocolectomy, most patients improve their nutritional status with improved health. The ileostomy patient seems to maintain nitrogen balance unless other reasons for malabsorption exist such as mucosal enzyme deficiencies, other resections, or recurrent disease.

The transit time of the small intestine is increased above normal in ileostomy patients.[18] The reason for this phenomenon is not apparent, but it may be partially explained by the ileal epithelial hypertrophy that occurs secondary to ileostomy construction. Sodium transport across the epithelium governs water absorption. Increased aldosterone levels have been proposed as "a means of mediating ileal fluid composition."[19] The total volume of body water and sodium is reduced in ileostomy patients. The average sodium losses are 60 mEq/day and are normally less than 10 mEq/day in the stool. Potassium losses are 6 to 12 mEq/day, and nitrogen losses are 1.5gm/day. Calcium and magnesium losses are generally not significantly affected.[19,20]

The bacterial count of the effluent in the ileostomy patient is increased many times, and the coliforms are increased 2,500 times but are still less than normal stool.[21] The systemic effects of ileostomies are known to include increased urinary calculi, particularly with high-output stomas. Approximately 60% of the calculi are composed of uric acid.

The incidence of gallstones remains controversial. Studies have suggested no difference in incidence[21] to a threefold increase.[22,23]

The physiologic changes of a continent pouch have been extensively studied and are beyond the scope of this chapter. Most patients have no major physiologic problems, but the pouch environment itself is one of continued study. The role of bacteria, short-chain fatty acids, ileal content, and stasis in short-term problems such as mucosal inflammation ("pouchitis") or long-term problems are yet to be well defined.[19,24]

CONSTRUCTION

The construction of a stoma should begin with good education of the patient. The possibility of a need for a stoma should be discussed. A nurse with a special interest or training in stoma care should be involved early in the process. Support groups (United Ostomy Association, Crohn's and Colitis Foundation) may be a good resource. Contact with other patients who have stomas is valuable. Involvement of other family members is of immense help in the education and adjustment process.

The location of the stoma greatly influences acceptance, quality of life, and management problems. Preoperatively, sites are marked with the patient lying, sitting, and standing. Multiple sites may be marked to cover eventualities. When a stoma is constructed unexpectedly, one should tend to place it cephalad, especially in the obese, to allow less difficulty visualizing it below a protuberance or fold. Paramedian incisions should be avoided, when possible, to avoid placing stomas in surgical scars. Placement of a stoma in the primary incision should be avoided when possible. Locations over flat, smooth skin and generally overlying rectus muscle are preferred (Fig. 48-1). Sites can be chosen with an effort to avoid scars, folds, ribs, iliac crests, the pubis, and the umbilicus. The quality of the skin is important; radiated areas and skin grafts should be avoided when possible.[25] Alternative sites include the upper rectus, umbilicus, and (rarely) the lumbar regions. Consideration should be given to issues of obesity, physical disability, and radiation. Continent stomas may be placed lower for cosmetic purposes.

Figure 48-1. Preferred sites for stoma formation.

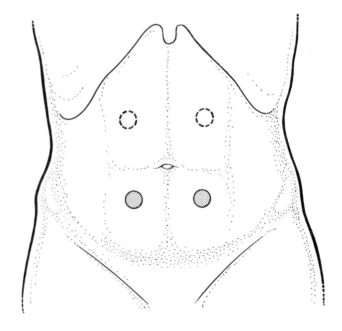

Basic surgical principles are observed, avoiding tension and ensuring good vascularity. The site should properly align openings in the skin, fascia, and peritoneum. The opening generally admits two fingers. Allowances may have to be made for larger intestinal diameters or excess pericolonic fat. The extremely obese may require a loop stoma instead of an end stoma to avoid tension and ensure better vascular supply.

Excess redundancy is to be avoided in the intraperitoneal portion. Controversy exists on the need for peritoneal fixation of the mesentery. I prefer to fix the ileal mesentery to the anterior abdominal wall toward the falciform ligament, to reduce torsion around the site and perhaps lessen prolapse. The end colostomy may be secured to the lateral peritoneum or tunneled under the peritoneum for the same reasons and perhaps to reduce herniation.[26,27]

Maturation of the stoma in the operation room helps to prevent serositis and subsequent stenosis. Three or four primary sutures are placed initially to create moderate eversion or a nipple in the ileostomy and mild eversion in the colostomy (Fig. 48-2). Liquid effluent in proximal stomas require more eversion. Appliances are affixed in the operating room or soon thereafter.

The construction of a good quality stoma requires time and attention to detail. This will provide a stoma that will fit better and will provide a better overall quality of life and acceptance.

TYPES

With the increasing use of resection for obstructive colonic disease, there has been less need for an initial loop stoma for fecal diversion. Stapling devices have facilitated subsequent closures of end stomas to rectal stumps. Better stoma appliances have facilitated stoma care and helped to advance the use of loop ileostomies for diversion. Loop ileostomies are generally easier for patients to manage than loop colostomies. Subsequent surgical options on the remaining colon are not as compromised with a loop ileostomy.

Diverting Stomas

Diverting stomas may be utilized at any point but are most common in the terminal ileum, transverse colon, and sigmoid colon. A portion of intestine with the involved segment or mesentery is exteriorized and matured. The resulting loop is utilized in surgery for inflammatory disease, trauma, and cancer. It allows easier control of distal disease or surgery and is generally used for temporary purposes. Common uses are for fecal diversion of obstructions, inflammatory conditions, or anastomoses. Such loops allow relatively simpler closure through a smaller incision. These advantages have popularized the loop stoma along with the realization that loop stomas divert fairly completely, at least for the first few months.[28–30]

Winslet et al.[31] showed that loop stomas do not generally spill over to the distal limb. Loop ileostomies had almost complete diversion, despite the relative orientation of the limbs. Retracted stomas tended to be less diverting, but only approximately 15% of the time. Similarly, colostomy stomas may be less diverting, as they tend to retract periodically. Loop stomas present longer than 3 months tend to divert less completely.[30]

Fecal diversion does not prevent subsequent complications, as demonstrated by Fielding et al.[32] in a large series of patients undergoing anterior resection. The diversion may reduce the level of septic complications and consequences and may allow earlier controlled corrective measures. The increased use of pri-

Figure 48-2. (**A & B**) Eversion technique for ileostomy.

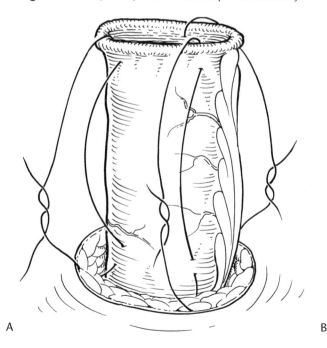

A

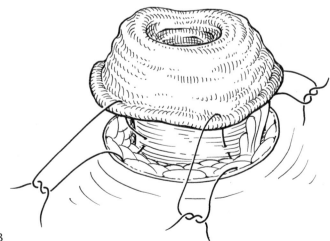

B

mary resection, colonic cleansing, and primary repair of trauma has reduced the need for diversion. Better controlled studies are needed to define the advantages or disadvantages of combined procedures with stomas.

Care in construction and selection of the site should be taken, as 40 to 60% of loop stomas may become permanent. The patient's medical condition, life expectancy, or personal preference may alter a decision for intended closure.[33-35]

If a choice is possible between loop ileostomy or loop colostomy, the ileostomy is preferred. It is less bulky, less odorous, and easier to manage. Ileostomy stoma closure may be associated with fewer complications and infections.[29]

Loop Stomas

The principles of construction of loop ileostomy or colostomy or end-loop stomas are similar. The easier construction and closure are part of their attraction. Loop stomas may be intentionally permanent when utilized to maintain blood supply through an obese or distended abdomen where an end stoma is not possible or where vascularity of an end stoma cannot be maintained. The distal end is closed and a convenient and easily advanced proximal loop is brought to the surface and matured.[36]

The principles of construction of a loop stoma are similar to those for any stoma. The abdominal opening is similar to that of end stomas but may have to be enlarged internally to accommodate large limbs. Efforts to minimize tension help to maintain vascularity. Only in circumstances of tension are stoma rods necessary under the loop. Some prefer to tunnel the rods under the skin to assist appliance adhesion or to use fascial bridges.

The loop stomas are matured where possible. Careful construction of a prominent and protruding stoma assists skin care and appliance application. By dividing the loop near the skin level on the distal aspect of the loop, the intestine can be folded back, producing a protruding stoma. Dividing the intestine from mesenteric surface to mesenteric surface, leaving a small intervening bridge, facilitates the formation of an appropriate nipple shape. Three or four sutures are placed as in end stoma construction, to evert the bowel, (Fig. 48-3) leaving the distal limb flush with the skin and inconspicuously at the margin of the stoma. This allows for smaller stomas and face plates, with improved appearance, skin control, and patient acceptance.

Construction of a loop colostomy differs little, and the principles are similar. Dissection of the omentum from the loop makes construction easier and less bulky. As the colon is already large, dividing near the skin level on the distal limb produces a smaller and less conspicuous limb and smaller stoma. A supporting rod may be necessary more often in loop colostomies because of their often heavy and dilated condition when obstruction is present.

In rare circumstances a "hidden" or subcutaneous loop colostomy is created proximal to a partially obstructing lesion. When further obstruction develops, the stoma is opened.

A "blow hole" stoma described by Rupert Turnbull for severe fulminating inflammatory bowel disease has few uses today. Skin level colostomies and a loop ileostomy have been utilized to decompress fulminating colitis with contained colonic perforations.[37]

End-Loop Stomas

The end-loop stoma as described by Prasad and Pearl[38] modifies the loop colostomy to a functioning end stoma and a small mucous fistula. The proximal end is matured as an end stoma and the distal segment is brought to the skin as only a portion of the diameter and sutured at skin level. A small unobtrusive mucous fistula is created and incorporated in the appliance. All the advantages of an end stoma and a loop stoma are incorporated (Fig. 48-4). This stoma is of use in the ileum or colon, or for an ileocolostomy.

The same term, *end-loop stoma*, is used for loop stomas necessitated by obesity. The end of the intestine is closed and a loop is brought up proximal to the closure. Technically, this is a loop ileostomy with a short-closed distal limb.

Complications of Loop Stomas

The metabolic complications of loop ileostomies are similar to those of end stomas. A more proximal stoma may be associated with more fluid and electrolyte losses and therefore greater risk of dehydration and sodium depletion.

The most common problems relate to skin irritation. A properly constructed loop with proper protrusion of the proximal limb will minimize the skin excoriation. Even if ileostomy output is greater, the colostomy may lead to more excoriation related to increased changes of the appliances, bulkier stomas, and less tendency to form loop colostomies with a proper spout.

Prolapse of loop stomas seems to be more common in long-standing loop colostomies. It more commonly involves the distal limb and may occur frequently with an end-loop stoma.[38] Treatment involves closure of the stoma where possible. Alternatively, continued conservative treatment, resection and separation of the limbs, or formation of an end-loop stoma may be attempted. Retraction of stomas leads to inadequate diversion and skin excoriation. Reconstruction or closure are surgical options. Small bowel obstruction may occur in 10% of patients but is infrequent with loop colostomies, in which the omentum and bulk of the mesentery and colon minimize local volvulus below the stoma or loops of intestine twisting around the stoma site.[38]

Loop Stoma Closure

Stoma closure is not a minor procedure and has significant risks and complications.[39,40] Complications of stoma closure may be as high as 50%, and wound infection rates are reported as high as 25%.[29,41,42] This is particularly the case with closure of separated limbs, for which a larger dissection, and resection are necessary. End and loop ileostomy closures both have comparable complication rates.[40] A large series of loop ileostomy closures shows an anastomotic leakage rate of 2.5% and a postoperative obstruction rate of 14% in the first month.[39] Loop ileostomy closure may have a lower complication rate when compared with loop colostomy closure.[29]

Closure of the stoma is elective, and ideal conditions should prevail. Preoperative evaluation to ensure that no distal obstruction or anastomotic leakage exists is important. Ensuring proper nutrition and resolution of all inflammatory processes is indicated. The optimal time for closure is individualized, but after 8 weeks from creation of the stoma is preferable.[42]

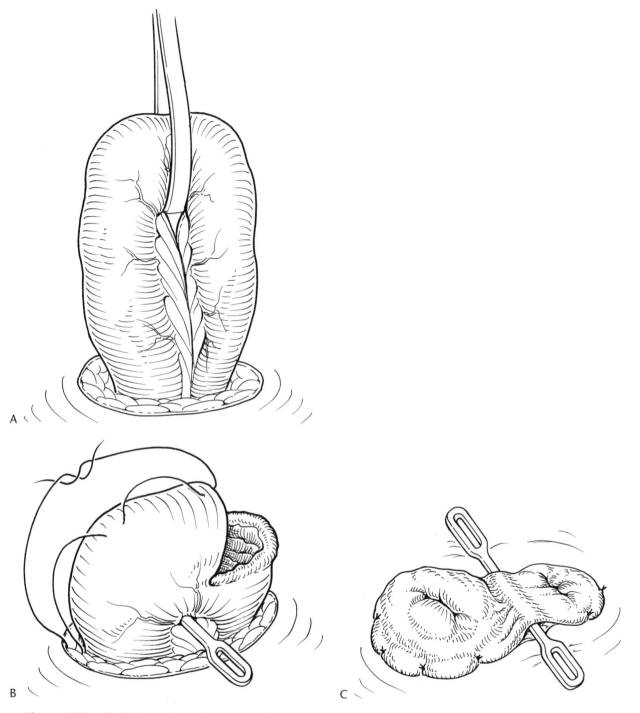

Figure 48-3. (**A–C**) Everted loop ileostomy technique.

Closure of loop ileostomies involves resection and anastomosis, which is accomplished with suturing or staples using a functional end-to-end technique. Colostomy closure involves the same technique or, alternatively, closing the anterior defect or enterostomy. Series vary on whether complications are less with either basic method. Techniques are probably less important than preserving basic principles of mobilization, good vascularity, and meticulous anastomotic technique. All methods are facilitated by closure of the stoma site early in the technique of mobilization to minimize contamination of the wound. Laparoscopic techniques currently seem to offer little assistance to what is usually a local procedure.

CECOSTOMY

Cecostomy was frequently advocated 40 to 50 years ago for a number of situations. These included distal colonic obstruction, cecal volvulus, proximal diversion for anastomoses or distal

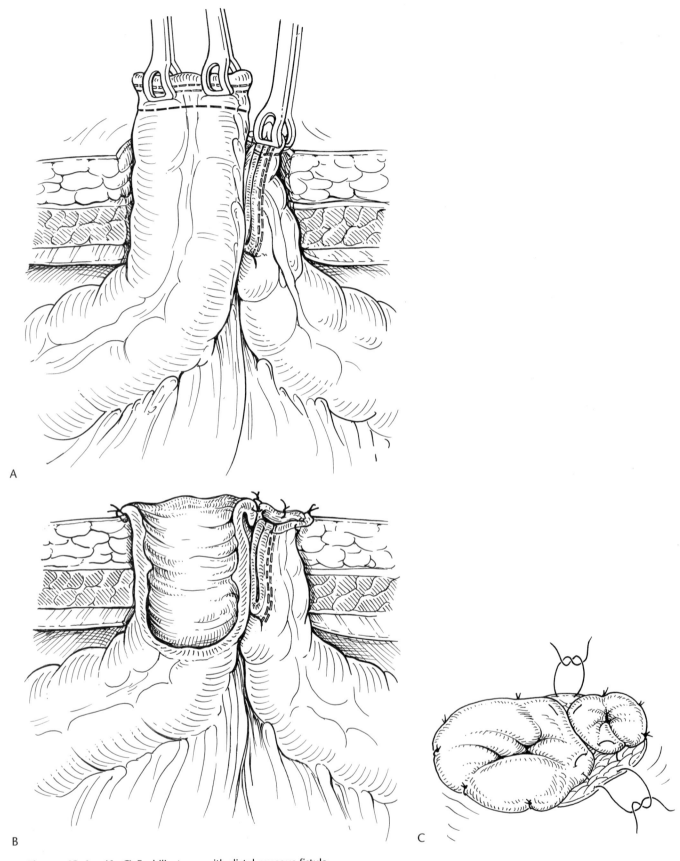

Figure 48-4. **(A–C)** End iliostomy with distal mucous fistula.

inflammation, or decompression of toxic megacolon or pseudo-obstruction. Cecostomy has had a less important role in the management of many of these clinical conditions. Resection for obstructing lesions and wider use of loop ileostomies has been partially responsible. Cecostomy, whether tube or open, rarely was diverting and was associated with significant complications.[43,44]

While series vary, cecostomy may play a role in fixation of reducible, viable cecal volvulus.[45] Decompression of pseudo-obstruction is generally accomplished endoscopically. When decompression is not possible, radiologic guided decompression cecostomy is an alternative.[46,47] Recurrent dilation may be controlled with endoscopically assisted placement, mimicking percutaneous endoscopic gastrotomy placement.

Open cecostomy with placement of a tube for exteriorization allows assessment of the integrity and vascularity of the cecum. Frequent irrigation of the tube to keep it open and functioning is required. A review of the subject by Senagore[48] gives the indications and options in detail.

MUCOUS FISTULA

The term mucous fistula refers to the use of defunctioning intestine brought to the skin as a nonfunctioning stoma. Loop stomas and end-loop stomas, by definition, have a mucous fistula. It is used for decompression of intestine with distal obstruction, to allow easier location of the efferent intestine for later resection or anastomosis, and for decompression in selected situations of questionably viable or inflamed intestine. Closed distal intestine occasionally breaks down, with leakage, particularly in severe inflammatory disease. Some surgeons prefer to decompress such intestine by creating a mucous fistula.

The separated limb of the mucous fistula should be placed well away from the primary stoma. While the mucosa fistula generally requires no appliance, if it is placed too close to an afferent functioning stoma the placement may be compromised. A small mucous fistula incorporated in a loop stoma provides no such compromise or problem. Prolapse and hernia are rare in areas of mucous fistula.

END ILEOSTOMY

End ileostomy most commonly results from proctocolectomy for inflammatory bowel disease or familial polyposis coli. Restorative ileoanal pouch procedures and continent ileostomies have lessened the need for permanent end ileostomy. Patients have no options for continent pouches in Crohn's disease with proctocolectomy. Others with particular situations, such as weak sphincters or desire to have a procedure with less complications, choose an end ileostomy. A permanent end ileostomy may be utilized rarely in severe acute ischemia or with multiple synchronous colonic carcinomas. A temporary end ileostomy may be performed when conditions of ischemia, infection, or poor nutrition do not allow anastomosis without increased risk. Occasionally the patient's overall condition does not warrant the possible anastomotic risks, and end ileostomy is performed.

The construction details of end stomas have been described in preceding sections. The obese may require an end-loop stoma to provide good vascular supply. A previous diverting loop ileostomy may be converted to an end-loop stoma with subse-

quent colectomy. End ileostomies created through areas of "backwash ileitis" may have a slightly thickened and larger appearance, but the mucosal inflammatory reaction reverts to normal mucosa in a few days. A technique of myotomies in two directions was described by Turnbull to create a quieter stoma and to lessen prolapse and retraction. This method is seldom employed but may occasionally be of use for assisting eversion of a thickened or dilated ileum.[49]

END COLOSTOMY

End colostomies are commonly sigmoid but occasionally wider resections necessitate a more proximal end stoma. An end stoma that is anticipated to be permanent and liquid, such as in the transverse colon, may be better accepted and managed as an ileostomy.

The permanent end colostomy is performed for (1) malignancy involving the distal rectum or anus or (2) benign conditions such as radiation proctitis, severe fistulae, trauma, or anal incontinence.

Temporary and colostomies may be performed for benign conditions such as inflammation, ischemia, trauma, hemorrhage, obstruction, or perforation for which anastomosis is not immediately indicated. Such conditions may be related to an inability to perform proximal bowel preparation, local conditions of infection or ischemia, or general patient conditions not warranting immediate anastomosis. Intraoperative colonic lavage has lessened some indications for temporary end colostomy. Subsequent medical conditions, patient acceptance of the stoma, or surgical difficulty with reanastomosis may force a temporary stoma to become permanent.[50,51]

The principles of stoma construction have been outlined above. Treatment of the intraperitoneal portion of the colostomy is up to the surgeon. Options include suture closure of the lateral paracolic gutter, simple suturing of the fascia to the colon, or extra-peritoneal tunneling of the distal portion as advocated by Goligher.[27] As with an ileostomy, immediate maturation of the colostomy is preferable using similar suture techniques but with less or minimal eversion. The use of skin staples and the end-to-end stapling device has been described but seems to offer little advantage.[52]

Complications of end colostomies are similar to those of all stomas, but less difficulty with skin irritation is seen. Patients with a distal colostomy and solid stool may be able to tolerate complications of hernia, stenosis, prolapse, and recession without the severe consequences that may occur with an ileostomy. End colostomies may lend themselves to good management with colostomy irrigation techniques to minimize gas, stool, and odor.[53,54]

CONTINENT COLOSTOMIES

Many different techniques and ideas for colostomy control or continence have been tried. Autogenous tissue grafting, implantable devices, external plug devices, or combinations of these have all been advocated.[55-61] Implantable devices generally have problems of tissue extrusion or infection. Plugging devices with expandable plugs may cause ischemic ulceration with prolonged usage. No satisfactory universal device has been devised. Patients with distal colonic stomas often have solid stool or infrequent movements, or manage the stoma with irrigation. By developing a pattern of "control" with the irrigation, many patents may opt for no appliance or a simple patch. The disadvantages of a continent device have discouraged many from their usage, particularly when they already have reasonable control with irrigation.

URINARY DIVERSION

Bricker[62] and Gilchrist et al.[63] introduced the concept of the intestine as a conduit to collect and divert urine to a stoma on the abdominal wall. Occasionally dilated ureters may be brought to the skin directly as temporary diversion. Intestinal conduits for urine collection with implantation of ureters into the intestinal segment have been created from ileum[62] or the ileal-cecal segment.[63] All the principles of a properly constructed and sited stoma pertain, to minimize irritation of the skin. Usually these procedures are performed as originally described, but any segment of the intestine may be utilized.[64] Cutaneous diversion with conduits is usually performed in patients with primary or secondary involvement of the urinary bladder with carcinoma. Neurologic or developmental disorders or radiation therapy may lead to the construction of an intestinal conduit. In the 1980s, using principles similar to those of the continent ileostomy, surgeons at the University of Indiana developed a continent collection device from an ileal-cecal segment. It is commonly termed an *Indiana pouch*.[65,66] Many others have developed other forms of continent devices.[64,67] This subject is large and beyond the scope of this chapter. Several excellent reviews are available.[64,67]

CLOSURE OF COLOSTOMIES

As previously discussed, stoma closures have significant complications. End stomas with separation of the proximal and distal ends may present a particularly difficult procedure. Reopening of the previous incision with dissection of adhesions from the previous resection or inflammation may be difficult. Waiting for maturation of scar tissue and adhesions and physiologic improvement of the patient with resolution of the underlying disorder is important. Long intervals between primary surgery and closure may lead to atrophy of the distal limb with narrowing or stenosis. The mucosal consequences of diversion colitis may be reversed using irrigation with short-chain fatty acids, which aids mucosal nutrition and integrity. Diversion colitis changes reverse spontaneously after anastomosis and bowel function.

The resected sigmoid with end colostomy and rectal stump (Hartmann's procedure) represented an even more difficult closure before the stapled end-to-end devices were introduced. Such devices have facilitated the closure. The proximal limb is closed and mobilized well and a fresh end prepared with the anvil portion of the stapling device in place. The distal end is identified and mobilized for a short distance, and the staple device is inserted transanally. The trocar is brought through the apex of the rectal stump and removed and the ends mated. The stapling device is closed, fired, opened, and removed in the usual fashion. Laparoscopy-assisted closure may offer some advantages in selected situations. Basic principles of timing, resolution of inflammation, and good technique pertain equally to laparoscopy-assisted closure.

QUALITY OF LIFE

In the modern era of surgery, with its lessened mortality rates, the mobidity of surgery and the quality of life are larger issues.[68] Close consultation and counseling may be necessary to advise patients of the need for a stoma and that a stoma will not usually be disabling. Improvements in stoma care, nursing techniques, appliances, adhesives, skin protectors, and supportive services have led to better quality of life and less morbidity. The choices must be well understood for patients selecting options in ulcerative colitis or even rectal cancer.

The issue of quality of life is a large one for which we do not have good studies or a good measuring device. Often the improved quality of life, particularly for patients with inflammatory disease, is a function of improved nutrition, energy, and well-being after resection. Patients with stomas for emergency conditions or for cancer may not have the same issues to confront. Sexual function and impotence may be more of an issue with resection for cancer.[69-71]

With an ileostomy, various studies have shown 70% to 90% satisfaction or "normal" lives.[69-71] However, restrictions of a severe nature were shown in 10% and moderate restrictions in 40% to 50% of patients with an ileostomy.[72] Restrictions were relative to preoperative condition or health. Patients choosing a continent ileostomy were happy with their quality of life despite a high complication or reoperation rate.[73,74] One study found only 10% with restrictions in any activities, and 97% would have undergone revisional surgery rather than conversion to an ileostomy. Many patients have improved body image and sexual life with a continent stoma.[74,75]

Patients with a permanent colostomy tend to be older and to have had surgery for rectal cancer. Such patients may have continuing concerns about their cancer, body image, sex lives, and stoma function and odor. Unfortunately, many had little time for education or to make decisions on alternative options. Very few studies have outlined quality of life with a permanent colostomy.[76-79] One study of patients followed for 10 years after surgery found 75% in good health.[76] Restrictions in social life were 24% in one study[79] and 40% in another study with end colostomies.[77]

Increasingly, patients need education and options. Better instruments for measuring quality of life and education are also needed. An extensive review of the subject has recently been published by McLeod and Cohen.[68]

COMPLICATIONS

Complications of colostomies and ileostomies are similar. Early complications may be compounded by emergency surgery, obesity, or decreased cardiac output or pulmonary function. Such conditions may increase the risk of ischemia, poor mucocutaneous healing, retraction, infection, and stenosis. Urgent surgery and abdominal distention may not allow for proper preoperative marking. Loop stomas placed temporarily may tend to prolapse, retract, or protrude unevenly, leading to increased difficulties with appliance adherence and skin problems. Less difficulties in siting may be encountered in the obese or distended patient, when the surgeon has not previously marked the or site is uncertain of the proper position, by selecting a site more cephalad. Patient ability to place the appliance will be improved, and fewer skin problems will ensue. This is preferable to a stoma placed low below a protuberant fold or pendulous abdomen. In questions of vascular supply, select a loop or end-loop stoma for better vascularity.

Ischemia, Retraction, Stricture, Stenosis, and Obstruction

Early ischemia produces a number of complications. As noted above, these may be transient or central in origin. Colostomies seem more likely to become ischemic, especially if the left colonic artery has been sacrificed. Similarly, colons may have fatty mesenteries and a large degree of pericolic fat and; mobilizing the colon to the skin without tension may be difficult.

The stoma should be pink and moist. Some slight superficial duskiness may be tolerated for short intervals. A dark or dry stoma should be inspected with a narrow sigmoidoscope or test tube to determine the depth of ischemia. If the ischemia is proximal to the fascia, then revision is needed. Such ischemia, even superficially, leads to a high incidence of mucocutaneous separation, infection, retraction, and ultimately stenosis.

Stenosis in a colostomy may lead to difficulty with emptying or irrigation. As in a narrowed anastomosis, it is surprising how narrow a colostomy may become before requiring revision. Patients requiring use of a colostomy cone for irrigation can revert to an irrigating catheter in some circumstances. In patients requiring revision, skin level circumferential or bilateral excisions of scar with resuturing to skin may be sufficient. With associated retraction or recession, further mobilization, usually through the stoma site and to the peritoneum, may be required.

Retracted or stenotic ileostomies present a much larger problem. These may lead to severe skin irritation and difficulty maintaining adhesion of the appliance. Frequent changes lead to further skin breakdown. A convex face plate is the best nonoperative option. Applying an extra ring of stoma adhesive paste or karaya paste or wearing a tight stoma belt may provide convexity and better fixation.

Stenotic ileostomies either at the skin or fascial level may lead to obstructive symptoms or ileostomy dysfunction. Increased blockage from food particles may similarly cause dysfunction. This is heralded by crampy pains and an increased watery stoma output. Food blockage and the dysfunction may be resolved with saline or water irrigation of the stoma using a catheter.[80] Patients with recurrent symptoms need to have recurrent Crohn's disease ruled out. With severe recurrence, complete mobilization, correction of the stenosis or resection, and construction of the stoma is required.

Obstructive symptoms may be related to adhesions or torsion of the intraperitoneal component. Ten percent of patients with proctocolectomy and ileostomy develop small intestinal obstruction. The incidence is even higher in patients with continent devices. Obstruction may be an early or late complication, but most occur in the first year.

Continent stomas may become obstructed at the valve, with slippage and inability to cannulate the pouch. The complete realm of complications with continent pouches is beyond the scope of this chapter.[81] Kock pouches, which cannot be cannulated, usually have slippage of the valve portion. Endoscopy will often allow entrance to the pouch and placement of a guide wire and catheter to decompress the pouch. The catheter should be left in place for several weeks or consideration given to revision of the pouch and nipple.

Prolapse

Prolapse of a stoma occurs in 1% to 16% of patients. There is very little difference between ileostomies and colostomies in incidence, symptoms, and presentation. Stomal prolapse occurs with and without an associated hernia. The subcutaneous or hidden form of prolapse occurs above the fascial opening but is often classified as a hernia. For practical purposes, both have a normal or slightly enlarged fascial opening and may or may not reduce spontaneously. Prolapse may require repair depending on the severity and progression of symptoms and the health of the patient.

The size and incidence of prolapse is related to obesity, ascites, pregnancy, and chronic obstructive lung disease. Although all prolapse is not preventable, certain measures may be taken to reduce the incidence, including

Preoperative site selection

Siting through rectus muscle

Proper sizing of the opening

Fixation of mesentery

Excision of redundancy

Retroperitoneal placement(?)

End stoma where possible

Most cases with mild and nonprogressive prolapse can be managed with reassurance and some adjustment of the appliance. Acute onset of symptoms with ischemia and pain may resolve with bed rest and observation. Operative therapy is indicated for gangrenous change, acutely painful and nonreducible prolapse, and progressive chronic prolapsing with ulceration, bleeding, and serous drainage.[82]

Operative therapy in high-risk patients, and perhaps as an initial procedure in many patients, may be sufficient with local excision and advancement of the redundancy along with reformation of the stoma. This is particularly true if the prolapse is fixed and not sliding.[83] In many cases, such therapy is insufficient because of the sliding component or associated hernia.

Temporary loop stomas with prolapse should be placed in continuity again, if possible. Otherwise, conversion to an end stoma with or without a mucous fistula is appropriate. Relocation with repair of the associated hernia is the best option for most prolapses. Occasionally high-risk patients may be managed with a modification of the Delorme operation.[84] We have no experience with a colopexy using a button, as recently revived. Fashioning an end loop with a mucous fistula, after local resection, may be a short-term solution.[38]

Parastomal Hernias

Some of the same issues of selection of surgery and nonoperative management for prolapse are appropriate for hernias. Combined defects are common. Etiologic factors and issues of prevention are similar. However, herniation may often be a consequence of emergency surgery or compromises on site selection and may be related to long-term stomas. Most patients with bulging around the stoma have minimal symptoms or problems. Examination with the patient standing and straining assists evaluation. Most hernias are a form of sliding hernia. It may be difficult to classify a peristomal hernia and whether its contents are intestine or omentum. A computed tomography scan may be of value in detecting hernias in the extremely obese.

The indications for surgical correction are similar to those of stomal prolapse. Acute symptoms of ischemia or infection require an acute surgical correction. Most hernias require careful assessment of the degree of disability and the severity of symptoms. Mildly symptomatic or asymptomatic hernias require no surgery. Paraileostomy hernias may require surgery more often because of special problems in maintaining an appliance and managing the effluent.

Nonoperative therapy requires reassurance, efforts at weight reduction when appropriate, the use of an elastic binder for support, or a flexible face plate and appliance.

Operative options include

1. Local repair—parastomal or intra-abdominal
2. Relocation
3. Local repair with prosthetic material
   Peritoneal
   Preperitoneal
   Extrafascial

An approach for each individual patient seems best. If a stoma is poorly situated, relocation is preferable. Mesh repair may be appropriate if the patient has no prior problems and likes the location. Multiple scars of the abdomen may lead to a local or mesh repair.[85,86] (Fig. 48-5).

No one large series with long-term follow-up is available. Resiting and mesh repairs have similar ranges of recurrences (5 to 35%).[87,88] Simple repair may recur in 70%. Infection with mesh occurs in less than 15% and is serious in less than 5%.[85,86] Associated complications such as bleeding, fistulae, or bowel injury are few.

Infection, Fistulae, and Ulcers

In instances of abscess and cellulitis in the parastoma skin, drainage should be undertaken either through the mucocutaneous junction of the stoma or with a parastomal incision outside the face plate of the appliance. While this may not always be possible, maintaining peristomal skin integrity and an adherent appliance will lessen complications.

Late occurrence of an abscess or fistula often indicates recurrent Crohn's disease in the proximal segment. Trauma or diverticulitis may lead to similar presentations. Fistulae created by sutures placed for eversion of the stoma or fixation to the fascia present early. I rarely use peritoneal or fascial sutures for stomas.

Parastomal ulceration secondary to appliances or Crohn's disease requires expert nursing and stomal therapy support. Treatment of the Crohn's disease usually requires steroids for control. Debridement and curettage and covering the ulcer with the appliance may support the medical management.[89] Good nutritional support or intravenous feeding may lessen effluent and assist healing.[90] Severe infections and ulcerations or fistulae may require innovative stomal care and skin protection.[91] Relocation of the stoma may be required, especially with fistulae and recurrent Crohn's disease.[92] If fistulae exit under a stomal face plate, relocation may be mandatory.

Ulcerations in parastomal skin in patients with inflammatory disease may represent pyoderma gangrenosum.[89,93] This extraintestinal manifestation of Crohn's disease or ulcerative colitis is particularly troublesome in this location. The clinical course of this disorder is often related to the disease activity. Medical or surgical remission of the inflammatory disease controls the skin disorder. Any refractory ulceration in patients with inflammatory bowel disease should be considered for pyoderma gangrenosum. A large review of the subject and local management may assist those with this rare complication.[94]

Ulcers occurring in stomas in a patient with a prior history of malignancy may indicate local implantation and possible widespread metastatic disease. A metachronous proximal cancer should be ruled out. Rarely, it represents a primary cancer located at the stoma.[95] Primary adenocarcinoma of the ileostomy has been reported. According to Loehner and Schoetz,[94] 11 cases have appeared in the literature. Ten of these cases arose in ileostomies performed for ulcerative colitis and the other in a polyposis coli patient.

Parastomal Varices

Recent reviews of parastomal varices, a rare complication clearly outline preventive measures and difficulties with local management of recurrent hemorrhages.[94,96–98] Patients with hepatic disease and portal hypertension are at risk of developing a shunting from the portal to systemic systems in the peristomal skin. Thin superficial varicosities develop under the face plate and at the mucocutaneous junction along with prominent stoma vessels. Recurrent bleeding may be severe and sudden.

Usually direct suture control is needed for control of the bleeding. Sclerosing injection has been utilized by a number of authors with varying degrees of short-term success. Relocation may be necessary.[99,100] Disconnection of the mucocutaneous junction with subsequent resuturing and scarring has been advocated.[101] Definitive portosystemic shunting or liver transplantation may be required to control the entire disease process and recurrent local hemorrhages.

Skin Conditions

The peristomal skin is subject to damage from the fecal effluent, occlusive appliances, and frequent appliance changes, which denude superficial skin layers. A well-sited stoma, properly fitting appliances, and good education by stomal therapists are essential to maintain the peristomal skin. A

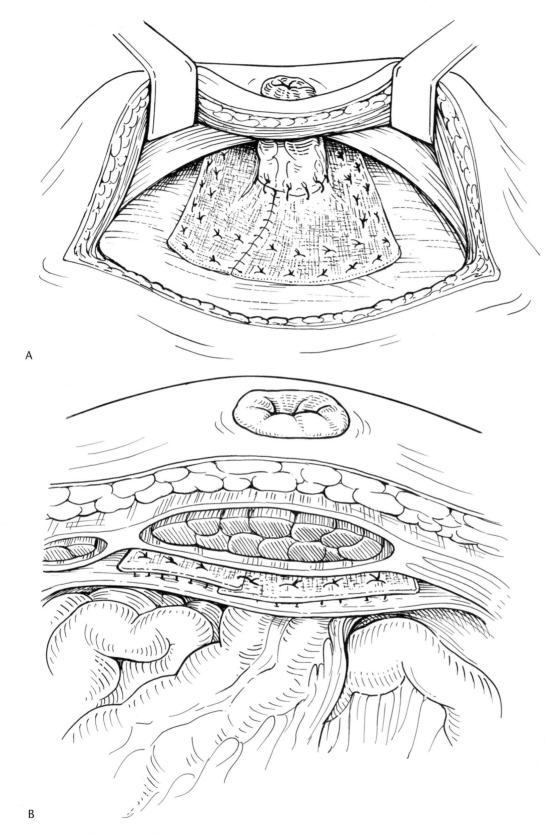

A

B

Figure 48-5. (**A & B**) Mesh repair for stomal hernia.

Common Peristomal Skin Problems

Infections
    Fungal
        Candida albicans
        Tinea corporis
    Bacterial
        Staphylococcus aureus
Chemical irritants
    Stomal effluents
        Erythema, ulcers
        Encrustations
        Pseudoepitheliomatous hyperplasia
    Chemicals
        Detergents, soaps
        Glues, solvents
Allergic responses
    Contact dermatitis
        Hydrogen peroxide
        Plastic, rubber, adhesives
        Tincture of benzoin
        Neomycin
Mechanical trauma
    Stripping of adhesives
    Pressure or friction from ill-fitted devices
    Folliculitis

(From Martin and Leal-Khouri,[102] with permission.)

major skin irritation will occur unless minor problems of fitting and leakage are aggressively attacked early. Some recurring problems require resiting or revision. Retraction and skin folds are particularly difficult management problems. Martin and Leal-Khouri,[102] have divided the commonest skin problems into four categories: chemical irritation, infection, allergy, and trauma.

Chemical Irritation

Contact chemical irritation from stool or urine contact with the skin is the most common skin problem. As noted, poorly fitting stomas lead to leakage under the face plate and subsequent skin inflammation. Such inflammation weeps fluid and may develop into open ulcerations.[103,104] Pressure sores from the edge of the face plate are more easily promoted. Inflammation also results from soaps, glues, and solvents applied to the peristomal skin. Rinsing off the soap well after use is very important. All these substances may leave residues, which are then held under the face plate of the appliance.

Many techniques and skills are required to reverse such skin changes. The use of adhesive face plates has lessened problems dramatically over the last few decades. Ulcerations may be filled with karaya or DuoDerm (Convatec, Princeton, NJ) and then Telfa (Colgate-Palmolive, Canton, MA) applied to fit the ulcer size. The wafer barrier with face plate can then be applied over the site.

Urine from leakage around the urostomy may cause triple phosphate or urine crystals to form in plaques. The alkalinity of the urine may be reversed with cranberry juice or vitamin C. Weak vinegar solutions applied to the area or to the appliance may help to dissolve the crystals. A heaped-up verrucous reaction under the face plate called pseudoepitheliomatous hyperplasia may occur in a number of situations. It resembles warts or a verrucous carcinoma but is benign. Chronic inflammation is the cause, but this reaction may be seen in Crohn's disease and in patients taking azathioprine or those undergoing organ transplantation. Fulguration may be required to reduce its size and to ensure proper fitting of the appliance.

Infections

The most common infection in the peristomal skin is *Candida albicans*, which is part of the normal intestinal and skin flora. With antibiotics, cleansing, and a moist environment under the face plate, *Candida* growth is facilitated. Less common are bacterial infections such as Staphylococcus *aureus*. Tinea corporis may occasionally develop in this area. Folliculitis may develop around the hair follicles. Trimming the hairs with scissors or electric razors minimizes the problem.

Candida infections cause erythema with satellite papules and pustules. Treatment with Nystatin powder, applied to the skin with each pouch change, will usually cure the problem.

Allergy

Allergic reactions to any one of a number of solvents, pastes, adhesives, or tapes used in stoma maintenance are possible.[105,106] The typical erythema and blistering at the contact site and in the distribution of the offending material are seen.

Secondary Problems in the Peristomal Skin

Dermatoses
    Psoriasis
    Eczema
    Pemphigus
    Crohn's disease
    Ulcerative colitis
    Pyoderma gangrenosum
    Fistulas
    Caput medusae
Radiation and chemotherapy
Primary skin cancers
    Squamous cell carcinoma
    Basal cell carcinoma
Metastatic malignancies
    Adenocarcinoma
    Anaplastic carcinoma
    Transitional cell carcinoma
Childhood and aging

(From Martin and Leal-Khouri,[102] with permission.)

Confirmation with skin patch testing may be needed to isolate and confirm the diagnosis. Topical steroids applied in spray form seem to control the conditions when they are applied under the face plate. Systemic steroids may be needed for severe reactions.[102]

Trauma

Skin trauma from repeated and frequent changes accentuates leakage problems related to poorly fitting appliances. Superficial skin is stripped, leading to skin irritation and inflammation. Adhesives and tapes compound the situation. Most well-fitting appliances can be maintained for 5 to 7 days, minimizing the skin trauma. Pressure ulcerations are a result of appliance fitting problems. Their treatment has been outlined earlier (Table 48-1).

Other Causes

Specific dermatoses such as psoriasis, eczema, and systemic lupus erythematosus may occur in the peristomal skin and may require specific therapy. Crohn's disease in the peristomal skin or fistulae requires specific medical or surgical treatment directed at inducing a remission of the disease. Pyoderma gangrenosum has been previously discussed. Primary and secondary carcinomas were addressed in a prior section. Radiation treatment can be performed with a stoma in place, but care is taken to observe the skin frequently. Appliances are removed during treatment to minimize scatter. A system that avoids adhesions and uses just a karaya ring pouch with a belt may be sufficient[102]. Skin problems are frequent. Good education and the advice of a stomal therapist are invaluable. Many problems

Table 48-2. Pouching Problems

Problem	(Nonsurgical) Solution
Flush or retracted stoma resulting in leakage or undermining of appliance	Appliances with convexity Pouches with convex design Convex inserts added to the flange of a two-piece system Belt may increase stability
Stoma located in a skin fold	Appliances with convexity Appliances with flexible design
Prolapsed stoma	Reduce prolapse prior to placing appliance with patient supine Apply prolapse belt if desired Appliance with flexible design
Peristomal hernia	Appliance with flexible design 4–6" hernia support ostomy belt
Changes in body contours (weight changes, pregnancy)	Change in appliance faceplate flexibility Accommodate changes in stoma size

(From Swatske et al.,[107] with permission.)

are then prevented or treated early, reducing the severity and complications (Table 48-1).

MANAGEMENT

The proper management of stomas is a large subject. Principles of proper construction, siting, and fitting of stomas have been addressed. The subject of the appropriate appliance and adhesive for each situation has been

Table 48-1. Common Peristomal Skin Conditions

Condition	Cause	Solution
Allergic	Sensitivity to skin barriers, adhesives, tapes	Use patch test to determine what patient can tolerate
Bacterial	Folliculitis	Trim peristomal hair with scissors or electric razor Use adhesive remover to ease release of adhesives
Fungal	Candida albicans	Apply Nystatin topical powder with each pouch change Dust off excess powder to allow appliance to seal
Chemical	Leakage of effluent under appliance	Determine cause of leakage Check for peristomal fistula Refit into proper appliance Dust skin with skin barrier powder prior to pouching Severe hyperplasia may require surgical debridement and use of nonadherent system until re-epithelialization occurs
Mechanical	Skin stripping from adhesive removal	Gently pull skin away from adhesive with warm, moist gauze square or adhesive remover
	Laceration of stoma from appliance due to shifting, improper sizing, or improper application	Remeasure stoma Observe appliance while patient is sitting, supine, and standing Observe patient system's technique
Other peristomal abscess	Commonly caused by recurrent Crohn's disease	Unroof ulcer If ulcer is <2 cm, cover with nonadherent gauze or hydrocolloid, apply pouch as usual, and change every 2–3 days If ulcer is >2 cm, apply nonadherent appliance

(From Lavery and Erwin-Toth,[53] with permission.)

addressed by others.[53,54,107] The support of ostomy associations may be valuable for patients both preoperatively and postoperatively. Common appliance or pouch problems are given in Table 48-2.

REFERENCES

1. LeClerc D (1699) History of Physick. p. 406, D Brown, London
2. Dinnick T (1934) The origins and evolution of colostomy. Br J Surg 22:142–153
3. (1800) System à Chirurque Hodierne. p. 688
4. Schmalkaldern CD (1798) Movum Methodum Intestina Continui Solutionc Factor Uniendi et Anum Artificialem Persanandi. Tzschiedrich, Wittenberg
5. Dupuytren G (1828) Memoir on a new method of treating accidental anus. Mem Acad R Med 259
6. von Mikulicz J (1903) Surgical experience with intestinal carcinoma. Arch Klin Chir 69:28–47
7. Bryant T (1882) A case of excision of a stricture of the descending colon through an incision made for a left lumbar colotomy. Proc Med Chir 9:149
8. Cromar CDL (1968) The evolution of the colostomy. Dis Colon Rectum 11:367–390
9. Cataldo PA (1993) History of stomas. pp. 3–37. Intestinal Stomas. In MacKeigan JM, Cataldo PA (eds): Principles, Techniques and Management. Quality Medical Publishers, St. Louis
10. Baum WG (1879) Resection sines carcinomatosen. Dickdarmstuckes. Zentralbl Chir 6:169–176
11. Brooke BN (1954) Ulcerative colitis and its surgical treatment. E&S Livingston, Edinburgh
12. Weir RF (1902) A new use for the useless appendix in surgical treatment of obstinate colitis. MRCC 62:201
13. Brown JY (1913) The value of complete physiologic rest of the large bowel in the treatment of certain ulcerative colitis and obstructive lesions of this organ. Surg Gynecol Obstet 16:610–613
14. Dragstedt LR, Dack GM, Kisner JB (1941) Chronic ulcerative colitis: a summary of evidence implicating *Bacterium neocrophorum* as an etiologic agent. Ann Surg 114:654
15. Brooke BN (1952) The management of an ileostomy including its complications. Lancet 2:102–104
16. Crile G Jr, Turnbull RB Jr (1954) The mechanism and prevention of ileostomy dysfunction. Ann Surg 140:459–465
17. Kock NG (1973) Continent ileostomy. Prog Surg 12:180–201
18. Soper NJ, Orkin BA, Kelly KA et al (1989) Gastrointestinal transit after proctocolectomy with ileal pouch-anal anastomosis or ileostomy. J Surg Res 46:300
19. Hill GT (1976) Ileostomy. Surgery, Physiology and Management. Grune & Stratton, New York
20. Grotz RL, Pemberton JH (1993) Stoma physiology. pp. 38–51. In MacKeigan JM, Cataldo PA (eds): Intestinal Stomas. Principles, Techniques and Management. Quality Medical Publishing, St. Louis
21. Gorbach SL, Nahas L, Weinstein L et al (1967) Studies of intestinal microflora. IV. The microflora of ileostomy effluent: a unique microbial ecology. Gastroenterology 53:874
22. Ritchie JK (1971) Ileostomy and excisional surgery for chronic inflammatory disease of the colon: a survey of one hospital region. I. Results of complications of surgery. Gut 12:528
23. Kurchin A, Ray JE, Bluth EI et al (1984) Cholelithiasis in ileostomy patients. Dis Colon Rectum 27:585
24. Phillips SF (1987) Biological effects of a reservoir at the end of the small bowel. World J Surg 11:763
25. Corman ML (1993) Preoperative considerations. pp. 52–57. In MacKeigan JM, Cataldo PA (eds): Intestinal Stomas. Principles, Techniques and Management. Quality Medical Publishing, St. Louis
26. Goligher JC (1958) Extraperitoneal colostomy or ileostomy. Br J Surg 46:97–103
27. Whittaker M, Goligher C (1976) A comparison of the results of extraperitoneal and intraperitoneal techniques for construction of terminal iliac colostomies. Dis Colon Rectum 19:342–344
28. Rombeau JL, Wilk PJ, Turnbull RB et al (1978) Total fecal diversion by the temporary skin-level loop transverse colostomy. Dis Colon Rectum 21:223–226
29. Williams NS, Nasmyth DG, Jones D et al (1986) Defunctioning stomas: a postoperative controlled trial comparing loop ileostomy with loop transverse colostomy. Br J Surg 73:566–570
30. Fontes B, Fontes W, Utiyama EM et al (1988) The efficacy of loop colostomy for complete fecal diversion. Dis Colon Rectum 31:298–302
31. Winslet MC, Drolc Z, Allan A, Keighley MK (1991) Assessment of the defunctioning efficiency of the loop ileostomy. Dis Colon Rectum 34:699–703
32. Fielding LP, Stewart-Brown S, Hittinger R et al (1989) Covering stoma for elective anterior resection of the rectum: an outmoded operation? Am J Surg 147:524–530
33. Winkler MJ, Volpe PA (1982) Loop transverse colostomy—the case against. Dis Colon Rectum 25:321–326
34. Boman-Sandelin K, Fenyo G (1985) Construction and closure of transverse loop colostomy. Dis Colon Rectum 28:772–774
35. Rutegard J, Dahlgren S (1987) Transverse colostomy or loop ileostomy as diverting stoma in colorectal surgery. Acta Chir Scand 153:229–232
36. Corman ML, Veidenheimer MC, Coller JA (1979) Loop ileostomy as an alternative to end stoma. Surg Gynecol Obstet 149:585–586
37. Turnbull RB, Weakley FL, Hawk WA et al (1970) Choice of operation for toxic megacolon phase of nonspecific ulcerative colitis. Surg Clin North Am 50:1151–1169
38. Pearl PK (1993) Diverting stomas. pp. 114–126. In MacKeigan JM, Cataldo PA (eds): Intestinal Stomas. Principles, Techniques and Management. Quality Medical Publishing, St. Louis
39. Feinberg SM, MacLeod RS, Cohen Z (1987) Complications of loop ileostomy. Am J Surg 153:102–107
40. Mileski WJ, Regs RV, Joehl RJ et al (1990) Rates of morbidity and mortality after closure of loop and end colostomy. Surg Gynecol Obstet 171:17–21

41. Sally RK, Butcher RM, Rodning CB (1983) Colostomy closure: morbidity reduction employing a semi-standardized protocol. Dis Colon Rectum 26:319–322

42. Pittman DM, Smith LE (1985) Complications of colostomy closure. Dis Colon Rectum 28:836–843

43. Westdahl PR, Russell T (1969) In support of blind tube cecostomy in acute obstruction of the descending colon. Analysis of ninety-three emergency cecostomies. Am J Surg 118: 577–581

44. King RD, Edelman S, Kirschner PA et al (1966) An evaluation of catheter cecostomy. Surg Gynecol Obstet 123: 779–786

45. Anderson JR, Welch GH (1986) Acute volvulus of the right colon: an analysis of 69 patients. World J Surg 10:336–342

46. Cran JR, Simmons RL, Frick MP et al (1985) Percutaneous decompression of the colon using CT guidance in Ogilve syndrome. AJR 144:475–476

47. Casola G, Withers C, van Sonnenberg E et al (1986) Percutaneous cecostomy for decompression of the massively distended cecum. Radiology 158:793–794

48. Senagore AJ (1993) Cecostomy. pp. 127–134. In MacKeigan JM, Cataldo PA (eds): Intestinal Stomas. Principles, Techniques and Management. Quality Medical Publishing, St. Louis

49. Kodner IJ (1978) Colostomy and ileostomy. Clin Symp 30: 2–36

50. Kodner IJ (1991) Colostomy: indications, techniques for construction, and management of complications. Semin Colon Rectal Surg 2:73–85.

51. Beck DE (1993) End sigmoid colostomy. pp. 97–106. In MacKeigan JM, Cataldo PA (eds): Intestinal Stomas. Principles, Techniques and Management. Quality Medical Publishing, St. Louis

52. Burke TW, Weiser EB, Hoskins WJ et al (1987) End colostomy using the end-to-end anastomosis instrument. Obstet Gynecol 69:156–159

53. Lavery IC, Erwin-Toth P (1993) Stoma therapy. pp. 60–84. In MacKeigan JM, Cataldo PA (eds): Intestinal Stomas. Principles, Techniques and Management. Quality Medical Publishing, St. Louis

54. Erwin-Toth P, Doughty DB (1992) Principles and procedures of stomal management. In Hampton BG, Bryant RA (eds): Ostomies and Continent Diversions. Mosby-Year Book, St. Louis.

55. Schmidt E (1982) The continent colostomy. World J Surg 6: 805–809

56. Khubchandani IT, Trimpi HD, Sheets JA et al (1981) The magnetic stoma device: a continent colostomy. Dis Colon Rectum 24:344–350

57. Alexander-Williams J, Amery AH, Devlin HB et al (1977) Magnetic continent colostomy device. BMJ 1:1269–1270.

58. Goligher JC, Lee PWR, McMahon MJ, Pollard M (1977) The Erlangen magnetic colostomy control device: technique of use and results in 22 patients. Br J Surg 64:501–507

59. Prager E (1984) The continent colostomy. Dis Colon Rectum 27:235–237

60. Burcharth F, Ballan A, Kylberg F, Rasmussen SN (1986) The colostomy plug: a new disposable device for a continent colostomy. Lancet 2:1062–1063

61. Cerdan FJ, Diez M, Campo J et al (1991) Continent colostomy by means of a new one-piece disposable device. Dis Colon Rectum 34:886–890

62. Bricker EM (1950) Bladder substitution after pelvic evisceration. Surg Clin North Am 30:1511

63. Gilchrist RK, Merricks JW, Hamlin HH et al (1950) Construction of a substitute bladder and urethra. Surg Gynecol Obstet 90:752

64. Dalton, DP (1993) Methods of urinary diversion. pp. 198–221. In MacKeigan JM, Cataldo PA (eds): Intestinal Stomas. Principles Techniques and Management. Quality Medical Publishing, St. Louis

65. Rowland RG, Mitchell ME, Bihrle R et al (1987) Indiana continent urinary reservoir. J Urol 137:1136

66. Bihrle R, Foster RS (1991) Continent ileocecal reservoirs: the Indiana pouch. p. 308. In King LR, Stone AR, Webster GD (eds): Bladder Reconstruction and Continent Urinary Diversion. Mosby-Year Book, St. Louis

67. King LR, Stone AR, Webster GD (1991) Bladder Reconstruction and Continent Urinary Diversion. Mosby-Year Book, St. Louis

68. McLeod RS, Cohen Z (1993) Quality of life with a stoma. pp. 85–94. In MacKeigan JM, Cataldo PA (eds): Intestinal Stomas: Principles, Techniques and Management. Quality Medical Publishing, St. Louis

69. McLeod RS, Lavery IC, Leatherman JR (1986) Factors affecting quality of life with a conventional ileostomy. World J Surg 10:474

70. Roy PH, Sauer WG, Beahrs OH, Farrow GM (1970) Experience with ileostomies. Evaluation of long-term rehabilitation in 497 patients. Am J Surg 119:77

71. Morowitz DA, Kirsner JB (1981) Ileostomy in ulcerative colitis. A questionnaire study of 1,803 patients. Am J Surg 141: 370

72. McLeod RS, Lavery IC, Leatherman JR (1985) Patient evaluation of the conventional ileostomy. Dis Colon Rectum 28: 152

73. McLeod RS, Fazio VW (1984) Quality of life with the continent ileostomy. World J Surg 8:90

74. Nilsson LP, Kock NG, Kylberg F et al (1981) Sexual adjustment in ileostomy patients before and after conversion to continent ileostomy. Dis Colon Rectum 24:287

75. Ojerskog B, Hallstrom T, Kock NG, Myrvold HE (1988) Quality of life in ileostomy patients before and after conversion to the continent ileostomy. Int J Color Dis 3:166

76. Wirsching M, Druner HU, Herrmann G (1975) Results of psychosocial adjustment to long-term colostomy. Psychother Psychosom 26:245

77. Devlin HB (1990) Colostomy: Past and present. Ann Coll Surg Phys 72:175

78. Coe M, Kluka S (1990) Comparison of concerns of clients and spouses regarding ostomy surgery for treatment of cancer: phase II. J Enterostom Ther 17:106

79. Von Smitten K, Husa A, Kyllonen L (1986) Long-term results of sigmoidostomy in patients with anorectal malignancy. Acta Chir Scand 152:211

80. Metcalf AM (1993) Ileostomy and pouch dysfunction. pp. 237–245. In MacKeigan JM, Cataldo PA (eds): Intestinal Stomas. Principles, Techniques and Management. Quality Medical Publishing, St. Louis

81. Gorfine SR, Bauer JJ, Gelernt IM (1993) Continent stomas.

pp. 154–187. In MacKeigan JM, Cataldo PA (eds): Intestinal Stomas. Principles, Techniques and Management. Quality Medical Publishing, St. Louis

82. Williams JG, Etherington R, Hayward MWJ et al (1990) Para-ileostomy hernia: a clinical and radiological study. Br J Surg 77:1355–1357

83. Nogueras JJ, Wexner SD (1993) Stoma prolapse. pp. 268–277. In MacKeigan JM, Cataldo PA (eds): Intestinal Stomas. Principles, Techniques and Management. Quality Medical Publishing, St. Louis

84. Abulafi AM, Sherman IW, Fiddian RV (1989) Delorme operation for prolapsed colostomy. Br J Surg 12:76

85. Bayer I, Kyzer S, Chaimoff CH (1986) A new approach to primary strengthening of colostomy with Marlex mesh to prevent paracolostomy hernia. Surg Gynecol Obstet 163:579–580

86. Sugarbaker PH (1980) Prosthetic mesh repair of large hernias at the site of colonic stomas. Surg Gynecol Obstet 150:577–578

87. Sugarbaker PH (1985) Peritoneal approach to prosthetic mesh repair of paracolectomy hernia. Am Surg 201:344–346

88. Rubin MS, Bailey HR (1993) Parastomal hernias. pp. 245–267. In MacKeigan JM, Cataldo PA (eds): Intestinal Stomas. Principles, Techniques and Management. Quality Medical Publishing, St. Louis

89. Last M, Fazio V, Lavery I, Jagelman D (1984) Conservative management of paraileostomy ulcers in patients with Crohn's disease. Dis Colon Rectum 27:779–786

90. Reynolds HM Jr, Frazier TG, Copeland EM III (1976) Treatment of paracolostomy abscess without proximal diverting colostomy: report of two cases. Dis Colon Rectum 19:458–459

91. Rolstad BS, Wong WD (1993) Nursing considerations with intestinal fistulas. pp. 307–328. In MacKeigan JM, Cataldo PA (eds): Intestinal Stomas. Principles, Techniques and Management. Quality Medical Publishing, St. Louis

92. Greenstein AJ, Dicker A, Meyers S, Aufses AH Jr (1983) Peri-ileostomy fistulae in Crohn's disease. Ann Surg 197:179–182

93. McGarity WC, Robertson DB, McKeown PP et al (1984) Pyoderma gangrenosum at the parastomal site in patients with Crohn's disease. Arch Surg 119:1186–1188

94. Loehner DL, Schoetz DJ (1993) Unusual problems in stoma management. pp. 339–349. In MacKeigan JM, Cataldo PA (eds); Intestinal Stomas. Principles, Techniques and Management. Quality Medical Publishing, St. Louis

95. Sigler L, Jedd FL (1969) Adenocarcinoma of the ileostomy occurring after colectomy for ulcerative colitis: report of a case. Dis Colon Rectum 12:45–48

96. Adson MA, Fulton RE (1977) The ileal stoma and portal hypertension: an uncommon site of variceal bleeding. Arch Surg 112:501–504

97. Goldstein WZ, Edoga J, Crystal R (1980) Management of colostomal hemorrhage resulting from portal hypertension. Dis Colon Rectum 23:86–90

98. Fucini C, Wolff BG, Dozois RR (1991) Bleeding from peristomal varices: perspectives on prevention and treatment. Dis Colon Rectum 34:1073–1078

99. Morgan TR, Feldshon SD, Tripp MR (1986) Recurrent stomal variceal bleeding: successful treatment using injection sclerotherapy. Dis Colon Rectum 29:269–270

100. Hesterberg R, Stahlknecht CD, Roher HD (1986) Sclerotherapy for massive enterostomy bleeding resulting from portal hypertension. Dis Colon Rectum 29:275–277

101. Beck DE, Fazio VW, Grundfest-Broniatowski S (1988) Surgical management of bleeding stomal varices. Dis Colon Rectum 31:343–346

102. Martin AG, Leal-Khouri S (1991) Principles of managing dermatologic and wound problems related to intestinal stomas. Semin Colon Rectal Surg 2:161–167

103. Rothstein MS (1986) Dermatologic considerations of stoma care. J Am Acad Dermatol 15:411–432

104. Bergman B, Knutson F, Lincoln K et al (1979) Chronic papillomatous dermatitis as a peristomal skin complication in conduit urinary diversion. Scand J Urol Nephrol 13:201–204

105. Camarasa JMG, Alomar A (1980) Contact dermatitis from a karaya seal ring. Contact Dermatitis 6:139–140

106. Beck MH, Burrows D, Fregert S et al (1985) Allergic contact dermatitis to epoxy resin in ostomy bags. Br J Surg 72:202–203

107. Swatske ME, Whittaker K, Young M (1991) Care of the intestinal stoma: preoperative, postoperative, long term. Semin Colon Rectal Surg. 2:148–155

INDEX

Page numbers followed by f refer to figures; those followed by t refer to tables.

895

metastases of colorectal carcinoma to, 355, 355f
survival rate in, 429, 430f
of rectum, 10
Venereal Disease Research Laboratory assay in syphilis, 288
Verapamil
in diarrhea, 684
in inflammatory bowel disease, 578
Villi, mucosal, countercurrent exchange mechanism in, 780
Vincristine therapy
in colon cancer, 494, 495t
in rectal cancer, 497
Viruses
in intestinal flora, 195
sexually transmitted, 286t, 289–293
HIV infection and AIDS in, 294–302. *See also* HIV infection and AIDS
Vitamins
absorption of, 21, 25, 26
deficiency in inflammatory bowel disease, 584, 585
Volume measurements of intestinal motility, 40, 41f, 42, 49, 50f
compared to pressure measures, 43

Volvulus, 1
cecostomy in, 885
in malrotation of intestines, 801–802, 803, 804, 807f
postoperative recurrence of, 804
sigmoidoscopy in, 73, 74
Vomiting in chemotherapy, 843
Von Recklinghausen's disease, neurofibromas in, 359, 531
V-Y anoplasty in anal fissure, 241, 241f

W
Waldeyer fascia, 6, 6f
in anterior resection of colorectal carcinoma, 443f, 444
in total rectal excision for carcinoma, 458, 460f
Warfarin, adverse effects of, 844
Warts, in condylomata acuminata, 291–293
Water, absorption of, 20, 21
colectomy and ileostomy affecting, 25
and stool consistency, 34
Water-soluble contrast studies, 90, 91f
in fistulography, 92–93
in pouchography, 91
Weight loss, 71
in inflammatory bowel disease, 584, 585

Western blot test in HIV infection and AIDS, 295
White blood cell scans in inflammatory bowel disease, 157–158, 159f, 159–160
Wound healing, perineal
in colorectal cancer, 459–460, 466
radiotherapy affecting, 483, 515
recurrent, 515, 517f
in total rectal excision, 459–460
in Crohn's disease, 630, 638
in pilonidal sinus, 250–253

Y
Yeasts, intestinal and fecal, 199
Yersinia infections, 649, 651
treatment of, 653, 655

Z
ZD 1694 in colorectal cancer, 499
Zileuton in inflammatory bowel disease, 578
Zinc
absorption of, 22
deficiency in inflammatory bowel disease, 585, 588
Z-plasty in pilonidal sinus, 249f, 250